GERIATRIC PHYSICAL THERAPY

Second Edition

GERIATRIC PHYSICAL THERAPY

Edited by

Andrew A. Guccione, PT, PhD, FAPTA
Senior Vice President for Practice and Research
American Physical Therapy Association
Alexandria, VA

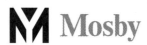 Mosby

A Harcourt Health Sciences Company

St. Louis   London   Philadelphia   Sydney   Toronto

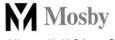
Mosby
A Harcourt Health Sciences Company

Publisher: John Schrefer
Editor: Kellie White
Developmental Editor: Christie M. Hart
Project Manager: Deborah L. Vogel
Senior Production Editor: Sarah E. Fike
Designer: Bill Drone

SECOND EDITION

Mosby, Inc.
A Harcourt Health Sciences Company
11830 Westline Industrial Drive
St. Louis, MO 63146

Printed in the United States of America

International Standard Book Number 0-323-00172-6

00 01 02 03 04 GW/MVY 9 8 7 6 5 4 3 2

CONTRIBUTORS

Dale L. Avers, PT, MSEd
Vice President of Academic Affairs
Rocky Mountain University of Health Professions
Los Angeles, California

John O. Barr, PT, PhD
Professor and Director
Department of Physical Therapy
St. Ambrose University
Davenport, Iowa

Mary C. Bourgeois, PT, MS, CCS
Program Coordinator
Rehabilitation Services
Beth Israel Deaconess Medical Center
Boston, Massachusetts

Marybeth Brown, PT, PhD
Associate Professor
Program in Physical Therapy
Washington University School of Medicine
St. Louis, Missouri

Julie M. Chandler, PT, PhD
Associate Director
Department of Epidemiology
Merck Research Laboratories
West Point, Pennsylvania

Charles D. Ciccone, PT, PhD
Professor
Department of Physical Therapy
Ithaca College
Ithaca, New York

Rebecca L. Craik, PT, PhD, FAPTA
Professor & Chair
Department of Physical Therapy
Beaver College
Glenside, Pennsylvania

Davis L. Gardner, MA
Professor Emerita
Department of Health Sciences
College of Allied Health Professions
University of Kentucky
Lexington, Kentucky

Lisa Giallonardo, PT, MS, OCS
Clinical Professor & MSPT Program Director
Department of Physical Therapy
Sargent College of Health and Rehabilitation Sciences
Boston University
Boston, Massachusetts

Andrew A. Guccione, PT, PhD, FAPTA
Senior Vice President for Practice and Research
American Physical Therapy Association
Alexandria, Virginia

John F. Knarr, PT, MS, ATC
Elite Physical Therapy
Los Angeles, California

Wendy M. Kohrt, PhD
Professor of Medicine
Department of Internal Medicine
University of Colorado Health Sciences Center
Denver, Colorado

Edmund M. Kosmahl, PT, EdD
Professor & Chair
Department of Physical Therapy
University of Scranton
Scranton, Pennsylvania

Toby Long, PT, PhD
Associate Director for Training
Director of Division of Physical Therapy
Child Development Center;
Associate Professor
Department of Pediatrics
Georgetown University
Washington, DC

Kathleen Kline Mangione, PT, PhD, GCS
Assistant Professor
Department of Physical Therapy
Beaver College
Glenside, Pennsylvania

Prudence D. Markos, PT, MS
Adjunct Assistant Professor
Graduate Program in Physical Therapy
MGH Institute of Health Professions
Boston, Massachusetts

Carol Miller, PT, MS, GCS

Assistant Professor
North Georgia College & State University
Graduate Program in Physical Therapy
Dahlonega, Georgia

Carolee Moncur, PT, PhD

Professor of Physical Therapy
Division of Physical Therapy
College of Health;
Adjunct Professor
Division of Rheumatology
School of Medicine;
Adjunct Professor
Department of Bioengineering
College of Sciences
University of Utah
Salt Lake City, Utah

Michael Moran, PT, ScD

Associate Professor
Department of Physical Therapy
College Misericordia
Dallas, Pennsylvania

Donald A. Neumann, PT, PhD

Department of Physical Therapy
Marquette University
Milwaukee, Wisconsin

Carolynn Patten, PT, PhD

Research Health Scientist
Rehabilitation Research & Development Center
VA Palo Alto Health Care System
Palo Alto, California;
Consulting Assistant Professor
Department of Functional Restoration
Stanford University School of Medicine
Stanford, California

Julie Pauls, PT, PhD, ICCE

Assistant Professor
School of Physical Therapy
Texas Women's University
The Woodlands, Texas

Nancy L. Peatman, PT, MEd

Clinical Associate Professor
Academic Coordinator of Clinical Education
Department of Physical Therapy
Sargent College of Health & Rehabilitation Sciences
Boston University
Boston, Massachusetts

Jean Oulund Peteet, PT, MPH

Clinical Assistant Professor
Department of Physical Therapy
Sargent College of Health & Rehabilitation Sciences
Boston University
Boston, Massachusetts

Marilyn D. Phillips, PT, MS

Director of Professional Development
American Physical Therapy Association
Alexandria, Virginia

Barbara Roberge, RNC, PhD, CS

Coordinator, Nurse Practitioner
Geriatric Nursing at Senior Health
Geriatrics Unit
Massachusetts General Hospital
Boston, Massachusetts

Carol Schunk, PT, PsyD

Vice President, Clinical Services
Therapeutic Associates Inc;
Director
Therapeutic Associates Outcomes Systems
Portland, Oregon

Ron Scott, PT, JD, MS, OCS

Associate Professor & Chair
Department of Physical Therapy
Lebanon Valley College
Palmyra, Pennsylvania

Lynn Snyder-Mackler, PT, ScD, SCS, ATC

Associate Professor
Department of Physical Therapy
University of Delaware
Newark, Deleware

Patricia E. Sullivan, PT, PhD

Associate Professor
Graduate Program in Physical Therapy;
Director
Center for International Health Care Education
MGH Institute of Health Professions
Boston, Massachusetts

LaDora V. Thompson, PT, PhD

Associate Professor
Department of Physical Medicine & Rehabilitation
University of Minnesota School of Medicine
Minneapolis, Minnesota

Kathleen H. Toscano, PT, MHS, PCS

Pediatric Rehabilitation Coordinator
Shady Grove Adventist Hospital
Rockville, Maryland

Mary Ann Wharton, PT, MS

Associate Professor & Curriculum Coordinator
Department of Physical Therapy
Saint Francis College
Loretto, Pennsylvania;
Adjunct Associate Professor
Physical Therapist Assistant Program
Community College of Allegheny County, Boyce Campus
Monroeville, Pennsylvania

Ann K. Williams, PT, PhD

Professor & Chair
Department of Physical Therapy
The University of Montana
Missoula, Montana

Rita A. Wong, PT, EdD

Professor & Chair
Department of Physical Therapy
School of Health Professions
Marymount University
Arlington, Virginia

Cynthia C. Zadai, PT, MS, CCS

Director
Rehabilitation Services
Beth Israel Deaconess Medical Center
Boston, Massachusetts

PREFACE

The purpose of the second edition of this textbook is to provide a comprehensive overview of current science and practice in geriatric physical therapy. Although the first edition of *Geriatric Physical Therapy* was designed primarily for physical therapist students and professional curricula, the text also was embraced by graduate physical therapists in post-professional programs and practicing clinicians. Therefore, the second edition addresses a wider scope of clinical issues than the first edition to meet the multiple needs of its readers in managing the geriatric patient. It is my strong belief that the current (and future) success of geriatric physical therapists lies in their ability to ground the practice of geriatric physical therapy in the foundational sciences and concepts and principles of general physical therapist practice. Similarly, it is hoped that this text assists readers to answer the question, "How does general physical therapist practice change when the patient is an older adult?" in order to draw upon the full extent of their knowledge and experience as physical therapists with all patients and clients as well as what is uniquely geriatric physical therapy.

The text is still organized into five parts. Part I concerns the fundamental process of the art of physical therapy, communication, and four fundamental areas of physical therapy science: clinical epidemiology, physiology, arthrokinesiology, and neuroscience. Part II contains seven chapters related to assessment. Chapter 6 in this part presents the concepts of health status, impairment, functional limitation, and disability, and explores application of the process of disablement model, as originally articulated by Nagi, to physical therapy. Chapters 7 and 8 detail clinical and formal functional assessments of basic and instrumental activities of daily living in the elderly and review sensory changes of aging and environments that facilitate independence. Cognitive loss and depression are two impairments known to influence elderly function, and Chapters 9 and 10 provide information on these conditions that is essential to physical therapist examination and evaluation of the geriatric patient. Chapters 11 and 12 promote an understanding of the medical workup and how medical evaluation and pharmacological treatment interface with physical therapist examination, evaluation, diagnosis, prognosis, and intervention.

Part III contains 13 chapters covering the clinical practice of geriatric physical therapy. These chapters present current research on the scientific basis of specific physical therapy interventions in key areas: functional training, ventilation and respiration, endurance training, muscle fatigue and endurance, posture, balance and falls, ambulation, lower extremity orthotics, lower extremity prosthetics, incontinence, pain management, wound healing, and patient-related instruction. These chapters highlight how physical therapy interventions with the older adult differ from treatment for younger individuals and in what instances examination strategies and intervention procedures and techniques need to be modified for the geriatric patient or client. Furthermore, contributing authors have attempted to draw some conclusions about what outcomes can realistically be achieved with an older adult with respect to a particular problem.

The chapters in Part IV consider the social context of geriatric physical therapy: reimbursement issues as well as the ethical and legal issues that surround the daily practice of geriatric physical therapy. Part V presents programmatic aspects of physical therapy services for elders who fall into one of four groups: those who live in nursing homes; those who live in the community and are generally well; those who continue to engage in athletics; and those with developmental disabilities. Each of these chapters outlines the characteristics of the target population and indicates how physical therapy services might be built around those needs.

The goal of geriatric physical therapy is to provide optimal clinical care and consultation to the thousands of individuals we see daily. The authors whose work is presented in this text rose to the challenge of defining geriatric physical therapy on the basis of the current evidence for practice; yet intellect alone does not ensure optimal care. The best thoughts must be translated into the best clinical actions. It is the hope of all the authors who contributed to this text that the reader will skillfully employ the principles that have been learned to perfect the practice of geriatric physical therapy.

Andrew A. Guccione, PT, PhD, FAPTA

ACKNOWLEDGMENTS

As with the first edition, the new and the continuing contributors to this second edition deserve the credit for its quality, and many thanks for making my task relatively easy once again.

Like most of us in health care, our colleagues in the publishing industry have undergone numerous acquisitions, mergers, consolidations, and configurations in the past 7 years. I am indebted to many staff at Mosby for ensuring continuity amid uncertainty, especially Christie Hart, whose efforts in bringing this new edition to press have earned my lasting gratitude. I am also grateful for the editorial precision Sarah Fike brought to this project.

In the years since the first edition, I had the opportunity to work closely with some extraordinary colleagues on the *Guide to Physical Therapist Practice*. No one at the time would have guessed at the profound impact that the Guide would have on the conceptualization of physical therapy. I am the grateful recipient of the insights of many colleagues whose intense passion for physical therapist practice has deeply influenced my own understanding of our discipline. I also would like to thank my former colleagues at the Beacon Hill Geriatric Primary Care Clinic of the Massachusetts General Hospital who graciously allowed me to practice with them as part of their team and refine theory through practice.

Seven years ago I noted:

> It is perhaps impossible to write a manuscript on any geriatric topic without pausing to reflect on aging, one's own mortality, and ultimately, a fundamental dimension of the universe: time itself. From a sociological perspective, time is not best measured by subtle deteriorations of physical matter. Rather, a person's own history is better understood as a sequence of interpersonal relationships in particular social contexts. Simply put, our family and friends allow us to mark where we have been, who we are now, and what we shall become.

I could not have known then how many of our colleagues, including a contributor to the first edition, would be lost to us well before they entered the ranks of older adults. Their memory lives on in our collective history and we must acknowledge their contributions to what we shall become as a profession.

Finally, I must recognize my wife, Nancy, and my daughters, Katie and Nicole, who have defined my own history, sustained me through many days, and without whom no future would be nearly as good.

Andrew A. Guccione, PT, PhD, FAPTA

CONTENTS

P A R T   I

Foundations of Geriatric Physical Therapy

IMPLICATIONS OF AN AGING POPULATION FOR REHABILITATION: DEMOGRAPHY, MORTALITY, AND MORBIDITY IN THE ELDERLY

ANDREW A. GUCCIONE, PT, PHD, FAPTA

INTRODUCTION

What are the implications of an increase in the number of older persons in American society, particularly as it affects rehabilitation specialists such as physical therapists? On the one hand, the "graying" of America has been portrayed as a social problem, one that particularly threatens to strip the current health care system of its scarce resources. On the other hand, we are aware of many healthy, active elderly, still very much engaged in life and, in fact, a resource to their families and their communities. Is it possible that these two contrasting representations of America's older persons refer to the same set of individuals?

The purpose of this chapter is to review the sociodemographic characteristics of the elderly, then relate these factors to mortality and morbidity in this population. In doing so,

we shall find that conflicting portrayals of older persons as active and healthy, or as sick and frail, are not incorrect, but more appropriately applied to only some segments of an entire population subgroup.

Although physical therapists implement interventions in a plan of care designed for individual patients or clients, each of us has physical, psychological, and social characteristics by which we can be categorized into groups. Knowing that individuals with certain characteristics—being a particular age or sex—are more likely to experience a particular health problem can assist therapists in anticipating some clinical presentations, placing an individual's progress in perspective, and even sometimes altering outcomes through preventive measures. It is also useful to know the prevalence of a particular condition (i.e., the number of cases of that condition in a population) and its incidence (the number of new cases of a condition in a population over a specified time period). Taken beyond examination of a single person, physical therapists can use this information to plan and develop services to meet the needs of an aging society whose members span a continuum across health, infirmity, and death.

DEMOGRAPHY
Definition of the "Elderly"
The first gerontologic question is, How does a particular segment of a population come to be categorized as "old?" The chronological criterion that is presently used for identifying the old in America is strictly arbitrary and usually has been set at 65 years. Yet the onset of some of the health

problems of elders may occur as soon as they enter their early 50s, and as detailed in Chapter 30, "older" athletes may be only in their 40s. As the mean age of the population increases each decade and more individuals live into their ninth decades, we can expect that our notion of who is old will change.

The number of Americans aged 65 and older continues to grow at an unprecedented rate. In 1996 there were 33.9 million people aged 65 or older,[77] reflecting the major changes in the population structure of the United States in this century. Individuals who had reached their 65th birthday accounted for only 4% of the total population in 1900. In 1940 they were 6.9% of the population, and by 1950, they were equal to 8.2%. Although they represented just fewer than 10% of the population in 1970, they currently account for approximately 13% of the U.S. population.[15] Individuals older than 85 currently represent about 10% of people older than 65. Although the number of elders aged 85 or older in 1990 accounted for just more than 1% of the population, their representation within the general populace is likely to quadruple by 2050.[75,77] The number of individuals older than 100 also continues to increase, even through the actual proportion of these elders among persons aged 65 and older (12 in 10,000) is relatively small.[77]

Two concurrent factors that have affected the increase in the proportion of aged in our society are a declining birthrate and a declining death rate.[57] With fewer births overall and more survivors at older ages, the age structure of the population changes from a triangular shape, with a larger number of younger individuals at the base, to a more rectangular distribution of the population by age, with a larger number of older individuals at the top. In 1996 the median age of the United States was 34.6 years (Fig. 1-1).[77]

Racial and nonwhite ethnic minorities are currently underrepresented among the nation's elders relative to the distribution of these subgroups in the general population. In the overall population, approximately 17% of the United States is nonwhite, and almost 75% of these individuals of all ages are black.[77] Although 87% of American elders were white, non-Hispanic individuals in 1990, it has been predicted that this proportion may decrease by as much as 20% in the next 50 years.[48] Among the oldest-old (85 years or older), the population of black elders is growing faster than that of their white counterparts.[75] Hispanic elders have the highest overall growth rate of any subgroup, and the number of Hispanic elders within the total population is expected to quadruple by 2015.[16] More recent immigrations in the 1990s of peoples from Southeast Asia will likely also result in increased representation of these groups among the elderly in the future, adding to the small number of American-born Asian elders.[46] Overall, the proportion of nonwhites among all American aged will grow. Therefore, the geriatric physical therapist must recognize that "the elderly" of the future will be more racially and culturally diverse than those elderly patients whom are currently served.

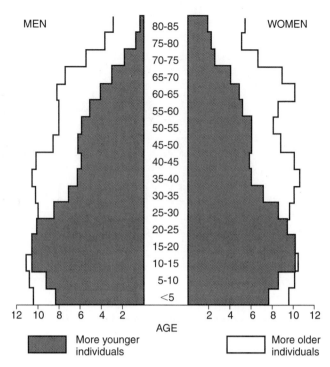

FIG. 1-1   Total population age structure by age group and sex showing shift in population from having more younger individuals (triangular shape) to a population having more older individuals (rectangular shape).

Sex Distribution and Marital Status

Because women usually live longer than men, the problems of America's elders are largely the problems of women. In 1996, there were just over 2 men for every 3 women older than 65; this ratio widened to about 1 man for every 3 women among individuals older than 85.[77] Older women have a significant probability of living longer than their mates. In contrast to the 46% of women aged 65 years or older who were widows, only 15% of their male counterparts had lost their spouses.[77]

Loss of a spouse or life partner poses its own set of challenges to the individual. Married women, in particular, may experience a severe disruption of typical social roles: wife, homemaker, confidant, and member of a couple. This disruption complicates the search for self-validation through the recognition, esteem, and affection of another that may have been present in marriage.

Living Arrangements

Although more than 70% of elders have surviving children, the proportion of elders living alone increases with age (Fig. 1-2).[34] Hispanic elders are less likely than whites or blacks to live alone.[76,85] Little is yet known about Asian elderly. When elders need assistance in basic and instrumental activities of daily living (ADL), spouses and children often provide the majority of help. Only a small portion of these services is usually provided by formal care-givers.[34] Decline in func-

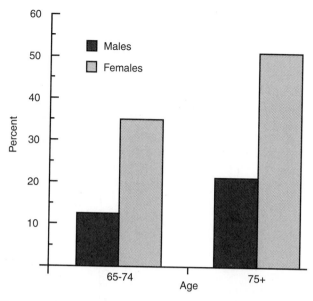

FIG. 1-2 Percentage of community elderly living alone, 1984. (Data from Kovar MG: Aging in the eighties, age 65 and over and living alone, contacts with family, friends, and neighbors. Preliminary data from the Supplement on Aging to the National Health Interview Survey: US, January–June 1984. *Advance Data From Vital and Health Statistics, No 116.* Hyattsville, Md, Public Health Service, DHHS No [PHS] 86–1250, 1986.)

tional abilities strongly predicts the likelihood that an elder living alone will seek other arrangements.[84] The unavailability of informal social support through family and friends has been implicated as a factor contributing to nursing home placement.[34]

Overall, just fewer than 5% of elders reside in a nursing home.[34] It has been suggested, however, that for every disabled elder in a nursing home there may be as many as three equally disabled elders who are able to continue living in the community with strong social support.[34] Furthermore, an analysis of the proportion of elderly in nursing homes by age reveals that nursing home utilization increases from 2% among those 65 to 74 years old to 20% for those 85 years and older.[34] In general, female nursing home residents outnumber males (Fig. 1-3, *A*), and white nursing home residents are more numerous than nonwhite residents (Fig. 1-3, *B*). Some evidence suggests that elders have as great as a 40% chance of spending at least some time in a nursing home in their lifetimes.[34] Many of these individuals will have short-term admissions and return to their premorbid living arrangements.

In 1995 elders in nursing homes were predominately female (75%); 75 years and older (82%); white (89%), non-Hispanic (92%); and widowed (62%).[9,73] Hing also had previously found that nursing home placement may be affected by functional dependency, cognitive impairment, marital status, and previous living arrangements.[30] Although comparisons made between nursing home usage in 1995, 1985, and 1973-1974 indicate some growth in minority place-

ments, black males and females use nursing homes substantially less than their white counterparts.[9] This underutilization pattern with respect to nursing homes may be balanced by broader utilization of community-based services and the presence of extensive informal care-giving networks among ethnic and racial subgroups of elders, even in the face of possibly greater activity limitations.[76] However, it is not clear that informal services make up for the care that would be provided formally in the community.[49,81] Data from the Asset and Health Dynamics Among the Oldest Old (AHEAD) study suggest that there may be a number of factors that influence the degree to which such networks are available to black elders.[56] This informal care-giving network may be a critical factor that will allow these elders to remain in the community in the future, given the likelihood that black elders will live alone as survivorship among blacks improves. Geriatric physical therapists may often need to expand their notion of "family" in their efforts to do patient-"family" teaching beyond the blood relatives of a minority elder.

Family Roles and Relationships

Despite many recent changes for younger generations of women, the degree to which current female elders are still bound by society to their traditional homemaking roles should not be underestimated.[51] A disabled male is able to retire from work, his primary socially ordained role, without taking on additional responsibility within the home. In contrast, a disabled woman, regardless of her employment status outside the home, is still expected to continue to do homemaking activities such as housekeeping and grocery shopping, whatever her level of physical function. Women are therefore more likely than men to report disability with respect to social roles.[32] The relative unavailability of assistance with home chores in comparison with other social support services may be a subtle discrimination against older women, although the level of unmet need in this area is not well-documented. These home services can often be the essential element in allowing an elder to remain living independently at home when functional abilities are compromised. Physical therapists will need to continue working with other health professionals to advocate for access to a wide range of services that support the highest level of independent living for the aged.

Although some anecdotes promote an image of American elders as abandoned by their children, ample evidence exists that elders do have frequent contact with their families.[2] Several factors that affect the amount of contact between elder and offspring have been cited. Daughters, particularly those who are middle-aged, tend to have more contact than sons. Widowed parents tend to have more contact with their children than their still-married peers, and unmarried children may be in contact with their parents more often than married children are. The simple fact is that the variability of family contact is very high and cannot easily be generalized, despite common wisdom about the nature of families, the

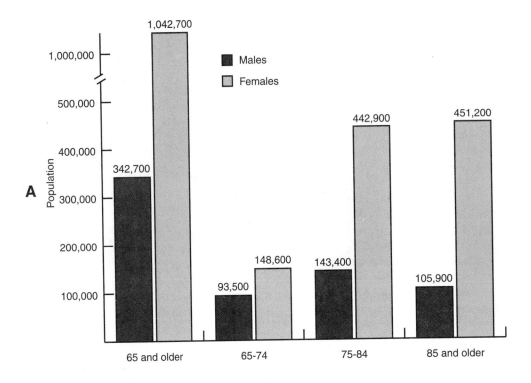

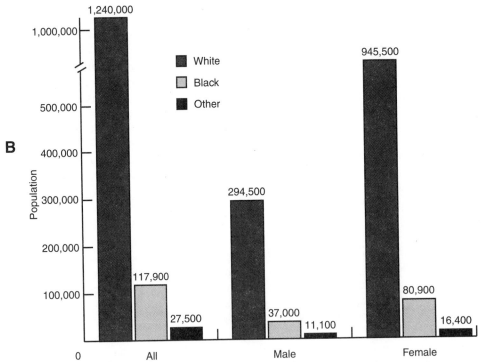

FIG. 1-3 A, Number of nursing home residents 65 years of age or older, by sex and age at admission: United States, 1995. **B,** Number of nursing home residents 65 years of age or older, by sex and race: United States, 1995. (Redrawn from Dey AN: Characteristics of elderly nursing home residents. Data from the 1995 National Nursing Home Survey. *Advance Data from Vital and Health Statistics, No 289.* Hyattsville, Md, Public Health Service, DHHS Publication No [PHS] 97–1250, 1997.)

influence of ethnicity, and gender-specific roles in caring for elders.

Elders who do live with family can often find themselves in multigenerational families, growing old with their children.[2] Whereas a sick elder is often the recipient of direct care and emotional support, healthy elders are often a source of financial and emotional support as well.[2] Spouses are the most likely individuals to care for their partners in old age and sickness. When a spouse is unable or unavailable to provide assistance, it is not always easily surmised who will do what for an aging parent in need. The actual provision of direct care to elders has traditionally been "women's work."[2,51] Research has not elucidated the role of men in caring for elderly parents as investigators have often assumed the common wisdom that care-giving falls to daughters and daughters-in-law, often to the exclusion of men as subjects in many studies.[2] Fewer children and increases in the number of women entering the work force have decreased the number of otherwise unemployed women available to take care of family elders.[2] Many of these middle-aged women find themselves caught with multiple and often competing obligations to their own children (some of whom may still be living at home), to their parents, and to themselves. Yet, research is lacking to substantiate that these "women-in-the-middle" regard this opportunity as a burden and do not derive satisfaction from this role.[11,59,64] Recommendations by physical therapists that increase the tasks of care-giving among family members (for example, assisting with a home exercise program) may be perceived as either a burden or as an opportunity to engage in a productive social role. Many stereotypes about different racial and ethnic groups exist, but the data do not support a facile conclusion that one group is more "predisposed" to offer assistance.[1] Physical therapists must evaluate each family situation for its unique characteristics.

The role of grandparent has also changed, especially for women.[2] Increased longevity increases the amount of one's life that might be spent being a grandparent. It is not unusual for an elder to witness a grandchild's movement through the life course from birth up to the grandchild's adulthood. Healthy elders still provide substantial financial and emotional support to their children. Many grandparents find themselves taking on additional baby-sitting and child-rearing responsibilities, particularly as their daughters remain employed outside the home. Therefore, an examination and evaluation of an elder's functional abilities in this social context might need to consider whether a grandparent has the dexterity to change a diaper, the strength to lift a toddler, and the stamina to walk young children home from the school bus.

Economic Status

Regarding the elderly as a single group with similar needs is a habit that is easy to acquire. The heterogeneity of the elderly as a group is perhaps best illustrated by considering how financially well-off economically the elderly are. If we treat the aged as a homogeneous group, they overall appear to be doing better economically than expected. This is due to the entrance of the youngest of the old, who benefit from private and workers' pension programs, into the ranks of the aged. Furthermore, the elderly are not generally as bad off as children, the other population subgroup that is largely dependent on society's resources. In comparison with poverty among children aged 17 years or younger, the elderly have experienced a relatively steady decline in poverty.[6] These group figures, however, obscure the realities of poverty among the elderly: poverty increases with age; women are more often in poverty than men; married males and females are better off than their nonmarried peers; elders living alone tend to show the highest poverty rate of all; and once poor, elders are likely to remain poor.[6,7] Furthermore, there is a substantial disparity in wealth between elders in the top 10% and the bottom 10% of wealth distribution.[71]

In 1995, the poverty line for a single person older than 65 was $7,309 per annum and was $10,259 per annum for an elderly couple.[77] Using this figure, 10.5% of the American population older than 65 were below the poverty line in 1995.[77] Disaggregating the poverty rate by race demonstrates additional disparities, with about one quarter of black elders and one quarter of Hispanic elders living in poverty.[77] These figures do not adequately portray the economic disadvantage of persons aged 65 or older who are between 100% and 200% of the poverty line. These individuals are in particular economic jeopardy: too "wealthy" to qualify for means-tested assistance and too poor to provide well for themselves.

It is worthwhile to inquire as to why women, even former working women, are especially prone to poverty in old age. Three reasons have been suggested.[82] First, women who did work usually held jobs in occupations and industries dominated by women and characterized by high rates of turnover, lack of unionization and pension coverage, and low wages and fringe benefits. Second, women have tended to have had interrupted careers that reduce their overall earnings histories. Therefore, because Social Security benefits are calculated on wage histories, average Social Security benefits for women are usually lower than those for men. Third, the reduction in benefits that occurs when a woman is widowed may hasten her slide into poverty, as a single income may be insufficient to meet basic needs. Although the market for physical therapy services will continue to increase with the growth of the geriatric population, the capacity of this predominantly female group to purchase physical therapy and other health care services "out of pocket" is likely to be limited. Given their overall economic resources, a substantial proportion of elderly income goes for medical insurance, deductibles, and co-insurance payments. The failure to remove these financial barriers could ultimately prevent access to physical therapy, despite the needs of this population.

MORTALITY

Life Expectancy

In addition to a declining birthrate, the other factor that accounts for the increasing number of elderly is an increase in average life expectancy. Life expectancy can be calculated from two points: at birth and a time closer to death. Taking the first approach, a child born in 1900 would have been expected to live only 49 years on the average, and only 41% of the children born that year would have been expected to reach age 65. By 1974 the average life expectancy of a child born that year had grown to 71.9 years, and 74% of that birth cohort is expected to reach age 65.[72] An American male born in 1995 is expected to live 72.6 years on the average and a female 6.3 years longer.[77]

Advancing age and gender are the two most important predictors of mortality in the elderly. Male death rates at every age are consistently higher than those for women.[4,15] On the positive side, there has been a consistent decline in the mortality rate in the general population and for persons aged 65 years or older. Older men have experienced a 33% decline in death rates over the course of the 20th century, whereas death rates among older women have dropped 45% in the same time period. However, racial disparities indicate that black men and women have not experienced declines in death rates that are similar to those of white elders.[15]

Despite recent medical advances in treating geriatric conditions, particularly cardiovascular disease, most of the changes in average life expectancy took place before 1955.[72] Since then, only a few years have been added to life expectancy calculations. Furthermore, the major gains in life expectancy in this century have occurred primarily due to advances in postnatal and infant care rather than advances in adult or geriatric health care.[72] The benefits of improved infant care, however, have not been distributed evenly throughout the population with respect to either race or gender. Male black children born in 1995 are expected to live 7.2 years less than their white counterparts. Although black females born in 1995 are generally expected to live longer than white males, these women will fall short of the life expectancy of white females by 4.9 years on the average.[77] Data on Hispanic and Asian elders have only begun to be routinely collected in national surveys. Initial analyses suggest that both of these groups of elders have lower death rates than their white counterparts.[10,47]

A slightly different picture of racial differences in longevity emerges if we consider life expectancy after age 65 rather than at birth, even though hypotheses about the life expectancy and health of minority elders are difficult to confirm and very dependent on the data source.[18] One of the most intriguing facts to emerge from studies of racial differences in mortality is a phenomenon called "black-white crossover."[83] Simply put, when comparing age-specific death rates, we find higher rates among young or elderly blacks compared with whites the same age and lower rates among very old blacks compared with very old whites (Fig. 1-4). Thus, if we include very old black elders in our frame of reference, their lower death rate counterbalances the higher death rate among younger blacks. Combining young blacks and old black elders into a single group statistically lowers the overall black mortality rate, even though younger blacks continue to have greater mortality than whites of the same age.[31] Crude generalizations of groups data, which underplay the heterogeneity of the elderly and differences among older persons across age-groups, can be misleading and should therefore be avoided.

Factors other than age itself have been hypothesized to influence death rates among elders. It is not clear, however, that what holds true for the overall population in general or for white elders in particular will hold true in studies of minority elders. For example, in their review of the physical

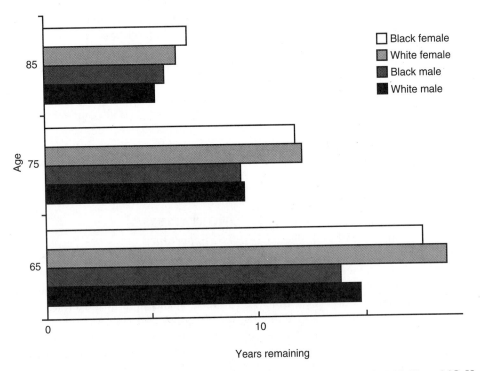

Fig. 1-4   Life expectancy of the elderly in 1984. (Redrawn from Havlik RG, Liu MG, Kovar MG: Health statistics on older persons, United States, 1986. *Vital and Health Statistics Series 3, No 25.* Washington, DC, Public Health Service, DHHS, No [PHS] 87–1409, 1987.)

health of middle-aged and aged blacks, Jackson and Perry found that there were no statistically significant differences in death rates between married and nonmarried blacks, despite the expectation that there would be such a difference based on other studies that have shown a direct relationship between survivorship and marital status.[31] They concluded that other factors such as income and education may be more important predictors of the life expectancy of black Americans. Gibson has proposed that risk factors for ill health in old age may be distinctly different for blacks than for whites.[17] While the racial disparity in average life expectancy has been persistent throughout this century, a percentage analysis reveals that minority gains have been substantial. Although fewer black males reached 65 than their white counterparts in 1977, this represents a 190% increase from 1900, double the increase documented for white males in the same time period. White females reaching their 65th birthday increased 91% from 1900 to 1977. Nonwhite females made an even more remarkable gain of a 230% increase in those reaching age 65 in comparison with their counterparts in 1900.[72]

Causes of Death

The three most common causes of death for all elderly are coronary heart disease (CHD), cancer, and stroke.[4,27] CHD accounts for 31% of all deaths in both men and women older than 65.[4] It is believed that declines in mortality from CHD in the past 30 years have been due to risk factor reduction earlier in the life span. Almost 20% of deaths in all elders are due to cancers.[4] Once again, however, it becomes important to distinguish between data on elders taken as a single group and data broken down by specific age-groups. Deaths from cancer rise through middle adulthood and decline with old age. Generally speaking, there are fewer deaths attributable to cancer in the elderly overall due to the prolonged survival of individuals with cancer to older ages. This contrasts with death from cardiovascular causes, which continues to increase rapidly with advancing years. Age-specific cancer death rates, however, show an increase in cancer mortality in each successive age-group.[27]

The death rate from stroke increases exponentially with age and is higher for men than women at every age.[5] Stroke mortality has declined in the United States for most of this century, most likely due to improvements in the detection and treatment of hypertension.

Morbidity

Active Life Expectancy

While gains in overall life expectancy are important indicators of a nation's well-being, active life expectancy, i.e., the years spent without and with a major infirmity or disabling condition, may provide more meaningful information for health professionals.[36] Using data from the Massachusetts Health Care Panel Study, Katz and colleagues calculated a score on each individual's overall level of independence in bathing, dressing, transfers, and eating.[36] They found that active life expectancy decreased with age, with the largest decrements for those older than 79 (Fig. 1-5). Elders who were 65 to 69 years old could anticipate another 10 years of independent ADL, whereas elders 80 to 84 years old would likely remain independent for only another 4.7 years. Indi-

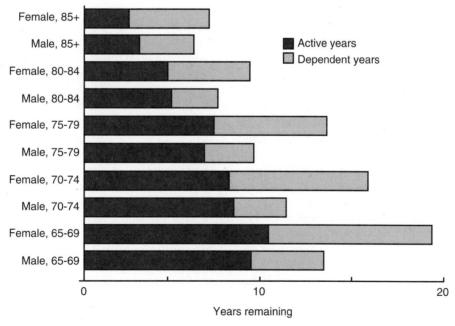

Fig. 1-5 Active versus dependent life expectancy in Massachusetts elderly, 1974. (Redrawn from Katz S, et al: *N Engl J Med* 1983: 309:1218-1224.)

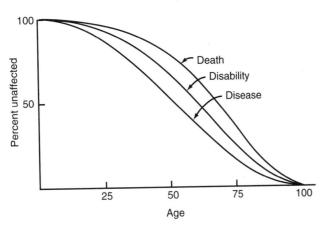

FIG. 1-6   Schematic relationships among disease, disability, and death.

viduals 85 or older who were independent in these four ADL were likely to enjoy an active life expectancy of a mere 2.9 years. Although active life expectancy did not differ in this study between men and women, there were substantial differences between the poor and nonpoor, especially at younger ages. Nonpoor elders aged 65 to 69 had 2.4 additional years of active life expectancy than poor elders. This difference narrowed dramatically to less than 1 year between poor and nonpoor groups for those 75 years or older.[36]

Fig.1-6 schematically depicts our current view of the life span. As an individual ages, the likelihood of onset of disease, followed by a period of disability and ultimately death, increases. Rowe and Kahn have proposed that human aging be classified into two categories: usual and successful.[66] Traditionally, geriatric research has focused on the pathologic changes associated with "normal" aging (disease and disability in Fig. 1-6), while ignoring the elders who do not exhibit these changes. Thus, "normal" aging has been used erroneously to mean "usual" aging. Although elders who are "successful" agers do not escape the eventuality of disease, disability, and death, they are able to decrease their overall morbidity and delay the onset of disability. Their success has been attributed to "intrinsic" factors such as heredity but also to extrinsic factors such as stress, diet, and exercise. Harris and Feldman have suggested a third category for "high-risk" or "accelerated" aging.[29] Their recommendations for the epidemiological study of aging are also applicable to health care.[29] Physical therapists can assist the promotion of successful aging by encouraging modification of some extrinsic factors, particularly in teenagers and young adults. Among usual agers, physical therapists can concentrate on reducing the disabling effects of disease and stopping a vicious cycle of "disease-disability-new incident disease." The goal of physical therapy for "accelerated" agers would be to maintain their current level of function and prevent further rapid deterioration.

The degree to which disease and disability can be "compressed" and postponed until the last years of life has been a source of great controversy. Fries had proposed that if the average age of onset of significant morbidity increased more rapidly than gains in life expectancy, both the proportion of one's life spent infirm and the overall length of infirmity would be shortened.[12-14]

Even though particular individuals might have experienced such a compression, the data generally did not support Fries' hypothesis for the entire population of this country's elderly.[23] Guralnik and his colleagues compared the prevalence of disability in 531 elders who had received three annual examinations to that of the 8821 survivors in the same cohort.[25] Their findings indicated that decedents in every age-subgroup group had more disability than survivors. Those dying at the oldest ages had more disability than those dying at younger ages. Thus, if more elders die at older ages, they will likely experience even greater functional deterioration for more years before their deaths than if they had died at younger ages.

Opposite to proposing a compression of morbidity, Olshansky and others have argued that there will be an expansion of morbidity as medical technology improves the likelihood of survival from previously fatal diseases without improving overall quality of life for these individuals.[58] Furthermore, the older individuals live, the more likely they are to experience functional decline. Thus, they appear to have traded death at an earlier age for more years spent with one of the nonfatal diseases of aging and its associated disability before death.

Prevalent Chronic Conditions

The proportion of elderly at any age without any chronic conditions is small.[24] More than one half of male elders older than 80 years and 70% of female elders of similar age have two or more chronic conditions. In 1991, arthritis was the most prevalent self-reported condition of the elderly, followed by high blood pressure, diabetes, hearing impairments, and heart disease.[50] Chronic conditions are not randomly dispersed throughout the population. Kingston and Smith analyzed data on 9744 men and women in the 1992 Health and Retirement Survey and found that blacks reported higher rates of hypertension, diabetes, and arthritis than white survey participants.[40] Hispanic participants reported higher rates of hypertension and diabetes but less heart disease.

Functional Limitations

In 1985 the total number of disabled elderly living in the community with any degree of chronic limitations in any basic or instrumental ADL was 5.5 million persons.[44] Limitations in functional activities increase with age. Elders in the 65- to 74-year-old group are thought to be healthier and generally better off than their counterparts aged 75 years or older, who are often termed the "frail elderly."

In 1984, data were gathered on 11,497 elders through the Supplement on Aging to the National Health Interview Survey.[8] More than three fourths of all these elders experienced no difficulty in self-care activities or walking. Age, however, did have a substantial effect on disability. Whereas 85% of elders between the ages of 65 and 69 experienced no difficulty in self-care activities or walking, only 66% of elders between 80 and 84 and 51% of elders older than 85 could report similar levels of well-being. While only 5.7% of elders aged 75 to 79 reported difficulty with four or more self-care activities, this figure almost doubled in the 80- to 84-year-old group and more than tripled in those 85 years or older. Preliminary data from the National Institute on Aging Established Populations for Epidemiologic Studies of the Elderly (EPESE) corroborated this finding that physical disability is most prevalent in the oldest-old.[5] The EPESE data also indicate that physical disability is more prevalent for elderly women than for men at every age.

It should be noted that while there is substantial evidence that function declines with age, there is also some evidence that some elders are able to maintain a high level of function. In a longitudinal study of physical ability of the oldest-old based on data from the Longitudinal Study on Aging, Harris and associates found that one third of elders older than 80 reported no difficulty in walking one-quarter mile; lifting 10 pounds; climbing 10 steps without resting; or stooping, crouching, and kneeling.[28]

As in the general population, it is generally agreed that physical disability overall increases with age among blacks.[31] The linearity of this increase has been challenged, as there is mounting evidence that younger blacks, that is, those 74 years old or younger, are more physically disabled than those aged 75 to 79, and that those aged 80 to 84 are more disabled than those 85 and older.[19]

Disease and Disability

Several studies have implicated cardiovascular diseases as a cause of disability in the elderly. We know from the Framingham studies, for example, that angina pectoris is related to disability in men and women. Furthermore, long-term and current hypertension, being overweight, and diabetes are associated with disability in women, but long-term hypertension is related to disability in men.[61,62] The demonstration of a relationship between angina and disability in women has been replicated in other studies as well.[55]

The Framingham Heart Study has also provided some insight into the relationships among stroke, mortality, and disability. Kelly-Hayes and colleagues reported on all incident strokes over a 10-year period in 3920 elders who were free of stroke at the start of the study in 1971.[38] Only 154 patients out of 213 incident cases of stroke survived more than 30 days. Of those who survived more than 30 days, 42 were living in institutions 1 year later. Factors predicting institutionalization were different in women than in men. Age, severity, and education were associated with institutionalization in women, whereas not being married was the only variable in men that predicted institutionalization after a stroke. These findings have been corroborated in a study of 1274 stroke cases in Australia. In addition to severity and side of paraly-

sis, Shah and colleagues found that age, sex, marital status, and ethnicity were associated with the outcome of rehabilitation.[69]

Kelly-Hayes replicated her previous finding of the high mortality rate of stroke in another analysis of new cases of stroke in a 4½-year period in the early 1980s.[39] Only 67 individuals out of 119 subjects who sustained a stroke were alive 1 year later. It is still unclear as to how long one can expect functional recovery after a stroke. Do patients reach a plateau of optimal function within 3 to 6 months of their stroke, or do they continue to make slow, progressive gains? Tangeman and associates found improvement in weight shifting, balance, and ADL in 40 individuals who were at least 1 year poststroke following an intensive rehabilitation program.[74] These subjects also demonstrated their new abilities at follow-up 3 months later. Although baseline measures were collected 1 month before the start of the study, these investigators were unable to determine whether the improvement demonstrated after intensive therapy represented a return to a previous plateau of optimal function or in fact demonstrated additional recovery. They could also not determine whether additional rehabilitation would benefit more severely impaired elders. All subjects could walk independently within the home when they entered the study. This research, however, does indicate that a short trial of therapy may be beneficial to some patients whose functional level has begun to fall or who may not have achieved their optimal functional level during rehabilitation immediately after their strokes.

Hip fractures in the elderly represent an enormous threat to well-being. Depending on the study, the mortality rate of hip fracture patients may be as high as 25%. Wolinsky and colleagues found that hip fracture almost doubled the risk of death in the first 6 months after fracture and was strongly associated with subsequent hospitalizations and a loss of function.[84] Estimates of recovery after a fracture have suggested that anywhere from 25% to 75% of these individuals will not achieve their premorbid level of function.[43] A study of 526 hip fracture patients over a 2-year period found that most recovery of the ability to walk and perform ADL occurred within 6 months. Poor recovery was associated with older age, prefracture dependency, longer hospital stay, dementia, postsurgical delirium in patients without dementia, and lack of contact with a social support network. It has also been shown that depression negatively affects outcomes in these patients[53] and that low levels of ambulatory ability will, in turn, engender depression in the months after hip fracture.[54]

Not all diseases affect function globally, as might be expected based on our understanding of the impacts of stroke or hip fracture. Some conditions have effects that are limited to activities that use the afflicted body part. For example, Satariano found that breast cancer, the most prevalent cancer of older women, limited activities that required upper body strength but did not affect other activities.[68] Similarly, in a study of knee osteoarthritis, a commonly afflicted joint in a highly prevalent disease, Guccione and co-workers found that limitations in only those activities that used the lower extremity were more likely among elders with this condition than elders without it.[20]

Few studies have attempted to establish the relationship between disease and disability in nursing home residents. Guccione and colleagues reported the functional status of 126 nursing home residents, of whom 51 had either rheumatoid arthritis or osteoarthritis.[21] Controlling for age, residents with arthritis had more pain and were more likely to require assistance dressing, bringing a glass to the mouth, turning a faucet, getting in and out of bed, bending down, and walking. They were also more likely to use a wheelchair daily than other residents without arthritis.

Comorbidity and Function

Guralnik and colleagues have provided ample evidence that an increase in the number of activities with which an elder has difficulty increases linearly with comorbidity, that is, co-existent medical conditions (Fig. 1-7).[24] Thus, it is not unusual for physical therapists to find that the most disabled patients are also likely to have a number of medical conditions that complicate not only understanding of the genesis of functional deficit but treatment as well. For example, the individual with a stroke, who also has degenerative changes in the foot and low tolerance for stressful activity secondary to angina with exertion, can present a particular challenge to the geriatric physical therapist's knowledge and skill.

Although there is an emerging body of knowledge on the effects of disease on function, less is known about the effects of co-existent disease on function. Elders vary a great deal in the degree to which their chronic comorbidity affects their functional capacities. Based on analyses of data from the 1984 Supplement on Aging, Verbrugge and co-workers concluded that relative to other diseases the most prevalent conditions do not appear to have the highest risks of physical disability in the elderly.[78] This conclusion should not be taken out of the context of its research aim to rank the relative impact of diseases on function. The impacts of prevalent conditions on function in the elderly are still considerable, even if somewhat less than rarer conditions, regardless of the rank order of their impacts. Guccione and colleagues analyzed the independent association of 10 different medical comorbidities with disability among 1769 community-based elders in the Framingham Heart Study cohort.[22] They found that disability in seven functional activities was most associated with stroke, hip fracture, and depression—three of the least prevalent conditions, even after controlling for age, gender, and the presence of any other medical conditions. The likelihood of disability associated with knee osteoarthritis and heart disease, the two most prevalent conditions, was substantial, even though these relationships were not as strong or consistent across all the functional activities as the less prevalent conditions. The combination of their prevalence and the magnitude of risk for disability that these two conditions pose for elders accounts for a larger percentage of disability in community-based elders than is attributable to more disabling, but less prevalent, diseases. Furthermore, even in stroke, which has a broad impact on function, dis-

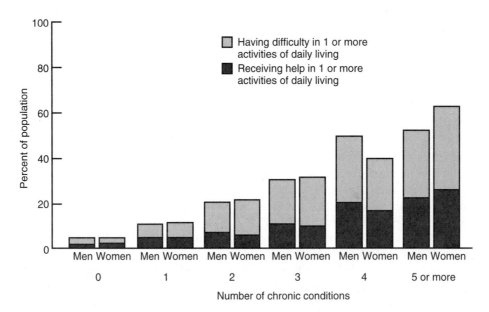

FIG. 1-7   Age-adjusted prevalence of men and women 60 years and older having difficulty and receiving help in one or more activities of daily living, by number of chronic conditions: United States, 1984. (Redrawn from Guralnik J, et al: Aging in the eighties: The prevalence of comorbidity and its association with disability. *Advance Data From Vital and Health Statistics,* Hyattsville, Md, Public Health Service, DHHS Publication No [PHS] 89–1250, 1989.)

ease-related disability may be attributable to different conditions in men and women.[33] Strategies to prevent diseases in younger adults and efforts to retard the effects of disease on function should ultimately alter the trajectory of disability in the elderly in a positive direction.[44]

Psychosocial Factors and Function

Physical therapists must also not forget that factors other than disease can modify disability in the elderly. Mor and colleagues found in a study of 1737 elders aged 70 to 74 years old that those who did not report exercising regularly or walking 1 mile were 1½ times as likely to decline functionally over 2 years; this is especially relevant to physical therapists.[52] Other research provides clues for other interventions involving life-style modifications before old age. In an analysis of data from the Alameda County Study, Kaplan found income, smoking, social isolation, and depression associated with trouble climbing stairs and getting outdoors in elders with incident of heart trouble, stroke, diabetes, or arthritis.[35] Using the same cohort, Guralnik and Kaplan compared the function of elders in the top 20% of functioning with that of the remainder elders at follow-up 19 years later.[26] They found several longitudinal predictors of good function: not being black; higher family income; absence of hypertension, arthritis, and back pain; being a nonsmoker; having normal weight; and consuming moderate amounts of alcohol. Although being male predicted higher levels of functioning in men, being female did not predict higher levels of functioning in women. This last finding highlights an important statistical problem in geriatric research: any population-based sample of elders is likely to contain more women, who, by virtue of living longer, are also more likely to be disabled. Thus, without controlling statistically for age and gender, any positive effect on functional outcome that might accrue to women at younger ages may be obscured.

Education is also linked to health and function. Manton and co-workers, using data from the 1982, 1984, and 1989 Long Term Care Surveys, found that increased mortality and decreased functional ability were strongly associated with fewer than eight years of schooling in both men and women.[45] In addition to finding that education was associated with functional level, Berkman and Gurland noted that income was also independently associated with functional limitations, even after controlling for a number of other variables.[3]

One of the most intriguing issues in minority health care is the effects of race on the health status of elders compared with the effects of income.[60,79] Wallace has suggested that race had effects on the health care of the black elderly living in St. Louis that were independent of income.[80] Satariano, on the other hand, could not find an independent effect for race in a sample of 906 black and white elders living in an economically depressed area of Alameda County.[67] When Keil and colleagues analyzed data on the elders in the Charleston Heart Study cohort, which included 71 high socioeconomic status (SES) black males, they found that black females had the highest rate of disability (55.8%), followed by white females, black men, and white males.[37] The high SES group of black males had the lowest prevalence of disability. Although further research is necessary to untangle the contributions of race and income to functional well-being in the elderly, it is important to consider the potential impact of these factors on the outcomes of rehabilitation, whether it be for the purposes of research or for clinical practice.

Factors that contribute to good function in the elderly may also differ between men and women. Using data from the Framingham Heart Study, Pinsky and co-workers found that age, alcohol use, smoking, ventricular rate, and education were all significantly related to function 21 years later in men but that only education predicted functional well-being in women.[63] Thus, in analyzing what factors may predispose an elder to functional decline, physical therapists should remember that what is generally known about the elderly may not apply equally to men and women.

Utilization of Services

Functional deficits are important markers for death, further functional decline, and increased utilization of services. In a 2-year follow-up study of 1791 white elders aged 80 or older, Harris and colleagues found that those who had received help with any ADL were four times more likely to have died.[28] Among those elders who survived, elders with functional limitations in any ADL were six times as likely to have used a nursing home in the intervening 2 years and two times as likely to have been hospitalized at least twice or to have had six or more physician visits in the year before follow-up. Data from the Medical Expenditure Panel Survey indicate that more than 80% of nursing home residents in 1996 needed assistance with three or more ADL.[41]

Although it was estimated that in 1987, 5.6 million noninstitutionalized elders had difficulty in walking or with at least one basic or instrumental ADL, many (3.6 million) received no formal services.[70] Almost 20% of these services were for professional or homemaking services provided in the home, except meals delivered to the home (Fig. 1-8). Adult day care accounted for less than 1%. When an elder received care at home, it was typically provided by a homemaker (Fig. 1-9). Functional limitations are strongly associated with the use of formal services. Elderly persons with three or more limitations in ADL are more likely to use home-based services rather than community-based services.

Rehabilitation specialists are quick to assume that merely offering their services to elders living in the community will delay functional decline and reduce the threat of institutionalization. Unfortunately, little evidence exists to support this assumption. Liang and co-workers provided intensive multidisciplinary care, including physical therapy, to frail elders living in the community and were unable to alter the long-range course of their physical decline.[42] This finding speaks to the multiplicity of factors that affect the disablement of older persons.

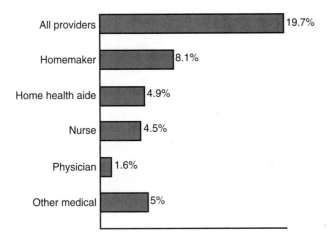

FIG. 1-8   Percentage of persons 65 and older with any functional difficulty who use particular services. (Redrawn from Short P, Leon J: Use of home and community services by persons ages 65 and older with functional difficulties. *National Medical Expenditure Survey Research Findings 5.* Rockville, Md, Agency for Health Care Policy and Research, Public Health Service, DHHS Publication No [PHS] 90–3466, 1990.)

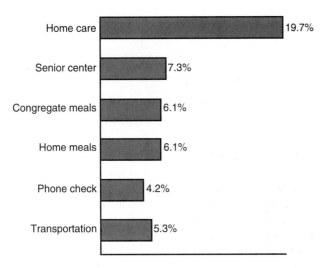

FIG. 1-9   Percentage of persons 65 and older with any functional difficulty receiving service from home care providers. (Redrawn from Short P, Leon J: Use of home and community services by persons ages 65 and older with functional difficulties. *National Medical Expenditure Survey Research Findings 5.* Rockville, Md, Agency for Health Care Policy and Research, Public Health Service, DHHS Publication No [PHS] 90–3466, 1990.)

SUMMARY

Changes in the demographic characteristics of the U.S. population represent a critical challenge to geriatric physical therapists. Elders are expected to live longer than ever before, but the quality of their lives in these added years is still a matter of conjecture. Aging with multiple diseases further aggravates a propensity toward physical decline with ad-

vanced age. Function deficits are the expected outcomes of disease; in turn, functional limitations predict increased utilization of services, further morbidity, and death. Future research must establish the ability of physical therapy to delay the onset of disease and disability and to prolong optimal function into old age.

REFERENCES

1. Allen-Kelsey GJ: Caregiver burden among African-American and Anglo-American family caregivers. *Topics Geriatr Rehabil* 1998; 14(1):63-73.
2. Bengston V, Rosenthal C, Burton L: Paradoxes of families and aging, in Binstock RH, George LK (eds): *Handbook of Aging and the Social Sciences,* ed 4. San Diego, Academic Press, 1996.
3. Berkman CS, Gurland BJ: The relationship among income, other socioeconomic indicators, and functional level in older persons. *J Aging Health* 1998; 10:81-98.
4. Bush TL, et al: Risk factors for morbidity and mortality in older populations: An epidemiologic approach, in Hazzard WR, et al (eds): *Principles of Geriatric Medicine and Gerontology,* ed 3. New York, McGraw-Hill, 1994.
5. Cornoni-Huntley JC, et al: Epidemiology of disability in the oldest-old: Methodologic issues and preliminary findings. *Milbank Mem Fund Q/Health Soc* 1985; 63:350-376.
6. Crystal S: Economic status of the elderly, in Binstock RH, George LK (eds): *Handbook of Aging and the Social Sciences,* ed 4. San Diego, Academic Press, 1996.
7. Crystal S, Waehrer K: Later-life economic inequality in longitudinal perspective. *J Gerontol* 1996; 51B:S307-S318.
8. Dawson D, Hendershot G, Fulton J: Aging in the eighties. Functional limitations of individuals age 65 and over. *Advance Data From Vital and Health Statistics, No 113.* Hyattsville, Md, Public Health Service, DHHS Publication No (PHS) 87-1250, 1987.
9. Dey AN: Characteristics of elderly nursing home residents: Data from the 1995 National Nursing Home Survey. *Advance Data From Vital and Health Statistics, No 289.* Hyattsville, Md, Public Health Service, DHHS Publication No (PHS) 97-1250, 1997.
10. Elo IT, Preston SH: Racial and ethnic differences in mortality at older ages, in Martin LG, Soldo BJ (eds): *Racial and Ethnic Differences in the Health of Older Americans.* Washington, DC, National Academy Press, 1997.
11. Farkas JI, Himes CL: The influence of caregiving and employment on the voluntary activities of midlife and older women. *J Gerontol* 1997; 52B:S180-S189.
12. Fries JF: Aging, natural death, and the compression of morbidity. *New Engl J Med* 1980; 303:130-135.
13. Fries JF: The compression of morbidity. *Milbank Mem Fund Q/Health Soc* 1983; 61:397-419.
14. Fries JF: The compression of morbidity: Miscellaneous comments about a theme. *Gerontologist* 1984; 24:354-359.
15. Furner SE, Brody JA, Jankowski LM: Epidemiology and aging, in Cassel CK, et al (eds): *Geriatric Medicine,* ed 3. New York, Springer-Verlag, 1990.
16. Gelfand DE: *Aging and Ethnicity.* New York, Springer Publishing Co, 1994.
17. Gibson RC: Age-by-race differences in the health and functioning of elderly persons. *J Aging Health* 1991; 3:335-351.
18. Gibson RC, Jackson JS: The black oldest-old: Health, functioning and informal support, in Suzman RM, Willis DP, Manton KG (eds): *The Oldest Old.* New York, Oxford University Press, 1992.
19. Gibson RC, Jackson JS: The health, physical functioning, and informal supports of the black elderly. *Milbank Mem Fund Q/Health Soc* 1987; 65(suppl 2):421-454.
20. Guccione AA, Felson DT, Anderson JJ: Defining arthritis and measuring functional status in elders: Methodological issues in the study of disease and physical disability. *Am J Public Health* 1990; 80:945-949.

21. Guccione AA, Meenan RF, Anderson JJ: Arthritis in nursing home residents: A validation of its prevalence and examination of its impact on institutionalization and functional status. *Arthritis Rheum* 1989; 32:1546-1553.

22. Guccione AA, et al: The effects of specific medical conditions on the functional limitations of elders in the Framingham Study. *Amer J Publ Health* 1994; 84:351-358.

23. Guralnik J: Prospects for the compression of morbidity: The challenge posed by increasing disability in the years prior to death. *J Aging Health* 1991; 3:138-154.

24. Guralnik JM, et al: Aging in the eighties: The prevalence of comorbidity and its association with disability. *Advance Data From Vital and Health Statistics, No 170.* Hyattsville, Md, Public Health Service, DHHS Publication No (PHS) 89-1250, 1989.

25. Guralnik JM, et al: Morbidity and disability in older persons in the years prior to death. *Am J Public Health* 1991; 81:443-447.

26. Guralnik JM, Kaplan GA: Predictors of health aging: Prospective evidence from the Alameda County Study. *Am J Public Health* 1989; 79:703-708.

27. Hadley EC: Causes of death among the oldest old, in Suzman RM, Willis DP, Manton KG (eds): *The Oldest Old.* New York, Oxford University Press, 1992.

28. Harris T, et al: Longitudinal study of physical ability in the oldest-old. *Am J Public Health* 1989; 79:698-702.

29. Harris TB, Feldman JJ: Implications of health status in analysis of risk in older persons. *J Aging Health* 1991; 3:262-284.

30. Hing E: Use of nursing homes by the elderly: Preliminary data from the 1985 National Nursing Home Survey. *Advance Data From Vital and Health Statistics, No 135.* Hyattsville, Md, Public Health Service, DHHS Publication No (PHS) 87-1250, 1987.

31. Jackson JJ, Perry C: Physical health conditions of middle-aged and aged blacks, in Markides KS (ed): *Aging and Health.* Newbury Park, NJ, Sage Publications, 1989.

32. Jette AM, Branch LG: Impairment and disability in the aged. *J Chronic Dis* 1985; 38:59-65.

33. Jette AM et al: The Framingham Disability Study: Physical disability among community-dwelling survivors of stroke. *J Clin Epidemiol* 1988; 41:719-726.

34. Kane RL, Ouslander JG, Abrass IB: *Essentials of Clinical Geriatrics,* ed 3. New York, McGraw-Hill, 1994.

35. Kaplan GA: Epidemiologic observations on the compression of morbidity. *J Aging Health* 1991; 3:155-171.

36. Katz S, et al: Active life expectancy. *New Engl J Med* 1983; 309: 1218-1224.

37. Keil JE, et al: Predictors of physical disability in elderly blacks and whites of the Charleston Heart Study. *J Clin Epidemiol* 1989; 42: 521-529.

38. Kelly-Hayes M, et al: Factors influencing survival and need for institutionalization following stroke: The Framingham Study. *Arch Phys Med Rehabil* 1988; 69:415-418.

39. Kelly-Hayes M, et al: Time course of functional recovery after stroke: The Framingham Study. *J Neuro Rehabil* 1989; 3:65-70.

40. Kingston RS, Smith JP: Socioeconomic status and racial and ethnic differences in functional status associated with chronic diseases. *Amer J Publ Health* 1997; 87:805-810.

41. Krauss NA, Altman BM: Characteristics of nursing home residents— 1996. *MEPS Research Findings No. 5.* Rockville, Md, Agency for Health Care Policy and Research, 1998, Pub No 99-0006.

42. Liang MH, et al: Evaluation of a rehabilitation component of home care for homebound elderly. *Am J Prev Med* 1986; 2:30-34.

43. Magaziner J, et al: Predictors of functional recovery one year following hospital discharge for hip fracture: A prospective study. *J Gerontol* 1990; 45:M101-107.

44. Manton KG: Epidemiological, demographic and social correlates of disability among the elderly. *Milbank Q* 1989; 67(suppl, pt 1):13-58.

45. Manton KG, Stallard E, Corder L: Education-specific estimates of life expectancy and age-specific disability in the U.S. Elderly Population: 1982 to 1991. *J Aging Health* 1997; 9:419-450.

46. Markides KS, Black SA: Race, ethnicity and aging: The impact of inequality, in Binstock RH, George LK: *Handbook of Aging and the Social Sciences,* ed 4. San Diego, Academic Press, 1996.

47. Markides KS, et al: Health status of Hispanic elderly, in Martin LG, Soldo BJ (eds): *Racial and Ethnic Differences in the Health of Older Americans.* Washington, DC, National Academy Press, 1997.

48. Martin LG, Soldo BJ: Introduction, in Martin LG, Soldo BJ (eds): *Racial and Ethnic Differences in the Health of Older Americans.* Washington, DC, National Academy Press, 1997.

49. Miller B, et al: Minority use of community long-term care services: A comparative analysis. *J Gerontol* 1996; 51B: S70-S81.

50. Mittlemark MB: The epidemiology of aging, in Hazzard WR, et al (eds): *Principles of Geriatric Medicine and Gerontology,* ed 3. New York, McGraw-Hill, 1994.

51. Moen P: Gender, age and the life course, in Binstock RH, George LK (eds): *Handbook of Aging and the Social Sciences,* ed 4. San Diego, Academic Press, 1996.

52. Mor V, et al: Risk of functional decline among well elders. *J Clin Epidemiol* 1989; 42:895-904.

53. Mossey JM, Knott K, Craik R: The effects of persistent depressive symptoms on hip fracture recovery. *J Gerontol* 1990; 45:M163-168.

54. Mutran EJ, et al: Social support, depression and recovery of walking ability following hip fracture surgery. *J Gerontol* 1998; 50B: S354-S361.

55. Nickel JT, Chirikos TN: Functional disability of elderly patients with long-term coronary heart disease: A sex-stratified analysis. *J Gerontol* 1990; 45:S60-68.

56. Norgard TM, Rodgers WL: Patterns of in-home care among elderly black and white Americans. *J Gerontol* 1997; 52B(Special Issue):93-101.

57. Olshansky SJ: The demography of aging, in Cassel CK, et al (eds): *Geriatric Medicine,* ed 3. New York, Springer-Verlag, 1990.

58. Olshansky SJ, et al: Trading off longer life for worsening health: The expansion of morbidity hypothesis. *J Aging Health* 1991; 3:194-216.

59. Pavalko EK, Artis JE: Women's caregiving and paid work: Causal relationships in late midlife. *J Gerontol* 1997; 52B:S170-S179.

60. Peck CW, et al: Differences by race in the decline of health over time. *J Gerontol* 1997; 52B:S336-S344.

61. Pinsky JL, et al: Framingham Disability Study: Relationship of disability to cardiovascular risk factors among persons free of diagnosed cardiovascular disease. *Am J Epidemiol* 1985; 122:644-656.

62. Pinsky JL, et al: The Framingham Disability Study: Relationship of various coronary heart disease manifestations to disability in older persons living in the community. *Am J Public Health* 1990; 80:1363-1367.

63. Pinsky JL, Leaverton PE, Stokes J: Predictors of good function: The Framingham Study. *J Chronic Dis* 1987; 40(suppl 1):159S-167S.

64. Rosenthal CJ, et al: Caught in the middle? Occupancy in multiple roles and help to parents in a national probability sample of Canadian adults. *J Gerontol* 1996; 51B:S274-283.

65. Rowe JW: Toward successful aging: Limitations of the morbidity associated with "normal" aging, in Hazzard WR, et al (eds): *Principles of Geriatric Medicine and Gerontology,* ed 2. New York, McGraw-Hill, 1990.

66. Rowe JW, Kahn RL: Human aging: Usual and successful. *Science* 1987; 237:143-149.

67. Satariano WA, et al: Race, socioeconomic status, and health: A study of age differences in a depressed area. *Am J Prev Med* 1986; 2:1-5.

68. Satariano WA, et al: Difficulties in physical functioning reported by middle-aged and elderly women with breast cancer: A case-control comparison. *J Gerontol* 1990; 45:M3-11.

69. Shah S, Vanclay F, Cooper B: Stroke rehabilitation: Australian patient profile and functional outcome. *J Clin Epidemiol* 1991; 44:21-28.

70. Short P, Leon J: Use of home and community services by persons ages 65 and older with functional difficulties. *National Medical Expenditure Survey Research Findings 5.* Rockville, Md, Agency for Health Care Policy and Research, Public Health Service, DHHS Publication No (PHS) 90-3466, 1990.

71. Smith JP: Wealth inequality among older Americans. *J Gerontol* 1997; 52B(Special Issue): 74-81.

72. Spence DL, Brown WW: Functional assessment of the aged person, in Granger CV, Gresham GE (eds): *Functional Assessment in Rehabilitation Medicine.* Baltimore, Williams & Wilkins, 1984.

73. Strahan GW: An overview of nursing homes and their current residents: Data from the 1995 National Nursing Home Survey. *Advance Data From Vital and Health Statistics, No 280.* Hyattsville, Md, National Center for Health Statistics, DHHS Publication No (PHS) 97-1250, 1997.

74. Tangeman PT, Banaitis DA, Williams AK: Rehabilitation of chronic stroke patients: Changes in functional performance. *Arch Phys Med Rehabil* 1990; 71:876-880.

75. Taeuber CM, Rosenwaike I: A demographic portrait of America's oldest old, in Suzman RM, Willis DP, Manton KG (eds): *The Oldest Old.* New York, Oxford University Press, 1992.

76. Tennstedt S, Chang B: The relative contribution of ethnicity versus socioeconomic status in explaining differences in disability and receipt of informal care. *J Gerontol* 1998; 53B:S61-S70.

77. US Bureau of the Census: *Statistical Abstract of the United States: 1997,* ed 117. Washington, DC, 1997.

78. Verbrugge LM, Lepkowski JM, Imanaka Y: Comorbidity and its impact on disability. *Milbank Q* 1989; 67:450-484.

79. Wallace SP: The political economy of health care for elderly blacks. *Int J Health Serv* 1990; 20:665-680.

80. Wallace SP: Race versus class in the health care of African-American elderly. *Social Problems* 1990; 37:517-534.

81. Wallace SP, et al: The persistence of race and ethnicity in the use of long-term care. *J Gerontol* 1998; 51B:S104-S112.

82. Warlick JL: Why is poverty after 65 a woman's problem? *J Gerontol* 1985; 40:751-757.

83. Wing JS, et al: The black/white mortality crossover: Investigation in a community-based study. *J Gerontol* 1985; 40:78-84.

84. Wolinsky FD, Fitzgerald JF, Stump TE: The effect of hip fracture on mortality, hospitalization, and functional status: A prospective study. *Amer J Publ Health* 1997; 87:398-403.

85. Worobey JL, Angel RJ: Functional capacity and living arrangements of unmarried elderly persons. *J Gerontol* 1990; 45:S95-101.

COMMUNICATION, VALUES, AND THE QUALITY OF LIFE

MARILYN D. PHILLIPS, PT, MS AND NANCY L. PEATMAN, PT, MED

INTRODUCTION

What we believe about human nature, perceive as valuable in our world, and identify as "quality of life" drive our decisions, our behavior, and our communication. Our personal and professional values guide and direct our behavior and choices based on what we perceive to be "most important" within a situation of conflicting demands. Health care professionals share some common professional values. These professional values must limit and define the parameters of our professional relationships and roles with clients and colleagues. As health care professionals, our role is to do no harm; to develop a trusting relationship based on honesty and truthfulness; to promote independence; to display an "unconditional positive regard"; and to promote a belief in each individual as unique, able, and capable of change.

Professional communication is a learned skill that promotes the establishment of a professional "helping" relationship. These relationships remain within the scope of our physical therapy skills, are directed toward the goals and independence of the client, and focus only on the client. Our professional communication is a tool consciously implemented to facilitate our physical therapy therapeutic interventions.

The purpose of this chapter is to highlight significant components of communication with the elderly, to address the parameters of one's professional role in relation to the elderly, and to identify the issues that commonly affect the quality of life of the elderly.

COMMUNICATION

Communication is commonly defined as the transmission of information or messages between individuals.[19] Communication is a learned, culturally based skill.[4] It is a complex process, conveyed in written, oral, and nonverbal forms. An effective communicator adapts the content of the message and the style of transmission of the message to the needs of the receiver.[19] For example, "That's HOT!"—a simple warning about a hot stove—would be communicated quite differently to a young child, to an adult, to a person with a hearing impairment, or to a person not fluent in the English language.

Similarly, effective communication with the elderly requires adaptation to the common physiological, psychological, and social changes that result from the aging process. These changes, when unrecognized in an elderly individual, are common barriers to effective communication. These changes present another barrier when they are incorrectly generalized to exist in all elderly persons. It must be remembered that the aging process produces a slowly progressing, yet individually unique, set of variations in physiological, psychological, and social functioning.[4,7] Thus, effective communication with an elderly individual considers the effects of the aging process on that individual and adapts accordingly.

Effects of Physiological Changes of Aging on Communication

Hearing

Hearing loss is the third most prevalent chronic condition affecting noninstitutionalized elders after arthritis and hypertensive disease.[22]

Presbycusis, the form of hearing loss due to age-related physiological changes of the inner ear, is one of the most widespread sensory deficits associated with aging.[26,30,31,35,36,49] The physiological changes in the inner ear may cause loss of high-frequency sounds and loss of sound localization; impairment of speech discrimination, especially for specific sounds of the alphabet (s, sh, ch, f, g, t, z); and distortion of received messages.

Auditory impairment is often gradual, with even mild to moderate hearing losses, resulting in significant communication and social dysfunction.[1] Auditory impairments are usually more severe in men than in women.[60] Elders with inner ear hearing loss have difficulty modulating the volume of their voice, may appear to be "not listening," may show confusion or puzzlement when being addressed, may respond slowly with repeated questions of "What?", and may complain of not "understanding." These behaviors common with inner ear hearing loss must be differentially diagnosed from dementia, depression, or impaired cognitive function.

Outer or middle ear hearing loss, commonly known as *conductive hearing loss,* is not limited to high-frequency sounds. Unlike the sensorineural hearing losses of the inner ear, conductive hearing loss may be corrected by increasing the volume of transmissions with a hearing aid. Hearing loss can have a devastating effect on an older adult's ability to communicate. Practitioners can learn to improve communication with the hearing impaired. Box 2-1 details common strategies that facilitate communication with the hearing impaired.[9,26,30,35,36,61,62]

Sight

Visual deficits affect receptive communication in the elder, especially when the visual deficit is only one of many sensory changes restricting communication. Low vision interrupts communication and social interaction for the elder who can no longer perceive nonverbal cues. All structures of the eye develop age-related changes to varying degrees.[7,30,31] These changes affect the ability to see in low light or to adapt to darkness or changes in light. Elders may also have difficulty in judging distances, seeing objects that are too close or located in peripheral fields of vision, or accommodating between close and distant objects. Colors, especially blue and green, may be poorly differentiated. Highly reflective surfaces will also challenge an elder. The maintenance of autonomy and the optimizing of visual reception are the key elements to effective communication with a vision-impaired individual. Box 2-2 suggests strategies for effective communication with a vision-impaired elder.[34]

Speech

Decreased respiratory efficiency and laryngeal function with aging results in a lower-pitched voice, a lower volume, and a shortened controlled expiration rate with speech production.

BOX 2-1
IMPROVING COMMUNICATION WITH THE HEARING IMPAIRED

- Move closer to the listener for increased ease of hearing and seeing.
- Face the listener with nonglaring light on the speaker's face.
- Signal before speaking to gain the listener's attention.
- Ask the listener what you can do to assist his/her hearing better.
- Assist in adjusting eyeglasses or hearing aids.
- Request permission to decrease background noise and music.
- Speak at eye level, facing the listener.
- Do not obscure your mouth or face because lipreading assists comprehension.
- Speak at a normal to slightly louder volume but not shouting.
- Speak at a normal to slightly slower rate, and articulate clearly.
- Watch the movement of the listener's head, which may indicate an ear with better hearing.
- Be concise because listening requires great concentration.
- Identify the topic of conversation and avoid sudden changes.
- Stress key words by increasing their duration.
- Pause after key words.
- Give the listener time to respond.
- Ask the listener to repeat information to ensure comprehension.
- Never use "baby talk."
- Use gestures to supplement speech.
- Rephrase rather than repeat missed statements.
- Use a notepad for messages as needed.
- Choose a voice pitch and sound frequencies within the individual's hearing range whenever possible.

BOX 2-2
IMPROVING COMMUNICATION WITH THE VISUALLY IMPAIRED

- Avoid startling an elder. Approach slowly and use verbal greetings and touch.
- Avoid positioning an elder in glaring light, and adjust levels of light to accommodate the elder's vision. This may be up to three times more light than a younger adult may require.
- Check the condition of eyeglasses. Request that the older adult use his/her eyeglasses while conversing with you.
- Position what needs attention in the center of the older adult's visual field.
- Provide large-print materials with high-contrast colors; for example, black print on yellow with 12-14 point type.
- Use tactile stimulation for cueing.
- Avoid moving personal belongings, and discuss any changes in placement of furniture or belongings.
- Wait for the elder's vision to adapt to changes in light.
- Reduce glare on surfaces including floors, bedside tables, and bathroom sinks.

These effects of aging may result in a softer, lower voice with breathiness, hoarseness, or vocal tremor. Sentences may shorten to accommodate a reduced, controlled expiration rate.[25] Communication with an elder with age-related speech changes is facilitated by a quiet environment, which permits the therapist and the patient to listen attentively. It is often helpful if the therapist watches the elder's lips and asks for clarification or repetition if the elder is not understood.

An increase in time between a stimulus and a response, or reaction time, is a manifestation of the gradual slowing of performance that is a normal physiological process. Increased reaction time is a phenomenon that begins early in life and becomes prominent only with age. Clinically, an increase in reaction time will contribute to a decrease in memory, especially recent memory; a decrease in the speed of processing information; a decrease in vocabulary; and a decrease in the rate of speech.[50] Promoting self-pacing and accommodating your rate of communication to match the elder's reaction time will significantly increase learning.[7]

Facial Expression

Facial expression is another normal age-related change that may affect expressive communication. Campbell and Lancaster note that sagging cheeks or jowls, which gives a resting appearance of "anger" or "crabbiness" to many elderly men and women, is actually the result of significant loss of fat in the muscle fibers of the face.[7] The assumption of mood or frame of mind from the resting facial expression of an elder could be misleading and impede effective communication.

Sleep Patterns

Age-related changes in sleep patterns begin in the fourth decade. Variability of sleep patterns is evident with an increase in the amount of time spent sleeping, a change in the stages of sleep, and an increase in the number of nighttime awakenings.[31] By the sixth decade, deep (stage 4) sleep is almost gone. With advancing age there is a gradual increase in the total amount of sleep time, in napping, in the amount of nap time, and in wake episodes after sleep onset.[6] After the age of 85 years, going to sleep often takes longer. An elder's mental acuity and overall ability to function are affected by problems of sleeplessness or changes in sleep patterns. Therefore, attention to sleep patterns may help a practitioner understand a patient's affect, communication style, and response to treatment.[32]

Strategies for Effective Communication

Communication is an essential component of the role of a health care professional. Effective interpersonal skills are *learned* skills that focus on the patient, promote trust and confidence, allow the expression of feelings and concerns, efficiently collect information, and effectively impart important information.

Research has shown that effective communication strategies improve patient outcomes as measured by patient satisfaction and compliance. Research on patient satisfaction, in general, and on older adults' satisfaction in particular, indi-

cates that communication between the practitioner and the client is improved when (1) the practitioner shows a warm, supportive interpersonal style and provides information; (2) the client is given the opportunity to explain his/her concerns and is an active participant in the decision making; and (3) the interaction is client-centered and addresses the client's needs.[20]

A variety of facilitative techniques exist that promote the effective treatment and overall well-being of one's patient or client when used appropriately. Several approaches to assist health professionals in developing the attitudes and interpersonal skills of an effective communicator have been developed.[17,19,33,43] All these strategies are founded on several commonly held professional values. Respect for the individual, the promotion of the patient's autonomy, and the nurturance of a trusting relationship are the guiding principles of all professional relationships. The strategies for improving communication with elders listed in Box 2-3 translate these principles into common actions.[8,40,51,58]

Facilitation of Communication and Socialization

Basic communication and interpersonal skills for the "helping professional" are outside the scope of this text. All health care providers should recognize the use of facilitatory communication skills and the establishment of a professional

---

Box 2-3

STRATEGIES FOR IMPROVING COMMUNICATION WITH ELDERS

- Do not stereotype. Do not assume a level of decreased mental function or confusion. Posture, gesture, and facial expressions can be deceiving.
- Be aware of, and adapt to, any age-related physical limitations that an elder may possess. Consider the sensory deficits in sight, hearing, speech, and reaction time, which may be barriers to communication.
- Secure the elder's attention by eye contact or a gentle touch.
- Identify yourself when greeting an elder. Request information from each elder on how best to communicate, e.g., "Should I speak louder?" or "Would you like your glasses?"
- Ask each individual what form of address is preferred. Do not use generic or pet names such as "Grampa" or "Mama." Each individual has a unique identity.
- Request permission to adjust the volume of the television or radio or to change the amount or angle of light.
- Maintain eye contact.
- Use topic cues. Identify the topic at the beginning of the conversation.
- Listen patiently to the older adult. Rephrase or repeat what was said, and encourage the older adult to elaborate.
- Watch facial expression and other nonverbal cues.
- Do not pretend to understand an elder's response. Request confirmation or clarification of a message you do not understand.
- Avoid speaking to elders as if they were children. Do not use a singsong voice or baby talk or give orders.
- Do not ignore individuals or talk about them in the presence of others as if they were not there.
- Respect an elder's routines and control of his life. Schedule and keep appointments at mutually agreed-on times.

"helping" relationship as essential vehicles to their provision of care. The essence of our professional interventions and effectiveness is our ability to respond to a human being as a unique, worthwhile individual. The use of touch, reminiscence, humor, and pets serve as effective stimuli to interaction and socialization with the elderly.

Touch

Touch has a significant effect in reinforcing our interactions with the elderly. Studies show touch to be a positive motivator that engenders a sense of trust, shows caring, and generally increases the duration of verbal responses from an elder.[23,24,59]

Reminiscence

Reminiscence is a useful communication approach that provides validation of the individual's place in the community, increases self-esteem, and assists in the resolution of losses. Reminiscence is a normal coping skill that begins in middle childhood. Reminiscence is defined as "the act or habit of thinking about or relating past experiences, especially those considered personally most significant."[38] Studies on reminiscence report an increase in communication, life satisfaction, and positive self-image.[3,42] The use of pictures; music; or topics such as "the Great Depression," FDR, hometowns, or favorite pastimes are examples that promote the expression of feelings and a sense of self-worth.[41]

Humor

Humor has numerous positive physiological and psychological effects on the body. Laughter "stimulates the production of catecholamines and hormones which enhance feelings of well being as well as pain tolerance. It decreases anxiety, increases the flow of endorphins, cardiac and respiratory rates, enhances metabolism and improves muscle tone."[55] Humor and laughter are very effective forms of communication that build trust, defuse anger or frustration, and promote shared experience. Humor is infectious and, similar to other types of communication, can be learned. The use of humor between a therapist and a patient requires three conditions: (1) a relationship that allows for the introduction of playfulness without misinterpretation; (2) a social environment that allows for playfulness without disrupting the serious business; and (3) a joker who provides clues to set the mood and takes the risk that the message will be ignored.[49,55] It must be remembered that healthy humor is not abusive or diminishing. Instead, healthy humor promotes understanding through positive shared experience, is life-affirming, and is stress-reducing.[47,48]

Pets

Communication can also be fostered by nonhuman means. Pets can play a significant role in combating loneliness and decreasing isolation by increasing verbalization and socialization among the elderly. Pets have been found to be natural "icebreakers," facilitating social interaction. The physical act of petting promotes a mutual relaxation, a therapeutic "caring for a living thing."[14] A pet is a companion, a "significant other," that provides structure to daily activities, gives and requires attention, and usually instigates a greater degree of physical exercise.

VALUES

Autonomy

Elders are people first and thus are entitled to be treated with respect and dignity and without bias. It is imperative that health care professionals respect and address the individuality of each elder they encounter, regardless of the circumstances in which they encounter them. It is not immediately important whether an older adult is living alone or is a resident of a nursing home; whether the person has multiple chronic illnesses or none; or whether the individual is cognitively alert or exhibits signs of dementia. A basic tenet of the geriatric physical therapist is that respect for the "person" is the paramount principle underlying all interactions.

The concept of respect implies preserving choice on the part of the older adult—freedom to actively participate in decision making, to the extent that he/she is capable, and to choose what is or what is not done to him/her, irrespective of chronological age.[5] The ability of older adults to retain this decision-making power and their enforceable right to make those decisions have been the impetus over the years for enacting legislation on informed consent and protection of patients' rights. When these legal requirements are enforced, the older adult is in control of the decision rather than subject to the imposition of decisions from external sources.

Societal and cultural beliefs, however, can significantly dilute the autonomy that is the right of the older adult. It is essential to explore how these influences, whether subtle or overt, affect therapeutic outcomes. For the geriatric physical therapist, it is not enough to be just aware of such factors. Rather, it is necessary that conscious attention be paid to these influences so that, whether patient or client, the older adult can be valued as a contributor to the health care team.

Ageism

Although awareness of the dangers of stereotyping elders is increasing, most would agree that conscious efforts to educate against negative generalizations need to continue since many older adults continue to be stigmatized. Unfortunately, we continue to live in an ageist society. *Ageism* has been variously described as the discriminatory treatment of the elderly, or a personal revulsion to growing older.[2,43] It fosters the development of erroneous assumptions about the capabilities, intelligence, and physical skills of the older adult, based purely on deep-seated beliefs about aging. It supports judgments about a person on the basis of chronological age and negates the concept of an individual approach to patient care by encouraging premature decisions regarding the older adult's status and potential. More important, in an era where collaboration between the health care provider and the client is being espoused, ageism effectively eliminates the older adult as the primary decision maker and significantly reduces the value of his/her contribution on any level.

One example of ageism can readily be seen in the words and language used when referring to older adults.[2] For example, the term "old people" connotes a more negative image than the word *elders*. In many cultures as well as in various religions, older adults are accorded positions of respect and authority. The council of elders in various churches is a positive image, implying a knowledgeable, decision-making group. And, in many native American cultures, elders are viewed in much the same way, commanding the respect of the tribe and dispensing wisdom collected through the years. Yet the uses of many demeaning and derogatory terms, such as "old biddy," "fogey," and "geezer," continue to flourish in our culture. If we accept the principle that the language we use is reflective of what we are thinking and that what we think is shaped by our values and beliefs, then the use of negative terminology when referring to the older adult population is more than a simple choice of words.[2] Rather, it is the verbalization of deeply held negative values and beliefs. Ageist language is common and is continually reinforced by the mass media. Over time, a term that was once offensive becomes less so, sometimes to the extent that it may become acceptable. The danger is that use, and eventual acceptance, of ageist language may contribute to maintaining the very stereotypes to be dispelled.[2] Although health care practitioners may consciously state that they do not subscribe to an ageist philosophy, they may in fact undermine their good intentions through the use of language with negative connotations of aging.

Older adults, themselves, can be guilty of ageism, conditioned through experience or observation of societal trends and behavior to expect, and then accept the words attributed to them as they age. Unfortunately, as Rodin and Langer have shown, continued labeling decreases feelings of self-worth and brings about negative changes in behavior and decrements in perceived control.[49] Real losses occur all around older adults by virtue of their life stage, e.g., loss of spouse; loss of friends; loss of home, and in some cases, even loss of children. These changes are adjustments in life that older adults can expect to occur as their chronological age increases. In general, adaptation to these life changes does not imply concomitant loss of control over decision making. However, older adults may be so conditioned to expect a loss of control as they age because of societal influences such as ageism that they unnecessarily and voluntarily give up additional control over their lives, self-imposing further loss. According to Ryden, loss of control over decision making can significantly affect an older adult's quality of life.[51] One way then to combat the possible effects of ageism in our society is to foster, in all cases, an elder's control of decision making, thereby improving the individual's quality of life.

Perceived Control vs. Helplessness/Hopelessness

Who controls the decision making for an older adult is especially pertinent to quality-of-life issues among our aging population. Perceived control of decision making is actually a very strong contributor to the level of morale of older

adults, and morale factors strongly into the overall equation of quality of life.[51] Conversely, loss of control and feelings of helplessness can lead to lack of motivation and withdrawal. Logically, then, fostering an older adult's control of decision making should be preserved if we are committed to retaining or improving the quality of life. However, just as ageist language has become accepted in society, so has the expectation that responsibility for decision making slowly, but automatically, shifts away from the older adult, presumably to someone who knows more or has the best interest of this person at heart. The presumption is faulty, especially in instances in which cognition and mental capacity are not in question; yet the practice of taking decision-making authority away from the older adult persists. The elder is robbed of the opportunity to contribute to the decision and relegated instead to the role of passive recipient of someone else's judgment. Because of the powerful role that control of decision making has in maintaining the morale, it is not surprising that loss of control may precipitate a lack of interest in interacting with people or the environment. These older adults may then be characterized as lacking motivation, or as apathetic, listless, and uncommunicative. They may engender a sense of helplessness and even hopelessness or despair.[56] Passive, withdrawn behavior, particularly in institutional settings, may be unconsciously reinforced by health care professionals who support the notion that the passive residents are the good residents, because they are not disruptive to the flow of work.[51] The likelihood of this occurrence is magnified in situations where the facility is consistently understaffed or where staffing patterns are irregular. Under these circumstances, as might be expected, quality of life for the older adult is further threatened, and therapeutic outcomes are seriously hampered.

Loss of control over decision making and its sequelae, as described in the preceding text, have devastating, but not irreversible, effects on the quality of life of an older adult. Research supports the reversible nature of such behavior. Strategies and techniques that address improving perceived control of decision making have been correlated with increased self-reports of happiness, morale, and enthusiasm as well as increased alertness and activity levels noted by others.[56] It is recommended that physical therapists and other health care practitioners interested in maintaining quality of life for older adults embrace strategies and plans that are designed to return control of decision making to the older adult. Teitelman and Priddy offer six basic therapeutic strategies that can be used to facilitate such control.[56] Although designed for use in long-term–care settings, their recommendations can be extrapolated to most environments and situations, including provision of therapy, whether it be hospital-based, subacute, home care, or provided in an outpatient setting.

1. *Promotion of choice and predictability.* Even small, or what may appear to others as insignificant, choices can have a positive impact on the older adult's perception of control and can be readily incorporated on a daily basis. For example, recognizing that elders, like all per-

sons, have preferences; for example, what they wear, what food they eat, and when they go to therapy . . . and allowing them to voice those preferences with the knowledge that their choices will be honored empowers them and can improve their mental as well as physical well-being. Predictability can be included by keeping the older adult informed of overall goals and expectations.

2. *Elimination of helplessness-engendering stereotypes.* Establishing effective, productive relationships with older patients and clients—respecting and valuing their worth and recognizing their potential contributions and decision-making abilities—is the most useful health care delivery model. Self-awareness, by the health provider, of ageism and the serious consequences of loss of control is paramount. Educating others to its devastating effects is the logical next step.

3. *Promotion of therapeutic attributions and a sense of responsibility.* This involves redirecting older adults' sense of guilt or blame for the cause of their problems and encouraging more personal responsibility for effecting a positive outcome or solution. Self-blame is destructive and has the potential to fuel existing feelings of helplessness/hopelessness, whereas taking a role in identifying/effecting a solution is generally therapeutic.

4. *Provision of success experiences early on in care.* Care needs to be taken early on not to overwhelm the older adult with demands and tasks that are intimidating. Less-challenging decisions (and activities) should be attempted first, while self-confidence is allowed to build. Negative results and errors need to be anticipated and minimized by the therapist, while praise and positive reinforcement are maximized.

5. *Modification of an elder's unrealistic goals for care.* The geriatric therapist's overall goal, individualized for each older adult, is to simultaneously maintain hope and promote a therapeutic relationship while modifying any unrealistic expectations.

6. *Use of control-enhancing communication skills.* Communication that is respectful and genuine and that values the patient's/client's views and feelings can reduce helplessness and improve collaboration and cooperation in the therapeutic environment.

Culture

Ensuring that older adults are in control of their own decisions has a positive influence on outcomes, quality of life, goal setting, motivation, willingness to collaborate with professionals, and to consider professional recommendations. However, cultural influence is a powerful factor that can effectively negate a positive outcome if overlooked. Wood describes ethnicity as "common history and shared culture," whereas culture itself refers to "socially transmitted beliefs, institutions and behavior patterns that are characteristic of a particular population group."[64] Culture and ethnicity have only recently begun to receive the attention that they deserve in the health care community. However, the potential impact of each of these factors on the eventual outcome of an older adult's care must be considered from the outset, if professionals are committed to providing the best possible care.

Ethnicity and culture can affect older adults' views of death, dying, the role of the family in illness, and the importance attached to folk beliefs and medicines as opposed to current technology and medical advances. Ethnic and cultural beliefs can significantly influence the level of respect bestowed on an elder, the dynamics of the family and support system in general, the development of provider-patient relationships, the need for control of decision-making power, and certainly the extent to which an older adult will adhere to professional recommendations.[18,64] In fact, an older adult may persist in rejecting professional recommendations despite efforts by the provider to increase his/her control of decision making if attention is not given to ethnic and cultural considerations. Wood cautions that elders may believe that their own assessments of their health, "often described in colorful folk medicine causalities," should be regarded by health care professionals as seriously as these opinions are taken within the ethnic subculture.[64] Furthermore, dismissal of long-standing, culturally based beliefs is not conducive to establishing a mutually rewarding, therapeutic relationship that is built on trust.

It is not realistic to expect that health care professionals have in-depth knowledge of all subcultures, but it is recommended that awareness of and sensitivity to cultural issues be encouraged and that empathy be practiced.[64] In the absence of in-depth knowledge of specific cultural beliefs, attention to the nonverbal signals of the older adult patient, such as body language, facial expression, and eye contact, can provide the health care professional with clues that perhaps further investigation into the cultural background of the patient is appropriate. Family members and colleagues can be exceptional resources and may be able to provide valuable insight into a particular cultural or ethnic group.

Of course, when providing health care in a region with known, strong cultural influences it is incumbent on the professional to become knowledgeable of local customs and beliefs and to be creative in working to incorporate them into the overall plan of care when possible. For example, in some subcultures, the individual is traditionally a passive recipient of care, dependent on a traditional healer and local customs to effect a change in health. In addition, these individuals may wait to consult with the traditional healer before accepting even minor professional recommendations. This oftentimes further delays the initiation of care. The health care professional who unknowingly expects full, active cooperation is likely to be frustrated by these practices but, once informed, can effectively plan a reasonable course of action. The professional must have a healthy respect and appreciation for ethnic and cultural differences among older adults and recognize that culture can be a powerful influence on the entire therapeutic process.

Advocacy

One way in which quality-of-life issues in older adults can be addressed is to emphasize the concepts of patient advocacy and informed consent. Informed consent may be simplistically defined and in effect misrepresented as meaning that the patient is part of the decision-making process. While this is true on a superficial level, this definition does not adequately explain the roles and responsibilities of other participants in the decision-making process. The original intent of informed consent legislation is that health care professionals provide the patient with sufficient information about the situation so that the patient can make an educated, and therefore, informed choice.[21] In other words, communication and discussion should provide the patient with all of the information required to actually make the decision and not simply to act as a contributor to the decision-making process.

Historically, however, a paternalistic attitude has been utilized and reinforced in the medical model of health care.[15,44,63] In paternalism, decisions regarding what is best for the patient are made by the professionals. Quill and Brody assert that 25 years ago, medical decisions were made almost exclusively by the physician, perhaps with the best of intentions, but certainly minus an open dialogue.[44] Today, this can occur when individuals are truly incapable of making independent decisions because of lack of consciousness or serious cognitive impairment.[63] However, in the case of older adults, a paternalistic approach is often taken even when there is no evidence to suggest that either of these conditions is present. Wetle has remarked that paternalistic attitudes use an ageist assumption that equates old age with incompetence.[63] Unnecessary paternalism perpetuates ageism and fosters dependent, hopeless, and helpless individuals.

On the opposite end of the spectrum from the more familiar practice of paternalism is what Gadow has called *consumerism* and what Quill and Brody have termed *independent choice*.[15,44] Rather than making all the decisions for the client, the consumerism model finds the health care professional providing the elder with factual information and then withdrawing, leaving the decision totally in the hands of the client. With this model, patients are left to make a decision without the opinion or recommendation of the physician or health care professional. While at first glance this model may appear to meet the requirements of patient self-determination, neither it nor paternalism provides a mechanism in which the client is assisted with the decision process itself. One model eliminates the patient from the equation (paternalism), whereas the other eliminates the professional (consumerism).[15] "Unfortunately, a generation of physicians has been trained under the 'consumerism' or 'independent choice,' model, creating new problems as serious as those posed by paternalism."[44] Advocacy is a third model and one that empowers the elder. It relies heavily on the dynamics of the patient-provider relationship and on the active participation by the professional in assisting the older adult to make a decision. As defined by Gadow, the advocacy model is "an effort to help individuals become clear about what they want in a situation, to assist them in discerning and clarifying their values, and to help them in examining options in light of their values."[15]

There are five components to the advocacy model. The first is that of self-determination, or autonomy. The more information that an older adult has, the more able the person will be to choose what course of action is right for a particular circumstance. In the absence of complete information, informed choice is not possible. The second component is that of the patient-provider relationship. The provider's role is to enable the patient to determine the amount and type of information to be presented.

The third component in this model is one that may be new to many health care professionals but one that is uniquely important to this model: providers need to share their own values with the patient. To be able to examine all options freely the patient is entitled to know what the provider's feelings and values are. This does not imply an imposition of the provider's values on the patient, nor a coercion to decide in a prescribed way. Rather, it is a sharing of perspective and opinion that serves to strengthen the patient-provider relationship by affirming that the provider is genuinely concerned with protecting the older patient's right to self-determination by providing all the information. Disclosing provider values also has the effect of assisting individuals to clarify their own values, the fourth component in the model. It is absolutely essential for the provider/professional to discern, through discussion, what is important to the older adult, in terms of quality-of-life issues, in order to provide appropriate information. For example, will a proposed intervention increase or decrease the quality of life that the patient values? Are proposed interventions in keeping with or discordant from strongly held cultural beliefs? This component emphasizes the need for the provider to be able to set aside personal values in deference to letting the patient's values be decisive.[15]

The final component of Gadow's model is the concept of individuality. Individuality includes considerations other than values that can be decisive in self-determination. How injury or insult to the body affects a person's perception of self can significantly influence the ability to exercise free choice. The perception of self and body may be so tightly intertwined that behavior after an injury will not be consistent with how the person might have been expected to behave before the illness. For example, depression after illness or injury can significantly influence decision making. Decisions made under these circumstances may not be in keeping with usual and customary behavior before the incident. To protect an older adult's right to free choice, it is critical that the health care professional be aware of the person's sense of individuality and how it may affect the capacity for self-determination. Most important, the provider needs to be prepared to actively assist the client in exploring these issues.

Gadow's advocacy model conceptualizes the compassionate health care provider as one who not only places the well-being of the older adult above all else but also recognizes that

TABLE 2-1
CHARACTERISTICS OF TWO MEDICAL DECISION-MAKING MODELS

ENHANCED AUTONOMY MODEL	INDEPENDENT CHOICE MODEL
Knowledge and expertise are shared between patients and physicians	Patients expertise and values dominate
Patient and physician collaborate	Patient has independence and control
Relationship-centered	Patient-centered
Physician serves as active guide	Physician serves as passive informer
Additive experience (win/win)	Zero-sum interaction (win/lose)
Competence-based	Control-based
Dialogue-based	Discussion-based
Physician is personally invested in outcome	Physician is detached operative
Patient and physician have joint responsibility for patient outcome	Physician abdicates responsibility to patient

From Quill TE, Brody H: Physician recommendations and patient autonomy: Finding a balance between physician power and patient choice. *Ann Intern Med* 125:763-769, 1996.

the individual is solely responsible for defining the conditions of "personal well-being." In this model, extensive consideration is given to the older adult as a unique being—an individual with a history of unique experiences, with values, needs, and desires that do not fade as age increases, and with a right to self-determination in all matters.

Quill and Brody use the term "enhanced autonomy" to describe Gadow's advocacy model and its recommended use in medicine. They contrast it with the "independent choice" model in Table 2-1. Enhanced autonomy is described as "relationship-centered," so that not only the physician and the patient but also family members and others can be included in the decision-making process. This is a model that uses open dialogue to explore patient and physician values, assumptions, and perspectives before the patient arrives at a decision. It requires that the physician be an active listener (a skill that must often be taught) as well as capable of leaving preconceived ideas behind in order to be open to new considerations. Above all, it requires a genuine concern about the patient's best interests. The underlying theme in the enhanced autonomy model is respect for the patient as a person. "It is not respectful to spare persons from advice or counsel just to maintain neutrality, nor is it respectful to treat persons according to rigid protocols . . ."[44] Quill and Brody make six recommendations for enhancing patient autonomy in medical care. These recommendations can be easily translated to the provision of physical therapy services in general and specifically to the care of the older adult.

1. *Share your expertise fully while listening to the patient's perspective.* Use understandable language and allow sufficient time for questions. Be prepared to explore differences in values and experiences.

2. *Recommendations must consider clinical facts as well as personal experience.* Most patients want to hear the physician's or other professional's perspective but need their values and perspectives to be heard and integrated. Make biases and past relevant experience part of the dialogue.

3. *Focus on general goals before specific treatment options.* This can help to avoid premature "choosing of" treatment that may not be in the patient's best interest.

4. *Carefully explore differences between your recommendations and the patient's wishes.* Dissecting the issue into component parts can help to identify areas in which there is agreement and those in which there is none. For example, agreeing on a treatment option can be difficult if there is disagreement as to the nature of the problem or the prognosis.

5. *Final choices belong to the informed patient.*

6. *Practice collaborating with patients in an open and honest way.* The skill required to know what to recommend and how to negotiate without dominating takes practice and gets better with experience.

Whether one uses the advocacy model described by Gadow or the enhanced autonomy model elaborated on by Quill and Brody, "patient compliance" becomes an obsolete phrase. Compliance, after all, is only an issue if one fails to abide by, obey, or do what someone else has deemed critical. As Ramsden so aptly states, "Failure of patients to comply with treatment may be related to failure of the health care professional to plan a strategy that is in tune with the individual's needs."[45]

ISSUES AFFECTING AN ELDER'S QUALITY OF LIFE

The Role of the Family

Family plays a significant role in the quality of life of the elderly. Families are sources of information, care-givers, and major sources of emotional support and socialization.[13] In turn, family members need support to fulfill these critical roles and to meet the needs of aging parents and relatives. Families require information on (1) the normal changes with aging, (2) available community resources, (3) knowledge and skills in the actual physical care of the elder, and (4) communication-skills training to deal with physiological changes and psychological changes of the aging elder.[10,37,45,46,52,53,59] When an elder becomes impaired, the family members are understandably grieved and often frustrated by the loss. Families require assistance in coping with their feelings, understanding the causes of impairment, and learning communication strategies that promote the elder's well-being and sense of control.[57] Thus, providing care for an elderly patient is usually a team approach that requires professional communication with the elder, the family, and other health care providers. Teaching the elder patient and the family is an important professional skill that directly affects the elder's quality of life.

Grief and Loss

Grief is a natural emotional response to an actual or impending loss.[11] The loss of physical function; loss of a limb; loss of a job; loss of life roles and their responsibilities and pleasures; loss of a loved one, especially a spouse; or imminent loss of one's own life all cause painful suffering. Grieving is a normal reaction for a patient and that patient's family. The grieving process, although recognized to have identifiable symptoms and phases, remains a unique, individual response strongly embedded in social and cultural values and beliefs.[11,16,39,54] Studies indicate that an individual's personality traits are the most powerful predictors of one's style of coping with grief.[16]

Symptoms of Grief

Somatic symptoms are a common response to grief. Tightness of the throat, shortness of breath, choking, frequent sighing, muscle weakness, tremors, an empty feeling in the abdomen, and chills are all common somatic symptoms present with grief. Sensory responses are known to be heightened or erratic. The grief-stricken individual may appear tense, restless, irritable, or hostile. Preoccupation with the image of the deceased or the lost object is common and often the only topic of conversation. Mental distress is often exhibited by disorientation to time, lack of ability to concentrate, restlessness, and a tendency to daydream. Similar to common depression, disturbances in sleeping; eating; and normal activity patterns, including hygiene, are common.

Phases of Grief

A number of models and theories of stages of grieving exist.[11,16,28] Each model attempts to delineate the gamut of human emotions associated with loss, including shock, disbelief, sadness, sorrow, anger, disgust, guilt, and relief. Although these models may assist our understanding of the complexity of the grieving process, none are meant to show a linear sequence of emotions or stages. The actual grief process is a total emotional response that is highly individualized.

Grief work does have some commonly recognized phases.[11,16,54] Shock, disbelief, and numbness are common initial reactions. Preoccupation with the loss of a person or object, intense pining, restlessness, irritability, intense loneliness, and overall anxiety are often-displayed initial responses. With time, intense grief work may display a wide range of emotional responses, from anger to apathy. The intensity of the grief response is related to the perceived significance of the loss, the bereaved individual's personality traits and coping methods, and the elder's accepted social and cultural norms. This time of grief work for the bereaved elder patient may be confused with a clinical depression. The apathy, mood swings, and aimlessness common in grief are similar to depression and may be treated like a major depressive episode. Caution is advised in the use of medications that may trigger additional mood swings or produce significant side effects that may actually prolong the grieving process.[54] Finally, a gradual reorganization and balance occur in the emotional and physical well-being of the grieving individual. It is important to recognize that significant new events or anniversary dates may continue to trigger grief reactions or mood swings. Health professionals have an important role in supporting their patients and their families through the grieving process. Verbal and nonverbal support, empathy, respect, and acknowledgment of their individual needs are all part of a comprehensive plan of care.

Fear of Dying

All individuals have fears related to dying and terminal illness. Some of the most common fears are isolation, pain, and dependence.[27,43] The health care provider has a decided role in supporting the dying patient by providing security, alleviating suffering, and providing as much control for the patient as possible. Continued physical and emotional support diminishes the fears associated with terminal illness and dying.

The fear of isolation is a fear of physical as well as emotional isolation. Family and health care providers confronted with the loss of the patient and their own inability to prevent the inevitable are known to retreat. This retreat is not only from the patient but also from the health care provider's own sense of loss or lack of control. The patient has the desire to be responded to as a living, worthwhile individual up to the time of death. A dying patient, facing the unknown, is supported by knowing that one will not be left alone.

The fear of pain is commonly expressed by dying patients. A decrease of, or freedom from, pain significantly increases an individual's quality of life. A clear commitment by health care providers to alleviate pain is a significant source of comfort for the dying patient.[27]

The dying patient's fear of dependence and of lack of control are compounded by fears of isolation and pain. With the loss of physical and mental functions, the dying patient faces loss of control of aspects of life. The health care provider's role is to empower the dying patient in whatever ways possible by promoting or sustaining an environment that is responsive to that patient's needs. All health care providers would do well by adopting the hospice philosophy of "affirming life and providing support and care" to dying patients so that they may live as fully and as comfortably as possible.[39] In addition, the adoption and promotion of living wills and Medical Directives could greatly enhance the dying patient's sense of control.[12]

COMMUNICATING WITH THE TERMINALLY ILL PATIENT

Communicating with a terminally ill patient should be no different than any other patient-therapist interaction. The uniqueness in our response to the patient with a terminal illness comes from our awareness of the significance and finality of death facing the patient and from the enormity of our own perceptions and fears of death and loss. These are complex issues that we face as individuals and as health care providers. The support of other health care providers is advisable when dealing with your own grief and loss for the dying patient. Our helping professional role is not automatic or easy; it requires significant practice and skill in communication and in the ability to listen, empathize, and consistently promote the well-being of an individual from that individual's own perspective. The key to all our professional interactions is the provision of care from the patient's perspective.

Maintaining Hope

Hope for a terminally ill patient may not necessarily be for a cure. Hope for a patient may be to see his/her next grandchild, to have time to settle the family finances, to have one more Thanksgiving with the family, or to ultimately have a quick and painless death. As illness progresses, patients' hopes may change. Your role is to facilitate the fulfillment of that patient's hope as realistically possible. Open, direct communication is required if the therapist is to learn what is important to the patient. The setting of mutual goals is essential.

Alleviating Suffering

Suffering is not a simple physiological response. Suffering—the lack of comfort or physical well-being—can be greatly reduced by the alleviation of fears. Patients need the support of knowing that they will not be abandoned or allowed to suffer as they approach death. Although a dying patient's decreasing physical capacity may greatly limit his/her independence, the role of the health care provider is to maintain that patient's dignity and self-control by promoting the patient's decision making as much as possible.

Saying Good-Bye

Saying good-bye to a patient, especially a patient with a terminal illness, can be very difficult. Ned Cassem[29] gives a clear perspective of what one may choose to say and why:

> What we often do because losses hurt so much is we don't say good-bye to anybody. The day comes and we disappear . . .What should be said is, 'I want you to know the relationship was meaningful, I'll miss this about you, or I'll find it hard to go down to the corner for a beer, it won't be the same, I'll miss the bluntness that you had in helping me sort out some things, or I'll miss the old bull sessions,' or something like that. Because those are the things you value. Now what does that do for the other person? The other person learns that although it's painful to separate it's far more meaningful to have known the person and to have separated than never to have known him at all. He also learns what it is in himself that is valued and treasured.

SUMMARY

Communication is an essential component of the role of the health professional. Communication and interpersonal skills are learned skills, which are driven by some commonly held professional values. Respect for the individual, promotion of the individual's autonomy, and nurturance of a trusting rela-

tionship are values that drive the communication approaches and interpersonal skills of health care professionals.

Effective communication with an elder requires adaptation to the common physiological, psychological, and social changes associated with the aging process. Changes in hearing, sight, speech, and facial expression alter the elder's communication intake and response. Effective communication with an elder considers the effects of the aging process on that individual and adapts to those physiological and social changes. Age-related learning, sight, hearing, and speech deficits in an elder require conscious adjustments in the communication approach of the health care provider. Effective communication with an elder may be facilitated through a variety of strategies and approaches including the use of touch, reminiscence, and humor.

An imperative for health care professionals is to respect and address the individuality of each elder they encounter. Ageism remains in our society and continues to foster erroneous assumptions about the capabilities, intelligence, and physical skills of the elder patient. Our use of language is a telling example of the insipid influence of ageism. Terms such as old biddy and geezer continue to thrive in our culture.

Our quality of life is directly related to our ability to control decisions and make choices. Ensuring that elders are in control of their own decisions has a positive influence on therapeutic outcomes, their quality of life, and adherence to professional recommendations. A significant variable when considering anyone's quality of life is the impact of culture and ethnicity. Sensitivity to cultural and ethnicity issues is essential. A model of advocacy embraces the principles of compassionate health care that truly empowers elders.

Grief, death, and dying are significant issues of life for all of us but are particularly prominent for the elderly. Communicating with the terminally ill patient and family is complex. Alleviating suffering, maintaining hope, and saying good-bye can be difficult skills for health care providers to learn. Health care professionals have an important role in supporting their patients. Communication is our tool.

REFERENCES

1. Anand JK, Court I: Hearing loss leading to impaired ability to communicate in residents of homes for the elderly. *Brown Med J* 1989; 298:1429.
2. Barbato C, Feezel J: The language of aging in different age groups. *Gerontologist* 1987; 27:527.
3. Bennett SL, Maas F: The effect of music-based life review on the life satisfaction and ego integrity of elderly people. *Br J Occup Ther* 1988; 51:433-436.
4. Brownlee AT: *Community, Culture, and Care: A Cross-Cultural Guide for Health Workers.* St Louis, Mosby, 1978.
5. Buehler D: Informed consent and the elderly. *Crit Care Nurs Clin North Am* 1990; 2:461-471.
6. Buysse DJ, et al: Napping and 24-hour sleep/wake patterns in healthy elderly and young adults. *J Am Geriatr Soc* 1992; 40(8):779-786.
7. Campbell JM, Lancaster J: Communicating effectively with older adults. *Fam Community Health* 1988; 11:74-85.
8. Caporael LR, Culbertson GH: Verbal response modes of baby talk and other speech at institutions for the aged. *Lang Communication* 1986; 6:99-112.

9. Cohen G, Faulkner D: Does "elderspeak" work? The effect of intonation and stress on comprehension and recall of spoken discourse in old age. *Lang Communication* 1986; 6:91-98.

10. Cohen PM: A group approach for working with families of the elderly. *Gerontologist* 1983; 23:248-250.

11. Despelder LA, Strickland AL: *The Last Dance: Encountering Death and Dying,* ed 2. Mountain View, Calif, Mayfield, 1987.

12. Emanuel LL, Emanuel EJ: The Medical Directive: A new comprehensive advance care document. *JAMA* 1989; 261:3288-3293.

13. Epstein JL: Communicating with the elderly. *J Market Res Soc* 1983; 25:239-262.

14. Erickson R: Companion animals and the elderly. *Geriatr Nurs* 1985; March-April:92-96.

15. Gadow S: Advocacy: An ethical model for assisting patients with treatment decisions, in Wong CB, Swazey JP (eds): *Dilemmas of Dying: Policies and Procedures for Decisions Not to Treat.* Boston, GK Hall Medical Publishers, 1981.

16. Gallagher DE, Thompson LW, Peterson JA: Psychosocial factors affecting adaptation to bereavement in the elderly. *Int J Aging Hum Dev* 1982; 3:79-95.

17. Gazda GM, Childers WC, Walter RP: Interpersonal Communication. Rockville, Md, Aspen, 1982.

18. Gelfand DE, Kutzik AJ (eds): *Ethnicity and Aging: Theory, Research and Policy,* vol 5. New York, Springer, 1979.

19. Gerrard BA, Boniface WJ, Love BH: *Interpersonal Skills for Health Professionals.* Reston, Va, Reston, 1980.

20. Greene, MG: Older patient satisfaction with communication during an initial medical encounter. *Social Science & Medicine* 1994; 38(9):1279-1288.

21. Guccione A: Compliance and patient autonomy: Ethical and legal limits to professional dominance. *Top Geriatr Rehabil* 1988; 3(3):62-84.

22. Hazard, WR, Andres R, Bieman EL, Blass JP: *Principles of Geriatric Medicine and Gerontology,* 2nd ed. New York, McGraw-Hill, 1990.

23. Hollinger LM: Communicating with the elderly. *Gerontol Nurs* 1986; 12:8-13.

24. Howard DM: The effects of touch in the geriatric population. *Phys Occup Ther Geriatr* 1988; 6:35-50.

25. Jackson MM: Aging and motor speech production, *Top Geriatr Rehabil* 1986; 1:29-43.

26. Kaplan H: Communication problems for the hearing impaired elderly: What can be done? *Pride Inst J Long Term Home Health Care* 1988; 7: 10-22.

27. Kinzel T: Relief of emotional symptoms in elderly patients with cancer. *Geriatrics* 1988; 43:61-65.

28. Kubler-Ross E: *On Death and Dying.* New York, Macmillan, 1970.

29. Langhorne J: *Vital Signs: The Way We Die in America.* Boston, Little, Brown, 1974.

30. Maloney CC: Identifying and treating the client with sensory loss. *Phys Occup Ther Geriatr* 1987; 5:31-46.

31. Mulrow CD, Aguilar C, et al: Association between hearing impairment and the quality of life of elderly individuals. *Am Geriatr Soc* 1990; 38:45-50.

32. Muncy JH: Measures to rid sleeplessness: 10 points to enhance sleep. *Gerontol Nurs* 1986; 12:6-11.

33. Navarro T, Lipkowitz M, Navarra JG: *Therapeutic Communication: A Guide to Effective Interpersonal Skills for Health Care Professionals.* Thorofare, NJ, Slack, 1990.

34. Null RL: Low-vision elderly: An environmental rehabilitation approach. *Top Geriatr Rehabil* 1988; 4(1):24-31.

35. Palumbo MV: Hearing Access 2000. Increasing awareness of the hearing impaired. *Gerontol Nurs* 1990; 16:26-31.

36. Patten PC, Piercy FP: Dysfunctional isolation in the elderly: Increasing marital and family closeness through improved communication. *Contemp Fam Ther Int J* 1989; 11:131-147.

37. Pfeiffer E: Some basic principles for working with older patients. *Am Geriatr Soc* 1985; 33:44-47.

38. Pincus A: Reminiscence in aging and its implications for social work practice. *Soc Work* 1970; 15:47-53.

39. Pizzi M: Hospice and the terminally ill geriatric patient. *Phys Occup Ther Geriatr* 1983; 3:45-54.

40. Portnoy EJ: Communication and the elderly patient. *Activ Adapt Aging* 1985; 7:25-30.

41. Price C: Heritage: A program design for reminiscence. *Activ Adapt Aging* 1983; 3:7-52.

42. Priefer BA, Gambert SR: Reminiscence and life review in the elderly. *Psychiatr Med* 1984; 2:91-100.

43. Purtilo R: *Health Professional and Patient Interaction,* ed 4. Philadelphia, WB Saunders, 1990.

44. Quill TE, Brody H: Physician recommendations on patient autonomy: Finding a balance between power and patient choice. *Ann Inter Med* 1996; 125:763-769.

45. Ramsden E: Compliance and motivation. *Top Geriatr Rehabil* 1988; 3(3):1-14.

46. Remnet VL: How adult children respond to role transitions in the lives of their aging parents. *Educ Gerontol* 1987; 13:341-355.

47. Richman J: The lifesaving function of humor with the depressed and suicidal elderly, *Gerontologist* 1995; 35(2):271-273.

48. Robinson VM: *Humor and the Health Professions.* Thorofare, NJ, Slack, 1977.

49. Rodin J, Langer E: Aging labels: The decline of control and the fall of self esteem. *J Soc Issues* 1980; 36:12-29.

50. Ryan EB, Giles H, et al: Psycholinguistic and social psychological components of communication by and with the elderly. *Lang Communication* 1986; 6:1-24.

51. Ryden MB: Morale and perceived control in institutionalized elderly. *Nurs Res* 1984; 33:130-136.

52. Santora G: Communicating better with the elderly: How to break down the barriers. *Nurs Life* 1986; 6:24-27.

53. Shulman MD, Mandel E: Communication training of relatives and friends of institutionalized elderly persons. *Gerontologist* 1988; 28: 797-799.

54. Stewart T, Shields CR: Grief in chronic illness: Assessment and management. *Arch Phys Med Rehabil* 1985; 66:447-450.

55. Sullivan JL, Deane DM: Humor and health. *Gerontol Nurs* 1988; 14: 20-24.

56. Teitelman J, Priddy J: From psychological theory to practice: Improving frail elders' quality of life through control-enhancing intervention. *Appl Gerontol* 1988; 7:298-315.

57. Thompson RF, Montalvo B: Psychosocial aspects of geriatrics: A six-point orientation scheme for training. *Fam Syst Med* 1989; 7:397-410.

58. Tobin SS, Gustafson JD: What do we do differently with elderly clients? *Gerontol Soc Work* 1987; 10:107-121.

59. Truglio LM, Hayes PM: Carers learn to cope. *Geriatr Nurs* 1986; 7: 310-312.

60. Van Wyk L: Hearing in the elderly. *JARD,* 1994; 3:22-23.

61. Walsh C, Eldredge N: When deaf people become elderly: Counteracting a lifetime of difficulties. *Gerontol Nurs* 1989; 15:27-31.

62. Washburn AD: Hearing disorders and the aged. Top Geriatr Rehabil 1986; 1:61-70.

63. Wetle T: Ethical issues in long-term care of the aged, *Geriatr Psychiatry* 1985; 18:63-73.

64. Wood J: Communicating with older adults in health care settings: Cultural and ethnic considerations. *Educ Gerontol* 1989; 15:351-362.

CHAPTER 3

PHYSIOLOGICAL CHANGES ASSOCIATED WITH AGING

LaDora V. Thompson, PT, PhD

INTRODUCTION

Age-related changes in the physiological organ systems of the human body are major public health problems in the rapidly expanding elderly population. It is unclear whether there are any reversible components in these aging problems. An understanding of the physiological changes and their impact on function is the crucial first step toward developing rational therapeutic or preventative measures to address these problems.

The physiological changes that occur with the passage of time do not include changes due to disease processes. Aging is not disease. The diseases that are commonly associated with the elderly are due to long-term abuse (abuse in the form of smoking, poor nutrition, inadequate exercise, exposure to noxious agents such as chemicals or ultraviolet radiation); however, this is not to say that all disease can be prevented by "clean and healthy living."

The decline in physical function associated with the reduced physical activity so commonly present in older adults does not describe aging. Older people become increasingly limited in their abilities to perform activities of daily living because of poor balance, reduced endurance, generalized weakness, or repeated falls. However, it is not clear whether these changes are due to the aging process *per se* or inactivity. For example, lean body mass, basal metabolic rate, aerobic capacity, and insulin sensitivity all decline with decreasing levels of physical activity and are also reduced with aging. Bortz[19] hypothesized that inactivity causes many of the functional losses attributed to aging, at every level from cellular and molecular to tissue and organ systems. Many of the physiological changes attributed to aging are similar to those induced by imposed inactivity and possibly could be attenuated, or even reversed, by exercise (Table 3-1).

Aging is associated with profound changes in *body composition.* With age, there is an increase in body fat mass, especially the accumulation of more internalized fat deposits (abdominal), and a decrease in lean body mass. This decrease in lean body mass occurs primarily as a result of losses in skeletal muscle mass.[50] The age-related loss in skeletal muscle mass has been termed "sarcopenia." The loss in muscle mass accounts for the age-associated decreases in basal metabolic rate, muscle strength, and activity levels, which, in turn are the cause of decreased energy requirements in the older adult. Daily energy expenditure declines progressively through adult life. The main determinant of energy expenditure is fat-free mass, which declines by about 15% between the third and eighth decades of life, contributing to a lower basal metabolic rate in the elderly.[29] Although body weight increases with age, the reasons are many. Chief among these causes are a declining metabolic rate and activity level coupled with an energy intake that does not match the declining need for energy.

These changes in body composition increase the older adult's risk of developing a wide range of chronic disorders, including hypercholesterolemia, atherosclerosis, hyperinsulinemia, insulin resistance, non–insulin-dependent diabetes (type II diabetes), and hypertension.[37] These changes, together with the age-associated decline in whole-body exercise tolerance (maximal oxygen consumption, $\dot{V}O_2max$), can substantially reduce the amount and intensity of physical activities performed by the older adult. This decline in physical activity also contributes to the loss of muscle mass and the accumulation of fat mass and is considered a major risk factor for the development of many age-related chronic diseases.[19] More importantly, these physical and metabolic impairments associated with aging and inactivity are reducing the quality of life for a rapidly expanding older population.

To the practicing therapist, it is largely irrelevant to simply discuss changes in the normal aging process, since the older patients are likely to have, in most cases, additional pathology underlying purely aging changes. However, a true understanding of the aging process is essential to fully understand how illness or chronic disease compounds an already compromised system. The objectives of this chapter are many. First, biological theories of aging are reviewed. Second, age-related changes in the physiological organ systems with special emphasis in the skeletal muscle system, cardiovascular system, and heart and peripheral vasculature at rest and during exercise are documented. Next, the adaptations to exercise are discussed followed by a discussion on the development of an exercise program for the older adult.

Aging Theories

The term *aging* is difficult to define because it has diverse meanings for different professionals.

Since this chapter will be reviewing the physiological changes that occur in the organ systems of the human body, biological aging will be emphasized. Developmental changes are irreversible normal changes in a living organism that occur as time passes. The changes that occur with development are neither accidental nor a result of abuse, inactivity, or disease. The developmental changes can be divided into three categories: development, maturation, and aging. *Development* refers to changes that occur before birth or during childhood. *Maturation* concerns the changes that result in the transformation of a child into an adult. *Aging* refers to the group of developmental changes that occur in the later years. Unlike development and maturation, changes associated with aging reduce a person's ability to function, maintain survival, and have a high quality of life. Thus, aging is a continuous set of time-dependent processes that generally mirrors chronological age but is highly variable and individualized. *Aged,* as generally used, can best be defined as a "state or condition" that may or may not correlate with chronological age and more often reflects the loss of a person's capacity to maintain independence.

Biological Aging
Aging includes several different kinds of changes. Age-associated changes that involve the physical structures and functioning of the body and that affect a person's ability to

Table 3-1

Physiological Characteristics Associated with Aging, Imposed Inactivity, and Exercise

Characteristic	Aging	Imposed Inactivity	Exercise
Body Composition			
Lean body mass	$\Downarrow$	$\Downarrow$	$\Uparrow$
Fat mass	$\Uparrow$	$\Uparrow$	$\Downarrow$
Bone mass	$\Downarrow$	$\Downarrow$	$\Uparrow$
Total body water	$\Downarrow$	$\Downarrow$	$\Uparrow$/-
Metabolism			
Basal metabolic rate	$\Downarrow$	$\Downarrow$	$\Uparrow$
Glucose tolerance	$\Downarrow$	$\Downarrow$	$\Uparrow$
Muscle glycogen	$\Downarrow$	$\Downarrow$	$\Uparrow$
Insulin responsiveness	$\Downarrow$	$\Downarrow$	$\Uparrow$
Calcium balance	$\Downarrow$	$\Downarrow$	$\Uparrow$
LDL cholesterol	$\Uparrow$	$\Uparrow$	-

$\Downarrow$ = Decrease; $\Uparrow$ = increase; - = no change.

function or survive are referred to as *biological aging.* The cells, critical components of each organ system of the human body, function at all times to build and maintain the structure of the body and carry out its function. The state of having proper and steady conditions is called *homeostasis.* Homeostasis involves many conditions, such as temperature, nutrient levels, and water content. Biological aging reduces the ability of the body to maintain homeostasis and therefore to survive. Numerous and diverse theories attempt to explain why and how biological aging occurs.

Biological aging of the different organ systems of the human body occurs at specific rates. The rates of biological aging are regulated by the following two general features:

1. A genetic component that imparts a species-specific capability to carry out basic biological processes necessary for life and reproduction
2. Environment and life-style components that are superimposed on the intrinsic genetic design and can influence the overall rates of aging and susceptibility to disease

The importance of the genetic component in the regulation of biological aging is demonstrated by the characteristic-longevity, or life span, of each animal species.[43] For example, humans live five times longer than cats, cats live five times longer than mice, and mice live twenty-five times longer than fruit flies. For humans and mammals, the genetic component in regulating the life span, defined as the *heritability of life span,* is small.

The small heritability of life span is strongly demonstrated by human twin studies.[43] When the twins are reared apart, the twins share less than 35% heritability of life span, i.e., the heritability of life span accounts for less than 35% of its variance. In contrast, the environment and life-style components in regulating life span is much greater and account for the remainder of the 65% observed variance. Thus the relative minor heritability of human life span implies that the choice of life-style and other environmental influences profoundly modify the outcome of aging.

General theories of aging have been proposed to explain the process of aging. However, even with extensive research, a good general theory of aging has not been presented. There are several theories of aging and the theories fall into two general categories: (1) the stochastic model of aging—the accumulation of damage to informational molecules and (2) the programmed model of aging—the regulation of specific genes. Most likely, aging is an integrated process that encompasses both general theories.

Accumulation of Damage to Information Molecules (Stochastic Model)

In general, the stochastic theories suggest that damage to cells and molecules underlie aging. Deoxyribonucleic acid (DNA) damage and damage to proteins from a variety of sources, with emphasis on free radicals and glycation, combine to produce manifestations of aging. Specifically, the accumulation of damage to informational molecules proposes that aging is the consequence of a progressive accumulation of errors in the makeup of the cells because the cells' repair processes do not keep up. The consequence of the error buildup is that the genetic foundation of the cell becomes altered and the expression of essential, functional protein is either limited or cannot proceed at all.

In functional cells, there are built-in mechanisms to repair minor DNA damage so that protein synthesis and cell homeostasis can be maintained. DNA damage is reflected in changes in the membranes and enzymes that are made by the cell. Manifestations of DNA damage are seen by cell membrane changes in its transport of ions and nutrients. With DNA damage, membrane-bound organelles, such as mitochondria and lysosomes, are present in reduced numbers. In addition, these organelles are less effective, presumably because of changes in their membranes and in the enzymes that regulate their reactions.

Random environmental events such as oxygen-free radical damage; somatic-cell–gene mutation; or cross-linkage among macromolecules, particularly proteins, alter the DNA's ability to function normally. *Normal function* is defined as the ability to transfer information from DNA to ribonucleic acid (RNA) to the synthesis of protein. Synthesis of aberrant protein or a failure to express essential, functional protein when required eventually leads to the cell's inability to contribute to tissue and organ homeostasis. Individual cell loss is not catastrophic to tissue or organ function because of the redundancy of cells. However, the tissue or organ fails when a significant complement of cells is altered.[57,107,122]

Collagen Cross-Linking

Collagen is the most abundant protein in body. With age, collagen is less soluble, rigid, and cross-linked. Free radicals, glucose, and ultraviolet light are thought to increase collagen cross-linking. Other substances in connective tissue (elastin) as well as DNA are subject to cross-linking. There is, at present, no knowledge on how to prevent collagen cross-linking from occurring. Functionally, the age-associated changes in collagen is observed in skin, loosened teeth, clouded lens, reduced kidney function, damaged lungs, reduced muscle capacity, reduced joint mobility, and altered circulatory effects.

Free-Radical Theory

Free radicals are highly reactive molecules with one or more unpaired electrons available for bonding. Oxidation of protein, fat, and carbohydrate results in free radical formation. The free radical theory of aging suggests that the highly reactive by-products of oxidative metabolism can react with key cellular constituents, including proteins, DNA, and lipids, to generate long-lived dysfunctional molecules that interfere with cellular function. Perhaps the most vulnerable biological structure damaged by free radicals is the plasma membrane, which is essential for homeostasis. Damage to mitochondrial DNA results in the body's inability to produce adequate energy for increased activity levels and may have a significant impact on skeletal muscle strength and endurance. Free-radical–induced damage of proteins in tendons and ligaments cause them to become excessively joined together and limit range of motion. Free radical damage can initiate inflammation; cause excess blood clotting; and promote several diseases, such as atherosclerosis. Clearly, free-radical damage alters essential organ function.

Vitamin E especially but also vitamins A and C are considered to be free-radical scavengers. Individuals with high levels of protection against free radicals (antioxidants) are thought to live longer. Older people, in general, have lower blood levels of vitamins A and C and perhaps E. It is still plausible that alterations in oxidant production and controls of oxidant-mediated damage may play significant roles in the rates of aging.

Glycosylation Theory

The glycosylation theory suggests that nonenzymatic glycosylation can create modified forms of proteins and perhaps other macromolecules that accumulate and cause dysfunction in aging. In this reaction, which does not require an enzyme, glucose joins with certain amino acids in proteins, rendering an altered amino acid, and ultimately a dysfunctional protein. The glycated proteins are damaged and are termed *advanced glycation end-products.* To date, there is no known benefit from glycation or advanced glycation end-products.

Glycated forms of human collagen do accumulate with age in tendon and skin. Adverse effects from glycation include body stiffening, reduced ability to control blood vessels and blood pressure, damage to blood vessel linings, increased blood clotting, eye damage, increased development of Alzheimer's disease, and amplification of most effects from diabetes. Glycation does not appear to cause aging. However, this cellular process has a significant impact on function and ultimately the quality of life for the older adult.

Pre-Programmed Gene Regulation

The regulation of specific genes proposes that the aging process is actively programmed by the cell's genetic machinery. This category of aging theories maintains that aging occurs because of intrinsic timing mechanisms and signals. For example, the programmed cell-death hypothesis during certain cell-lines during development and maturation support this theory. Deliberate programmed death of cells is called *apoptosis* and occurs during development to remove unwanted or extra cells, e.g., webbing between toes and fingers.

Telomere

Cells fall into three types: continuously replicating, replicating in response to a challenge, and nonreplicating. Although some cells continuously replicate in vivo, they have a finite replicative life. With each cell division, a portion of the terminal end of the chromosome (the telomere) is not replicated and therefore shortens. It is proposed that telomere shortening is the signal that results in the shift to a senescent pattern of gene expression and ultimately cell senescent.[47] Functionally, this process may activate detrimental genes that cause aging.

Master Clock

The most plausible of the genetic regulation theories of aging center around the theme of a "master clock." The master clock theme suggests that humans have an organ, cell type, or perhaps an intracellular molecule that *loses function over time* and that is coupled to and assists time- or age-dependent changes in the other organs and cell types. The difficulty with this master clock theory is that there is no good evidence as to where this master clock or timing mechanism might lie or how it might control aging in so many diverse organ systems.

Potential master timers for the aging process have been nominated and incorporate the other theories of aging. Master timers include somatic mutations in DNA; telomere shortening; cross-linking of extracellular connective tissue fibers; changes in the composition and fluidity of the plasma membrane; changes in mitochondrial function; alterations in immune surveillance; alterations in the rate of protein degradation and synthesis; programmed loss of mitotic capacity in fibroblasts; speed of DNA repair enzymes; and changes in hypothalamic, pineal, or pituitary cell function.

It is not easy to find the master clock because there are so many age-associated alterations in the diverse physiological systems. Among the age-related changes it is difficult to determine whether the changes in the extracellular, intracellular, and multicellular function are primary, i.e., tightly linked to some fundamental control system or whether the changes occur secondarily as a consequence of other age-dependent changes.

In conclusion, the number and diversity of theories attempting to explain biological aging can be perplexing. It is evident that the aging process or processes are multifactorial in origin and may be different in the various organ systems. Further, it appears that in the absence of disease, the ability of an individual to maintain homeostasis through protective mechanisms or repair is key to longevity and quality of life. Understanding the aging process may assist in providing appropriate care for the older adult and through good nutrition, exercise, and appropriate health care, it may be possible to retard the negative manifestations of aging.

FUNCTIONAL PERFORMANCE THRESHOLD

The ability to perform activities of daily living is important in maintaining independence for the older adult. There is a minimum criteria of physical functioning, e.g., strength, range of motion, endurance, balance, required to perform activities of daily living; this is defined as the *functional performance threshold.* Young adults have considerable physiological capacity and reserve that enable them to perform activities and exercise well in excess of the metabolic and physical demands required by routine daily activities of living. They function well above the functional performance threshold and possess a large reserve. With aging, however, changes to the various organ systems, particularly the heart

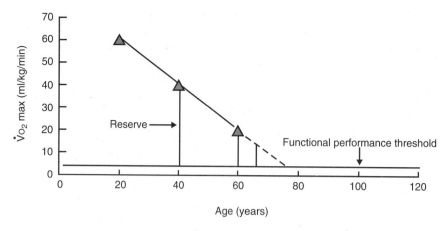

FIG. 3-1 Functional capacity, measured as V̇o₂max, declines with aging. The functional performance threshold is the minimum criterion required to perform activities of daily living. The amount of reserve decreases with age, such that the older individual functions closer to the minimal threshold.

and skeletal muscles, reduce the physiological capacity and reserve (Fig. 3-1). Thus the older adult performs daily routines closer to the functional performance threshold. The physiological reserve of the older adult is limited. If a decline in health status results in a functional capacity below this critical threshold of functioning, the older adult will be unable to do self-care activities and live independently. Falling below this critical threshold can result from progressive age-related changes or an extended period of immobility or illness sufficient to lower an older adult's already minimal reserves. Thus the loss of physiological reserve increases the risk of disability.

An objective of rehabilitation for older adults is to maintain physiological capacity and reserve well above the functional performance threshold. A person's ability to perform functional activities is primarily dependent on the integrity of the *cardiovascular system* and its ability to influence oxygen transport and tissue oxygenation. Both the structural and the physiological changes that occur in the cardiovascular system with aging influence the reserve capacity and bring the older adult closer to the functional performance threshold. Specifically, the age-related changes in the cardiovascular system decrease cardiac functional reserve capacity; limit the performance of physical activity; and lessen the ability to tolerate a variety of stresses, including cardiovascular disease. The following is an example of this concept of functional performance threshold and the cardiovascular system.

First, consider that in steady-state measures of oxygen consumption, walking on a level grade at 5 km/h requires 3.2 metabolic equivalent values (METS) (1 MET = 3.5 ml O₂/kg/min). With illness or inactivity, aerobic capacity falls below the level required for daily tasks. Because exercise can increase aerobic capacity, it should improve functional status when aerobic capacity is below the threshold needed for normal daily function. However, aerobic exercise would not affect ability to walk at 5 km/h in most adults, whose aerobic capacity already greatly exceeds 3.2 METS.

Physiologically, aging is associated with a variety of alterations in cardiovascular function, yet despite these changes, the cardiovascular system continues to function reasonably well in supplying the needs of tissues, at least at rest.[20,32,33,100,104] When the cardiovascular system is stressed, during exercise or in response to situations imposing an increase in metabolic demand for oxygen, age-related alterations are evident and limit function.[4,5,12,16,18,117,118] The age-related changes in the cardiovascular system and the impact on function are summarized in Table 3-2.

Ultimately, it is possible that older persons perceive activities associated with a relatively low metabolic demand as physically demanding. Certain activities may no longer be able to be performed whereas others may require frequent rest periods.

A person's ability to perform functional activities, such as walking, stair climbing, and carrying packages, is also dependent on the integrity of the *skeletal muscle system*. Activities of daily living require a minimum amount of muscle strength and muscle endurance. The required muscle strength and endurance can be referred to as a *functional performance threshold*. As men and women grow older, however, these simple activities of daily living may become difficult because of a reduction in muscle mass and muscular strength. Table 3-3 describes alterations in muscle and function with aging. Weakness of the lower extremities has been implicated with difficulties in rising from a chair and getting out of bed, in slow gait speed, and in balance problems and falls.[1,2,66,120]

Thus the lack of functional capacity or falling below the functional performance threshold of muscle strength and endurance can lead to a more dependent life-style and earlier entry into long-term care facilities. The decrease in functional capacity of muscle strength and endurance also contributes to the risk of falls, a decline in bone density, and the incidence of hip fractures and orthopedic injury in older adults.[3,8,15,83,111] As observed in the cardiovascular system, the

Table 3-2

Age-Related Changes in the Cardiovascular and Arterial Systems and Their Functions

Morphological and Structural Changes	Functional Significance
Heart	
↑ Fat constituents (adipose)	↓ Excitability
↑ Fibrous constituents	↓ Cardiac output
↑ Mass and volume	↓ Venous return
↑ Lipofuscin (by-product of glycogen metabolism)	↑ Cardiac dysrhythmias
↑ Amyloid content	
↓ Specialized nerve conduction tissue	
↓ Intrinsic and extrinsic innervation	
↑ Connective tissue and elastin	
↑ Calcification	
Blood Vessels	
↑ Loss of normal proportion of smooth muscle to connective tissue and elastin constituents	↓ Blood flow to oxygenate tissues
↑ Rigidity of large arteries	↓ Blood flow and risk of clots in venous circulation
↑ Atheroma arterial circulation	↓ Cardiac output
↑ Calcification	↓ Venous return
↑ Dilation and tortuosity of veins	

↓ = Decreased; ↑ = increased

Table 3-3

Age-Associated Changes in Skeletal Muscle

Morphological and Structural Changes	Functional Significance
↓ Muscle mass	↓ Strength and power
↓ Type I fiber number	↓ Fast and strong movements
↓ Type II fiber number	↑ Injury
↓ Type II fiber area	
↑ Connective tissue	
↑ Fat content	
↓ Oxidative capacity	↓ Endurance and sustained power
↓ Capillary density	
↑ Contraction time	Slowing of movements
↑ Relaxation time	Altered coordination
↓ Maximal shortening velocity	Altered ability to perform rapid, changing movements
↓ Motor unit number	↓ Fine, controlled movements
↑ Motor unit size	↓ Excitability
↓ Number of anterior horn cells	
↓ Nerve conduction velocity	
↓ Number of dihydropyridine receptors and ryanodine receptors	↓ Excitability, altered electromechanical transduction

↓ = Decreased; ↑ = increased

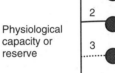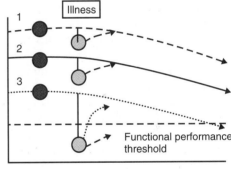

Fig. 3-2 Numbers *1, 2, 3* represent three older adults with different amounts of physiological reserve. Each adult experiences an illness, resulting in a hospitalization. The amount of physiological reserve may have a significant impact on the recovery potential.

change in functional capacity or reserve is not noticed until the individual is stressed due to exercise or an illness.

A person's rehabilitation potential depends on many factors, e.g., age, cognition, strength, co-morbidities, depression, and medications. Since there is an age-related decline in physiological capacity, bringing the older person closer to the functional performance threshold may influence his/her rehabilitation potential. For example, an older adult with a large physiological capacity who falls and breaks a hip may recover immediately with therapeutic intervention. The opportunity to return to independent living for this individual is great because he/she did not fall below the threshold of functioning. In contrast, an individual with a minimal physiological capacity has the potential to drop below the threshold of functioning after a hip fracture. The rehabilitation process may be hindered due to the poor health status, and the benefits of therapeutic intervention resulting in independent living are unknown (Fig. 3-2).

PHYSIOLOGICAL CHANGES

Many of the physiological changes associated with aging result from a gradual loss. These losses may begin in early adulthood, but due to the redundant make-up of the organ systems, these losses do not become functionally significant until the decline is extensive. For example, the kidney can show an increase in number of abnormal glomeruli without any change in creatinine clearance. However, at some point, when the number of abnormal glomeruli increases to a substantial amount, kidney function fails. Based on cross-sectional studies, most physiological organ systems seem to lose function at about 1% a year beginning around age 30. In contrast, longitudinal studies suggest that the changes are less dramatic and do not occur until after the age of 70.[6,108] Two systems—the cardiovascular and skeletal muscle, which demonstrate gradual declines in function with age—are discussed after a short review of their anatomy.

REVIEW OF THE CARDIOVASCULAR SYSTEM AND FUNCTION

Anatomy

The heart is a pump that provides the force necessary to circulate the blood to all the tissues in the body. Three layers of tissue form the heart wall: an outer epicardium, a middle myocardium, and an inner endocardium. The epicardium is a serous membrane that consists of connective tissue and provides a thin protective layer. *Blood vessels* that nourish the heart wall are located in the epicardium. The thick middle layer is the myocardium. It forms the bulk of the heart wall and is composed of cardiac muscle tissue. *Contraction* of the myocardium provides the force that ejects blood from the heart and moves it through the blood vessels. The smooth inner lining of the heart wall is endocardium, which permits blood to move easily through the heart. The endocardium also forms the valves of the heart and is continuous with the lining of the blood vessels.

The internal cavity of the heart is divided into four chambers: right atrium, right ventricle, left atrium, and left ventricle. The two atria are thin-walled chambers that receive blood from the veins. The two ventricles are thick-walled chambers that forcefully pump blood out of the heart. The valves keep the blood flowing in the correct direction. The valves between the atria and ventricles are called *atrioventricular valves,* whereas those at the bases of the large vessels leaving the ventricles are *semilunar valves.*

Function

The major function of the cardiovascular system is to pump blood through the systemic and pulmonary circulations and thereby transport respiratory gases (oxygen), nutrients, and metabolic products (carbon dioxide) to and from tissues. Thus, cardiac function must be sufficient to meet the demands of the working tissues. The overall expression of cardiac function is *cardiac output,* i.e., the amount of blood pumped by the heart into the circulation per unit of time (in the healthy adult, cardiac output is 5.5 L/min). Cardiac output depends on two main factors—stroke volume and heart rate (Fig. 3-3)—and is calculated by the following formula:

$$\text{Cardiac Output} = \text{Stroke Volume} \times \text{Heart Rate}$$
$$\text{(ml/min)} \qquad \text{(ml/cycle)} \qquad \text{(cycles/min)}$$

Stroke volume is the amount of blood pumped from a ventricle each time the ventricle contracts. Stroke volume depends on the amount of blood in the ventricle when it contracts (end-diastolic volume) and the strength of contraction. The end-diastolic volume, the amount of blood in the ventricle at the end of diastole (or beginning of systole), is directly related to venous return. The more blood returned by the veins, the greater the volume in the ventricle to be pumped out again. In this way, increased venous return increases end-diastolic volume, which increases stroke volume.

The amount of blood in the ventricle also affects contraction strength. There is a direct relationship between venous return, end-diastolic volume, and contraction strength; this relationship is known as the *Frank-Starling relationship of the heart.* As blood fills the ventricles, the cardiac muscle fibers stretch to accommodate the increasing volume. In response to this stretch, the fibers contract with a greater force, which increases the amount of blood ejected from the ven-

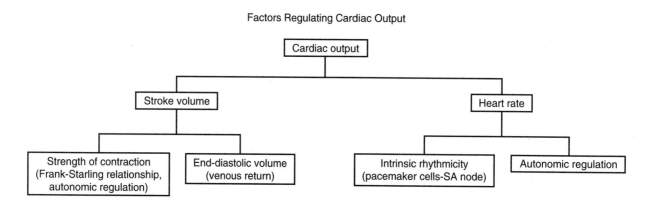

FIG. 3-3 Factors regulating cardiac output.

tricle (stroke volume). Conversely, if venous return decreases, end-diastolic volume decreases, there is less stretch in the muscle fibers, and contraction strength decreases. The autonomic nervous system also affects stroke volume by altering the contraction strength. Sympathetic stimulation increases the contraction strength of the ventricular myocardium. When sympathetic stimulation is removed, the contraction strength decreases.

Heart rate depends on the autonomic innervation and the intrinsic rhythmicity of the specialized pacemaker cells. The pacemaker cells, located in the sinoatrial node (SA), acting alone produce a constant rhythmic heart rate. Regulating factors act on the sinoatrial node to increase or decrease the heart rate to adjust cardiac output to meet the changing needs of the body. Most changes in the heart rate are mediated through the cardiac center in the medulla oblongata of the brain. This center has both sympathetic and parasympathetic components to regulate the action of the heart. Factors such as blood pressure levels and the need for oxygen determine which component is active. Generally, the sympathetic impulses increase the heart rate and cardiac output, whereas the parasympathetic impulses decrease the heart rate.

Baroreceptors are stretch receptors in the wall of the aorta and in the wall of the internal carotid arteries, which deliver blood to the brain. As blood pressure increases, the vessels are stretched, which increases the frequency of impulses going from the receptors to the medulla oblongata. This prompts the cardiac center to increase parasympathetic stimulation and to decrease sympathetic stimulation so heart rate, cardiac output, and blood pressure decrease. As blood pressure decreases, the frequency of baroreceptor impulses also decreases. In response, the cardiac center increases sympathetic impulses and decreases parasympathetic impulses to increase the pressure.

Blood pressure is produced by the pumping action of the heart and influences cardiac output. The term *blood pressure* refers to arterial blood pressure, the pressure in the aorta and its branches. The pressure in the arteries is greatest during ventricular contraction (systole) when blood is forcefully ejected from the left ventricle into the aorta; this is called *systolic pressure.* Arterial pressure is lowest when the ventricles are in the relaxation phase (diastole) of the cardiac cycle just before the next contraction; this is referred to as *diastolic pressure.* Pulse pressure is the difference between systolic and diastolic pressures. Four major factors interact to affect blood pressure. These factors are cardiac output, blood volume, peripheral resistance, and viscosity. Each one has a direct relationship to blood pressure.

Cardiac output is the amount of blood pumped by the heart in 1 minute (5.5 L/min). Anything that increases either the heart rate or the stroke volume will increase cardiac output and also increase blood pressure. When either heart rate or stroke volume decreases, cardiac output decreases, which decreases blood pressure.

The volume of blood in the body directly affects blood pressure. Although blood volume varies with age, body size,

and gender, the normal average is more than 5 L for adults. Any changes in blood volume—severe hemorrhage, vomiting, or reduced fluid intake—are accompanied by corresponding changes in blood pressure. When blood volume decreases, blood pressure also decreases. If the body retains too much fluid, blood volume and blood pressure increase.

Peripheral resistance is the opposition to blood flow caused by friction of the vessel walls. Increased peripheral resistance causes an increase in blood pressure. Vasoconstriction decreases the vessel diameter and increases resistance, which subsequently increases blood pressure. When blood vessels lose their elasticity, their resistance increases and so does blood pressure. An increased peripheral resistance results in increased blood pressure because the heart has to pump more strongly against this increased resistance to flow. This increased resistance to flow is defined as the *afterload* and refers to the work carried out by the heart in pumping against the arterial resistance.

Viscosity is a physical property of blood that refers to the ease with which the molecules and cells slide across each other. Viscosity opposes the flow of a fluid. Normally the viscosity of blood remains fairly constant, but it changes when either the number of blood cells or concentration of plasma proteins changes. If the number of erythrocytes increases, the blood becomes more viscous and blood pressure increases.

The arterial blood pressure is maintained within normal ranges by changes in cardiac output and peripheral resistance as expressed in the following formula:

Blood Pressure = Cardiac Output × Total Peripheral Resistance

As previously stated, baroreceptors respond when the walls are stretched by sudden increases in pressure. The impulses of the baroreceptors are transmitted to the cardiac and vasomotor centers in the medulla oblongata. The centers respond by sending out signals that decrease heart rate (decrease cardiac output) and cause vasodilation (decrease peripheral resistance). These actions return blood pressure toward normal. The baroreceptors are important for moment-by-moment blood pressure regulation. Thus, both the sympathetic and parasympathetic divisions of the autonomic nervous system innervate the heart, whereas blood vessels are predominantly innervated by the sympathetic nervous system (Fig. 3-4).

With exercise, increased skeletal muscle activity results in an increased demand for oxygen. The accumulation of metabolites in the working skeletal muscle dilate blood vessels in the active skeletal muscle tissue, thus increasing blood flow and oxygen supply to that tissue. This increase in blood flow to the active tissue is at the expense of blood flow to other tissues unless the cardiac output is increased. However, cardiac output is increased reflexively. Specifically, vascular dilation and increased blood flow to the active skeletal muscle tissue result in a decreased total peripheral resistance. The decreased total peripheral resistance is sensed as a fall in blood pressure, resulting in a reflex increase in cardiac out-

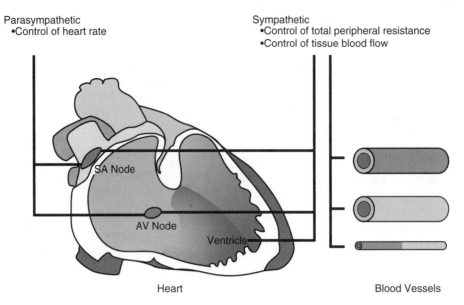

FIG. 3-4   The heart is innervated by both the sympathetic and parasympathetic fibers, whereas the blood vessels are predominantly innervated by sympathetic fibers.

put. Hence, working skeletal muscles or tissue demands determine cardiac output.

The *cardiac cycle* refers to the alternating contraction and relaxation of the myocardium, coordinated by the conduction system, during one heartbeat. The atria contract at the same time, then they relax while the two ventricles simultaneously contract. The contraction phase of the chambers is called *systole;* the relaxation phase is called *diastole.* When the terms systole and diastole are used alone, they generally refer to action of the ventricles. With a normal heart rate of 72 beats per minute, one cardiac cycle lasts 0.8 second. The cycle begins with atrial systole when both atria contract. During this time, the atrioventricular valves are open, the ventricles are in diastole, and blood is forced into the ventricles. Atrial systole lasts for 0.1 second, then the atria relax (atrial diastole) for the remainder of the cycle, 0.7 second. When the atria finish their contraction phase, the ventricles begin contracting. Ventricular systole lasts for 0.3 second. Pressure in the ventricles increases as they contract. This closes the atrioventricular valves and opens the semilunar valves, and blood is forced into the pulmonary trunk and ascending aorta that carry blood away from the heart. During this time, the atria are in diastole and are filling with blood returned through the venae cavae. After ventricular systole, when the ventricles relax, the semilunar valves close, the atrio-ventricular valves open, and blood flows from the atria into the ventricles. All chambers are in simultaneous diastole for 0.4 second, and about 70% of ventricular filling occurs during this period. The remaining blood enters the ventricles during atrial systole. The most widely used index of overall cardiac pump performance is ejection fraction. The ejection fraction is determined with the end-diastolic volume (preload), the resistance to emptying (afterload), and the intrinsic muscle performance (contractility).

Aging has a direct effect on each component of the cardiovascular system including the heart muscle, blood vessels, and autonomic nervous system. When considering the cardiovascular system of an older adult, it is necessary to consider how the system is able to meet the demands of the working tissues despite altered cardiac and arterial function.

Age-Related Structural Changes in the Heart

Structural changes with aging involve the myocardium, the cardiac conduction system, and the endocardium. There is a progressive degeneration of the cardiac structures with aging, including a loss of elasticity, fibrotic changes in the valves of the heart, and infiltration with amyloid.

The age-associated structural characteristics that have the greatest impact involve the contractility of the heart's left ventricular wall (the largest chamber of the heart and the one from which blood is pumped into the aorta) and the ability of the *arteries to distend* in response to the heart's pumping action (aorta). The heart's left ventricular wall affects the heart's pumping capacity because of its ability to contract quickly, and it fully determines the force and rate at which blood is pumped into the arteries. The pumping capacity of the heart is reduced with age due to a variety of changes affecting the structure and function of the heart muscle.

Heart Mass and Myocytes

For decades, it was thought that the heart undergoes atrophy with advancing age, but evidence suggests that, if anything, the opposite may be true. The use of echocardiography has made it possible to measure accurately left ventricular wall thickness and chamber size, thus allowing noninvasive and accurate assessment of left ventricular mass. An age-related increase in the left ventricular posterior wall thickness of approximately 25% has been found between the second and the seventh decades.[53,69,106] An increase in heart mass with aging, for the most part, is due to an increase in the average *myocyte size,* whereas the *number of myocardial cells* declines.[114]

The increase in ventricular wall thickness may represent both cellular hypertrophy and an increase in *noncellular components.* Increases in myocardial collagen, fibrosis, and lipofuscin take place with aging. Collagen content within the myocardium increases, and there is a change in physical properties of collagen (due to altered cross-linking).[54] The pericardium, composed of bundles of collagen, becomes stiffer, which contributes to the decrease in compliance of the left ventricular wall. *Lipofuscin,* a brownish lipid-containing substance, accumulates at the poles of the nuclei of myocardial cells. Lipofuscin is thought to arise by the peroxidation of lipid/protein mixtures, and in the myocardium increases at a rate of about 0.3 percent per decade (as a result of free radicals). Thus, at the age of 90, the pigment occupies 6% to 7% of the intracellular volume. Basophilic degeneration, probably a by-product of glycogen metabolism, is found within the sarcoplasmic reticulum (due to glycation).

The progressive deposition of amyloid in the myocardium, usually in the atria, occurs in up to one third of elderly people. This histologic feature of aging, amyloidosis, is observed in the vasculature and many organs, too.[68] This protein infiltrates tissue, rending it dysfunctional. Adipose deposition between muscle cells is also common, resulting in fattier heart tissue in the ventricles and the interatrial septum. Fat deposits in the interatrial septum may displace conduction tissue in the sino-atrial node and lead to conduction disturbances.

Stimulus for Ventricular Hypertrophy (Increased Mass)

In younger adults, ventricular hypertrophy occurs in response to an increased cardiac volume or pressure work load, e.g., during high-resistant weight training. However, the stimulus for the increase in left ventricular wall thickness in the older adult is unclear. Age-associated ventricular hypertrophy may result from altered systolic blood pressure and aortic compliance that occur with aging. For example, with age the volume of blood in the ascending aorta increases due to age-related aortic dilatation. This increase in volume of blood must be advanced by the heart for ejection to occur; thus there is an increase in work load (afterload) that has to be performed by the heart. The increase in work load acts as the stimulus for muscle hypertrophy.

Valves

An age-related increase in valvular circumference has been reported in all four cardiac valves (aortic semilunar valve, pulmonary semilunar valve, bicuspid valve, tricuspid valve), with the greatest changes occurring in the aortic valve (the valve between the left ventricle and the aorta). The aortic

valvular circumference approaches that of the mitral valve (bicuspid valve located between the left atrium and left ventricle) by the tenth decade of life.[69] The age-associated increase in valvular circumference does not appear to be associated with valvular incompetence. Other valvular changes with aging include thickening and calcification of the cusps and leaflets. These changes do not usually cause significant dysfunction, although in some older adults, severe aortic valvular stenosis and mitral valvular insufficiency are related to degenerative changes with age. Clinical heart murmurs are detected more frequently.

Myocardial Subcellular Changes

Subcellular changes take place within the myocardial cells. The nucleus, containing DNA, becomes larger and may show invagination of its membrane. Nucleoli (the dense body within the nucleus that contains a high concentration of RNA) increase in size and number. The chromatin shows clumping, shrinking, fragmentation, or dissolution, and there is an increased likelihood of finding chromosomal abnormalities (due to DNA damage). The mitochondria show alterations in size, shape, cristal pattern, and matrix density, which reduce their functional surface (due to accumulation of damage). The cytoplasm is marked by fatty infiltration or degeneration, vacuole formation, and a progressive accumulation of pigments such as lipofuscin. The combined age-related changes in the subcellular compartments of the cells result in decreased cellular activities such as altered homeostasis, protein synthesis, and degradation rates.

Cardiac Muscle Compliance

In general, the walls of the heart become less compliant with age. The decreased capacity of the left ventricular wall to expand during diastole results in a reduced and delayed filling of the left ventricle. Subsequently, during the systolic (emptying) phase of the cardiac cycle, the left ventricle contracts less and ejects less blood (Frank-Starling relationship). Increased left *atrial* size is another age-related change that is thought to be related to an age-related decrease in left ventricular compliance, resulting in a decreased rate of left ventricular filling. Again, the decline in left ventricular compliance provides an increase work load on the atria, resulting in hypertrophy of the atria.

Age-Related Structural Changes in the Blood Vessels

In addition to the changes in the heart muscle itself, there are effects of aging on the arteries that further compromise the system's ability to distribute blood to the working tissues. Blood vessels require varying degrees of distensibility or compliance depending on their specific function. The forward motion of blood on the arterial side of the circulation is a function of the elastic recoil of the vessel walls and the progressive loss of pressure energy down the vascular tree. The peripheral vasculature provides the delivery system by which blood pumped by the heart reaches the various body tissues, therefore age-related changes in the blood vessels may limit the maximal perfusion of these tissues and affect cardiac performance as well. The decrease of elasticity of the arterial vessels with aging may result in chronic or residual increases in vessel diameter and vessel wall rigidity, which impair the function of the vessel.

One important set of changes involves the *aorta*, the chamber into which blood is ejected at each contraction of the heart muscle. In general, the wall of the aorta becomes less flexible, or shows an increase in wall stiffness, so that the blood leaving the left ventricle of the heart is faced by more resistance and cannot travel as far into the arteries. This change in wall stiffness can be attributed to changes in the elasticity of the vessel. There is a decrease in the amount of elastic fibers and an increase in collagen fibers. The collagen fibers are altered and less flexible (possibly due to an increase in cross-linking).

Second, the aorta acts as a buffer for the total blood volume in the arterial system because about one half of the stroke volume is stored in the aorta.[11] Up to the age of 60, the aortic buffering capacity is not decreased by the increased aortic wall stiffness. This is possible because the increase in aortic volume accommodates a given volume injected into it with less change in radius. This factor is known as *volume elasticity* (change in pressure for a given volume change). Thus the volume elasticity shows no age-associated changes up to about 60 years. However, after the age of 60, there is a marked decrease in volume elasticity. As the aorta stiffens with age, less diastolic aortic recoil occurs and results in a decreased aortic contribution to forward flow. Functionally, the aorta will not be able to propel the blood volume toward the systemic circulation.

Age-associated changes also occur in the more peripheral vessels (arteries and capillaries) and have a significant influence on the ability to propel the blood toward the capillaries and working tissues. In general, the walls of the arteries throughout the body become thicker so that they, too, are less flexible and stiffer (altered elasticity). Changes in the arterial stiffness with aging are accompanied by an increase in arterial diameter.[26,121] The stiffness of large arteries is associated with a loss in capacity to increase in diameter when needed to accommodate larger blood volumes. Thus, there is a decrease in arterial distensibility and compliance.[55,73,95]

The age-associated increase in arterial stiffness is thought to result from a diffuse cellular process that occurs in the vessel wall. There is an increase in chondroitin sulfate and heparin sulfate and a decrease in hyaluronate and chondroitin content. There is a relative loss of elastin fibers and an increase of collagen and collagen cross-linking.[96] The glycoprotein component of elastin fibrils decreases and eventually disappears, becomes frayed, and its calcium content increases.[97]

Impedance of blood flow through the arteries is further influenced by the accumulation of lipids that occurs over the individual's lifetime. The normal effects of aging include an increase in the concentrations of total plasma cholesterol, triglycerides, and the low- and very–low-density lipoproteins (LDLs and VLDLs) that transport these substances through circulation of the blood. Table 3-2 identifies the changes in arterial structural and functional properties with aging.

The walls of veins may become thicker with age because of an increase in connective tissue and calcium deposits. The valves also tend to become stiff and incompetent. Varicose veins develop. Because of low blood pressure in veins, these changes probably are not significant for cardiovascular function. They may be of concern because of the possibility of phlebitis and thrombus formation.

Function

The structural changes in the aorta and other large arteries are reflected clinically in a rise of the systolic pressure and widening of pulse pressure with advancing age. These histological, morphological, and stiffness changes found in the aging aorta and arteries are similar to those seen with essential hypertension.

The age-related increase in arterial stiffness may have an important impact on myocardial performance. The stiffer aorta with no change in heart rate can result in higher systolic ventricular pressure and decreased aortic diastolic pressure. Increases in ventricular diastolic pressure and volume may be observed. Such hemodynamic changes occurring in the older heart due to increased aortic stiffness require greater left ventricular stroke work and result in increased wall tension and myocardial oxygen consumption during systole. Thus, these findings suggest that the resistance to ventricular emptying increases with age; this increase in afterload may explain, at least in part, the age-related increase in left ventricular mass. The age-associated increases in arterial stiffness and pressure can be modified by life-style and diet because arterial stiffness varies inversely with aerobic capacity.[115]

Venous Circulation

The venous circulation is dependent on its being highly compliant to accommodate the greatest proportion of the blood volume at rest. Although the mechanical characteristics of venous smooth muscle have been less well-studied compared with arterial smooth muscle, the efficiency of its contractile behavior can be expected to be reduced with aging. Further, its electrical excitability and responsiveness to autonomic nervous systems tend to be less rapid and less pronounced.

Blood

The blood appears to be rather resistant to the aging process and under normal conditions blood values remain normal. The volume and composition remain consistent. Blood cells retain their normal size, shape, and structure.

The amount of red bone marrow decreases with age so the capability for blood cell formation decreases, but the hemopoietic mechanisms are still adequate for normal replacement so that blood counts and hemoglobin levels stay within normal ranges. Unusual circumstances, such as hemorrhage, may put a strain on the hemopoietic mechanism so it takes longer to rebuild after a hemorrhagic event.

In summary, arteries increase in diameter and wall thickness with aging, and these changes are associated with an increase in arterial wall stiffness and with a reduction in volume elasticity. Age-related alterations in the blood vessels do not appear to limit function and only are manifested upon stressful situations.

Age-Related Changes in the Electrical Conduction System of the Heart

With aging, the heart's conduction system changes such that the frequency and regularity of cardiac impulses may become abnormal (dysrhythmia). First, cardiac conduction is affected by the decrease in the number of pacemaker cells in the sinoatrial node with age.[67] Beginning by age 60 there is a pronounced "falling out," or decrease, in the number of pacemaker cells in the sinoatrial node, and by age 75 less than 10% of the cell number found in the young adult remains. A less dramatic cellular decrease is noted in the atrioventricular node and the intraventricular bundle of His.

Although this loss in specialized conduction cells is moderate, it is also associated with fibrotic changes in the specialized nerve conduction system.[109] With advancing age, there is an increase in elastic and collagenous tissue in all parts of the conduction system. Fat accumulates around the sinoatrial node, sometimes producing a partial or complete separation of the node from the atrial musculature. This occurrence in extreme cases may be related to the development of sick sinus syndrome. Fibrous infiltration of the bundle of His and bundle branches is common. A variable degree of calcification of the left side of the cardiac skeleton, which includes the aortic and mitral anuli, the central fibrous body, and the summit of the interventricular septum, occurs. Because of their proximity to these structures, the atrioventricular node, A-V bundle, bifurcation, and proximal left and right bundle branches may be damaged or destroyed by this process, resulting in so-called primary or idiopathic block.

Several features of the electrocardiogram are altered by normal aging based on the structural changes with age (Fig. 3-5). Although resting heart rate is not age-related, the P-R and Q-T intervals show small increases with age.[102] The age-related increase in the P-R interval has been shown to be due to conduction delay occurring proximal to the bundle of His.[31] The conduction time from the bundle of His to the ventricle is not altered. There is a leftward shift of the QRS axis with advancing age, perhaps reflecting a variable degree of fibrosis in the anterior fascicle of the left bundle branch as well as mild left ventricular hypertrophy. The S-T segment becomes flattened, and the amplitude of the T wave diminishes.

Fifty percent of older persons have been reported to have electrical conduction abnormalities at rest, which has considerable implications for the mechanical behavior of the

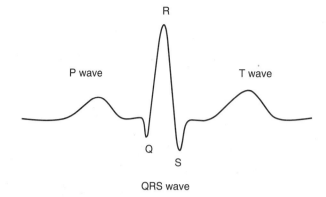

FIG. 3-5 The electrocardiogram shows age-related changes as described in the text.

_____

heart and the regulation of cardiac output, particularly when stressed during activity and exercise.[24]

In summary, the heart pumps less effectively with age. Additionally, changes with age in the integrity of the valves and those changes in the ventricles result in less efficient pumping action of the heart.[58] The age-related anatomical and physiological changes of the heart and blood vessels result in reduced capacity for oxygen transport at rest and, in particular, in response to situations imposing an increase in metabolic demand for oxygen. Therefore, older individuals may experience fatigue with minimal exertion and may no longer be able to perform certain activities. The functional capacity and reserve decrease, bringing the older individual closer to the minimum criterion of functioning.

Age-Related Physiological Changes of Heart Rate, Stroke Volume, Ejection Fraction, Cardiac Output, and Blood Pressure

Heart Rate

Heart rate is determined by the influence of the autonomic nervous system on the intrinsic pacemaker activity of the sinoatrial node. The parasympathetic and sympathetic nervous systems interact in controlling heart rate, the parasympathetic system acting through the vagus to slow the heart and the sympathetic system acting to increase heart rate. In young adults, the resting heart rate is normally reported to be about 70 beats/min and to be under predominantly vagal inhibitory control at rest.

Since resting heart rate is controlled by the autonomic nervous system, it can be affected by emotional factors and by changes in posture. Resting heart rate is also determined by fitness, so a very fit individual may have a low resting heart rate with a concomitantly higher resting stroke volume. Hence, resting heart rate changes with age may be relatively difficult to interpret.

Supine resting heart rate is widely reported to be unchanged by aging.[38,45,101] In contrast, sitting-position heart rate decreases with age.[101] Respiratory sinus arrhythmia, which is the variations in heart rate due to respiration (during inspiration heart rate increases), and heart rate variability decrease with aging.[36,105]

The diminished heart rate variability is observed during postural stress with a simultaneous diminished change in diastolic blood pressure (even in the absence of overt postural hypotension). The interaction of age and posture on heart rate suggests that age-associated changes occur in mechanisms that regulate heart rate. Hence, diminished heart rate variability and respiratory sinus arrhythmia with age may represent altered autonomic reflex function, including reduced vagal control. A shift in the balance of autonomic control of the heart from vagal to sympathetic occurs with age.

In addition, the number of pacemaker cells in the sinoatrial node declines with age, so that by the age of 70 years only about 10% of the number found in young adults are present.[32] This decline in pacemaker cell number may, in part, explain the decreased heart rate.

In contrast to resting heart rate, maximum exercise heart rate is a much more constant parameter. Maximum heart rate, which is the heart rate achieved at the point when no further increase in maximum oxygen consumption is observed despite increases in the intensity of the work load, shows a linear decrease with age.[30,65,70] For example, the maximum exercise heart rate in young adults is 200 beats/min compared with 150 to 160 beats/min in the older adult (Fig. 3-6). The decline in maximal heart rate with age is independent of habitual activity status,[44] whereas the maximal oxygen uptake reflects the level of physical fitness as well as the effects of cardiovascular disease.

Stroke Volume

Stroke volume is changed little by aging; at rest in healthy individuals, there may even be a slight increase.[30,98] Earlier studies note a decrease in left ventricular end-diastolic volume, but the screening of individuals was not stringent. In contrast, left ventricular end-diastolic volume may increase slightly with age when no cardiovascular disease is present.[75]

Ventricular performance or left ventricular contractility (*ejection fraction*) does not show any age-related change. However, there are several age-related changes in the left ventricle, including increases in afterload, a reduction in peak diastolic filling rate, and the increase in wall thickness and overall mass (described previously).

With increasing age, there is a reduction in the rate of left ventricular filling during early diastole as reflected by the rate of closure of the mitral valve. This impairment of left ventricular filling may derive at least in part from age-related increases in left ventricular wall thickness, which diminish ventricular diastolic compliance. To support this, there is myocardial stiffness and prolongation of isovolumetric relaxation. Perhaps as a result of this reduction of ventricular compliance, the left atrium is enlarged with age (increased work by the atrium). There is evidence of an increase in mitral inflow velocity during atrial systole.[82]

Because of these changes a greater proportion of blood must enter in late diastole. These changes do not have an impact at rest, whereas they have a significant impact during exercise, limiting maximum cardiac output in exercise when diastole will be shortened and limiting coronary blood flow. The decreased left ventricular compliance or increased ventricular stiffness may be due to increased amounts of connective tissue.

Cardiac Output

Cardiac output at rest is unaffected by age.[70,74,94] Maximum cardiac output and aerobic capacity are reduced with age. There is a linear decline through the adult years, so the average 65-year-old has 30% to 40% the aerobic capacity of a young adult.[30]

Resting Blood Pressure

Blood pressure is a measure of cardiovascular efficiency. Although blood pressure is characteristically heightened among older adults,[53,54] there is evidence suggesting that there are no effects of aging on this index of cardiovascular

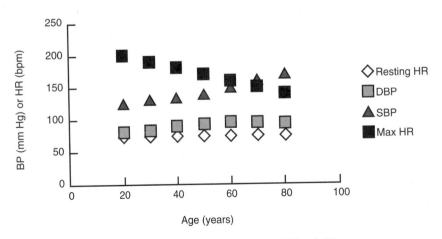

Fig. 3-6   Effects of increasing age on BP and HR.

functioning in healthy individuals[87] or when physiological indicators of physical fitness are statistically controlled. A lack of consistency across different investigations is most likely related to variations across samples in the incidence of hypertension, a chronic cardiovascular disorder that involves elevated blood pressure. The inclusion of individuals with hypertension in samples of older adults tested for normal aging effects presents an obvious confounder of the effects of aging with the effects of disease.

Blood pressure is determined by cardiac output and by total peripheral resistance. Since cardiac output is little altered by age in the healthy older adults, blood pressure increases with age are likely to reflect mainly alterations in total peripheral resistance and diminished aortic compliance. Remember the equation:

$$\text{Blood Pressure} = \text{Cardiac Output} \times \text{Total Peripheral Resistance}$$

Systolic Blood Pressure vs. Diastolic Blood Pressure

Both systolic and mean blood pressures significantly increase from 20 to 80 years. Specifically, systolic blood pressure tends to increase with age throughout life, whereas diastolic pressure increases until the age of about 60 years and then stabilizes or even falls.[71]

The main cause of isolated systolic hypertension in the elderly, where the systolic pressure increases with age[92] (as depicted in Fig. 3-7), is a decreased arterial compliance (Fig. 3-8). The compliance of the aorta falls by a factor of three to four over the age range of 20 to 80 years.[36] Even in normotensive, rigorously screened volunteers, age-related increases in arterial stiffness occur,[116] and aortic stiffening correlates with LDL cholesterol levels.[61]

In summary, increased left ventricular stiffness, diminished compliance with resulting prolongation of relaxation, and a reduced rate of early diastolic rapid filling occur with age. Ventricular diastolic function, therefore, is compromised by aging changes, and diastolic filling becomes more dependent on atrial contraction in older persons. The degree of ventricular diastolic impairment due to aging alone, however, is not usually severe enough to cause clinical heart failure.

Older adults do not appear to have cardiac limitations at rest. They are at risk of developing heart failure if hypertension or ischemic heart disease is present even though ventricular systolic function is normal. Some studies have reported that 45% to 55% of patients older than 65 years with clinical heart failure have normal systolic ventricular function.[9]

Age-Related Cardiovascular Response During Exercise

The preceding section addressed aging changes in cardiac performance evident at rest. In many organ systems, functional impairments may become manifest only under conditions that tax the capability of the system—that is, stress, such as exercise. The following section centers on the age-related changes in the cardiovascular system in response to aerobic exercise.

Exercise performance is determined by a multistage continuous treadmill or bicycle test, each successive stage requiring greater energy expenditure than the preceding one. The cardiovascular system supports this exercise by distributing increasing amounts of blood to the working muscles. The working muscles need sufficient oxygen to satisfy their increased metabolic requirements. The ability to deliver oxygen to the working muscles is quantified by measuring the maximal oxygen consumption ($\dot{V}O_2max$), which is the product of the maximal cardiac output (heart rate and stroke volume) and maximal systemic arteriovenous oxygen (a-$\bar{v}O_2$) difference. The term *maximal systemic a-$\bar{v}o2$ difference* is the difference in the oxygen content of arterial and mixed venous blood. At rest, a-$\bar{v}O_2$

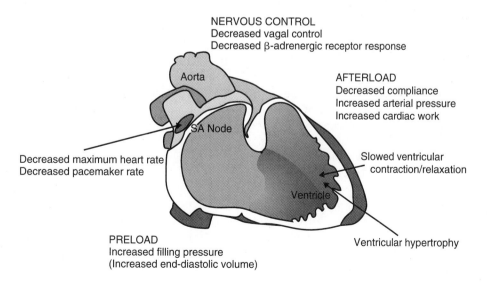

NERVOUS CONTROL
Decreased vagal control
Decreased β-adrenergic receptor response

Aorta

SA Node

AFTERLOAD
Decreased compliance
Increased arterial pressure
Increased cardiac work

Decreased maximum heart rate
Decreased pacemaker rate

Slowed ventricular
contraction/relaxation

Ventricle

PRELOAD
Increased filling pressure
(Increased end-diastolic volume)

Ventricular hypertrophy

FIG. 3-7 Schematic representation of the effects of age.

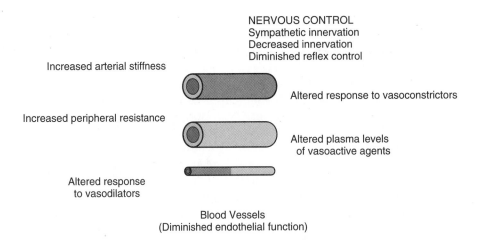

FIG. 3-8   Schematic representation of age-related alterations in vascular function.

difference is normally 4 to 5 ml of oxygen per 100 ml of blood. The large quantity of oxygen still remaining with hemoglobin provides an automatic reserve by which cells can immediately obtain oxygen should the metabolic demands suddenly increase. $\dot{V}O_2$max is considered an indicator of cardiovascular fitness.

Heart Rate and Exercise

During exercise, the expected rise in cardiac heart rate necessary to increase cardiac output in order to provide for the increased oxygen consumption by the exercising muscles is much lower in the elderly than in the young. The maximum achievable heart rate with exercise decreases linearly with age and may be calculated empirically, using 220 beats per minute as the maximum in the adult. The age changes can be calculated by subtracting the age of the individual from the 220 values. Thus, in an 80-year-old the maximal heart rate that can be achieved while exercising is $220 - 80 = 140$ beats/min. Although the decline is progressive, the change is more precipitous after 50 years of age. The age-associated changes in heart rate influence the maximal cardiac output, significantly influencing $\dot{V}O_2$max.

Mechanisms for Heart Rate Changes During Exercise

The increase in heart rate during various types of physical activity is a function of the relative (% of maximum) load or power output rather than the absolute exercise intensity. Therefore, to determine possible changes in the regulation of heart rate, the same relative exercise stimulus must be applied. In older adults, there is a consistent smaller tachycardia (increase in heart rate) during both isometric and dynamic exercise compared with younger adults.

One possibility for the lower response in heart rate in the older adult is that there is a reduction in cardiac vagal influence on heart rate under resting conditions and that this limits the degree of reduction in vagal tone possible in response to exercise. The other possibility is that older adults

have some impairment in β-adrenergic activation of heart rate during exercise. For example, there could be lower synaptic concentration of norepinephrine in older subjects (due to a diminished neural activation, impaired neuronal release, and/or enhanced neuronal reuptake); circulating levels of epinephrine may rise less during exercise in older adults; or older adults may have impaired β-adrenergic receptor and/or postreceptor responsiveness.

Stroke Volume and Exercise

At light work loads there is no age-associated difference in stroke volume, but the stroke output diminishes as effort is increased toward a maximum. The stroke volume during exhausting work is thus 10% to 20% percent smaller than in a young adult. The ability to increase stroke volume in the older adult during exercise is achieved with an increase in end-diastolic volume through the Frank-Starling relationship.[74,98] The Frank-Starling relationship links the volume and pressure of blood in the ventricle (filling pressure) to the force of contraction of the ventricular muscle so that an increased filling of the ventricle causes an increased stretch of the wall and results in an increased force of contraction.

Cardiac Output and Exercise

Cardiac output increases similarly with increasing work loads in various age groups; however, the mechanism of augmentation of cardiac output is different between the age groups. The young adults demonstrate a large increase in heart rate from rest to exercise. In young adults, stroke volume increases with exercise because of a large decrease in end-systolic volume compared to rest. For example, a cardiac output of 15 L/min is achieved by a heart rate of approximately 135 beats/min and a stroke volume of 115 ml in the young and a heart rate of 115 beats/min and a stroke volume of 135 ml in the elderly.[98]

Therefore, exercise cardiac output is maintained with age. Importantly, the mechanisms that account for the increase in exercise cardiac output differ according to age. In the young adult, through β-adrenergic stimulation, there is a large increase in heart rate and decrease in end-systolic volume. Older adults, likely because of the age-associated decreased responsiveness to catecholamines, show a failure of end-systolic volume to decrease and a decreased chronotropic response to exercise. End-diastolic volume increases in the older adult, with a consequent increase in exercise stroke volume. This shift to the Frank-Starling relationship suggests some impairment of the exercise response in the older adult.

Role of Afterload

One major determinant of afterload, the characteristic aortic impedance to flow, is derived from the relationship between pressure and flow during the cardiac cycle. At low exercise levels in younger individuals, there is a stepwise increase in stroke volume with increasing work load and no change in impedance from resting values. In contrast, the older subjects demonstrate a striking increase in impedance during exercise, with minimal augmentation of stroke volume. These differences persist through maximal work loads. Thus, the increased afterload imposed by the vasculature of older subjects during exercise may be a factor in stroke volume responses (altered ejection fraction). The increased afterload in the older population may reflect an impaired vasodilator response to catecholamines on the heart and peripheral vasculature.

The diminished effect of catecholamines with advancing age could be secondary to a decrease in impaired target organ responsiveness to catecholamines, since plasma catecholamine levels during maximal treadmill exercise increase in the older adult.

Left-Ventricular Contractility and Exercise

Left ventricular systolic performance is well-maintained with aging under resting conditions but is reduced even in healthy older subjects during strenuous exercise. Thus the impaired "pump" performance during exercise appears to be mediated, at least in part, by age-associated reductions in β-adrenergic function or responsiveness on the heart.

$\dot{V}O_2MAX$—MAXIMAL AEROBIC POWER

The best physiological measure of an individual's endurance work capacity is the amount of oxygen consumed at maximal exercise (maximal aerobic power, or $\dot{V}O_2max$). $\dot{V}O_2max$ is determined by the capacity of the cardiovascular system to deliver O_2 to the working skeletal muscles and the capacity of the muscles to extract O_2 from the blood to generate energy (adenosine triphosphate [ATP]). $\dot{V}O_2max$ is determined by maximal heart rate and stroke volume (cardiac output) and maximal arterio-venous oxygen difference. Therefore any age-related change in these factors could alter $\dot{V}O_2max$. For more than 50 years, cross-sectional studies have repeatedly demonstrated a significant age-related decrement in

$\dot{V}O_2max$. Together, these data suggest that exercise capacity or aerobic performance declines by approximately 1% per year.[35] Most of the oxygen consumption takes place in skeletal muscle during heavy exercise. The age-related decline in skeletal muscle mass, however, does not entirely explain the decline in $\dot{V}O_2max$.

Aerobic performance capacity is most likely determined by functional integrity in respiration, circulation, and muscle metabolism. Part of the age-related decline in aerobic performance capacity may, therefore, result from a decline in the quality of skeletal muscle as reflected in the decreased oxidative capacity, as described in the following.

In early studies, the observed decline in $\dot{V}O_2max$ with age was attributed to a decrease in both maximal cardiac output and maximal a-$\bar{v}O_2$ difference. The decrease in maximum cardiac output was due to a decrease in both maximum heart rate and maximum stroke volume.[30] However, systolic blood pressure and right ventricular end-diastolic pressure were greater at peak exercise in the older men compared with younger men. The conclusions drawn from early studies are tentative because they may have included subjects with coronary artery disease. In addition, maximum aerobic capacity may have been limited in these studies by noncardiovascular factors, such as body composition, physical activity status, and respiratory function.

Thus, the decline in $\dot{V}O_2max$ or physical work capacity can be attributed to, at least partly, age-related reductions in maximum heart rate, contractility, and cardiac output in exercise and partly to decreased muscle mass and quality of skeletal muscle.[48]

Therapists need not be so concerned about the separation of aging from its confounding factors. Perhaps their most important realization is that because of these factors—i.e., deconditioning, latent coronary artery disease, and multiple organ system pathology acting on a substrate that has already been altered by time per se—the presentation of disease may be modified. The potential for rehabilitation may be limited due to the lack of physiological reserve or capacity. Indeed, it is this multifaceted characteristic of human illness that requires the therapist to treat the whole patient—not just the disease or the aging process.

In conclusion, the primary age-associated cardiovascular changes include a decrease responsiveness of myocardium and vascular smooth muscle to β-adrenergic stimulation and an increase in arterial stiffness with resultant increase in afterload. Whether these changes are inherent to the aging process or due to a secondary change, such as the increasing sedentary life-style, is unknown. The older adult appears to have adequate cardiac reserve or adaptation, such as the Frank-Starling relationship or the increased contribution of atrial contraction to end-diastolic volume, which maintain normal cardiac function at rest and exercise. However, these age-associated changes make the older adult more prone to develop symptoms in the setting of disease, such as hypertension, coronary artery disease, or atrial fibrillation.

REVIEW OF THE SKELETAL MUSCLE SYSTEM AND FUNCTION

Skeletal muscles contract in order to perform four major functions: movement, posture, joint stability, and heat production. An individual skeletal muscle may be made up of hundreds, or even thousands, of muscle fibers bundled together by specific connective tissue covering. Muscles are attached to bones by tendons.

Anatomy

Each skeletal muscle fiber is a single cylindrical muscle cell composed of typical cellular organelles (nucleus, sarcoplasmic reticulum). The sarcoplasm of muscle cells is packed with myofibrils composed of actin and myosin myofilaments. Actin and myosin are considered the major force-producing proteins in skeletal muscle. The arrangement of the actin and myosin myofilaments form the basic unit of muscle, the sarcomere. The individual muscle fibers are arranged in parallel to form fasciculi, which in turn make up muscle. Skeletal muscles have an abundant blood and nerve supply.

Skeletal muscle contraction is the result of a complex series of events, based on chemical reactions and mechanical reactions, at the individual muscle fiber level. This chain of reactions begins with stimulation by an alpha motor neuron and ends when the muscle fiber is again relaxed. Skeletal muscles are stimulated to contract by special nerve cells called *alpha motor neurons*. As the axon of the alpha motor neuron penetrates the muscle, the axon branches, so there is an axon terminal for each muscle fiber. A single alpha motor neuron and all the muscle fibers it stimulates is a called a *motor unit*.

The region in which an axon terminal meets a muscle fiber is called the *neuromuscular junction*. Acetylcholine, a neurotransmitter, is contained within synaptic vesicles in the axon terminal and diffuses across the synaptic cleft to acetylcholine receptors. Receptor sites for the acetylcholine are located on the sarcolemma. Acetylcholinesterase rapidly inactivates the acetylcholine. This ensures that one nerve impulse will result in only one muscle impulse and only one contraction of the muscle fibers. Skeletal muscle contraction is produced by simultaneous and synchronized contraction of muscle fibers.

The energy source for muscle contraction is ATP. Energy from ATP is needed for the actin and myosin to generate force. Muscles have limited storage capacity for ATP, thus the ATP supply is replenished by creatine phosphate, glucose, and fatty acids. Fatty acids and glucose become the primary energy sources when muscles are actively contracting for extended periods of time. Oxygen is required for the breakdown of fatty acids and glucose to ATP. When adequate oxygen is available, glucose is metabolized via aerobic metabolism or respiration to produce ATP. If adequate oxygen is not available, the mechanism for producing ATP from glucose is anaerobic metabolism (glycolysis). Aerobic metabolism produces nearly 20 times more ATP per glucose than the anaer-

obic pathway, but anaerobic metabolism occurs at a faster rate. Limited amounts of oxygen can be stored in muscle fibers. Myoglobin contains iron groups (hemoglobin) that attract and temporarily bind with oxygen. When the oxygen levels inside the muscle fiber diminish, the oxygen can be supplied from myoglobin.

Skeletal muscle is composed of two main skeletal fiber types. The type II, fast-twitch fibers, have a lower oxidative capacity, little myoglobin, greater glycolytic potential, and a faster twitch response than the slow-twitch, type I fibers. The type I fibers are also known as *fatigue-resistant fibers* because of their metabolic qualities that include greater mitochondrial density, capillary density, and myoglobin content. With the exception of postural muscles, most human skeletal muscle is composed of both fiber types. During slow, low-intensity exercise, most of the muscle force is generated by the type I fibers. During higher intensity exercise, both type I and type II fibers are recruited.

The sarcoplasmic reticulum is a specialized form of smooth endoplasmic reticulum that stores calcium ions in muscle. The properties of the sarcoplasmic reticulum are the strongest determinants of the speed of contraction of the isometric twitch. The rates of sarcoplasmic reticulum calcium uptake are strongly correlated with the contraction time of the isometric twitch.

Two proteins participate in sarcolemmal excitation-sarcoplasmic reticulum calcium release: dihydropyridine receptor, a voltage-gated calcium channel, and a calcium release channel, a ryanodine receptor. The dihydropyridine receptor is expressed in the transverse tubule, and it elicits calcium release from the sarcoplasmic reticulum through a hypothetical mechanical interaction with the ryanodine receptor.

Function

Muscle force or strength, is proportional to the cross-sectional area of the muscle fibers. Speed of contraction is an important characteristic of muscle performance. This property is important because the velocity of movement and the power generated by muscle can have greater relevance than absolute muscle strength in the ability to perform a number of activities of daily living, to independence, and to functional capacity. Maximal shortening velocities in a muscle depend on several factors. First, total shortening and shortening velocity are the sum of the movements of actin and myosin filaments. The velocity also depends on the load on the muscle; the force-velocity relationship stresses this concept. Muscles lift a heavy load slowly but can shorten rapidly when lightly loaded. Velocity of shortening is also dependent on the molecular properties of the myosin isoform synthesized within the muscle fiber. There is a direct proportionality between the ATPase activity, ability to hydrolyze ATP, and shortening velocity. Type II skeletal muscle fibers hydrolyze ATP faster than type I fibers, resulting in faster shortening velocities. Power, or work/time, is the product of force and velocity. Muscular endurance is the ability to perform exercise over a prolonged period of time. The endurance of a muscle is a function of the fiber composition and the oxidative capacity of the muscle. The endurance capability of a muscle depends on the balance between energy output and energy supply. The ability of the blood flow to supply oxygen to the mitochondria in skeletal muscles and the capacity of the muscle fibers for oxidative metabolism determine endurance.

Aging has a significant effect on the components of the skeletal muscle system, including the alpha motor neurons, neuromuscular junction, excitation-contraction coupling, and contractile proteins. When examining the skeletal muscle system of an older adult, it is important to consider how this system is able to meet the demands required for activities of daily living.

Age-Related Changes in Skeletal Muscle

Skeletal muscle undergoes major structural and functional adaptations in response to physical inactivity, just as it does in response to disease, nutritional status, and obesity, and these effects must be considered when examining the independent effects of aging on muscle structure and function. Age-related reductions in muscle mass are a direct cause of declines in muscle strength with aging. This reduction in muscle strength is a major cause of disability in the older adult since strength and power are major components of gait, balance, and the ability to walk.[13]

Reductions in Muscle Mass

Aging is associated with decreases in total muscle cross-sectional area, amounting to approximately 40% between the ages of 20 and 80 years (Fig. 3-9). Reductions in leg muscle cross-sectional area have been observed to begin in early adulthood and accelerate beyond 50 years of age.[17] This reduction in muscle cross-sectional area is accompanied by increases in noncontractile structures such as fat and connective tissue.[88,95] Thus, the girth or volume measurements of muscle, used commonly in the clinic, may not show the actual reduction in the contractile proteins responsible for force generation (actin and myosin). Net growth or the maintenance of muscle mass occurs as a result of the balance

between protein synthesis and degradation. The rates of skeletal muscle protein synthesis decline with age and may also contribute to muscle atrophy and repair process after injury.[46]

Reduction in Muscle Fiber Number

The total number of muscle fibers is significantly *reduced* with age, beginning at about 25 years and progressing at an accelerated rate thereafter.[77] The decline in muscle cross-sectional area is most likely due to decreases in total fiber number, especially type II fast-twitch glycolytic fibers.[77] The loss of muscle fibers is followed by a replacement with fat and fibrous tissue and a gradual increase in non-muscle tissue.

Changes in Muscle Fiber Size

The size of the individual fast-twitch type II fibers decreases with age (vastus lateralis, tibialis anterior, and biceps brachii), whereas the slow-twitch type I fiber size does not change.[56,77] For example, in the third or fourth decade of life, the mean cross-sectional area of individual fast-twitch type II fibers in the quadriceps femoris muscle exceeds that of slow-twitch type I fibers by approximately 20%. By the age of 85 the area of individual fast-twitch type II fibers is less than 50% of that of slow-twitch type I fibers.[21,113] In addition, small, angulated fibers and grouped atrophy are commonly seen in muscles of older men and women. These morphological changes are similar to changes that are observed in skeletal muscle diseases.

The reduction in number of muscle fibers contributes more to the decrease of whole muscle cross-sectional area than does the reduction in area of individual fibers. The findings that individual fast-twitch type II fibers decrease in cross-sectional area suggest that the relative contribution of fast-twitch type II fibers to force generation is less in the older adult.

It is not surprising that most reduction in muscle fiber cross-sectional area is seen in type II fibers, particularly the IIb fibers (fast-twitch, predominantly glycolytic and readily fatigable). Order of recruitment of motor units and therefore muscle fibers dictates that type I fibers will remain in relatively regular use, even in older adults, whereas the type II fibers and particularly the IIb fibers will rarely be recruited and therefore are subject to disuse atrophy. These changes have a significant impact on force production and sustained power production.

Motor Unit Number and Size

There is a decrease in total number of motor units with age.[22,24] The average motor neuron loss from the second to tenth decade is approximately 25%. The loss of motor neurons seems to be uniform within and between the segments.[112] The decrease in motor unit number is accompanied by an increase in size or innervation ratio, such that on average, each motor neuron innervates more muscle fibers in the older adult. The increase in size of the motor unit is found primarily in the muscles of the lower limb, particu-

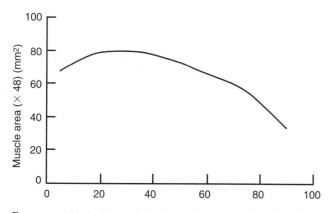

FIG. 3-9   The decline in skeletal muscle mass as a function of age.

larly in persons 60 years old, and more in distal than in proximal muscles.

Electrophysiological studies have shown a reduced number of functioning motor units with increasing age, mainly after age 60 in both proximal and distal muscles. Loss and dysfunction are observed among the largest and fastest motor units, i.e., type II motor units.[39]

Axon

The loss of motor neurons is accompanied by a reduction in both the numbers and diameters of motor axons. There is an age-related reduction in the numbers of large and intermediate myelinated ventral root fibers but no significant reduction of the small nerve fibers. This preferential loss is estimated to be approximately 5% from young age to old age. Quantitative electromyography (EMG) has shown changes in both duration and amplitude of motor unit action potentials with increasing age.[62] Axonal nerve conduction velocities of all motor nerve fibers are uniformly slowed with aging. This suggests that with aging, the alterations in conduction velocities could reflect a variety of changes in the nerve fibers, such as a dropout of the largest fibers, a segmental demyelination, and a reduced internodal length. In addition, the mean soma size of motor neurons is reduced with age with accumulation of lipofuscin.

Neuromuscular Junction

The neuromuscular junction is the crucial link between the motor neuron and the muscle. Normally, the junction has a high safety factor, meaning that the arrival of an action potential at the nerve terminal results in an action potential in the muscle fiber. The motor end plates have been noted to undergo continuous remodeling during normal development, maturation, and aging, with gradual changes in both presynaptic and postsynaptic components.

The number of preterminal axons entering an end plate increases, and there is increased incidence of branches or boutons. The convolutions in the motor end plate decrease, and the sarcolemma becomes smoother. The length of end plates increases and is composed of a greater number of smaller conglomerates of acetylcholine receptors. The significance of these changes on the transmission of the action potentials and excitation-contraction coupling is, however, not fully understood. It is possible that these changes are compensatory rather than the result of degeneration per se, thereby preserving neuromuscular function with increasing age. However, these changes may alter the surface area of the postsynaptic terminal, resulting in a diminished ability of the muscle cells to be activated by the motor neuron.

Altered Motor Unit Remodeling

Motor unit remodeling is the natural cycle of turnover of synaptic connections occurring at the neuromuscular junction by the process of denervation, axonal sprouting, and reinnervation of the muscle. In aging, however, it appears that motor unit remodeling is altered. Aging of skeletal muscle is associated with a combination of changes in nerve and muscle cells, resulting in weakened neural influences and a shift toward "functional denervation" concomitant with senile muscle atrophy. Motor unit remodeling is altered such that type II fibers are selectively denervated and reinnervated by collateral sprouting of axons from fibers of the slow motor units. This is an attractive theory that accounts for many observed functional and morphological age-related changes in skeletal muscle. The reason for altered motor unit remodeling is unclear; it might result from faster axonal growth in slow motor units or from their superiority in establishing permanent connections with both type I and II muscle fibers. It has been suggested that the type II fibers, which become reinnervated by slow motor unit axons, actually become type I fibers, with respect to physiological and biochemical properties.[72] The fast motor unit axons degenerate when they no longer innervate muscle fibers.

Terminal sprouting is a mechanism that maintains neuromuscular contact and is persistent through life. This process decreases with advancing age. Motor end plate–associated choline acetyltransferase (a marker enzyme for synapse integrity) and acetylcholinesterase (which is necessary for transmitter breakdown) activity also decline with age.[14] Age-associated motor unit remodeling is a consequence of alterations in the normal turnover of synaptic junctions that results from a cycle of denervation, axonal sprouting, and reinnervation. In young adults, the turnover occurs without any alteration in the type of innervation reaching fibers. With age, however, it is common to observe an aggregation of type I fibers. This age-associated change reflects some denervated type II fibers becoming reinnervated by axonal sprouting from adjacent innervated type I fibers.

Age-Related Changes in Motor Neurons

Aging beyond 60 years is associated with a reduction in number of lumbosacral spinal cord motor neurons.[112] These decreases appear to be caused by losses of the largest alpha motor neurons and their myelinated axons in lumbar ventral roots, with preservation of smaller motor neurons. The surviving segmental neurons increase in branching complexity and exhibit additional collateral growth, perhaps as a compensatory mechanisms for the loss of motor neurons and an increased load due to increased innervation ratios to the muscle fibers they innervate. With age, the size of slow motor units increases. The number of fibers and the total fiber area in a given motor unit also increase.

The collected evidence strongly suggests that as age increases beyond 60 years, muscle undergoes continuous denervation and reinnervation, due to an accelerating reduction of functioning motor units. This is mediated through a loss of motor neurons in the spinal cord and myelinated ventral root fibers. Initially, reinnervation can compensate for this denervation. However, as this neurogenic process progresses, more and more muscle fibers become permanently denervated and subsequently replaced by fat and fibrous tissue.

Sarcoplasmic Reticulum, Dihydropyridine Receptor, Ryanodine Receptor

An age-related change in the properties of the sarcoplasmic reticulum appears to be the most probable explanation for the altered twitch contractile properties with age. The age-related slowing of the isometric twitch (prolonged twitch contraction duration) is, in part, related to an impairment of the calcium uptake activity of the sarcoplasmic reticulum.

The dihydropyridine receptor and the ryanodine receptor are key molecules involved in skeletal muscle excitation-contraction coupling. With age there are *decreases* in the number of dihydropyridine receptors, ryanodine receptors, and the dihydropyridine/ryanodine receptor ratio in both fast- and slow-twitch muscles.

The dihydropyridine receptor is a voltage-gated calcium channel, and its activation by transverse-tubule membrane depolarization evokes calcium release from the sarcoplasmic reticulum through the ryanodine receptor. Contractile proteins on binding calcium initiate muscle contraction and force development. Hence, the dihydropyridine and ryanodine receptors play a central role in skeletal muscle contraction. The reduction in the number of receptors alters the electromechanical transduction leading to muscle force development, resulting in muscle weakness in the elderly.

Age-Related Changes in Muscle Performance

Strength

Age-related decreases in strength have been well-documented. A variety of limb muscles have been tested during isometric strength tasks and demonstrate that reductions in isometric and dynamic voluntary strength become substantial by the seventh decade of life and may accelerate thereafter. Arm, leg, and back strength decline at an overall rate of 8% per decade, starting in the third decade of life.[10] The rate of decline is not linear but is slightly lower early in the decline and accelerated late in life. Healthy men and women in their seventh and eighth decades of life demonstrate average reductions of 20% to 40% in maximal isometric strength in various muscles.

The age-associated reduction of quadriceps muscle strength is such that the average 80-year-old is at or near the minimum level of strength required to rise from a chair. Leg muscle strength also appears to be related to maximum and sustainable walking speeds in ambulatory older populations (Fig. 3-10).

There is evidence to indicate that the muscles in the arms and legs are affected disproportionately. Loss of muscle strength in leg muscles is greater than loss in arm muscles between the ages of 30 and 80 (40% compared with 30%). Weight-bearing muscles showed greater changes than non–weight-bearing muscles.[110]

These age-related reductions are relatively similar for both male and females. Because of its functional importance in gait and fall prevention, as well as the accumulated morphological, histochemical, and biochemical data, a great deal

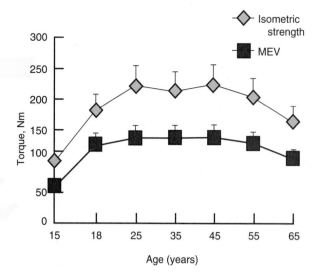

FIG. 3-10 Maximal isometric strength (Nm) and maximal knee extension velocity (MEV) with age.

of work has focused on the strength of the quadriceps femoris group. Studies using concentric isokinetic contractions of the knee extensors and ankle plantar flexors have shown that aging is associated with a 20% to 40% loss in strength in both males and females. It has been reported in both the elbow and knee extensor muscles in men, and the knee extensors and flexors in women, that age-related decrements in strength are less remarkable during isokinetic eccentric contractions than during concentric contractions.[90,91]

Muscle weakness may be due to a decline in the ability to activate the existing muscle mass. It is conceivable that age-related weakness may be caused partly by decreased central drive and thus a decrease in ability to voluntarily activate a muscle. The threshold of excitability of the corticospinal tract increases progressively with age and is significantly higher in the elderly.[99] The weakness may, in part, be due to loss of muscle mass and therefore in the number of force-generating crossbridges interacting between actin and myosin. Lastly, the reduction in strength could be attributed to changes in the intrinsic properties of the remaining skeletal muscle fibers, a decrease in the force developed by each actin and myosin crossbridge. There may be a combination of all three factors contributing to the decline in strength. The conclusion may be drawn that unknown factors in addition to a loss of muscle mass must explain the age-associated loss of strength.

Power and Endurance

The power output is governed by (1) the velocity of shortening and (2) the force-generating capacity of the muscle. Aging reduces the peak forces that can be generated by muscles at fast contraction speeds, resulting in a decrease in peak power output. Peak power output declines by about 20%

with age. The decrease in power output results, at least in part, from motor unit remodeling, which reduces the fast-to-slow-fiber ratio.

The importance of understanding the mechanisms underlying these particular muscle properties is supported by the close association between age-related reductions in lower extremity power output and functional abilities such as maximal walking speed and stair climbing ability. This reduced capacity for rapid-force generation might also limit the ability to respond quickly to a loss of balance and increase the risk of falling.

A decline in muscular endurance is a feature of old age that contributes to functional loss and disability. Alterations in muscle, both contractile and metabolic, with advanced age may contribute to the decrease in muscle endurance. The alterations include reduced blood supply and capillary density and impairment of glucose transport and therefore of substrate availability, lower mitochondrial density, decreased activity of oxidative enzymes, and decreased rate of phosphocreatine repletion.

Velocity

The maximal speed of muscle contraction decreases with age. This decrease is reflected in a decrease in the actin-activated myosin ATPase activity and may in part explain the slowing of movement with age.

With age, the muscle twitch is characterized by prolonged contraction and one-half relaxation times. Thus, fused tetanic forces occur at lower stimulation frequencies (an adaptation that increases muscle efficiency). This adaptation also lengthens the time for muscle relaxation, thus impairing the ability to perform rapid and powerful alternating movements.

Metabolic Pathways: Glucose Uptake

Aging is associated with decreased glucose tolerance and a greatly increased incidence of noninsulin-dependent diabetes mellitus (NIDDM). The decreasing glucose tolerance of aging is linked to the age-associated changes in body composition and activity levels. Improved fitness as a result of aerobic exercise improves glucose tolerance, and exercise prevents the onset of NIDDM.[60]

Specifically, glucose tolerance is impaired in persons older than 60. Insulin resistance is primarily due to defects in skeletal muscle with age. Levels of Glut-4 protein, the insulin-regulated glucose transporter in plasma membranes, decrease in skeletal muscle during maturation but not during aging. Although the pool of intracellular transporters does not change, there is an age-associated decline in the insulin-receptor signaling system. There is a down-regulation of tyrosine kinase activity of the insulin receptor, which explains why there is an age-associated reduction in the translocation of transporters from the intracellular compartment to the sarcolemmal membrane. This change in the insulin-receptor signaling system at the cellular level has a significant impact on function.

Enzyme Activity

Age-related impairments in skeletal muscle metabolism take place. However, the glycolytic enzymes (phosphorylase, phosphofructokinase, and lactate dehydrogenase) do not show age-associated changes. With exercise in the older individual, there is a greater metabolic stress and a decreased rate of phosphocreatine repletion after exercise.

In contrast, the aerobic enzymes (succinate dehydrogenase, citrate synthase, and β-hydroxyacyl-CoA-dehydrogenase) decline with age. With age, mitochondrial decay occurs. This mitochondrial decay includes decreased mitochondrial content, decreased oxidative capacity, decreased enzyme activities, and increased mitochondrial DNA deletions or mutations.

In addition to the decrease in skeletal muscle mitochondrial capacity, there is a decline in capillary density.[27,81] These changes have a significant impact on aerobic metabolism, limiting fatty acid oxidation, glucose and lipid metabolism, and glycogen storage.[57] Functionally, these changes decrease oxygen uptake by muscle during exercise and contribute to the decline in $\dot{V}O_2max$ in older people by reducing the $a\text{-}\bar{v}O_2$ difference maximum.[78,86] In addition, the decline in mitochondrial content and function impairs muscle oxidative and endurance capacity and is, therefore, likely to contribute to the increase in muscle fatigability that occurs with aging.

Blood Flow and Capillarity

Sustained muscular performance requires a proper balance between energy supply and demand. The decreased endurance capacity of muscle with age likely reflects decreased blood flow and decreased oxidative capacity, possibly impairing energy balance.[25,63] Capillary density decreases with age and appears to be due to an actual reduction in the total number of blood capillaries, as both capillary-to-fiber ratio and the number of capillaries in contact with each muscle cell is lower in the aged.[28] The reduction in capillarity has major importance for the ability of muscle to sustain power output over time.

In summary, maintenance of muscle mass and strength may be critical for maintaining independent function in the elderly. Muscle mass and muscle strength decline with advancing age, and the underlying mechanisms responsible for the altered muscle performance are unclear but most likely involve multiple levels.

AGE AND EXERCISE

Skeletal and cardiac muscle adaptations occur because of changes in intensity, duration, and frequency of physical activity (increase or decrease). The adaptations include alterations in morphological, biochemical, and molecular properties. These adaptations that are associated with altered physical activity lead to altered functional characteristics from the cellular to the whole tissue and functional performance levels.

Exercise training (increase in physical activity) is very specific.[4] The principle of *specificity* refers to adaptations in the metabolic and physiological systems, depending on the type of overload imposed. It states that strength training induces specific strength adaptations and that specific aerobic exercise elicits specific endurance-training adaptations. Exercise specificity results in enhanced capacity to develop maximal power after strength training, whereas maximal endurance is improved after aerobic training. Strength and endurance training adaptations may occur independently or concurrently if appropriate training programs are used.

Benefits of Strength Training

Strength training, or *resistance exercise,* is generally defined as training in which the resistance against which a muscle generates force is progressively increased over time. The maximal weight or resistance a person can lift or move to complete the movement is defined as *one repetition maximum (1 RM).* Muscle strength has been shown to increase in response to training between 60% and 100% of the 1 RM. The changes in strength-trained muscles are generally limited to adaptations in the muscle itself (Box 3-1). Strength training increases muscle size, defined as *hypertrophy.* The fast-twitch type II fibers show greater hypertrophy than slow-twitch type I fibers with strength training. This increase is largely the result of an increase in contractile protein content. The process of muscle hypertrophy is directly related to an increase in the synthesis rates of myosin. The increase in total contractile protein with strength training occurs without a parallel increase in the total volume of mitochondria within the cell (decrease in the ratio of mitochondria to cell volume). This adaptation may have an impact on the capability of the muscle to sustain power output. The changes in the muscle with strength training may increase the fatigability of the muscle.

Neurologic factors (neural facilitation) are involved in strengthening; however, they are observed in the early phases of a training program before muscular hypertrophy occurs.

Strength Training and the Older Adult

The very old and frail elderly experience skeletal muscle atrophy, a decrease in muscle mass, as a result of disuse, disease, undernutrition, and the effects of aging per se. Muscle weakness that accompanies advanced age has been related to the risk of falling and fracture in these older individuals. Studies demonstrate that frail elderly men and women, well into their tenth decade of life, retain the capacity to adapt to resistance exercise training with significant and clinically relevant muscle hypertrophy and increases in muscle strength.

Results from the resistance training studies performed in the young, middle-aged, elderly, and the oldest old indicate that it is the intensity of the stimulus, not the underlying fitness or frailty of the individual, that determines the magnitude of the gains in strength and muscle size. For example, when the intensity of the exercise is low, only modest increases in strength are achieved by older persons.[7,76] Whereas, if given an adequate training stimulus (>60% of 1 RM), older men and women show similar or greater strength gains compared with young individuals as a result of resistance training.

Progressive resistance exercise, defined as periodically increasing the exercise intensity, is the key element in the success of the training program with the older adult. For example, older men responded to a 12-week progressive resistance training program (80% of the 1 RM, three sets of eight repetitions of the knee extensor and flexors, 3 days per week, reevaluation of 1 RM every 2 weeks) by more than doubling extensor strength and more than tripling flexor strength. The increases in strength averaged approximately 5% per training session, similar to strength gains observed in younger men.[51,52]

The muscle hypertrophy and increased strength, along with the changes in body composition and hormonal and nervous system adaptations associated with strength training, have a substantial impact on the daily activities of living and functional independence of the elderly. In frail elderly living in a nursing home, a high-intensity progressive resistance training program of 8 weeks' duration increased strength on the average of 174%, with a mean increase in muscle cross-sectional area of 15%.[41] These increases in muscle size and strength were associated with clinically significant improvements in gait speed, balance, and functional independence.

Strength training can also have substantial benefits for protection from injury in the elderly, as falling is strongly related to hip weakness, poor balance, and postural sway. Exercise training in the form of therapeutic rehabilitation that is instituted after hospitalization due to disease, acute illness, or surgery has the potential to prevent disability and institutionalization in the elderly by enhancing muscle function.[40]

Total food intake, and perhaps selected nutrients, can affect muscle hypertrophy during a strength-training program. Progressive resistance training seems to have profound anabolic (to build up) effects in the older adult. Resistance training is therefore an effective way to increase energy requirements, decrease body fat mass, and maintain metabolically active tissue mass in older people. Resistance training may be an important adjunct to weight loss inter-

---

BOX 3-1

CHANGES THAT OCCUR WITH RESISTANCE TRAINING

Skeletal Muscle
- Increases in resting levels of anaerobic substrates (ATP, CP, glycogen)
- Increase in fiber size (fast-twitch type II fibers)
- Increase in activity of anaerobic enzyme function (glycolysis)
- Increased capacity for levels of blood lactic acid
- Improved motivation
- Improved pain tolerance

vention in the older adult. In addition to its effect on energy metabolism, resistance training improves insulin action in older adults.

It is clear that the capacity to adapt to increased levels of physical activity is preserved even in the oldest old. Regularly performed exercise, in the form of resistance training, results in a remarkable number of positive changes in elderly men and women. Because sarcopenia and weakness may be almost universal characteristics of advancing age, strategies for preserving or increasing muscle mass in the elderly should be implemented. With increasing muscle strength, increased levels of spontaneous activity have been seen in both healthy, free-living older subjects and in very old and frail men and women. Thus, resistance training, in addition to its positive effects on skeletal muscle, insulin action, bone density, energy metabolism, and functional status, may also be an important way to increase overall levels of physical activity in the elderly.

Benefits of Aerobic Exercise

Aerobic exercise takes place in the presence of oxygen and involves aerobic metabolism of glucose. The exercise is relatively comfortable and can be sustained for 20 minutes to many hours. Regularly performed aerobic exercise increases $\dot{V}O_2$max, and the extent of change is dependent on the baseline fitness level of the individual and the intensity of the aerobic training.[34]

The fundamental adaptations of the heart to aerobic training include a resting and submaximal exercise bradycardia, increased maximal stroke volume, an increase in left ventricular end-diastolic volume, improved myocardial contractile function, and subtle to moderate increases in myocardial mass (Box 3-2). The adaptive response of $\dot{V}O_2$max is rapid.

The absolute gains in aerobic capacity after aerobic exercise training are similar between young and older individuals.[59,81] However, the mechanism for adaptation to regular submaximal exercise appears to be different between old and young people. Older individuals show a greater increase in oxidative capacity of the skeletal muscles after training. The skeletal muscle glycogen stores in the older adults are lower than those of the young adults initially but increase significantly with exercise. The skeletal muscles of older adults increase in capillary densities, mitochondrial enzyme levels, and ability of muscles to extract oxygen from the blood.[28,81] These skeletal muscle adaptations contribute to the rise in $\dot{V}O_2$max in the elderly with training. These skeletal muscle enzyme adaptations and the increase in blood flow to muscle with exercise training raise the $\dot{V}O_2$max in the older person by increasing the a-$\overline{v}O_2$ difference maximum, a major determinant of $\dot{V}O_2$max.[78]

The other major determinant of $\dot{V}O_2$max is cardiac output. In older adults, left ventricular systolic performance and diastolic filling dynamics improve with endurance exercise training. The mechanisms involved for the improvement in left ventricular systolic performance and diastolic filling in

---

BOX 3-2
CHANGES THAT OCCUR WITH AEROBIC TRAINING

Skeletal Muscle
- Increases in capacity to generate ATP aerobically
- Increase in the number of mitochondria
- Increase in the size of mitochondria
- Increase in activity of aerobic enzyme function
- Increase in skeletal muscle myoglobin content (increase quantity of oxygen available)
- Increase in blood flow within the muscle
- Selective skeletal fiber hypertrophy (slow-twitch type I fibers)
- Increase in muscle's capacity to mobilize fat, oxidize carbohydrate

Cardiac Muscle
- Increase in weight and volume (increase in the size of the left ventricle wall and cavity)
- Increase in total hemoglobin and plasma volume
- Decrease in resting and submaximal exercise heart rate
- Increase in stroke volume at rest and during exercise
- Increase in diastolic filling
- Increase in maximal cardiac output
- Increase in capacity to extract oxygen from the circulating blood
- Decrease in systolic and diastolic blood pressure at rest and submaximal exercise

---

response to training are complex. The mechanisms may involve the integration of cardiac loading conditions, i.e. hypertrophy, Frank-Starling relationship, a reduction in vascular stiffness, and enhanced contractile function in response to β-adrenergic stimulation in the trained state.

Although both older men and women respond to endurance training with an increase in $\dot{V}O_2$max, the mechanism of adaptation is also different. In older men, two thirds of the increase in $\dot{V}O_2$max is due to an augmented cardiac output and one third is due to a wider a-$\overline{v}O_2$ content difference. On the other hand, in older women, there is a similar increase in $\dot{V}O_2$max with training; however the changes in left ventricular systolic performance and diastolic-filling dynamics do not occur. Thus, the increase in $\dot{V}O_2$max in older women is due to peripheral adaptations that lead to the enhanced a-$\overline{v}O_2$ content difference. Peripheral adaptations include increases in skeletal muscle capillarization and activity of mitochondrial marker enzymes, e.g., citrate synthase. The underlying reasons for this gender-specific adaptation are unclear but most likely reflect the difference in hormonal patterns.

The fact that aerobic exercise has significant effects on skeletal muscle may help explain its importance in the treatment of glucose intolerance and NIDDM. A moderate intensity aerobic exercise program at 50% maximal heart rate (HR) reserve, 55 min/day, 4 days/week for 12 weeks without weight loss results in improved glucose tolerance and rate of insulin-stimulated glucose disposal and an increase in skeletal muscle GLUT 4 levels. So, endurance training and dietary modifications are generally recommended as the primary treatment in the non–insulin-dependent diabetic older person.

Reversing Decline

Although both aerobic and resistance training are recommended to improve muscular function in the elderly, only resistance training can reverse or delay the decline in muscle mass and strength with aging. Increased strength and mass can be important steps in maintaining daily functional activities of independence in older persons in whom "disuse" atrophy has limited their daily activities. Aerobic exercise has long been an important recommendation for those with many of the chronic diseases typically associated with old age. These include non–insulin-dependent diabetes mellitus, hypertension, heart disease, and osteoporosis. The incorporation of aerobic and resistance exercise training into the life-style of older individuals can have a considerable impact on the functional capacity, physiological reserve, and independence. Exercise enhances the functional capacity, bringing the older adult physically well above the threshold of performance.

The opposite spectrum of exercise training is inactivity, or immobilization (a decrease in physical activity). With immobilization, there is a significant decline in muscle strength and endurance. Skeletal muscle mass declines rapidly (atrophy). In the cardiovascular system, resting and submaximal heart rates and blood pressure increase, and maximal oxygen consumption is reduced. Total blood and plasma volumes are reduced, and blood viscosity is increased along with the risk of thromboembolism. The rate of deconditioning during immobilization has been reported to exceed that of exercise training, which has particular consequences in the older individual with less physiological reserve. The effects of immobilization are accentuated in older people.

DEVELOPING EXERCISE INTERVENTIONS FOR THE OLDER ADULT

In a program of exercise for the older adult, it is important to include aerobic exercise, strengthening, and flexibility components.[89] In evaluating the older adult for exercise, several factors need to be considered. First, it is unrealistic to totally depend on an exercise tolerance test to develop the exercise program or prescription.[119] Second, a good history, systems review, and appropriate use of tests and measures are essential to determine risk factors and associated medical conditions.[49,85] Third, it is critical to establish goals conjointly with the older adult and to obtain commitment of participation.[103] Both physiological changes and psychosocial problems impact the older adult's exercise prescription and how the program is conducted (Box 3-3).

Exercise Program

The exercise prescription or program should contain aerobic exercise and resistance training. Increasing evidence indi-

---

> **BOX 3-3**
> ## PHYSICAL CHANGES THAT ALTER THE EXERCISE PROGRAM FOR THE OLDER ADULT
>
> Reduction in the following:
> Maximal aerobic power
> Cardiovascular reserve
> Elasticity of peripheral vasculature
> Heat tolerance
> Muscular strength
> Elasticity of connective tissue
> Musculoskeletal flexibility

---

cates the benefits of both forms of exercise for the older adult. The exercise prescription, tailored to the individual older adult, describes the type, frequency, duration, and intensity of the proposed activity. It includes information on the warm-up, conditioning, and cool-down components of each exercise session.

Resistance Exercise

A decrease in functional mobility and recurrent falls are associated with the well-documented decline in muscle strength in older adults. This age-related muscle weakness may be related to physical inactivity (disuse syndrome), nutritionally inadequate diet, comorbid disease, and the biological aging process. Several clinical trials of healthy community-dwelling older adults younger than 80 have reported increases of 17% to 70% over baseline maximum isometric strength after 6 weeks of static exercise.[84] A long-term program of strength training is necessary to sustain improvements in muscle function. This is particularly important in the elderly, in whom loss of muscle mass and weakness are prominent deficits. Resistance training of both the upper extremities and lower extremities can be accomplished with precautions and supervision and be of significant value in maintaining basic self-care activities and increasing strength and muscle mass.[42,80]

Resistance exercise, or muscle strength training, can be accomplished by virtually anyone. Many health care professionals have directed their older adult patients away from resistance training in the mistaken belief that it can cause undesirable elevations in blood pressure. With proper technique, the systolic pressure elevation is minimal. Muscle strengthening exercises are rapidly becoming a critical component to rehabilitation programs, e.g., cardiac, as clinicians realize the need for strength as well as endurance for many activities of daily living. Strength training is an effective method for developing musculoskeletal strength and is often prescribed for fitness, health, and the prevention and rehabilitation of orthopedic injuries.

Definition and Benefits

Strength conditioning, or *progressive resistance exercise,* is generally defined as training in which the resistance against which a muscle generates force is progressively increased over time. Progressive resistance training involves few contractions against a heavy load. Muscle strength has been shown to increase in response to training between 60% and 100% of the 1RM (the maximum amount of weight that can be lifted with one contraction). For example, lifting weight requires that a muscle shorten as it produces force; this is called a *concentric contraction*. Lowering the weight, on the other hand, forces the muscle to lengthen as it produces force; this is an *eccentric muscle contraction*. These lengthening muscle contractions have been shown to produce ultrastructural damage that may stimulate increased muscle protein turnover. The metabolic and morphological adaptations from resistance and endurance exercise are quite different. Strength conditioning will result in an increase in muscle size, and this increase in size is largely the result of increased contractile proteins.

The physiological adaptations most often associated with strength training include increases in muscle mass, bone mass, and connective tissue thickness and associated increases in muscle strength and endurance. In addition to its effect on increasing muscle mass and function, resistance training can also have an important effect on energy balance. When participating in a resistance-training program, a person needs more calories to maintain body weight. This increase in energy need is due to increases in resting metabolic rate and in protein metabolism. Thus, resistance training can preserve or even increase muscle mass during weight loss. This aspect of resistance training may be perceived as a benefit. Strength training, as part of a comprehensive fitness program, may reduce the risk of coronary heart disease, non–insulin-dependent diabetes, and certain types of cancer. It improves function and reduces the probability of falls in the elderly. These benefits can safely be obtained when exercise program variables (frequency, volume of training, and model of training) are manipulated to meet the needs of the individual.

Risks of Exercise

The possible adverse effects of exercise that are most worrisome are sudden death, injury, and osteoarthritis. The most serious but least common of these is *sudden death,* defined as death occurring either during the actual activity or within 1 hour after it. Although reported rates of sudden death vary from 4 to 56 times greater than chance, the absolute risk is low: one cardiac death per 396,000 hours of jogging or one death per 15,000 to 18,000 exercises per year.[64]

There are few data on the risks of injury associated with the physical activities performed by older adults, such as walking and gardening. Injuries sustained by participants in organized exercise programs, which are primarily due to overuse, are relatively common. The ankle is the joint most likely to be injured. Most nontraumatic musculoskeletal injuries in runners are directly related to distance run and increasing mileage. Age and obesity do not appear to be contributing factors in current studies. There are no good studies of nontraumatic musculoskeletal injuries related to walking, cycling, or gardening.

Pre-existent musculoskeletal problems may be a deterrent to beginning an exercise regimen. More than 50% of older adults involved in a variety of new activities developed injuries that were exacerbations of preconditions.[79] For previously healthy persons, injury rates ranging from 10% to 50% for both novice and experienced exercisers have been reported. Significantly lower rates of injury are associated with low-impact exercise, such as walking, than with higher-impact activities, such as aerobic dance and jogging. Almost all organized walk/jog exercise programs reporting injuries cite the primary involvement of the lower extremities. Because most participants recover from the injury and maintain training intensity by substituting for example an uphill treadmill walk for jogging, high impact rather than intensity has been implicated as the cause of injury.

The fear that the physical activity may stimulate osteoarthritis or exacerbate a pre-existing condition has kept some older adults from participating in an exercise program and may prevent health care professionals from recommending that they do so. Because osteoarthritis affects 85% of all persons 70 years and older, it is important to know whether activities limit this population.

Physical inactivity may in fact promote osteoarthritis through repetitive stress placed on joints supported by weak muscles and stiff tendons. Regular weight-bearing exercise may help prevent osteoarthritis by improving muscle strength, increasing bone density, and reducing obesity.

Compliance

Dropout rates as high as 50% from recommended exercise programs have been documented.[23] Older adults are more likely to participate in such a program if advised to do so by their health care provider. Clearly defining the expected health benefits of exercise, such as lowering blood pressure and improving longevity, improves compliance. Older persons are also more likely to participate in activities that easily fit into their daily schedule. Any proposed activity that requires transportation, someone to exercise with, special equipment, or high cost will limit participation. Regular, stepwise low-level exercise is preferable to infrequent bouts of strenuous physical activity. Encouragement by health care professionals by phone may promote compliance with an exercise regimen.

Thus, some of the declines in cardiovascular and muscular function with aging can be reversed or prevented by aerobic and resistance exercise training. The adaptations that occur in response to training are usually related to the initial exercise capacity of the older adult, because exercise training improves functional declines that are related to being sedentary. Hence, functional improvements in response to exercise training can be large in older persons and, in relative terms (percent of basal), comparable to that in younger subjects.

SUMMARY

Lack of functional capacity leads to a more dependent lifestyle and earlier entry into nursing homes. Decreased functional capacity also contributes to the risk of falls and a decline in the physiological organ system. From a health care point of view, the increased risk of hospitalization is a costly health problem.

REFERENCES

1. Alexander NB, et al: Healthy young and old women differ in their trunk elevation and hip pivot motions when rising from supine to sitting. *J Am Geriatr Soc* 1995; 43:338-343.
2. Alexander NB, Schultz AB, Warwick DN: Rising from chair: Effects of age and functional ability on performance biomechanics. *J Gerontol* 1991; 46:M91-M98.
3. Aloia, JF, Vaswani AN, Yeh J, Cohn SH: Premenopausal bone mass is related to physical activity. *Arch Intern Med* 1988; 148:121-123.
4. American College of Sports Medicine: *Guidelines for Exercise Testing and Prescription,* ed 4. Philadelphia, Lea & Febiger, 1991.
5. American Heart Association: Medical/Scientific Statement, Exercise Standards, A Statement for Health Professionals, Writing group: Fletcher GF, et al: Dallas, American Heart Association, 1991.
6. Andres R, Tobin JD: Endocrine systems, in Finch, CE, Hayflick, L (eds): *Handbook of the Biology of Aging.* New York, Van Nostrand Reinhold, 1977.
7. Aniansson A, Gustafsson E: Physical training in elderly men with special reference to quadriceps muscle strength and morphology. *Clin Physiol* 1981; 1:87-98.
8. Aniansson A, Zetterberg C, Hedberg M, Komi PV: Impaired muscle function with aging. A backward factor in the incidence of fractures of the proximal end of the femur. *Clin Orthop Relat Res* 1984; 191:193-200.
9. Aronow WS, Ahn C, Kronzon I: Prognosis of congestive heart failure in elderly patients with normal and abnormal left ventricular systolic function associated with coronary artery disease. *Am J Card* 1990; 66:1257-1259.
10. Asmussen E: Aging and exercise, in Horvath SM, Yousef MK (eds): *Environmental Physiology: Aging, Heat and Altitude* (Sec 3). New York, Elsevier, North Holland, 1980.
11. Bader H: Dependence of wall stress in the human thoracic aorta on age and pressure. *Circ Res* 1967; 20:354-361.
12. Balady G, Weiner D: Exercise testing in healthy elderly subjects and elderly patients with cardiac disease. *J Cardiopulmonary Rehabil* 1989; 9:35.
13. Bassey EJ, et al: Leg extensor power and functional performance in very old men and women. *Clinical Science* 1992; 82:321-327.
14. Berman HA, Decker MM: Changes with aging in skeletal muscle molecular forms of butyrocholinesterase and acetylcholinesterase. *Fed Proc* 1985; 44:1633.
15. Bevier WC, et al: Relationship of body composition, muscle strength, and aerobic capacity to bone mineral density in older men and women. *J Bone Miner Res* 1989; 4:421-432.
16. Blumenthal DS, Weiss JL, Mellits ED, Gerstenblith G: The predictive value of a strongly positive stress test in patients with minimal symptoms. *Am J Med* 1981; 70(5):1005-1010.
17. Booth FW, Weeden SH, Tseng BS: Effect of aging on human skeletal muscle and motor function. *Med Sci Sports Exerc* 1994; 26:556-560.
18. Borg G: Perceived exertion: A note on history and methods. *Med Sci Sports Exerc* 1973; 5:90.
19. Bortz WM: Disuse and aging. *JAMA* 1982; 248:1203-1208.
20. Brandfonbrener M, Landowne M, Shock NW: Changes in cardiac output with age. *Circulation* 1953; 12:557-566.
21. Brooke MH, Engel WK: The histographic analysis of human muscle biopsies with regard to fiber types 1: Adult male and female. *Neurology* 1969; 19:221-233.

22. Brown WF: A method for estimating the number of units in thenar muscles and the changes in motor unit counting with aging. *J Neurol Neurosurg Psychiatry* 1972: 35:845-852.
23. Buskirk EF: Exercise, fitness, and aging, in Bouchard C, et al (eds): *Exercise, Fitness and Health: A Consensus of Current Knowledge.* Champaign, Il, Human Kinetics, 1990.
24. Campbell MJ, McComas AJ, Petito F: Physiological changes in aging muscles. *J Neurol Neurosurg Psychaitry* 1973; 36:174-182.
25. Cartee GD, Farrar RP: Muscle respiratory capacity and VO$_2$max in identically trained young and old rats. *J Appl Physiol* 1987; 63:257-261.
26. Cliff WJ: The aortic tunica media in aging rats. *Exp Mol Pathol* 1970; 13:172-189.
27. Coggan AF, et al: Histochemical and enzymatic comparison of the gastrocnemius muscle of young and elderly men and women. *J Gerontol* 1992; 47:71-76.
28. Coggan AF, et al: Skeletal muscle adaptations to endurance training in 60- to 70- y-old men and women. *J Appl Physiol* 1992; 72:1780-1786.
29. Cohn SH, et al: Compartmental body composition based on total body nitrogen, potassium and calcium. *Am J Physiol* 1980; 239:E524-E530.
30. Conway J, Wheeler R, Sannerstedt R: Sympathetic nervous activity during exercise in relation to age. *Cardiovasc Res* 1971; 5:577-581.
31. Das DN, Fleg JL, Lakatta EG: Effect of age on the components of atrioventricular condition in normal man. *Am J Cardiol* 1982; 49:1031.
32. Davies MJ: Pathology of chronic A-V block. *ACTA Cardiol* 1976; 21:19-30.
33. Davies MJ: The pathology of myocardial ischemia. *J Clin Path* 1977; 11:45-52.
34. DeBusk RF, Stenestarnd U, Sheehan M, Haskell WL: Training effects of long versus short bouts of exercise in healthy subjects. *Am J Cardiol* 1990; 65:101-113.
35. Dehn MM, Bruce A: Longitudinal variations in maximal oxygen uptake with age and activity. *J Appl Physiol* 1972; 33:805-807.
36. DeMeersman RE: Aging as a modular of respiratory sinus arrhythmia. *J Gerontol* 1993; 48:B74-B78.
37. Depres JP, et al: Regional distribution of body fat, plasma lipoproteins, and cardiovascular disease. *Arteriosclerosis* 1990; 10:497-511.
38. Docherty JR: Cardiovascular responses in ageing: A review. *Pharmacol Rev* 1990; 42:103-125.
39. Doherty TJ, Brown WF: The estimated numbers and relative sizes of thenar motor units as selected by multiple point stimulation in young and older adults. *Muscle Nerve* 1993; 16:355-366.
40. Felsenthal G, Garrison SJ, Steinberg FU: *Rehabilitation of the Aging Patient.* Baltimore, Williams and Wilkins, 1994.
41. Fiatarone MA, et al: High intensity strength training in nonagenarians: Effects on skeletal muscle. *JAMA* 1990; 263:3029-3034.
42. Fiatarone MA, et al: Exercise training and nutritional supplementation for physical frailty in very elderly people. *N Engl J Med* 1994; 330:1769-1775.
43. Finch CE, Tanzi RE: Genetics of aging. *Science* 1997; 278:407-411.
44. Fleg JL, Lakatta EG: Role of muscle loss in the age-associated reduction in VO$_2$max. *J Appl Physiol* 1988; 65:1147-1151.
45. Fleg JL, Das DN, Wright J, Lakatta EG: Age-associated changes in the components of atrioventricular conduction in apparently healthy volunteers. *J Gerontol Med Sci* 1990; 45:M95-M100.
46. Florini JF: Biosynthesis of contractile proteins in normal and aged muscle, in Kaldor G, DiBattista WJ (eds): *Aging in Muscle,* vol 6. New York, Raven, 1978.
47. Fossel M: Telomerase and the aging cell. *JAMA* 1998; 279:1732-1735.
48. Fowlie S: Aging, fitness and muscular performance. *Rev Clin Gerontol* 1991; 1:323-336.
49. Frishman W, DeMaria A, Ewy G: Clinical assessment. *J Am Coll Cardiol* 1987; 10:48A.
50. Frontera WR, Hughes VA, Evans WJ: A cross-sectional study of upper and lower extremity muscle strength in 45-78 year old men and women. *J Appl Physiol* 1991; 71:644-650.
51. Frontera WR, Meredith CN, O'Reilly KP, Evans WJ: Strength training and determinants of VO$_2$max in older men. *J Appl Physiol* 1990; 68:329-333.

52. Frontera WR, et al: Strength conditioning in older men: Skeletal muscle hypertrophy and improved function. *J Appl Physiol* 1988; 64:1038-1044.

53. Gerstenblith G, et al: Echocardiography assessment of a normal adult aging population. *Circulation* 1977; 56:273-278.

54. Gerstenblith G, Lakatta EG, Weisfeldt ML: Age changes in myocardial function and exercise response. *Prog Cardiovasc Dis* 1976; 19:1-21.

55. Gozna ER, Marble AE, Shaw A, Holland JG: Age-related changes in the mechanics of the aorta and pulmonary artery of man. *J Appl Physiol* 1974; 36:407-411.

56. Grimby G, Aniansson A, Zetterberg C, Saltin B: Is there a change in relative muscle fiber composition with age? *Clin Physiol* 1984; 4:189-194.

57. Hayflick L: Current theories of biological aging *Fed Proc* 1975; 34:9-13.

58. Higginbotham MB, et al: Regulation of stroke volume during submaximal and maximal upright exercise in normal man. *Circ Res* 1986; 58:281-291.

59. Holloszy JO, Coyle EF: Adaptations of skeletal muscle to endurance exercise and their metabolic consequences. *J Appl Physiol* 1984; 56:831-838.

60. Holloszy JO, et al: Effects of exercise on glucose tolerance and insulin resistance. *ACTA Med Scand Suppl* 1986; 711:55-65.

61. Hopkins KD, et al: Biochemical correlates of aortic distensibility in vivo in normal subjects. *Clin Sci* 1993; 84:593-597.

62. Howard JE, McGill KC, Dorfman LJ: Age effects on properties of motor unit action potentials: ADEMG analysis. *Ann Neurol* 1988; 24:207-213.

63. Irion GL, Vasthare VS, Tuma RF: Age-related change in skeletal muscle blood flow in the rat *J Gerontol* 1987; 42:660-665.

64. Johnson RJ: Sudden death during exercise *Postgrad Med* 1992; 92:195-206.

65. Jones AD, Stitt F, Collison D: The effects of exercise and changes in body temperature on the intrinsic heart rate in man. *Am Heart J* 1970; 7:488-498.

66. Judge JO, Underwood M, Gennosa T: Exercise to improve gait velocity in older persons. *Arch Phys Med Rehabil* 1992; 74:400-406.

67. Kantelip JP, Sage E, Duchene-Marullaz P: Findings on ambulatory electrocardiographic monitoring in subjects older than 80 years. *Am J Cardiol* 1986; 57:398-401.

68. Kantrowitz A: Restoring cardiac function: an emerging spectrum of therapeutic options. *J Biomaterial Appl* 1986; 1:13-38.

69. Kitzman DW, et al: Age-related changes in normal human hearts during the first ten decades. Part II (maturity): a quantitative anatomic study of 765 specimens from subjects 20 to 99 years old. *Mayo Clin Proc* 1988; 63:137-146.

70. Kostis JB, et al: The effects of age on heart rate in subjects free of heart disease. *Circulation* 1982; 65:141-145.

71. Kotchen JM, McKean HE, Kotchen TA: Blood pressure trends with aging. *Hypertension* 1982; 4:128-134.

72. Kugelberg E: Adaptive transformation of rat soleus motor units during growth. *J Neurol Sci* 1976; 27:269-289.

73. Lagrue G, Ansquer JC, Meyer-Heine A: Peripheral action of spironolactone: Improvement in arterial elasticity. *Am J Cardiol* 1990; 65:9-11.

74. Lakatta EG: Do hypertension and aging have a similar effect on the myocardium? *Circulation* 1987; 75(Suppl I):I-69-I-77.

75. Lakatta EG: Cardiovascular regulatory mechanisms in advanced age. *Physiological Rev* 1993; 73(2): 413-467.

76. Larsson L: Physical training effects on muscle morphology in sedentary males at different ages. *Med Sci Sports Exerc* 1982; 14:203-206.

77. Lexell J, Taylor CC, Sjostrom M: What is the cause of ageing atrophy? Total number, size and proportion of different fiber types studied in whole vastus lateralis muscle from 15- to 83-year old men. *J Neurol Sci* 1988; 84:275-294.

78. Makrides L, Heigenhauser GJF, Jones NL: High-intensity endurance training in 20- to 30- and 60- to 70-y-old healthy men. *J Appl Physiol* 1990; 69:1792-1798.

79. Matheson GO, et al: Musculoskeletal injuries associated with physical activity in older adults. *Med Sci Sports Exerc* 1989; 21:379-385.

80. McCartney N, McKelvie RS, Haslam DRS, Jones NL: Usefulness of weightlifting training in improving strength and maximal power output in coronary artery disease. *Am J Cardiol* 1991; 67:939-945.

81. Meredith CN, et al: Peripheral effects of endurance training in young and old subjects. *J Appl Physiol* 1989; 66:2844-2849.

82. Miyatake K, et al: Augmentation of atrial contribution to left ventricular flow with aging as assessed by intracardiac Doppler flowmetry. *Am J Cardiol* 1984; 53:586-589.

83. Myers AH, et al: Risk factors associated with falls and injuries among elderly institutionalized persons. *Am J Epidemiol* 1991; 133:1179-1190.

84. Nichols JF, Omize DK, Peterson LL, Melspum LP: Efficacy of heavy-resistance training for active women over sixty: muscular strength, body composition, and program adherence. *J Am Geriatr Soc* 1993; 41:205-210.

85. O'Rourke R, Chatterjee K, Wei J: Coronary heart disease. *J Am Coll Cardiol* 1987; 10:52A-56A.

86. Ogawa T, et al: Effects of aging, sex, and physical training on cardiovascular responses to exercise. *Circulation* 1992; 86:494-503.

87. Ordway GA, Wekstein DR: The effect of age on selected cardiovascular responses to static isometric exercise. *Pro Soc Exp Biol Med* 1979; 161:189-192.

88. Overend TJ, Cunningham DA, Paterson DH, Lefcoe MS: Thigh composition in young and elderly men determined by computed tomography. *Clin Physiol* 1992; 12:629-640.

89. Pollock ML, Wilmore JH: *Exercise in Health and Disease*, ed 2. Philadelphia, WB Saunders, 1990.

90. Porter MM, Myint A, Kramer JF, Vandervoort AA: Concentric and eccentric strength evaluations in older men and women. *Med Sci Sports Exerc* 1994; 25:S189.

91. Porter MM, Myint A, Kramer JF, Vandervoort AA: Concentric and eccentric knee extension strength in older and younger men and women. *Can J Appl Physiol* 1995; 20:429-439.

92. Probstfield JL, et al: The systolic hypertension in the elderly program (SHEP): An intervention trial on isolated systolic hypertension. *Clin Exp Hypertens* 1989; A11:973-989.

93. Pruitt LA, Jackson RD, Bartels RL, Lehnhard HJ: Weight-training effects on bone mineral density in early postmenopausal women. *J Bone Miner Res* 1992; 7:179-185.

94. Reneman RS, Van Merode T, Hick P, Hoeks APG: Flow velocity patterns in and distensibility of the carotid artery bulb in subjects of various ages. *Circulation* 1985; 71:500-509.

95. Rice CL, Cunningham DA, Paterson DH, Lefcoe MS: Arm and leg composition determined by computed tomography in young and elderly men. *Clin Physiol* 1989; 9:207-220.

96. Roach MR, Burton AC: The effect of age on the elasticity of human iliac arteries. *Can J Biochem Physiol* 1959; 37:557-570.

97. Robert L, Robert B, Robert AM: Molecular biology of elastin as related to aging and atherosclerosis. *Exp Gerontol* 1970; 5:339-356, 1970.

98. Rodeheffer FJ, et al: Exercise cardiac output is maintained with advancing age in healthy human subjects: Cardiac dilatation and increased stoke volume compensate for a diminished heart rate. *Circulation* 1984; 69:203-213.

99. Rossini PM, Desiato MT, Caramia MD: Age-related changes of motor evoked potentials in healthy humans: Non-invasive evaluation of central and peripheral motor tracts excitability and conductivity. *Brain Res* 1992; 593:14-19.

100. Schulman SP, Gerstenblith G: Cardiovascular changes with aging: The response to exercise. *J Cardiopulmonary Rehabil* 1989; 9:12-16.

101. Schwartz JB, Gibb WJ, Tran T: Aging effects on heart rate variation. *J Gerontol* 1991; 46:M99-M106.

102. Shephard RJ: Habitual physical activity levels and perception of exercise in the elderly. *J Cardiopulmonary Rehabil* 1989; 9:17-23.

103. Shephard RJ, et al: Exercise compliance of elderly volunteers. *J Sports Med Phys Fitness* 1987; 27:410-418.

104. Simonson E: The effect of age on the electrocardiogram. *Am J Cardiol* 1972; 29:64-73.

105. Simpson DM, Wicks R: Spectral analysis of heart rate indicated reduced baroreceptor-related heart rate variability in elderly persons. *J Gerontol* 1988; 43:M21-M24.

106. Sjogren AL: Left ventricular wall thickness in patients with circulatory overload of the left ventricle. *Ann Clin Res* 1972; 4:310-318.

107. Starke-Reed PE: The role of oxidative modification in cellular protein turnover and aging. *Prog Clin Biol Res* 1989; 287:269-276.

108. Svanborg A, Bergstrom G, Mellstrom D: *Epidemiological Studies on Social and Medical Conditions of the Elderly.* Copenhagen, World Health Organization, 1982.

109. Tammaro AE, Casale G, deNicola P: Circadian rhythms of heart rate and premature ventricular beats in the aged. *Age Ageing* 1986; 15:93-98.

110. Thompson LV: Effects of age and training on skeletal muscle physiology and performance. *Phys Ther* 1994; 74(1):71-81.

111. Tinetti ME, Speechley M, Ginter SF: Risk factors for falls among elderly persons living in the community. *N Engl J Med* 1988; 319:1701-1707.

112. Tomlinson BE, Irving D: The numbers of limb motor neurons in the human lumbosacral cord through life. *J Neurol Sci* 1977; 34:213-219.

113. Tomonaga M: Histochemical and ultrastructural changes in senile human skeletal muscle. *J Am Geriatr Soc* 1977; 25:125-131.

114. Unverferth DV, et al: Human myocardial histologic characteristics in congestive heart failure. *Circulation* 1983; 68:1194-1200.

115. Vaitkevicius P, et al: The age-associated increase in arterial stiffness is attenuated by chronic exercise. *Circulation* 1991; 84(Suppl II):II29, 1991.

116. Vaitkevicius PV, et al: Effects of age and aerobic capacity on arterial stiffness in healthy adults. *Circulation* 1993; 88:1456-1462.

117. Wenger N: The elderly patient with cardiovascular disease, in Chatterjee K, et al (eds): *Cardiology: An Illustrated Text/Reference,* vol 2. Philadelphia, JB Lippincott, 1991.

118. Williams M: *Exercise Testing and Training in the Elderly Cardiac Patient.* Champaign, IL, Human Kinetics Publishers, 1994.

119. Williams MA, Sketch MH: Guidelines for exercise training of elderly patients following myocardial infarction and coronary bypass graft surgery. *Geriatr Cardiovasc Med* 1988; 1:107-110.

120. Wolfson L, Judge J, Whipple R, King M: Strength is a major factor in balance, gait, and the occurrence of falls. *J Gerontol* 1995; 50A:64-67.

121. Wolinsky H: Long-term effects of hypertension on the rat aortic wall and their relation to concurrent aging changes. Morphological and chemical studies. *Circ Res* 1972; 30:301-309.

122. Zs-Nagy I, Nagy K: On the role of cross-linking of cellular proteins in ageing. *Mech Age Dev* 1980; 14:245-281.

CHAPTER 4

ARTHROKINESIOLOGIC CONSIDERATIONS IN THE AGED ADULT

Donald A. Neumann, PT, PhD

INTRODUCTION

Arthrokinesiology is the study of the structure, function, and movement of skeletal joints. This term combines the word *kinesiology,* which is the science of movement, with the Greek prefix *arthro,* which means "joint." The purpose of this chapter is to address specific arthrokinesiologic issues that

are unique to the musculoskeletal system of the aged adult. The chapter focuses on the age-related changes in periarticular connective tissue and not the neuromuscular system per se. This chapter assumes that natural age-related changes can occur in joint function even in the absence of disease.

A strict chronological classification of the "aged" adult is not given since so much variation exists in the manner that adults actually grow old. *Aged,* however, is not synonymous with *aging,* since technically the aging process begins immediately after conception. The *aged adult* therefore will refer to the adult whose biological systems have already matured, and owing to their advanced age, structural and functional joint changes have occurred or are imminent. These changes may be extremely subtle and pose virtually no disability, or they may be extremely profound and result in total disability.

This chapter is organized into three parts. In the first part the principles and terminology unique to communicating concepts of arthrokinesiology are reviewed. The basic structure and related function of each major joint tissue is then considered. This brief review is followed by the main topic of the second part, which covers the specific age-related changes that are known or hypothesized to occur in periarticular connective tissues. Finally, this chapter describes how age-related changes at the tissue level can cause changes in movement at the joint level.

This chapter should enhance the ability to observe a typical aged adult and relate some movement or postural dysfunction to specific mechanical age-related causes within the joint. This ability should ultimately enhance the therapist's ability to evaluate and treat the specific physical needs of the elderly.

REVIEW OF BASIC PRINCIPLES OF ARTHROKINESIOLOGY

The first part of this chapter describes the mechanical principles of arthrokinesiology that govern normal joint function. These principles serve as a foundation for the third part, which describes changes in joint mobility and stability that may be likely in the aged individual.

Bone and Joint Kinematics

Kinematics, as defined with respect to arthrokinesiology, is the study of the motion within a joint or between bones, without regard to forces or torques that have caused the motion.[82] *Osteokinematics,* therefore, describes the motion of a rotating *bone* about an axis of rotation that is oriented perpendicular to the path of the moving bone. For example, if elbow flexion occurred from the anatomical position, the osteokinematic motion of the forearm would take place in the sagittal plane about a mediolateral (ML) axis (Fig. 4-1). When we move our limbs, the distal bone of an articulation may move in relation to a fixed proximal bone (see Fig. 4-1), or the proximal bone may move in relation to a fixed distal bone. An *open kinematic chain* describes the linkage of two bones where the distal bone rotates in relation to a more stable proximal bone. In contrast, a *closed kinematic chain* describes the movement of a proximal bone rotating in relation to a more stable distal bone. Regardless of which bone is performing most or all of the rotation, a given bone's osteokinematic motion is determined by the mechanical events that have occurred *between* joint surfaces.

Arthrokinematics describes the relative rotary and translatory movements that occur between joint surfaces.[93] *Translation,* in this context, refers to the glide (or slide) of an articular surface where all points along the bone glide in a direction somewhat parallel with each other. For example, *glenohumeral abduction* may be described as an action of the convex humeral head *rolling* (or rotating) superior and simultaneously gliding (or sliding) inferior on the concave surface of the glenoid fossa. The rotary motion of the humeral head may be likened to a large marble rolling up a slight depression on the glenoid fossa. In order for the marble to remain within the confines of the concave fossa, the rolling marble must simultaneously glide inferior to compensate for any distance the marble may have gained "rolling" up the glenoid surface (Fig. 4-2). In this present example, these "roll and glide" arthrokinematics must occur if full glenohumeral abduction is to be accomplished. Full abduction may be limited in the aged person if the joint's connective tissue resists either the translation or the rotation of the bone. This example is discussed in greater detail in the final part of this chapter.

Bone and Joint Kinetics

In the scope of arthrokinesiology, *kinetics* describes the joint forces and torques that cause potential motion at a joint. In order to fully understand potential motion about a joint, one must appreciate the difference between a force and a torque. Think of a force as a "push or a pull" that originates from muscle activation, the pull of gravity, the push from a therapist, or connective tissue's inherent resistance to stretch. Forces cause bones to translate in space and/or rotate in a plane about an axis. In this chapter, *active forces* refers to forces produced by muscle contraction through active effort. *Passive forces,* on the other hand, are the forces produced purely by the resistance generated when periarticular structures are stretched. As subsequent discussions will suggest,

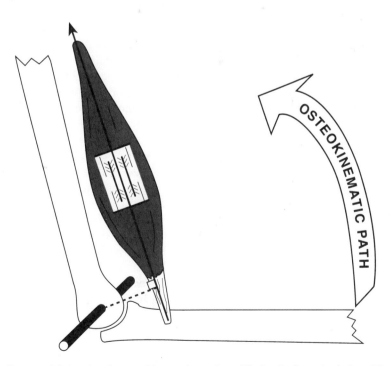

FIG. 4-1   Elbow model showing the osteokinematic motion of flexion in the sagittal plane. The *dark rod* is the axis of rotation, and muscle's force line is the *dark, thin arrow.*

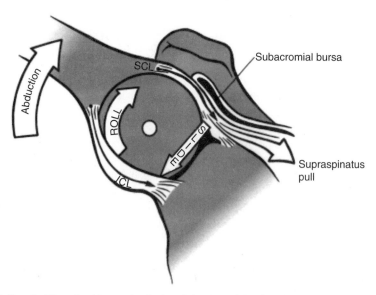

FIG. 4-2   Roll-and-slide arthrokinematics during abduction of the glenohumeral joint. The supraspinatus is shown contracting to direct the roll of the humeral head. The taut inferior capsular ligament *(ICL)* is shown supporting the head of the humerus. (SCL = superior capsular ligament.) *Stretched tissues* are depicted as thin, elongated arrows. (Reprinted with permission from Neumann DA: *Human Kinesiology: Applications to Physical Rehabilitation.* St. Louis, Mosby, in press.)

increased stiffness in "aged" connective tissues may contribute to decreased range of motion in the elderly.

As depicted in Fig. 4-1, forces acting on a bone may cause the bone to rotate within a plane about an axis of rotation. This "turning effect" of a bone is called a joint *torque.* This torque, or moment, may be estimated by the product of the force multiplied by a given moment arm. In this chapter, an *internal moment arm* (*dashed line* in Fig. 4-1) is defined as the length of a line that extends from the axis of rotation (*dark rod* in Fig. 4-1) to the perpendicular intersection of the muscle's force line (*dark, thin arrow* in Fig. 4-1). Furthermore, the product of an active muscle force and internal moment arm is referred to as an *internal torque.* The modifier *internal* is used since the torque was produced by a force *internal* to the musculoskeletal system. The torque effect of a muscle group's contraction is often measured by various "isokinetic" testing devices.[82]

In this chapter, an *agonist* muscle is considered the muscle or muscle group that is primarily responsible for producing the active forces that direct bone movement. The *antagonist* muscle, in contrast, is considered the muscle or muscle group that has an action opposite to the agonist muscle. Realize that as the agonist muscle contracts and shortens, the antagonist muscle must elongate while creating a passive force that would not significantly inhibit the intended movement.

In most joint systems, large active muscle forces are required to "drive" the movement or provide joint stability. These forces have been referred to as *myogenic,* since they are produced by action of muscle.[66] Myogenic joint forces most often compress joint surfaces and assist with certain physio-logical activities such as joint stability and cartilage nutrition. In the case of disease or weakened articular tissue secondary to advanced age, large myogenic joint forces can cause joint damage, pain, and dysfunction.

To illustrate the concept of a compression force between joint surfaces, consider the model in Fig. 4-3, which shows the kinetics about the right hip during single-limb standing. Since the pelvis is assumed to be fixed about the right femur, the model assumes a condition of static equilibrium. The "external" torque caused by body weight is prevented from rotating the pelvis clockwise due to an equivalent counterclockwise torque produced by the hip abductors. Since the external moment arm used by body weight is about twice as long as the internal moment arm used by the hip abductors (*D1* vs. *D* in Fig. 4-3), the hip abductor force must equal twice the body weight.[67] As Fig. 4-3 shows, body weight and hip abductor force produce a combined force that must be matched by an equivalent joint force oriented in an opposite direction. This force, often called a *joint reaction force,* most often compresses the joint together (*JRF* in Fig. 4-3). Normally, in the healthy young joint, this large force is transferred across the joint without problem. In certain pathological or osteoporotic conditions, however, the joint reaction forces exceed the physiological tolerance of the weakened bone, and hip fracture may result.

Posture and Positions of Natural Joint Stability

In order to fully appreciate the implications of faulty posture in the aged population, a brief review of the mechanical interactions between joint tissue and the pull of gravity on body segments is required. Consider that a pair of articular

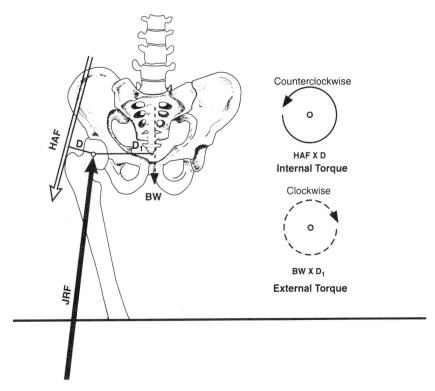

FIG. 4-3　Closed-chain action of the right hip abductor muscle when the pelvis is held stationary about the right femoral head. Assume that the pelvis is only free to rotate *within the frontal plane* about an anteroposterior *(AP)* axis that pierces the right femoral head. The hip abductors must generate an internal torque that stabilizes the pelvis and trunk about the right hip during single-limb support. This stability requires that the internal torque equal the external torque. *HAF* = hip abductor force; *D* = internal moment arm; D_1 = external moment arm; *BW* = body weight; *JRF* = joint reaction force. NOTE: The external moment arm is equal to the length of a line that extends from the axis of rotation to a point of right-angle intersection with body weight's force vector. (Modified from Neumann DA, Cook TM: *Phys Ther* 1985; 65:306.)

surfaces assume a position of maximal congruency (or fit) at one unique position within a joint's range of motion. This position of natural stability has been referred to as the joint's *close-packed position.*[93] In this position, the ligaments and joint capsule may be relatively elongated and stretched slightly. The resistance to this stretch may be temporally stored as a passive force that may provide an element of transarticular stability.

In the hip and knee joints, the major component of each joint's close-packed position corresponds to positions where stability is required during standing, i.e., in hip and knee extension. While standing in hip and knee extension, the force line of gravity usually falls posterior to the hip and anterior to the knee. This force line produces a series of external torques that *maintain* these stable joint positions. Active muscle force while standing may therefore be minimized, subsequently reducing energy expenditure as well as myogenic joint force. Gaining useful force through noncontractile and metabolically "inexpensive" tissues for certain static, low-torque stability functions may have certain physiological advantages.[68] This discussion resumes in the third part of

this chapter with specific clinical significance to the aged person.

AGE-RELATED CHANGES IN JOINT CONNECTIVE TISSUE

Growing old is usually associated with a reduced level of physical activity. In fact, the body's physiological responses to both are quite similar.[12] Furthermore, as one reaches an advanced age, the chance of being affected by a disease increases. The interaction of these facts requires that three points be considered when studying the arthrokinesiologic aspects of geriatric physical therapy. First, changes in the structure and function of joint connective tissue may occur simply as a natural process of growing old. The manner in which these natural "age-related" changes affect joint function is the main focus of this chapter. Second, the type and degree of physical activity one engages in also have a significant influence on the structure and function of connective tissues.[85] The third point to consider is that pathology can affect the joint's connective tissue *at any age* and lead to profound functional limitations and disability. The effects of disease, reduced physical activity, and advanced age often occur simultaneously and may have a combined effect on joint function. Countless other factors, such as genetics, previous postural habits, and earlier injury, also interact and influence an aged person's arthrokinesiologic function. The exact nature of the interaction is very complicated and not fully understood.

This part of the chapter proceeds with a brief review of the structural and functional aspects of the various joint connective tissues. This review will set the stage for an overview of the functional changes that are believed to occur in aged joint tissue.

Periarticular Connective Tissue (PCT)
Review of Tissue Structure and Function

Periarticular connective tissue includes ligament, associated joint capsule, aponeurosis, tendon, intramuscular connective tissue, and skin. All these tissues are physically linked to joints, and therefore their extensibility influences a joint's range of motion. The predominant histological components of all PCT are fibroblasts and fibrous proteins, namely, collagen and elastin, extracellular ground matrix, and water.[86,93] The ground matrix resembles a viscous gel that consists of large, branching proteoglycan molecules. Although terminology is inconsistent and often confusing, these macromolecules are often referred to as *acid glycosaminoglycans* (*AGAGs*).[80] AGAGs consist of repeating disaccharides, each attached to negatively charged carboxylate and/or sulphate esters.[93] This material and water act as filler and cementing substance for the embedded fibrous protein.

Collagen provides most of the structure and tensile strength to all connective tissues in the body. At least 14 types of genetically different collagen have been identified in the body, most in connective tissue. Subsequent discussion in this chapter refers to type I collagen since this is the main protein in PCT.

Collagen fibers strongly resist stretch and are capable of providing great strength to the tissue in which they reside. The mechanical stability of collagen is maintained through life by a complex mechanism referred to as *intermolecular cross-bridging*. The tropocollagen molecules, the building blocks of the collagen fibril, are strongly linked together at regular parallel intervals. Many fibrils are grouped together to form the collagen fiber and ultimately the collagen fasciculi. Once collagen fibers are formed, their rate of turnover is very slow. The protein should not be considered inert or static. Collagen metabolism can be influenced by physical and chemical stimuli. This can be observed in tissues that are in the process of producing a scar or after periods of decreased physical activity.[48]

Elastin is another protein found in most PCT. Connective tissues with abundant elastin stretch easily with almost perfect recoil. The physical alignment and relative proportions of collagen and elastin determine the PCT's ability to limit, guide, or stabilize joint motion.

Ligaments are a type of dense connective tissue composed chiefly of thick, longitudinal bands of collagen with relatively few cells and extracellular gel substance. Macroscopically, ligaments resemble thick cords that connect bone to bone and thereby provide structural stability across a joint. Each collagen fiber within a ligament best resists elongation in the direction parallel to the long axis of the fiber. Significant elongation of the ligament itself is restricted by the inherent stiffness in the collagen. The stiffness within the ligament stabilizes and protects a joint against unnatural motion that may injure other joint structures, including muscle. Ligaments often blend in with, and are structurally part of, each joint's *articular capsule*. The collagen fibers within ligaments and capsule may be arranged slightly oblique to the long axis of the ligament or capsule. This arrangement provides resistance to the multidirectional elongations that may arise due to various joint movements.

Collagen fibers provide a limited amount of elasticity to capsular ligaments. This is based on the fact that unstretched collagen fibers are oriented in a wavy or coiled manner. Significant ligamentous resistance to stretch is delayed slightly until the collagen fibers are pulled straight. After the stretch is removed, the elastin fibers may aid in recoiling the collagen fibers back to their prestretched appearance.[59] As stated earlier, forces that stretch collagen and elastin may be temporally stored and used to perform joint stability functions.

A *tendon* transfers muscle force to bone. The fibrous tissue within the tendon is mostly white collagenous bands of dense connective tissue with limited amounts of elastin. The collagen bundles are thick, tightly packed, and aligned parallel with each other and to the long axis of the tendon. The parallel fiber arrangement allows tendons to resist elongation even in the presence of very high stretching forces. This characteristic high stiffness of the tendon reflects a function of transmitting large muscular forces to bone.[42] Since tendons contain a limited amount of elastin, they elongate slightly due to muscle pull but return to their original length after the removal of the muscle force.

Skeletal muscle is composed chiefly of contractile proteins that are wrapped in a continuous sheath of *intramuscular connective tissue*. This tissue surrounds each muscle fiber, muscle fasciculi, and external surface of the individual whole muscle. The intramuscular connective tissue ultimately blends with the connective tissue fabric of the tendon and periosteum. The intramuscular connective tissues contain both collagen and elastic fibers.[20] When these tissues are stretched beyond a specific length, the inherent elasticity within these tissues may assist in the production of forces that move and/or stabilize our joints. Internal torques produced about a joint may therefore be the result of *both* active and passive forces.[7] Active forces may be considered *neurogenic* since the nervous system "actively" initiates the coded impulses that cause contractile proteins to shorten and exert a pull on adjacent intramuscular connective tissues. Passive forces generated from stretched muscle, on the other hand, do not require any volitional neural input. These forces may be considered *elastogenic* since they are produced by the forces that are stored within the stretched elastic connective tissue elements of a whole muscle.[68]

Finally, the basic structure of *skin* must be considered since this tissue surrounds all joints and must deform slightly to allow the extremes of a joint's range of motion. The dermis, a deeper skin component, is a form of connective tissue that contains large amounts of collagen. The majority of the thickness of the dermis is a dense, irregular connective tissue that consists of collagen fibers oriented in a wavy and coiled pattern. Elastin fibers are also present in the dermis, but to a much lesser extent than collagen. As is well-known by watching a joint move through full motion, the dermis can be stretched quite a distance before any significant resistance is encountered. The eventual resistance is due to the straightening out of the coiled collagen fibers. When the stretch of the skin is removed, young, healthy skin returns to its original position by the rebound action of the elastic fibers. The wavy and multidirectional physical orientation of all the fibrous elements in the dermis allows the skin to resist forces in many directions.

Review of Mechanical Properties of Connective Tissues

Before proceeding further with the discussion of age-related changes in PCT, a few selected mechanical properties that are relevant to the study of connective tissue need to be reviewed.

Researchers may deform connective tissues in vitro, and the resistance the tissue produces to the deformation may be measured as a force. A deformation-force curve may be plotted and yield information about the tissue's ability to tolerate certain biological or environmental factors. Ligaments or tendons are often tested for their ability to produce a tensile force, that is, a force generated as a resistance to stretch. Hyaline cartilage, on the other hand, is often tested to determine its ability to resist compression. Elasticity and viscosity each describe a unique property of a tissue's resistance to deformation.[96] Connective tissues are partially *elastic* and therefore temporally store a component of the force that originally caused their deformation. Like a spring, stretched elastic tissues tend to return to their original prestretched length after the removal of the force. *Viscosity* describes the extent to which a tissue's resistance to deformation depends on the *rate* of the deforming force. Viscosity is a time-dependent property, whereas elasticity is not. Realize that most connective tissues demonstrate a *viscoelastic property* since both the rate of deformation *and* instantaneous tissue length determine the amount of resistance the tissue generates when deformed. Usually the greater the amount and rate of deformation, the greater the resistance offered by the tissue.

Connective tissues may be excised from animals of different ages and subjected to various forms of mechanical testing. As an example, Fig. 4-4 shows a plot depicting the results of a typical "stress vs. strain" test on an excised tendon of a

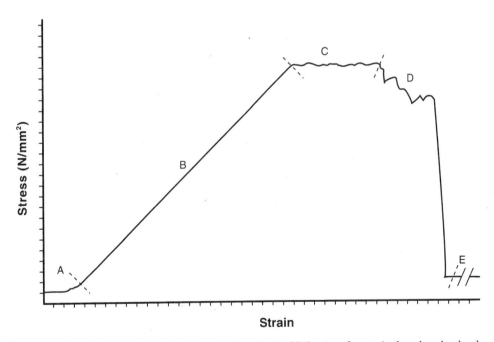

FIG. 4-4 Hypothetical data showing the typical mechanical behavior of an excised tendon that has been stretched to a point of rupture. Tissue *stress* (or force per unit cross-sectional area) has been plotted against a constant *strain* (stretch) rate. *Region A* shows the length where the slack is taken up from the tendon and little, if any, stiffness is recorded. *Region B* shows the length where the tendon shows a linear elastic stiffness. *Region C* depicts the length where the tissue starts to exhibit permanent deformation. *Region D* shows the length at which the tendon actually starts to rupture, and *Region E* shows complete structural failure of the tissue.

rabbit.[90] The terms *stress* and *strain* are somewhat analogous to the terms *force* and *deformation*, respectively. For purposes of normalization, the force developed in the deformed tissue is divided by the tissue's cross-sectional area and thus presented as a pressure measurement called *stress*. The deformation, either in elongation or compression, that is applied to the tissue is often normalized to a percent change in original length and referred to as *strain*. The plot in Fig. 4-4 illustrates several mechanical characteristics common to many viscoelastic tissues that are stretched to a point of rupture. This graph shows five regions that each show specific information about mechanical properties of connective tissue. *Region A* shows that at the beginning of the stretch the increase in length in the tendon does not result in a significant increase in stress in the stretched tendon. This region of low resistance is reportedly due to the straightening out of the unloaded coiled collagen fibers.[1] Once the fibers have been stretched out straight, the stress-strain relationship becomes linear due to the parallel arrangement of the fibers *(Region B)*. The slope of the stress vs. strain curve in Region B is a measure of the tissue's *stiffness*. Region B is often referred to as the *elastic region*, since at this length removal of the stretch force would result in the tissue recoiling back to its original length. *Region C* shows a property of stretched tissue known as *plasticity*. This is evident by continued elongation of the tissue without an increase in resistance from within the tissue. Connective tissue that is stretched to a length where plasticity actually begins may remain permanently deformed. In fact, this is part of the logic used in a therapeutic stretching program in physical therapy. *Region D* shows a stretch length that causes actual structural failure within the tendon. In this case, the force of the stretch exceeded the ability of the collagen to transmit the force. Continued elongation of the tissue will eventually cause complete tissue failure, as evident by a complete lack of resistance to increased stretch *(Region E)*. It is important to realize that the characteristics of the plot in Fig. 4-4 would most likely vary as a function of tissue age, specific type, and rate of the stretch.

Age-Related Changes in PCT

The mechanical properties of PCT change with advanced age. The structural and functional changes in the collagen protein account for most change; however, the precise physiological mechanisms are not known or universally accepted.[20,73] Much of the research literature presented in this chapter regarding the effects of advanced age on human PCT is based on animal research. Human research in this area obviously cannot be conducted with rigid experimental control for variables such as previous physical activity, earlier tissue trauma, nutrition, or breeding. Making direct inferences to human aged tissue based on animal data may be done, however, with caution. Extensive research is needed before definitive descriptions can be given to account for purely age-related changes in the structure of human PCT.

Age-related animal research suggests that ligaments and tendons increase in stiffness and demonstrate a decrease in the maximal length at which rupture occurs.[18] A biochemical analysis of aged tissue usually shows an increase in the relative amount and diameter of collagen;[87] an increase in fibril size and aggregation; and a relative decrease in water, elastin, and proteoglycan content.

A mechanism to account for the increase in stiffness in age-related PCT may be the fact that aged collagen shows increased numbers of cross-links between adjacent tropocollagen molecules.[5,35] Increased rates of cross-linking would increase the mechanical stability of collagen and may explain the increased stiffness in the tissue.[75]

The unique structure of collagen provides a natural element of stiffness and rigidity to connective tissue. Increased amounts of collagen in PCT may partially explain the increased PCT stiffness shown in aged animals and perhaps humans.[35] Increased collagen content in the endomysium of the rat's intramuscular connective tissue has been shown to correlate with increased stiffness of the whole muscle.[4] Increased numbers of cross-linkages may increase collagen's resistance to degradative enzymes, therefore increasing the relative content of the protein in aged PCT.[60] Reduced physical activity tends to be a natural part of advanced aging in animals and humans. Understanding the *interactive* effect of advanced age and reduced physical activity on connective tissue stiffness would be very beneficial. Williams and Goldspink[94] monitored the changes in muscle's connective tissue in relatively *young* animals following rigid limb immobilization. They reported marked increases in relative intramuscular collagen as well as stiffness after 4 weeks of immobilization, particularly evident if the muscles were immobilized in a shortened length. The immobilized "young" muscles appeared to show qualitative and quantitative changes similar to what has been observed in aged tissue. These results suggest that physical activity, regardless of age, has a very important influence on muscle stiffness. Further research is needed to understand the precise manner in which physical activity influences the stiffness of aged PCT in general.

Hyaline Cartilage

Review of Tissue Structure and Function

Hyaline cartilage lines the articular ends of bone and protects the joint from damaging transarticular forces. Without this shock-absorbing and lubricating function, normal everyday joint forces would exceed the compression limits of underlying subchondral bone, thus causing fracture.[92] The elastic quality of articular cartilage dissipates high loads as well as decreases the rate of the compression on the joint surfaces.

Hyaline cartilage consists of a small population of chondrocytes widely dispersed in a relatively dense extracellular matrix.[61] The matrix is chiefly composed of water, collagen fibers, and long, branching proteoglycan macromolecules.[52,78] The collagen fibrils within the matrix provide "scaffolding" to the cartilage, lending both shape and tensile strength. The negative electrochemical charges on the proteoglycan side chains cause adjacent chains to repel, adding additional stiffness to the collagen-proteoglycan mesh. The structure of the matrix is further reinforced by the presence of water molecules that bind to and fill the spaces between the hydrophilic proteoglycans.[28] The "crowded" extracellular matrix of articular cartilage may be visualized as a "stuffing" that supports the collagen network. This structure provides healthy articular cartilage the ability to deform repeatedly and re-form after an exceedingly large number of compressions throughout a lifetime. The rate of the deformation of the articular cartilage is controlled somewhat by the action of water slowly oozing through the impedance offered by the matrix. The water under pressure flows toward the relatively unloaded areas of the cartilage. As the joint is unloaded, the water returns to its original location by the swelling pressure produced by the hydrophilic macromolecules within the matrix.[15] The amount of swelling is physically restrained by the tensile properties of the collagen network.

Age-Related Changes in Articular Cartilage

Histological observation of healthy articular cartilage in the aged adult shows that the density of chondrocytes and the amount of collagen within the extracellular matrix remain essentially unchanged.[29] The water content in the tissue, however, does reduce with advanced age. The hydrophilic proteoglycans have been shown to become shorter in aged tissue and therefore lose their ability to hold water in the matrix.[16] Dehydrated articular cartilage may have a reduced ability to dissipate forces across the joint.

Aged articular cartilage may become more susceptible to mechanical failure. Freeman and Meachim[29] have hypothesized that the loss of physical strength of aged cartilage may be due to fragmentation of the collagen network and/or ruptures of the interfiber bonding. This collagen fragmentation and weakening may, in part, explain the high incidence of localized structural disintegration often observed on the surface of aged articular cartilage. Cartilage lesions, often referred to as *fibrillated* cartilage, are commonly observed with the naked eye during a joint dissection. Fig. 4-5, *A* through *C*, shows a scanning micrograph of the articular surface of a femoral condyle in a 71-year-old male cadaver. Fig. 4-5, *A*, shows the surface of what appears to be healthy but aged articular cartilage. Fig. 4-5, *B* and *C*, demonstrates samples taken from fibrillated articular tissue from a different location of the same knee. Fibrillated articular tissue may be limited to superficial layers of articular cartilage, or the tissue may show vertical splitting and fragmentation that reach and expose subchondral bone.

The literature supports the notion that some amount of fibrillation in articular cartilage is normal and a natural age-related process.[57] Of course, the increased fibrillation may be partially due to the reduced physical activity that often accompanies advanced age. Fig. 4-6 shows data that suggest that many joints exhibit natural degeneration with increased age.[37] According to Freeman and Meachim, histological

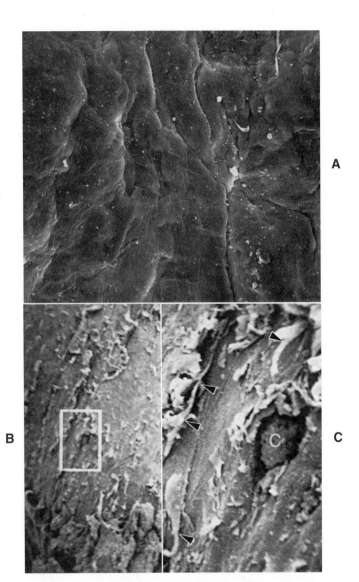

FIG. 4-5 A scanning electron micrograph of the articular surface of a femoral condyle of a knee in a 71-year-old embalmed cadaver. **A,** Articular cartilage from an apparently "normal" looking region of the lateral femoral condyle. The wavy but smooth surface texture represents the normal aging process in hyaline cartilage (200×). **B,** Fibrillated articular cartilage from a fragmented and pitted region of the medial femoral condyle from the same knee as above (225×). **C,** Higher magnification of *B* (600×) showing the fragmented regions of the cartilage (*arrow heads*). The lower case *c* indicates an exposed chondrocyte, which is usually concealed within the matrix. (Micrographs courtesy Dr. Robert Morecraft, University of South Dakota, School of Medicine.)

analysis of fibrillated tissue reveals rupture of the collagen network and an associated weakness in the tissue.[29] Fibrillated cartilage does not tolerate compression and tensile forces nearly as well as intact aged cartilage. Freeman suggests that the collagen structure of aged fibrillated cartilage experiences mechanical fatigue that causes the proteoglycans to "leak out" of the tissue.[28] Decreased proteoglycans within the matrix would diminish the natural dampening effect of

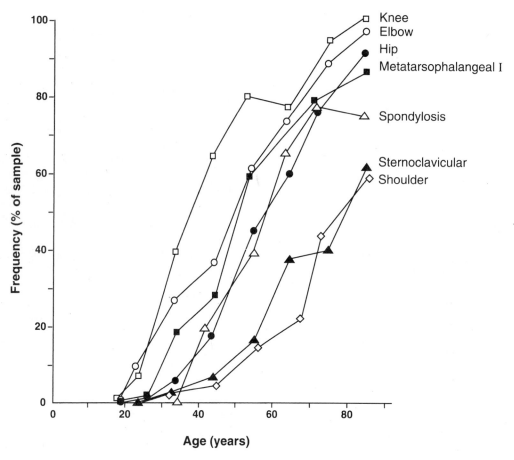

FIG. 4-6   Plot showing the frequency of location of degenerative joint disease as a function of age. Th joints were inspected during 1000 necropsies. (Redrawn from Heine J: *Virchows Arch Pathol Anat Physiol Klin Med* 1926; 260:521-663. Used by permission.)

cartilage. The cumulative mechanical wear of advanced age may cause, or is strongly associated with, a weakening of articular cartilage.[29]

In summary, some degree of mechanical degeneration of aged human articular cartilage should be considered a normal process. The wear may be from repeated loading of joints over the good part of a lifetime. The ability of even "healthy" articular cartilage to dissipate transarticular forces may diminish in the aged population.

Any discussion of aged articular cartilage should include the point that osteoarthritis is not an imminent consequence of the natural fragmentation of collagen. Fibrillated tissue does not always lead to the disease of osteoarthritis. The link between the hypothesized wear-and-tear theory of fibrillated cartilage and the development of osteoarthritis has not been shown conclusively. Granted, osteoarthritis does occur with greater frequency in the elderly. As a matter of fact, by age 60, more than 60% of the population may have some degree of cartilage abnormality in certain joints.[83] Nevertheless, one cannot assume that the disease of osteoarthritis is purely a mechanical result of aging. If this logic were true, then *all* old persons should develop osteoarthritis, and this is not the case. Genetic, biochemical, traumatic, and morphological factors may also be interrelated with the effect of aging and development of osteoarthritis.[29,49]

Due to the relatively high incidence of osteoarthritis in the aged population, the physical therapist should be aware of the basic clinical consequences of the disease.[33] Osteoarthritis often presents with severely degenerated and thinned articular cartilage. The severe collagen weakening and proteoglycan depletion observed in advanced osteoarthritis markedly reduce the cartilage's ability to resist tensile and compressional forces. As a consequence, undampened joint forces may cause a reactive hardening or sclerosis of the unprotected subchondral bone.[72] This reactive response is in accord with the Wolff's law (1892) that bone is laid down in areas of stress and reabsorbed in areas of nonstress. Degenerated cartilage and stiffer subchondral bone are not able to adequately attenuate high transarticular forces. Osteophytes and various remodeling may occur as a further progression of Wolff's law, and the entire morphology and geometry of the joint surfaces may change. Physical therapists need to understand the deleterious consequences of having their patient's arthritic joints subjected to large and repetitive joint forces. Concepts of "joint protection" need to be used with these patients.[63]

Bone

Review of Tissue Structure and Function

Bone contains widely dispersed specialized cells that manufacture and secrete a dense, fibrous extracellular matrix. Compact bone's characteristic rigidity and stiffness are due to the presence of the dense collagen network within the extracellular matrix. This collagen lattice is structurally reinforced by calcium phosphate-based minerals. Bone would be a very soft and pliable material if it were not for the mineralization of the calcium salts on the collagen and matrix material.

The collagen fibers within compact bone possess some degree of elasticity and therefore are well-suited to resist tensile forces.[25] Calcium phosphate, in contrast, is very good at resisting compression forces. The interaction of these two materials provides bone with a unique ability to resist forces in multiple directions. The outer cortex shell of bone is very dense to withstand the high forces produced by muscle pull and weight-bearing activities. The inner, more spongy, cancellous bone is porous, which allows bone to flex slightly under a load.

Despite bone's inert appearance, the tissue is physiologically very dynamic and hence possesses a rich blood supply.[51] Osteocytes constantly differentiate into active osteoblasts that produce new bone. Simultaneously, the osteoclasts act as macrophages and reabsorb unneeded or extra bone. The net result of this constant process of syntheses and reabsorption is to change the shape, density, and ultimate weight-bearing ability of bone. This dynamic process allows bone to remodel and heal itself in response to mechanical stress and trauma. Bone, by being a reactive tissue, can alter geometrical shape to withstand the force demands imposed by muscle contraction and gravity. The exact mechanism by which bone cells actually sense and alter cellular synthesis in response to mechanical stress is not known for sure. One popular theory suggests that as a bone bends slightly from a mechanical stress, small piezoelectrical charges induce an electrical field that stimulates osteoblastic activity.[43]

Age-Related Changes in Bone

The precise shape and density of bone are maintained through life by a balance of mechanical and physiological mechanisms. Mechanical stress stimulates the formation of new bone, whereas the endocrine system functions to ultimately reabsorb bone.[51] Increased internal stress stimulates a net increase in bone density so that the bone can withstand higher forces. As an individual advances in age and becomes less active, a loss of bone mass per unit volume usually occurs. If the bone becomes excessively brittle and prone to fracture, the condition may be classified as *osteoporosis*. This process is characterized by a progressive loss of both fibrous matrix and mineral content;[53] new bone is not made at a rate to replace the natural rate of bone absorption. De-

creased bone mass results in a decreased ability of bone to support loads and resist external forces.[17,54] As an example, consider the relatively common incidence of avulsion fracture of the tibial tuberosity in the aged population. This fracture occurs when the ligamentum patella and tibial tuberosity are pulled free from the shaft of the tibia due to excessive force produced in the quadriceps muscle. The large tensile force developed through the ligamentum patella exceeds the capability of the bone to maintain an intact tibial tuberosity.

The medical impact of osteoporosis in the elderly is significant, particularly evident by the high incidence of fracture of the hip.[24,58,97] Hip fracture can lead to significant loss of functional status in the elderly. One study showed that at 1 year after hip fracture, only 33% of persons regained their prefracture status in performing basic activities of daily living.[40] According to a longitudinal study by Gallagher and colleagues, the rate of hip fracture doubles each decade after age 50.[32] There are also gender differences. Hip fracture affects 32% of women and 17% of men by age 90. The strength of the proximal osteoporotic femur is often not able to withstand the high forces that result from a fall and/or vigorous muscle contraction. Hip fracture in the elderly often results from high torsional forces created about the shaft of the femur during a twisting motion.[30] Interestingly, the aged femur has demonstrated increased stiffness when stressed at high force levels. The femur therefore would lose some ability to "give" under high forces. This may partially account for the fact that older bones fracture at significantly lower force levels than younger bones.[38]

The decline in physical activity and subsequent diminished stress placed on bone are often associated with growing old.[36] Therefore, the loss of bone mass and increased susceptibility to fracture should be considered a normal age-related process. Experiments have shown that males lose about 3% of their cortical bone mass each decade after age 40.[53] Women, on average, lose cortical bone at a similar rate but show an accelerated rate of bone loss after menopause. The postmenopausal loss of bone in women reflects the normal physiological role of estrogen in the maintenance of cortical bone mass. One should keep in perspective, however, that diminished physical activity from bedrest may have a more significant demineralizing effect on bone than does the decrease in estrogen after menopause.[38] Fortunately, bone loss in postmenopausal women can be minimized somewhat through active dynamic exercise.[81] Furthermore, according to a review by Prior and colleagues, regular moderate physical activity in persons with osteoporosis can reduce the risk of falls and bone fracture.[70]

ARTHROKINESIOLOGIC IMPLICATIONS OF AGING

Joints in the elderly display a subtle decrease in both angular velocity and displacement.[84] This observation may be made even in the absence of overt pathology such as stroke, arthritis, or Parkinson's disease. The following discussion suggests reasons why the elderly tend to reduce the speed and amount of extremity movement from primarily an arthrokinesiologic perspective. This discussion closes by analyzing the effects that torques and forces may have on the structure and function of the aged joint system.

Kinematic Considerations of the Joints in the Aged
Reduction in Joint Angular Velocity

Reduced Physical Activity. Decreased velocity of joint movement in the aged seems to parallel a natural decline in overall physical activity. The exact reason why the elderly slow down is multifaceted and not as obvious as would first appear. Consider that the elderly often assume a more sedentary life-style. This life-style may be chosen due to a combination of personal, family, cultural, or socioeconomic reasons. The decline in physical activity may also be related to actual age-related physiological changes in the sensorimotor systems, such as decreased muscle strength or decreased vision. Excessive medication; debilitating medical problems or poor nutrition; and a general overcautiousness, coupled with a fear of falling, are additional factors that may contribute to the decreased physical activity.

The elderly often experience major life stresses that may have a subtle effect on their psychological as well as physiological ability to engage in physical activity. For example, the elderly woman who has just lost her husband may not feel as comfortable taking evening walks on her own. This decreased daily level of physical stress placed on her cardiovascular system, for example, would reduce her system's aerobic capacity. Eventually, an attempt at any significant physical exertion becomes an uncomfortable experience rather than a rewarding one. The cycle of inactivity, decreased physical fitness, and continued inactivity tends to perpetuate itself in the elderly as well as in the young.

Sensorimotor Changes. The general responsiveness of the nervous system tends to slow with advanced age (see Chapters 3 and 5). This slowing may partially account for a decline in physical activity and subsequent slowed joint movement.[50] Age-related changes in the nervous system include decreased reaction times; increased rate of loss of brain cells; altered level of neurotransmitter production; and a decreased acuity of the auditory, vestibular, and visual systems.[25,41,47,69,79,84] Possibly, the slowed movement displayed by many elderly is simply a natural mechanism that provides additional time to adequately interpret and process incoming environmental stimuli. Many people have experienced the situation of driving behind a slow-moving automobile with an elderly person at the wheel.[74] The person may not be acting inconsiderately, but rather driving at a "top" speed at which his/her slowed neuromuscular system can safely process and react to multiple streams of sensory input.

A subtle decline in sensorimotor processing in the elderly is certainly just one of many possible explanations that may account for their reduced level of physical activity. Skeletal muscle fibers atrophy with age, and this atrophy may be more prevalent in the fast-twitch muscle fibers.[34] Also, a research study has shown that the conduction velocity of motor nerves decreases with advanced age.[26] These factors, coupled with the factors previously mentioned, would theoretically decrease the rate or magnitude of force generated by muscle and partially account for diminished joint angular velocity.[44]

Stiffness in Periarticular Connective Tissue

Increased PCT stiffness may be another contributor to slowed movement in the aged. Increased levels of resistance to joint motion has been measured directly in the elderly.[96] To discuss the implications of this concept, consider an example where an elderly person demonstrates slowed neck rotation to the left, let us say, in response to the call of his/her name. The motion of left cervical rotation requires a concentric contraction of the left rotators. These muscles must provide sufficient force to rotate the neck as well as elongate the antagonistic right rotator muscles. Increased intramuscular connective tissue stiffness in the right rotator group, for example, could act as a resistance to the left rotation motion. Since most connective tissues demonstrate viscoelastic properties, the passive resistance generated by the right rotators would be dependent on these muscles' length as well as the rate of their elongation. Attempts at increasing the velocity and subsequent amount of left cervical rotation may increase the resistance offered by the right muscle group's intramuscular connective tissue. Significant resistance offered by these tissues would reduce the productive power output of the intended motion of left rotation. Recall that power output about a joint is the product of internal joint torque multiplied by the average angular velocity of the movement.

A Natural Adaptive Mechanism

Regardless of specific physiological mechanisms, consider the hypothesis that the slowing of extremity motion in the aged may be, in part, simply a natural biological process intended to ensure the safety and well-being of the individual. For example, age-related changes in the nervous system may slow extremity movement, which would, in effect, protect painful joints, reduce the likelihood of a fall, or protect a skeletal system with osteoporosis from large forces. This adaptive mechanism may be similar to that of the young child's soft and pliable skeletal system. A child's pliable bones are able to bend and therefore give slightly to the potentially damaging forces that occur as the young child learns to interact with the relentless pull of gravity.

Reduction in the Extremes of Joint Range of Motion

The loss of passive range of motion in the elderly is often progressive and subtle, occurring usually at the extremes of a joint's potential movement. This reduced magnitude of joint movement may exist even in the absence of pathology.

In general, the magnitude of passive joint range of motion declines with advancing age.[11,39,91] Healthy adult men and women tend to have greatest joint mobility in their 20s, with a gradual decrease thereafter.[10] The loss of range of motion is highly variable across joint and subject; however, joint flexibility is clearly inversely related to age. Bell and Hoshizaki have shown that females tend to lose range of motion at a slower rate than males and that joints of the upper extremity remain more flexible than the joints of the lower extremities.[10]

What factors could account for this rather strong association between advanced age and a progressive decrease in joint range of motion? To consider this question, a few prerequisites for full active range of joint motion should be recognized. First, full range of motion requires that the articular surfaces allow a tracking for movement without undue physical interference. Second, a sufficient motor drive with adequate sensory feedback is needed from the neuromuscular system. Third, the PCT must possess a stiffness level that does not inhibit a joint's full range of motion.

Several factors may impede full active or passive range of motion in the elderly. Age-related changes may occur in the joint from previous injury, occupation, or poor posturing. Subsequent excessive joint wear may predispose osteophyte formation and incongruities at the articular surfaces. These factors, in conjunction with increased viscosity of the synovium, calcification of articular cartilages, and increased fatigability of muscle, could all interfere with full joint motion.

Increased Stiffness in PCT

Stiffness in PCT certainly needs to be considered as a prime factor in the reduced range of joint motion in the elderly. In all joints, aged or otherwise, the extremes of movement are resisted slightly due to the inherent stiffness provided by the PCT. Wright and Johns have determined from in vivo human experiments that articular capsule and muscle combine to account for about 90% of the total passive stiffness in a healthy joint.[96] The resistance generated by tendon and skin accounted for most of the remaining natural stiffness. Human joints of aged individuals have shown significant increases in passive resistance to movement.[13,96] This phenomenon may be partially explained by increased stiffness in local joint PCT. As reviewed previously in this chapter, the increased stiffness in the PCT may be due to alterations in the structure of the collagen. Increased stiffness may also result from a reduction in physical activity in the elderly and subsequent lack of natural stretch applied to PCT.[2,9]

Knowledge of the relative influence of each specific PCT to stiffness in the human aged joint would enhance the planning and implementation of physical therapy programs aimed at maintaining overall joint mobility. Clinical evidence suggests that the intramuscular connective tissues may account for a significant amount of the limitation of joint motion in the aged. James and Parker measured passive ankle dorsiflexion in subjects older than 80.[39] Significantly less passive ankle dorsiflexion was available when the knee was in full extension as compared with full flexion. The extended knee evidently placed additional stretch on the aged

and somewhat stiff connective tissue within the multijointed gastrocnemius muscle. The increased stiffness in the muscle was only fully realized when the muscle was stretched over both ankle and knee joints simultaneously.

Another aspect of increased stiffness in intramuscular connective tissues of the aged relates to total metabolic efficiency. The increased resistive "drag" provided by stiff intramuscular connective tissue within antagonist muscle may limit the effectiveness of work output of the agonist muscle. This passive resistance, albeit relatively small when expressed over any particular single joint, may be rather significant when *multiple* joint actions are attempted, particularly at the extremes of motion. The increased muscular effort of the agonists may contribute to general fatigue when the elderly engage in physical activity. Poor nutrition or compromised function of the cardiopulmonary system may further compound the problem.[77]

Age-Related Influences in Joint Mechanics

Increased stiffness in PCT in the aged may have significant influence on joint arthrokinematics. Consider the motion of active glenohumeral abduction to full range. To achieve this motion, all PCT and muscle that have the potential to produce a glenohumeral *adduction* torque (either through active or passive means) must be elongated. Furthermore, the head of the humerus must be able to stretch a pouch formed by the inferior aspect of the glenohumeral capsule. The inferior slide of the humeral head is part of the natural arthrokinematic pattern of full abduction (see Fig. 4-2). Significant capsular and ligamentous stiffness may interfere with the natural translations that constitute the arthrokinematics of abduction. Increased tissue resistance to any expansion of the capsule, for example, would inhibit the descent of the humeral head. This may cause the head of the humerus to roll superior on the glenoid *without* the necessary compensatory inferior glide. The head of the humerus may impinge on the supraspinatus tendon or make contact with the coracoacromial arch, thus limiting further abduction (Fig. 4-7). Increased transarticular forces may result since greater muscle forces may be needed to rotate and/or translate the bones against the resistance imparted by the stiffer capsule. Abnormal muscle synergies may also result over time, since, as in the previous abduction example, the serratus anterior may have to develop greater and longer duration forces to upward rotate the scapula on the thorax in efforts to assist the shoulder abduction.

Practical and Clinical Significance of Decreased Joint Mobility

The functional impact a limitation of joint motion has on aged individuals depends on which joint is limited, the degree of the limitation, and the overall health and mobility of the person. Consider the following research study. Shoulder abduction range of motion was measured in 1000 persons who were still relatively mobile and living in their homes.[9] The subjects were considered healthy but did possess a wide

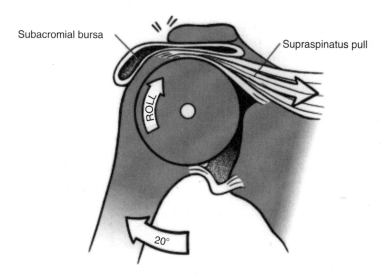

FIG. 4-7   Biomechanics of shoulder "impingement syndrome." Note that abduction *without* a sufficient inferior slide causes the humeral head to impinge against the acromion of the scapula, blocking further abduction. Calculations show that without the slide, the superior roll would result in impingement after only about 20 degrees of abduction. (Reprinted with permission from Neumann DA: *Human Kinesiology: Applications to Physical Rehabilitation*. St. Louis, Mosby. In press.)

range of typical age-associated medical problems. The authors found that more than 50% of the subjects older than 75 years could not actively abduct their shoulder up to 120 degrees. Also, the mean shoulder abduction range of the 75-year-old group was about 30 degrees less than that of a group of subjects with an average age of 39 years. From a practical standpoint, a maximal range of 120 degrees of shoulder abduction should be considered a significant impairment, since many functional activities that require the hand to be brought above the head would be limited.[8] The person who could only actively abduct a shoulder to 110 degrees would, for example, have difficulty returning items to a top shelf in the kitchen. Besides the obvious practical limitations imposed from this lack of mobility, consider other more subtle implications. The elderly person may eventually respond to progressive loss of motion by moving the contents of kitchen cupboards to a lower level. From a practical standpoint, this modification is certainly a sensible one. From an arthrokinesiologic standpoint, however, the modification would reduce the number of abduction efforts attempted each day. The tightness in the shoulder may become self-perpetuating. A simple home exercise program may delay when the cupboards have to be modified and therefore allow the natural demands of the functional task to maintain required joint flexibility.

Loss of range of motion in the aged may inform the physical therapist of other aspects of a person's overall health. In the study by Bassey and colleagues, the amount of shoulder motion deficit was positively correlated with an index of the subject's health.[9] Of interest was a statistically significant correlation between a 10% loss of mean shoulder abduction for women and the presence of arthritis, lack of (overall)

mobility, and incontinence. The therapist must be aware that a reduction in joint motion may be an indirect symptom of some other more significant medical problem. According to the multiple regression equation determined from the Bassey study, the therapist should be alerted to a greater statistical likelihood of systemic health problems if the active shoulder abduction motion in 60-year-old persons is less than about 140 degrees.[9]

A distinction should be made between loss of joint motion associated with a disease process and a loss of motion due to the natural process of growing old. Often this distinction is not clear. An interesting example may be made in this regard by considering the data from Bell and Hoshizaki.[10] These researchers measured the range of motion in several joints and correlated this measurement to subject's gender and age. When considering the 17 joint motions tested, cervical motions showed generally the steepest and most consistent decline with age across both genders. One may speculate that this specific loss of motion may, in part, parallel the natural age-related decline in the acuity of some of the special senses. An important function of the cervical spine is to allow the special senses of vision, hearing, smell, and balance to be placed in a wide range of positions. Even a small decline in the acuity of these afferent systems may reduce the functional demand placed on the cervical joints and theoretically contribute to their loss of passive motion. Research could not be found to substantiate this speculation; however, the logic appears to be sound and worthy of study.

Two final points will be made as a conclusion to this discussion on limitation of joint motion in the elderly. First, it is essential to realize that *not all* elderly individuals lose significant range of motion as they age. Exceptions will always exist, and the reasons for such exceptions should be analyzed as clues to effective treatment principles. The literature does report cases of very athletic aged individuals who have significantly greater range of motion than younger or more sedentary persons.[27] Furthermore, significant increases in range of motion can be gained in the elderly through regular stretching programs.[21,45,71] Further research is needed to decipher the complex interaction between aging, mental attitude, and physical activity on the mechanical behavior of PCT in the human. Why certain persons maintain full range of motion and others do not is an important research question in the field of geriatric physical therapy. The importance of such a question will only increase as the active elderly occupy an even greater percentage of living persons in our society.

Finally, consider the idea that an age-related "limitation" in extremity mobility may lend a subtle element of safety to aged persons and, therefore, in this regard may be beneficial. For example, aged persons tend to walk at reduced velocities and with a broader and shorter stride length.[62] This gait pattern seems to favor stability and security during walking. This slowed and cautious gait pattern may reduce stride length as well as the amount of ankle dorsiflexion required during the stance phase. The reduced magnitude and/or frequency of heel cord stretch may eventually limit the maximal range of available ankle dorsiflexion. In the larger picture, the small reduction in ankle range of motion may be considered beneficial if the altered gait actually prevents a fall and a subsequent scenario of hip fracture and prolonged bedrest.

Joint Mobility and Influence on Whole Body Posture

As just discussed, in certain conditions, subtle restrictions in joint motion may provide a physiological benefit to the overall health of the elderly. As a contrast to this argument, consider how a moderate limitation in joint motion may have a potentially negative physiological effect, particularly in regard to standing posture.

Previously in this chapter, we discussed that in erect standing the body's force line of gravity creates multiple external torques that favor stability of various joints of the lower extremity. Fig. 4-8 shows this same concept, but with a focus on the external (flexor) torque at *the hip*. Note that in erect standing, the ability to achieve full hip extension places the superincumbent force line of gravity *posterior* to the mediolateral axis at this joint (Fig. 4-8, *A*). Gravity now acts with an external moment arm that is posterior to the hip and therefore produces an extensor torque. This extensor torque helps maintain the stable position at this joint. Furthermore, full hip extension stretches and elongates the hip's capsular ligaments, producing transarticular hip forces that may assist with the stability of the extended hip. The extensor torque can be balanced by a passive flexor torque produced by the natural stiffness in the taut iliofemoral ligament. Therefore, in theory, the sagittal plane stability at the hip

during standing can be achieved with minimal hip muscle contraction.

In contrast to the relative ease of standing when the hip joint is fully extended, consider the effect of a hip flexion "contracture" on standing (Fig. 4-8, *B*). Lack of full hip extension in the elderly is relatively prevalent[76] and may be predisposed by periods of prolonged sitting. The forward placement of the pelvis and trunk shown in Fig. 4-8, *B*, may shift the force line of gravity slightly anterior to the hip. The force line of gravity acts now *as a hip flexor,* not as an extensor as shown in Fig. 4-8, *A*. Increased extensor muscle force would be required to maintain the standing position. The subsequent increase in myogenic hip joint force may exacerbate existing hip pain or increase cartilage wear. Also, standing with a hip flexion contracture may direct the larger muscular forces toward *thinner* regions of articular cartilage. Furthermore, the increased metabolic requirements of maintaining low levels of hip extensor muscle contraction may add to general fatigue. This situation may encourage increased sitting, which may perpetuate the cycle of continued or increased PCT tightness.

Kinetic Considerations of the Joints in the Aged

In earlier sections of this chapter, the concepts of joint forces and torques are briefly discussed. This section focuses exclusively on these concepts with continued specific attention on the elderly. Arthrokinesiologic implications that relate to *internal torque* about the joint are discussed first. The remainder of this section reviews a clinical example in which connective tissue about the joint fails to resist the deforming postures created through external torques.

Internal Joint Torque Considerations

Maximal internal torque about a joint is defined as the product of the maximal volitional muscle force multiplied by the length of the associated internal moment arm. Aging and various changes in structure and function of connective tissue can alter these variables, and each is discussed separately.

Reduced Ability to Generate Muscle Force. Clinically, the elderly patient often shows a reduced "muscular strength" as tested through a dynamometer, isokinetic device, or manual muscle testing. More precisely stated, the maximal internal torque produced about joints tends to decline with advanced age.[3,6,55,89] Assuming that the length of the internal moment arm at any given joint angle remains constant as one reaches an advanced age, the lowered peak internal torque generation must be due to reduced peak muscle force. Skeletal muscle mass declines with advanced age, and this factor alone could account for a significant amount of the loss of force production. The loss of muscle mass may be in part due to simple disuse atrophy secondary to a reduction in physical activity. Other factors that may contribute to the reduced peak muscular force in the aged are a loss in the number of functioning motoneurons,[19] a preferential atrophy of fast-twitch (type II) muscle fibers,[34,46] decreased quality of

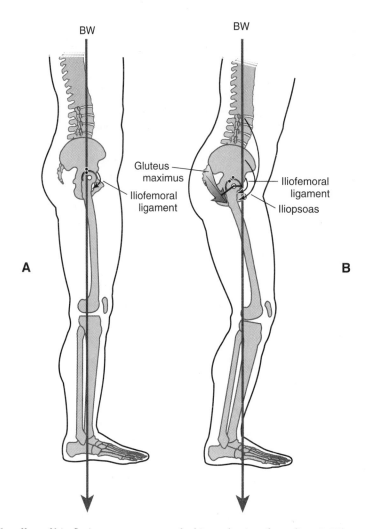

FIG. 4-8 The effect of hip flexion contracture on the biomechanics of standing. **A,** When a person stands with hips fully extended, the body weight *(BW)* force is directed slightly *posterior* to the axis of rotation at the hip. Due to the external moment arm, the force of body weight causes an *extensor torque* at the hip. The taut anterior capsule of the hip (shown as the iliofemoral ligament) prevents further hip extension. **B,** With a flexion contracture, attempts at standing upright are resisted by passive tension in the stretched iliopsoas muscle and iliofemoral ligament. This posture redirects body weight *anterior* to the hip joints, causing a hip *flexor torque.* The gluteus maximus is shown contracting to prevent the hip joint from flexing further into a squat position. (The external moment arms used by the gluteus maximus and body weight are shown by dark black lines.) In **A** and **B,** the dots at the hip show the regions of thickest cartilage. (Courtesy C. Wadsworth, Editor, Orthopedic Section of APTA: Arthritis Home Study Course "The Synovial Joint: Anatomy, Function, and Dysfunction," by Neumann DA, 1998.)

synapses at the neuromuscular junction,[56] or simply a decreased motivation to produce large forces. Additional factors on sensorimotor changes in the elderly are reviewed elsewhere.

Evidence exists that the natural decline in active muscle force in the elderly may be reduced with exercise programs that increase levels of physical activity.[22,31,88] Earlier in this chapter, we discussed that joint range of motion can also be maintained or improved with exercise. Exercise programs that strive to increase or maintain muscle active force production, as well as maintain joint flexibility and angular velocity, are as rational for elderly persons as those designed for the younger persons. Safe levels of stress imposed on bone during properly designed exercise may decelerate osteoporosis, which offers an additional benefit to exercise for the elderly.

Work vs. Power Considerations. Relating concepts of work and power to this discussion may add a deeper layer of understanding to the physiological and practical limitations of an aged musculoskeletal system. The work that is performed about a joint during concentric muscle contraction is equal to the product of the average internal torque multiplied by the degrees (or radians) of joint rotation. The difficulty an elderly person may have in thoroughly cleaning a

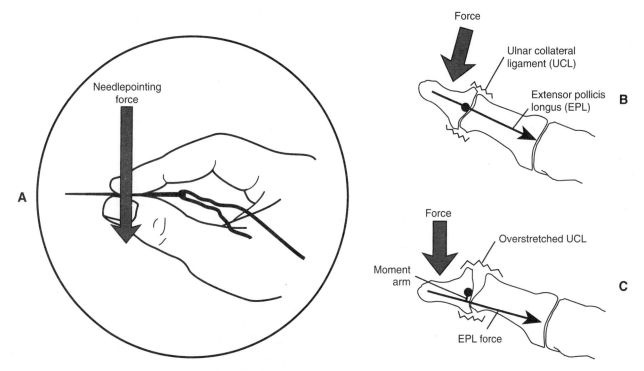

FIG. 4-9   Drawing showing the mechanics involved with thumb interphalangeal *(IP)* radial deviation deformity secondary to needlepointing activity. **A,** Note the "radial" direction of needlepointing force exerted from index finger to the thumb's distal phalanx. **B,** The long-term force causes an excessive and chronic radial deviation torque about the thumb's IP joint. **C,** Throughout the years, the radial deviation torque overstretches the ulnar collateral ligament (UCL) at the IP joint. The IP deformity created an internal moment arm, so the extensor pollicis longus *(EPL)* muscle force can now actively radially deviate the IP joint. Axis of rotation for radial deviation torque is shown as a *dark circle*.

window, for example, may arise from both variables that define work, since both are expected to naturally decline in the elderly. This is why both "strengthening" and range-of-motion exercises are usually recommended for the elderly.

Power is defined as the rate of performing work. In the example above, the *time* required to clean the window becomes a relevant variable. The average power produced about a joint during a task is determined by the product of the average internal torque multiplied by the average velocity of the joint movement. Decreased velocity of movement, either from increased resistance from antagonist muscle or increased central processing time, would result in reduced power. When practical, reducing the time element of a task performance reduces some of the limitations imposed by the diminished ability of the elderly person to generate significant power. Often, however, the time element of a task cannot be removed, such as the time required to respond with sufficient muscle force to catch oneself from a fall. In this case, the rate of muscle contraction and subsequent speed of joint rotation may be of greater physiological importance than the amount of peak muscle force.

Change in Length of Internal Moment Arm. Joint posture may be defined as the habitual position of a joint or series of joints. The length and orientation of the internal moment arm may change in the elderly and subsequently alter

joint posture. The fact of having lived and worked to old age often provides the time needed for forces to significantly influence the length and therefore effectiveness of the internal moment arm. To illustrate this point, consider the case of a 92-year-old female who has been needlepointing for several hours a day for the last 40 years. She presents with a substantial radial deviation deformity at the interphalangeal (IP) joint of her dominant hand. An analysis of the needlepointing activity in a healthy young hand shows that the index finger produces a radial deviation force that causes the deviation of the IP joint (Fig. 4-9, *A-C*). Year after year, the chronic tensile forces placed on the IP's ulnar collateral ligament have caused the ligament to elongate beyond its natural length due to the action of a constant external force. The elongated ligament now acts more like a plastic material than an elastic one. The elongated ulnar collateral ligament would offer little resistance to the omnipresent radial deviated (external) torque. What is essential to understand in this scenario is that the radial deviated deformity at the IP joint mechanically displaced the tendon of the extensor pollicis longus (compare Fig. 4-9, *B*, with Fig. 4-9, *C*). The force line of pull of the thumb extensor now acts with an internal moment arm that can generate a radial deviation internal torque. Any active IP extensor muscle activation will now maintain or increase the pathomechanics of the deformity.

This self-perpetuating cycle of joint deformity is not limited to the aged population, but this group is particularly susceptible since long periods of time have been available for forces to act on the joints.

The presence of disease may interact with aging and further influence the biomechanics of joint posture. Consider both rheumatoid arthritis and osteoarthritis. Chronic synovitis from rheumatoid arthritis may reduce the ability of the articular capsule to provide resistance to large external torques. A deformity called ulnar drift at the metacarpophalangeal joint serves as a prime example of this situation.[14] Also, consider when severe hip osteoarthritis involves a remodeling of the proximal femur such that the distance between the greater trochanter and femoral head diminishes (compare Fig. 4-10, *A,* with Fig. 4-10, *B*). The result of this remodeling is a decrease in length of the internal moment arm that the hip abductors use to produce frontal plane stability during the stance phase of walking.[63] The hip abductors must therefore produce greater amounts of force during the stance phase to offset the loss of length of the internal moment arm. Hip joint forces would therefore increase and possibly stimulate continued bony remodeling with possible continued re-

duction in internal moment arm length. Once again, a pathomechanical situation is shown to be self-perpetuating. In this case, the deleterious effects of the pathomechanics may be alleviated by orthopedic surgery or instruction from physical therapy in the proper use of a cane.[64,65]

External Joint Torque Considerations

Joint posture is determined by the net effect of all internal and external torques acting about the joint. Recall that external torque is the product of a force multiplied by the length of the external moment arm (see Fig. 4-3). The force component of an external torque may arise from gravity, from a weight applied to a limb, or through some other source that is external to the joint. The external moment arm is the distance from the axis of rotation to the perpendicular intersection with the external force.

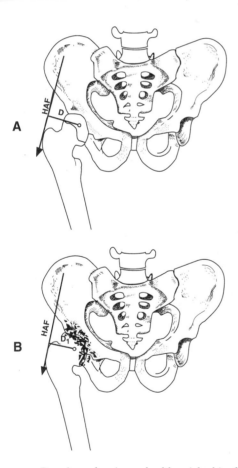

FIG. 4-10 Drawings showing a healthy right hip free of osteoarthritis (**A**) with hip abductor force *(HAF)* and associated internal moment arm *(D)*. Right hip with osteoarthritis is shown (**B**) with diminished internal moment arm *(D₁)* secondary to partial disintegration of femoral head. (From Neumann DA: *Arthritis Care Res* 1989; 2:146-155. Used by permission.)

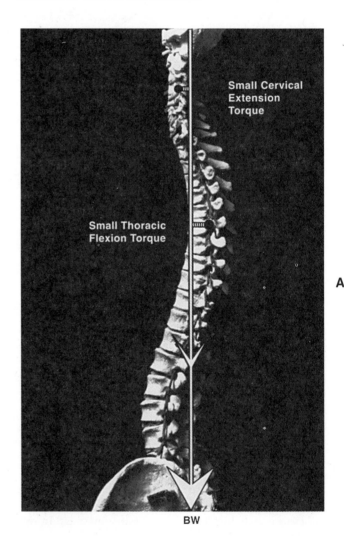

FIG. 4-11 Model showing the orientation of the force line of gravity from body weight *(BW, arrow)* at the cervical and thoracic spines. **A** through **C** show a progression in severity of kyphosis. Each model demonstrates the mediolateral axis at the midpoint of the thoracic and cervical regions *(dark circles)* and the associated external moment arms *(hatched lines)*. **A,** Patient with ideal standing posture and *normal thoracic kyphosis.* BW creates a small cervical extension torque and a small thoracic flexion torque.

Pathomechanics of Senile Kyphosis. Accentuated kyphosis in the elderly is quite common and may sometimes result in significant disability. This sagittal plane postural asymmetry usually develops gradually over time and is partially responsible for loss of body height in the elderly. Relatively large external (gravitational) torques may develop about the spine of the aged person as a consequence of changes in the mechanics of the connective tissues. To describe the associated pathomechanics, consider the ideal posture of an aged person's spinal column (Fig. 4-11, *A*). Note that in ideal standing posture, the force line of gravity is directed on the concave side of the cervical and thoracic curvatures. This allows the force line to act with an external moment arm that maintains the natural posture of these spinal regions. For purely comparison purposes, assume that a small cervical extension torque and a small thoracic flexion torque are constantly present in the ideal posture shown in Fig. 4-11, *A*. To limit the extent of these natural cervical and thoracic curvatures, restraining forces must be produced from adjacent tissues. In the thoracic spine, the anterior side of the intervertebral discs are compressed as a result of the natural anterior concavity in the thoracic curve. Since intervertebral discs become more dehydrated and less elastic with advanced age, their effectiveness in resisting compression forces would diminish.[95] A small flexor external torque, acting over long time periods, could compress and deform the anterior margins of intervertebral thoracic discs, thereby accentuating the local kyphosis. As the thoracic flexion posture increases, the force line of gravity shifts further anterior, thus increasing the length of the external moment arm and magnitude of the flexed posture (Fig. 4-11, *B*).

Sagittal plane x-rays of aged adult spines with moderate kyphosis often show an anterior translation or shift of the upper thoracic and cervical regions. This anterior shift, observed by comparing Fig. 4-11, *A*, with Fig. 4-11, *B*, increases the lengths of the external moment arms, which produce a moderate thoracic and cervical flexor torque. As a result, increased back extensor muscle force may be needed to hold

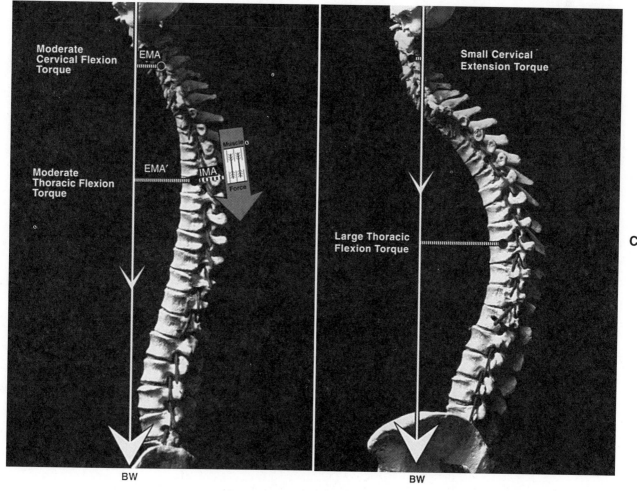

FIG. 4-11, CONT'D **B,** Patient with *moderate thoracic kyphosis.* BW creates a moderate cervical and thoracic flexion torque. *EMA'* = external moment arm at the thoracic spine midpoint; *EMA* = external moment arm at cervical spine midpoint; *IMA* = internal moment arm for back extensor muscular force. **C,** Patient with *severe thoracic kyphosis.* BW causes a small cervical extension torque and a *large* thoracic flexion torque.

the person's trunk and head upright. Increased muscle force would increase the magnitude of intervertebral joint forces and possibly predispose arthritic changes, compression fractures, and/or disc injury.[23]

A simple biomechanical principle may be used to estimate the amount of myogenic joint force transferred across a midthoracic intervertebral segment of a moderately kyphotic spine. Based on an assumption of static equilibrium, the sum of the internal and external torques about a joint equals zero.[63] For sagittal plane rotary equilibrium about a midthoracic region in the spine (see Fig. 4-11, *B*), the product of body weight (BW) and the length of the external moment arm (EMA') equals the product of the muscle force multiplied by the length of the internal moment

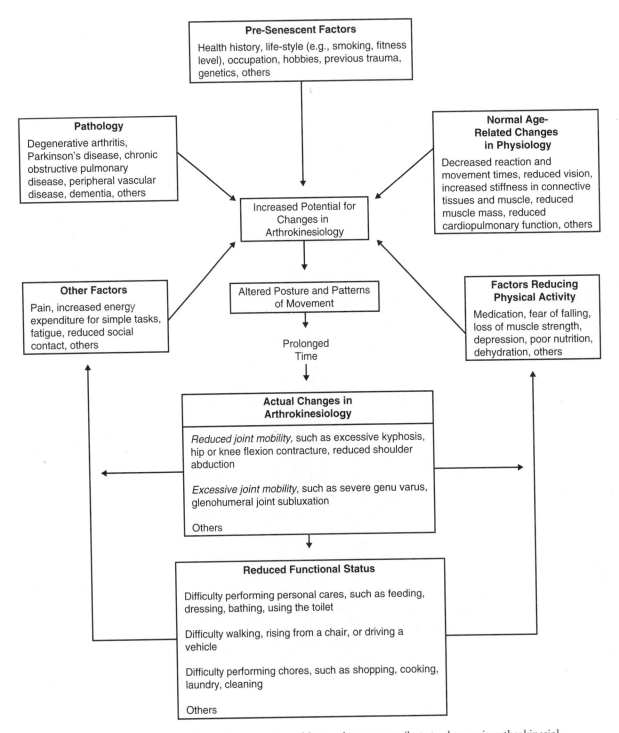

FIG. 4-12 This diagram shows the interaction of factors that can contribute to changes in arthrokinesiology in the elderly.

arm (IMA). To estimate the myogenic joint force across the dark circle shown in Fig. 4-11, *B*, the extensor muscle force required to maintain the kyphotic spine upright must be determined. Observe that the length of the EMA' is about twice as long as the associated IMA. The required muscle force therefore can be estimated by multiplying body weight above the chosen axis of rotation by the ratio of EMA' to IMA. Assuming BW above the midthoracic vertebra to be 90 pounds and moment arm ratio about 2, then at least 180 pounds of muscle extensor force would be needed to hold the sagittal plane posture in Fig. 4-11, *B*. This force, transferred across a small intervertebral surface area, would result in a relatively large physical pressure that must be supported by adjacent tissue.

Applying this same biomechanical equation to the ideal posture shown in Fig. 4-11, *A*, one can estimate an approximate 67% reduction in myogenic joint force at the thoracic spine. This reduction is based on the ideal posture having an external moment arm of only one third the length of that present in the moderately kyphotic posture. This simple mathematical calculation emphasizes the concept that posture and the subsequent length of the external moment arms have a profound effect on forces produced across a joint.

The thoracic posture shown in Fig. 4-11, *B*, may, in extreme cases, progress to that shown in Fig. 4-11, *C*, which was modeled after an actual x-ray of a standing elderly person. During standing, this patient showed a small cervical extension torque and a large thoracic flexion torque. Note that despite the large thoracic kyphosis, this particular patient was able to hold her head in enough extension so that the weight of her head assisted in the maintenance of the normal cervical lordosis. However, the main point in Fig. 4-11, *C*, to appreciate is the impact that the large external flexor torque would have in the midthoracic region. This large torque will continue as long as the force line of gravity acts with such a large external moment arm. The increased compression forces produced on the anterior side of the thoracic vertebrae may stimulate bony remodeling with a continued decrease in height of the anterior side of the thoracic bodies. This loss in thoracic "height" is responsible for most of the loss in overall body height in the elderly. Compression fractures from osteoporosis may augment the kyphosis by increasing the anterior concavity of the middle thoracic spine. This case of severe senile kyphosis should be a reminder of the important role connective tissue has in absorbing the relentless forces of gravity. When aged tissues lose their ability to resist deformation from external forces, gravity wins the ultimate "tug of war" and dominates the clinical course of the posture.

SUMMARY

Arthrokinesiology, or the study of the structure, function, and movement of skeletal joints, is one component of the scientific basis of physical therapy. Age-related changes in joint function can, and do, occur in the elderly, even in the absence of disease. When the effects of disease are coupled with reduced physical activity, the elderly may experience substantial decrements in function. Successful treatment of joint impairments and abnormal posture in the elderly is based on a careful analysis of the pathomechanics of the affected joints.

In conclusion, Fig. 4-12 shows a model of the complex interaction among factors that may lead to *changes in arthrokinesiology* within the elderly. An important role of the physical therapist is to understand when or how physical therapy can diminish the effect these factors have on an individual's function and ultimately his/her quality of life. This figure is certainly not complete, but is intended to serve as a starting point to analyze a very complex topic. Readers are encouraged to expand and modify this model based on additional information and/or clinical and personal experiences.

ACKNOWLEDGMENTS

I would like to thank the following persons for critiquing, illustrating, or in other ways helping this chapter: Joan Holcomb, Nick Schroeder, Elisabeth Rowan, Peter Blandpied, PT, PhD; Robert Morecraft, PhD; Richard Jensen, PT, PhD; and Michelle Schuh, PT, MS. I am also indebted to Marquette University and Lawrence Pan, PT, PhD, for allowing me the time and resources to continue my intellectual pursuits.

REFERENCES

1. Abrahams M: Mechanical behavior of tendon in vitro. *Med Biol Eng* 1967; 5:433-443.
2. Adrian MJ: Flexibility in the aging adult, in Smith EL, Serfass RC (eds): *Exercise and Aging: The Scientific Basis*. Hillside, NJ, Enslow, 1981.
3. Alexander NB, et al: Muscle strength and rising from a chair. *Muscle Nerve* 1997; S5:S56-S59.
4. Alnaqeeb MA, Al Zaid NS, Goldspink G: Connective tissue changes and physical properties of developing and ageing skeletal muscle. *J Anat* 1984; 139:677-689.
5. Amiel D, et al: Age-related properties of medial collateral ligament and anterior cruciate ligament: A morphologic and collagen maturation study in the rabbit. *J Gerontol* 1991; 46:159-165.
6. Aniansson A, et al: Muscle morphology, enzymatic activity, and muscle strength in elderly men: A follow up study. *Muscle Nerve* 1986; 9: 585-591.
7. Asmussen E, Bonde-Peterson F: Apparent efficiency and storage of elastic energy: Human muscle during exercise. *ACTA Physiol Scand* 1974; 92:537-545.
8. Badley EM, Wagstaff S, Wood PHN: Measures of functional ability (disability) in arthritis in relation to impairment of range of joint movement. *Ann Rheum Dis* 1984; 43:563-569.
9. Bassey EJ, et al: Flexibility of the shoulder joint measured as range of abduction in a large representative sample of men and women over 65 years. *Eur J Appl Physiol* 1989; 58:353-360.
10. Bell RD, Hoshizaki TB: Relationships of age and sex with range of motion of seventeen joint actions in humans. *Can J Appl Sport Sci* 1981; 6:202-206.
11. Boone DC, Azen SP: Normal range of motion of joints in male subjects. *J Bone Joint Surg* 1979; 61A:756-759.
12. Bortz WM: Disuse and aging. *JAMA* 1982; 248:1203-1208.
13. Botelho SY, Cander L, Guiti N: Passive and active tension-length diagrams of intact skeletal muscle in normal women of different ages. *J Appl Physiol* 1954; 7:93-95.
14. Brand PW: *Clinical Mechanics of the Hand*. St Louis, Mosby, 1985.

15. Brandt KD, Fife RS: Ageing in relation to the pathogenesis of osteoarthritis. *Clin Rheum Dis* 1986; 12:117-130.
16. Buckwalter JA, Kuettner KE, Thonar EJ-M: Age-related changes in articular cartilage proteoglycans: Electromicroscopic studies. *J Orthop Res* 1985; 3:251-257.
17. Burstein AH, Reilly DT, Martens M: Aging of bone tissue, mechanical properties. *J Bone Joint Surg* 1976; 58A:82-86.
18. Butler DL, et al: Biomechanics of ligaments and tendons, in Hutton RS (ed): *Exercise and Sports Sciences Reviews*, vol 6. Philadelphia, Franklin Press, 1979.
19. Campbell ML, McComas AJ, Petito F: Physiological changes in aging muscle. *J Neurol Neurosurg Psychiatry* 1973; 36:174-182.
20. Caplan A, et al: Skeletal muscle, in Woo SL-Y, Buckwalter JA (eds): *Skeletal Muscle Injury and Repair of the Musculoskeletal Soft Tissues.* Park Ridge, Ill, American Academy of Orthopaedic Surgeons, 1988.
21. Chapman EA, deVries HA, Swezey R: Joint stiffness: Effects of exercise on young and old. *J Gerontol* 1972; 27:218-221.
22. Charette SL, et al: Muscle hypertrophy response to resistance training in older women. *J Appl Physiol* 1991; 70:1912-1916.
23. Cook TM, Neumann DA: The effects of load placement on the EMG activity of the low back muscles during load carry by men and women. *Ergonomics* 1987; 30:1413-1423.
24. Craik RL: Disability following hip fracture. *Phys Ther* 1994; 74:387-398.
25. Diamond MC, et al: Plasticity in the 904-day-old male rat cerebral cortex. *Exp Neurol* 1985; 87:309-317.
26. Downie AW, Newell DJ: Sensory nerve conduction in patients with diabetes mellitus and controls. *Neurology* 1961; 11:876-882.
27. Dummer GM, Vaccaro P, Clarke DH: Muscular strength and flexibility of two female Master's swimmers in the eighth decade of life. *J Orthop Sports Phys Ther* 1985; 6:235-237.
28. Freeman MAR: The fatigue of cartilage in the pathogenesis of osteoarthritis. *Acta Orthop Scand* 1975; 46:323-328.
29. Freeman MAR, Meachim G: Ageing and degeneration, in Freeman MAR (ed): *Adult Articular Cartilage*, ed 2. Kent, England, Pitman Medical Publishing, 1979.
30. Freeman MAR, Todd RD, Pirie CJ: The role of fatigue in the pathogenesis of senile femoral neck fractures. *J Bone Joint Surg* 1974; 56B:698-702.
31. Frontera WR, et al: Strength conditioning in older men: Skeletal muscle hypertrophy and improved function. *J Appl Physiol* 1988; 64:1038-1044.
32. Gallagher JC, et al: Epidemiology of fractures of the proximal femur in Rochester, Minnesota. *Clin Orthop* 1980; 150:163-171.
33. Ghosh P: Articular cartilage: What it is, why it fails in osteoarthritis, and what can be done about it. *Arthritis Care Res* 1988; 1:211-221.
34. Grimby G, et al: Is there a change in relative muscle fibre composition with age? *Clin Physiol* 1984; 4:189-194.
35. Hall DA: *The Ageing of Connective Tissue.* New York, Academic Press, 1976.
36. Hawker GA: The epidemiology of osteoporosis. *J Rheumatol - Supplement* 1996; 45:2-5.
37. Heine J: Uber die Arthritis deformans. *Virchows Arch Pathol Anat Physiol Klin Med* 1926; 260:521-663.
38. Hogan DB: Imposed activity restriction for the elderly. *Am Coll R Med Clin Can* 1985; 18:410-412.
39. James B, Parker AW: Active and passive mobility of lower limb joints in elderly men and women. *Am J Phys Med Rehabil* 1989; 68:162-167.
40. Jette A, et al: Functional recovery after hip fracture. *Arch Phys Med Rehabil* 1987; 68:735-740.
41. Kennedy R, Clemis JD: The geriatric auditory and vestibular systems. *Otolaryngol Clin North Am* 1990; 23:1075-1082.
42. Kirkendall DT, Garrett WE: Function and biomechanics of tendons. *Scand J Med Sci and Sports* 1997; 7:62-66.
43. Lanyon LE, Hartman W: Strain related electrical potentials in vitro and in vivo. *Calcif Tissue Res* 1977; 22:315-327.
44. Larsson L: Morphological and functional characteristics of the ageing skeletal muscle in man. *Acta Physiol Scand [Suppl]* 1978; 457:1-29.
45. Levarlet-Joye H, Simon M: Study of statics and litheness of aged persons. *J Sports Med* 1983; 23:8-13.
46. Lexell J, et al: Distribution of different fiber types in human skeletal muscle: Effects of aging studied in whole muscle cross sections. *Muscle Nerve* 1983; 6:588-595.
47. Lipsitz LA, Goldberger AL: Loss of complexity and ageing. *JAMA* 1992; 267:1806-1809.
48. Liu SH, et al: Collagen in tendon, ligament, and bone healing. A current review. *Clin Orthop* 1995; 318:265-278.
49. Lohmander LS: Articular cartilage and osteoarthrosis. The role of molecular markers to monitor breakdown, repair, and disease. *J Anat* 1994; 184:477-492.
50. Maki BE, McIlroy WE: Postural control in the older adult. *Clin Geriatr Med* 1996; 4:635-655.
51. Martin AD, McCulloch RG: Bone dynamics: Stress, strain, and fracture. *J Sports Sci* 1987; 5: 155-163.
52. Mayne R, Buckwalter JA: Collagen types in cartilage, in Kuettner KE, Schieyerbach R, Hascall VC (eds): *Articular Cartilage Biochemistry.* New York, Raven Press, 1986.
53. Mazess RB: On aging bone loss. *Clin Orthop* 1982; 165:239-252.
54. McCalden RW, McGeough JA, Court-Brown CM: Age-related changes in the compressive strength of cancellous bone. The relative importance of changes in density and trabecular architecture. *J Bone Joint Surg* 1997; 79A: 421-427.
55. McDonagh MJN, White MJ, Davies CTM: Different effects of ageing on the mechanical properties of human arm and leg muscles. *Gerontology* 1984; 30:49-54.
56. McMartin DN, O'Conner JA: Effect of age on axoplasmic transport of cholinesterase in rat sciatic nerves. *Mech Ageing Dev* 1979; 10:241-248.
57. Meachim G: Cartilage fibrillation on the lateral tibial plateau in Liverpool necropsies. *J Anat* 1976; 121:97-106.
58. Melton LJ: Epidemiology of hip fractures: Implications of the exponential increase with age. *Bone* 1996: 121S-125S.
59. Minns RJ, Soden PD, Jackson DS: The role of the fibrous components and ground substance in the mechanical properties of biologic tissues. A preliminary investigation. *J Biomech* 1973; 6:153-165.
60. Mohan S, Rahada E: Age related changes in rat muscle collagen. *Gerontology* 1980; 26:61-67.
61. Muir H: The chondrocyte, architect, of cartilage. Biomechanics, structure, function and molecular biology of cartilage matrix macromolecules. *Bioessays* 1995; 17:1039-1048.
62. Murray MP, Kory RC, Clarkson BH: Walking patterns in healthy old men. *J Gerontol* 1969; 24:169-178.
63. Neumann DA: Biomechanical analysis of selected principles of hip joint protection. *Arthritis Care Res* 1989; 2:146-155.
64. Neumann DA: Hip abductor muscle activity in persons with a hip prosthesis while walking carrying loads in one hand. *Phys Ther* 1996; 76:1320-1330.
65. Neumann DA: Hip abductor muscle activity in persons who walk with a hip prosthesis with different methods of using a cane. *Phys Ther* 1998; 78:490-501.
66. Neumann DA, Cook TM: Effect of load and carry position on the electromyographic activity of the gluteus medius muscle during walking. *Phys Ther* 1985; 65:305-311.
67. Neumann DA, Soderberg GL, Cook TM: Comparison of maximal isometric hip abductor muscle torques between hip sides. *Phys Ther* 1988; 68:496-502.
68. Neumann DA, Soderberg GL, Cook TM: Electromyographic analysis of hip abductor musculature in healthy right-handed persons. *Phys Ther* 1989; 69:431-440.
69. Peress NS, Kane WC, Aronson SM: Central nervous system findings in a tenth decade autopsy population. *Prog Brain Res* 1973; 40:473-483.
70. Prior JC, et al: Physical activity as therapy for osteoporosis. *Can Med Assoc J* 1996; 155:940-944.
71. Raab DM, et al: Light resistance and stretching exercise in elderly women: Effect upon flexibility. *Arch Phys Med Rehabil* 1988; 69: 268-272.
72. Radin EL, Paul IL, Tolkoff MJ: Subchondral bone changes in patients with early degenerative joint disease. *Arthritis Rheum* 1970; 13:400-405.
73. Rauterberg J: Age-dependent changes in structure, properties, and biosynthesis of collagen, in Platt D (ed): *Gerontology, 4th International Symposium.* New York, Springer-Verlag, 1989.

Piezoelectric

74. Retchin SM, Anapolle J: An overview of the older driver. *Clin Geriatr Med* 1993; 2:279-297.

75. Rigby BJ: Aging pattern in collagen in vivo and in vitro. *J Soc Cosmet Chem* 1983; 34:439-451.

76. Roach KE, Miles TP: Normal hip and knee active range of motion: The relationship to age. *Phys Ther* 1991; 71:656-665.

77. Roberts SB: Energy requirements of older individuals. *Eur J Clin Nutrition* 1996; 50:S112-S118.

78. Rosenberg LC, Buckwalter JA: Cartilage proteoglycans, in Kuettner KE, Schieyerbach R, Hascall VC (eds): *Articular Cartilage Biochemistry.* New York, Raven Press, 1986.

79. Schmidt RF, Wahren LK, Hagbarth KE: Multiunit neural responses to strong finger vibration. I. Relationship to age. *Acta Physiol Scand* 1990; 140:1-10.

80. Scott JE: Supramolecular organization of extracellular matrix glycosaminoglycans in vitro and in the tissues. *FASEB J* 1992; 6:2639-2645.

81. Smith EL, Reddan W, Smith PE: Physical activity and calcium modalities for bone mineral increase in aged women. *Med Sci Sports Exerc* 1981; 13:60-64.

82. Soderberg GL: *Kinesiology: Applications to Pathological Motion,* ed 2. Balitmore, Williams & Wilkins, 1997.

83. Sokoloff L: *The Biology of Degenerative Joint Disease.* Chicago, University of Chicago Press, 1969.

84. Spirduso WW: Physical fitness, aging, and psychomotor speed: A review. *J Gerontol* 1980; 35:850-865.

85. Staff PH: The effects of physical activity on joints, cartilage, tendons, and ligaments. *Scand J Soc Med Suppl* 1982; 29:59-63.

86. Stevens A, Lowe J: *Human histology,* ed 2. St. Louis, Mosby, 1997.

87. Strocchi R, et al: Age-related changes in human anterior cruciate ligament (ACL) collagen fibrils. *Italian J Anat Embroy* 1996; 101: 213-220.

88. Thompson LV: Effects of age and training on skeletal muscle physiology and performance. *Phys Ther* 1994; 74:71-81.

89. Vandervoot A, Hayes KC, Belanger AY: Strength and endurance of skeletal muscle in the elderly. *Physiother Can* 1986; 38:167-173.

90. Viidik A: Functional properties of collagenous tissues. *Int Rev Connect Tissue Res* 1973; 6:127-215.

91. Walker JM, et al: Active mobility of the extremities in older subjects. *Phys Ther* 1984; 64:919-923.

92. Weightman B, Kempson GE: Load carriage, in Freeman MAR (ed): *Adult Articular Cartilage,* ed 2. Kent, England, Pitman Medical Publishing, 1979.

93. Williams PL, et al: *Gray's Anatomy,* ed 38. Churchill Livingston, New York, 1995.

94. Williams PR, Goldspink G: Connective tissue changes in immobilized muscle. *J Anat* 1984; 138:343-350.

95. Woo SL-Y, Buckwalter JA: *Injury and Repair of the Musculoskeletal Soft Tissues.* Park Ridge, Ill, American Academy of Orthopaedic Surgeons, 1988.

96. Wright V, Johns RJ: Physical factors concerned with the stiffness of normal and diseased joints. *Bull Johns Hopkins Hosp* 1960; 106:215-231.

97. Yano K, et al: Bone mineral measurements among middle-aged and elderly Japanese residents in Hawaii. *Am J Epidemiol* 1984; 119:751-764.

SENSORIMOTOR CHANGES AND ADAPTATION IN THE OLDER ADULT

CAROLYNN PATTEN, PT, PHD AND REBECCA L. CRAIK, PT, PHD, FAPTA

INTRODUCTION

Aging is typically characterized by notable declines in the control and organization of movement. Most prominent among these are slowing of movement (both movement initiation and execution), deterioration in the quality of executed movement, and loss of muscular strength and power. Loss of motor function that supports fundamental activities of daily living such as the muscular power to climb stairs or the locomotory speed to cross the street before the traffic light changes progressively denies an elder of his/her independence and autonomy. Moreover, many of the most meaningful roles and activities in life, such as playing a musical instrument, painting, participating in sports activities, or operating a vehicle, involve tasks requiring skilled motor performance. Thus, inability to participate in these fulfilling activities robs an elder of a rich aspect of his/her life. From the larger perspective of societal costs, it is important to appreciate changes in motor function with aging as demographers propose that by the year 2025 one in five persons will be older than 65 years.[90] This statistic portends a consistent trend toward a greater proportion of the population evidencing physical disablement with concomitant dependency on family members, institutions, and public resources.

While a public health perspective on aging is sobering, extension of the human life span is an important opportunity for disciplines in science and medicine to advance understanding of biological mechanisms and explore their limits. Historically the aging process has been characterized as one of progressive decline across biological systems. In refreshing contrast, more than a decade ago an insightful commentary on aging was rendered by Rowe and Kahn.[181] Ordinary descriptions of the aging process promoted, to use their term, "a gerontology of the usual," despite the fact that examples of individuals who continue to function at levels commensurate with lesser chronological age are not uncommon. This now-classic notion has inspired extensive investigation regarding the determinants of aging in the absence of pathology and concomitantly has occasioned change in the accepted definition of normal aging.[36] In both the basic sciences and the practice of geriatric medicine, it has become accepted that portrayal of aging as a chronic, progressive deterioration or as affected with insidious pathologies is simply not accurate. Rather, it has been established that aging, in and of itself, is not synonymous with pathology nor the inability to forestall pathology. Normal (biological) aging is what Rowe and Kahn termed "successful" aging, whereas the more "typical" degenerative view of aging is what they termed "usual" aging. The semantic argument is justified when we realize that "usual" aging incorporates many pathologies—some subtle, some frank.

Complicating historical descriptions of aging are the major longitudinal studies of aging in this country. The Baltimore Longitudinal Study on Aging (BLSA) and the Boston Normative Aging Study were initiated with the intention of developing an accurate description of the aging process. The Framingham Heart Study, initiated as a longitudinal study of cardiac function, naturally evolved into a study of normal aging as the cohort aged. The advent of these three longitudinal studies was, however, well in advance of our ability to make clear differentiation between normal aging and pathology. At the inception of these studies, Alzheimer's disease, for example, had yet to be identified and defined as a clinical and pathological entity. Due to descriptions emanating from these epidemiological efforts, the common wisdom became that with aging decline could be expected across physiological systems, including increased blood pressure, impaired memory, and loss of cortical neurons. Currently, it has been established that none of these familiar biological impairments is a characteristic of normal aging. Hence, the seminal longitudinal studies merely *describe* an increasingly heterogeneous population in which pathology becomes more prevalent with advancing age. It is important to emphasize that increased prevalence of pathology *accompanies* secular trends of aging, but these pathologies do not constitute aging per se.

Across biological and behavioral domains, a common theme with aging is variability. With increasing age, biological variability increases much more rapidly than performance declines.[172] From the perspective of "successful aging,"[181] this is simply evidence of the need to separate the biological process attributable to aging and that or those attributable to pathology. Moreover, with each additional decade, the survivors are likely to be the most healthy, most successful, most able to forestall deleterious sequelae of aging. It is also not clear that aging is a unitary phenomenon affecting all physiological systems equally or in like chronology. Rather, there is more evidence of greater vulnerability in certain systems (e.g., certain aspects of the central nervous system), impairment in which is likely to be responsible for the characteristic manifestations of "usual" aging. The study of aging then is multifactorial, which in the context of motor behavior, involves scrutiny of the interaction between an organism and its environment, including perception; motivation; integration of activity across physiological systems; and only finally execution of motor action.

Appreciation of age-related changes in movement function requires understanding of both sensorimotor control and the biological correlates of aging. The complexity surrounding decline in the quality and quantity of movement is focused on a number of factors that may contribute to a decline in sensorimotor performance. These factors could be the result of changes intrinsic to the individual, factors extrinsic to the individual, or a combination of both. Some intrinsic factors associated directly with the integrity of the individual's cognitive status and also with the neuromusculoskeletal system include changes in such variables as neurons, central or peripheral synaptic mechanisms, peripheral nerve, peripheral receptors, muscle, bone, or joints. Other intrinsic factors, such as the status of hormones, the cardiovascular system, respiratory system, and basal metabolism, play an indirect but critical role in guaranteeing the integrity of the sensory and muscular systems. Extrinsic factors that can affect the normal function of the neuromusculoskeletal system include death of a spouse, retirement from an occupation, retirement from community involvement, loss of income, change in nutritional status, decline in physical activity level, and inadequate health care. Indeed, altered motor control with aging is complex and multifactorial.

The perfect theory of motor control would offer a framework or model that proposes the interaction within and between intrinsic and extrinsic factors to produce movement. Age-related change in any variable would then lead to a predictable change in behavior that could be confirmed by measurement. A variety of motor control theories have been proposed to account for movement, discussion of which can be found in two recent publications.[234,235] These contemporary perspectives on motor control view the biological organism as "complex" and its behavior as "adaptive."[103] *Complexity* belies the multitude of levels, including the cell, organ, system, and organism, at which observation can be made; *adaptive* suggests the utility of behavioral action that, for example, enables feeding, communication, and locomotion (all movement activities) essential to the function and survival of the organism—in this case the person. Change subserving adaptive behaviors can then be found at various biological and physiological levels. In the specific context of aging, change over time has typically been viewed as a progressive and deteriorating process. It is a significantly different point of view to consider that change across the life span may, in fact, involve compensations in support of preserving adaptive movement function, thereby enabling the organism to respond to environmental and task demands.

The scope of this chapter is limited to addressing some of the intrinsic changes that occur in the sensorimotor system, including the brain. The assumption is made that sensation must be intact for the individual to learn and to execute the myriad of motor behaviors produced by the human. Since any model of motor control assumes integrity of the neuromusculoskeletal system, the information presented in this chapter should be relevant regardless of the motor control model assumed.

The purpose of this chapter is to present the kinds of changes that occur in the sensorimotor system of the aging human. A commonly uttered classroom phrase is "Who cares?" In this case, the question should be more specific: "Why should a physical therapist care about biological, cellular, or systems changes associated with aging?" Perhaps the most important reason to care is to emphasize the multiple factors that influence the older person's ability to produce a particular movement in either the clinical situation or the context of daily life. As more knowledge about performance is gained, it is important to remember the impact of the systems involved in producing the performance. If the nervous system or muscle is incapable, less capable, or uses different strategies to respond to external stimuli, then clinicians need to incorporate such information into their decision-making to provide effective treatment. For the individual who presents in the clinical situation with another primary diagnosis, age-related changes in function must be considered as a background upon which this new diagnosis is superimposed. For example, due to age-dependent changes in the sensorimotor system, the older adult who has suffered a stroke may recover differently from the younger person who has had a stroke. This chapter highlights the changes that occur with aging in the sensorimotor system in order to integrate this knowledge with that of various disease processes and provide a more comprehensive view of clinical expectations for the older adult.

A variety of research techniques used by individuals in a number of different disciplines are presented in this chapter. Since individual researchers focus on a specific aspect of aging, it is necessary for the physical therapist practitioner to gather information collected from a variety of laboratories that used different techniques to construct the integrated "picture" of age-related effects on the whole system—the person. The student who is interested in the impact of aging on sensorimotor changes is, therefore, faced with information from a variety of disciplines that are all relevant to what initially may have seemed to be a simple question.

This chapter assumes a working knowledge of neuroscience, and the reader is encouraged to use a neuroscience textbook as a companion to the material presented. Several illustrations of normal anatomy have been included to remind the reader of names and locations of some of the nervous system structures referred to in the text.

The chapter is subdivided into five major sections. The first section focuses on neuroanatomical and neurochemical changes that have been reported to occur in the central nervous system (CNS) with primary emphasis on the brain; in the second section, changes in various sensory systems including the visual, auditory, vestibular and somatosensory systems are reviewed; section three examines the age-related changes reported in the motor unit, including the muscle and its peripheral efferent connections; section four examines changes in the sensorimotor system and includes a discussion of reflex and reaction time testing; section five discusses the potential for adaptation in the older individual.

Neuroanatomical Changes with Aging

One theory associated with the process of aging is that mitotic cells undergo a programmed number of cell doublings until cell division ceases in the senescent cell.[83] Loss of the ability to replicate is, therefore, thought to be a primary mechanism in the aging process. How does this theory apply to the neuron? Most neurons are postmitotic cells, i.e., cells that do not divide. What causes the loss of neurons and synapses? Is there an indication that the morphology of the aging brain is different from the younger brain? When is the neuron considered an aged cell? Clinically, the assumption has been made that loss of synapses and, therefore, loss of communication among neurons leads to the development of dementia.[102] These are the types of questions that this section addresses.

Morphology and Physiology
Neuroanatomical Changes in the CNS

Gross Brain Changes. A linear, age-related decrease in adult brain weight has been well-documented.[95] The general trends noted from earlier studies in which autopsy materials were used to study brain weight have been confirmed by more recent studies that have used computer tomography (CT), positron emission tomography (PET), or magnetic resonance imaging (MRI) to examine the brain.

Peress, Kane, and Aronson,[164] using 7579 brains from autopsies of subjects from the third to the tenth decades, concluded that both males and females showed a steady linear decline in brain weight and that the decline was in both the supratentorial and infratentorial areas. Miller, Alston, and Corsellis[137] studied 91 brains from ages 20 to 98 years and found no change until age 50, and then a 2% decrease per decade. The progressive decrease in brain weight and volume begins in middle life, and the current estimates are a total loss through the life span of about 15% of adult brain weight.[56] More recent efforts in which brain weight was normalized to body weight and careful screening was performed to select mentally intact individuals continues to support the phenomenon of an age-related decline in brain weight and volume.[102]

Changes in gross morphology accompany the decrease in overall brain weight and volume. The two most prominent age-related features are a decline in the physical dimensions of gyri, known as *gyral atrophy,* and ventricular dilation (Fig. 5-1). Gyral atrophy describes a decrease in the gray or white matter or both. The term "gyral atrophy" is preferred to "cortical atrophy" because it remains unclear whether this morphological change occurs in the cortex, its underlying white matter, or both.[105] Postmortem investigations and in vivo studies using CT support the finding that gyral atrophy occurs as an age-related phenomenon. Significant gyral atro-

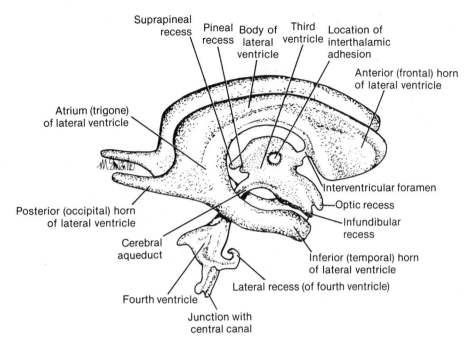

FIG. 5-1 The ventricular system is projected into a hemisected brain to show its location. The anterior horn, body, posterior horn, inferior horn, and atrium are the subdivisions of the lateral ventricles. (From Nolte J: *The Human Brain: An Introduction to Its Functional Anatomy,* ed 2. St. Louis, Mosby, 1988. Used by permission.)

phy, when present on autopsy, is not found throughout the cerebral cortex but appears to be limited to specific regions, including the convexities of the frontal lobes, the parasagittal region, and the temporal and parietal lobes.[58,105] It appears that gyral atrophy begins in the parasagittal region, evidenced by a strong statistical correlation between chronological age and atrophy in this region.[107] In a study of healthy men ranging from 31 to 87 years of age, atrophy was present in the postcentral gyrus (Brodmann's areas 1, 2, 3) of the left parietal lobe and in the association areas (Brodmann's areas 5 and 7) of the right parietal lobe in older adults (Fig. 5-2, *A* and *B*, and Fig. 5-3).[184] Noticeably, involvement of the temporal lobe is more likely to occur on the left and to be exaggerated in the polar region.[105] There is some significant individual variation in gyral atrophy, and there is also a significant linear correlation between gyral thickness and chronological age.[61] Interestingly, when examined using MRI, not all aged subjects show brain atrophy. Observations made by MRI suggest that brain atrophy is not an inevitable consequence of advancing age.[56] Moreover, such findings invite question regarding the association between gross morphological changes in brain tissue and cortical function.

Ventricular dilation has been reported to accompany both aging and decreased brain weight (see Fig. 5-1).[106] The lateral ventricles are most commonly examined in this regard. In general, a progressive increase in the size of the ventricles occurs up to the seventh decade, followed by a marked ventricular increase in individuals in the eighth and ninth decades and a plateau in ventricular enlargement thereafter. It remains unclear whether an increase in ventricular size is a significant or reliable predictor of intellectual function. Fluid volume in the ventricles and subarachnoid space has been found to increase after the sixth decade. This increase in cerebrospinal fluid in the ventricles has been found to correlate highly with impairments of higher intellectual function, including naming and abstract reasoning.[105]

Some evidence suggests a relationship between a specific area of atrophy and function.[68,140] For example, enlargement of the left lateral sulcus (fissure of Sylvius), suggesting loss of cortical tissue, has been correlated with decreased cognitive performance.[68] Atrophy of specific brain regions is now being used in the diagnosis of neurodegenerative diseases such as Alzheimer's disease (AD). Much additional study using neuropsychological protocols is required to define the relationship between cognitive or functional status and clinical tests, the results of which characterize cortical atrophy. In general, gyral atrophy, decreased brain weight, and increased ventricular dimensions are quite exaggerated in the brains of individuals affected with Alzheimer's disease.[105] As is the case in the aging population, there is a considerable *interindividual* variation in these morphological features, with some overlap demonstrated between normal individuals and those affected with pathologies including Alzheimer's disease.

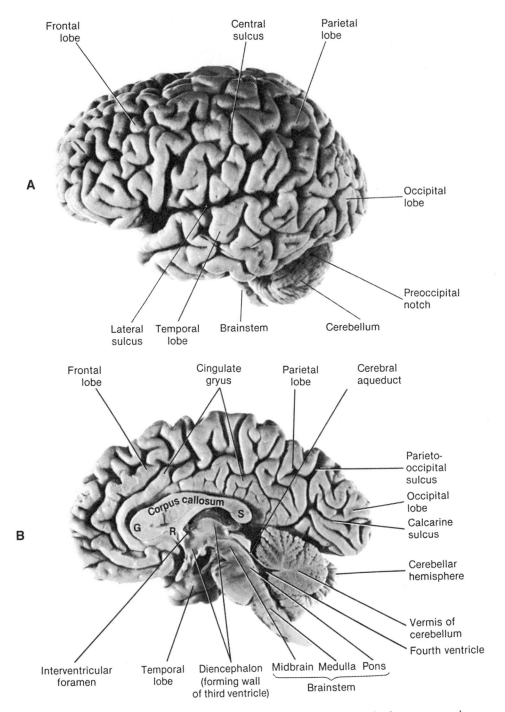

FIG. 5-2   **A,** Major regions of the brain are seen in a lateral view. The central sulcus separates the precentral gyrus from the postcentral gyrus. **B,** Regions of the cerebrum, cerebellum, and brainstem shown in a sagittal plane. The portions of the corpus callosum, the major pathway for communication between the left and right hemispheres, are the rostrum *(R)*, splenium *(S)*, and genu *(G)*. (From Nolte J: *The Human Brain: An Introduction to Its Functional Anatomy,* ed 2. St. Louis, Mosby, 1988. Used by permission.)

CNS Metabolism and Cerebral Blood Flow

The classic view is that cerebral blood flow (CBF) is regulated to meet the requirements of cell metabolism. Glucose is the main energy source for cerebral metabolism, and thus various studies have demonstrated the relationship among the rate of cerebral glucose utilization, oxygen requirements to support glucose metabolism, and the integrity of CNS function[195] Metabolic rates of glucose utilization in the intact human can now be examined using radioactive glucose analogues and dynamic imaging techniques.[176] The assump-

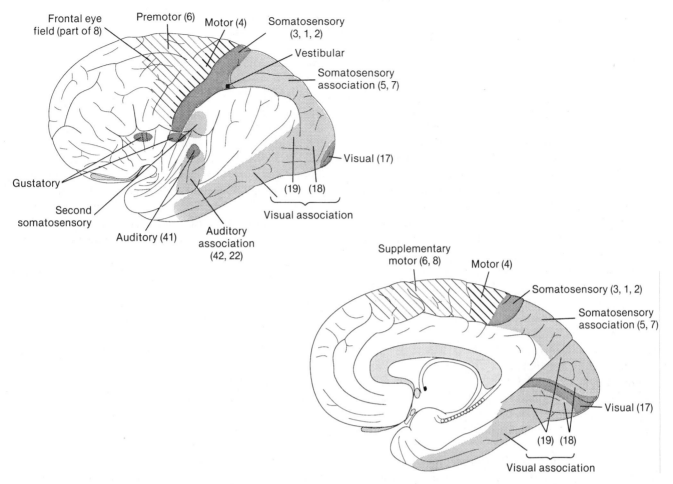

FIG. 5-3 These two diagrams illustrate some of the functional areas of the cerebral cortex and their approximate associations with Brodmann's areas. Brodmann's areas 9 and 10 are not depicted here but are found anterior to the premotor cortex in the frontal lobes and are associated with cognition and other higher functions. (From Nolte J: *The Human Brain: An Introduction to Its Functional Anatomy,* ed 2. St. Louis, Mosby, 1988. Used by permission.)

tion that cerebral atherosclerosis is associated with the aging process has led to the suggestion that poor CBF may be a primary mediator of brain tissue deterioration.[211]

However, the belief that compromised CBF leads to less oxygen and glucose delivery and thus compromising neurons and leading to neuronal death has been challenged. CBF and cerebral metabolic rate of oxygen utilization diminish with normal aging. Rapid declines in CBF and cerebral metabolism have been observed between the first and third decades of life, whereas a more gradual decline occurs between the third and tenth decades.[109] Significantly, the rates of decline in CBF and metabolism are not regarded as important, and it has been noted that CBF and metabolism may change at different rates.[95] The age-related rates of decline in blood flow, oxygen requirements, or glucose utilization by the brain are not profound enough to account for the extent of gyral atrophy that accompanies aging. Thus, other factors must be explored to account for degradation in the cerebrum.

CORTICAL CELL LOSS ABSENT WITH NORMAL AGING

As recently as a decade ago the common teaching was of progressive neuronal loss with aging (Wickelgren, 1996). This representation of neuroanatomical decline was apparently consistent with the model of psychomotor and behavioral deterioration typically manifested with aging. More recent efforts at understanding the neurobiology of aging have demonstrated that tissue samples from which these historical data were obtained often included specimens that today would be considered reflective of pathology. Moreover, the prevalent tissue processing techniques of the time were such that shrinkage of tissue in fixation was not only considerable, but due to age-related differences in water content, more dramatic in the case of young than old tissue. Excessive tissue shrinkage rendered increased cell density per unit volume of tissue, and since the typical criterion measure of the day was neuronal density, the findings reported significantly greater cell numbers in young than older individuals.

Accordingly, the notion of cortical neuronal loss with aging, i.e., the maxim that between 50 to 100,000 neurons are lost each day, became the accepted construct.[105]

More recently, research using contemporary neuroanatomical techniques, including more careful tissue fixation and stereological evaluation of cellular parameters, has demonstrated across species that cortical neuronal loss is not evidenced with normal aging.[81,166,167] This recent finding is in stark contradiction to prevailing thinking,[43] which emphasizes the need to differentiate biological effects due to normal aging and progressive, pathological changes that become more prevalent with advancing age. Moreover, this finding necessarily changes the neuroanatomical focus with normal aging from the cellular to subcellular level.

It is the case, however, that loss of cortical neurons is manifest with dementing processes and, importantly, that approximately 5% of individuals older than 65 years and 50% of individuals older than 85 years are affected with dementia. At one time those few, elite individuals who apparently defied our expectation of aging were considered remarkable and fortunate. There is now in science and medicine growing consensus[36] that these individuals must be acknowledged as representative of "normal," not usual, aging in order to gain insightful differentiation between the ill-defined changes of late life, which often resemble subclinical cases of not only dementia, but Parkinsonism, and numerous other systemic pathological conditions.[36,181]

Subcortical Nuclei: Neurotransmitter Systems

If cortical cell loss is not directly related to aging, what then are neurobiological changes that can truly be attributed to aging? Evidence points to significant neuronal loss in subcortical regions, including the thalamus, striatum, and locus coerelus[105] and notable cell loss from the basal forebrain and hippocampus.[104,105,141,180] It is noteworthy that these regions project to and function as modulators of higher cortical function acting through a variety of neurotransmitters. Further, the "reticular core"—the diffuse network of neurons and fibers that projects from the spinal cord, through the brainstem, throughout the brain, and ultimately to the cortex—is dramatically affected with aging. Due to its ubiquity, function of this system cannot be discretely defined, although it can safely be described as a system for incorporating large amounts of information and hence subserves important integrative function for behavior.[105]

In apparent conjunction with neuronal loss at the subcortical level, thinning is evidenced in cortical regions receiving subcortical projections. For example, cortical layer I in area 46 of prefrontal cortex demonstrates significant signs of degeneration in dendritic extent and demonstrable increases in both neuroglia and pericytes.[166] The grave significance of cell loss in subcortical areas is the depletion of neurotransmitter functions. All affected subcortical systems (i.e., substantia nigra, the midbrain raphe system, and basal forebrain) are significant sources of neurotransmitters, i.e., respectively, dopamine, serotonin, acetylcholine, choline acetyltransferase, and of projections to cortical association areas.[105,167] Consequently the most significant neurobehavioral loss with aging is the ability to modulate activity. Thus, there are anatomical substrates that explain the frequent assessment of important nervous function with aging as a "loss of flexibility."[1]

Another age-related change evidenced across species is the pervasive loss of Purkinje cells from the cerebellum (2.5% per decade).[104] From the perspective of motor control, this CNS structure plays a critical role in regulating the execution of a wide variety and multiple aspects of movement, including control of posture and balance, locomotion, sequencing of movement, repetitive and alternating movements, and smooth pursuit eye movements. The cerebellum is also important in controlling critical parameters of movement, including temporal patterning, velocity/acceleration, and scaling of force magnitude.[72] Aside from Purkinje cell loss, cerebellar dysfunction may be inferred because it is highly myelinated. Age-related impairments in myelin are notable, as will be discussed in the following text. In addition, whereas regional metabolic activity of the cerebellum appears significantly unchanged with aging, CO_2 reactivity is clearly impaired, reflecting the degree of vascular responsiveness to dilation/constriction.[204] Importantly, age-related loss of motor coordination is directly correlated with oxidative damage in the cerebellum. Declines in motor and cognitive function occur at different rates but reflect regionally specific levels of oxidative damage.[66] Further, loss of noradrenergic modulation important to cerebellar plasticity, e.g., motor learning, by acting as a GABA-ergic agonist, correlates directly with rate of learning a novel motor task in old rats. However, noradrenergic modulation is improved in caloric-restricted 24-month-old rats. The significance of this finding is that caloric restriction is the only model known to reliably forestall the oxidative cellular damage that accumulates with aging.[14,15,75] Hence we are presented with of a body of evidence indicating significant age-related impairment in modula-tory activity, plasticity, and global cerebellar regulation of movement.

Cellular and Subcellular Components

Myelin. As discussed earlier, among the most salient neural changes with aging is a progressive decrease in brain weight beginning in the third decade and totaling approximately 100 grams, or 7%, across the life span.[81,205] Whereas this gross anatomical feature was once attributed to cell loss,[25] it is now evident that much of the loss in brain mass occurs in white matter, or myelinated structures. This suggestion is made from results of both histochemical[219] and dynamic imaging techniques,[5] both of which evidence retention of the "cortical ribbon" comprised of gray matter or neuronal structures (Fig. 5-4). Deterioration of myelin affects the cortex, evident through gyral atrophy; the long cortico-cortico fibers; and the reticular core previously discussed. Not only does volume and mass of myelin diminish, but the integrity of myelin is also impaired. Swelling and

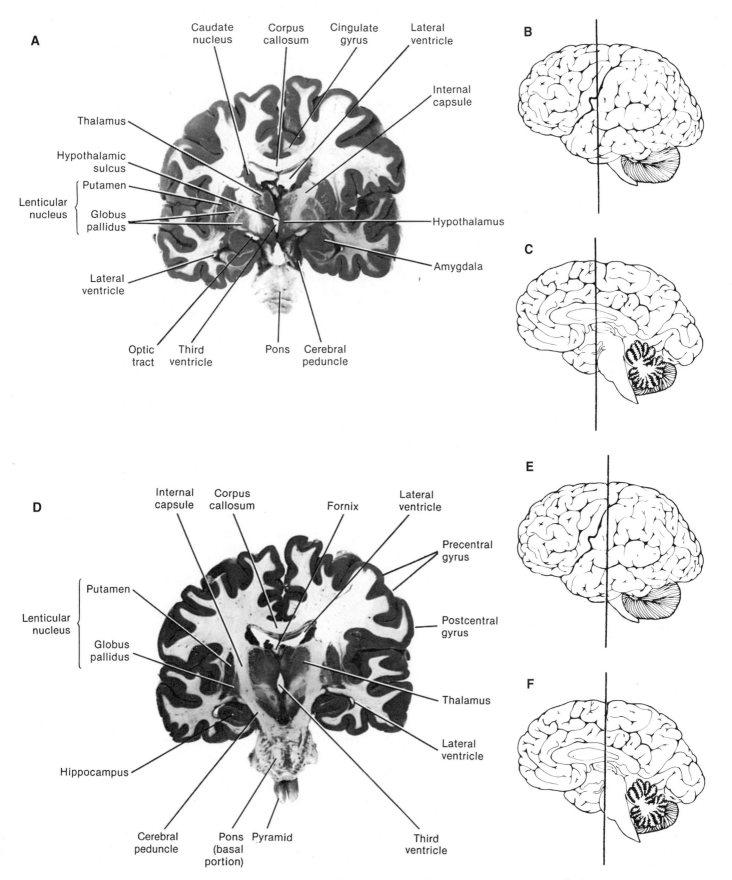

FIG. 5-4 **A,** A coronal (frontal plane) section through the brain. The position of the section in the intact brain is indicated by the *vertical line* in **B** and **C.** The section is through the anterior portion of the diencephalon, so that parts of the thalamus are seen. The caudate, putamen, and globus pallidus are components of the basal ganglia. **D** is posterior to the coronal section in **A.** The location of the section within the brain is indicated by the *vertical line* in **E** and **F.** Note the position of the hippocampus, which is a portion of the limbic system. (From Nolte J: *The Human Brain: An Introduction to Its Functional Anatomy,* ed 2. St. Louis, Mosby, 1988. Used by permission.)

"blebbing" of myelin are commonly observed, which needless to say, affect the rate and quality of axonal conduction.[219] While loss of myelin, in and of itself, is a significant neuroanatomical effect, it appears that the structures that take the longest to myelinate with development, i.e., cortex, long intercortical pathways, and corticospinal pathways, are the first to be affected with aging.[104,105]

In the context of neural function, deterioration of myelin is important for rapid, accurate, and effective transmission of signals. Importantly, the ability of individual cells and nuclei within the CNS to communicate depends heavily on myelinated structures. Thus, slowing of psychomotor speed, delayed processing with increasing complexity of information requiring communication and activity of cortical association areas, and transmission of motor responses via corticospinal and peripheral neural pathways can easily be understood on the basis of compromise to myelinated structures.

Cellular Components and Processes

Survival of cortical neurons does not guarantee their uncompromised function. Impairment has been documented in a number of important cellular features, including membrane properties, neurotransmitter synthesis, integrity of neurotransmitter receptors, and oxidative metabolism. In addition, notable inclusions in the cytoplasm, lipofuscin, and phagocytic debris become increasingly prevalent while clumping of mitochondria occurs in the nucleus. Decreased levels of cytochrome oxidase, the final step in the oxidative metabolic pathway leading to ATP synthesis, has been noted, inferring compromised cerebral metabolism. To concur with this cellular phenomenon, decreases in regional cerebral blood flow have been widely documented.[96,167] It is noteworthy that nonpyramidal cells are more prone to these cellular inclusions.

The most common reported age-related changes at the cellular level are the presence of lipofuscin, the senile or neuritic plaque, and the neurofibrillary tangle (NFT). Lipofuscin is a dark, pigmented lipid found in the cytoplasm of aging neurons.[24] The effect of this pigment on cell function remains unclear. There is speculation that an excessive accumulation of lipofuscin may interfere with the function of the neuron, although its primary role at this time is as a biological marker of aging.[58] Neuritic (senile) plaques are discrete structures located outside of the neuron[58] and comprised of degenerating small axons, some dendrites, astrocytes, and amyloid. Plaques have been nicknamed "tombstones" in evidence of their association with neuronal degeneration.[105] Although the senile plaque is found in human disease (e.g., in Parkinson's disease and dementias),[225] it is also reported as a normal age-related change.[143] Plaques have been reported to occur beginning in the fifth decade; to be located primarily deep in the sulci of the neocortex, hippocampus, and amygdala; and to increase in number with advancing age. A significantly increased number of plaques is clearly observed in dementia.[101,102]

Whereas the neuritic plaque is thought to occur most often in the neocortex, NFTs have been reported to occur in the hippocampal formation and in specific brainstem nuclei in the healthy aging brain.[7] The origin of the NFT is unknown, but it is distinguished in structure and location from the plaque.[226] The NFT appears to occur within the perikaryon and is first identified with silver stain as a darkly stained, thick band that later increases and becomes twisted. The NFT often displaces the nucleus and distorts the cell body. Like the plaque, the NFT is noted more commonly with advancing age, but its presence is quite exaggerated, particularly in the neocortex, in dementia. The presence of neurofibrillary tangles in the cortex is a hallmark of dementia.

Also at the cellular level are signs of degeneration in dendritic number and extent. Loss of dendritic branches from the basal/apical trees are most notable, as is a frank decrease in overall dendritic population.[43] Dendritic proliferation typically accompanies improvements in learning, memory, and performance, thus loss of these delicate and sensitive structures portends decreased capacity for important neural processing and performance. Decreased synapses between cells also appears to be an age-related phenomenon and an important mechanism subserving integrated neural function (Fig. 5-5).[20]

Taken together, the evidence regarding cellular degeneration with aging points to alterations in overall integrity of CNS functioning on a more global level. Interestingly, behavioral performance directly parallels age-related alterations in white matter and cellular integrity. By way of example, aged primates trained to perform a recall task that involved choosing a nonmatching stimulus following a temporal delay demonstrated performances that corresponded in rank-order to the qualitative state of both neuronal structure and myelin integrity in layer I of Brodmann's cortical area 46.[166] In the specific context of motor control, Haug recognized fewer signs of aging in cortical sensory areas 7 and 17 but striking deterioration of motor area 6, critical to motor planning and programming, which is targeted by striatal pathways from the basal ganglia.[81]

Summary: Neuroanatomy

At the gross level, brain structure becomes progressively changed with chronological age. In contrast to historical perspectives, however, evidence from current research suggests that these changes that include gyral atrophy, decreased brain weight, and ventricular dilation fail to map directly to functional change in higher cortical function in normal aging. Importantly, evidence has been presented refuting the traditional canon that cortical neurons are lost progressively with age. Thus, age-related change in the central nervous system shifts its focus to selective cell loss in specific subcortical formations, including the substantia nigra, the basal forebrain (nucleus basalis of Meynert), locus ceruleus, brainstem, and cerebellum. Neuronal loss in these subcortical regions appears to occur most in regions projecting to the cortex, thus compromising modulation of higher corti-

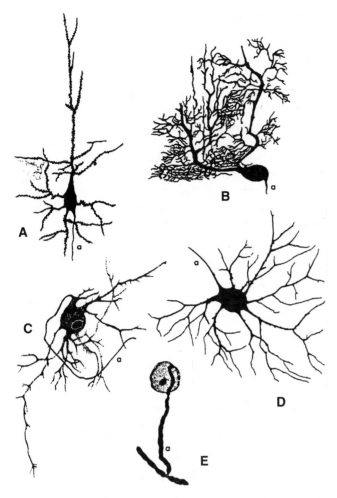

FIG. 5-5 There are a variety of forms of neurons. The neuron in **A** is a pyramidal cell and typical of the cerebral cortex. The bumps on the dendrites are dendritic spines, which appear to enhance synaptic contact area. The axon is labeled *a* in each of the illustrations. The Purkinje cell, the neuron depicted in **B**, may be viewed as the final common pathway leaving the cerebellar cortex. **C**, A sympathetic postganglionic neuron. **D**, An alpha motoneuron; a motor unit consists of this neuron and all the muscle fibers it innervates through its branching axon. The neuron depicted in **E** is a dorsal root ganglion cell. (From Willis WD, Grossman RG: *Medical Neurobiology: Neuroanatomical and Neurophysiological Principles Basic to Clinical Neuroscience,* ed 3. St. Louis, Mosby, 1988. Used by permission.)

cal function. Age-related decrease in brain weight and dimension is very closely associated with deterioration of myelin.

Rather than frank neuronal loss, normal aging of the brain results from general deterioration at the cellular level and decline in the ability of individual cells within a region to work together to produce integrated action. Lipofuscin accumulates intracellularly with aging but at this time is remarkable only as a biological marker of aging. Other cellular level features of normal aging are inclusions of phagocytic debris, clumping of mitochondria, and deterioration of neurotransmitter receptors. Cell function becomes diminished,

as evidenced by reduced metabolic activity. Importantly, synthesis of neurotransmitters is reduced.

It is now possible to differentiate normal aging from the numerous pathological conditions that accompany aging. Moreover, it is tremendously important to differentiate normal aging from pathology. In pathologies, including Alzheimer's disease and other dementias, cortical neuronal loss is remarkable and accompanied by exaggerated neuronal loss throughout the brain. Neurofibrillary tangles (neuronal inclusions) and neuritic plaques (extracellular bodies, scarring) are widely prevalent in the brains of individuals with Alzheimer's disease. Thus the contrast can be drawn between subtle slowing and deterioration of the highest levels of function in normal aging and remarkable neuronal loss, leading to wholesale impairment of executive function including memory, reasoning, language, and integrative function.

NEUROCHEMICAL CHANGES IN THE CNS WITH AGING

Morphological changes in the aging brain described in the preceding text are accompanied by significant neurochemical changes. Primary neurotransmitters (NTs) include acetylcholine, dopamine, norepinephrine, serotonin, gamma-aminobutyric acid (GABA), excitatory amino acids, opioid peptides, and other peptide neurotransmitters. Detailed reviews of the age-related changes for the neurotransmitters and the intracellular action of NTs are available.[129,177] Since most of the research related to NTs and aging was derived from animal models, caution must be exercised in generalizing the research findings to humans. This section focuses only on acetylcholine and dopamine as examples of the kinds of research relating to aging changes in neurotransmitters.

Acetylcholine

Acetylcholine (ACh) is essential to the function of the central and peripheral nervous systems and is utilized in both the somatic and autonomic nervous systems. Acetylcholine has been the focus of extensive research during the past 20 years because of the location of cholinergic neurons in the basal forebrain and the neural connections with structures associated with learning and memory. The "cholinergic hypothesis" attributes learning and memory deficits to a decline in the cholinergic systems of the forebrain.[147] A primary site for ACh is in the basal forebrain, where the cholinergic system innervates the hippocampus, neocortex, and amygdala. Since the hippocampus is one of the structures associated with memory and learning, many investigators have tried to establish a link between the presence of ACh and the integrity of short-term memory and learning. Extensive research using animal models has involved assaying whole brains for ACh content, producing lesions and observing behavioral responses, introducing fetal tissue to replace lost cholinergic neurons, and introducing specific ACh excitotoxins or ACh uptake blockers. Research in humans who display Alzheimer's disease (AD) has enabled correlation between the behavioral correlates of ACh deficits seen in the animal models and the patients.[147] For example, animal models that demonstrate a loss of cortical acetylcholine display a selective memory loss of recent events and information.[13] Other investigators have reported reduced cortical ACh content in the aging human and a profound loss of acetylcholine in specific cortical sites in patients with Alzheimer's disease.[71]

A variety of studies using both animals and humans suggest that appropriate pharmacological or dietary manipulation improves short-term memory losses under certain conditions. Rogers and Bloom reviewed a series of experiments in animals and humans suggesting that the acetylcholinesterase (ACE) inhibitor physostigmine or dietary supplements using one of the precursors for acetylcholine, choline, or lecithin showed some promise for delaying or improving senile cognitive deficits.[177] The results remain controversial at this time, and additional work is necessary before its therapeutic efficacy is embraced. A review of the vast literature related to the role of ACh suggests that there are age-dependent changes in the cholinergic system and that ACh plays a critical role in cognitive function. Damage to the cholinergic neurons that connect with more rostral portions of the basal forebrain structures disrupts learning and memory; damage to regions of the neocortex that receive the basal cholinergic neurons results in deficits in attentional function.[147] Much more research is necessary to elucidate the specific mechanisms associated with a decline in the cholinergic system with aging.

Dopamine

Although dopamine (DA) is widespread in the CNS, the most frequently studied dopaminergic neurons are those located in the substantia nigra that project to the striatum of the basal ganglia.[177] The dysfunction of these neurons is directly related to Parkinson's disease. DA is also located in the diencephalon and the medulla. Changes in the synthesis, inactivation, catabolism, content, and receptors have all been reported with aging. The synaptic actions of DA are terminated by presynaptic reuptake and by actions of enzymes such as monamine oxidase. Again, the research identifying age-related change to each of the aspects of metabolism and catabolism is incomplete and controversial.

In general, there is consensus that the amount of DA present and the number of receptors in the striatum of the basal ganglia decrease after the fourth decade. On the other hand, the number of receptors increases in persons with Parkinson's disease. Rogers and Bloom explain this disparity by suggesting that the person with Parkinson's disease may still be able to compensate for the decreased amount of neurotransmitter, whereas the aging individual may have lost this compensatory capacity.[177] The administration of L-Dopa, a precursor of DA that crosses the blood-brain barrier, has been shown to improve motor function in aged rats and in humans with Parkinson's disease. Much additional research

is needed, particularly in regard to the role of DA in motor function of aging humans.

Summary: Neurotransmitters

Evidence exists to suggest that age-related changes occur in each of the major neurotransmitter systems, but the precise mechanism that produces a change in NT content remains unclear. Aging can affect a variety of steps between synthesis of the NT to the final production of a response in the postsynaptic cell. It is difficult to relate the loss of a specific NT to a decline in functional performance. Loss of function may be related to the synergistic effect of multiple neurotransmitters or may reflect an age-related lack of balance among neurotransmitters. At this time the role of neurotransmitters and behavior remains at the descriptive level. Currently emerging research on the role of estrogen in preventing neuronal circuit degeneration emphasizes the need for better understanding of the neuroendocrine changes that accompany aging.[145] Much work needs to be completed before it will be obvious whether dietary or pharmacological supplementation will increase the synthesis or action of a particular neurotransmitter or retard changes in neuronal circuitry and thereby retard age-related change or improve function.

SENSORY CHANGES WITH AGING

It is a generally accepted concept that sensory integrity declines with aging. The clinician is interested in learning which sensory systems are affected and which part of the system is affected. Are there specific targets of the pathway that are more susceptible to the process of aging? Is there a decrease in the speed with which the nervous system responds to external stimuli in the older individual? If so, where is the change occurring? Are the afferent, central, and efferent systems equally affected by age?

The Visual System

There is a gradual decline in visual acuity before the sixth decade followed by a rapid decline in many patients from 60 to 80 years of age.[3] Visual acuity may decline as much 80% by the ninth decade. Impairment of visual accommodation has been noted.[23] By age 40 to 55, visual correction is necessary in most people for accurate near vision. Common ophthalmological disorders in the older person include cataracts, glaucoma, and macular degeneration.

Visual acuity is a measure of visual discrimination of fine details.[42] The macula lutea, located in the posterior pole of the human eye, is only about 6 mm in diameter, but it is the most important part of the eye for contrast discrimination because of the high concentration of cone receptors in this area. The innermost part of the macula is the fovea, and it is about 1.85 mm in diameter. Age-related maculopathy (ARM) is an age-related degenerative disorder of the macula that occurs with a rising prevalence in persons 50 years and older.[108] The late stages of ARM are called *age-related macular degeneration (AMD)*. The prevalence of AMD is up to 15% in persons older than 85 years, and AMD is the most common cause of blindness in the elderly. At this time there is no adequate therapy for the majority of people disabled by AMD. A standard eye chart examines the integrity of the cones in the macula and their connection with the visual pathway. Testing for visual acuity with an eye chart assumes that the ability of the eye to resolve the smallest letter demonstrates the eye's ability to resolve larger objects and that contrast is not important.[42] Such assumptions are valid for reading; letters are small and there is high contrast between the letters on the written page and the background. The need to resolve fine details of high contrast may not be meaningful for other visual tasks, such as recognizing a step in a dimly lit hallway or recognizing a larger object such as a face in a crowd of faces. Therefore, traditional acuity testing may describe the person's ability to read but may not test "functional" vision.

Traditionally, changes in visual acuity have been related to a change in the optical portion of the visual system—the structures within the eyeball.[42] The small pupil that occurs with aging and the clouding of the lens and its inability to change its shape (accommodation) were the primary targets for visual correction in the older individual. The most common visual problem among older adults is presbyopia, or difficult focusing on near objects. It is important to recognize the complexity of the visual system and to note that investigators are examining the effect of aging on each aspect. For example, the causes of loss of age-related changes in accommodation (presbyopia) are a source of multiple lines of investigation. Among the possible causes for presbyopia are increased stiffness in the lens substance, decreased stiffness in the lens capsule, decreased effectiveness of the ciliary muscle, increased stiffness of the choroid, and a changing geometric relationship among the components of the accommodative system.[233] Recognizing the lack of understanding related to the underlying mechanisms associated with presbyopia should assist the clinician in recognizing that detection of visual acuity problems in patients may not lead to correction and that compensatory strategies are critical to ensure maintained functional ability.

Impairment in other aspects of the visual system also accompany aging so that *if* correction of the optical system in the aging individual *is possible*, the correction may not lead to improved functional vision. Presentation of a visual stimulus such as a reversing checkerboard pattern to the human eye will reliably evoke consistent electrocortical activity. The visual evoked response (VER) has a characteristic deflection pattern and predictable latency, and results of using this technique have been reviewed.[169] After maturation, there is a general slowing in the latency of the VER to stimuli with high spatial frequency that appears age-related. The slowing has been proposed to occur due to a decrease in the number of axons in the optic nerve and changes in processing in the thalamus and occipital cortex. Therefore, glare and abrupt changes in light are problems for the older adult. This difficulty may explain some of the factors that lead the older person to give up night driving and may increase his/her risk of

falling. Although additional research is necessary to correlate the electrical with physical findings, some of the changes in the visual system will be reviewed that may account for the increased latency in the visual pathway.

Aging affects more than just the optical system. Age-related changes in the sensory components of the visual system have been demonstrated beginning at the retina. Photoreceptors demonstrate an age-related loss as does the function of the ganglion cells within the retina and of their axons that project to the thalamus.[67] The number of neurons in portions of the primary visual cortex (Brodmann's area 17) is significantly reduced with aging.[52] A loss of one half of the cells that process information has been proposed based on the comparison of neuronal density at age 20 to neuronal density at age 80.

Other age-related deficits in the visual system have been noted.[42,189] Aging affects the integrity of the visual fields, dark adaptation, and color vision. Color discrimination changes also take place with aging. In particular, older adults have more difficulty identifying blues and greens. There is a differential loss of sensitivity to blue, but there is also some loss of sensitivity over the entire spectrum by the fourth decade. Spatial visual sensitivity decreases in the older adult, especially to low spatial frequencies and slow moving targets.

The motor integrity of the visual system is not spared during aging. Pupillary responses are diminished, or even absent, and the size of the resting pupil decreases markedly.[128] The corneal touch threshold increases throughout life, although the decline is more rapid after the fifth decade. By the ninth decade, corneal sensitivity is reported to be only one half to two thirds as great as in the second and third decades.[139] The corneal reflex may be entirely absent in elderly normal patients.

The ocular motor system also undergoes a progressive loss.[42] Convergence is compromised, ptosis occurs, and there is a symmetrical restriction in upward gaze. Smooth pursuit, saccades, and optokinetic nystagmus are each reduced in the elderly.

In summary, corrected visual acuity in the older individual may not lead to enhanced functional vision. There are a variety of changes that occur along the visual sensory and visual motor pathways that lead to a host of age-related changes in the visual system. Careful functional visual screening is essential for elderly persons who are having difficulty maneuvering in the environment.

The Auditory System

Although changes in the auditory system have been demonstrated as early as the fourth decade, functional impairment is not typically evident until the seventh decade.[82] More than one half of all Americans who suffer significant hearing loss are 65 or older. Hearing has been related to independent lifestyle: 39% of individuals 75 or older and living in the community have been reported to have a hearing loss, whereas as many as 70% of institutionalized older adults have difficulty hearing.[175]

Presbycusis, age-related decline in auditory function, is the most common cause of hearing loss in adults.[18] Presbycusis is characterized by the gradual, progressive onset of bilateral hearing loss of high-frequency tones. This age-related change can reflect cellular aging in the auditory and CNS pathways as well as acoustic trauma, cardiovascular disease, and the cumulative effects of ototoxic medications. Presbycusis can occur for at least two distinct reasons: (1) changes in the peripheral sensory organ; the outer, middle and inner ear; or changes in the central pathway or (2) changes in the auditory portions of the cerebral cortex. The peripheral structures are related to hearing sensitivity, whereas the central systems are related to understanding speech, especially under difficult listening conditions.

Age-related changes in hearing include a slowly progressive, bilateral hearing loss, affecting high-frequency sensitivity first and later involving loss across the entire spectrum.[82] These changes are related to age-related alterations in the cochlea. Word recognition and sentence identification tasks both show an age-related exponential decline, suggesting a decrease in perceptual processing of the temporal characteristics of speech. A build-up of ear wax, i.e., cerumen, in the external auditory canal can also impair hearing.[164] As the individual ages, the cerumen glands atrophy and produce drier cerumen.

The data just presented are supported by results from a study in which 1662 men and women were examined between the ages of 60 to 90 years.[70] Pure-tone thresholds increased with age, but the rate of change with age did not differ by gender, even though men had poorer threshold sensitivity. Maximum word recognition ability declined more rapidly in men than in women. Hearing aids were being used in only 10% of subjects likely to benefit from this device.

The relationship between satisfaction with hearing aid use and the site of auditory lesion was studied in another investigation.[134] As the site of lesion moved from peripheral to central, subjects' satisfaction with the hearing aid declined. In subjects with purely peripheral, conductive hearing loss, satisfaction with hearing aid use was as high as 84%. In subjects with damage to a central site, i.e., sensorineural hearing loss, satisfaction declined to less than 15%.

In a study designed to determine some of the factors that may affect spoken-word recognition in hearing-impaired older listeners, the findings suggest that there are distinct age-related changes in speech recognition.[196] A reduced ability to distinguish talkers or voice characteristics by age, race, or gender was associated with normal aging and in the older adults with presbycusis. The ability to accommodate for alterations in speaking rate was not an age-related phenomenon but only present in older subjects affected by age-related hearing impairment. Finally, age, but not age-related hearing loss, reduced the older person's ability to ignore irrelevant aspects of speech waveforms, i.e., reduced signal-to-noise ratio. The findings of this study support the clinical observation that older persons may have difficulty recognizing the talker and that accelerated speech and shouting can increase the distortion for the older listener.

In summary, aging can produce different hearing disorders that interfere with social interaction. Since a primary mode of communication with our patients is verbal, appreciation of any impairment to the auditory system is critical for the clinician.

The Vestibular System

Complaints of dizziness and disequilibrium are common in older persons. Since other chapters in this book address the functional aspects of the vestibular system, this section focuses on neuroanatomical or physiological changes and some functional correlates that have been cited for the vestibular system during aging.

The vestibular end organs are responsible for transforming the forces associated with head acceleration into action potentials, producing awareness of head position in space (orientation), and motor reflexes for postural and ocular stability.[8] The utricles and saccule sense linear acceleration, and the semicircular canals monitor angular acceleration. At rest, the afferent nerves from these structures maintain a balanced tonic rate of firing. The tonic activity and its change in level with head movement are used in cortical, brainstem, and spinal centers to elicit the appropriate vestibuloocular and vestibulospinal responses.

Presbyastasis is the term to describe age-related disequilibrium when no other pathological condition is noted.[106] Studies of the vestibular system indicate an age-related 20% decline in hair cells of the saccule and utricle and a 40% reduction in hair cells in the semicircular canals.[97] A recent report of changes in the vestibular nuclear complex of persons aged 40 to 93 years suggests a 3% neuronal loss per decade.[127] Neuronal loss was greatest in the superior vestibular nucleus, a nucleus that receives most of its input from the semicircular canals, and least in the medial vestibular nucleus. Age-related changes in the morphology of the vestibular system correspond to changes in vestibular function using caloric testing, i.e., bathing the auditory canal with warm or cold water and examining ocular responses.[106] Young patients respond with involuntary eye movements of high frequency and large amplitude when warm or cold water is placed in the auditory canal compared with persons older than 60 years. Age-related changes in the vestibulospinal system are more difficult to assess because of the prominent overlap in function with other descending sensory-motor pathways. It is not clear whether these changes reflect a change in the integrity of the labyrinth, diminished CNS modulation, or vascular changes.

Presbyastasis must be distinguished from pathology of the vestibular system in older individuals. Vertigo, nystagmus, and postural imbalance may be symptoms of age-related decline if underlying vestibular pathology is ruled out. The incidence of presbyastasis in the healthy aging population is not available.

The literature suggests that disequilibrium may be attributed to the normal aging of the vestibular system in addition to other factors that include vestibular pathology, changes in other sensory systems, and changes in the motor system. Differentiating the causes for disequilibrium may lead to more successful treatment intervention.

The Olfactory and Gustatory Systems

Decrements in the chemical senses of smell and taste are common aspects of aging.[186] Hyposmia, a diminished sensitivity to smell, and hypogeusia, a diminished sensitivity to taste, are both reported as age-dependent changes in the olfactory and gustatory systems, respectively. The mechanisms that account for the age-related changes in the two systems remain equivocal. Age-related rather than trauma-related hypotheses for hyposmia include changes beginning in the structure and function of the upper airway and include changes in the olfactory bulb and nerves, hippocampus, amygdala, and hypothalamus. The current hypothesis for age-related hypogeusia is a change in the taste cell membranes with altered functioning of ion channels rather than a decreased number of taste buds. Such deficits can alter food choices and intake of food, leading to exacerbation of disease states, impaired nutritional status, and weight loss that interferes with a program of physical therapy designed to enhance functional capacity. From a more holistic perspective, decreased taste and smell sensitivity may put the older person at risk to toxic chemicals and poisons since cues for chemical safety are dampened with aging. A comprehensive anatomical and physiological review of these systems is available in the literature.[190]

The Somatosensory System

Anatomical Changes

What indication is there that the morphological and physiological changes of the peripheral receptors, afferent pathways, and CNS affect the integrity of the somatosensory sensation? Birren and Schaie cite more than 4000 references on age-related changes in normal human function.[18] The problem with many of these studies is that they isolate a single variable for testing, such as position sense. It is difficult, therefore, to gain an understanding of how the sensorimotor system changes within one individual.

A number of age-related changes in the peripheral nervous system (PNS) have been documented.[182] Morphological changes in the nerve cells, roots, peripheral nerves, and specialized nerve terminals have been linked with the aging process. Meissner's corpuscles, which detect touch and are limited to hairless skin, decrease in concentration with age (Fig. 5-6).[21] In old age, the corpuscles become sparse, irregular in distribution, and highly variable in size and shape. Pacinian corpuscles, responsible for sensing repetitive features of touch such as vibratory stimuli, undergo age-related change in morphology and decrease in density. Merkel cells, which are also touch receptors, do not appear to demonstrate significant age-related change.[187] In addition to an age-related decline in some of the receptors, an age-related decline in afferent nerve fibers also occurs. A 32% loss of fibers in both the dorsal and ventral roots of T8 and T9 at age 90 years has been reported.[47] The degeneration of the dorsal columns that occurs with aging may reflect the loss of centrally directed axons of the dorsal root ganglion cells. The longer fibers comprising the gracile nucleus of the dorsal columns are most affected in this process.[146]

The peripheral nerves also show a similar degree of dropout with aging.[159] Age-related loss of nerves in cranial and spinal nerve roots affect thick fibers more than thin fibers.[203] The anatomical site of the nerve may be important since preferential large fiber loss has been reported in the sciatic, anterior tibial, and sural nerves, for example, but not in the superficial radial nerve.[158,203]

Aging is also associated with a gradual shortening of the internodal length. The distance between the nodes of Ranvier is normally greater in fibers of larger diameter. Irregularities of internodal length occur in the nerves of older individuals.[78,119,220] Abnormally short internodes for a given axon diameter might result either from segmental demyelination and remyelination or as a result of complete degeneration of fibers followed by regeneration. Since the longer the distance between nodes the faster the saltatory conduction, the shortened internodes contribute to an increased conduction velocity and, therefore, the action potentials may take longer than usual to reach the CNS.

Physiological Changes

Physiological age-linked alterations in the PNS have also been documented.[116] Whereas a gradual decline in maximal nerve conduction velocity has been described in some studies[55,57] no significant change in normal sensory and motor conduction velocity has been reported in other studies.[136] Table 5-1 lists conduction velocities for peripheral nerve fibers. The collective data on age-related changes in conduction velocity do not suggest that changes are substantial enough to account for the degree of sensory loss reported in older individuals.

The integrity of the sensory pathway from the periphery to various regions within the CNS has been examined using the somatosensory evoked potential (SEP).[51] Peripheral nerve stimulation produces a variety of potentials that can be recorded from the scalp, over the spine, or in the periphery. The SEP has components that are focally restricted to the somatosensory area contralateral to the stimulated side. Electrical stimulation is most often used to elicit SEPs, but a mechanical stimulus can also be used. Commonly used peripheral nerves are the median and the peroneal.

SEPs change with maturation and with age.[156] Normative data are still being collected but, in general, the latencies appear to increase with age. The amplitude of the SEP recorded from the scalp appears to decrease with age. Evoked potentials to peroneal nerve stimulation recorded from surface

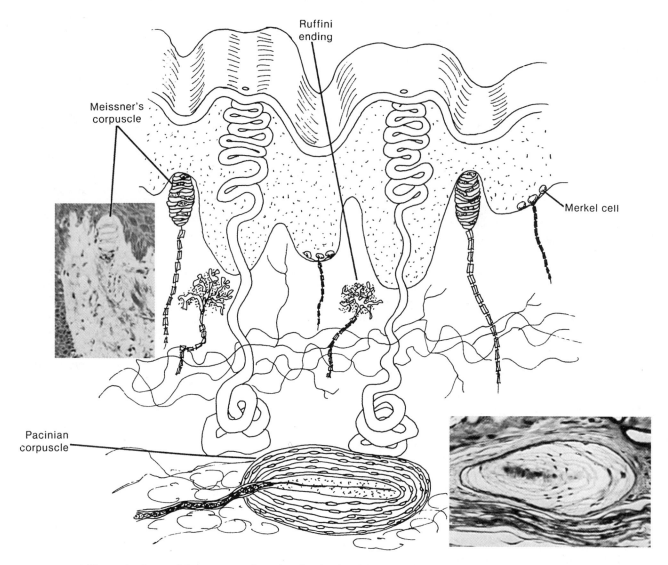

FIG. 5-6   Some of the sensory endings found in hairless (glabrous) skin are illustrated. Note the position of the various mechanoreceptors. Meissner's corpuscles are limited primarily to hairless skin. (From Nolte J: *The Human Brain: An Introduction to Its Functional Anatomy,* ed 2. St. Louis, Mosby, 1988. Used by permission.)

electrodes placed over the spine also show an age-related increase in latency from the lumbar to the cervical region. The delay in central rather than peripheral somatosensory axons is proposed by some investigators as the primary site for the age-related slowing in the SEP.

When sensory detection is studied quantitatively, a progressive impairment with age is noted in many, but not all, peripheral cutaneous modalities. Every student learns that spatial acuity varies from one body region to another; the acuity of the tongue, for example, is 50 times better than that of the back.[202] The common clinical method of testing is to have the subject report that he/she feels the stimulus and to locate it (point localization) or to detect whether one or two points of stimulation are applied simultaneously (two-point discrimination). Point localization and two-point resolution

are highly correlated. Touch-pressure perception approaches a fourfold reduction in males older than 40.[60] The sensory threshold increases the more distal the stimulus application site.[73] Schmidt used microneurography to record from median nerve fibers in 12 subjects ranging from 18 to 64 years old.[187,188,] An age-related decline to flutter and tap (light touch) was reported, which appeared due more to changes in the peripheral sensory units rather than conduction along the afferent nerves. Methods used in research have revised the procedures for assessing spatial acuity. Stevens and Choo, for example, revised the method for two-point discrimination to reduce detection errors. Rather than responding to the application of two distinct points, the subject responds to two lines, each 5 mm in length. Spatial acuity was assessed over 13 regions in 122 male and female

TABLE 5-1
CONDUCTION VELOCITIES, DIAMETERS, AND FUNCTIONS ASSOCIATED WITH VARIOUS PERIPHERAL NERVE FIBERS

ROMAN NUMERAL CLASSIFICATION	DIAMETER	LETTER CLASSIFICATON	CONDUCTION VELOCITY	MYELINATED	TYPES OF STRUCTURES INNERVATED
Ia	12–20 μm	Not Used	70–120 m/sec	Yes	Muscle spindle primary endings
Ib	12–20 μm	Not Used	70–120 m/sec	Yes	Golgi tendon organs
Not used	12–20 μm	α	70–120 m/sec	Yes	Efferents to extrafusal muscle fibers
II	6–12 μm	Aα*	30–70 m/sec	Yes	Other encapsulated endings and endings with accessory structures: Meissner's corpuscles, Merkel endings, muscle spindle secondary endings, and so on
Not used	2–10 μm	γ	10–50 m/sec	Yes	Efferents to intrafusal muscle fibers
III	1–6 μm	Aδ	5–30 m/sec	Yes	Some nociceptors; some cold receptors; some hair receptors
Not used	<3 μm	B	3–15 m/sec	Yes	Preganglionic autonomic efferents
IV	<1.5 μm	C	0.5–2 m/sec	No	Most nociceptors; some cold receptors; warmth receptors; some mechanoreceptors; postganglionic autonomic efferents

From Nolte J: *The Human Brain: An Introduction to Its Functional Anatomy*, ed 2. St Louis, Mosby, 1988.
*Some afferents in nonmuscle nerves, particularly joint afferents, range up to 17 μm in diameter. Some investigators refer to these larger fibers, in the 12–17 μm range, as Aα and call those in the 6–12 mm range Aβ. Others refer to all nonmuscle afferents larger than 6 mm as Aα.

subjects between 8 and 87 years of age. An age-related decline in acuity in males and females characterized all regions; however, the hands and feet demonstrated the greatest decline compared with more central regions, including the lips and tongue. Compared with the younger subjects, the older subjects demonstrated a 400% deterioration in spatial acuity in the great toe and 130% decrease in the fingertip. Stereognosis and graphesthesia usually remain intact with aging. Although an increase in the thresholds for light touch and pinprick has been reported from laboratory investigations, similar loss is not reported consistently in clinical studies. Two possibilities may explain the discrepancy between laboratory and clinical results: (1) the loss of touch is not a functional loss, and (2) clinical testing is not sensitive enough to detect a significant loss. No data exist to support either explanation at this time.

Cutaneous threshold for vibration is more affected in the lower extremities than the upper extremities.[114,136] Diminished or lost vibratory sensation in the lower extremities has been reported to be present in 10% of individuals at age 60 and in approximately 50% of individuals beyond the age of 75.[89]

Cutaneous pain threshold increases with age, but limited research exists on age-related changes in pain sensitivity and perception and the results are ambiguous.[38] Research studies suggest an age-related increase in thresholds to thermal pain but no age-related change in pain threshold when electrical stimulation is used to produce pain. There is some indication that the changes in thermal pain threshold may be related to central rather than peripheral mechanisms, i.e., the central processing of pain information may be reduced in the older person. A recent investigation suggests that there is a selective age-related change in Aδ mediated pain and not in

C-fiber–mediated pain. The Aδ fibers are believed to mediate the pain associated with early warning that is sharp and pricking in nature while the C fibers have been implicated in the pain that is often described as dull, burning, or aching and results in protective behaviors. This finding is consistent with the anatomical changes previously described in the age-related changes in myelinated fibers.

Increased thresholds to thermal sensitivity, i.e., temperature detection rather than painful thermal detection, have been reported in laboratory testing, but clinical testing has not indicated an age-related functional decline in thermal modalities. It is not uncommon, however, to see an older person wearing a sweater on a hot summer day. The clinician must remember that successful ability to detect non-painful thermal stimuli applied to the skin does not assess the thermoregulation of the older person.[232] Thermoregulation, or the ability to maintain the body's core temperature in the range of 99.0° to 99.6° F, is centrally mediated and therefore affected by aging.

Proprioception has undergone relatively little study in the aging population, and the results are controversial. Perception of passive motion in the metacarpophalangeal and metatarsophalangeal joints was reported to be similar in young and older subjects.[89] Although older subjects detected motion less well at low frequencies of movement, no major decline was reported in joint motion sensation. Similarly, impairment of proprioception rarely occurred in a neurological screening of a sample of subjects ranging from 67 to 87 years old.[12] However, passive movement thresholds were reported to be twice as high for the hip, knee, and ankle with no change in upper extremity perception in subjects older than 50 compared with subjects younger than 40.[115] Skinner and colleagues examined joint position sense of the knee in

29 subjects ranging in age from 20 to 82 years.[193] Both the abilities to reproduce passive knee position and to detect motion were assessed. Joint position sense deteriorated with increasing age as measured by both tests. A more recent study compared the subjects' perception of a passively positioned knee angle using a visual analogue scale to the actual angle and reported an age-related decline in position sense.[10] The perception was reported to increase by 40% by applying an elastic bandage around the knee. The research to date on position sense suggests that age-related loss of position sense may be joint sensitive.

Potvin and colleagues assessed neurological status on 61 right-hand–dominant men ranging from 20 to 80 years old.[171] One hundred and thirty-eight tests were used to measure cognition, vision, strength, steadiness, reactions, speed, coordination, fatigue, gait, station, sensation, and tasks of daily living. Tests were excluded if reliability was not demonstrated. Age-related linear decreases were reported for many neurological functions. The declines throughout the age span varied from less than 10% to more than 90% depending on the function. Larger losses of function were observed on the dominant body side.

For the upper and lower extremities, vibratory sensibility showed the greatest decline. The greatest vibratory loss was reported in the toes and ankle. Vibratory loss in the toes and the ankle was also the variable most highly correlated with aging, i.e., the oldest subjects demonstrated the poorest ability to detect a vibratory stimulus. Touch of face and upper arm, two-point discrimination, and position sense in upper and lower limbs showed no variance with age. Since the actual testing procedures were not described, it is difficult to compare the results of this study with other research findings. This study serves as a background for additional research since the results address the integrity of the sensorimotor system in a large sample of subjects.

Summary: Sensory Systems

There remains a paucity of data to describe age-related changes in somatosensory sensation. The literature is not conclusive because samples remain small, the oldest subjects in some studies are only 65 years old, different modalities of sensation are not studied in the same population, and protocols differ. Very little attention has been paid to the age-related changes in skin, which could also affect the older person's ability to detect a stimulus without directly altering the peripheral receptor or the afferent pathway.[191] Another important deficit in the literature to date is that integrity of one sensation is not studied throughout the body. It is common, for example, to study change in sensation in the knee alone rather than to report changes in proprioception throughout multiple major joints of the body. This research approach makes it difficult to summarize age-related changes in sensation that occur throughout the body. Some investigators have used very sophisticated laboratory techniques to document changes in sensation, but the results have not been supported by investigators using standard clinical neurological screening techniques. Caution must be exercised in generalizing findings about sensory changes reported in one body region to the whole body or changes reported in one study to the population of healthy older individuals.

Which portion of the sensory system is primarily responsible for changes in sensation remains unclear. Since age-related cutaneous deficits are more often reported in the lower extremities than the upper extremities, age-related changes in the long afferent pathways are likely to play some role in the sensory changes. The numbers of peripheral receptors decrease and there is a loss of 5% to 8% of nerve fibers per decade after age 40.[182] An increasing number of abnormalities in myelination are reported with increasing age; longer fibers and larger fibers are most affected. A progressive slowing of maximal sensory and motor conduction velocities at a yearly rate of 0.12 to 0.16 m/s has been proposed, and conduction along central afferent pathways to the cerebral cortex is prolonged. It appears that the relatively small changes in the conduction velocity along peripheral afferent fibers do not contribute significantly to loss of sensory perception. The combined loss of peripheral receptors, changes in central afferent pathways, and changes in central processing sites are more likely to be responsible for observed age-related changes in behavior.

The consistent findings across studies are that sensation in the lower extremity appears more affected by aging than the upper extremity and that vibratory sensation is consistently reported to decline with age. Since the integrity of each sensory system is most often tested under static conditions rather than during functional behavior, it is very difficult to predict whether seemingly small changes in separate systems will aggregate to produce a profound loss during the execution of a task. Such an assumption needs to be tested under carefully controlled conditions.

A review of a study by Waite and colleagues highlights the issues raised in this section.[221a] Standardized neurological examinations were completed on 537 community-dwelling men and women 75 or older. The physical examination included a standardized assessment of the various neurological signs scored on a 4-point scale. Their study included a subgroup of 154 persons without diagnoses of stroke, dementia, cognitive impairment, gait slowing, gait ataxia, and Parkinsonism. The only significant correlations with age in this group were impaired vibration sense in the thumbs and gait instability. None of the other classical clinical neurological signs were significantly changed. Therefore, it may not be aging, per se, that accounts for changes in neurological signs but rather the neurodegenerative syndromes that accompany aging. Clinical and functional significance of the effects of age-related sensory changes on motor performance clearly remain a rich area for future research.

NEUROMUSCULAR FUNCTION WITH AGING

It is difficult to focus on changes in movement control without considering changes in the function of the muscle or the activity level of the individual. This section focuses on the integrity of the neuromuscular apparatus with aging: changes in the rate or quality of movement and the effect of physical activity on muscle are addressed in a subsequent section of this chapter and in other chapters. The *motor unit* (*MU*) is defined as the single alpha motoneuron and all the muscle fibers it innervates. It is therefore important to examine changes in the muscle, the neuromuscular junction, and the efferent neuron to completely discuss changes with aging. A commonly reported clinical finding is that older individuals demonstrate decreased strength when compared with younger individuals.[29,41,149,217] *Strength* has been defined operationally in a number of ways. For the purpose of this chapter, strength is defined as some measure of the muscle's force-producing capability such as torque, work, or force. Research related to age-related decreases in voluntary muscle strength suggests that healthy persons in their seventh and eight decades are weaker than young adults by an average of 20% to 40% during isometric and concentric testing of the knee extensors and that those older than 80 show reductions of greater than 50%.[179] What is the reason for such a decline in force-producing capability with age? This section examines changes at the motor neuron level, incorporates effects at the neuromuscular junction and in skeletal muscle, and finally discusses effects on spinal segmental pathways.

Muscle and Muscular Strength

Among the earliest age-related observations of altered muscular strength and function are declines in both isometric and dynamic strength, beginning with the 50- to 59-year age interval.[118] Although decreases in muscle girth are not always readily apparent, biopsy data demonstrate significant loss of type II muscle fibers, coupled with connective tissue infiltration of the muscle. Quadriceps muscle performance assessed either as isometric force; dynamic (isovelocity) peak torque at 30, 60, 120 and 180°/sec; or as maximal extension velocity (MEV) can be significantly predicted through stepwise regression analysis by three independent variables: chronological age, fat-free soft tissue mass, and type II fiber area. Importantly, even without the factor of type II fiber area, a strong correlation has been demonstrated between age and muscular strength. Declines in strength range between 24% and 36% depending on the aspect of muscular performance assessed. Subsequent studies concur with Larsson's early findings with acceptable variability between muscles, genders, and methods. It is significant that isometric and dynamic strength appear to decline similarly[178] and that decline in the rate of tension development can be accounted for by the loss of fast-twitch muscle.[41]

Since Larsson's seminal observations, interest in muscle performance with aging has remained keen, producing elaboration on his early findings (see Porter, Vandervoort, and Lexell, 1995 for a recent review).[171] Recent data obtained from autopsy specimens concur with this now-accepted body of data and reveal more complex changes in fiber distributions with age.[123] Significant grouping or "clumping" of muscle fibers attributed to a given motor unit is evidenced.

This clumping disrupts the mosaic, or heterogeneous, distribution of types I and II fibers and their respective motor units across a muscle's cross-sectional area. The phenomenon of enclosed muscle fibers, evidenced as a high proportion of fibers surrounded completely by fibers with like histochemical properties, resembles the collateral reinnervation process that occurs after peripheral nerve injury or poliomyelitis.[135,209] Thus, grouping of muscle fibers in aging is considered to be direct evidence of a neurogenic process with the degree of enclosure correlating to the degree of denervation and reinnervation a muscle has sustained. Once the reinnervation capacity of the muscle has been sufficiently diminished so that fibers are permanently denervated, the muscle fiber is lost and the tissue volume becomes replaced by fat and fibrous tissue.

The degree of atrophy does not fully account for the observed loss of strength, an observation suggesting that factors other than simple loss of tissue mass are involved. A wide range of morphological changes within both types I and II fibers have been reported. Changes have been reported in mitochondria, sarcoplasmic reticulum, and the transverse tubular system.[79,214] The physiological effects of these changes are not known but have been suggested to be coupled with an impaired activation of the myofibrils.[79] Muscle satellite cells that transform into myoblasts may also be metabolically less active, and therefore the aged muscle may not be able to respond to injury as well as young muscle. Only modest decreases in high-energy metabolites (ADP, ATP, and phosphocreatine) have been reported in the aged muscle.[142] Other enzymes necessary for glycolysis are reduced, however, suggesting a specific disturbance in cytoplasmic glycolysis and gluconeogeneses.[148] Patterns of fatty acid metabolism appear unchanged in the aged.[210]

Whereas electrophysiological[37] and histological[77] studies support a preferential type II atrophy with aging, results from studies that use histochemistry have produced conflicting data. A common histochemical technique is staining muscle biopsies for actomyosin myofibrillar ATPase because type I and type II fibers contain different ATPases.[26] Larssen reported an age-related decrease in the relative proportion of type II fibers,[118] but other investigators have not confirmed these findings with histochemical techniques.[4,63] The myosin heavy chain composition (MHC) of a fiber determines its contractile characteristics, and it is MHC that reacts with ATPase stain to yield a muscle fiber type.[49] Recent work suggests that the conflict among investigators using histochemical techniques may be because older fibers are in transition from one type to another and that the transition is undetected by ATPase stain. For example, examination of MHC within single fibers suggests that older subjects have a higher number of single fibers that contain two forms of MHC, types I and IIa, within one fiber than is seen in the younger subjects.[110]

Although muscular strength may decline with aging, it is notable that the relationship between strength and muscle cross-sectional area (CSA) is not direct.[173] Discrepancies between CSA and strength can be as large as 15% in the quadriceps.[178] The ratio of strength/CSA has been reported as 30% lower in aged versus young adults.[30] The significance of differential loss of motor unit/muscle fiber types and concomitant changes in muscle tissue composition is in the contractile or force-generating capacity of the muscle that appears to be altered by the remodeling that accompanies aging. However, work performed by Frontera and co-workers that initially indicated significant age-related differences in strength of the elbow and knee extensors and flexors (as assessed by isovelocity testing) demonstrated minimal to no differences between young and older individuals once corrections were made for diminished muscle mass with age.[69] The corpus of work performed on muscle performance and muscle morphology has thus led to the conclusion that declines in muscular strength are primarily due to losses in muscle mass.[178] The loss of the mosaic or interdigitated distribution of motor units and muscle fibers may, however, have a qualitative effect on force development and smooth force modulation.

Motor Neurons Are Lost with Aging

As early as the third decade of life, anterior horn cells in the spinal cord demonstrate significant accumulation of lipofuscin.[111] By the fifth decade, loss of anterior horn cells (α-motor neurons) begins, and by age 60 loss of these neurons can be as high as 50%.[37,111] In conjunction with motor neuron (MN) loss are notable changes in the electrophysiological properties of the motor unit. The significance of MN and MU loss lies in their role to generate and modulate muscular force through recruitment of MUs and rate coding of already active MUs.[39,84]

However, the literature presents controversy related to which neurons are lost. A selective loss of large anterior horn cells that subserve the largest motor units has been reported in lumbar ventral roots.[179] However, a different investigation indicated that the total number of neurons in the whole ventral horn decreased significantly with aging but the loss of small neurons, considered to be interneurons, was predominant while medium-sized and large neurons were spared.[205] Axonal counts reveal a significant decrease in both anterior and posterior roots beginning after age 30. By age 89, a 32% reduction in anterior root axons has been reported.[59] The reduction includes both large and small myelinated fibers. The remaining axons demonstrate demyelination and remyelination. The results of these studies emphasize the need for more extensive research in the ventral horn to characterize age-related change. The use of small samples over a wide age range, i.e., 14 to 100, without simultaneous measurement of morphology and function have failed to address the issue completely.

Peripheral Structures

With aging, peripheral nerves demonstrate a progressive reduction in myelinated fibers, most notably in the largest diameter fibers.[111] Ventral roots appear to be more affected than dorsal roots and lumbosacral segments more than cer-

vical segments. Interestingly, while the epineurial and perineurial sheaths thicken, the endoneurial sheath demonstrates fibrosis due to an increased presence of collagen. The microcirculation of peripheral nerve is particularly vulnerable to aging, and atherosclerosis has been suggested as a mechanism. Accordingly, there appears to be a direct relationship between dysfunction of the vasa nervosum and the loss of myelinated fibers.

Peripheral nerve motor conduction velocities decrease progressively with advancing age.[97] Changes in motor nerve conduction velocity (MNCV), an average of 9% in a population of apparently healthy elders, are suggestive of a segmental demyelinating process. In the ulnar nerve, a reduction of 1 $m \cdot s^{-1}$ per decade from age 20 to 55 and 3 $m \cdot s^{-1}$ per decade thereafter has been reported.[31] Impairments in the integrity of myelin and consequent function of myelinated structures as previously discussed more thoroughly are consistent with the global mechanisms of deterioration throughout the CNS and consequent deterioration in communication between CNS structures. However, such slowing may not be as significant as the other age-related changes in the muscle.

The neuromuscular junction (NMJ) also demonstrates degeneration with aging[6,111] beginning as early as the third decade. Fragmentation and degeneration are prevalent in the endplate region, with an increase noted in the number of preterminal axons. In middle age (~50-59 year interval), motor neurons appear to adjust for small losses by sprouting and adding new synaptic sites; however, this compensatory ability declines with age. In old age, neuromuscular junctions appear notably deteriorated, or dismantled.[5] Alignment of presynaptic and postsynaptic elements of the NMJ becomes progressively disrupted as these structures constantly remodel through neuron-target interaction. It is quite noteworthy that changes in the integrity of the NMJ occur well in advance of loss of motor neurons, motor units, or muscle fibers and therefore reflect one of the critical mechanisms that underlie age-related change in neuromuscular system function. In this light it is especially interesting that human laryngeal neuromuscular junction demonstrates little, if any, age-related change between ages 4 and 95.[111] Whether preservation of neuromuscular integrity in this particular structure is preserved due to activity or is somehow attributable to parent innervation is unclear, but it remains an interesting question.

Synaptic transmission is obviously affected by impaired NMJ integrity; by late age many synaptic transmissions are subthreshold for activating muscle fiber contraction. Interestingly, NMJ remodeling appears to reflect the degenerative state of the postsynaptic muscle fiber. It is the case that interaction of presynaptic and postsynaptic structures are necessary for synaptic maintenance—an observation that stresses the importance of trophic factors in maintenance of integrity of neural transmission. Muscle-derived trophic factors acting on MNs appear to affect nerve endings in muscle, whereas MN-derived trophic factors appear to play an important role in the maintenance of muscle fibers. The role of reciprocal influences between nerve and muscle appears particularly significant in the context of age-related change.[138]

Sensory nerve conduction (NCV) appears to deteriorate in advance of motor nerve conduction and is manifest as early as ages 30 to 50. In both motor and sensory domains, NCV decreases and action potential amplitudes diminish. The net result of peripheral nervous decline includes elevated thresholds to all modalities of sensation, diminished tendon jerk reflexes (monosynaptic) in a distal-to-proximal pattern, and moderate progressive delays of motor nerve conduction.[111]

The Motor Unit

Age-related loss of motor neurons, previously discussed, results in significant effects at the level of the motor unit.[37,135] Initially, a debate raged regarding whether the mechanism underlying change at the motor unit level is myopathic or neuropathic. Since these early findings were published[37] there has grown general agreement that the process is neuropathic with myopathic symptoms following as a secondary sequela.[117] Regression analysis of MU counts demonstrates a linear relationship throughout the sixth decade (50 to 59 years) with considerable variability about the mean and then a dramatic downward trend from the seventh to tenth decades.[37,135] Muscular function declines beginning in the sixth decade and is accompanied by considerable remodeling in the peripheral musculature.

Another salient characteristic of age-related change in the motor unit is a predominance of slow-twitch muscle fibers or type I motor units. It was previously suggested that neuronal loss may selectively affect the largest α-motoneurons, presumably those innervating type II muscle and comprising high threshold motor units. For some time, the common wisdom suggested that type II fibers are selectively denervated and reinnervated from slow (type I) motor units through collateral sprouting, and evidence exists to support this notion.[179] More recently, however, it has been suggested that the shift toward slower motor unit properties with aging results from de-differentiation between slow- and fast-twitch muscle as a result of lower concentrations of circulating hormones, including thyroid hormone (T_3).[117]

The electrophysiology of the MU demonstrates a significant increase (59%) in the motor unit action potential (MUAP), indicating that the territory of the MU includes more muscle fibers. *Collateral sprouting,* the process wherein muscle fibers orphaned by dying motor neurons are reinnervated by collateral axon fibers from neighboring motor neurons,[107] is highly prevalent with aging[135] and contributes to explanation of both the increased MUAP and to encapsulated muscle fibers or "clumping" of motor unit territories in the muscle. With iterative denervation and reinnervation, individual muscle fibers are progressively "shed" from a motor unit since the neuron is no longer able to provide it metabolic support.[135] Finally, contractile responses are consistent with retention of slow-twitch motor units.[53]

Motor Unit Mechanical Properties

At the level of muscle and the motor unit there are several important adaptations serving to ameliorate the decline of muscular strength that occurs with motor neuron loss. In the older group ($\geq$60 years, ranging to 96 years) from the Campbell, McComas, and Petito survey,[37] the M-response (a measure of excitable muscle mass) declined 53%, whereas the muscular-twitch tension declined only 32% as compared with young subjects. Here, an obvious mismatch is evidenced between apparent potential (CSA) and measured deficit in performance. Furthermore, electrophysiological properties of the MU demonstrated a 45% longer contraction time, a 206% increase in half-relaxation time, and an increase in MU twitch tension that was not directly quantified but clearly evident in the plotted relationship (see Fig. 5-5).[37] Subsequently, similar results have been demonstrated to corroborate these findings.[53,54,218]

Collateral reinnervation of orphaned muscle fibers by remaining motor neurons increases the force response for any given functional unit of activation. According to McComas, "as much as 80% to 90% of motor units can be lost before weakness and atrophy supervene."[135] McComas' statement agrees with that of Perry who routinely finds in post-polio patients upwards of 50% loss of motor units before noticeable muscle weakness can be appreciated.[165] Thus, there appears to be considerable reserve in physiological systems subserving neuromuscular function, and therefore considerable loss can occur before remarkable declines in functional performance can be appreciated.

The average amplitude of the MUAP is 60% greater in aged subjects—reflecting the increased motor unit territories that result from collateral reinnervation. The duration of the action potential is 9% longer—a small, but statistically significant change that serves to prolong the twitch duration and either support the enlarged motor unit territory or extend the muscle active state.[86] Taken together, the typical interpretation of these results is consistent with a shift to slow-twitch muscle fibers and motor unit contractile properties. More insightfully, it is evident that the adaptations in the motor unit all occur in favor of maintaining an optimal tradeoff of force response per unit of active metabolic muscle tissue.

Motor Unit Discharge Properties

With regard to motor unit discharge behavior, there is strong evidence suggesting impaired central drive (the maximal rate of MU discharge) under isometric conditions in older adults.[100,122,162] A tendency toward decreased motor unit rate discharge (MUDR) has been evidenced in submaximal force conditions.[93,194] A substantial decrease is noted, however, in maximal MUDR during maximal effort muscular contractions.[100] Notably the impairment in central drive is substantially greater than that in maximal voluntary force when compared with young adults (39% versus 16%) and is not evidenced unequivocally at 50% of maximal voluntary force. Considerable evidence has been presented in the literature suggesting that MU discharge properties are matched to the mechanical properties of muscle in order to optimize force production.[16,17] Thus, decreased maximal motor unit discharge rates might be easily explained by recalling that mechanical properties of muscle are substantially altered toward slow-twitch characteristics with aging.[150]

Older adult weightlifters appear to maintain central drive, suggesting the importance of physical activity on integrity of neural function.[122] This investigation was, however, performed without comparison with a young control group; therefore, the extent of preservation in central drive cannot be determined on an absolute scale. An additional finding regarding motor unit function with aging is observation of cases of motor unit derecruitment against the order prescribed by Henneman's size principle.[85,98] It is suggested that antagonist co-contraction may explain this unusual observation. Accuracy was required to perform the experimental task, and older adults with fewer motor units may use an alternative strategy to achieve sufficient stability for accurate force production.[98,197]

Impaired central motor unit drive might be directly related to subtle deterioration of cortical function, or conduction. Motor neurons are activated through corticospinal pathways, and the central nervous system coding of force is modulated through the activity of pyramidal cells in cortical areas 4 and 6 by their discharge rate.[62,72] In subsequent investigation, however, Patten and co-workers demonstrated significant increases in MUDR as an early response to strength training in both young and older subjects, with discharge rates matching for both age groups at the second training session.[162] During the remainder of a 6-week training period, however, MUDR returned to baseline in older adults while remaining somewhat elevated in young controls. These adaptations occurred in the face of significant increases in MVC in both groups. This finding has subsequently been replicated in a separate group of subjects and a different muscle group.[99] The obvious question regarding corticomotoneuronal discharge rate is then answered: maximal MUDR is not impaired due to aging. Rather, altered maximal MUDR may serve as a neuromuscular adaptation to optimize the contractile response of muscle.

Spinal Segmental Pathways

The spinal segmental motor system is comprised of numerous reflex pathways integrating peripheral afferent information with descending supraspinal signals. The integrative nature and locus of this aspect of the motor system suggest its response is likely to reflect substantial age-related change. In general, spinal segmental responses dictate the balance of muscular activity in antagonist muscle pairs (co-contraction). A foremost role of the segmental motor system is to compensate the non-linear contractile characteristics of muscle and provide the central nervous system a mechanism through which to regulate muscle stiffness. Segmental reflexes control muscle stiffness over a broad range of muscle

lengths. Co-activation of antagonist muscle pairs, increasing joint stiffness, increases the range over which stiffness can be varied—an important function, given the limited variation in the stiffness of individual muscles[126,155] and the notable alterations in stiffness of muscle and tendon with aging.[2,117]

Spinal segmental pathways have demonstrated their susceptibility to both long- and short-term adaptation, or plasticity, to task-specific training.[64,215,227-229] Importantly, notable alteration in the degree of presynaptic inhibition on spinal segmental pathways has been evidenced,[35,112,144] indicating deterioration in the ability to modulate task-dependent motor output, e.g., development of muscular force and postural responses with aging. Chronic changes in spinal segmental pathways may be responsible for increased demonstration of antagonist muscle co-contraction observed across a broad range of motor activities in older adults.

Summary: Musculoskeletal System

Considerable age-related change has been documented in the neuromuscular system. While at one time, these changes appeared to paint a picture of chronic, progressive decline, current evidence suggests that the majority of age-related changes in neuromuscular function might be viewed as compensatory. This detail is important to the clinician who wishes to understand the biological processes that underlie age-related change in order to plan interventions well-suited to the adaptive potential of the aging neuromuscular system. Age-related change may not be all negative. Rather, it appears to serve a significant role in preserving function in a broad range of systems. Quite pertinent to the interests of the rehabilitative clinician, however, is preservation of muscular control and movement function.

Muscular strength, whether assessed in an isometric or dynamic context, declines after the fifth decade but fails to demonstrate direct correspondence with changes in muscle cross-sectional area. The most salient change is loss of type II, or fast-twitch, muscle fibers coupled with increased prevalence of type I, or slow-twitch, fibers. As early as the fifth decade, anterior horn cells that innervate skeletal muscle die off, and by age 60 their loss can be as great as 50%. It would indeed be elegant if large ventral horn neurons corresponding directly to large motor units with fast-twitch contractile characteristics were preferentially lost; however, current data indicate that neuronal loss involves both small- and large-motor neurons. Accordingly, the notion that fast-twitch fibers are selectively lost has been revised with evidence indicating that instead muscle fiber types undergo dedifferentiation with aging, probably as a result of significant changes in hormonal regulation.

With loss of motor neurons, the morphology of the motor unit and the innervation of skeletal muscle become dramatically altered. Motor neuron loss leaves muscle fibers behind such that orphaned fibers become incorporated into remaining motor units through collateral reinnervation.

This process results in larger motor units that are less heterogeneously distributed throughout the muscle. The mechanical response of aging muscle demonstrates a 32% reduction in twitch force; however, contraction time is increased by 45%, and half-relaxation time is increased by 206%. This significant slowing in the contractile motor unit response maintains the active state for an extended period and prolongs force production. The significant changes in muscle fiber composition in conjunction with alterations in the contractile response and the redistribution of motor unit territories suggest that the transfer of force to the tendon will be conspicuously altered with potential effects on the quality of muscular force production.

Important age-related changes have been observed in subcellular structures affecting both metabolic and regenerative function of muscle. The neuromuscular junction, a highly dynamic structure due to its constant remodeling, demonstrates progressive impairment in alignment of presynaptic and postsynaptic elements. Understandably, synaptic transmission becomes compromised, affecting the responsiveness and potential to activate muscle. Hence the "wisdom" of prolonging the muscle contractile state begins to become evident. Motor unit discharge rates appear to be altered. Although this finding is equivocal at submaximal force levels, it has been demonstrated in several muscles that MU discharge rates are reduced in typical, sedentary elders at maximal force. This finding, however, appears to be further evidence of compensatory change matching MU discharge properties with the altered contractile response of muscle and potentially, too, with altered synaptic transmission. In extremely active individuals and in response to strength training, however, maximal MU discharge rates in elders have been observed to be comparable with those of young individuals. This finding is strong evidence that observed change in neuromuscular function with age results from compensations to promote efficient, optimal muscular function. Finally, changes in segmental pathways are notably altered with aging, affecting the ability to modulate motor activity in response to task demands. Remodeling of these pathways may be triggered by motor neuron loss and may also be responsible for the frequent observation of antagonist muscle co-contraction in elders.

SENSORIMOTOR CHANGES WITH AGING

Paucity of movement is a common observation in old animals and humans.[198,199] The limited movement becomes hesitant and slow. Even when the speed of movement is retained, the initiation of movement is delayed. Sensorimotor integrity has been examined using a variety of protocols including the study of reflexes, the time it takes the subject to respond to and execute a task, and functional performance. Since other chapters in this text address age-related decline in functional activities, this section will focus on studies that have been designed to determine why movement time changes, rather than describing the decline in coordinated movement patterns that accompany aging.

Reflex Testing

Reflex testing is performed to assess the integrity of the sensorimotor pathways without the influence of cognitive processing. The latency of a reflex response can, therefore, be used to assess the integrity of the simplest sensorimotor connection. Investigators who postulate that the Achilles tendon tap elicits a monosynaptic response in the agonist MUs purport to study the simplest sensorimotor connection.

The reflex change most commonly noted with aging is diminution or absence of the Achilles tendon response, which has been reported to occur in 10% of older subjects.[92] Other investigators note only small increases in the latency of the Achilles and patellar tendon reflexes. These latter findings are consistent with the research findings suggesting a small but unremarkable decline in conduction velocity in sensory and motor nerves.[12,183] Comparison between the latency associated with the Achilles tendon reflex and the latency in a known polysynaptic reflex response reveals the same small age-related increase in latency, rather than a longer latency for the polysynaptic response.[27] Such results suggest that the Achilles tendon reflex may be more than a monosynaptic response[33] or that central synapses are preserved in the polysynaptic pathway. If the latter hypothesis is correct, the increased latency in both monosynaptic and polysynaptic reflexes can be attributed to changes in conduction velocity of the afferent and efferent pathways. The lack of significant changes in the integrity of reflexes with aging suggests that other factors must be examined to account for older individuals' slow movement.

The Central Efferent Pathway

Magnetic and electrical stimulation of the motor cortex through the scalp are two recently developed, non-invasive techniques used to study the integrity of motor pathways in the human.[22] Motor evoked potentials (MEPs) are recorded from a muscle contralateral to the stimulated motor cortex. Conduction times can be recorded within the CNS by recording over the spinal cord at the level of the relevant motoneurons. For example, conduction time can be recorded between the cortex and the L4-5 level of the spinal cord, and the MEPs can be recorded from the tibialis anterior. Although data indicating age-related changes in MEPs in the sixth through tenth decades are still unavailable, the MEP technique is mentioned here because preliminary data on age-related changes are exciting. Results from subjects ranging from 19 to 50 years old indicate a trend for decline in central conduction time with age.

Reaction Time

Cited changes in the peripheral systems might account for some slowing in stimulus encoding and execution of movement. Are there changes in central decision, comparison, and response selection as well? In other words, what role does cognition play in producing a slowed movement? Aspects of cognitive processing have been studied using reaction time with the assumption that the time it takes to perform a response reflects the stages of processing involved. *Reaction time (RT)* is defined as the time required to initiate a movement after stimulus presentation. In a simple RT test, the subject knows that a single response is required for the stimulus. Simple RTs have been shown to increase with age.[201] Birren summarized the results from a variety of studies and reported a 20% increase in RT in 60-year-old subjects compared with 20-year-old subjects.[19] However, several investigators have suggested that physically active older subjects have faster RTs than sedentary older individuals.[40,198]

Measurement of RT includes the time for electromechanical transduction from muscle activity to movement. Some investigators have used EMG activity to separate premotor time (PMT) and motor time (MT). *PMT* is defined as the time between stimulus onset to EMG activity, and *MT* is defined as the time from EMG activity to the initiation of the movement. By subdividing reaction times, the assumption is that insight can be gained into the extent to which muscular factors slow performance.

The effect of age on PMT and MT appears dependent on the task involved.[224] Although both PMT and MT are affected by aging, different tasks demonstrate more slowing in PMT or MT. For example, when the subject is merely required to move the hand, the PMT seems particularly affected by age.[222] When the subject is required to move the arm against resistance[191] or to jump,[157] the main slowing is in the MT, which includes the time needed for the muscle contraction. While movements against resistance may increase pain or fatigue and therefore require new compensatory strategies, the results of this research suggest that as age increases there is a progressively slower buildup of muscular contraction when action is required. This change is particularly evident when substantial force has to be exerted either to overcome resistance or to produce a very rapid movement. In a recent review of the effect of exercise on improving PMT and MT, the authors conclude that substantial training does not significantly improve the time necessary to complete a task and suggest that slowness of movement reflects a change in the neural pathways that does not appear to improve significantly with increased physical activity.[161]

A two-choice RT test requires selection between two responses instead of one response in simple RT. The two-choice RT is therefore a more complex task. As movement complexity increases, the RT increases in the older adults.[125,201] Older individuals are more sensitive to small changes in movement complexity than younger individuals and also experience more difficulty when tasks demand both accuracy and speed. Choice of accuracy over speed can lead to problems when a whole body response is required quickly to prevent a fall, for example.

To summarize, premotor and movement times are significantly related to chronological age. Premotor time is slower in older individuals regardless of the task. Motor time appears to depend on the amount of muscle activity required to produce the task, i.e., the higher the required muscle force, the longer the motor time. In both speed of reaction and movement, fastest responses are reported for subjects in their second decade. Consistency of response is greatest in the third decade. Beyond age 60, the variability in premotor and movement times increases greatly compared with the younger subjects' performance.[224] More complicated tasks are more sensitive in indicating age-related decline. Collectively, the results indicate the importance of the CNS when considering the effects of age on sensorimotor capacity.

VOLUNTARY MOVEMENT
Movement Organization
With aging, significant and demonstrable alterations in the organization of movement range from isometric force control tasks to locomotion. Regardless of the goal or constraints, there appear to be some common themes across tasks: slowing of movement and increased co-contraction of paired antagonist muscles. These alterations have been separately attributed to dysfunction of specific central nervous system structures[46] and impaired efficiency of the muscle contractile process.[206,207] Moreover, they are suggestive of the potential need to (re-)learn movement control due to the dramatic age-related alterations in both the neural and biomechanical systems.

Although intuitively increased movement duration might be explained by impaired psychomotor speed, a higher proportion of slow contracting muscle, muscular weakness, deterioration of neural conduction pathways, or some combination of these, older adults are capable of producing movements of comparable velocity and duration as young adults. Rather, it appears to be the temporal structure of movement that is altered with aging.[46] In uniaxial arm movements, older subjects are unable to produce symmetrical bell-shaped velocity profiles typical of normal constrained movements.[28,60] The deceleration phase is significantly longer than the acceleration phase and often clear decomposition of movement is apparent after peak velocity. Hypermetria may also be present at movement endpoint. Further, the parameter of peak velocity/average velocity (V_m/V_{av}) is lower in older subjects and remains lower than in young subjects across multiple amplitudes of movement. Rather than scaling movement on a particular parameter such as V_m/V_{av}, as young subjects do, older adults appear unable to generalize a particular scalar process[46] to different movement conditions. Finally, as has been frequently demonstrated in reaching, gait, and constrained isometric ramp contractions, older adults appear to produce movements of rather similar duration, regardless of movement amplitude.[46,121] In the specific context of gait, a habitual history of sedentary life-style has been directly associated with a narrowing of the range of available gait velocities in older women (60 to 70 years).[121]

On more careful scrutiny of reaching movements, Darling and co-workers concluded that movement trajectories were less accurately controlled in older subjects.[50] Rather than the characteristic tri-phasic burst of EMG between agonist and antagonist muscles,[80] significant tonic antagonist pair co-contraction is demonstrated throughout the movement. With practice, some change is evidenced in the EMG pattern; however, the antagonist burst remains ill-timed, producing phasic co-contraction rather than the reciprocal pattern characteristic of skilled movement.[221] Consequently control of force output is less precisely graded and is accompanied by increased trial-to-trial variability. Significant antagonist muscle pair co-contraction with aging is not only characteristic of arm movements with clear constraints on amplitude and accuracy, but also affects postural tasks,[132] isometric force tasks,[76,197] and gait.[65,120]

Posture and Balance

Among the most serious concerns with advancing age is the fear of falling and sustaining serious injury. Thirty percent of community-dwelling individuals aged 65 or older fall; half of these individuals fall more than once per year.[174] Between 1% and 5% of these falls result in fractures, most commonly of the hip.[88] More significant, however, is the loss of self-efficacy associated with falling because fear of falling can typically cause an elder to self-limit activities, initiating a downward spiral of physical activity and physical abilities.[212,213] Critical to prevention of falling are the contributions of physiological systems subserving the functions of balance and postural control.

The focus thus far has been on involuntary and voluntary movement of the moving limb. Since this review has demonstrated changes in the CNS, including loss of neurons, impaired cerebral metabolism, and altered neurotransmitter activity, one may speculate that such changes disrupt the activation of postural responses to unexpected motion.[131] The literature suggests that there are age-related changes in the control of spontaneous postural sway, suggesting an increase in the amount of correction activity required to maintain stability. Is there evidence that aging affects trunk and interlimb coordination? For example, is the ability to produce preparatory postural adjustments before the onset of voluntary movement altered with increased age? Older subjects have been reported to fail to produce the normal postural adjustments before performing a voluntary movement.[92,198] For example, when asked to perform a unilateral knee flexion during standing, the lack of necessary postural adjustments in trunk and contralateral limb musculature leads to a loss of balance.[133] Loss of balance is increased when the subjects are asked to make the movements more rapidly. Such data suggest a change in coordination of movement and posture that is age-related. Moreover, preliminary evidence suggests that in the older person lateral stability is more affected than stability in the sagittal plane. It is tempting to speculate that these changes correlate with age-related impairment in the vestibular system, hip proprioception,

and integrity of sensation from the plantar surface of the foot as previously discussed in the context of age-related sensory changes.[131] However, such speculation remains to be grounded in sound research associating impairments in sensory system function with behavioral outcomes at the level of movement.

The sensitivity of balance/postural control to impairment with aging lies in its multi-system nature. A comprehensive description of the task of balancing includes detection of body motion by the sensory systems, integration of this sensory information by the central nervous system, and finally execution of appropriate motor responses.[153] Accordingly, at least three major physiological systems and their subcomponents contribute to balance: sensory-perceptual, central integrative, and neuromusculoskeletal.[92,151]

Sensory-Perceptual Component

Control of posture and balance is governed by inputs from three systems: visual, vestibular, and proprioceptive—each of which is referenced to a separate external coordinate system and none of which senses the body's center of gravity directly.[132,154] Three sensory contributions afford redundancy in the perceptual task, allowing a margin for errors endemic to the proprioceptive and visual systems and for response latencies of the vestibular system.[153] Proprioception, which provides information relative to support surface conditions, is in normal, healthy populations considered the dominant sensory guide to balance, followed by vision and finally vestibular inputs.[230] With aging, however, declines in proprioception are common due to peripheral neuropathic processes typical of aging and to declines in joint range of motion that limit sensory contributions from joint receptors.[111,231] With diminished proprioceptive capacities, it is typical for the elderly subject to become reliant on vision. Vision, which senses body position relative to the surrounding environment, is not only quite error prone, but a slow perceptual system at best, demonstrating significant deterioration with age.[201] Elders are most impaired in their perception of low frequency visual phenomena, e.g., slowly moving targets and spatial sensitivity. It is significant then that postural control and locomotion depend on low-frequency visual information.[230] Finally, function in the vestibular system, which senses body position relative to the individual's inertial-gravitational reference, is quite variable with aging.[200,230] The importance of vestibular contributions to posture and balance is to resolve sensory conflicts when one or more systems signal erroneous information.

Central Integrative Component

As should be evident, contributions from multiple sensory systems require integrative action of the central nervous system to choose and weigh correct versus incorrect perceptual information. This process of sorting out the varied sensory inputs has been termed by Nashner[152] "sensory organization," and the environmental situation in which the balance task occurs—e.g., perturbation while standing, slip or trip, etc.—the "sensory context."[130] Either term is suggestive of a contextually dependent[216] and perhaps self-organizing[103,192] process within the CNS simplifying the integrative process and speeding the onset of motor response.

As previously discussed, reaction times (motor responses) can be delayed with aging and are slowed more remarkably as the complexity of the situation increases.[124,223] Evaluation with the sensory organization component of the dynamic posturography test has evidenced elders responding at normal or very near normal levels for all conditions except the visual conflict. When presented with both inaccurate proprioceptive and visual information, the integrative task is to suppress the inappropriate perceptual information, rely on appropriate vestibular guides to orientation, and maintain standing posture. Approximately 40% of elderly individuals fall in the visual conflict condition. Impaired performance in this task has been attributed to physiological slowing at the highest level of motor control.[92] A modicum of evidence documenting improvements in postural control under challenging sensory contexts made through training suggests adaptive potential in the aging nervous system.[94,163]

Neuromusculoskeletal Component

The primary task of the motor effector system is to maintain the body's center of gravity (CG) within its base of support, whether the context of the task involves sitting, standing, or locomotion and, if perturbed, to restore the CG within the base of support. In standing conditions the motor responses subserving posture and balance have been called *muscle synergies*,[153] implying a functional organization of musculoskeletal components organized to minimize the on-line neural decision making. Postural adjustments are not thought of as hard-wired, stereotyped reflex responses, but as behavioral responses that are functionally adaptive in a context-specific mode.[91,216]

Effective postural responses require appropriate timing or response latency to the given task, scaling of the particular response amplitude, and suitable intersegmental coordination to produce an effective kinematic pattern for maintenance or restoration of posture.[92] In standing conditions, older subjects demonstrate increased sway or CG displacement; however, the increased magnitude of sway magnitude does not appear to place the elder directly at risk for injury. In fact, the relationship between increased sway magnitude and falling is unclear because the tendency to fall increases more distinctly with chronological age.[76] Rather, in elders, postural responses to perturbation or to trips are manifest too late or are of insufficient magnitude to enable regaining balance.[231] The scaling and intersegmental coordination of postural responses are also frequently disrupted, leading to ineffective strategies that are often destabilizing rather than restorative.[92]

Locomotion and Gait

The phenomenon of "slowing down" often observed in older individuals has also been attributed to the aging process. Gait speed is reported to decline 1% to 2% per decade for individuals younger than 62 years and 16% per decade for individuals aged 63 years and older.[87] Common changes in gait associated with aging include a slower speed of walking, decreased step length, and increased time spent in double support.[149] The causal relationship between the age-related changes in walking and the age-related changes in the neuromusculoskeletal system remain unknown at this time. For example, a diminished step length may relate to an age-related diminished pelvic rotation, decreased knee extension at heel strike, diminished plantar flexion at toe-off, or a combination of these and the myriad other factors reviewed in this chapter. It is therefore not possible to say that age-related changes in the basal ganglia, cerebellum, or spinal cord; slowed reaction times; or diminished muscle function lead to a shortened step length and a slower walking speed. At this time, we are only able to provide careful descriptions of the changes in performance that accompany aging and through continued research proceed toward the goal of associating changes at the cellular and system levels with those in observed behavior.

Functional Movement

There is a significant gap in understanding between laboratory studies of human movement and outcome studies that report an older person's ability to perform activities of daily living (ADLs). Whereas laboratory studies attempt to quantify movement parameters and provide a comprehensive description of the quality of movement and mechanisms that may be interacting to produce the movement, outcome studies focus on the person's ability to complete a task successfully without regard to the quality of the movement. The Potvin study cited previously emphasizes this gap in knowledge.[171]

In Potvin's study, neurological status was assessed in 61 men ranging in age from 20 to 80 years. In addition to examining sensory status, tests of sensorimotor status and ADL were examined. Simple reaction times for the upper and lower extremities showed significant age-related effects. In examining movement using quasi-laboratory conditions, the greatest age-related declines in function in the upper extremity were in hand-force steadiness and speed of hand-arm movements. The most difficult task involving the lower extremities was standing on one leg and maintaining balance with the eyes closed. Although the RT demonstrated age-related effects, the declines were far less than those reported for hand-force control and one-legged standing—two tasks in which an age-related decline of at least 50% was observed. Average loss of function for 10 ADL tasks was 30%. The most age-sensitive ADL tasks were donning a shirt and cutting with a knife.

Therefore, while well-controlled laboratory studies provide insight into the mechanisms responsible for age-related decline in specific movements, the results may not reflect the severity of deterioration in functional movement. When subjects are observed functioning under more natural conditions, additional factors may increase the complexity of the task and result in more significant declines in function. Evidence to support the need to consider the interaction of the neural and muscular systems is exemplified in a study conducted by Kinoshita and Francis.[107a] The control of precision grip force during lifting and holding objects with slippery and nonslippery surface textures was compared in young, older (69 to 79 years), and very old (80 to 93 years) subjects. The very old subjects held on to the object longer, held the objects with more force, and demonstrated more fluctuations in grip force compared with the younger subjects. The authors concluded that aging affects the programmed force production capacity by causing alterations in the preparatory force action during the lifting task, adjustments in the grip force during the holding task, and increases in the variability of performance. These declines in performance of functional movement suggest that age-related changes in skin properties, cutaneous sensibility functions, and central nervous system function are factors that contribute significantly to force production and must be considered in addition to the age-related changes in the properties of the muscle, changes in neuromuscular control, and alterations in the neural organization of movement.

ADAPTATION

The dictionary defines *plasticity* as the capacity to change. However, the term has come to have very specific meaning in the scientific literature. Neuroscientists use the term plasticity to explain structural or physiological change in the CNS. Plasticity is demonstrated, for example, by morphological evidence that suggests an altered neural organization or by a change in the efficiency of a synapse. Therefore, plasticity can be defined as a response of neurons to perturbations in their local environment.[44] Plasticity is viewed as an "adaptive" response to a perturbation. Although the changes may be the nervous system's attempt to adapt, it is not clear whether the changes in neural networks correlate with functional adaptation.

The term *mutability*, rather than plasticity, is often used to describe the muscle fiber's ability to change in response to a new demand. The clinician does not, therefore, observe plasticity or mutability. Rather, the clinician observes the behavioral consequences of plasticity that may result from the sparing of function, substitution of function, or recovery of some lost function. Despite the lack of correlation between cellular and functional changes, in the aged individual it is important to know whether the nerve and muscle possess the ability to respond to perturbation.

Plasticity

Perturbation of a neuron may be in the chemical composition of the neuron's immediate surrounding, its afferent supply, its targets, or in its neighboring neurons and glia. The plastic responses to such perturbations may include alteration in dendritic or axonal morphology, synapses, receptors, or metabolism.[44]

Dendrites account for as much as 95% of the receptor surface, which allows for contact with other neurons.[185]

Dendrites are important in the neuron's ability to receive and process information. Most studies of the aged nervous system have focused on the cerebral cortex, hippocampus, and olfactory bulb. Little information exists about the cerebellum, brainstem, and spinal cord. Therefore, any evidence presented here cannot be generalized to changes in the entire nervous system. As stated earlier a loss of synapses, dendritic branches, and dendritic spines occurs with age. There is also evidence in the human brain of an age-related increase in the number of dendritic branches and dendritic spines in the aging brain.[32,48] The presence of increased dendritic growth of remaining neurons, coupled with the loss of other neurons, suggests that the dendritic growth is a compensatory response to the death of neighboring neurons. The mechanism to account for the proliferation of dendrites is speculative. One theory is that the glial cells, particularly the astrocytes, in the CNS and the Schwann cells in the PNS serve as sources of a trophic factor.[9] Another possibility in the CNS is that norepinephrine (NE) serves as a trophic (nourishing) system.[74] The relationship between the structural changes in the dendrites and changes in neurochemistry has not been established at this time.

New synapses (synaptogenesis) have been demonstrated to form in the adult brain.[48] In the CNS, partial denervation results in sprouting by the remaining fibers. Sprouting continues to be demonstrated in the aging animal brain, but the rate and magnitude of sprouting appear to decline. It is assumed that sprouting can occur in the aging human brain and can be adaptive or maladaptive. The return or maintenance of function depends on which connections are formed. The relationship between sprouting and functional ability in the human has also not been established.

The factors that accelerate the plastic changes include the environment and diet. There is little evidence in the human to suggest a cause-and-effect relationship among these factors. Research in aged animals suggests that dendritic spine density increases with an enriched environment.[45] There is some evidence, although it is controversial, to suggest that dietary supplements that include the precursors for acetylcholine may delay memory loss in older human subjects.[48] Although the research on human plasticity is scant, there are early indications that plasticity is possible in the aging human and that the clinician may be able to potentiate this process through activities performed in the clinical environment.

Mutability

The possibility of preventing age-related decline in motor unit function is theoretically greater than for age-related changes in other tissues. This assumption is justified because of the well-documented ability of muscle to respond to physiological stimulation by improving its functional capacity and by correcting certain types of structural and chemical damage. In response to appropriate stimuli, muscle fibers can enlarge several-fold, as well as increase oxidative capacity. Are age-related functional changes in part a result of disuse? Can activity prevent or reverse these regressive changes? Aging is associated with an evolving reduction of physical activity, and deconditioning occurs fairly rapidly.[11] Other chapters address the literature that suggests that the older individual is capable of regaining strength.

Larsson studied the effect of physical training on vastus medialis morphology in 18 sedentary males ranging in age from 22 to 65 years.[118] Subjects were involved in a 60- to 80-minute strength training program two times per week for 15 weeks. Muscle biopsies were taken and strength measurement was performed before and after the training period. Maximal isometric and dynamic torque were evaluated using an isokinetic device. Age-related muscle fiber atrophy seen before training diminished after the training period because of an increase in fiber size in older subjects. The increase in fiber size was more marked in the older subjects. Increased torque was noted in all subjects, but the training effect was more marked in older subjects. Such data suggest that older muscle is mutable. However, the oldest subject was only 65 years old.

Knee extension and elbow flexion have also been studied in young and elderly individuals[113]: seven sedentary young subjects who were an average of 28 years old and 26 older subjects who were an average of 69 years old. The older subjects were subdivided into four groups: sedentary, swimmers, runners, and strength-trained individuals. The older physically active subjects had trained an average of 15 years, three times per week. Maximal isometric torque for knee extension was 44% lower and elbow flexion was 32% lower in the sedentary elders compared with the young subjects. Speed of movement was 20% and 26% slower in the knee and arm movement, respectively, in the sedentary elders compared with the young subjects. Cross-sectional area for the vastus lateralis and biceps brachii was reduced, and a preferential type II atrophy was demonstrated for the vastus lateralis and the biceps brachii. The only active older group who did not show age-related decline were the strength-trained older men who demonstrated no significant difference on any of the variables tested when compared with the sedentary young subjects. This study suggests that muscle mutability may be retained in certain muscles in some older individuals through the age of 69 and that retention may be dependent on intensity and specificity of physical activity, e.g., strength training in this case, rather than general conditioning. The relationship between muscle fiber types and the quality or quantity of functional performance was not addressed in this study. Since the sample size for this study was small and the older subjects were younger than 70 years old, additional work is necessary to generalize these findings.

In his review of the literature of how physiological systems change with exercise, Buskirk concludes that a general adaptation occurs with exercise.[34] Although the adaptation is age-dependent, he suggests that regular exercise retards the downward trends in systems of the body that are commonly associated with aging. The two studies previously cited support the hypothesis that muscle retains mutability with age.

Changes in this retention need to be studied within active, sedentary individuals over time.

SUMMARY

This chapter has presented material that highlights age-related changes throughout the sensorimotor system. Based on the knowledge of various pathologies and disease processes, the clinician can then develop a more comprehensive view and more appropriate expectations for the course of clinical recovery in the older adult. With increasing evidence that encroachment of subtle disease and pathology are not tantamount to aging, it has become essential to revisit our cultural expectation of normal aging. Accordingly, investigators of human subjects and consumers of the research literature reporting findings obtained from human subjects must screen for subtle pathology in the "normal" or "healthy" older individual. A body of research is now accumulating with evidence that behavioral outcomes differ significantly between "usual" and "successful" elders.

Although the majority of investigators agree that reported nervous system or muscle changes are a natural part of the aging process, there remains no consensus regarding the rate of age-related change within or across systems, nor regarding what factors are primary in accelerating or retarding the aging process. Many investigations have selected a particular region of the brain, a specific sensation, or a particular body region for study. It is important to recognize this limitation and not generalize findings from one region to the whole body. Where possible, studies have been cited that correlate age-related function in an anatomical or physiological substrate with behavioral function. Little research has been performed in this regard, thus we remain without clear evidence demonstrating the relationship between age-related change in neuromusculoskeletal function and age-related movement performance. Regardless of one's preferred model of motor control, age-related changes in nervous system and musculoskeletal function present a complex interaction requiring additional research.

Recent evidence across domains of neuroscience, physiology, and biology indicate that age-related decline of neural function is non-linear and may be attributed to more subtle mechanisms than loss of cortical neurons. The ability of nuclei and association areas within the brain to communicate becomes compromised due to impaired cellular integrity, loss of dendritic extent, and deterioration of myelinated structures. At the periphery of the motor system, muscle undergoes dramatic changes including loss of fast-twitch fibers and infiltration with connective tissue. Tendon connective tissue also remodels, leaving tissues in the muscle-tendon system with significantly increased stiffness. Motor neurons are lost from the spinal cord ventral horn at a relatively linear rate after age 60.

Current thinking holds that altered motor behavior demonstrated with aging may reflect compensations on the part of the neural control system for physiological alterations across multiple systems, as have been previously described. Many direct adaptations may occur in the segmental motor system; however, there is evidence of compensations made throughout the neuraxis. An important compensation is the increase in motor unit territory due to collateral reinnervation from remaining motor neurons. Significant additional changes may include decreased maximal motor unit discharge rates in order to match mechanical properties of remodeled muscle and to prevent synchronization of motor unit discharge in a diminished MN population. Alterations in the mechanical properties of the muscle-tendon system may adjust the length-tension relationship of muscle favorably and therefore alter the conditions under which the development of muscular force is optimized.

At the segmental level, adaptations in the stretch reflex gain may serve to increase muscle stiffness in the immediate response to perturbations while increases in joint stiffness achieved through co-contraction may bolster this early response. Additional adaptations in segmental pathways reinforce the manifestation of decreased reciprocal control of muscle pairs and increased co-contraction; these include increased pre-synaptic inhibition of the Ia pathway, and potentially increased recurrent inhibition through the Renshaw cell. An image emerges of a system with maintained, but substantially less flexible, control of movement.

An oft-described behavioral phenomenon with aging is regression from mature to immature patterns of movement, including increasing dependence on co-contraction and difficulty with sensory conflicts. In development, many of these patterns have traditionally been attributed to immaturity of myelinated neural pathways.[208] It is perhaps significant that central nervous structures that were slowest to myelinate are the first to deteriorate with aging.[105] Evidence of similar responses and mechanisms governing movement in development and aging suggest that rather than attrition and deterioration alone, age-related alterations in motor control may represent adaptive responses across multiple biological systems affording the organism compensatory mechanisms for continued function. Improved understanding of normal, physiological processes attributable to aging lies in our ability to uncover the transitions between normal (adult) movement and these compensatory strategies. Particular promise lies in careful comparisons between "usual" elders—those who evidence "old" behaviors—and "successful" (normal) older adults—those whose function remains more like their younger chronological age peers.

As it has for the authors, this chapter on the sensorimotor system may lead initially to readers' concern for their own potential age-related decline in function. More recent and exciting research on plasticity, mutability, the effects of exercise, and the long-term results of lifetime habits of physical activity should, however, buoy the spirit. Additional research is needed to determine whether early evidence demonstrating proposed plasticity of the aging nervous system is functional and can be significantly altered through extrinsic factors. It is quite encouraging to propose that qual-

ity and vigor of movement performance might be improved through exercise.

Functional change in the aging neuromusculoskeletal system as measured by the physical therapist occurs in conjunction with anatomical, physiological, and neurochemical changes in the sensorimotor system. Research evidence to corroborate this belief and elucidate the critical mechanisms is becoming available. Accordingly, full understanding of factors affecting functional performance in the older adult involves knowledge across domains of science and medicine and efforts of a multidisciplinary health care team. Above all, care and treatment of the aging individual begins with differentiation between physiological factors attributable to aging and pathological influences superimposed on aging physiological systems.

REFERENCES

1. Albert M: Neuropsychological and neurophysiological changes in healthy adult humans across the age range. *Neurobiol Aging* 1993; 14:623-625.
2. Alnaqueeb MA, Al Zaid NS, Goldspink G: Connective tissue changes and physical properties of developing and ageing skeletal muscle. *J Anat* 1984; 139(4):677-689.
3. Anderson B, Palmore E: Longitudinal evaluation of ocular function, in Palmore E (ed): *Normal Aging II, Reports From the Duke Longitudinal Studies, 1970-1973.* Durham, NC, Duke University Press, 1974.
4. Aniansson A, et al: Muscle morphology, enzyme activity and muscle strength in elderly men and women. *Clin Physiol* 1981; 1:73-86.
5. Balice-Gordon RJ: Age-related changes in neuromuscular transmission. *Proceedings of NIA Conference, Sarcopenia and Physical Function in Old Age,* 1996.
6. Balice-Gordon RJ: Schwann cells: Dynamic roles at the neuromuscular junction. *Curr Biol* 1996; 6(9):1054-1056.
7. Ball MJ: Histopathology of cellular changes in Alzheimer's disease, in Nandy K (ed): *Senile Dementia: A Biomedical Approach.* New York, Elsevier, 1978.
8. Baloh RW: Neurotology of aging: Vestibular system, in Albert ML (ed): *Clinical Neurology of Aging.* New York, Oxford University Press, 1984.
9. Banker GA: Trophic interactions between astroglial cells and hippocampal neurons in culture. *Science* 1980; 209:809-810.
10. Barrett DS, Cobb AG, Bently G: Joint proprioception in normal, osteoarthritic and replaced knees. *J Bone Joint Surg* 1991; 73B:53-56.
11. Bassey EJ: Age, inactivity and some physiological responses to exercise. *J Gerontol* 1978; 24:66-77.
12. Benassi G, et al: Neurological examination in subjects over 65 years: An epidemiological survey. *Neuroepidemiology* 1990; 9:27-38.
13. Beninger RJ, et al: Animal studies of brain acetylcholine and memory. *Arch Gerontol Geriatr Suppl* 1989; 1:71-89.
14. Bickford P: Motor learning deficits in aged rats are correlated with loss of cerebellar noradrenergic function. *Brain Res* 1993; 620(1):133-138.
15. Bickford P: Aging and motor learning: A possible role for norepinephrine in cerebellar plasticity. *Annu Rev Neurosci* 1995; 6(1):35-46.
16. Bigland-Ritchie B, et al: Changes in motoneurone firing rates during sustained maximal voluntary contractions. *J Physiol* 1983; 340:335-346.
17. Binder-Macleod SA: Variable-frequency stimulation patterns for the optimization of force during muscle fatigue, in Gandevia SC, et al (eds): *Fatigue: Neural and Muscular Mechanisms.* New York, Plenum, 1995.
18. Birren J, Schaie KW: *Handbook of the Psychology of Aging.* New York, Van Nostrand Reinhold, 1977.
19. Birren JE, Woods AM, Williams MV: Speed of behavior as an indicator of age changes and the integrity of the nervous system, in Hoffmaister F, Miller C (eds): *Brain Function in Old Age.* New York, Springer-Verlag, 1979.

20. Black JE, et al: Learning causes synaptogenesis, whereas motor activity causes angiogenesis, in cerebellar cortex of adult rats. *Proc Natl Acad Sci* 1990; 87:5568-5572.

21. Bolton CF, Winkelmann RK, Dyck PJ: A quantitative study of Meissner's corpuscles in man. *Neurology* 1966; 16:1-9.

22. Booth KR, et al: Motor evoked potentials and central motor conduction: Studies of transcranial magnetic stimulation with recording from the leg. *Electroencephalogr Clin Neurophysiol* 1991; 81:57-62.

23. Botwinick J: *Aging and Behavior.* New York, Springer, 1978.

24. Brody H, Vijayashanker N: Anatomical changes in the nervous system, in Finch CE, Hayflick L (eds): *Handbook of the Biology of Aging.* New York, Van Nostrand Reinhold, 1977.

25. Brody H: Organization of the cerebral cortex III. A study of aging in the human cerebral cortex. *J Comp Neurol* 1955; 102:511-556.

26. Brooke JD, et al: Aging human segmented oligosynaptic reflexes for control of leg movement. *Neurobiology of Aging* 1989; 10:721-725.

27. Brooke MH, Kaiser KK: Muscle fiber types: How many and what kind? *Arch Neurol* 1970; 23:369-379.

28. Brooks VB, Cooke JD, Thomas JS: The continuity of movements, in Stein RB, Pearson KG, Smith RS, Redford JB (eds): *Control of Posture and Locomotion.* New York, Plenum Press, 1973.

29. Bruce RA: Exercise, functional capacity, and aging—Another viewpoint. *Med Sci Sports Exerc* 1984; 16:8-13.

30. Bruce SA, Newton D, Woledge RC: Effects of age on voluntary force and cross-sectional area of human adductor pollicis muscle. *Q J Exp Physiol* 1989; 74:359-362.

31. Buchtal F, Rosenfalck A: Evoked action potentials and conduction velocity in human sensory nerves. *Brain Res* 1966; 3:1.

32. Buell SJ, Coleman PD: Quantitative evidence for selective dendritic growth in normal human aging but not in senile dementia. *Brain Research* 1981; 214:23-42.

33. Burke D: Spasticity as an adaptation to pyramidal tract injury. *Advances in Neurology* 1988; 47:401-423.

34. Buskirk ER: Health maintenance and longevity: Exercise, in Finch C, Schneider EL (eds): *Handbook of the Biology of Aging.* New York, Van Nostrand Reinhold, 1985.

35. Butchart P, Farquhar R, Part NJ, Roberts RC: The effect of age and voluntary contraction on presynaptic inhibition of soleus muscle Ia afferents in man. *Exp Physiol* 1993; 78:235-242.

36. Calne DB, Eisen A, Meneilly G: Normal aging of the nervous system. *Ann Neurol* 1991; 30:206-207.

37. Campbell MJ, McComas AJ, Petito F: Physiological changes in aging muscles. *J Neurol Neurosurg Psychiatry* 1974; 37:131-141.

38. Chakour MC, Gibson SJ, Bradbeer M, Helme RD: The effect of age on A- and C-fibre thermal pain perception. *Pain* 1996; 64:143-152.

39. Clamman HP: Motor unit recruitment and the gradation of muscle force. *Phys Ther* 1993; 73(12):830-843.

40. Clarkson PM: The effect of age and activity level on simple and choice fractionated response time. *Eur J Appl Physiol* 1978; 40:17-25.

41. Clarkson PM, Kroll W, Melchionda AM: Age, isometric strength, rate of tension development and fiber type composition. *J Gerontol* 1981; 36:648-653.

42. Cohen MM, Lessell S: The neuro-ophthalmology of aging, in Albert ML (ed): *Clinical Neurology of Aging.* New York, Oxford University Press, 1984.

43. Coleman PD, Flood DG: Neuron numbers and dendritic extent in normal aging and Alzheimer's disease. *Neurobiol Aging* 1987; 8:521-545.

44. Coleman PD, Flood DG: Is dendritic proliferation of surviving neurons a compensatory response to loss of neighbors in the aging brain?, in Finger S, et al (eds): *Brain Injury and Recovery: Theoretical and Controversial Issues.* New York, Plenum Press, 1988.

45. Connor JR, Diamond MC, Johnson RE: Aging and environmental influences on two types of dendritic spines in the rat occipital cortex. *Exp Neurol* 1980; 79:371-379.

46. Cooke JD, Brown SH, Cunningham DA: Kinematics of arm movements in elderly humans. *Neurobiol Aging* 1989; 10:159-165.

47. Corbin KB, Gardner ED: Decrease in number of myelinated fibers in human spinal roots with age. *Anat Rec* 1937; 68:63-74.

48. Cotman CW, Holets VR: Structural changes at synapses with age: Plasticity and regeneration, in Finch C, Schneider EL (eds): *Handbook of the Biology of Aging.* New York, Van Nostrand Reinhold, 1985.

49. Danieli-Betto D, Zerbato E, Betto R: Type 1, 2a, and 2b myosin heavy chain electrophoretic analysis of rat muscle fibers. *Biochem Biophys Res Commun* 1986; 138:981-987.

50. Darling WG, Cooke JD, Brown SH: Control of simple arm movements in elderly humans. *Neurobiol Aging* 1989; 10:149-157.

51. Desmedt JE, Brunko E: Functional organization of far-field and cortical components of somatosensory evoked potentials in normal adults, in Desmedt JE (ed): *Progress in Clinical Neurophysiology.* Basel, Karger, 1980.

52. Devaney KO, Johnson HA: Neuron loss in the aging visual cortex of man. *J Gerontol* 1980; 35:836-841.

53. Doherty TJ, Brown WF: Age-related changes in the twitch contractile properties of human thenar motor units. *J Appl Physiol* 1997; 82(1):93-101.

54. Doherty TJ, Vandervoort AA, Taylor AW, Brown WF: Effects of motor unit losses on strength in older men and women. *J Appl Physiol* 1993; 74(2):868-874.

55. Dorfman LJ, Bosley TM: Age related changes in peripheral central nerve conduction in man. *Neurology* 1979; 29:38-44.

56. Double KL, et al: Topography of brain atrophy during normal aging and Alzheimer's disease. *Neurobiol Aging* 1996; 17:513-521.

57. Downie AW, Newell DJ: Sensory nerve conduction in patients with diabetes mellitus and controls. *Neurology* 1961; 11:876-882.

58. Duara R, et al: Cerebral glucose utilization, as measured with positron emission tomography in 21 resting healthy men between the ages of 21 and 83 years. *Brain* 1983; 106:761-775.

59. Dyck, PJ: Pathologic alterations of the peripheral nervous system of man, in Dyck PJ, et al (eds): *Peripheral Neuropathy.* Philadelphia: WB Saunders, 1975.

60. Dyck PJ, Schultz PW, O'Brien PC: Quantitation of touch-pressure sensation. *Arch Neurol* 1972; 26:465.

61. Earnest MP, et al: Cortical atrophy, ventricular enlargement and intellectual impairment in the aged. *J Neurol* 1979; 29:1138-1143.

62. Eccles JC: *The Understanding of the Brain,* New York, McGraw-Hill, 1977.

63. Essen-Gustavsson B, Borges O: Histochemical and metabolic characteristics of human skeletal muscle in relation to age. *ACTA Physiol Scand* 1986; 126:107-114.

64. Evatt ML, Wolf SL, Segal RL: Modification of human spinal stretch reflexes: preliminary studies. *Neurosci Lett* 1989; 105:305-355.

65. Finley FR, Cody KA, Finzie RV: Locomotion patterns in elderly women. *Arch Phys Med Rehabil* 1969; 50:140-146.

66. Forster MJ, et al: Age-related losses of cognitive function and motor skills in mice are associated with oxidative protein damage in the brain. *Proc Natl Acad Sci* 93 1996; (10):4765-4769.

67. Fozard JL, et al: Visual perception and communication, in Birren JE, Schaie KW (eds): *Handbook of the Psychology of Aging.* New York, Van Nostrand Reinhold, 1977.

68. Freedman M, et al: Computerized axial tomography in ageing, in Albert ML (ed): *Clin Neurol Aging.* New York, Oxford University Press, 1984.

69. Frontera WR, et al: A cross-sectional study of muscle strength and mass in 45 to 78 year old men and women. *J Appl Physiol* 1991; 71:644-650.

70. Gates GA, et al: Hearing in the elderly: The Framingham cohort, 1983-1985. Part 1. Basic audiometric test results. *Ear Hear* 1990; 11:247-256.

71. Geula C, Mesulam MM: Cortical cholinergic fibers in aging and Alzheimer's disease: A morphometric study. *J Neurosci* 1989; 33:469-481.

72. Gilman S, Newman SW: *Manter and Gatz's Essentials of Clinical Neuroanatomy and Neurophysiology.* Philadelphia, FA Davis, 1996.

73. Goldberg JM, Lindblom U: Standardized method of determining vibratory perception thresholds for diagnosis and screening in neurological investigation. *J Neurol Neurosurg Psychiatry* 1979; 42:793-803.

74. Goldman-Rakic PS: Circuitry of the prefrontal cortex and regulation of behavior by representational memory, in Mountcastle B, et al (eds): *Handbook of Physiology.* Baltimore, Williams & Wilkins, 1987.

75. Gould TJ, et al: Effects of dietary restriction on motor learning and cerebellar noradrenergic function in aged F344 rats. *Brain Res* 1995; 684(2):150-158.

76. Grabiner MD, Enoka RM: Changes in movement capabilities with aging. *Exerc Sport Sci Rev* 1995; 23:65-104.

77. Grimby G, Saltin B: The ageing muscle. *Clin Physiol* 1983; 3:209-218.

78. Gutmann E, et al: The rate of regeneration of nerve. *J Exp Biol* 1942;19:14-44.

79. Gutmann E, Hanzlikova V: Fast and slow motor units in aging. *J Gerontol* 1976; 22:280-300.

80. Hallett M, Shahani BT, Young RR: EMG analysis of stereotyped voluntary movements in man. *J Neurol Neurosurg Psychiatry* 1975; 38:1154-1162.

81. Haug H: Brain sizes, surfaces, and neuronal sizes of cortex cerebri: A stereological investigation of man and his variability and a comparison with some mammals (primates, whales, marsupials, insectivores, and one elephant). *Am J Anat* 1987; 180(2):126-142.

82. Hayes D, Jerger J: Neurotology of aging: The auditory system, in Albert ML (ed): *Clinical Neurology of Aging.* New York, Oxford University Press, 1984.

83. Hayflick L: The cellular basis for biological aging, in Finch CE, Hayflick L (eds): *Handbook of the Biology of Aging.* New York, Van Nostrand Reinhold, 1977.

84. Henneman E, Mendell LM: *Handbook of Physiology, Section I: The Nervous System, Volume II: Motor Control, Part I.* Bethesda, Md, American Physiological Society, 1981.

85. Henneman E, Somjen G, Carpenter DO: Excitability and inhibitability of motoneurons of different sizes. *J Neurophysiol* 1965; 28:560-580.

86. Hill AV: The mechanics of voluntary muscle. *The Lancet* 1951; Nov. 24:947-951.

87. Himann J, et al: Age-related changes in speed of walking. *Med Sci Sports Exerc* 1987; 20:161-166.

88. Hindmarsh JJ, Estes EH: Falls in older persons. *Arch Intern Med* 1989; 149:2217-2222.

89. Hobson W, Pemberton J: *The Health of the Elderly at Home.* London, Butterworth, 1955.

90. Holden C: Live long and prosper? *Science* 1996; 273:42-48.

91. Horak FB: Clinical measurement of postural control in adults. *Phys Ther* 1987; 67(12):1881-1885.

92. Horak FB, Shupert CL, Mirka A: Components of postural dyscontrol in the elderly. *Neurobiol Aging* 1989; 10:727-738.

93. Howard JE, McGill KC, Dorfman LJ: Age effects on properties of motor unit action potentials: ADEMG analysis. *Ann Neurol* 1988; 24: 207-213.

94. Hu M, Woollacott MH: Multisensory training of standing balance in older adults I: Postural stability and one-leg stance balance. *J Gerontol: Med Sci* 1994; 49(2):M52-M61.

95. Itoh M, et al: Stability of cerebral blood flow and oxygen metabolism during normal aging. *J Gerontol* 1990; 36:43-48.

96. Jagust WJ: Neuroimaging in normal aging and dementia, in Albert ML, Knoefel JA (eds): *Clinical Neurology of Aging.* New York, Oxford University Press, 1994.

97. Kaeser HE: Nerve conduction velocity measurements, in Vinken PJ, Bruyn AW (eds): *Handbook of Clinical Neurology.* Amsterdam, North Holland, 1970.

98. Kamen G, De Luca CJ: Unusual motor unit discharge behavior in older adults. *Brain Res* 1989; 482:136-140.

99. Kamen G, Knight CA, Laroche DP, Asermley DG: Resistance training increases vastus lateralis motor unit firing rates in young and old adults. *Med Sci Sports Exerc* 1998; 30(5):S337.

100. Kamen G, Sison SV, Du CCD, Patten C: Motor unit discharge behavior in older adults during maximal-effort contractions. *J Appl Physiol* 1995; 79(6):1908-1913.

101. Katzman R, Terry R: *The Neurology of Aging.* Philadelphia, FA Davis, 1983.

102. Kawamura YI, et al: Effect of age on glucose utilization and responsiveness to insulin in forearm muscle. *J Am Geriatr Soc* 1977; 28: 304-307.

103. Kelso JAS: *Dynamic Patterns: The Self-Organization of Brain and Behavior.* Cambridge, Mass, The MIT Press, 1995.

104. Kemper TA: The relationship of cerebral cortical changes to nuclei in the brainstem. *Neurobiol Aging* 1993; 14:659-660.

105. Kemper TA: Neuroanatomical and neuropathological changes during aging and dementia, in Albert ME, Knoefel JA (eds): *Clinical Neurology of Aging.* New York, Oxford University Press, 1994.

106. Kennedy R, Clemis JD: The geriatric auditory and vestibular systems. *Otolarygol Clin North Am* 1990; 23:1075-1082.

107. Kimura J:. *Electrodiagnosis in Diseases of Nerve and Muscle.* Philadelphia, FA Davis, 1989.

107a. Kinoshita H, Francis PR: A comparison of prehension force control in young and elderly indivduals. *J Appl Physiol* 1996; 74:450-460.

108. Kliffen M, et al: Morphologic changes in age-related maculopathy. *Microscopic Research and Technology* 1997; 36:106-122.

109. Klitgaard H, et al: Function, morphology and protein expression of ageing skeletal muscle: A cross-sectional study of elderly men with different training backgrounds. *ACTA Physiol Scand* 1990; 140:41-54.

110. Klitgaard H, et al: Ageing alters the myosin heavy chain composition of single fibres from human skeletal muscle. *ACTA Physiol Scand* 1990; 140:55-62.

111. Knox CA: Neuroanatomical changes associated with aging in the peripheral nervous system, in ME Albert, Knoefel JA (eds): *Clinical Neurology of Aging.* New York, Oxford University Press, 1992.

112. Koceja DM, Marcus CA, Trimble MH: Postural modulation of the soleus H-reflex in young and old subjects. *Electroencephalogr Clin Neurophysiol* 1995; 97:387-393.

113. Kokmen E, Bossemeyer RW, Williams WJ: Neurological manifestations of aging. *J Gerontol* 1977; 32:411-419.

114. Kokmen E, Bossemeyer RW, Williams WJ: Quantitative evaluation of joint motion perception in an aging population. *J Gerontol* 1978; 33:62.

115. La Fratta CW, Canestrari RE: A comparison of sensory and motor nerve conduction velocities as related to age. *Arch Phys Med Rehabil* 1966; 47:286-290.

116. Laidlaw RW, Hamilton MA: A study of thresholds in perception of passive movement among normal control subjects. *Bull Neurol Institute* 1937; 6:268-340.

117. Larsson L, Ansved T: Effects of aging on the motor unit. *Prog Neurobiol* 1995; 45:397-458.

118. Larsson L, Grimby G, Karlsson J: Muscle strength and speed of movement in relation to age and muscle morphology. *J Appl Physiol* 1979; 46(3):451-456.

119. Lascelles RG, Thomas PK: Changes due to age in internodal length in the sural nerve of man. *J Neurol Neurosurg Psychiatry* 1966; 29:40-44.

120. Lassau-Wray ER, Parker AW: Neuromuscular responses of elderly women to tasks of increasing complexity imposed during walking. *Eur J App Physiol* 1993; 67:467-480.

121. Leiper CI, Craik RL: Relationships between physical activity and temporal-distance characteristics of walking in elderly women. *Phys Ther* 1991; 71(11):791-803.

122. Leong B, Kamen G, Patten C, Burke JR: Maximal motor unit discharge rates in the quadriceps muscle of older weight lifters. *Med Sci Sports Exerc,* 1999; 31(11):1638-1644.

123. Lexell J: Ageing and human muscle: Observations from Sweden. *Can J Appl Physiol* 1993; 18(1):2-18.

124. Light KE: Information processing for motor performance in older adults. *Phys Ther* 1990; 70(12):820-826.

125. Light KE, Spirduso WW: Effects of adult aging on the movement complexity factor of response programming. *J Gerontol* 1990; 45:107-109.

126. Loeb GE: The control and responses of mammalian muscle spindles during normally executed motor tasks. *Exerc Sport Sci Rev* 1984; 12:157-204.

127. Lopez I, Honrubia V, Baloh RW: Aging and the human vestibular nucleus. *J Vestib Res* 1997; 7:77-85.

128. Lowenfeld IE: Pupillary changes related to age, in Thompson HS (ed): *Topics in Neuro-Opthalmology.* Baltimore, Williams & Wilkins, 1979.

129. Magnoni MS, et al.: The aging brain: Protein phosphorylation as a target of changes in neuronal function. *Life Sci* 1991; 48:373-385.

130. Maki BE, Fernie GR: A system identification approach to balance testing. *Prog Brain Res* 1988; 76:297-306.

131. Maki BE, McIlroy WE: Postural control in the older adult. *Clin Geriatr Med* 1996; 12:635-658.

132. Manchester D, Woollacott MH, Zederbauer-Hylton N, Marin O: Visual, vestibular and somatosensory contributions to balance control in the older adult. *J Gerontol* 1989; 44:118-127.

133. Mankovskii N, Mints YA, Lysenyuk UP: Regulation of the preparatory period for complex voluntary movement in old and extreme old age. *Hum Physiol* 1980; 6:46-50.

134. McCandless G, Parkin J: Hearing aid performance relative to site of lesion. *Otolaryngol Head Neck Surg* 1979; 87:871-875.

135. McComas AJ, Galea V, De Bruin H: Motor unit populations in healthy and diseased muscles. *Phys Ther* 1993; 73(12):868-877.

136. Merchut MP, Toleikis SC: Aging and quantitative sensory thresholds. *Electromyogr Clin Neurophysiol* 1990; 30:293-297.

137. Miller AKH, Alston RL, Corsellis JAN: Variations with age in the volumes of grey and white matter in the cerebral hemispheres of man: Measurements with an image analyzer. *Neuropathol Appl Neurobiol* 1980; 6:119-132.

138. Miller JB, Stockdale FE: What muscle cells know that nerves don't tell them. *Trends Neurol Sci* 1987; 10(8):325-329.

139. Millodot M: The influence of age on the sensitivity of the cornea. *Invest Opthalmol Vis Sci* 1977; 16:240-242.

140. Milner B, Petrides M: Behavioural effects of frontal-lobe lesions in man. *Trends Neurosci* 1984; 7:403-407.

141. Mishkin M: Neural circuitry underlying behavioral deficits in aging. *Neurobiol Aging* 1993; 14:615-617.

142. Moller P, et al: Effects of aging on energy-rich phosphagens in human skeletal muscles. *Clin Sci* 1980; 58:553-555.

143. Morimatsu M, Hirai S, Muramatsu A: Senile degenerative brain lesions and dementia. *J Am Geriatr Soc* 1975; 23:390-406.

144. Morita H, et al: Progressive decrease in heteronymous monosynaptic Ia facilitation with human ageing. *Exp Brain Res* 1995; 104:167-170.

145. Morrison JH, Hof PR: Life and death of neurons in the aging brain. *Science* 1997; 278:412-418.

146. Mufson EJ, Stein DG: Degeneration in the spinal cord of old rats. *Exp Neurol* 1980; 70:179-186.

147. Muir JL: Acetylcholine, aging and Alzheimer's disease. *Pharmacol Biochem Behav* 1997; 56:687-696.

148. Munsat TL: Aging of the neuromuscular system, in Albert ML (ed): *Clinical Neurology of Aging.* New York, Oxford University Press, 1984.

149. Murray MP, et al: Age related differences in knee muscle strength in normal women. *Phys Ther* 1980; 60:412-419.

150. Narici MV, Bordini M, Cerretelli P: Effect of aging on human adductor pollicis muscle function. *J Appl Physiol* 1991; 71(4):1277-1281.

151. Nashner LM: Adapting reflexes controlling the human posture. *Exp Brain Res* 1976; 26:59-72.

152. Nashner LM: Sensory, neuromuscular, and biomechanical contributions to human balance, in Duncan P (ed): *Balance: Proceedings of the APTA Forum.* Alexandria, Va, American Physical Therapy Association, 1989.

153. Nashner LM, McCollum G: The organization of human postural movements: A formal basis and experimental synthesis. *Behav Brain Sci* 1985; 8:135-173.

154. Nashner LM, Shupert CL, Horak FB: Head-trunk movement coordination in the standing posture. *Prog Brain Res* 1988; 76:243-251.

155. Nichols TR, Houk JC: Improvement in linearity and regulation of stiffness that results from actions of the stretch reflex. *J Physiol* 1976; 39:119-142.

156. Noel P, Desmedt JE: Cerebral and far-field somatosensory evoked potentials in neurological disorders involving the cervical spinal cord, brainstem, thalamus, and cortex, in Desmedt J (ed): *Progress in Clinical Neurophysiology.* Basel, Karger, 1980.

157. O'Sullivan DJ, Swallow M: The fibre size and content of the radial and sural nerve. *J Neurol Neurosurg Psychiatry* 1968; 31:464-470.

158. Ochoa J, WPG Mair: The normal sural nerve in man: II. Changes in the axons and Schwann cells due to aging. *ACTA Neuropathol (Berl)* 1969; 13:217-239.

159. Onishi N: Changes of jumping reaction time in relation to age. *J Sci Labour* 1966; 42:5-16.

160. Ostry DJ, Cooke JD, Munhall KG: Velocity curves of human arm and speech movements. *Exp Brain Res* 1987; 68:37-46.

161. Panton LB, Graves JE, Pollock ML: Effects of aerobic and resistance training on fractionated reaction time and speed of movement. *J Gerontol* 1990; 45:M26-31.

162. Patten C, Kamen G: Adaptations in human motor unit discharge behaviour to strength training. *Soc Neurosci Abstracts* 1996; 22:130.

163. Patten C, Kamen G, Sison SV, Du CC: Improvements in balance in young and older adults documented by accelerometry. *Med Sci Sports Exerc* 1993; 25(5):S198.

164. Peress NS, Kane WC, Aronson SM: Central nervous system findings in a tenth decade autopsy population. *Prog Brain Res* 1973; 40:473-483.

165. Perry J: *Gait Analysis.* New York, Slack, 1992.

166. Peters A, Leahu D, Moss MB, McNally KJ: The effects of aging on Area 46 of the frontal cortex of the Rhesus monkey. *Cereb Cortex* 1994; 6:621-635.

167. Peters A, et al: Neurobiological bases of age-related cognitive decline in the Rhesus monkey. *J Exp Neurol Exp Pathol* 1996; 55(8):861-874.

168. Pikna JK: Concepts of altered health in older adults, in *Pathophysiology: Concepts of Altered Health States.* Philadelphia, JB Lippincott, 1998.

169. Polich J, Starr A: Evoked potentials in aging, in Albert ML (ed): *Clinical Neurology of Aging.* New York, Oxford University Press, 1984.

170. Porter MM, Vandervoort AA, Lexell J: Aging of human muscle: Structure, function and adaptability. *Scand J Med Sci Sports* 1995; 5:129-142.

171. Potvin AR, et al: Human neurologic function and the aging process. *J Am Geriatr Soc* 1980; 28:1-9.

172. Powell DH: *Profiles in Cognitive Aging.* Harvard University Press, 1994.

173. Pyka G, Lindenberger E, Charette S, Marcus R: Muscle strength and fiber adaptations to a year-long resistance training program in elderly men and women. *J Gerontol: Med Sci* 1994; 49(1):M22-M27.

174. Redford JB: Preventing falls in the elderly. *Hosp Med* 1991; 27(2):57-71.

175. Rees TS, Kuckert LG, Milezuk HA: Auditory and vestibular dysfunction, in Hazzard WR, et al: *Principles of Geriatric Medicine and Gerontology.* New York, McGraw-Hill, 1994.

176. Reivich M, et al: The [18F] fluorodeoxyglucose method for the measurement of local cerebral glucose utilization in man. *Circ Res* 1979; 44:127-137.

177. Rogers J, Bloom FE: Neurotransmitter metabolism and function in the aging central nervous system, in Finch C, Schneider EL (eds): *Handbook of the Biology of Aging.* New York, Van Nostrand Reinhold, 1985.

178. Rogers MA, Evans WJ: Changes in skeletal muscle with aging: Effects of exercise training. *Exerc Sports Sci Rev* 1993; 21:65-102.

179. Roos MR, et al: Age-related changes in motor unit function. *Muscle Nerve* 1997; 20:679-690.

180. Rosene DL: Comparing age-related changes in the basal forebrain and hippocampus of the rhesus monkey. *Neurobiol Aging* 1993; 14:669-670.

181. Rowe JW, RL Kahn: Human aging: Usual and successful. *Science* 1987; 237:143-149.

182. Sabin TD, Venna N: Peripheral nerve disorders in the elderly, in Albert ML (ed): *Clinical Neurology of Aging.* New York, Oxford University Press, 1984.

183. Sagar HJ, et al: Remote memory function in Alzheimer's disease and Parkinson's disease. *Brain* 1988; 111:185-206.

184. Sandor T, et al: Symmetrical and asymmetrical changes in brain tissue with age as measured on CT scans. *Neurobiol Aging* 1990; 11:21-27.

185. Schade JP, Baxter CF: Changes during growth in the volume and surface area of cortical neurons in the rabbit. *Exp Neurol* 1960; 2:158-178.

186. Schiffman SS: Taste and smell losses in normal aging and disease. *JAMA* 1997; 278:1357-1362.

187. Schmidt RF, Wahren LK: Multiunit neural responses to strong finger pulp vibration. II. Comparison with tactile sensory thresholds. *ACTA Physiol Scand* 1990; 140:11-16.

188. Schmidt RF, Wahren LK, Hagbarth KE: Multiunit neural responses to strong finger pulp vibration. I. Relationship to age. *ACTA Physiol Scand* 1990; 140:1-10.

189. Sekuler R, Hutman LP, Owsley CJ: Human aging and spatial vision. *Science* 1980; 209:1255-1256.

190. Silverberg N, Silverberg L: Aging and the skin. *Postgrad Med* 1989; 86:131-136.

191. Singleton WT: The change of movement timing with age. *Br J Psychol* 1954; 45:166-172.

192. Skarda CA, Freeman WJ: How brains make chaos in order to make sense of the world. *Behav Brain Sci* 1987; 10:161-195.

193. Skinner HB, Barrack RL, Cook SD: Age-related decline in proprioception. *Clin Orthop* 1984; 184:208-211.

194. Soderberg GL, Minor SD, Nelson RM: A comparison of motor unit behaviour in young and aged subjects. *Age Ageing* 1991; 20:8-15.

195. Sokoloff L, et al: The ^{14}C deoxyglucose method for the measurement of local cerebral glucose utilization: Theory, procedure, and normal values in the conscious and anesthetized albino rat. *J Neurochem* 1977; 28:879-916.

196. Sommers MS: Stimulus variability and spoken word recognition. II. The effects of age and hearing impairment. *J Acoust Soc Am* 1997; 101:2278-2288.

197. Spiegel KM, et al: The influence of age on the assessment of motor unit activation in a human hand muscle. *Exp Physiol* 1996; 81: 805-819.

198. Spirduso WW: Physical fitness, aging, and psychomotor speed: A review. *J Gerontol* 1980; 35:850-865.

199. Spirduso WW: Exercise and the aging brain. *Res Q Exerc Sport* 54: 208-218, 1983.

200. Spirduso WW: *Physical Dimensions of Aging.* Champaign, Ill, Human Kinetics, 1995.

201. Stelmach GE, Worringham CJ: Sensorimotor deficits related to postural stability. *Clin Geriatr Med* 1985; 1:679-725.

202. Stevens JC, Choo KK: Spatial acuity of the body surface over the life span. *Somatosens Mot Res* 1996; 13:153-166.

203. Takahashi J: A clinicopathologic study of the peripheral nervous system of the aged: Sciatic nerve and autonomic nervous system. *J Am Geriatr Soc* 1966; 21:123-133.

204. Tamaki K, Nakai M, Yokota T, Ogata J: Effects of aging and chronic hypertension on cerebral blood flow and cerebrovascular CO_2 reactivity in the rat. *Gerontology* 1995; 41(1):11-17.

205. Terao S, et al: Age-related changes in human spinal ventral horn cells with special reference to the loss of small neurons in the intermediate zone: A quantitative analysis. *ACTA Neuropathol* 1996; 92:109-114.

206. Thelen DG, Ashton-Miller JA, Schultz AB, Alexander NB: Do neural factors underlie age differences in rapid ankle torque development? *J Am Geriatr Soc* 1996; 44:804-808.

207. Thelen DG, Schultz AB, Alexander NB, Ashton-Miller JA: Effects of age on rapid ankle torque development. *J Gerontol: MEDICAL SCIENCES* 1996; 51A(5):M226-M232.

208. Thelen E, Ulrich BD, Jensen JL: The developmental origins of locomotion, in Woollacott MH, Shumway-Cook A (eds): *Posture and Gait.* Columbia, SC, University of South Carolina Press, 1989.

209. Thomas CK, et al: Patterns of reinnervation and motor unit recruitment in human hand muscles after complete ulnar and median nerve section and resuture. *J Neurol Neurosurg Psychiatry* 1987; 50:259-268.

210. Thomas TR, et al: Fatty acid pattern and cholesterol in skeletal muscle of men aged 22-73. *Mech Ageing Dev* 1978; 8:429-434.

211. Thompson LW: Cerebral blood flow, EEG and behavior in aging, in Terry RD, Gershon S (eds): *Neurobiology of Aging.* New York: Raven Press, 1976.

212. Tinetti ME, Speechly M: Prevention of falls among the elderly. *N Engl J Med* 1989; 320(16):1055-1059.

213. Tinetti ME, Speechly M, Ginter SF: Risk factors for falls among elderly persons living in the community. *N Engl J Med* 1988; 320(16): 1055-1059.

214. Tomanga M: Histochemical and ultrastructural changes in senile human skeletal muscle. *J Am Geriatr Soc* 1977; 25:125-131.

215. Trimble MH, Koceja DM: Modulation of triceps surae H-reflex with training. *Intern J Neuroscience* 1994; 75:293-303.

216. Turvey MT, Fitch HL, Tuller B: The Bernstein perspective I: The problems of degrees of freedom and context-conditioned variability, in Kelso JAS (ed): *Human Motor Behavior.* Hillsdale, NJ, LEA, 1982.

217. Vandervoort A, Hayes KC, Belanger AY: Strength and endurance of skeletal muscle in the elderly. *Physiother Can* 1986; 38:167-173.

218. Vandervoort AA, McComas AJ: Contractile changes in opposing muscles of the human ankle joint with aging. *J Appl Physiol* 1986; 61: 361-367.

219. Vincent SL, Peters A, Tigges J: Effect of aging on the neurons within area 17 of the rhesus monkey cerebral cortex. *Anat Rec* 1989; 223: 329-341.

220. Vizoso AD: The relationship between internodal length and growth in human nerves. *J Anat* 1950; 84:342-353.

221. Vorro J, Hobart D: Kinematic and myoelectric analysis of skill acquisition: I. 90 cm group. *Arch Phys Med Rehabil* 1981; 62:575-582.

221a. Waite LM, et al: Neurological signs, aging, and the neurodegenerative syndromes (abstract). *Arch Neurol* 1996; 53(6):498-502.

222. Weiss AD: The locus of reaction time change with set, motivation, and age. *J Gerontol* 1965; 20:60-64.

223. Welford AT: Motor skills and aging, in Mortimer JA, Pirozzolo FJ, Maletta GJ (eds): *The Aging Motor System.* New York, Praeger Scientific, 1982.

224. Welford AT: Between bodily changes and performance: Some possible reasons for slowing with age. *Exp Aging Res* 1984; 10:73-88.

225. Wisniewski HM, Soiser D: Neurofibrillary pathology: Current status and research perspectives. *Mech Ageing Dev* 1979; 9:119-142.

226. Wisniewski HM, Terry RD: Morphology of the aging brain, human and animal, in Ford DH (ed): *Neurobiological Aspects of Maturation and Aging.* Amsterdam, Elsevier, 1973.

227. Wolf SL, Segal RL: Conditioning of spinal stretch reflexes: Implications for rehabilitation. *Physical Therapy* 1990; 70:652-656.

228. Wolpaw JR, Carp JS: Adaptive plasticity in spinal cord, in Seil J (ed): *Advances in Neurology.* New York, Raven, 1993.

229. Wolpaw JR, Herchenroder PA, Carp JS: Operant conditioning of the primate H-reflex: factors affecting magnitude of change. *Exp Brain Res* 1993; 97:31-39.

230. Woollacott MH: Aging, posture control, and movement preparation, in Woollacott MH, Shumway-Cook A (eds): *Development of Posture and Gait Across the Life Span.* Columbia, SC, University of South Carolina Press, 1991.

231. Woollacott MH, Shumway-Cook A, Nashner LM: Postural reflexes and aging, in Mortimer JA, Pirozzolo FJ, Maletta GJ (eds): *The Aging Motor System.* New York, Praeger Scientific, 1982.

232. Worfolk JB: Keep frail elders warm! The thermal instabilities of the old have not received sufficient attention in basic educational programs. *Geriatr Nurs* 1997; 18:7-11.

233. Wyatt HJ, Fisher RF: A simple view of age-related changes in the shape of the lens of the human eye. *Eye* 1995; 9:772-775.

234. Winstein CJ, Knecht HG (eds): Movement science. *Physical Therapy* 1990; 70(12):759-907.

235. Lister ML: Contemporary management of motor control problems: Proceedings of the II Step Conference. Alexandria, Va, Foundation for Physical Therapy, 1991.

236. Wickelgren I: For the cortex, neuron loss may be less than thought. *Science* 1996; 273:48-50.

PART II

PRINCIPLES AND CONCEPTS OF ASSESSMENT

HEALTH STATUS: A CONCEPTUAL FRAMEWORK AND TERMINOLOGY FOR EXAMINATION, EVALUATION, AND DIAGNOSIS

ANDREW A. GUCCIONE, PT, PhD, FAPTA

INTRODUCTION

Many different concepts are required to capture the broad dimensions of an elder's eventual experience with disease and illness. Terms such as *health status, well-being,* and *quality of life* have all been used at various times to describe a facet of the human condition of individuals as they age. Physical therapists direct a substantial proportion of their clinical attention toward understanding the relationships among health, disease, and function, especially how the processes of normal aging and medical morbidity interact to alter a person's physical ability to do even the simplest activities of daily living (ADL) and fulfill the role obligations associated with living independently as an adult.

The preceding chapters have reviewed in great detail the multiple changes that occur with aging or result from certain medical problems that an elder is likely to face. When evaluating data on an individual geriatric patient, who may present clinically with almost any combination of these changes, a therapist may feel overwhelmed by all the abnormal results noted on the initial examination. One of the greatest challenges of geriatric physical therapy is to collect complete, but only pertinent, data and to categorize these clinical findings in a way that helps the therapist to understand what the patient's problems are; how they have come about; and what, if anything at all, could be done by a physical therapist to remedy the patient's situation. This chapter has three purposes. The first purpose is to present a model of health status that can be used by physical therapists to categorize the data they might collect during an initial examination. Second, we will explore how the parts of the model interconnect and may be used to assist the physical therapist to understand the patient's problems in functional terms that also suggest what a physical therapist might do to maintain or improve the patient's level of function. Finally, this chapter outlines factors that are relevant to designing a physical therapist plan of care that is tailored to the specific needs of an older individual and to implementing interventions that will produce a positive outcome.

THE CONCEPT OF HEALTH STATUS
Definition of Health

The World Health Organization (WHO) defined *health* as a state of complete physical, psychological, and social well-being, and not merely the absence of disease or infirmity.[28] According to this definition, "health" is best understood as

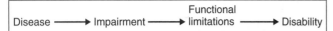

FIG. 6-1   Schematic representation of the four components of health status and the process of disablement in the model developed by Nagi.

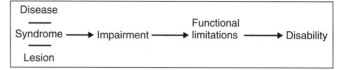

FIG. 6-2   Expansion of the Nagi model to include conditions other than disease or active pathology that may result in impairments.

an end point and pertains to the psychological and social domains of human existence—not just the physical state of the human being. In contrast to "complete health" as an end point, there is health that most physical therapists recognize: an objective state between wellness and death. *Illness,* in comparison with "objective" health, refers to the internal subjective experience of the individual who is aware that personal well-being has been jeopardized and how that person responds to that experience.

Sociologist Saad Nagi constructed a model of health status that furthers our understanding of the relationship between health and functional status, especially in the elderly, by describing the process of disablement.[15-18] In this model, health status is parceled out into four distinct components that evolve sequentially as an individual loses well-being: disease or pathology, impairments, functional limitations, and disability (Fig. 6-1). Each of these terms is discussed in the text that follows. Taken together, these concepts describe the essential elements of an overall framework for physical therapist examination, evaluation, and diagnosis.

Disease

In Nagi's model, the term *disease* refers to an ongoing pathological state that is delineated by a particular cluster of signs and symptoms and is recognized externally by either the individual or a practitioner as abnormal. Nagi's concept of disease is rooted in the principle of homeostasis: the human organism responds to an active pathological state by mobilizing its resources to respond to a threat and to return to its normal state.[18] Disease may be the result of infection, trauma, metabolic imbalance, degenerative processes, or other etiological factors. Whatever the cause, Nagi's concept of disease emphasizes two features: (1) an active threat to the organism's normal state and (2) an active response internally by the organism to that threat, which may be aided externally by therapeutic interventions.

The term disease in Nagi's model does not cover all of the conditions of many elders that necessitate the services of a physical therapist. There are also numerous medical conditions that affect an individual's ability to function but are not related to any *single* active pathology. Congestive heart failure (CHF), for example, is a medical syndrome that is a recognized cluster of signs and symptoms. Although CHF evolves from active pathological factors over time, it is the co-existence of these pathological factors over the same time period that may explain CHF in the elderly.[27] Osteoarthritis, which is neither active nor progressive in all cases, may also be a medical condition that is best understood as a cluster of pathological processes, not a single disease.[26] A physical ther-

apist's caseload may also include individuals whose medical diagnoses indicate fixed lesions, which identify previous insults to a body part or organ and sites of dysfunction but are not presently associated with any active processes. A patient who has had a stroke is a common example of an individual with a fixed neuroanatomical lesion that is no longer associated with any ongoing pathological process. Therefore, Nagi's original model can be developed further to include threats to health, other than disease, that can lead to impairment (Fig. 6-2).

Impairment

The second term in Nagi's model is *impairment.* Impairments, many of which evolve as the consequence of disease, pathological processes, or lesions, can be defined as alterations in anatomical, physiological, or psychological structures or functions that are the results of underlying changes in the elder's normal state and also contribute to an elder's illness. Physical impairments, such as pain and decreased range of motion (ROM) in the shoulder, may be the overt manifestations (or symptoms and signs) of either temporary or permanent disease or pathological processes. This will not be true, however, for every geriatric patient. The genesis of some impairments can often be unclear. Poor posture, for example, is neither a disease nor a pathological state, yet the resultant muscle shortening and capsular tightness may present as major impairments in a clinical examination. Thus, not all older patients are patients because they have a disease. Some elders are treated by physical therapists because their impairments are sufficient cause for concern. Our efforts with geriatric patients are directed primarily at impairments of the cardiopulmonary, integumentary, musculoskeletal, and neuromuscular systems.

Physical therapists are recognized experts in the measurement of impairments through the application of test procedures such as goniometry and manual muscle testing. Given that much of physical therapy is directed toward remediating or minimizing impairments, some additional elaboration of the concept of impairment is particularly useful in geriatric physical therapy. Schenkman and Butler have proposed that impairments can be classified in two ways.[24,25] Some impairments are the direct effects of a disease, syndrome, or lesion and are relatively confined to a single system. For example, they note that weakness can be classified as a neuromuscular impairment that is a direct effect of a peripheral motor neuropathy in the lower extremity. There may also be impairments in other systems that can be regarded as indirect effects of the underlying problem. For example, attempts to ambulate a patient with a peripheral motor neuropathy may put unnecessary strain on joints and ligaments that may be detected on clinical examination as musculoskeletal impairments. The combination of weakness and ligamentous strain may lead to a composite effect, the impairment of pain.

Although Schenkman and Butler expanded the concept of impairment around individuals with neurological dysfunction, categorizing clinical signs and symptoms into impairments that are direct, indirect, or composite effects can help to bring together the data of the medical history and the findings of the clinical examination into a cohesive relationship. For example, consider a 79-year-old female with severe peripheral vascular disease (PVD). Upon clinical examination, the physical therapist notes that this individual has lost sensation below the right knee. Sensory loss is an impairment that would be classified as a direct effect of PVD. As the individual is ambulating less and cannot sense full ankle ROM, loss of ROM may be an indirect effect of the patient's PVD on the musculoskeletal system. The combination of the direct impairment—sensory loss below the knee—and the indirect impairment—decreased ROM in the ankle—may help to explain another clinical finding, poor balance, which can be understood as a composite effect of other impairments. Piecing clinical data together in this fashion allows the therapist to uncover the interrelationships among a patient's PVD, loss of sensation, limited ROM, and balance deficits. Without a framework that sorts the patient's clinical data into relevant categories, the therapist might never comprehend how the patient's problems came to be and thus how to intervene. Treatment consisting of balance activities alone would be inappropriate, since the therapist must also address the loss in ROM as well as teach the patient to compensate for the sensory loss in order to remediate the impairments.

Functional Limitations

While most of us anticipate that our body systems will deteriorate with time as we age, an inability to do for one's self from day to day perhaps most clearly identifies when elders are losing their health. Nagi proposed that functional limitations were the results of impairments and consisted of an individual's inability to perform the tasks and activities that constitute usual activities for that individual, for example, reaching for something on an overhead shelf or carrying a package. As measures of behaviors at the level of a person, and not anatomical or physiological conditions, limitations in functional status should not be confused with diseases or impairments that encompass aberrations in specific tissues, organs, and systems that present clinically as the patient's signs and symptoms.

Functional limitations occur in distinct categories of tasks and activities: physical, psychological, and social. *Physical function* covers an individual's sensorimotor performance in the execution of particular tasks and activities.

Rolling, getting out of bed, transferring, walking, climbing, bending, lifting, and carrying are all examples of physical functional activities. These sensorimotor functional abilities underlie the fundamental daily organized patterns of behaviors that are further classified as basic ADL such as feeding, dressing, bathing, grooming, and toileting. The more complex tasks associated with independent community living, for example, using public transportation or grocery shopping, are categorized as "instrumental" ADL, often abbreviated as "IADL." Successful performance of complex physical functional activities, such as personal hygiene and housekeeping, typically requires integration of cognitive and affective abilities as well as physical ones.[6]

Psychological function has two components: mental and affective. *Mental function* covers a range of cognitive activities, such as telling time and performing money calculations, that are essential to living independently as an adult. Attention, concentration, memory, and judgment are all elements of mental function. An elder's emotional state and effectiveness in coping with the stresses attributable to disease or negative impacts of the aging process are indicators of the patient's affective function. *Affective function* broadly refers to both the everyday "hassles" of daily existence that are part of every elder's experience as well as the more traumatic events such as death of a spouse. Self-esteem, anxiety, depression, and coping are also represented in the construct of affective functioning.

Social function encompasses an individual's social activities such as church attendance or family gatherings as well as performance of social roles and obligations. Grandparenting and being employed outside the home are two examples of social role functioning relevant to an older individual and therefore are potential problems to be considered in the physical therapist's initial examination. Although physical therapists are chiefly concerned with physical functional activities, individuals typically conceive their personal identities in terms of specific social roles: worker, father, grandmother, wife, community volunteer. All of these roles demand a certain degree of physical ability. Many opportunities for social interaction for retired elders occur around volunteer and leisure activities, even if it means only the manual dexterity required to dial a telephone. Therefore, the positive effects of physical therapy with the elderly may not be strictly limited to improvement in physical functional status. Improved social functioning may accompany changes in physical ability as well.

Although every geriatric patient can be expected to carry at least two medical diagnoses, each of which will manifest itself in particular impairments of the cardiopulmonary, musculoskeletal, or neuromuscular systems, impairment does not always entail functional limitation. One cannot assume that an individual will be unable to perform the tasks and roles of usual daily living by virtue of having an impairment alone. For example, an elder with osteoarthritis (disease) may exhibit loss of range of motion (impairment) and experience great difficulty in transferring from a bed to a chair (function). Another individual with equal loss of ROM may use a method for transferring without any difficulty, perhaps by using available joint motion to the best advantage or by using assistive devices. Sometimes patients will overcome multiple, and even permanent, impairments by the sheer force of their motivation. In the first case, a decrease in difficulty while bathing after remediation of the joint impairment would usually be accepted as clinical evidence of a causal relationship between impairment and functional loss.

The degree to which any of these limitations in physical functional activities may be linked to impairments has not been fully determined through research. The few studies that have been reported in the literature support a relationship between impairments and functional status. Bergstrom and colleagues have studied a group of 79-year-old men and women.[2,3] They found that lower extremity joint complaints were more common than upper extremity complaints. Among those elders who had upper extremity complaints, ROM was most restricted in the wrists or shoulders. Hip motion was limited in 84% of the individuals who had lower extremity complaints. When elders with symptoms and joint complaints were compared with elders without such problems, significant differences were found in the ability to use public transportation and climb stairs. Elders with musculoskeletal impairments were also more likely to use ambulation aids. Badley and co-workers conducted a study of 95 patients with arthritis whose mean age was 61.[1] If an individual could not flex the knee more than 70 degrees, the researchers noted that their subjects had difficulty walking to a toilet, transferring to a toilet, getting in and out of a bath, and walking up and down stairs. In a panel of elders in Massachusetts, Jette and colleagues found that musculoskeletal impairments in the hand influenced limitations in basic ADL over a 5-year period.[13] Progression of impairment in the lower extremity had similar significant impact on the progression of deficits in IADL. It has also been noted that the relationship between lower extremity impairment and functional performance is not always linear. Ferruci and colleagues found that strength above a certain threshold did not account for lower extremity function among 1.0002 women in the Women's Health and Aging Study.[5]

Functional assessment, which is covered elsewhere in this text, allows the therapist to determine whether the manner in which tasks and activities are done represents an important quantitative or qualitative deviation from the way in which most people of similar age would perform them. In the absence of norms for elderly functional performance, the therapist must bring previous experience with adults, who are similar to the patient, to bear on this judgment, rather than compare functionally limited elders with healthier and younger adults. Furthermore, even if the therapist concludes that the patient's performance is other than "normal," this does not imply that an elder cannot meet socially imposed expectations of what it means to be independent or that an elder is permanently disabled.

Disability

Nagi reserved the term *disability* for patterns of behavior that emerged over long periods of time during which an individual experienced functional limitations to such a degree that they could not be overcome to create some semblance of "normal" overall role and task performance. Thus, the concept of disability includes deficits in the performance of ADL and IADL that are broadly pertinent to many social roles. The person with limited shoulder motion who is fully able to bathe independently by using the range of motion available at other joints to their best mechanical advantage and a shower mitt cannot accurately be described as "disabled," even though functional performance may be extremely limited without the use of an altered movement pattern and an assistive device. Although each of the terms that have been presented so far involves some consensus about what is "normal," the concept of a "disability" is socially constructed. Disability is characterized by discordance between the actual performance of an individual in a particular role and the expectations of the community of what is "normal" for an adult. The meaning of "disabled" is taken from the community in which the individual lives and the criteria for "normal" within that social group. The term disabled connotes a particular status in society. Labeling a person as disabled requires a judgment, usually by a professional, that an individual's behaviors are somehow inadequate based on the professional's understanding of the expectations that the activity should be accomplished in ways that are typical for an elder's age and gender as well as cultural and social environment.

The evidence suggests that functional limitations and disability in a geriatric population change over time, and not all elders exhibit functional decline[7,14,21] If we follow any cohort of elders over time, there will be more disability overall within the group, but some individuals will actually improve and others will maintain their functional level. Restricting the use of the term *disabled* to describe only long-term overall functional decline in geriatric populations encourages us to understand a particular elder's functional limitations and disability in a dynamic context subject to change, particularly after therapeutic intervention. Disability depends on both the capacities of the individual and the expectations that are imposed on the individual by those in the immediate social environment, most often the patient's family and care givers. Physical therapists who apply a health status perspective to the assessment of patients draw on a broad appreciation of an elder as a person living in a particular social context as well as having individual characteristics. Changing the expectations of a social context—for example, explaining to family members what level of assistance is appropriate to an elder after stroke—may help to diminish disability as much as supplying the patient with assistive devices or increasing the physical ability to use them.

Granger notes that while the pathways from disease to disability are thought to be unidirectional, disability may itself initiate further impairments and functional limitations that foster disease.[8] Perhaps no clearer example of disability in the elderly exists than the person who has been crippled by cardiac disease because rehabilitation has not encouraged resumption of a level of activity that is "normal" for that person. Lack of activity may result in further impairment in both the cardiopulmonary and musculoskeletal systems, which may further put the individual at risk of recurrent cardiac episodes.

Another model of the process of disablement can be found in the International Classification of Impairments, Diseases and Handicaps (ICIDH). The ICIDH is currently under extensive revision. Revisions of the ICIDH that have been circulated for review internationally in 1998 continue using the term *impairment* but abandon the terms *disability* and *handicap* in favor of the terms *activity limitation* and *participation restriction,* respectively.[12] These proposed changes in ICIDH terminology, if adopted, would be closer to the concepts of functional limitation and disability used in the Nagi model and greatly reduce the overall differences between the two models.

Nagi's model has never had a term to cover the concept of handicap, a term which is more often found in the European literature, but less frequently used nowadays by clinicians and researchers in the United States. *Handicap* is a term that describes the social disadvantage of disability and is a function of a society's response to needs of people with different abilities.[8] In some instances, even a person who is functioning independently may still be "handicapped" by the social stigma of using an assistive device such as a wheelchair. Physical therapists can help change social attitudes and environmental restrictions such as architectural barriers that stigmatize individuals and restrict participation in all aspects of society.

THE RELATIONSHIP BETWEEN IMPAIRMENT AND FUNCTIONAL STATUS

Nagi's model describes the major concepts of a diagnostic process that is potentially useful to physical therapists to plan and direct treatment.[10] Although additional research is necessary to elaborate the relationship between impairments and function suggested by the research cited in the preceding text, the domain of the physical therapist's expertise is found in the ability to identify cardiopulmonary, integumentary, musculoskeletal, and neuromuscular impairments that may underlie physical functional limitations. To provide physical therapy interventions that will achieve the goal of restoring or improving function, the physical therapist must know more than the patient's signs and symptoms, which are expressions of the individual's disease and impairments. The clinician must also attempt to discern which impairments affect the patient's ability to function. Physical therapy is a complex clinical art and science, but the primary question of the discipline is simple and has two parts: What is the patient's current functional level and, which impairments contribute to the patient's functional limitations (Fig. 6-3)?

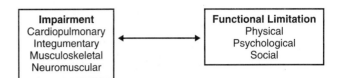

FIG. 6-3   The primary focus of a physical therapy evaluation is to determine the relationship between a patient's impairments and functional limitations.

When the therapist's attention turns toward planning intervention, the key question is, Of the impairments that are related to the patient's functional limitations, which ones can also be remedied by physical therapy treatment? Furthermore, if the patient's impairments cannot be remedied, the physical therapist then seeks to determine how the patient may compensate by using other abilities to accomplish the task and how can the task be modified so that it can be performed within the restrictions the patient's condition imposes on the situation? This latter process may be referred to as the *process of enablement* and encapsulates the rehabilitation specialist's response to the process of disablement.[4] In the next section, the process of diagnosis in physical therapy is reviewed using the terminology of *health status* and the *process of disablement.*

APPROACHES TO CLINICAL DIAGNOSIS

Physical therapists engage in the diagnostic process every time they assess a patient, cluster findings, interpret data, and label patient problems.[10,19,23] Sackett and colleagues point to four different approaches that are used by practitioners to arrive at a clinical diagnosis.[22]

One approach to clinical diagnosis uses a *decision tree* to progress the initial examination along one of a large number of potential paths. A patient's response to each inquiry or clinical assessment procedure automatically determines the next inquiry. The major disadvantage of this approach is that all contingencies have to be worked out explicitly in advance. If a patient's response or clinical presentation has not been included on the tree, then the next step of the examination remains unknown. Matching all the possible responses that could be exhibited by an older adult to specific routines of clinical examination is a daunting challenge. Furthermore, as the profession of physical therapy seeks to establish its scientific credibility, each step of the decision tree must be validated empirically.

A second strategy for clinical diagnosis is the *complete history and physical,* which has also been termed the *strategy of exhaustion:* "the painstaking invariant search for, but paying no immediate attention to, all medical facts about the patient followed by sifting through the data for the diagnosis."[22] Generally, this is the method of the novice and is abandoned with experience. Sackett and colleagues have commented that all medical students should be taught (1) how to do both a complete history and physical and (2) then once they have mastered its components, never to do one. A similar admonition may be appropriate for physical therapy students and clinicians, especially those with an interest in caring for the elderly. Students and clinicians must have mastery of all the components of a complete history and physical examination. Performing every clinical test and measure that a practitioner knows as an initial examination is, however, time-consuming, fiscally irresponsible, and likely to yield an uninterpretable catalog of abnormal findings. This does not mean that only cursory clinical examinations of the elderly are indicated. On the contrary, optimal clinical examination may require in-depth tests and measures of certain aspects of a patient's clinical presentation in order to understand the factors contributing to the patient's functional deficits. The salient point is that examination will be limited to only those aspects.

A third approach to clinical diagnosis is called *pattern recognition,* which can be defined as the "instantaneous realization that the patient's presentation conforms to a previously learned picture." Two examples of patterns recognized by many physical therapists are the upper extremity position of the adult with spastic hemiplegia and the bilateral swelling and ulnar deviation of the metacarpals of an individual with rheumatoid arthritis. These patterns represent something immediately identifiable to the experienced therapist that has been learned over time. It has been suggested that pattern recognition is increasingly used as a diagnostic strategy as clinical experience grows.[22]

Unfortunately, pattern recognition is a reflexive approach to categorizing a patient's problems that is not always a reflective process as well. The drawback of pattern recognition is that it can place too much reliance on the therapist's previous experience and lead to a narrow set of premature conclusions. If, for example, we are examining someone with shortened bilateral step length in a shuffling pattern, previous clinical experience might suggest that this is a neuromuscular impairment. On the other hand, previous exposure to patients with the bony changes associated with rheumatic diseases, who may exhibit the same nonspecific gait abnormalities, may lead to concerns about structural deformities of the metatarsals and pain (metatarsalgia). Neither conclusion would be correct without further corroborating evidence. Experienced clinicians can develop a tendency to see patterns and assign a diagnostic interpretation to the patient's signs and symptoms prematurely. There is, however, great value to pattern recognition as part of a clinical diagnostic strategy, especially at the start of the diagnostic process. By suggesting that a patient's clinical presentation might conform to some previously encountered pattern, the therapist is able to limit the search for corroborating evidence to substantiate the clinical impression.

The fourth diagnostic method is called the *hypothetico-deductive strategy,* which is defined as the formulation of a short list of potential diagnoses or actions from the earliest clues about the patient, followed by performance of specific clinical tests and measures that will best reduce the length of the list. This method corrects for the flaw in pattern recognition by not structuring the search for corroborating evidence too narrowly. Neither does it open the search too widely, requiring the therapist to consider every abnormal clinical finding that might be identified through a "complete" history and physical, especially one performed on a geriatric patient. In the next section, the essential steps of the hypothetico-deductive method are presented as a schema for evaluation and treatment planning.

SCHEMA FOR PATIENT MANAGEMENT

The *Guide to Physical Therapist Practice* describes a patient/client management model comprised of five components: examination, evaluation, diagnosis, prognosis, and intervention.[11] The Guide has two underlying premises: (1) the process of disablement is a useful model for understanding and organizing physical therapist practice and (2) diagnosis by physical therapists is an essential element of practice requiring a classification scheme that directs intervention. Each component of the model makes a vital contribution to the achievement of positive outcomes whereby functional limitations and disability are diminished or eliminated, patient satisfaction is attained, and secondary prevention is successful.

Examination

As defined in the Guide, examination has three parts: history, systems review, and specific tests and measures. Before meeting the patient, a physical therapist should organize the data collection. Owing to the reimbursement requirements currently imposed on physical therapists, many elders enter physical therapy with a referral that may contain a few useful facts about the patient's medical history or the reason for the referral. In these circumstances the first question to ask oneself is, Given the facts about the patient that are available before the examination, have any impairments or functional limitations been identified even before the patient is seen for the first time?

The collection of two kinds of clinical data should be integrated into the format for the first clinical encounter. First, there are a number of factors identified in the literature and reviewed elsewhere in this text that may influence the trajectory of a patient from disease to disability that need to be taken into account (Fig. 6-4). Specifically, these include a patient's age, gender, education, and income. With respect to the geriatric patient in particular, the therapist must also consider other medical conditions, overall health habits, cognitive ability, mood, and the patient's physical and psychosocial environments. Additional information that would assist in setting goals and designing intervention and information from other disciplines can also be very helpful. Data on the individual's current medical conditions and medications, for example, are extremely relevant. If the overall goal is to optimize patient function, then one of the first steps is

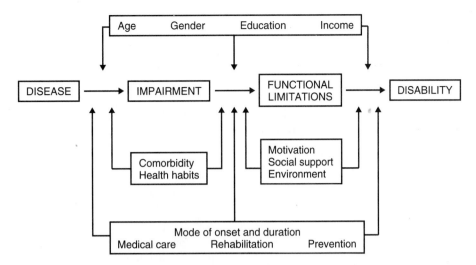

FIG. 6-4 Expansion of Nagi model to account for the influence of personal, social, and environmental factors and health care services on the process of disablement. (From Guccione AA: Arthritis and the process of disablement. *Phys Ther* 1994; 74:408-414. Used by permission of the American Physical Therapy Association.)

to ascertain the patient's current level of function. Whenever the patient's communication ability is intact, the initial interview begins by allowing patients to identify what they see as the primary functional limitations that have prompted the need for physical therapy. In their formulation of a hypothetico-deductive strategy for clinical diagnosis, Rothstein and Echternach emphasize the value of listening as patients identify their problems and allowing the individuals to express the desired goal of treatment in their own terms.[20] By talking with the patient the therapist begins to develop not only a professional rapport but also an understanding of the patient's appreciation of the situation. Listening to the patient also permits the therapist to address an ethical dimension of practice. Allowing the patient to identify the goals of treatment is one way to ensure that a person's autonomy has been respected.[9] This is especially pertinent to care provided to older individuals who may find their ability to control their own personal destinies compromised by professional judgments made "in their best interests."

When the patient is unable to communicate effectively, the therapist may turn to proxy information. The patient's family and friends may be able to give some insight as to what the patient would regard as the goals of intervention. The therapist may also hypothesize about a patient's functional deficits based on previous experience with similar patients.

Data from the history, as well as data on how the patient's problems have been treated in the past, allow the therapist to hypothesize that certain impairments or functional limitations might exist by virtue of the individual's medical condition(s) and sociodemographic and other personal characteristics. For example, suppose that the physical therapist learns from the patient's history that the patient has a medical diagnosis of Parkinson's disease, that she is 81 years old, and that she lives alone. The diagnosis of Parkinson's disease suggests the possibility of the following impairments: loss of motor

control and abnormal tone, ROM deficits, faulty posture, and decreased endurance for functional activities. Using epidemiological research about what functional limitations are likely for females living alone, specific questions about independence in IADL, with specific tests and measures as indicated, would be appropriate to include in the examination. Social isolation, for example, may lead to depression, which could further aggravate a person's functional difficulties.

After organizing one's thoughts around whatever historical information about the patient is available, the therapist begins the "hands-on" component of the clinical encounter. The systems review is a brief examination of the anatomical and physiological status of the cardiopulmonary, integumentary, musculoskeletal, and neuromuscular systems, especially as each of these affects a person's ability to initiate and sustain purposeful movement directed toward performance of a task or activity pertinent to the patient's function. The data generated by the systems review is then used by the physical therapist to select specific tests and measures that, in turn, will be used to establish a diagnosis and prognosis and to develop the plan of care. The tests and measures that are done as part of an initial examination should only be those necessary to confirm or reject a hypothesis about the factors that contribute to making the patient's current level of function less than optimal.

Evaluation

After the examination, the therapist evaluates the data by making clinical judgments about their meaning and their relevance to the patient's condition. It is not unusual for geriatric patients to have multiple impairments and functional limitations, many of which can be identified by a physical therapist and could be treated using physical therapy procedures. However, the purpose of evaluation is twofold: (1) to indicate which deficiencies in function are essential to a person's optimal well-being and (2) to identify the impairments that are most associated with the patient's current level of function and must be remediated for the patient to reach an optimal functional level.

Specific tests and measures are used in the examination to clarify the extent of functional limitation and disability and to identify impairments. Tests and measures will vary in the precision of measurement, yet useful data may be generated through various means. Data generated from either a gross test, such as "break" test for strength, or from a very precise manual muscle test could be used to reject the hypothesis that muscle performance is a contributing factor to the patient's functional deficit, depending on particular circumstances. Similarly, a functional assessment instrument may quantify a large number of ADL or IADL, yet fail to detect a particular task and activity that is most important to the patient. The "correct" test or measure is the one that yields data that are sufficiently accurate and precise to allow the therapist to make a correct inference about the patient's condition. Therefore, the therapist must consider the quality of the data; the likelihood of error; and, most importantly, the risk to the patient associated with making a clinical judgment with less-than-acceptable certainty when evaluating the meaning of the data collected on examination.

Diagnosis

The relationship between impairment and function forms the tentative basis for a system of classification for diagnosis by physical therapists.[10] The Guide established, through an extensive consensus process, preferred practice patterns that describe a cluster of impairments associated with health conditions that impede optimal function.[11] After evaluation of the examination data, the therapist first uses the classification scheme of the preferred practice patterns to complete the diagnostic process that began with the collection of data in the examination, then proceeds through the organization and interpretation of data during evaluation, and culminates with the application of a label for the patient's clinical presentation, that is, the diagnosis. As constructed on the basis

of impairments, the preferred practice patterns fulfill a major requirement of professional diagnosis, i.e., the label (diagnosis) applied as the end result of the diagnostic process directs intervention within the scope of practice of the professional applying the label.[10]

Prognosis and Treatment Planning

The next task of the physical therapist is to state a prognosis, which is a prediction about the optimal level of function that the patient will achieve and the time that will be required to reach that level. Having done that, the patient can then indicate the anticipated goals of treatment, which generally are related to the change in impairment anticipated at discharge as well as the expected outcomes of care. Physical therapy intervention will end when the expected outcomes are achieved. Therefore the functional outcomes of treatment should be stated in behavioral terms. On the basis of these anticipated goals and expected outcomes, the physical therapist then completes a plan of care that specifies the interventions to be implemented, including their frequency, intensity, and duration.

When it is decided that an individual's impairments and functional limitations are amenable to physical therapy intervention, the therapist should establish a schedule for evaluating the effectiveness of the intervention. If the patient achieves the anticipated goals for changes in impairments but does not also achieve the expected functional outcomes, this is an indication that the therapist has incorrectly hypothesized the relationship between the patient's impairments and functional status.[20] In this instance, the therapist may re-examine the patient to modify the plan of care.

Intervention

Intervention, as explicated by the Guide, has three components: (1) coordination, communication, and documentation; (2) patient-related instruction; and (3) direct intervention. Effective and comprehensive care that addresses the patient's needs is promoted through the processes of coordination, communication, and documentation. The range of

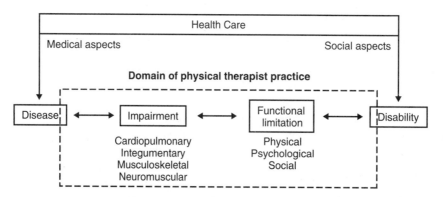

FIG. 6-5   The scope of physical therapist practice within the continuum of health care services. (Modified from Guccione AA: Physical therapy diagnosis and the relationship between impairments and function. *Phys Ther* 1991; 71:499-504. Used by permission of the American Physical Therapy Association.)

an elder's needs can be very broad and often exceed a physical therapist's scope of practice. Health care can be conceived of as a continuum of services. At one end are medical and nursing care to deal with the patient's disease and illness. At the other end of the continuum is social care and a system to facilitate re-entry of a patient with a permanent disability into the community. Although some overlap will always exist, each of these professionals has a primary relationship with the patient that is predicated on the professional's domain of expertise. Superimposing the continuum of health care onto the patient's clinical needs may provide some clues as to which other practitioners should be consulted in a well-coordinated plan of care (Fig. 6-5). Patient-related instruction, which includes teaching family, care-givers, and other professionals, is a critical therapeutic intervention for many geriatric patients and is discussed in Chapter 25.

The Guide describes nine major groups of direct interventions, all of which are relevant to geriatric physical therapy: therapeutic exercise; functional training in self-care and home management; functional training in community and work integration or reintegration; manual therapy techniques; prescription, application and as appropriate, fabrication of devices and equipment; airway clearance techniques; wound management; electrotherapeutic modalities; and physical agents and mechanical modalities. Specific applications of these direct interventions are discussed at length in Part III of this text.

Although a host of procedures and techniques might be used to remediate an impairment or minimize a functional limitation, only those that are most likely to promote the outcome in a cost-effective manner should be chosen for inclusion in the plan of care. The combination of direct interventions used with any particular patient will vary according to the impairments and functional limitations that are addressed by the plan of care for that individual. Most of the direct interventions used by physical therapists are aimed directly at remediating impairments that underlie functional limitations; however, two of the direct interventions listed in the preceding text consider the functional limitation itself. Although physical therapists sometimes apply therapeutic exercise in the position of function—for example, standing balance exercises—or try to simulate the environment in which the functional activity is performed—for example, a staircase—the functional activity in and of itself should not be confused with the core elements of a physical therapist's plan of care, that is, therapeutic exercise and functional training. It is particularly helpful for the therapist working with geriatric patients to appreciate that there are some impairments that will not change, no matter how much direct intervention is provided. This realization will diminish unnecessary treatment. In these instances, physical therapists may still achieve positive patient outcomes by teaching patients how to compensate for their permanent impairments by capitalizing on other capabilities or by modifying the environment to reduce the demands of the task.

SUMMARY

The process of disablement is a conceptualization of health status with four components that form a framework for geriatric examination, evaluation, and diagnosis supported by the *Guide to Physical Therapist Practice*. Physical therapists have particular expertise in the clinical analysis of the relationship between impairments and functional limitations and in the application of direct interventions to remediate impairments. In general, the expected outcome of physical therapy for geriatric patients is to maintain or improve their functional status.

REFERENCES

1. Badley EM, Wagstaff S, Wood PHN: Measures of functional ability (disability) in arthritis in relation to impairment of range of joint movement. *Ann Rheum Dis* 1984; 43:563-569.
2. Bergstrom G, et al: Prevalence of symptoms and signs of joint impairment at age 79. *Scand J Rehabil Med* 1985; 173-182.
3. Bergstrom G, et al: Functional consequences of joint impairment at age 79. *Scand J Rehabil Med* 1985; 17:183-190.
4. Brandt EN, Pope AM (eds): *Enabling America: Assessing the Role of Rehabilitation Science and Engineering*. Washington, DC, National Academy Press, 1997.
5. Ferruci L, et al: Departures from linearity in the relationship between measures of muscular strength and physical performance of the lower extremities: The Women's Health and Aging Study. *J Gerontol* 1997; 52A:M275-M285.
6. Gill TM, et al: Impairments in physical performance and cognitive status as predisposing factors for functional dependence among nondisabled older persons. *J Gerontol* 1996; 51A:M283-M288.
7. Gillen P, et al: Functional and residential status transitions among nursing home residents. *J Gerontol* 1996; 51A:M29-M36.
8. Granger CV: A conceptual model for functional assessment, in Granger CV, Gresham GE (eds): *Functional Assessment in Rehabilitation Medicine*. Baltimore, Williams & Wilkins, 1984.
9. Guccione AA: Compliance and patient autonomy: Ethical and legal limits to professional dominance. *Top Geriatr Rehab* 1988; 3(3):62-73.
10. Guccione AA: Physical therapy diagnosis and the relationship between impairments and function. *Phys Ther* 1991; 71:499-504.
11. Guide to physical therapist practice. *Phys Ther* 1997; 1163-1650.
12. *ICIDH-2: International Classification of Impairments, Activities and Participation. Manual of Dimensions of Disablement and Functioning. Beta-1 draft for field trials*. World Health Organization, Geneva, 1997.
13. Jette AM, Branch LG, Berlin J: Musculoskeletal impairments and physical disablement among the aged. *J Gerontol* 1990; 45:M203-208.
14. Manton KG: A longitudinal study of functional change and mortality in the United States. *J Gerontol* 1988; 43:S153-161.
15. Nagi SZ: Some conceptual issues in disability and rehabilitation, in Sussman MB (ed): *Sociology and Rehabilitation.* Washington, DC, American Sociological Association, 1965.
16. Nagi SZ: *Disability and Rehabilitation*. Columbus, Ohio State University Press, 1969.
17. Nagi SZ: An epidemiology of disability among adults in the United States. *Milbank Mem Fund Q/Health Soc* 1976; 54:439-467.
18. Nagi S: Disability concepts revisited: Implication for prevention, in Pope AM, Tarlov AR (eds): *Disability in America: Toward a National Agenda for Prevention.* Washington, DC, National Academy Press, 1991.
20. Rose SJ: Musing on diagnosis. *Phys Ther* 1988; 68:1665.
21. Rothstein JM, Echternach JL: Hypothesis-oriented algorithm for clinicians: A method of evaluation and treatment planning. *Phys Ther* 1986; 66:1388-1394.
22. Rudberg MA, et al: Functional limitation pathways and transitions in community-dwelling older persons. *Gerontologist* 1996; 36:430-440.
23. Sackett DL, et al: *Clinical Epidemiology: A Basic Science for Clinical Medicine*, ed 2. Boston, Little, Brown, 1991.

24. Sahrmann SA: Diagnosis by the physical therapist—prerequisite for treatment. *Phys Ther* 1988; 68:1703-1706.

25. Schenkman M, Butler RB: A model for multisystem evaluation, interpretation, and treatment of individuals with neurologic dysfunction. *Phys Ther* 1989; 69:538.

26. Schenkman M, Butler RB: A model for multisystem evaluation and treatment of individuals with Parkinson's disease. *Phys Ther* 1989; 69:932-943.

27. Sorensen LB, Blair JM: Rheumatologic diseases, in Cassel CK, et al (eds): *Geriatric Medicine,* ed 3. New York, Springer-Verlag, 1997.

28. Wei JY: Disorders of the heart, in Hazzard WR, et al (eds): *Principles of Geriatric Medicine and Gerontology,* ed 3. New York, McGraw-Hill, 1994.

29. World Health Organization: *The First Ten Years of the World Health Organization.* Geneva, World Health Organization, 1958.

CHAPTER 7

FUNCTIONAL ASSESSMENT OF THE ELDERLY

ANDREW A. GUCCIONE, PT, PhD, FAPTA

INTRODUCTION

There can be little dissension that the ultimate goal of all physical therapy interventions with the elderly is to restore or maintain the highest level of function possible for the individual, particularly function associated with movement. Whenever physical therapists take on this challenge, they assist elders in maintaining their identities as competent adults. Very young children begin to define themselves, in part, through their independence and mastery over the physical environment, and their pleasure in these achievements is self-evident. Disease and illness threaten more than

an older person's physical health. By altering the ability to function, disease and its effects curtail the customary activities that a person identifies as essential to meaningful living. Therefore, functional assessment, in its broadest sense, is particular to the individual and a measure of those activities by which an individual judges the quality of life.

The four purposes of this chapter are to review what is currently known about the physical functional status of the elderly, describe the elements that may be included in a physical functional assessment, discuss some of the methodological aspects of administering a functional assessment, and describe some of the formal functional assessment instruments that have been used broadly in geriatric clinical practice and research.

As has been described in Chapter 6 and elsewhere in this text, the data of a functional assessment alone cannot determine the interventions included in the plan of care. The physical therapist must review functional limitations in light of other clinical findings that identify the patient's impairments and other psychological, social, and environmental factors that modify function in determining whether a patient will become disabled.[45] The therapist then hypothesizes which findings contribute to the patient's functional deficits and will be the focus of patient-related instruction and direct intervention. Three patients may have the same limitation, i.e., inability to transfer independently from bed to chair, yet require entirely different programs of intervention. If the first individual lacked sufficient knee strength to come to a standing position, then the plan of care would incorporate strengthening exercises to remedy the impairment and improve the patient's function. If the second patient lacked sufficient range of motion (ROM) at the hip due to flexion contractures to allow full upright standing, then intervention would focus on increasing ROM at the hip to improve function. The third individual may possess all the musculoskeletal and neuromuscular prerequisites to allow function but still require appropriate instruction to do it safely and with minimal exertion. Each individual may achieve a similar level of functional independence, yet none of the three would have received the exact same treatment to achieve the same outcome.

Physical Functional Limitations and Disability in the Elderly

As elaborated in Chapter 6, physical, psychological, and social function are all dimensions of function that are included in the measurement of a person's overall health status.[49] Physical therapists are most often concerned with evaluating and diagnosing physical functional limitations and then remediating the impairments that underlie them. Physical functional activities, the focus of this chapter, can be subdivided into five areas: mobility, which includes transfers and ambulation; basic self-care and personal hygiene activities of daily living (ADL); more complex activities essential to an adult's living in the community, known as instrumental ADL (IADL); work; and recreation.

Epidemiological studies of functional limitations in the elderly provide a group context into which a physical therapist can place an individual patient's level of function.[8] In general, we know that the ability to function independently declines with age and that this decline is influenced by a host of biological, psychological, and social factors.[36] There are several major sources of epidemiological data on function in the elderly.[54] These include the Supplement on Aging (SOA) to the 1984 National Health Interview Survey,[14] the 1985 National Nursing Home Survey (NNHS),[28] the 1987 National Medical Expenditure Survey (NMES),[38] the 1982 and 1984 National Long Term Care Surveys (NLTCSs),[40] and the Establishment of Populations for the Epidemiologic Study of the Elderly (EPESE) project begun in 1982.[6] Function is not a static phenomenon in the elderly. It is important to note that each of these data sets yields somewhat different rates on the incidence and prevalence of functional limitations and disability in the elderly that indicate transitions in functional status are more the norm than the exception.[7]

Community-Dwelling Elders

The SOA data indicate that as few as 19% of the 26.4 million noninstitutionalized persons older than 65 in 1984 had difficulty walking (Fig. 7-1).[26] Gender-specific rates of difficulty in walking, however, were different. Just over 20% of women older than 65 had difficulty walking, whereas only 15.5% of their male counterparts did. Slightly more than 77% of those surveyed in the SOA reported no difficulty in any of basic ADL, which is not surprising in a noninstitutionalized population. Difficulty in bathing and in getting outside were reported by 10% of these elders, whereas 6% experienced difficulty in dressing. Almost one quarter of these elders had trouble with a single home-management task, heavy home chores (Fig. 7-2). Nearly 27% had difficulty with at least one of six IADL: preparing meals, shopping, managing money, using the telephone, doing heavy home chores, and per-

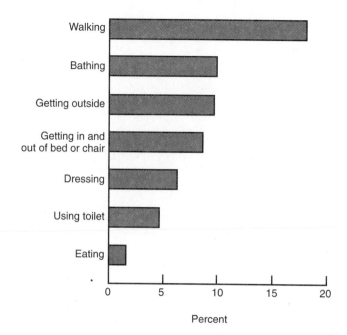

FIG. 7-1 Percentage of the noninstitutionalized population 65 years of age or older who have difficulty with activities of daily living, by type of activity: United States, 1984. (Redrawn from Havlik RJ, et al: Health statistics on older persons, United States, 1986. *Vital and Health Statistics, Series 3, No 25.* Hyattsville, Md, Public Health Service, DHHS No (PHS) 87–1409, 1987.)

forming light housework. Male elders reported less difficulty in almost all these tasks than female elders did.

Data on elders who participated in a longitudinal follow-up to the SOA, known as the LSOA, suggest that there may be a hierarchy of disability with a definite sequence: walking, bathing, transferring, dressing, toileting, and feeding.[11] If this hierarchy is confirmed in subsequent studies, it supports the importance of lower extremity functional limitations as an early marker of disability in the elderly.[22] Despite the fact that advancing age increases the risk of functional limitations, there are still a substantial number of old-old who remain physically independent. Harris and her colleagues examined physical ability in 80-year-olds who participated in LSOA.[25] Using four items from Nagi's measure of work disability, they found that 67% of all white persons aged 80 or older had no difficulty lifting 10 pounds; 57% had no difficulty climbing up 10 steps; 49% had no difficulty walking a quarter of a mile; and 47% had no difficulty with stooping, crouching, or kneeling (Fig. 7-3). The order in which the activities became more difficult was the same for men as for women. Women, however, reported more difficulty with each of these tasks than men did. Differences between men and women in the incidence of disability have been demonstrated in other studies as well.[11]

Given that any sample of elderly will most likely contain a larger proportion of older and therefore more functionally disabled women than men, a difference in the rates of functional deficits between men and women is not unexpected.[12] The differential rates of disability in IADL between men and

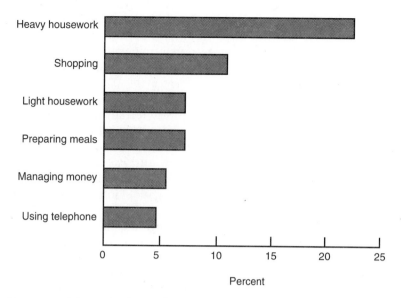

FIG. 7-2 Percentage of the noninstitutionalized population 65 years of age or older who have difficulty with instrumental activities of daily living, by type of activity: United States, 1984. (Redrawn from Havlik RJ, et al: Health statistics on older persons, United States, 1986. *Vital and Health Statistics, Series 3, No 25.* Hyattsville, Md, Public Health Service, DHHS No (PHS) 87–1409, 1987.)

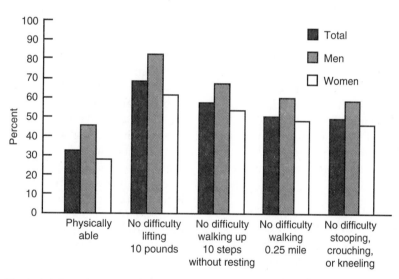

FIG. 7-3 Physical ability of noninstitutionalized white persons, age 80 or older. (Redrawn from Harris T, et al: Longitudinal study of physical ability in the olders-old. *Am J Public Health* 1989; 79:698–702.)

women are also partially explained by a gender bias in the items of many surveys. Among present-day elders, many men do not perform housekeeping and other similar activities. Therefore, men may not report having any difficulty at all performing these tasks because they did not perform them at the time of the interview. Neither have many male elders generally ever performed these tasks, a reflection of the arbitrary notion of what is "proper" for a man or a woman in general society or a particular sociocultural environment. A similar finding was obtained in the EPESE study of elders with low back pain.[35] Although elderly women with low back pain reported modestly higher rates of disability in

basic ADL than men, the rate of limitation in doing household chores for women was more than double the rate for men.

Besides underscoring the gender bias of some items that might be included in a functional assessment, differences in functional status between men and women remind us that function is also a sociological phenomenon. Functional assessment does not only measure the individual's abilities to perform tasks that are personally meaningful to the individual. Functional assessment also depends on social expectations of what is "normal" functioning for an adult. In some social groups, a man might never be expected to do house-cleaning nor would anyone anticipate that a woman would shovel snow, because performing these activities runs counter to what a man or a woman "should" do. It is therefore necessary that the overall approach to functional assessment of an elder include items that take into account what is "normal" in that person's social and cultural sphere.

A judgment about whether an elder's functional level is normal also draws heavily on cultural and ethnic attitudes. If there is a certain expectation in the family that debilitation in old age is a normal occurrence and that elders are entitled to have even the simplest ADL done for them, then there is little likelihood that the goal of independence in all ADL will be supported when the episode of care ends. Therefore, physical therapists working with elders from specific groups should have an understanding of different cultural and ethnic expectations regarding independent function.

Institutionalized Elders

The substantial difference in functional limitations and disability between elders still living in the community and those who reside in a nursing home has been known for some time. Inability to perform simple self-care activities typically places an elder at risk for admission to a nursing home. Data from the NNHS that compare nursing home residents with their noninstitutionalized peers clearly indicate the disparity in functional levels between these two groups of elders. Whereas more than 90% of elders in nursing homes required assistance in bathing, only 6% of community-dwelling elders needed help in this activity. Similarly, just more than 40% of nursing home residents needed assistance to eat, whereas only 1.1% of their peers outside the nursing home were similarly limited (Table 7-1).

Data on the differences in disability between community-dwelling and institutionalized elders provide direction for physical therapists planning a functional assessment for an individual patient. The relationship between ADL and IADL is generally hierarchical; that is, limitations in ADL usually predict limitations in IADL.[3,51] For example, we know that most elders living in the community are generally independent in all ADL and may experience limitations in a few IADL. Thus, a home-care physical therapist working with a patient recently returning home from an acute care hospital after a hip fracture would first explore the individual's ability to do the tasks and activities encompassed by basic ADL, such as transfers, ambulation, and toileting. If deficits were found, independence in these activities would serve as the first goals of intervention. If the patient was independent in basic ADL upon initial examination, or became independent through the physical therapist's intervention, the therapist would then examine the elder's limitations in performing IADL, which supports a person's ability to live independently in the community.

Physical therapists should be wary, however, of assuming too quickly that there is a need for institutionalization merely on the broad epidemiological evidence supporting a relationship between limitations in basic ADL and the ability to remain living in the community. Epidemiological data summarize various facts about a group, but a particular fact need not apply to every member of that group. Furthermore, despite the fact that most elders living in the community generally function at a higher level than their institutionalized peers, many elders with functional limitations do manage to remain outside of institutions with formal services or through the efforts of families and friends. Physical therapists play an important role in identifying an elder's needs for formal care-givers, such as homemakers and home health aides, and in teaching families how to manage an elderly patient's limitations well enough so that the individual may continue to reside in the community.

At least two other factors also influence whether an elder limited in the most basic ADL continues to live in the community. First, there are not enough nursing home beds in some areas to accommodate the need of the community for such placements. Thus, an elder might benefit from admission to a nursing home but will continue to live at home. Second, even if nursing home beds are available, some elders lack the appropriate insurance coverage or the financial means to claim them. These individuals will therefore remain in the community, sometimes under the most distressing circumstances. Therapists working in the community should anticipate that elders who are disabled enough to require human assistance around the clock will constitute at least a small portion of their caseloads from time to time.

TABLE 7-1

PERCENTAGE OF PERSONS 65 YEARS OF AGE AND OVER, BY WHETHER NURSING HOME RESIDENT OR NONINSTITUTIONALIZED AND TYPE OF DEPENDENCY IN SELECTED ADL: UNITED STATES, 1984 AND 1985

TYPE OF DEPENDENCY	NURSING HOME RESIDENTS, 1985(%)	NONINSTITUTIONALIZED POPULATION*† 1984(%)
Requires assistance in		
Bathing	91.2	6.0
Dressing	77.7	4.3
Using toilet room	63.3	2.2
Transferring‡	62.7	2.8
Eating	40.4	1.1

*From Dawson D, Hendershot G, Fulton J: Aging in the eighties. Functional limitations of individuals age 65 years and over. *Advance Data From Vital and Health Statistics. No 133.* DHHS Publication No (PHS) 87–1250. Hyattsville, Md. Public Health Service. April 30, 1987.
†Percentage of the noninstitutionalized elderly dependent in activities of daily living is a measure of those who *received* help rather than those needing it.
‡Transferring refers to getting in or out of a bed or chair.

COMPONENTS OF PHYSICAL FUNCTIONAL ASSESSMENT

Functional assessment data can be useful to physical therapists in several ways.[34] On the individual level, a functional assessment can be used as a quick screen to identify the need for more extensive evaluation by a physical therapist or other practitioners. If an elder who has functional deficits becomes a patient, these data determine the overall goals of physical therapy treatment. Such goals serve as indicators of a patient's progress and validate the success (or failure) of the therapist's intervention. Finally, organizing and analyzing functional data by types of patients or patients' problems can provide valuable documentation of the needs of a group for treatment, the benefits of a particular treatment approach, or the success of an innovative program.

Mobility

A primary concern of physical therapists in performing a physical functional assessment of an elderly individual is to identify any functional limitations in mobility: ambulation on level surfaces within the home, stair climbing, negotiating uneven terrain, and walking for longer distances in the community.

Basic Activities of Daily Living (ADL)

Basic ADL include all of the fundamental tasks and activities necessary for survival, hygiene, and self-care within the home. A typical ADL battery, which may be administered by a physical therapist alone or cooperatively with other health professionals, covers eating, bathing, grooming, dressing, bed mobility, and transfers. Incontinence and the ability to use a bathroom are especially important elements in the assessment of physical function in some older individuals. The ability of an elder in three aspects of toileting may each require exploration: to get to the bathroom in an appropriate time period, to move safely on and off the receptacle, and to perform self-hygiene tasks.

Instrumental Activities of Daily Living (IADL)

An examination and evaluation of IADL addresses multiple areas that are essential to living independently as an adult: cooking, shopping, washing, housekeeping, and ability to use public transportation or drive a car. For some individuals, it may also be appropriate to investigate the ability to perform home chores such as shoveling snow or yardwork.

Work

One measure of adult competence is employment. Previously, it has been assumed that elders did not need to or want to work. Changes in federal regulations during the 1980s raised the minimum age at which individuals may receive full Social Security benefits and also removed a mandatory retirement age for most occupations.[32] Therefore, elders who want to, or need to, remain in the work force may do so if they are physically able to perform the tasks of their employment. The ability to work may be investigated in two ways. One approach is to consider the conditions of work itself: whether an individual is working the anticipated number of hours each week; whether the requirements of the job have been modified in any respect to allow the individual to work; and whether the quantity or quality of work done has met the anticipated standard of performance. Another approach to assessing work is to examine the ability to perform 10 particular physical tasks, first described by Nagi,[45] that are associated with work disability: (1) walking up 10 steps without resting; (2) walking a quarter of a mile; (3) sitting for 2 hours; (4) standing for 2 hours; (5) stooping, crouching, or kneeling; (6) reaching up overhead; (7) reaching out to shake hands; (8) grasping with fingers; (9) lifting or carrying 10 pounds; and (10) lifting or carrying 25 pounds. Using these data on "advanced" mobility, one can infer what an elderly individual's capacity to work would be.

Recreation

Recreational activities are no less important than work to maintain a sense of well-being. Clearly, more older men and women today are maintaining interests in recreational sports that they developed earlier in life. Other elders are just discovering the pleasures of physical exertion. Functional assessment of recreational activities, however, is not limited only to sports. Many elders enjoy dancing and gardening, which require a relatively high degree of balance, flexibility, and strength. Even sedentary activities, such as stamp collecting or playing chess, require a certain degree of physical ability in the hand and upper extremity and therefore may be functional measures of the outcomes of intervention for some patients.

METHODOLOGICAL ISSUES

There are three methodological issues that are germane to the discussion of functional status measurement: reliability, validity, and clinical utility.[2,4,18,19,42,48] It is sometimes erroneously assumed that measurement issues are relevant only if a clinician uses a formal instrument to measure function. This is simply not the case. All physical therapist examination involves tests and measures that provide data used by the physical therapist to render an evaluation of the patient's condition. The certainty of that professional judgment is a function of the quality of the data. It is important to know whether apparent improvement in a patient's level of function is a real change in performance or merely a variation in measurement due to the nature of the test or the skill of the tester in administering the test. These are issues of reliability. It is also important to know whether the therapist actually gathered the information that was intended to be gathered and what inferences about the patient's status or prognosis are appropriate based on the data. These are the central questions of the validity of a measurement.

Reliability

There are several forms of reliability, each of which is pertinent to judging the value of the information derived from a particular test. The first kind of reliability is termed *internal consistency* and is a measure of the degree to which items on a test purportedly measure the same thing and yield similar results.[48] Internal consistency is important in judging the value of assessment instruments that use a battery of multiple items to cover a component of function such as basic ADL, IADL, or mobility. Internal consistency is an indicator of how well the items within a segment "hang together" and measure the same kind of thing. If a battery contains too many questions all measuring the same thing, it may be possible to drop some items and examine a patient more efficiently.

Two other kinds of reliability indicate how much variability in test scores is due to the tester. The first of these, *intra-rater reliability,* attests to the degree to which a measurement will change when the same tester administers the test on two separate occasions when no real change has occurred between administrations. This form of reliability is often taken as an indicator of the stability of a test between administrations. *Inter-rater reliability* indicates the agreement of test results when two or more testers measure the same thing. Both of these forms of reliability are critical to clinical practice, especially in geriatric physical therapy because multiple care-givers may repeat measurements on the same patient over a period of time and use these data to determine a patient's improvement or deterioration.

Validity

There are several kinds of validity that are pertinent to functional assessment.[48] The first is *face validity,* which requires the judgment that the assessment appears on the face of it to be a test of what is to be measured. For example, an IADL test should measure activities such as cooking, grocery shopping, and housekeeping in some way. If the test consisted of only sociodemographic data and goniometric measurements, we would conclude that this test lacked face validity as a measure of IADL.

Content validation establishes the degree to which test measures adequately sample a domain of activities. For example, a formal measure of recreational activity might only mention two of the more strenuous sports—hiking and kayaking, list only running and jogging under cardiovascular training activities, and omit more sedentary pastimes altogether. Such an instrument would not have adequately sampled the multitude of activities that constitute "recreation," especially for older adults. Therefore, we would conclude that this instrument lacked content validity.

Although *construct validity* often involves statistical approaches that are far beyond the scope of this text, it is a critical dimension of functional assessment. Construct validation answers the question: Does a test yield measurements that represent the underlying concept of what we want to measure? All the questions posed to a patient during an initial examination and all the measurements taken during assessment do not fall into the same category. Some formal functional assessment instruments were developed before there was much concern about the psychometric properties of physical therapy tests and measures. These instruments tend to combine disease severity, impairment, and functional limitations under a single category of "function." Several even combine scores on various subsections of the test to give an overall "functional" score. A single number appears to be a useful and reliable summary of the patient's sta-

tus, but it can be difficult to determine exactly what construct has been measured by this sort of score. Although these scores may be reliable, their validity is a separate question. Physical therapists should use them thoughtfully because they may often reflect more than a person's functional status.

Sometimes the results of a test can be compared with a "gold standard," which is accepted as an unimpeachable measure of whatever is being tested. This comparison demonstrates that the test has concurrent validity. For example, the results obtained from a formal ADL instrument that uses a patient's self-report might be shown to be similar to the results obtained from having the patient actually perform the activities listed in the instrument. We might then compare the patient's self-report to that of another individual who knows the patient well. We might also demonstrate that elders who are judged as being independent by this self-report measure also have fewer impairments in ROM, strength, and balance.

Physical therapists are also responsible to establish a prognosis, or the likelihood of achieving anticipated goals and expected outcomes, as part of the process of physical therapist patient/client management.[20] Often, we base these judgments on a combination of the patient's clinical presentation and our prior clinical experience. What we lack as often is a clear understanding of the predictive validity of our measurements, which allows us to know that a certain score on a test at the initiation of treatment predicts the outcome of intervention. Knowing the predictive validity of a baseline functional assessment would greatly facilitate the formulation of achievable goals and increase the efficiency of discharge planning from the beginning of intervention.

Clinical Utility

The ultimate value of any clinical data is their usefulness to the task at hand. Reliable and valid data are necessary but not sufficient conditions for test results to have clinical utility. If a test or instrument has clinical utility, all necessary data will be gathered completely and in the shortest time period. Too many questions and too many complicated steps increase respondent burden. If an elder becomes annoyed, fatigued, or distracted by the examination, then the therapist may have hindered the development of professional rapport with the patient, an important factor in the success of any rehabilitation program.

Is it necessary to use a formal, structured instrument to conduct a functional assessment? It is doubtful that a single instrument will contain all the activities that would constitute a complete examination of any one person's function. Therefore, a therapist may wish to combine a formal instrument with unstructured assessment and open-ended questions as part of the overall examination. This will ensure that there are similar baseline data with known reliability and validity on all patients as well as data that capture information unique to the individual. Given that some formal instruments may not be well-suited to particular clinical needs, it is tempting to "mix and match" from several instruments.

Extrapolating items from a variety of instruments may provide the kind of data desired, but it may be at the expense of reliability and validity. Further methodological problems may arise when instruments are not administered in the format for which they were developed and tested. Users may prefer or need to gather data in some instances by using trained interviewers. This requires that explicit instructions for the interviewers have been developed to ensure comparability of results.

PARAMETERS OF MEASUREMENT
Independence

The concept of functional independence may be conceived in several ways. These include dependence or the degree of assistance needed to perform a task, how much pain accompanies the task, the amount of time it takes to perform the activity, or whether an individual uses an assistive device or aid to perform the task. The amount of difficulty an individual has when attempting to perform functional activities is another way to operationalize independence. The concept of difficulty is composite of several criteria to assess how functional activities are performed and summarizes the degree of effort expended in performing the task. It involves elements of how long the activity takes, how much discomfort the individual experiences, and to what degree assistive devices are required.

In order to collect the appropriate information on an elder's functional status, the therapist must consider the way in which functional limitations are identified and the kind of data needed. Merely using an assistive device and performing an activity with difficulty are appropriate criterion levels of disability for some clinical or research purposes, but each parameter alone may not identify the same individuals as limited. The difficulty of an activity may be diminished, in fact, by using an adaptive device.[53] The need for human assistance may be a more meaningful criterion of dysfunction when the data will be used to plan an elder's need for services or to make public policy decisions.

Therapists must also consider what constitutes a clinically meaningful change in function. If an individual's behavior may be graded only as "independent or dependent," then the scoring system may not be sensitive to real changes that indicate a patient's progress. For example, progression from being totally nonambulatory to requiring only moderate assistance to ambulate can represent substantial improvement in function. However, if the patient can only be rated as "independent/dependent," then treatment might erroneously be judged as ineffective. Careful consideration of the precision of descriptors is essential to capture subtle yet noticeable improvements in a patient's condition.

Capacity vs. Habit

A second dimension of the examination and evaluation of function involves the degree to which the therapist wishes to determine the patient's capacity to function, or, in contrast, the patient's habitual function. Clinical care may be likened in some respects to a scientific inquiry of behavior. In some instances, data about the behavior under controlled conditions is more useful than data obtained from a natural, uncontrolled environment in revealing the capacity of a person to achieve a certain level of performance and to identify the threshold for failure in performance. Data of this sort indicate how a person will function at full potential. On the other hand, data that account for task performance in terms of one's daily habits tell us a great deal about what someone is likely to do, even though it may fall short of the individual's full potential to function. Thus, depending on how the functional assessment is implemented, there may be some disparity between what elders demonstrate or perceive as their capabilities and what they will habitually perform at home. It may also be very frustrating for the clinician when an individual demonstrates awareness of the full potential for function but does not habitually engage in that level of performance. Therefore, therapists must recognize that even if an elder has the capacity to perform the activity but will not do it, treatment to achieve a higher level of function may be inappropriate because it will not be one of the goals of intervention accepted by the patient.

MODES OF ASSESSMENT
Direct Observation

There are three primary methods to measuring functional status. Data on an individual's level of physical function may be collected by observing, by asking the subject to perform a function under a specific set of conditions, or gathered from a self-report or interviewer-administered questionnaire. Therapists are most familiar with direct observation of the activity. The major advantage of this approach is that the professional judgment of functional status is based on clear-cut objective evidence of the ability to perform the task.[24] Physical performance measures are also not limited by language barriers.[21] If the therapist and the patient do not speak the same language, the therapist may act out the activity and signal that the patient should do the same. Observations of performance have some disadvantages. This method assumes that the controlled environment of a structured situation in the clinic is reasonably similar to the environment in which a person functions. An individual may not be able to transfer out of a chair in the clinic but may be totally independent in transferring using any chair in that person's home. Physical performance measures are also time-consuming for the therapist and therefore costly.

There are a number of tests that are sometimes also referred to as *performance measures,* including the 6-minute walk test,[5] the Physical Performance and Mobility Examination,[55] the Functional Reach Test,[9,10] the Get Up and Go test,[41] the Timed "Up and Go" test,[47] and the Physical Performance Battery.[23] Typically, these instruments record quantitative data and may also generate a single score. In some instances, these instruments have been shown to correlate closely the success or failure of an individual in performing goal-directed functional activities or tasks or some key indicators such as falls, hospitalizations, or need for services.

Although these tests use the same method of direct observation as may be used to document abilities in ADL or IADL, they most typically measure performance limitations at the levels of impairment and functional limitations. On review, the broad object of measurement in these tests is the quantification of the complex integration of systems that permits an individual to maintain a posture, transition to other postures, or sustain safe and efficient movement. Furthermore, the data from such tests characterize a person's performance limitations under controlled conditions. It is critical to appreciate that even though each of these performance tests can contribute to an overall understanding of a person's functional limitations because they help to identify the movement dysfunction that may underlie physical disability, they do not assess disability in any particular ADL or IADL, even when a test contains elements that mimic everyday life. They generally do not capture function as it actually occurs in a natural environment. Furthermore, they do not always account for factors that may positively or negatively modify a person's function, given that the functional task or activity must be accomplished in the "real" world of the patient, which is also influenced by cognition, motivation, social support, and physical environment.

Self-Report

While direct observation may have stood as the gold standard for some time, self-report approaches have become well-accepted in research and have been increasingly integrated into clinical practice. Self-report is now considered the most feasible and cost-effective means of gathering standardized functional status data on large numbers of individuals.[42] Self-assessment is a valid method of assessing function and may be preferable to performance-based methods in some circumstances.[34,44,52] One further consideration in using a self-report mode of assessment is whether to use a trained interviewer to administer the instrument or to allow the respondent to read and answer a questionnaire. There appears to be little difference in the quality of the data obtained by self-report or a face-to-face interviewer.[43] However, it may be the case that visual loss or shorter attention spans recommend the use of trained interviewers for some elders.

Some self-report instruments phrase questions as "Could you . . . ?" whereas another may query the same activity by asking "Do you . . . ?" As previously explained, these are not equivalent forms of the same question and do not yield the same information. The first way of phrasing a question taps into an elder's beliefs about personal abilities, which may be based only partially on empirical evidence. The second approach establishes whether the individual does the activity. Thus, an elder might respond to a question about stair climbing in the following way: "I could climb the stairs to the second floor of my home (if I had to), but I do not climb the stairs (because it hurts my knee and I don't want to)."

The time frames of particular items vary from questionnaire to questionnaire. The period of inquiry may be for the same day, the past week, or even the past month. Therapists must decide in advance what is the appropriate time period in which to sample behavior, given the fluctuating nature of many geriatric problems.

Selected Instruments for Geriatric Functional Assessment

A considerable number of functional assessment instruments with particular relevance to geriatric physical therapy have been presented in the literature. Comprehensive reviews of these instruments have been published elsewhere.[1, 18,19,42] A few of these instruments are reviewed in the following text. They were selected on the basis of being representative of the current state of the art in geriatric functional assessment as well as for their predominance in geriatric clinical practice and research.

Katz Index of Activities of Daily Living

Katz's index is the prototypic instrument for measuring basic ADL in geriatric patients.[30,31] The index covers activities in six categories: bathing, dressing, toileting, transfers, continence, and feeding. Unfortunately, this instrument does not address ambulation and other components of mobility, which are particularly pertinent to physical therapy. Although designed for use among institutionalized elders, the theoretical foundation of the Katz index is actually taken from a developmental model of children. According to this model, feeding is designated as the "lowest" and most easily acquired function, whereas bathing represents the developmentally "highest" level of function. Each item on the Katz is rated according to the degree of assistance needed to do the task. Responses in each category of activity are then dichotomized as independent or dependent, according to predetermined criteria. The pattern of responses is then converted to a cumulative letter grade from A through G, which denotes a particular pattern of dependency in the hierarchy of function. For example, an "A" means independent in all six functional categories; a "C" indicates independent in bathing, dressing, and one other function; and a "G" denotes dependence in all activities. The psychometric properties of the Katz are sufficient to justify its widespread use in both clinical care and research.

Functional Independence Measure

The Functional Independence Measure (FIM) is an 18-item measure of physical, psychological, and social function that is part of the Uniform Data System for Medical Rehabilitation.[16,17] The FIM uses the level of assistance an individual needs to grade functional status from total independence to total assistance. A person may be regarded as independent if a device is used, but this is recorded separately from "complete" independence. The instrument lists six self-care activities: feeding, grooming, bathing, upper body dressing, lower body dressing, and toileting. Bowel and bladder control, aspects of which some may consider as impairments rather than function, are categorized separately. Mobility is tested only through three items on transfers. Under the category of locomotion, walking and using a wheelchair are listed equivalently, whereas stairs are considered separately. The FIM also includes two items on communication and three on social cognition.

The FIM measures what the individual does, not what that person could do under certain circumstances. The interrater reliability of the FIM has been established at an acceptable level of psychometric performance. The face and content validity of the FIM as well as its ability to capture change in a patient's level of function have also been determined. A trained clinician must administer the FIM because the response for each item requires a professional judgment.

OARS Multidimensional Functional Assessment Questionnaire

The Older American Resources and Services (OARS) was one of the first formal approaches developed explicitly to assess the function of elders in multiple domains.[13,15] The OARS, which was developed and tested at the Duke Center for the Study of Aging and Human Development, is composed of an instrument to assess functional activities (the Multidimensional Functional Assessment Questionnaire [MFAQ]) and a questionnaire to identify the resources that an elder uses. The MFAQ is designed to be administered by a trained interviewer. To ensure the reliability and validity of the responses given to the interviewer, the MFAQ begins with an assessment of the elder's cognitive function. The Services Assessment Questionnaire (SAQ) records both an elder's use of services and the perceived need for services. A total of 24 generic services are covered, e.g., nursing and homemaker services, legal and protective aid, and recreation.

The items on the MFAQ cover basic and instrumental ADL, social interaction and resources, economic resources, physical health, and mental health. After reviewing the responses, the interviewer rates the elder in each of the five dimensions using a six-point scale. The scale's end points are "excellent functioning" and "total or complete impaired function." The MFAQ's reliability and validity have been established and meet acceptable levels of psychometric performance. It has also been shown that the MFAQ is sensitive enough to detect gross changes over time and can discriminate among elders who live independently in the community, require adult day care, or are institutionalized.

Philadelphia Geriatric Center Multilevel Assessment Instrument

The Multilevel Assessment Instrument (MAI) is based on Lawton's conceptual model of adult behavior, which is hierarchically organized by the complexity of the behavior.[37] There are five behavioral domains represented in the MAI: physical health, cognition, self-care, and instrumental ADL; time use (employment, hobbies, recreation); social interaction; personal adjustment (morale, psychiatric symptoms); and perceived environment (housing, neighborhood, per-

sonal security). The items on ADL investigate the perceived ability of an individual—i.e., "Can you . . . ?"—rather than actual performance of the task—i.e., "Do you . . . ?" Limitations are graded by the degree of human assistance required rather than the quality of the performance. As discussed elsewhere in this text, the psychological dimension of health status is composed of mental and affective function. The MAI is an excellent example of an instrument that differentiates cognition, morale, and psychiatric symptoms.

The MAI is available in full, midlength, and short forms. The MAI in all its forms had extensive testing of its reliability and validity. In general, the MAI has demonstrated acceptable psychometric characteristics, particularly in its long form. The instrument was designed to be administered by an interviewer and can be completed in less than 1 hour.

Minimum Data Sheet for Nursing Home Resident Assessment and Care Screening

The Omnibus Budget Reconciliation Act of 1987 (OBRA '87) mandated a number of changes in nursing home regulations, which were meant to guarantee quality of care for nursing home residents. One mechanism to monitor care to all Medicare or Medicaid nursing homes, developed subsequent to the enactment of OBRA '87, was the Resident Assessment Instrument (RAI), which was revised in 1995 (version 2.0).[39] The RAI has three parts: the Minimum Data Set (MDS), Resident Assessment Protocols (RAPs), and Utilization Guidelines. The MDS is used to assess the patterns of a patient's function in multiple dimensions: cognitive, communication/hearing, vision, physical functioning and structural problems, continence in the last 14 days, psychosocial well-being, mood and behavior, and activity pursuit. The MDS is also used to collect basic demographic data, disease diagnoses, health conditions, oral/nutritional status, oral/dental status, skin condition, medication use, and special treatment and procedures—an area that specifically lists physical therapy.

After the initial admission of the patient to a facility, the MDS must be completed by the 14th calendar day of residency including weekends. After this initial administration, the resident must be reassessed using the full MDS annually. A subset of MDS items must also be assessed on each resident every 3 months. If there is a significant change that appears to be permanent, a resident should be assessed using the MDS within 14 days after the change has occurred, in addition to any quarterly or yearly reassessments. The law requires that each assessment be conducted or coordinated by a registered nurse, who may choose to assign parts of the assessment to other health professionals, including physical therapists.

Physical therapists are part of an MDS assessment team and are most typically involved with the MDS section on physical functioning and structural problems. This section considers nine different areas: ADL (bed mobility, transfers, walking and locomotion, dressing, eating, toilet use, personal hygiene); bathing; balance; range of motion; modes of locomotion; modes of transfer; the need to have tasks broken down into component parts; rehabilitation potential; and change in ADL in the last 90 days. The first three of these items are coded according to the degree of human assistance a resident needed to perform the task and the type of support provided by staff, if assistance was required. The time frame for assessment on each ADL, balance, range of motion, modes of locomotion, and modes of transfer is the 7 days before the assessment.

After the MDS is completed, the data are reviewed to determine whether the patient has any of the 18 common problems identified by the RAPs. The RAPs address the following clinical problems: delirium, cognitive loss/dementia, visual function, communication, ADL function/rehabilitation potential, urinary incontinence and indwelling catheter, psychosocial well-being, mood state, behavior problem, activities, falls, nutritional status, feeding tubes, dehydration/fluid maintenance, dental care, pressure ulcers, psychotropic drug use, and physical restraints. The RAP review will determine the plan of care for each patient.

The MDS was developed with extensive field testing to ensure its clinical utility. Available data on its inter-rater reliability suggest that the instrument meets minimum criteria in this regard.[27] Further clinical use and research will be necessary to determine whether its developers succeeded in producing a clinically relevant and psychometrically sound instrument. A derivative instrument for use across the inpatient spectrum of postacute care (PAC), the MDS-PAC, has been under development and will likely supplant the MDS 2.0 after its completion.

The Outcome and Assessment Information Set

The Outcome and Assessment Information Set (OASIS) was designed as a data collection tool to gather information on the adult patient in the home care setting and allow home health agencies to assess the quality of care by measuring pertinent outcomes of care.[33,46,50] During its development, use of the OASIS by home health agencies was voluntary. However, beginning on Jan. 1, 1999, home health agencies were mandated to use the OASIS as a Condition of Participation in the Medicare program by the Health Care Financing Administration. Developed over a 10-year period, the current version of OASIS, known as *OASIS-B*, contains 79 core items covering sociodemographic characteristics, environmental factors, social support, health status, and functional status. Future revisions of OASIS, which will be ongoing, will be labeled OASIS-C, OASIS-D, and so on. Created as part of a research program to develop outcomes measures applicable to home health, it is critical to appreciate that OASIS was not designed to be a comprehensive assessment of a patient, nor should it be used as an "add-on" assessment. Unlike any other instrument discussed here, items from the OASIS are meant to be integrated into an agency's existing clinical assessments to highlight various aspects of a patient's status that identify particular needs for care at various stages: upon admission into the home health

service, whenever the patient's condition requires a comprehensive assessment, at follow-up at least every 57 to 62 days and at discharge.

The OASIS was intended to be a "discipline-neutral" instrument, administered by any health professional including physical therapists. Ease of administration increases with familiarity with the instrument. Unlike most other instruments, the response sets that are attached to each item are specifically matched to the item. Some response sets have only two descriptors to choose between, whereas other items list as many as nine different descriptions of behavior to select. Therefore, the user must be familiar with the possible response set to each item and anticipate that comfort level in using this instrument will increase over a gradual learning curve. The ADL/IADL section is comprised of 14 different items including grooming, dressing the upper body, dressing the lower body, bathing, toileting, transfers, ambulation/locomotion, feeding, meal preparation, transportation, laundry, housekeeping, shopping, and the ability to use the telephone. The format of the instrument in this section allows recording of both prior and current functional status on each of the items. The OASIS was field-tested through demonstration projects and refined by a panel of experts. Reliability testing is ongoing.

SUMMARY

The purpose of geriatric physical therapy intervention is to improve or maintain the functional status of the individual. Previous studies of the functional status of elders have indicated that age alone is a risk factor for functional decline. When normal aging is coupled with the effects of disease, an elder may experience a severe deterioration in quality of life. A functional assessment is therefore an essential component of the physical therapist's examination and evaluation. Regardless of whether the functional assessment is conducted with a formal structured instrument, an unstructured interview, or direct observation of performance, the results must be reliable, valid, and clinically useful.

REFERENCES

1. Applegate WB, Blass JP, Williams TF: Instruments for the functional assessment of older patients. *N Engl J Med* 1990; 322:1207-1214.
2. Arnold SB: The measurement of quality of life in the frail elderly, in JE Birren, et al (eds): *The concept and measurement of quality of life in the frail elderly.* San Diego, Academic Press, 1991.
3. Asberg KH, Sonn U: The cumulative structure of personal and instrumental ADL. *Scand J Rehabil Med* 1989; 21:171-177.
4. Bombardier C, Tugwell P: Methodological considerations in functional assessment. *J Rheumatol Suppl* 1987; 14(suppl 15):6-10.
5. Cahalin LP, et al: The six-minute walk test predicts peak oxygen uptake and survival in patients with advanced heart failure. *Chest* 1996; 110:325-332.
6. Cornoni-Huntley JC, et al: Epidemiology of disability in the oldest-old: Methodologic issues and preliminary findings. *Milbank Mem Fund Q/Health Soc* 1985; 63:350-376.
7. Crimmins EM, Saito Y, Reynolds SL: Further evidence of recent trends in the prevalence and incidence of disability among older Americans from two sources: The LSOA and the NHIS. *J Gerontol* 1997; 52B:S59-S71.

8. Dawson D, Hendershot G, Fulton J: Aging in the eighties. Functional limitations of individuals age 65 years and over. *Advanced Data From Vital and Health Statistics, No 133.* Hyattsville, Md, Public Health Service, DHHS Publication No (PHS) 87-1250, 1987.

9. Duncan PW, et al: Functional reach: A new clinical measure of balance. *J Gerontol* 1990; 45:M192-197.

10. Duncan PW, et al: Functional reach: Predictive validity in a sample of elderly male veterans. *J Gerontol* 1992; 47:M93-98.

11. Dunlop DD, Hughes SL, Manheim LM: Disability in activities of daily living: Patterns of change and a hierarchy of disability. *Am J Publ Health* 1997; 87:378-383.

12. Ferrucci L, et al: Progressive versus catastrophic disability: A longitudinal view of the disablement process. *J Gerontol* 1996; 51A:M123-M130.

13. Fillenbaum GG, Smyer MA: The development, validity and reliability of the OARS Multidimensional Functional Assessment Questionnaire. *J Gerontol* 1981; 36:428-434.

14. Fitti JE, Kovar MG: The Supplement on Aging to the 1984 National Health Interview Survey. *Vital and Health Statistics, Series 1, No 21.* Washington, DC, Public Health Service, DHHS Publication No (PHS) 87-1323, 1987.

15. George LK, Fillenbaum GG: OARS methodology: A decade of experience in geriatric assessment. *J Am Geriatr Soc* 1985; 33:607-615.

16. Granger CV, et al: Advances in functional assessment for medical rehabilitation. *Top Geriatr Rehabil* 1986; 1(3):59-74.

17. Granger CV, et al: Functional assessment scales: A study of persons with multiple sclerosis. *Arch Phys Med Rehabil* 1990; 71:870-875.

18. Guccione AA, Jette AM: Assessing limitations in physical function in patients with arthritis. *Arthritis Care Res* 1988; 1:170-176.

19. Guccione AA, Jette AM: Multidimensional assessment of functional limitations in patients with arthritis. *Arthritis Care Res* 1990; 3:44-52.

20. Guide to Physical Therapist Practice. *Phys Ther* 1997; 1163-1650.

21. Guralnik JM, et al: Physical performance measures in aging research. *J Gerontol* 1989; 44:M141-146.

22. Guralnik JM, et al: Lower-extremity function in persons over the age of 70 years as a predictor of disability. *New Engl J Med* 1995; 332:556-561.

23. Guralnik JM, et al: A short physical performance battery assessing lower extremity function: Association with self-reported disability and prediction of mortality and nursing home admission. *J Gerontol* 1994; M85-94.

24. Harris BA, et al: Validity of self-report measures of functional disability. *Top Geriatr Rehabil* 1986; 1(3):31-41.

25. Harris T, et al: Longitudinal study of physical ability in the oldest-old. *Am J Public Health* 1989; 79:698-702.

26. Havlik RJ, et al: Health statistics on older persons, United States, 1986. *Vital and Health Statistics, Series 3, No 25.* Hyattsville, Md, Public Health Service, DHHS Publication No (PHS) 87-1409, 1987.

27. Hawes C, et al: Reliability estimates for The Minimum Data Set for Nursing Home Resident Assessment and Care Screening. *Gerontologist* 1995; 35:172-178.

28. Hing E: Use of nursing homes by the elderly: Preliminary data from the 1985 National Nursing Home Survey. *Advance Data From Vital and Health Statistics, No 135.* Hyattsville, Md, Public Health Service, DHHS Publication No (PHS) 87-1250, 1987.

29. Jette AM, et al: Interrelationships among disablement concepts. *J Gerontol* 1998; 53A:M395-M404.

30. Katz S, et al: Studies of illness in the aged. The index of ADL: A standardized measure of biological and psychosocial function. *JAMA* 1963; 185:914-919.

31. Katz S, et al: Progress in the development of the index of ADL. *Gerontologist* 1970; 10:20-30.

32. Kovar MG, LaCroix AZ: Aging in the eighties: Ability to perform work-related activities. Data from the Supplement on Aging to the National Health Interview Survey, United States, 1984. *Advance Data From Vital and Health Statistics, No 136.* Hyattsville, Md, Public Health Service, DHHS Publication No (PHS) 87-1250, 1987.

33. Krisler KS, Campbell BM, Shaughnessy PW: *OASIS basics: Beginning to use the outcome and assessment information set.* Denver, Center for Health Services and Policy Research, 1997.

34. Lachs MS, et al: A simple procedure for general screening for functional disability in elderly patients. *Ann Intern Med* 1990; 112:699-706.

35. Lavsky-Shulan M, et al: Prevalence and functional correlates of low back pain in the elderly: The Iowa 65 + Rural Health Study. *J Am Geriatr Soc* 1985; 33:23-28.

36. Lawrence RH, Jette AM: Disentangling the disablement process. *J Gerontol* 1996; 51B:S173-S182.

37. Lawton MP, et al: A research and service oriented multilevel assessment instrument. *J Gerontol* 1989; 37:91-99.

38. Leon J, Lair T: Functional status of the non-institutionalized elderly: Estimates of ADL and IADL difficulties. *National Medical Expenditure Survey Research Findings 4.* Agency for Health Care Policy and Research. Rockville, Md, Public Health Service, DHHS Publication No (PHS) 90-3462, 1990.

39. *Long term care facility resident assessment instrument (RAI) user's manual.* Washington DC, American Health Care Association, 1995.

40. Manton KG: A longitudinal study of functional change and mortality in the United States. *J Gerontol* 1988; 43:S153-161.

41. Mathias S, Nayak USL, Issacs B: Balance in elderly patients: The "Get Up and Go" test. *Arch Phys Med Rehabil* 1986; 67:387-389.

42. McDowell I, Newell C: *Measuring health: A guide to rating scales and questionnaires,* ed 2. Oxford, Oxford University Press, 1987.

43. Morris WW, Boutelle S: Multidimensional functional assessment in two modes. *Gerontologist* 1985; 25:638-643.

44. Myers AM, et al: Functional performance measures: Are they superior to self-assessments? *J Gerontol* 1996; 48:M196-M206.

45. Nagi SZ: An epidemiology of disability among adults in the United States. *Milbank Mem Fund Q/Health Soc* 1976; 54:439-467.

46. *Outcome and Assessment Information Set implementation manual: Implementing OASIS at a home health agency to improve patient outcomes.* Baltimore, Department of Health and Human Services Health Care Financing Administration, 1998.

47. Podsiadlo D, Richardson S: The timed "Up and Go": A test of basic functional mobility for frail elderly persons. *J Am Geriatr Soc* 1991; 39:142-148.

48. Rothstein JM: Measurement and clinical practice: Theory and application, in Rothstein JM (ed): *Measurement in Physical Therapy.* New York, Churchill Livingstone, 1985.

49. Rubenstein LV, et al: Health status assessment for elderly patients. Report of the Society of General Internal Medicine Task Force on Health Assessment. *J Am Geriatr Soc* 1988; 37:2-569.

50. Shaughnessy PW, Crisler KS: *Outcome-based quality improvement. A manual for home care agencies on how to use outcomes.* Washington, DC, National Association for Home Care, 1995.

51. Sonn U, Asberg KH: Assessment of activities of daily living in the elderly. A study of a population of 76 year olds in Gothenburg, Sweden. *Scand J Rehabil Med* 1991; 23:193-202.

52. Tager IB, Swanson A, Satariano WA: Reliability of physical performance and self-reported functional measures in an older population. *J Gerontol* 1998; 53: M295-300.

53. Verbrugge L, Rennert C, Maddans JH: The great efficacy of personal and equipment assistance in reducing disability. *Am J Publ Health* 1997; 87:384-392.

54. Wiener JM, et al: Measuring activities of daily living: Comparisons across national surveys. *J Gerontol* 1990; 45:S229-237.

55. Winograd CH, et al: Development of a physical performance and mobility examination. *J Am Geriatr Soc* 1994; 42:743-749.

CHAPTER 8

ENVIRONMENTAL DESIGN: ACCOMMODATING SENSORY CHANGES IN THE ELDERLY

MARY ANN WHARTON, PT, MS

INTRODUCTION

The ability to function in the everyday environment is essential to older individuals. Maintaining independence, however, may be compromised by sensory changes that individuals experience over their life span. Changes in vision, hearing, taste, smell, and touch may deprive older persons of necessary sensory cues to perceive the environment and may influence both their behavior and the behavior of others toward them. The ability of physical therapists to recognize the relationship between sensory changes and environmental interaction, to recommend adaptations to accommodate those changes, and to teach intervention strategies will promote continued independent functioning of older individuals.

Most individuals experience gradual sensory loss with age. Such changes are normal and irreversible and may not be uniform within the same individual. For example, visual loss may occur primarily in one eye, or an individual may have poor vision but excellent hearing. Moreover, loss of the different senses may be experienced at different ages. Hearing loss generally accelerates after age 40, vision and smell after 50, and taste after 55.[88] The important point is that the sensory declines experienced with aging are highly individualized, with some elderly people experiencing relatively minor declines and maintaining optimal functional ability and other individuals experiencing significant declines with resultant increased functional dependency. Typically, the declines occur gradually and may be unnoticed until elderly individuals are no longer capable of independent functioning within the environment.

Throughout life, individuals rely on sensory cues to perceive and interpret information from their surroundings. As sensory declines occur with aging, older persons may misinterpret cues from the environment or may experience sensory deprivation. The consequences may be loss of independence by older individuals. Therefore, individuals may need higher thresholds of stimulation to continue to function in the environment. As individuals experience loss in functional ability, they may also become increasingly reliant on sensory cues from the environment. An interdependence develops between the senses and the environment: one relies on one's senses to perceive and derive pleasure from the environment, and one relies on the environment to promote and support functional ability as age-related sensory declines are experienced.

As physical therapists interact with the elderly, it is critical to recognize the importance of the balance between sensory perception and ability to function effectively in the en-

Table 8-1
Examples of Accommodations to Enhance Functioning for Older Individuals Experiencing Sensory Loss

Sensory Change	Examples of Accommodations
Vision	
Visual field	Lower height for directional and informational signs
Acuity	Visual aids (glasses, contact lenses); magnifiers; large-print books and devices; large-print computer software
Illumination	UV-absorbing lenses; increased task illumination; gooseneck lamps; 200-300 watt light bulbs
Glare	Lamp shades, curtains, or blinds to soften light; cove lighting to conceal light source; non-glare wax on vinyl floors; carpeting; wallpaper or flat paints; avoid shiny materials such as glass or plastic furniture and metal fixtures
Dark adaptation	Night-lights with red bulbs; pocket flashlights, automatic light timers, light switches at point of entry to a room
Color	Bright, warm colors (reds, oranges, yellows); avoid pastel hues; avoid monotones
Contrast	Bright detail on dark backgrounds (white lettering/black background); warm colors to highlight handrails, steps; placemats or table coverings that contrast with plates, floor
Depth perception	Avoid patterned floor surfaces
Hearing	Hearing aids; pocket amplifiers; increasing bass and turning down treble on radios, televisions; smoke alarms, telephones, and doorbells with visual cues such as flashing lights; insulating acoustic materials to minimize background noise
Taste and Smell	
Taste	Color to increase perceived flavor intensity; use of spices, herbs, and flavorings to enhance foods; feel for bulges in canned goods to detect spoilage; date stored and frozen foods
Smell	Adapt smoke detectors with loud buzzers; safety-spring caps for gas jets on stoves; vent kitchens in institutions to allow residents to experience cooking aromas, and place flowers in living areas
Touch	
Tactile sensitivity	Introduce texture into the environment through wall hangings, carpet, textured upholstery; use soft blankets and textured clothing
Thermal sensitivity	Avoid temperature extremes from air conditioning, hot bathwater, heating pads

vironment. Therapists need to evaluate elderly individuals for sensory changes and to recommend appropriate interventions and modifications to enhance optimal functional performance in an environment without creating dependence (Table 8-1).

Sensory Changes: Relationship to Functional Ability within the Environment

Vision
Vision is important in identifying environmental cues and distinguishing environmental hazards. As people age, changes in vision and visual perception may lead to misinterpretation of visual cues and result in functional dependence.

Physiologically, this decline in vision can result from age-related changes in the structures of the eye and in external ocular structures. Neuronal changes, perceptual changes, and pathological conditions also contribute to vision and visual perceptual changes in the elderly. The ability to function in the environment, in spite of changes in vision and visual perception, is dependent on the ability to adapt to visual impairment, including decreasing visual efficiency and low vision. Older individuals must adapt to problems such as decreased visual field, changes in visual acuity, increased needs for illumination balanced by needs to reduce glare, delayed dark-light adaptation, increased needs for contrast, decreased power of accommodation, and changes in color vision and depth perception.

Visual Field
A decrease in both peripheral and upper visual fields accelerates with aging. Decreased pupil size, resulting in admittance of less light to the peripheral retina, may be responsible for early changes. Later changes may result from decreased retinal metabolism. Mechanical causes are due to relaxation of the upper eyelid and loss of retrobulbar fat, which results in the eyes sinking more deeply into the orbits. As a result, upper gaze can be compromised by as much as 20 degrees in a 70-year-old.[51,70,87,88]

Within the environment, this decrease in upper visual field may cause older individuals to miss cues above head level. Common examples of cues found above head level may include traffic and street signs, direction or information signs in public buildings (Fig. 8-1), hanging light fixtures, and environmental hazards such as hanging tree limbs.[88]

Lateral field, or peripheral vision, deficits—described as the inability to detect motion, form, or color on either side of the head while looking straight ahead—are particularly significant for elderly persons. For safety in the environment, older persons must be able to detect people or objects in the lateral field, and elderly drivers must possess adequate lateral awareness.[22]

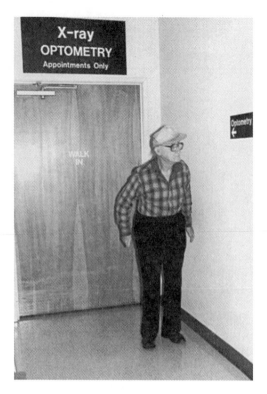

Fig. 8-1   Placement of signs is an important consideration for older individuals. The wall sign is placed at eye level to accommodate changes in visual field. The door sign is a better size and has better contrast, but it is too high for an older individual to see clearly. (From Melore GG: Visual function changes in the geriatric patient and environmental modifications, in Melore GG (ed): *Treating Vision Problems in the Older Adult.* St Louis, Mosby, 1997. Used with permission.)

Visual Acuity

Visual acuity, the capacity of the eye to discriminate fine details of objects in the visual field, generally declines with age, although this decline is not universal or inevitable. The 20/20 standard for "normal" vision occurs around age 18 and remains unchanged until age 50. Slight diminution of visual acuity occurs between the ages of 50 and 70 and at a greater rate after age 70. Factors responsible for decreased visual acuity include increased thickness of the lens, which affects the amount of light allowed to reach the retina, and the loss of elasticity of the lens. These changes result in decreased ability to see clearly and particularly affect near objects. Additionally, changes in the iris and pupil may decrease acuity. As one ages, the iris loses its ability to change width, and pupil size remains small in both dim and bright light. One specific consequence is decreased night vision. It is likely that optical factors alone are insufficient to account for acuity loss and that age-related changes in the retina and brain are also contributing factors. These include a loss of photoreceptors, bipolar cells, or ganglion cells within the retina and anatomical or functional changes in the geniculostriate pathway.[22,23,51,68,87,88]

Visual aids can be beneficial in improving visual acuity for the elderly. Glasses and contact lenses can enhance vision

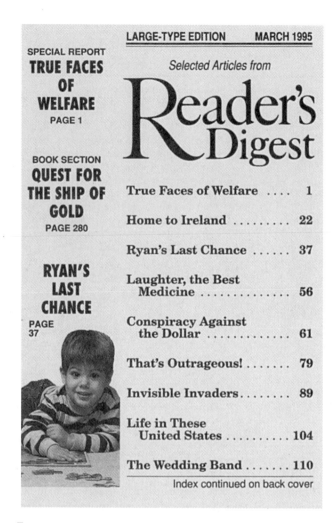

Fig. 8-2   Large-print *Reader's Digest.* The 18-point type provides 2.0 × relative size magnification compared with the 9-point type of a standard edition. (From Williams DR: Functional adaptive devices, in Cole RG, Rosenthal BP (eds): *Remediation and Management of Low Vision.* St Louis, Mosby, 1996. Used with permission.)

when worn properly, especially in the early stages of vision loss. Hand-held magnifiers are adequate for use over short periods, e.g., when reading a telephone book. Table stand magnifiers are beneficial when a person is reading books or newspapers because they cause less eye fatigue by maintaining a constant distance between the object being magnified and the magnifier. Illuminated magnifiers that hang from the neck are useful when a person is sewing or performing craft work. Other low-vision aids can be obtained at low-vision clinics.[49,73]

In addition to visual aids, certain modifications to environmental stimuli can enhance visual functioning for older persons. Use of large print is suggested for signs and labels, including medication schedules, telephone lists, and home programs. Large-print books (Fig. 8-2) and newspapers are also available, as are other large-print devices such as measuring tapes and rulers, measuring cups and spoons, cookbooks, wristwatches, phone dialers, and games. Local agencies for the blind are helpful in identifying such resources.[3,9,47,62,73,81,88]

Large-print typewriters are available that provide an effective means of personal communication for visually impaired older adults. The technology is less intimidating than computers for some older individuals, and they are more cost-effective. The National Braille Association has recommended three single space lines per vertical inch as the maximum acceptable pitch for large-print typewriters. To be considered "large print," lowercase letters should measure at least ⅛ inch to approximate 18-point type.[81]

Computer adaptations are available for older individuals who are visually impaired. Hardware programs are available that magnify images on a computer screen. These programs require installation of a specific type of computer board. Full-page monitors are another computer adaptation available for the visually impaired individual. Additionally, IBM- and Macintosh-compatible onscreen software programs are available, but these may have specific hardware requirements; compatibility with the computer system to be used should be determined before purchase. An advantage of using large-print software is that the font of the print can be selected to fit the needs of the viewer. It is recommended that "silent software" be used when dealing with large-print computer access software. Once loaded into the computer, this type of software will enlarge any program the viewer is using without interfering with that program. The exception is that some graphic-oriented programs may not be compatible with some computer enlargement programs. One barrier to the use of software programs is that enhancements are developed so rapidly that the application software may be obsolete within 2 to 3 months after it is purchased (Fig. 8-3). For visually impaired individuals whose needed magnification limits the number of characters on the screen to six or fewer, voice or braille computer displays may be indicated.[25,48,81]

Illumination

Within the environment, declining visual acuity necessitates a stronger stimulus or light source. This was originally thought to be primarily related to senile miosis (an age-related decrease in pupillary size), changes in the refractory media, and a reduction in retinal cones and rods. More recent studies, conducted under varying light conditions, argue that the effects of aging are neural rather than optical in origin. These studies further suggest that it is the neural changes that have the greatest effects on vision under low illumination.

Studies speculate that a link exists between the light history of an individual and aging, although direct evidence is not firmly established. It is hypothesized that aging of the visual system represents accumulated deteriorative changes that exceed the capacity of cells to renew their parts. Exposure to ultraviolet radiation (UVR) and short-wave light appears to accelerate this deterioration. As a result of this speculation, it is suggested that increasing light levels to meet the demands of the aging visual system be done at wavelengths that prevent or minimize further photoreceptor aging. It is further suggested that additional protection be obtained by using UV-absorbing chromophores in prescription lenses, contact lenses, intraocular lens implants, and sunglasses.[23,80]

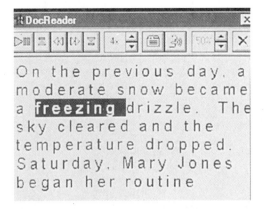

Fig. 8-3 Computer with software for producing enlarged text. (From Berger JW, Fine SL, Maguire MG: *Age-Related Macular Degeneration.* St Louis, Mosby, 1999. Used with permission.)

As a result of these optical and neural changes, it has been estimated that older individuals require as much as two to three times more light than their younger counterparts. Wall-mounted light fixtures and peripheral lighting from floor lamps are superior to a central ceiling source because they do not foster formation of shadows on critical corner and furniture areas. Background lighting should not be as bright as that in the area on which attention is directed. Lighting that focuses directly on the task, rather than overhead lighting, is recommended to meet the needs of older individuals for reading, task performance, and other close work. Using 200- or 300-watt light bulbs in reading lamps instead of the more typical 100-watt bulb is one of the simplest ways to provide adequate task illumination. Another way to modify the necessary amount of illumination independent of light bulb wattage is to simply move the light source closer to the task material, since the effective amount of illumination is inversely proportional to the distance of the light source to the surface. Gooseneck lamps (Fig. 8-4) or small, high-intensity lamps with three-way switches are also helpful in achieving the proper ratio of background-to-task lighting.[5,9,22,23,31,51,56,68,73,78,80,88]

Glare

When illumination is increased, care must be exercised to avoid excessive and intensive illumination, which can create a hazard for older persons in the form of glare. Glare results from diffuse light scattering on the retina as it passes through mildly opaque refractive media, inhibiting clear vision. A primary cause of glare sensitivity is the increasing opacity of the lens, which diffuses the incoming light. Degenerative changes that take place in the cornea also contribute to glare.[5,86,88]

Direct glare occurs when light reaches the eye directly from its source. An example of direct glare is uncontrolled natural light that enters a darkened room through a window. Another example of direct glare is excessive light from exposed light bulbs. Indirect glare can be the result of light reflecting off another surface. Examples include light reflecting

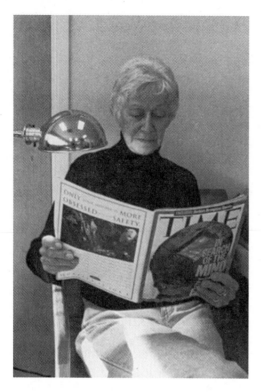

Fig. 8-4   Use of a gooseneck lamp to increase effective task lighting without increasing light bulb wattage. (From Melore GG: Visual function changes in the geriatric patient and environmental modifications, in Melore GG (ed): *Treating Vision Problems in the Older Adult.* St Louis, Mosby, 1997. Used with permission.)

off highly polished surfaces including waxed floors; plastic-covered furniture; polished silverware; or stainless steel assistive devices, including grab bars and walkers.[5,9,49,88]

Glare can be lessened by modifying light sources. Diffuse, soft lighting is preferable to single-light sources. Lamp shades should be used to soften the light. Glare from windows can be minimized by use of sheer curtains, venetian blinds, tinted-glass windows, or drapes. Wall-mounted valance or cove lighting that conceals the light source is also recommended. Fluorescent fixtures can be used to reduce glare, but they must be checked to ensure that they do not create another hazard for elderly individuals in the form of flickering. Also, "white" fluorescent lights are recommended because they make it possible to choose a "cool" light to eliminate the harshness and minimize accentuation of the blues, greens, and yellows created by typical fluorescent lights.[31,78,81]

Another method of controlling glare is reducing the number of reflective surfaces. Positioning light sources to avoid reflection from shiny surfaces, such as waxed floors, is helpful. Use of carpeting, wallpaper, flat paints, and paneling is preferable to use of high-gloss paints. Glass, plastic, and glossy furniture should be avoided or covered with textured surfaces to minimize the effects of glare. Gleaming metal fixtures can be replaced with wood or plastic fixtures. Assistive devices, including grab bars and walkers, should not be constructed of shiny materials.

Care should be taken to control the sources of glare in public areas. For example, mall directories and bus signs should be covered with nonglare materials rather than highly reflective plastics. Grocery stores and drugstores should refrain from displaying products wrapped in plastic. Name tags, street signs, and publicity for older individuals should be prepared on dull surfaces to minimize glare.

Outdoor areas are also vulnerable to glare, especially with bright sunlight or with wet, shiny surfaces on rainy or snowy days. Sunscreens and adequate shade from trees are recommended to limit glare from direct sunlight. If it is not possible to provide adequate control for glare, older individuals should be encouraged to use sunglasses, visors, brimmed hats, or umbrellas. Glare that occurs at dusk as poorly illuminated objects are contrasted against a bright, post-sunset sky can be particularly troublesome for older individuals. Night glare that occurs from oncoming headlights can also be hazardous. Use of well-lit routes and divided highways can minimize this hazard for older individuals.[9,29,51,57,58,73,88]

Dark Adaptation

Dark adaptation, or the ability of the eye to become more visually sensitive after remaining in darkness for a period of time, is delayed in older persons. One reason for this visual change is the smaller, miotic pupil, which limits the amount of light reaching the periphery of the retina. It is this area of the retina that contains the rods, which are sensitive to low-light intensities. Another reason for delayed dark adaptation in the elderly is the metabolic changes in the retina. The oxygen supply to the rod-dense area of the retina diminishes as a result of vascular changes, which, in turn, affect the efficiency of the rods to respond to low levels of illumination. As a result of these changes, older persons have difficulty adapting to darkness and to abrupt and extreme changes in light.[51,87,88]

Use of a night-light is recommended to assist in overcoming the decreased ability for the eyes to adapt to the dark. A red bulb is suggested since it reduces the time required for adaptation to the dark and permits older individuals to see well enough to function. It is also recommended that older individuals carry a pocket flashlight to aid in transition to dimly lit environments. Improving lighting at the point of entry to an area, through pull cords or light switches near the entrance to a room, is also recommended. Automatic timers or keeping a light on at all times in dimly lit areas can prevent older individuals from having to enter a darkened room.[38,45,49,51]

Accommodation

Accommodation, the ability of the eye to focus images on the retina independent of object distances, is impaired with aging. Functionally, this results in the inability to focus clearly over a range of distances. The decrease in this ability, referred to as *presbyopia*, occurs gradually and affects near vision first.

Loss of accommodation is the result of several factors. Both the cornea and lens lose transparency with aging. In

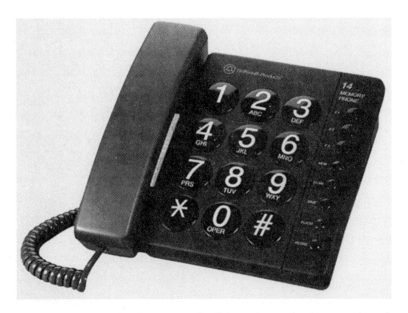

FIG. 8-5 Black telephone with white lettering on the dial to enhance visual contrast. Large-button phone numbers also enhance visual acuity. (From Williams DR: Functional adaptive devices, in Cole RG, Rosenthal BP (eds): *Remediation and Management of Low Vision.* St Louis, Mosby, 1996. Used with permission.)

addition, the lens thickens, flattens, and yellows and becomes rigid. The ciliary muscle weakens and relaxes. As a result, the lens gradually loses its ability to change shape and focus at varying distances. Difficulty is encountered by older individuals when they attempt to read small print or detail, unless the material is held at a distance. Reading glasses are initially indicated. Later, bifocals are needed to compensate for the inability of the lens to change shape and focus on objects of varying distances.[5,41,52,87,88]

Color

The ability to perceive, differentiate, and distinguish colors declines with aging as a result of changes in retinal cones, the retinal bipolar and ganglion cells, the visual pathways that terminate in the occipital cortex, and the lens. As the lens thickens and yellows with age, it becomes less sensitive to colors that have shorter wavelengths. The ability to distinguish cool colors—blues, greens, and violets—is particularly impaired since they have the shorter wavelengths. Hue and saturation levels are particularly affected by aging, but brightness appears to be spared. Warm colors with longer wavelengths, including the reds, oranges, and yellows, are easier to differentiate and should therefore be used as focal points against sharply contrasting backgrounds. In addition to loss of color discrimination at the blue end of the color spectrum, a loss of sensitivity over the entire spectrum occurs. As a result, light pastel colors may be difficult to distinguish. Monotones also provide difficulty for older individuals, as may dark shades, which tend to blend into shadows. As a result, older persons may have trouble negotiating around dark furniture or in areas where dark floor surfaces and dark walls or doorways come together. Optimal lighting is needed to minimize this hazard.

Both warm and cool colors can be included in a color scheme when living environments are designed for the el-

derly. Even though cool colors are more difficult to distinguish, they may be preferred for their soothing effects, particularly with agitated older individuals. The use of bright, warm colors, which are better seen, should be encouraged for sensory stimulation. Contrasting bright yellows, reds, and oranges with cool blue, green, and violet colors may help minimize difficulties associated with loss of depth perception. The goal with the use of color is to use contrast to assist elderly individuals in distinguishing objects from their backgrounds. It is also important that the use of color be aesthetically pleasing.[5,9,18,19,20,22,29,32,51,83,87,88]

Contrast

The ability to discriminate between degrees of brightness appears to decrease in individuals age 60 and older. In particular, contrast sensitivity to medium and high spatial frequencies declines progressively with age, and contrast sensitivity to low spatial frequencies remains unchanged. Typically, older individuals have difficulty seeing objects that have low contrast, especially with a bright background. Elderly persons require greater than two times as much light to see low-contrasting objects with the same degree of clarity as younger people. Earlier studies attributed this decreased ability to discriminate between degrees of brightness to be the result of an increase in light scatter secondary to age-related eye changes. More recent studies indicate that changes in the retina and the brain or neuronal loss within the visual pathways are responsible.[18,20,22,23,51,68,87]

Use of sharp contrast enhances the visual performance of older individuals. Bright detail on dark backgrounds is easier to distinguish than low contrast or dark detail on light background. Recommendations include white lettering on the telephone dial of a black telephone (Fig. 8-5) or white lettering on a black background for reference dials on appliances. Use of warm colors—reds, oranges, and yellows—is recommended to highlight important visual targets such as handrails, steps, intersections, and traffic signs. Floors and rugs should contrast with woodwork and walls. To enhance eating, plates should contrast with tablecloths or tabletops. Colored rims on dishes and glasses can provide sufficient contrast to avoid spills. The table covering should also contrast with the floor to enhance the reference point of older individuals and help prevent falls.[33,49,54,62,69,88]

Depth Perception

Related to loss of color discrimination is change in depth perception, or the ability to estimate the relative distance and relief of objects. Lack of color contrast results in a flat visual effect, or decreased depth perception and inability to judge distances. As a result of the inability to judge distances, older persons may have difficulty estimating the height of curbs and steps and may have difficulty with activities of daily living that require distance judgment, including feeding tasks.

Related to depth perception is figure-ground, which is the object of focus from a diffuse background. It is difficult for older individuals to recognize a simple visual figure when it is embedded in a complex figure background. Specific implications for the elderly are in selection of floor coverings. When a pattern is present on a floor surface, it may create a hazard as older individuals perceive it as one object or several objects. The avoidance of patterns is therefore recommended for floor surfaces, particularly in hallways or living areas.[9,42,70,87,88]

Hearing

Hearing provides a primary link that allows individuals to identify with the environment and communicate effectively. Age-related hearing loss can lead to decreased awareness of environmental cues; poor communication skills; and ultimately, social isolation. With aging, there are both physiological and functional changes in the auditory system. Both the peripheral auditory system, which includes the structures of the ear itself, and the central nervous system, which integrates and gives meaning to sound, are affected. Age-related hearing loss can be attributed to three factors: conductive loss, sensorineural loss, and combined conductive and sensorineural loss. Changes that typically occur with aging and are detrimental to the older individual's ability to function independently in the environment include high-tone hearing loss, decreased speech discrimination, and difficulty in detecting and appropriately filtering background noise.

Conductive Hearing Loss

Conductive hearing loss results from dysfunction of the external ear, the middle ear, or both. Factors responsible for this type of hearing loss include impacted cerumen, perforation of the tympanic membrane, serum or pus in the middle ear, and otosclerosis. Conductive hearing loss occurs when sound transmission to the inner ear is lost because the intensity of the signal is not sufficient. Even though the signal is weakened, sound received by the inner ear can still be an-

alyzed since the inner ear itself is not affected. Therefore, increasing the intensity of the signal through louder speech or through mechanical amplification, such as a hearing aid, may help restore the ability to hear.

With a conductive loss, some impairment will occur in the ability to hear sounds of all frequencies. The specific pattern is dependent on the etiology of the hearing loss. An appropriate intervention when speaking to older individuals with a conductive hearing loss is to increase the speaker's volume to enable the elderly to hear the signal more clearly and to understand the speech. For individuals with profound hearing loss, an appropriate strategy may be to speak directly into the individual's ear. Devices such as timers, alarm clocks, smoke detectors, and doorbells can be modified or changed so that the signal is within the hearing range of older persons.[1,5,9,29,35,44,47,49,87,88]

Sensorineural Hearing Loss

Sensorineural hearing loss occurs when there is a dysfunction in conversion of sound waves to electrical signals by the inner ear or dysfunction in transmission of nerve impulses to the brain. Age-related sensorineural hearing loss is referred to as *presbycusis*. *Sensory* presbycusis is due to a loss of hair cells at the basal end of the organ of Corti and results in loss of high-frequency hearing. *Neural* presbycusis is due to degenerative changes in nerve fibers of the cochlea. It leads to loss in speech discrimination but not in pure-tone thresholds. As a result, the person continues to hear tone but cannot understand what is heard. Amplifications may be of little benefit, since these devices can amplify unintelligible sounds. *Metabolic* presbycusis results from atrophy of blood vessels in the wall of the cochlea. It is most likely the result of arteriosclerotic vascular changes. It results in a relatively uniform reduction in pure-tone sensitivities for all frequencies and is accompanied by recruitment, which is a rapid increase in loudness as the sound intensity increases. *Mechanical* presbycusis is the result of atrophic changes in the structures involved with vibration of the cochlear partition. The result is increasing hearing loss from low to high frequencies. The ability to understand speech is affected. High-pitched consonants such as *s, t, f,* and *g* are increasingly difficult to understand, especially in the presence of background noise, which masks the weak consonant sounds, or with rapid articulation.[14,23,38,44,66]

Older individuals with a sensorineural hearing loss may have significant difficulty maintaining independent function in the environment. In addition to difficulty in hearing and/or understanding speech, these individuals may have great difficulty hearing and interpreting key signals from the environment. Recommendations to assist these individuals incorporate strategies to address the hearing loss. Lower frequency and pitch of signals from television, stereo systems, or radio can be achieved by adjusting the treble and bass to compensate for loss of high frequency, i.e., by tuning the bass up and the treble down. Use of microphones by speakers and entertainers will also cut out some of the high-frequency sound, making it easier for individuals to hear. Devices that have high-frequency sound, such as smoke alarms, telephones, and doorbells, should also have a visual cue, such as a flashing light.

For individuals with presbycusis, a hearing aid may be of limited benefit, since this device may only amplify a distorted signal. Some assistive listening devices, such as pocket amplifiers with external earphones, microphones, and earphones, may be beneficial[48,49,66] (Fig. 8-6). As with profound conductive loss, speaking directly into the individual's ear may be of benefit for the person without a device.

Environmental background noise that competes with the older person's ability to hear can be minimized by use of acoustic materials such as drapes, upholstered furniture, and carpets, which absorb noise. Insulating sheet rock should be installed in noisy areas such as kitchens or maintenance rooms. Tight window seals can minimize exterior noise.

In institutions and public buildings, noise from telepages, radios, televisions, dishwashers, and air conditioners should be eliminated where possible. Background music should be eliminated, since it contributes to the older individual's in-

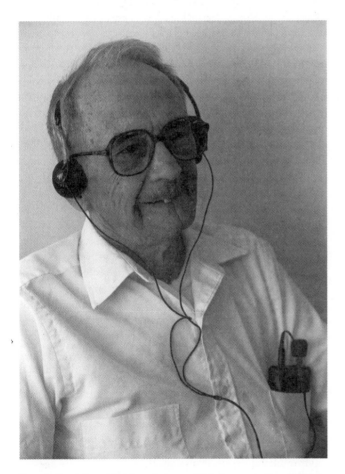

Fig. 8-6 A hand-held pocket amplifier increases the ability to communicate with a hearing-impaired individual. (From Lohman H, Padilla RL, Byers-Connon S: *Occupational Therapy with Elders: Strategies for the COTA*. St Louis, Mosby, 1998. Used with permission.)

ability to hear. Fluorescent lighting should be used with discretion, since the buzzing sound that is produced may also interfere with hearing.[9,29,35,49,71,87,88]

Taste and Smell

Taste and smell intertwine to provide additional links with the environment. These senses allow individuals to appreciate foods and pleasant odors in the environment, such as fresh-baked bread, the smell of newly cut grass, and roses. They also allow detection of unpleasant odors that can serve as warning to environmental hazards. Examples include unsafe drink and foods, fire, and noxious gases. Research on age-related changes in these senses is limited and often contradictory, but there is evidence that they are diminished. Current research indicates that smell has more significant change and that taste changes are relatively minimal. This decline in taste and smell can affect the older individual's behavior, safety in the environment, and nutrition.

Taste

Although there is no agreement on the cause, it is known that the number of taste buds decreases with age. By age 60, most people have lost approximately half of their taste buds. This loss further accelerates after age 70. This loss of functioning taste buds, combined with neuron reduction in taste centers, may account for changes in taste with aging. Other age-related changes that affect taste may include changes in the elasticity of the mouth and lips, decreased saliva flow, changes in oral secretions, increased incidence of gingivitis and periodontitis, and tongue fissures. Smoking and illness may also contribute to the decline of taste sensitivity.

Regardless of cause, age-related changes in taste acuity are thought to be small. Taste buds located in the front of the tongue that are responsible for sweet and salty tastes are the first to atrophy. Stronger stimuli are needed to appreciate these tastes, and older people may use excessive amounts of salt or may prefer sweets. This can pose problems for older individuals suffering from hypertension or diabetes. Taste buds located on the posterior surface of the tongue that are responsible for bitter tastes and allow rejection of bitter toxins are lost later. Additionally, older persons may experience an increased sensitivity to bitterness, with the resultant complaint that food tastes bitter or sour.

Recommendations to enhance the taste experience include suggestions to compensate with other senses. One study demonstrated that an increase in color caused a significant increase in the perceived flavor intensity of beverages for older individuals. This study speculated that the elderly depend heavily on visual cues to determine characteristics of food products because they are less sensitive to changes in flavor.[15] Other suggestions include encouraging older individuals to stimulate smell with the aroma of cooking foods since smell is so closely intertwined with taste and to prepare meals using a variety of aromas, temperatures, and textures. Oral hygiene should be encouraged before eating to rid the mouth of unpleasant tastes. Spices, herbs, flavor extracts, and sugar and salt substitutes can be used to enhance the flavor of foods.[5,14,35,87,88]

When dealing with canned foods, older persons should be taught to feel for any bulges in the can and to discard any suspicious cans. Stored foods should be dated and checked for spoilage. Defrosted foods should be used promptly, since thawing and refreezing affects flavor and texture.[14,87,88]

Smell

Research on olfactory sensitivity and smell is contradictory, but sensation appears to decline as a result of age, as well as a result of other factors associated with age. These factors may include continuous exposure to odor, leading to decreased acuity, or exposure to environmental pollutants or smoking. Structural causes may include fiber loss in the olfactory bulb, with a loss of approximately three-fourths of the olfactory fibers by age 80 or 90. Alterations in nasal anatomy and physiology may also occur secondary to diseases of the respiratory system.

A critical function of the sense of smell is to warn individuals of environmental dangers, including smoke or gas fumes. For elderly persons who experience a decline in the ability to smell and are living alone, it is critical that environmental adaptations be considered. One recommendation is to use smoke detectors with loud buzzers. Since declining sensitivity to odor may limit the individual's ability to detect mercaptans (foul-smelling additives) used to warn of natural gas leaks, safety-spring caps for gas jets of a stove are also recommended. If the sensory loss is profound, switching from gas to electrical appliances may be indicated.

Social interaction of older persons may be affected by a declining sense of smell. Individuals may not be able to detect body odor, so particular attention must be given to bathing patterns. Perfumes may be overutilized, making the scent overpowering and offensive to others.

For the institutionalized elderly person, unpleasant odors from cleaning equipment, sanitizing sprays, and substances designed to mask offensive odors abound. Pleasant odors associated with positive life experiences are often overlooked. Absence of "good" smells adversely affects the quality of life for these individuals. Opportunities should be created to stimulate positive life experiences with pleasant smells. Kitchens can be vented to allow the aroma of cooking food to permeate residential hallways and dining areas. Flowers with fragrant scents can be placed in living areas to enhance the older person's sensory experience.[9,14,28,29,35,87]

Touch

The sense of touch is a complicated human response that involves many separate processes—including touch, temperature, pain, as well as vibration sensitivity, kinesthesia, and stereognosis. Sensory input is subdivided into touch and tactile systems. Touch is used for awareness and protective responses. It can be determined culturally and is often lacking in the older person's environment, contributing to the individual's diminished sensorium. Tactile input is used to inter-

act with the environment and allows individuals to perceive multiple characteristics of an object.[9,37,85] For example, a surface may feel smooth or rough, soft or hard, warm or cold.

Little conclusive research has been done on the sense of touch. However, evidence suggests that touch decreases with age and varies from individual to individual. Many of the losses in somatesthetic sensitivity are the result of diseases that occur with greater frequency in the elderly, rather than a result of aging per se. Increased thresholds for touch, especially textures, temperature, and kinesthesia, have implications for the older individual's ability to obtain needed sensory input from the environment.

Tactile Sensitivity

Degenerative changes in Meissner's corpuscles may result in decreased sensitivity of the skin on the palm of the hand and sole of the foot but not of hairy skin. The resultant decrease in touch acuity can affect the ability of older individuals to localize stimuli. As a result, older individuals may have problems differentiating or manipulating small objects, including buttons and coins. The decrease in speed of reaction to tactile stimulation can cause harm to older persons, as they take longer to become aware of harmful or noxious stimuli such as temperature extremes, chemical irritants, or simple pressure from a stone in a shoe.[87]

Introducing texture into the environment can be valuable in assisting independent function of older individuals, especially if there is impairment in other senses. Wall hangings, carpet, and textured upholstery on furniture can enhance tactile input and add warmth. Use of texture on handrails or doorknobs can give environmental cues and enhance safety. Tactile deprivation can be minimized by the use of soft blankets and sheets and textured clothing.[9,29]

Thermal Sensitivity

Changes in vascular circulation and loss of subcutaneous tissue in older individuals may result in changes in thermal sensitivity and impaired ability to cope with extreme environmental temperatures. One consequence is that older persons may feel cold and uncomfortable, even on a day that seems warm to a younger person. Air conditioning may not be tolerated, especially in the institutional environment.

Additionally, extremes in hot temperatures, e.g., from hot bathwater or a heating pad, may not be readily detected by older individuals. As a consequence, individuals may suffer a burn from the inability to react quickly to the temperature extreme.[9,29,35]

GENERAL PRINCIPLES OF DESIGN

Environmental design principles that accommodate age-related changes in sensation can enhance independent functioning of elderly individuals. The ideal environment will vary according to the needs of individuals but should be supportive of sensory changes while promoting satisfaction, safety, and security. Design that accommodates sensory changes that occur with age should enhance the ability of individuals to function at the maximum level of competence. Overuse and underuse of sensory cues should be avoided, since both create dependence and result in a mismatch between the individual and the environment.*

The extent to which an environment demands a behavioral response is defined as *environmental press*. The ability of the individual to respond adaptively in areas of functional health, social roles, sensory-motor and perceptual functions, and cognition is referred to as *competence*. As the demanding physical environment fails to support aging individuals, safety, self-image, and interactions with others may be adversely affected, and stress may result. In this circumstance of high environmental demand, individuals with high competence levels will withstand greater levels of press, whereas individuals with the least capabilities will likely exhibit maladaptive behavior. Individuals in such situations must either change their competence through rehabilitation or alter their physical environment. Although rehabilitation to improve competence may be a sound solution, it is acknowledged that environmental adaptations are generally easier. Simple environmental changes, such as increased lighting, easily identifiable landmarks for cuing, or decreased background noise, may foster meaningful changes in behavior and interaction within the environment.[9,39,46,84,86]

Recommending too many changes in sensory stimuli within the environment may lead to sensory distortion, resultant overload, and decreased environmental press. This excessive decrease in environmental press may result in lack of challenge for some individuals, leading to marginal performance and dependent behavior. The optimal environment for the elderly is one that provides a measure of challenge and, at the same time, provides the necessary supports for the individual.[46]

Numerous environmental checklists can be found in the literature that address physical barriers in the home and institution. However, special consideration must also be given to accommodating sensory changes.[11,64,74,75] Each area of the physical environment in which older persons function must be addressed, with a focus on this interdependence of sensory loss, functional ability, and reliance on the environment for support. In addition to recommendations cited previously in this text, several areas deserve further emphasis. These include comments on personal/living space, long-term–care residencies, physical therapy departments, stairs, escalators, and driving.

Personal/Living Space

Since the home is the hub of most activity for older individuals, creating an environment to support sensory loss and enhance maximum functional independence is critical. Incorporating the previously outlined design principles that accommodate losses in vision, hearing, taste, smell, and touch will not only facilitate independence but may also minimize the occurrence of accidents leading to death or disability. Ex-

amples include use of enhanced lighting and provision of contrast in personal living space to deter falls that result from decreased vision and the use of smoke detectors with visual cues to decrease vulnerability to death from fires in older individuals with decreased ability to hear and smell.[86]

Long-Term–Care Residencies

Long-term–care residencies that were designed using traditional concepts derived from the medical model may fail to meet the needs of today's frail elderly population who suffer from multiple chronic conditions. To enhance the quality of life for these older individuals, architects and administrators are challenged to incorporate design principles that create environments to support age-related changes and enhance functional performance of individuals with sensory losses.

Appropriate lighting can support greater independence and enhance the safety of older individuals with visual deficits. Although direct, incandescent lighting adds warmth, it may not provide adequate illumination and may also create light pools and shadows. Therefore, direct lighting is not recommended for use in corridors. It is, however, appropriate as supplemental task lighting. Desk lamps and table lamps by chairs should be provided for reading and close work. Indirect "white" fluorescent lighting is recommended for use in corridors, since this type of lighting provides adequate, even illumination and minimizes glare. Warm white bulbs are recommended because they give a softer tint. Care should be taken to minimize flickering, which can be a hazard for the elderly. A regular schedule for checking ballasts on fluorescent lights and replacing worn-out bulbs can minimize this problem.[13,79,81]

Long-term–care facility design should be attentive to choices in materials for window coverings, ceilings, wall coverings, and floors. Window treatments should be chosen to minimize the effect of glare, since this is often a problem in residential facilities. Curtains or blinds can be used for this purpose. Draperies should be considered since they not only minimize glare but also serve to absorb extraneous background noise and assist in lowering energy costs.[7,13,56,79]

Ceilings and wall coverings in residential facilities should be chosen to support sensory deficits of elderly residents. Ceilings should be covered with acoustic tile specially designed to absorb noise and extraneous sounds that interfere with speech discrimination. Use of these materials is particularly recommended in corridors, dining rooms, and other areas where background noise is prevalent. Wall coverings can be chosen to serve multiple purposes. Color can be used for resident orientation and cuing. Choosing paint or fabric of different colors for various areas within the facility can provide meaning, especially for confused or demented residents. Use of contrast on door frames can serve as added landmarks and assist residents in locating their personal room. Color contrast between walls and floors can provide valuable sensory information to minimize falls in ambulatory individuals. Textured wall coverings that are soft to touch have the added benefit of providing tactile cues for

---

References 4,6,9,16,26,27,36,40,43,60,63,76,86

older individuals deprived of touch and for visually impaired residents. Repetitive, random, and vivid patterns that create visual illusions and unstable figure-ground relationships should be avoided.[7,13,56,59]

Floor coverings should be selected to enhance the mobility of older residents. Vinyl or linoleum is often chosen since it is easy to clean and provides little resistance for wheelchair mobility. One problem with vinyl surface is that it is a major source of glare. This can be controlled to an extent with use of nonglare wax. An alternative to vinyl is the use of carpet, which has traditionally been avoided because of stains and odor. Newer design, including solution-dyed fibers and liquid-barrier backing, has minimized these problems.

One study recommends the use of carpeting to enhance walking in elderly hospital inpatients. This study determined that gait speed and step length were significantly greater on carpeted than on vinyl surfaces.[82] Mobility of wheelchair-bound elderly need not be hampered by use of carpeting, since low-looped pile that is very tightly woven can minimize friction.[7,13]

Another study looked at the role of carpeted and vinyl floors in relation to injuries older individuals received as a result of a fall in a hospital. The study retrospectively reviewed a random sample of accident forms. Out of the group of patients who fell on carpet, only 17% sustained injuries. In the group of patients who fell on vinyl, 46% sustained injuries. Statistical analysis indicated less than 1% probability that the reduced rate of injury for those patients who fell on carpet was owed to chance. Results of this study support the hypothesis that individuals who fall on carpet are less likely to be injured than those who fall on vinyl flooring.[30] However, results of this investigation should be viewed in light of a more recent study that investigated the effects of flooring on standing balance among older persons. The results of this study indicate that the more compliant—i.e., the softer—the floor covering, the greater the effect on sway during moving visual environments. This may be a function of the sensitivity of older individuals to visual and proprioceptive inputs and of difficulty in handling sensory conflicts to the postural control system. The results of this study suggest that the type of floors could effect the potential for falling. High softness (plush) flooring modules increase the potential for destabilizing balance and increase risk of a fall, even though these more compliant floors are more comfortable and may reduce the potential for hip fracture in the event of a fall. The fact that the moving environments were particularly destabilizing with highly compliant surfaces suggests that floor compliance will cause even greater instability during walking. However, additional studies are needed to verify this assumption.[61] This study supports the use of low-pile carpeting in geriatric residences to improve balance of older individuals.

Furniture selected for residential facilities should be functional and, at the same time, supportive of sensory changes. Use of fabric upholstery can provide tactile cues and eliminate problems of glare created by vinyl upholstery. Choosing

color that contrasts with flooring can serve as a valuable visual cue for residents with visual deficits. Repetitive and illusionary patterns should be avoided.[13]

Particular consideration should be given to design of resident rooms in long-term–care facilities. Beds and chairs should be comfortable and stable and support functional ability of residents.[10,21,50] Adequate illumination should be provided, with provisions included for task lighting. Glare should be controlled through use of appropriate window treatments, floor surfaces, and furniture choices. Color and contrast should be considered during the selection of wall coverings, and even furniture coverings. For example, bedspreads should be chosen to contrast with floor coverings so that a visually impaired resident will be able to safely transfer on and off the bed.[65]

Special considerations for personal bathrooms and central bathing areas focus on features to enhance resident safety. One important consideration is to control glare, which is a particular problem with vinyl flooring, porcelain sinks, bathtubs, toilets, chrome towel bars, and grab bars. Suggestions to minimize glare include use of colored fixtures that can additionally provide contrast with floor and wall coverings. These are aesthetically pleasing and can serve as an important safety feature for older individuals with visual deficits and who may experience difficulty in judgment when the toilet, bathtub, or grab bar is of the same color as the floor.[13]

Communal dining areas can pose several design challenges in residential facilities. In addition to the usual problems with lighting and control of glare, there is the added problem of noise control. Since dining areas are commonly located adjacent to the kitchen, background noise from dishwashers and food processors can contribute to difficulty with hearing-impaired residents and can cause further social isolation of these individuals. Use of good insulating materials or locating dining areas away from kitchens is recommended to minimize this problem. Further reduction in background noise can be attained through use of tablecloths and placement of paper pads between cups and saucers.[7,13]

Physical Therapy Departments

If the elderly are to receive maximum benefit from physical therapy intervention, it is crucial that design principles incorporating recommendations to accommodate for sensory loss with aging be utilized when new facilities are built or existing space is renovated. Concepts previously discussed that accommodate sensory changes must be implemented. These include controlling light sources; minimizing glare; and choosing appropriate ceilings, wall coverings, and floor coverings. Specific recommendations for physical therapy departments include choosing walkers and other assistive devices that are constructed of non-shiny materials in an effort to control glare. Some pieces of equipment, such as parallel bars, some whirlpools, and various other modalities, are, by design, constructed of shiny material. When using this equipment, light sources should be controlled to minimize the effect of glare.

When mat tables and treatment tables are being chosen, the overall design of the physical therapy department should be considered. These surfaces should be covered with material that provides contrast to floor coverings, so that elderly clients are afforded a specific visual cue that will enhance safety in transfers.

One significant problem in most physical therapy departments is background noise. Suggestions to minimize this noise include confining whirlpool areas to separate rooms that are insulated with acoustic material. Another recommendation is to provide individual treatment booths rather than sectioning treatment areas with curtains. Not only will this afford privacy for older individuals, it will also serve as a means of limiting background noise. Background music from radios and use of intercom devices should be discouraged, since they serve as further distracters for the elderly with hearing loss.

Finally, use of texture is encouraged to enhance tactile sensation. When possible, linens should be used on mats and treatment tables rather than paper coverings. These should also contrast with floor coverings to enhance visual perception. Low-pile carpeting should be considered to enhance ambulation, absorb sound, and minimize glare.

Stairs

Stairs are one area within the environment not previously discussed that require special consideration, since they are common sites of accidents leading to injury, hospitalization, and even death. Safe negotiation of stairs requires integration of visual and kinesthetic tests of the conditions of the stairs. This is particularly critical for descent, which is generally more hazardous than ascent. Successful stair negotiation requires that individuals make a transition from free-form movement on level surfaces to the highly circumscribed foot placement that is required on stairs. Visual feedback is used initially in order to judge the position of the stair treads and maximize accuracy of foot placement. Looking at the steps then allows the user to scan the flight of steps for hazards, including broken treads, irregularities, or other obstacles. Once the visual test is accomplished, individuals rely on kinesthetic tests to obtain a feel of the treads and ensure accurate foot placement. In elderly individuals, visual distractions drawing the user's attention away from the stairs as well as visual deceptions built into the design of the stairs were identified as two leading causes of stair accidents. Furthermore, the most critical piece of visual information for successful descent of steps was identified as a singular and unambiguous indication of the edge of each step. Optical illusions created by patterned carpeting overpower the ability of individuals to detect tread edges and create a significant hazard. Similar hazards are created by three-dimensional textures, including shag carpeting, since these textures cause treads to appear to merge into a continuous surface.[2]

Other environmental considerations on stairs include use of adequate lighting to enhance visual feedback. Light switches should be located at both the top and bottom of the flight of steps. Night-lights should also be located near the first and last steps to provide cuing during darkness. Glare reflecting from floor surfaces should be minimized by the use of nonglare surfaces, including appropriate types of carpeting. Light from windows located near stairs should be controlled with window coverings. Glare derived directly from light sources should be minimized by positioning and by avoiding exposed lightbulbs. Kinesthetic feedback may be enhanced by use of carpeting; however, the addition of ribbed vinyl or rubber stair nosing of a contrasting color should be considered to aid in reducing the risk of falls by enhancing detection of the edge of the step. Stairs without carpeting can be marked by a strip of paint or tape in a contrasting color.[51,55,57,75]

Escalators

Escalators have been identified as a hazardous environment for the elderly since their use may result in accidents involving falls. It is thought that the repeated optical image that is a critical design feature of escalators may induce visual depth illusion, resulting in disorientation. More research is needed to determine whether the illusion adversely affects postural stability of older individuals more than that of younger people. However, it is theorized that the higher proportion of falls on escalators for older people may be a result of age-related declines in vision and a suspected relationship to postural stability. Older individuals should be alerted to the potential hazards of escalator use, and individuals with vision and visual perceptual deficits should be encouraged to avoid use of escalators. Additionally, these individuals should be cautioned to avoid similar surfaces such as carpeting or linoleum that use repeated patterns.[17]

Driving

Since driving is a privilege that enhances independent functioning in the environment, it is important to consider the impact that age-related sensory changes might have on this skill. Vision is a critical sensory modality that undergoes changes with age. Older drivers must learn to give careful consideration to this system in relationship to specific skills needed for driving.

Although it seems logical that good vision is necessary for safe driving, there are no data to support the idea that poor vision results in unsafe driving. Studies linking vision and accident involvement have provided mixed results and are based more on theoretical considerations rather than empirical data. It is generally believed that there is a weak relationship between visual performance and accident involvement for multiple reasons. These reasons include facts such as most accidents have multiple causes (the most frequently cited human causes of accidents are attentional or higher-order perceptual failings), many large scale studies rely on relatively unreliable vision data obtained from gross driver screenings, and drivers with reduced capacities may restrict driving to times when light conditions are favorable. Nevertheless, several studies link specific visual impairments and theoretically related driving tasks or accident-causing behaviors. These studies have found positive relationships between driver skills and visual acuity, depth perception, and contrast sensitivity.[34,67]

It is generally recognized that age-related decline in visual acuity is highly individualistic and that deterioration in static acuity under optimal illumination, reduced illumination, and glare is not significant before the age 60. Studies have found small but consistent correlations between photopic static acuity, or day vision, and accident involvement, particularly for older drivers. Between 5% and 10% of 60- to 65-year-old drivers have corrected acuity worse than the 20/40 minimum acuity level required by 38 states and the District of Columbia. Although not as extensively studied, static acuity under reduced illumination may be more relevant to the visual requirements of older drivers. One study indicated that low-level static acuity was one of the best predictors of accident involvement among older drivers. This is particularly relevant, since the onset is earlier and magnitude much larger than decline in photopic static acuity.[67] Older drivers should recognize the importance of adequate visual correction with glasses or contact lenses and may need to modify driving patterns in low-light conditions.

Dynamic visual acuity, or the ability to detect a moving object, is a more complex task than static visual acuity. Deterioration in this ability begins earlier and accelerates faster with increasing age. Studies have demonstrated a significant relationship between dynamic visual acuity and amount of driving and accident involvement. It is theorized that this correlation is due to the fact that this skill requires the combination of multiple visual sensory and motor skills that are necessary for safe driving, including fine oculomotor control. Another skill that is conceptually critical to safe driving is motion perception. The ability to detect movement relative to the driver is critical to detecting imminently dangerous situations. This ability is primarily limited by neural mechanisms, although the ability of the eye to effect smooth tracking also involves the oculomotor system. Studies have shown that visual training can be effective in enhancing motion discrimination in the elderly and that some effects can be generalized to driving situations.[67] Older drivers should be encouraged to participate in visual training sessions that include complex, dynamic visual skills.

Declining visual field is another factor that must be given consideration. Older individuals must be aware of pedestrians or vehicles in the lateral field, and individuals who experience declines in peripheral vision must be taught to compensate by turning their heads or by using car mirrors. Similarly, drivers who have experienced loss in the upper visual field must be alerted to the need to look upward to avoid missing overhead road signs and traffic signals.[22]

Depth perception is also known to decline with age and is additionally affected by increased susceptibility to glare, loss of visual acuity, dark adaptation, changing needs for illumination and contrast, and altered color perception. Older drivers need the ability to judge distances between their vehicle and other moving or stationary objects. This is critical for judging distances from oncoming cars, maintaining appropriate distances, safely passing other vehicles, merging onto a highway, or braking before reaching an intersection.[22] Older drivers who experience difficulty with depth perception and are unable to compensate for this loss should be strongly cautioned to avoid driving.

Since older individuals have problems with dark adaptation, they may experience difficulty with changes in illumination coming from oncoming headlights or streetlights. As a result, night driving may pose a safety hazard, and older individuals may need to confine driving to daylight hours.[38] Additionally, older drivers may be limited in night driving by glare intolerance. They should be instructed to compensate for this by avoiding looking at oncoming headlights, traveling on divided highways, or traveling on well-lit roads.[72] Vehicle design modifications introduced on 1986 models have proved beneficial for older drivers who experience decreased night vision and difficulty with glare. These include changes in headlights, rear lights, and directional signals that can be seen on the side of the vehicle. They also include design concepts that result in reduction in windshield and dashboard glare and installation of rear window defrosters and wipers.[67,77]

The impact of diminished color discrimination on driving is questionable. However, it has been suggested that it may take some older drivers twice as long as younger drivers to detect the flash of a brake light since red colors may appear dimmer as individuals age.[22] The high-mounted rear brake light introduced in 1986 vehicle models may serve as an accommodation for older drivers.[77]

In addition to visual loss, older drivers may experience difficulty because of age-related changes in hearing. Specifically, they may be unable to hear horns from other motorists warning of oncoming hazards, or they may be unable to localize the source of such signals. Vehicle malfunction warnings, such as brake sensors, may also go undetected with diminished hearing. Older drivers can compensate for this loss by adhering to a strict vehicle maintenance schedule.

The final deterrents to safe driving for older individuals that must be given consideration are hazards specific to the road environment itself, e.g., poorly placed and poorly designed road signs. Signs should be of sufficient size and should provide adequate color contrast to be seen by older drivers. Traffic lights pose another difficulty. Hazards pertaining to traffic light changes at intersections occur when older drivers react slowly to light changes from green to red. It has been suggested that older drivers would benefit if engineering slowed the speed at which a traffic light changes to 10% less the current recommended speed of change. Since night drivers rely on median and roadside delineator lines as visual cues, increasing the width of these markers from 4 to 8 inches has also been speculated to be of benefit to older night drivers. Older drivers with visual deficits may have difficulty on two-lane highways and older highways that have closely placed on-ramps and off-ramps. Newer highway design that includes four-lane highways with wide separation and better delineation of on-ramps and off-ramps should prove valuable for older drivers.[67,77] Finally, because older individuals are thought to have difficulty with visual depth illusion created by repeated optical patterns, repetitive patterns that occur in bridges, tunnels, and expressways may pose hazards.[17] Some older drivers should avoid these environments to foster safe driving.

TEACHING/CONSULTING STRATEGIES

Physical therapists working with the elderly are challenged to incorporate teaching strategies to accommodate sensory loss into treatment programs. Their unique knowledge of sensory changes that accompany aging, coupled with knowledge of appropriate interventions, will maximize the rehabilitation experience and afford the elderly an opportunity to utilize newly acquired skills in an environment that maintains reasonable control over functional ability and enhances quality of life.

Simply indicating which changes accompany normal aging may encourage older individuals to seek appropriate interventions and avoid the resignation that often accompanies a sense of helplessness at thoughts of "growing old." The physical therapist should encourage use of adaptive equipment and assistive technology to compensate for specific sensory loss. For example, individuals with visual loss should be supported in use of glasses and other low-vision aids, and persons with hearing loss should be encouraged to use hearing aids or other amplification devices that have been prescribed. Where indicated, physical therapists should support and encourage referral to appropriate specialists for evaluation of specific deficits and prescription of needed devices. They should also be knowledgeable of service agencies within the community that specialize in assistive technologies and support services for older individuals with sensory loss and assist individuals in contacting and using these agencies. Additionally, therapists should instruct the elderly in environmental modifications that are unique to their individual needs.

Physical therapists can use their knowledge and skills related to movement dysfunction and ergonomics to further enhance the functional independence of older individuals who require accommodations for sensory changes. For example, physical therapists can be particularly helpful in providing recommendations to utilize correct posture to enhance comfort for older individuals who use accommodations for low vision. This is important because the maintenance of focal distance, line of sight, head tilt, back position, and body posture determine the comfort and efficiency of many recommended low-vision systems. Suggestions may include modification of head position and line of sight to successfully use the device. Similar suggestions may be made

for computer users who are visually impaired. Additionally, therapists may serve a valuable role in recommending adaptations to prescribed devices that address concurrent problems often experienced by older, visually impaired patients. These may include the use of adjustable reading stands to hold large-print reading material or special ring stands, clamps, or headbands to position magnifying devices for individuals with arthritis, stroke, or Parkinson's disease, who may otherwise have difficulty using the prescribed device. Finally, physical therapists can be essential in assisting with mobility training for individuals who require the use of mobility assistive devices such as canes or dog guides.[53,81]

Specific teaching strategies that incorporate instruction in techniques to strengthen the sensory stimulus should be part of the physical therapy intervention for older individuals with sensory impairment. Examples might include adjustments to volume and tone of radios and televisions for hearing-impaired individuals or use of large-print books for the visually impaired. Another technique is to teach older individuals to compensate with other senses. For example, individuals with a diminished sense of smell can be taught to inspect food visually for signs of spoilage, or individuals with visual impairments can be encouraged to use auditory substitutions, including talking books and other talking products. The final strategy is to teach the elderly to modify behavior. One example is to teach older individuals with the visual problem of dark adaptation to pause when entering a darkened room from a bright, outdoor environment.[29,81,88]

Because of their knowledge of age-related sensory changes and environmental modifications, physical therapists should assume active roles as consultants. Providing information to architects and designers will foster safe access of facilities by older individuals. This is particularly important in public buildings, including churches, hospitals, outpatient clinics, and senior centers. Additionally, independence of individuals in retirement complexes, senior housing, and long-term–care facilities can be enhanced when design principles are incorporated. Therapists should assist in plans for construction of new facilities and renovation of existing facilities. Encouraging architects and builders to incorporate universal design concepts and design considerations to allow adaptability of structures to accommodate sensory changes related to age and disability may allow older individuals to remain in their own homes, and may be more economically feasible than renovating structures that do not incorporate such principles. Also, therapists should take an active role in purchase of supplies for existing facilities. Quality of life for older residents can be maximized by selecting such items as furniture, wall and floor coverings, and window treatments that enhance, rather than impede, functional performance. Finally, physical therapists can encourage development of appropriate products to meet the needs of older individuals with sensory loss by serving as consultants to companies that design and manufacture these devices.[8,24,33,48]

SUMMARY

It is important for physical therapists who work with the elderly to recognize sensory changes that occur with aging and to understand the effects that these changes have on the ability of older individuals to function in the environment. Knowledge of adaptations within the environment to accommodate and support losses that occur in vision, hearing, taste, smell, and touch can maximize the rehabilitation experience for the elderly and promote optimal functional independence.

Physical therapists should be able to apply this information concerning sensory losses and environmental adaptations to general principles of design in order to create meaningful environments for older persons. Consideration should be given to all aspects of the environment in which older individuals function. These include personal living space and long-term–care residencies. Specific attention should be given to architectural barriers found in physical therapy departments and on stairs and escalators. Since driving is a skill that allows access to other activities of daily living, special consideration must also be given to this function.

The roles of physical therapists as teacher and consultant should be emphasized. Physical therapists have unique knowledge of the needs of the elderly, and they should be encouraged to share this knowledge with architects, designers, administrators, and others who deal with facilities and products used by older individuals.

Finally, physical therapists should recognize that there is a critical need for further research on age-related sensory changes and on the relationship between these changes and the use of environmental adaptations, assistive technology, and adaptive devices. A limited number of studies have been done to address these considerations, and the majority of the recommendations are based more on theory than controlled studies. Furthermore, many of these recommendations are based on assumptions about the older individual's perceptions related to aging, the environment, and the motivation to preserve maximum function within the environment through appropriate modifications. Qualitative studies are needed to support such assumptions. Physical therapists should be willing to participate in or support such research efforts in order to further this science, and benefit the older individuals that they serve.

REFERENCES

1. Anderson RG, Meyerhoff WL: Otologic disorders, in Calkins E, Davis PJ, Ford AB (eds): *The Practice of Geriatrics.* Philadelphia, WB Saunders, 1986.
2. Archae JC: Environmental factors associated with stair accidents by the elderly. *Clin Geriatr Med* 1985; 1:555-569.
3. Arditi A: Topography, print legibility, and low vision, in Cole RG, Rosenthal BP (eds): *Remediation and Management of Low Vision.* St. Louis, Mosby, 1996.
4. Barrowclough F: Design for geriatric care. *Nurs Times* 1976; 72: 1330-1331.
5. Brant BA: Sensory disorders, in Stone JT, Wyman JF, Salisburg SA (eds): *Clinical Gerontological Nursing, A Guide to Advanced Practice,* ed 2. Philadelphia, WB Saunders, 1999.
6. Brennan PL, Moos RH, Lemke S: Preferences of older adults and experts for physical and architectural features of group living facilities. *Gerontologist* 1988; 28:84-90.
7. Brown WJ: Planning considerations for resident-oriented long-term care settings. *Contemp Longterm Care* 1987; 10:53-55.
8. Christenson MA: The therapist as geriatric environmental consultant. *Top Geriatr Rehabil* 1987; 3:79-83.
9. Christenson MA: Adaptations of the physical environment to compensate for sensory changes. *Phys Occup Ther Geriatr* 1990; 8:3-30.
10. Christenson MA: Chair design and selection for older adults. *Phys Occup Ther Geriatr* 1990; 8:67-85.
11. Christenson MA: Designing for the older person by addressing environmental attributes. *Phys Occup Ther Geriatr* 1990; 8:31-48.
12. Christenson MA: Enhancing independence in the home setting. *Phys Occup Ther Geriatr* 1990; 8:49-65.
13. Christenson MA, Gieneart D: Redesigning the long-term care facility. *Phys Occup Ther Geriatr* 1990; 8:87-111.
14. Cleary BL: Age-related changes in the special senses, in Matteson MA, McConnell ES, Linton AD (eds): *Gerontological Nursing: Concepts and Practice,* ed 2. Philadelphia, WB Saunders, 1997.
15. Clydesdale FM: Changes in color and flavor and their effect on sensory perception in the elderly. *Nutr Rev* 1994; 52:S19-S21.
16. Cohen JJ, et al: Establishing criteria for community ambulation. *Top Geriatr Rehabil* 1987; 3:71-77.
17. Cohn TE, Lasley DJ: Visual depth illusion and falls in the elderly. *Clin Geriatr Med* 1985; 1:601-620.
18. Cooper BA: A model for implementing color contrast in the environment of the elderly. *Am J Occup Ther* 1985; 39:253-258.
19. Cooper BA, et al: The use of the Lanthony New Color Test in determining the effects of aging on color vision. *J Gerontol* 1991; 46:320-324.
20. Cronin-Golomb A, et al: Visual dysfunction in Alzheimer's disease: Relation to normal aging. *Ann Neurol* 1991; 29:41-52.
21. Fernie GR: CAD/CAM approaches to the development of seating and mobility aids for the elderly. *Can J Public Health* 1986; 77(suppl 1): 114-118.
22. Fox MD: Elderly drivers' perceptions of their driving abilities compared to their functional visual perception skills and their actual driving performance. *Phys Occup Ther Geriatr* 1988; 7:13-49.
23. Fozard JL: Vision and hearing in aging, in Birren JE, Schaie KW (eds): *Handbook of the Psychology of Aging,* ed 3. San Diego, Academic Press, 1990.
24. Frain JP, Carr PH: Is the typical modern house designed for future adaptation for disabled older people? *Age Ageing* 1996; 25:398-401.
25. Goodrich GL, Sacco T: Visual function with high-tech low vision devices, in Cole RG, Rosenthal BP (eds): *Remediation and Management of Low Vision.* St. Louis, Mosby, 1996.
26. Goodwin S: Not so grand design. *Nurs Times* 1986; 82:26.
27. Gray G: Design of new building for the elderly. *J R Soc Health* 1989; 109:18-20.
28. Grisso JA, Mezey MD: Preventing dependence and injury: An approach to sensory changes, in LaVizzo-Mourey R, et al (eds): *Practicing Prevention for the Elderly.* Philadelphia, Hanley and Belfus, 1989.
29. Hayter J: Modifying the environment to help older persons. *Nurs Health Care* 1983; 4:265-269.
30. Healey F: Does flooring type affect risk of injury in older in-patients? *Nurs Times* 1994; 90:40-41.
31. Hiatt LG: Is poor lighting dimming the sight of nursing home patients? *Nurs Homes* 1980; 29:32-41.
32. Hiatt LG: The color and use of color in environments for older people. *Nurs Homes* 1981; 30:18-22.
33. Hiatt LG: Roles for gerontologists, the future of aging and technology. *Generations* 1986; 11:5-8.
34. Higgins KE: Low vision driving among normally-sighted drivers, in Cole RG, Rosenthal BP (eds): *Remediation and Management of Low Vision.* St. Louis, Mosby, 1996.
35. Hooper CR: Sensory and sensory integrative development, in Bonder BR, Wagner MB (eds): *Functional Performance in Older Adults.* Philadelphia, FA Davis, 1994.

36. Horwitz J: Residents' response to retirement community architecture. *Contemp Longterm Care* 1987; 10:92-93.

37. Howard DM: The effects of touch in the geriatric population. *Phys Occup Ther Geriatr* 1988; 6:35-50.

38. Kee CC: Sensory impairment: Factor X in providing nursing care to the older adult. *J Community Health Nurs* 1990; 7:45-52.

39. Kiernat JM: Environmental aspects affecting health, in Maguire GH (ed): *Care of the Elderly: A Health Team Approach.* Boston, Little, Brown, 1985.

40. Kiernat JM: Promoting independence and autonomy through environmental approaches. *Top Geriatr Rehabil* 1987; 3:1-6.

41. Kollarits CR: The aging eye, in Calkins E, Davis PJ, Ford AB (eds): *The Practice of Geriatrics.* Philadelphia, WB Saunders, 1986.

42. Kosnik W, et al: Visual changes in daily life throughout adulthood. *J Gerontol* 1988; 43:63-70.

43. LaBuda DR: Bringing gerontologists and technologists together. *Generations* 1986; 11:8-10.

44. Leibowitz HW, Shupert CL: Spatial orientation mechanisms and their implications for falls. *Clin Geriatr Med* 1985; 1:571-580.

45. Liang MH, et al: Rehabilitation management of homebound elderly with locomotor disability. *Clin Geriatr Med* 1988; 4:431-439.

46. Maguire GH: The changing realm of the senses, in Lewis CB (ed): *Aging: The Health Care Challenge,* ed 3. Philadelphia, FA Davis, 1996.

47. Maloney CC: Identifying and treating the client with sensory loss. *Phys Occup Ther Geriatr* 1987; 5:31-46.

48. Mann WC: Technology, in Bonder BR, Wagner MB (eds): *Functional Performance in Older Adults.* Philadelphia, FA Davis, 1994.

49. McConnell ES, Murphy AT: Nursing diagnoses related to physiological alterations, in Matteson MA, McConnell ES, Linton AD (eds): *Gerontological Nursing: Concepts and Practice,* ed 2. Philadelphia, WB Saunders, 1997.

50. McGilloway FA: A chair is a chair, or is it? *Nurs Mirror* 1980; 151:34-35.

51. Melore GG: Visual function changes in the geriatric patient and environmental modifications, in Melore GG (ed): *Treating Vision Problems in the Older Adult.* St. Louis, Mosby, 1997.

52. Meltzer DW: Ophthalmic aspects, in Steinberg FU (ed): *Care of the Geriatric Patient in the Tradition of EV Cowdry,* ed 6. St Louis, Mosby, 1983.

53. Musick JE: Clinical strategies for the visually impaired computer user, in Cole RG, Rosenthal BP (eds): *Remediation and Management of Low Vision.* St. Louis, Mosby, 1996.

54. Null RL: Low-vision elderly: An environmental rehabilitation approach. *Top Geriatr Rehabil* 1988; 4:24-31.

55. Owen DH: Maintaining posture and avoiding tripping. *Clin Geriatr Med* 1985; 1:581-599.

56. Parsons HM: Residential design for the aging (for example, the bedroom). *Hum Factors* 1981; 23:39-58.

57. Pease JA: Carpeting, new advances in technology provide more functional homelike environments. *Generations* 1986; 11:41-44.

58. Pinto MR, et al: Reduced visual acuity in elderly people: The role of ergonomics and gerontechnology. *Age Ageing* 1997; 26:339-344.

59. Rapelje DH, Schiff MR: Homes for the aged—:improving their interiors. *Dimens Health Serv* 1984; 61:22-24.

60. Raphael CC: An architect's viewpoint. *Top Geriatr Rehabil* 1987; 3:19-25.

61. Redfern MS, Moore PL, Yarsky CM: The influence of flooring on standing balance among older persons. *Hum Factors* 1997; 39:445-455.

62. Rosenthal BP: The function-based low vision evaluation, in Rosenthal BP, Cole RG (eds): *Functional Assessment of Low Vision.* St. Louis, Mosby, 1996.

63. Rouse DJ: Technology transfer, aerospace technology put to earthly use for elders, *Generations* 1986; 11:15-17.

64. Satariano WA: The disabilities of aging: looking to the physical environment [editorial comment]. *Am J Public Health* 1997; 87:331-332.

65. Schwartz S: Chronic care: Improving the quality of design. *Dimens Health Serv* 1982; 59:10-13.

66. Senturia BH, Goldstein R, Hersperger WS: Otorhinolaryngologic aspects of geriatric care, in Steinberg FU (ed): *Care of the Geriatric Patient in the Tradition of EV Cowdry,* ed 6. St Louis, Mosby, 1983.

67. Shinar D, Schieber F: Visual requirements for safety and mobility of older drivers. *Hum Factors* 1991; 33:507-519.

68. Spear PD: Neural basis of visual deficits during aging. *Vision Res* 1993; 33:2589-2609.

69. Steen R, et al: Age-related effects of glare on luminance and color contrast sensitivity. *Optom Vis Sci* 1994; 71:792-796.

70. Stelmach GE, Worringham CJ: Sensorimotor deficits related to postural stability. *Clin Geriatr Med* 1985; 1:679-694.

71. Stone R, Sonnenschein MA: Can you hear me? Technology for coping with hearing loss. *Generations* 1986; 11:39-40.

72. Sullivan N: Vision in the elderly. Part 2, Coping with declining visual function. *J Gerontol Nurs* 1983; 9:231-235.

73. Sullivan N: Vision in the elderly. Part 1, Declining visual function in old age. *J Gerontol Nurs* 1983; 9:228-231.

74. Tiedskaar R: Geriatric falls, in Gambert SR (ed): *Contemporary Geriatric Medicine,* vol 2. New York, Plenum, 1986.

75. Tiedskaar R: Fall prevention in the home. *Top Geriatr Rehabil* 1987; 3:57-64.

76. Walker JM, et al: Walking velocities of older pedestrians at controlled crossings. *Top Geriatr Rehabil* 1987; 3:65-70.

77. Waller JA: The older driver, can technology decrease the risks? *Generations* 1986; 11:36-37.

78. Walls MAK: Low vision and the elderly, in Melore GG (ed): *Treating Vision Problems in the Older Adult.* St. Louis, Mosby, 1997.

79. Wells TJ: Major clinical problems in gerontologic nursing, in Calkins E, Davis PJ, Ford AB (eds): *The Practice of Geriatrics.* Philadelphia, WB Saunders, 1986.

80. Werner JS, Peterzell DH, Scheetz AJ: Light, vision, and aging. *Optom Vis Sci* 1990; 67:214-229.

81. Williams DR: Functional adaptive devices, in Cole RG, Rosenthal BP (eds): *Remediation and Management of Low Vision.* St. Louis, Mosby, 1996.

82. Willmott M: The effects of a vinyl floor surface upon walking in elderly hospital in patients. *Age Ageing* 1986; 15:119-120.

83. Winters RK: Adapting the environment to age-related sensory losses. *J Am Acad Nurse Pract* 1989; 1:106-111.

84. Wister AV: Environmental adaptation by persons in their later life. *Res Aging* 1989; 11:267-291.

85. Wolfson LI, et al: Gait and balance in the elderly: Two functional capacities that link sensory and motor ability to falls. *Clin Geriatr Med* 1985; 1:649-659.

86. Yerxa EJ, Baum S: Environmental theories and the older person. *Top Geriatr Rehabil* 1987; 3:7-18.

87. Yurick AG, et al: *The Aged Person and the Nursing Process,* ed 2. Norwalk, Conn., Appleton-Century-Crofts, 1984.

88. Zegeer LJ: The effects of sensory changes in older persons. *J Neurosci Nurs* 1986; 18:325-332.

CHAPTER 9

COGNITIVE IMPAIRMENT

CAROL SCHUNK, PT, PsyD

INTRODUCTION

Decline in cognitive ability from a previous higher level of function brings multiple problems that influence rehabilitation of the older individual. While therapists may focus on physical disability, it is impossible to reach treatment goals without an awareness of the normal cognitive changes that accompany aging and the changes that occur with a specific illness. Consideration of the mental condition influences the therapeutic plan and results in setting appropriate goals and achieving a successful outcome.

Definition

The terms *confusion, dementia,* and *senility* are commonly used to describe mental function of the elderly. Although many people consider "getting old" to be the reason for mental decline, actual changes attributed to normal aging are minimal. Cognitive changes that are severe enough to interfere with function are part of a cluster of dementing illness— not old age. Dementia is a Latin word and means "pathological condition of the mind."[39] Senility is a term often used with mental deterioration in the elderly. However, these are not diagnostic terms and are not based on specific organic causes.[36] Chronic encephalopathy, characterized by global in-

tellectual deterioration severe enough to interfere with social and personal activities, is also commonly referred to as dementia. Properly defined, dementia is characterized by persistent observed cognitive changes resulting from an illness. The key terminology in the definition of dementia are *acquired* and *persistent.* "Acquired" implies abilities that were once within the behavioral domain of the individual are now dysfunctional. "Persistent" differentiates dementia from delirium, which produces a fluctuating state of dysfunction.

Prevalence

Since some of the dementing illnesses progress slowly, early detection is difficult because the person retains social skills and the ability to compensate for any deficits. An individual may be quite functional within the structure of the family home and with familiar objects and routines. Not until this person is out of his/her natural environment, such as in a new grocery store, will symptoms become noticeable. A spouse may unconsciously begin to help the affected mate, therefore prolonging the identification of dementia. In the United States only the prevalence of dementia is estimated because of the lack of a solid data base and problems with accurate diagnosis. Based on European studies, the prevalence of dementia is between 10% and 20% of all elders, depending on the sample and the criteria of dementia that were used. Although published data for the United States are minimal, approximately 15% of the population older than 65 is estimated to be cognitively impaired.[36] Risk for deterioration increases with advancing age, ranging from 3% of those 65 to 74 years old, 18.7% of those 75 to 84 years old, and more than 47% of those aged 85 or more.[9] The prevalence in nursing home residents older than 65 has been estimated as high as 50%.[38] Of elders with an organic mental disorder, an estimated 10% to 20% have reversible or partly reversible conditions.

CHANGES ASSOCIATED WITH NORMAL AGING

Predictable changes in patterns of some cognitive functions are common with normal aging. The health care practitioner should be able to differentiate between normal and abnormal patterns in order to plan the appropriate treatment approach. The change associated with old age that brings a cognitive decline is referred to as *aging associated cognitive decline (AACD)*. This term characterizes subjects with cognitive decline that falls short of dementia.[15] Criteria include subjective gradual cognitive decline for at least 6 months, and objective criteria as measured by performance one standard deviation below age and education norms as identified in neuropsychological testing. All domains of cognitive performance are considered, including memory and learning, attention and concentration, thinking, language, and visuospatial functioning. Prevalence for AACD in a population aged 68 to 78 years was 26.6%.[15]

Often the therapist may be in the initial position to detect the onset of dementia symptoms when assessing the individual's ability to participate in therapy. With normal aging, there may be some change in functional activity. There is also a cognitive component to performance of many physical activities of daily living (ADL). Consequently, if a cognitive decline is not correctly identified, change in functional activity may be misinterpreted as a physical condition. If cognitive deficits co-exist with functional changes, early identification provides an advantage in developing strategy to assist with daily activity and in maintaining independence. Given that approximately 20% of cases of dementia are reversible, this differentiation is important.[42]

Memory and Learning

Memory loss is the cognitive component most often associated with aging. This has undoubtedly contributed to the perceptions that the elderly cannot remember basic information and have severe lapses in memory—two of the many myths of growing old. Although lapses in memory may occur as one ages, the ability to recall with cues is common. In healthy individuals, this kind of memory problem usually does not interfere with social or personal activities. Age-associated memory impairment (AAMI) is the condition proposed by the National Institute of Mental Health that describes memory loss in the elderly not sufficient to warrant a diagnosis of dementia. Hanninen reports studies showing prevalence of AAMI ranging from 34.5% to 38.4%, although some researchers estimate that most individuals older than 50 are affected to some degree.[15] Criteria are based on a score of one standard deviation below the norm in a standard memory test. However, the data are normed on the mean of younger adults, making the condition and the diagnosis controversial.[15]

The most prominent structural theory of memory describes three distinct types: sensory memory; short-term, or primary, memory; and long-term, or secondary, memory.[16] Sensory memory is the initial momentary memory in which there is brief registration of the physical characteristics of stimulus, such as pain with an injection. Short-term, or primary, memory is a brief repository for conscious processing of small amounts of information. Recognition of a street-

light changing from green to red is a result of primary memory. Both of these types of memory are relatively unaffected by aging. Changes that have been documented are of little practical importance, given normal demands.[16]

Long-term, or secondary, memory is the level in which documentation of age-related decline is most prominent. Providing for unlimited long-term retention of the information, secondary memory is responsible for analysis and organization of information, for storage, plus future retrieval.[16] Recall seems to be the primary activity affected by aging, with free recall being more involved than cured recall and recognition—the "Why did I come into this room?" phenomenon. Older individuals may not recall why they walked into the kitchen until the memory is cued by the sight of the phone and the recollection that they intended to make a call. While reduction in effectiveness is gradual, the most notable transition of decline is between ages 50 and 70 years. Poor performance with secondary memory tasks is caused by multiple reasons as well as intervening variables. In some memory theories, a tertiary level dealing with remote memory has been described. Research in this area is minimal but does not substantiate the common belief that older individuals are superior in remembering the past but inferior in remembering the present.

Memory loss associated with the normal older person has been termed *benign senescent forgetfulness* (BSF). Early stages of a mental disorder may often be mistaken for BSF. However, functional decline that is evident as the mental disorder progresses is unique to dementia and is not present with BSF. Therefore, physical therapists may have a crucial role in differentiating between BSF and other mental disorders. BSF is identified as a slowly progressive, mild impairment of cognitive functioning and is not severe enough to interfere with daily activities. While still under investigation, BSF is currently being viewed as a variant of aging that occurs in one third of individuals older than 85.[28]

Another common, but inaccurate, belief is that the capacity to learn new information declines with age. While there is some evidence that age-related changes in learning occur, problems inherent to the research limit interpretation. These include comparisons across studies and multiple factors that contribute to cognitive changes, response time, interference of prior material, and retrieval. Also complicating the research are isolating factors such as learning new motor skills, sensory changes, cognitive reorganization of material between stimulus and response, dividing attention between several tasks simultaneously, and highly speeded tasks. Despite these variables, the capacity for cognitive reserve has been demonstrated in the older person. While more limited than a younger person's capability to learn, the ability exists in older persons to improve performance.[2]

Intelligence

Age-related deterioration in intelligence is difficult to study because of the cohort effects, generational bias of tools, and selective attrition. While consistent longitudinal studies over many decades can eliminate some of these variables, there still exist factors particular to one generation that are difficult to eliminate. The measurement tools are not sensitive to the variety of educational and cultural conditions that influenced the current older person. Actual documented declines are minimal and do not affect daily functioning. The Wechsler Adult Intelligence Scale (WAIS) is the most common tool for measuring intelligence. WAIS studies show that verbal and performance scores peak by ages 18 to 30 and stabilize until the mid-50s to early 60s.[16] Based on data from the Seattle Longitudinal Study, Hertzog and Schaie determined 55 to 70 years as the transition time from stability to decline in general intelligence.[17] While decline in performance on many cognitive tests is evident, substantial decline in the older person is generally limited to those older than 75. Performance skills that are time-related and influenced by decrease in reaction time tend to change more drastically than verbal skills. This phenomenon is known as the *classic aging pattern* and is the basis for age-graded intelligence quotient (IQ) scores.

The difference between fluid and crystal intelligence is also relevant to understanding cognitive dysfunction in the elderly. Fluid intelligence involves the capacity to use unique kinds of thinking to solve unfamiliar problems and is believed to decline with age. Crystallized knowledge, acquired through education and acculturation, remains stable through age 70. Creativity is often researched as a component of intelligence, with the assumption that declines are universal with age. Clinically, this can be interpreted as meaning, "If you haven't done it, forget it." While some studies suggest that creativity peaks by about 35 years, enough exceptions exist to encourage patients to take on new challenges and to personally keep us all inspired.[16] Additional factors that must be considered are the lack of reinforcement for creativity in old age and environmental issues, which geriatric clinicians can positively influence.

Executive Functioning

Executive functioning, or executive abilities, involves complex behavior that combines memory, intellectual capacity, and cognitive planning. Activities of executive functioning include planning, active problem-solving, working memory, anticipating possible consequences of an intended course of action, initiating an activity, inhibiting irrelevant behavior, and being able to monitor the effectiveness of one's behavior.[13] Working memory is the core of executive functioning and incorporates complex attention, strategy formation, and interference control. There is evidence of a mild decline of executive functioning with normal aging; however, this decline is greater when a neurological disorder, such as a cerebrovascular accident (CVA) or dementia, is also present. Executive function is measured by the Minnesota Mental State Exam (MMSE) and the Behavioral Dysfunction Scale.

The interesting aspect of executive functioning is its relationship to motor function. Grigsby studied the contribution of executive cognitive abilities and ADL to executive functioning.[13] He concluded that executive functioning is an important factor for self-reported and observed performance of complex, independent ADL, such as managing money and medications. Intact executive functioning can actually serve as a fall prevention measure by minimizing behavior that jeopardizes safety despite motor or sensory impairment. Conversely, executive dysfunction should trigger the therapist's awareness of the risk for falls.[33]

Personality

Stereotypical beliefs about personality development, such as theories about stages of personality and an aged personality profile, are generally inaccurate. The best available evidence suggests that personality types remain fairly stable throughout life.[16] Therefore, younger individuals who are characterized by an internal locus of control or who believe they have the ability to control the events in their lives will continue to react accordingly as they age. Those who experience a severe mid- to late-life crisis tend to react similarly to the way they reacted to situations throughout life. Activity also follows this model: elders who were active stay active. In his research on the trait theory of personality, Hartke concluded, "consistency in personality is more the rule than change in personality as one ages."[16] The change that does occur is promoted as a continuation of individuality of the person. Traits that have been predominant will continue to be influential as a person ages. Clinically, this means patients who display a negative outlook about therapy have probably always had a negative attitude about a variety of situations.

The area that does warrant additional exploration is personality changes related to illness. Evidence is minimal that specific changes do occur, but research itself is lacking. The distinction between the influence of aging or the illness process on personality is inconclusive, making any generalizations to aging inappropriate.[16]

DIFFERENTIAL DIAGNOSIS

Diagnostic Criteria

The fourth revised edition of the *Diagnostic and Statistical Manual of Mental Disorders* (*DSM-IV-R*) of the American Psychiatric Association provides a universal reference of diagnostic criteria for cognitive disorders. When there is no reference to an etiological condition, the cognitive disorder is classified as a mental symptom. Delirium, intoxication, withdrawal, and dementia are the most common mental symptoms. A mental disorder designates a mental symptom for which the etiology is known or presumed and is characterized by a "psychological or behavioral abnormality associated with transient or permanent dysfunction of the brain."[1] Therefore, a patient is correctly diagnosed as having a mental disorder by the presence of an organic mental syndrome plus the presence of an organic factor etiologically related to the decline in mental function.

Delirium and dementia characterize patients as having global cognitive impairment as opposed to select dysfunction. Differential diagnosis between delirium and dementia is often difficult, because one may be superimposed on the other. Impairment in sensorium or level of consciousness is the distinguishing feature of delirium.[22] Specific features of delineating delirium, depression, and dementia are described in Table 9-1.[22] Dementia cannot be accurately diagnosed in the presence of delirium; in order to have a co-existing diagnosis, it would be necessary for the dementia to have been identified prior to symptoms of delirium.

There is no specific course or pattern for mental symptoms. When associated with a specific episode of a neurological disease, onset may be sudden but remain stable. This may be in contrast to a gradual onset with a progressive course of involvement, such as that found in patients with dementia of the Alzheimer type. In some cases, onset may be gradual, such as an organic brain tumor. In this case, symptoms may subside with treatment.

Dementia

The *DSM-IV-R* describes dementia as a group of disorders characterized by the development of multiple cognitive deficits. The contributing factors may be physiological effects of a medical condition or the effects of a substance. The essential feature of dementia is impairment in short- and long-term memory, associated with a decline in abstract thinking, judgment, and other disturbances of higher cortical function. These factors must be severe enough to interfere significantly with work, social activities, or relationships with others. Memory is the most classic feature, with retaining the ability to perform new tasks showing greater decline than remembering remote material. As the case progresses, both recent and remote memory may be affected, with the person reaching the stage in which recognition of familiar people is impaired. Disorientation may be missed early on, because the individual will attempt to compensate for the loss. Disorganized thinking is apparent in the person's inability to follow directions or tolerate changes in routine.[1]

A 25-year time trend study looked at the incident of dementing illness.[19] While the results supported an increasing incidence of dementing illness among the elderly, the study was not balanced among all groups, and environmental factors could have contributed to the results. The awareness of the public and the medical community may have led to the diagnosis and identification of individuals whose cognitive decline might have been erroneously attributed to "old age." The primary increase was noted in primary degenerative dementia of the Alzheimer type (DAT), with a decrease in dementia due to unknown causes.

Making an accurate diagnosis of dementia requires that the practitioner understand the normal process of cognitive changes with aging. Although research on cognitive changes associated with normal aging is not definitive, a diagnosis of dementia is applicable only when there is demonstrable evidence of memory impairment and other features to the degree in which there is interference with social or occupational function. One characteristic of dementia is the decline in intellectual functioning from a previous level; therefore, knowing a person's baseline cognitive ability is essential.

Unfortunately, clinical assessment of premorbid cognitive function is not always possible and is complicated in the elderly when family input is unavailable. Consideration of educational, occupational, and socioeconomic levels can provide information in determining a previous level, but often the clinician must piece together a picture of the individual's prior status. Irreversible dementia disorders cluster into several categories, with primary neuronal degeneration of the Alzheimer type and multi-infarct dementia being the most common. In a study of dementia mortality, Lanska found that only 4% of those in their last year of life did not receive facility based care, the majority being in skilled- or intermediate-care–nursing facilities. Although dementia was present in those studied, it was not responsible for the deaths; however, it certainly affected the quality of life in their last year.[21]

TABLE 9-1
COMPARATIVE FEATURES OF DELIRIUM, DEMENTIA, AND DEPRESSION

	DELIRIUM	DEMENTIA	MAJOR DEPRESSION
Definition	Impaired sensorium (reduced level of consciousness)	Global decline in cognitive capacity in clear consciousness	Disturbance in mood, with associated low vital sense and low self-attitude
Core symptoms	Inattention, distractibility, drowsiness, befuddlement	Amnesia, aphasia, agnosia, apraxia, disturbed executive functioning	Sadness, anhedonia crying
Common associated symptoms	Cognitive impairment, hallucinations, mood lability	Depression, delusions, hallucinations, irritability	Fatigue, insomnia, anorexia, guilt, self-blame, hopelessness, helplessness
Temporal features	Acute or subacute onset	Chronic onset, usually gradual	Episodic subacute onset
Diurnal features	Usually worse in the evening and night	No clear pattern	Usually worse in the morning

From Lyketosos CG: Diagnosis and management of delerium in the elderly. *JCOM* 1998; 5(4): 54.

Alzheimer's Disease

DAT, accounting for 60% of those with dementia, is the category of organic mental disorder for individuals with Alzheimer's disease. A definitive diagnosis is usually made postmorbidly through autopsy. However, the trend is shifting from a diagnosis of inclusion rather than exclusion, as evident in a consensus statement sponsored by the Alzheimer Association, the American Geriatrics Society, and the American Association for Geriatric Psychiatry.[10] *DSM-IV* diagnostic criteria recognize memory impairment as the cognitive deficit required for diagnosis. The memory loss is accompanied by aphasia, apraxia, or disturbance in executive functioning. McKhann and colleagues published clinical criteria that have been widely adopted for the probable diagnosis of Alzheimer's disease.[25] Their criteria include typical insidious onset of progressive dementia that is not caused by any other disease and has produced memory loss and cognitive decline. Heredity does play a role but seems to be a separate classification, accounting for only a minority of cases. Inherited episodes are characterized by early onset with symptoms beginning about age 50.[10] While genetics may play a strong role, the contribution of a family history overall continues to be studied. Classification by subtypes is possible with the identification of the presence of delirium, delusions, or depression; contribution of family history; rapid or slow progression; and early or late onset.[7]

Diagnosis is difficult in the early stages, because the individual may present very well socially with no physical appearance of a problem. The relationship of education and occupational level to dementia is often studied.[35,40] It has been hypothesized that advanced education and high occupational experience create a reserve against the manifestations of DAT—the theory being that educational and occupational attainment may provide a reserve that allows an individual to cope longer before a positive diagnostic criteria are apparent. This makes an early diagnosis even more difficult. Stern considered these two factors simultaneously and found that the risk of DAT was greatest in the group with both low education and low occupation levels. When the clinical severity was constant, the decline from premorbid levels was greater in those with more education.[35]

Forgetfulness is often the first characteristic expressed subjectively by the individual and not evident on clinical assessment. Memory impairment as demonstrated by difficulty with acquisition of new information is the first obvious symptom. The actual loss in the process of memory involves poor encoding and retrieval and poor recognition recall. The course of the disease is usually divided into stages, with the middle stage being identified by cognitive deficits that are quite obvious, such as intellectual decline and language disturbance. Premorbid personality and behavior changes occur along with the cognitive decline, presenting a very difficult situation for family members. Awareness of the cognitive decline is often accompanied by depression. In the late stage the person is incapable of self-care, often becoming mute and inattentive. Research shows that physicians often overlook dementia of this type, even in patients with whom they are familiar.[8]

Behavioral problems are also evident in the clinical presentation, although there are minimal empirical data to support the clinical observations of behavioral problems associated with the cognitive deficits of persons with DAT. Teri and colleagues surveyed 55 families who had a member with irreversible dementia, including 60% with DAT, in order to identify the "biggest problem" of patient care.[37] In a list of 22 behaviors, more than half the care-givers described four problems: memory disturbance, catastrophic reactions, suspiciousness, and making accusations. Clarification of the associated behavioral problems and associated cognitive and functional factors were also investigated. Results showed that the most common patient problems were cognitively oriented memory loss (84%), confusion (82%), and disorientation (64%). The next most common problems reported by more than 20% of the participants were related to activity and emotional distress, decreased activity, loss of interest, tension, apathy, depression, and bodily preoccupation. Despite these results, there was no support for a relationship between overall cognitive impairment and behavioral problems in patients with comparable cognitive impairments. The association between rate of decline and various health and behavioral factors was studied to determine the influence on deterioration. While the results indicated that there was an association between some factors and rate of decline, the progression of the disease is variable.[36]

Multi-Infarct Dementia

The *DSM-IV-R* classifies multi-infarct dementia as an organic mental disorder, with the essential feature being cerebrovascular disease. The cognitive disorder is the result of the additive effects of small and large infarcts that produce a loss of brain tissue. Deterioration is select, with some functions left completely intact. While the location of the infarction is relevant, predicting the exact course of the mental dysfunction based on site is often misleading. This may be in part because multiple strokes have occurred, obstructing a clear attribution of the deficit to a particular lesion. Common disturbances include problems with memory, abstract thinking, judgment, impulse control, and personality. Three forms of multi-infarct are most common: large vessel disease, strokes, and multiple microcerebral infarcts.[8] While the clinical presentation may resemble some features of Alzheimer's disease, the signs of abrupt onset, step-by-step deterioration, fluctuating course, and emotional lability are specific to multi-infarct dementia.[1]

Reversible Dementia

Dementia was once regarded as a permanent, irreversible, and progressive disorder. It is now known that many cases of dementia are not related to an irreversible pathology of the central nervous system but to a cognitive disorder that can be treated. Estimates show that 10% to 30% of those presenting with dementia symptoms can be treated to correct a metabolic or structural condition, also resulting in restoration of intellectual function.[28] Without investigating the potential medical causes of dementia, a true diagnosis cannot be made. Several of the conditions that can mask the diagnosis of a reversible dementia include drug complications; infectious diseases; nutritional, psychiatric, and metabolic disorders; and trauma. Change in cognitive status secondary to drugs is possibly the most common cause of reversible dementia. The complication may be a result of drug-drug interaction either from self-medicating or inattentiveness by the physician on the drug combinations being prescribed. Because of the multiple medical problems of the elderly, there may be several physicians involved in the person's care, each being unaware of the medications prescribed by the other. Psychosocial factors such as depression, social isolation, anxiety, grief, or communication disorders can also be manifested by a decrease in cognitive function. Without exploration of other factors, a misdiagnosis of irreversible dementia is possible.

Data are limited in documenting a relationship between increased incident of dementia and psychosocial factors such as bereavement, isolation, relocation, stress, or life-style changes.[41] However, once dementia is documented, there is evidence that environmental and psychosocial variables do have an impact on severity and progression. Factors may include inadequate stimulation, diet, and medical care.

Pseudodementia

The relationship between depression and dementia presents a complicated diagnostic picture in the elderly. Although dementia is an organic disorder with cognitive disturbance as the main symptom and depression is an affective disorder, cognitive deficits caused by depression simulate dementia.[11] *Pseudodementia* is the term used when dementia-like behavior is actually the result of a major depressive episode. Characteristics of depression, sometimes estimated as affecting 25% of the older population to some degree, include psychomotor retardation, flattened affect, and disinterest in events around them. Patients presenting in this fashion could be labeled as having a decline in mental ability simply because they do not have the interest in answering questions intended to establish a cognitive level. Also termed *dementia syndrome of depression*, the presenting symptoms of memory impairment—decline in intellectual function and poor performance on mental status examinations—can be diagnostically confusing. A comparison of depression in demented and non-demented population showed a greater incident in those with dementia (11.8% to 3.9%, respectively). *DSM-IV* depression criteria that were more commonly found in the demented group were lack of energy, thinking/concentration difficulties, loss of interest, and psychomotor disturbance. Of note to rehabilitation professionals is the fact that disability in daily life was the only variable associated with both the demented and non-demented group. Since the two conditions can co-exist, there is a contemporary trend not to use the term pseudodementia, which may imply that the individual must be either depressed or demented but not both.[14]

Although persons with dementia or depression may present similarly, observation of behavioral characteristics is revealing. Even though depressed patients may respond to testing in a slow, labored manner, they are aware of content and provide accurate responses.[39] Those with true dementia are unable to produce the correct response, even when they are pressed for an answer. Dysphoria is a distinguishing characteristic in depression, as evident in profound sadness, apathy, and feelings of helplessness and hopelessness. Social contact and activity are lessened, and a low self-esteem and an increase of self-blame are present.

A study by Pearson and colleagues examined the relationship between depressive diagnosis and cognitive and functional limitations in DAT patients.[29] They found that depression did affect functional status beyond the effects of cognitive impairment. Therefore, if depression is an overlying condition, functional status may improve with successful treatment of the depressive episode. A trial regimen of antidepressants may provide information for a clear diagnosis. If the mood improves as the depression is resolved, cognitive function will return to pre-depressive level. Should the individual continue to display characteristics of decline in mental ability, then investigation for dementia would be initiated. Some evidence exist that depression in the elderly is a predictor or possible causal factor of dementia.[5] Therefore, a diagnosis of pseudodementia may still be related to an eventual onset of dementia.

Given change in functional status, involvement of the physical therapist is appropriate. The focus will not only be on physical training but on monitoring the cognitive orientation to therapy. Since improvement in functional activities requires aspects of cognition such as attention and memory, the therapist may be the primary practitioner to note decline or improvement in mental function.

Anxiety

Because of the number of stressful situational changes that occur as one ages, anxiety-type behavior may be more common than it is in a person's younger years. Early stage dementia can be a cause of anxiety as the person becomes aware of his/her deteriorating mental capacity. If the dementia is related to organic causes, a diagnosis of organic anxiety syndrome may be appropriate.[1] Common diseases in the older person that may be the etiological cause of an anxiety syndrome include pulmonary embolus, chronic obstructive pulmonary disease, and alcohol withdrawal. According to the American Psychiatric Association, the primary diagnostic criterion is prominent, recurrent panic attacks or generalized anxiety with evidence of specific organic factors related to the disturbance. Anxiety disorders have a similar symptomatic picture as presentation to an anxiety syndrome but without similar etiology. In the elderly, situational factors such as relocation may precipitate an anxiety disorder.

Coping Behavior

As a result of the multiple changes in later life, the older individual's ability to cope may influence behavior. Coping styles are closely related to personality styles, developed throughout life as one confronts challenges and changes. Stress is often the by-product of factors and situations occurring later in life. Although the stresses may occur more frequently, there is no indication that the ability to cope with stressful events declines with age. Economic, health, and social resources may be minimized with old age and therefore compromise the individual's ability to deal with stressful life events. However, if all is constant, the notion of declining ability to cope in later life has not been validated.

Given pain as a major stress for many older persons, Keefe and Williams were prompted to conduct a comparison study of coping strategies for different age-groups.[18] Results showed that chronic pain patients of different ages tend to rely on similar coping strategies to deal with pain and rate the effectiveness of their pain in a similar fashion. Those who used a catastrophizing or an emotional non-participatory reaction had higher levels of pain and psychological distress, whereas those who indicated a high ability to deal with the pain reported lower levels of pain and depression. Given the lack of differences in coping strategies, a study by Middaugh and colleagues concluded that there is no reason why older persons would not be good candidates for chronic pain programs, because they were able to benefit as much as younger patients.[27] Subjects showed decrease in level of pain and the ability to enhance functional activity regardless of age.

ASSESSMENT

There are no neurodiagnostic procedures or electrophysiological techniques that unequivocally confirm the presence of primary degenerative dementia. Therefore, diagnosis is often made on clinical grounds.[41] Because of the number of individuals with possible cognitive deficits in long-term–care facilities and home care, there is a need for a rapid bedside assessment tool.[32] One commonly used instrument is the Pfeiffer Short Portable Mental Status Questionnaire, which contains 10 questions and can be used to screen for moderate to severe cognitive impairment.[31] The Mini-Mental Status Examination (MMSE) seems to be the most accepted of the brief standardized tests, providing the most information in the greatest number of domains.[10,23] In addition, the MMSE provides specific norms for older adults.[3] The MMSE is viewed as a screening tool rather than a diagnostic tool, and a score of less than 24 out of the 30 possible points indicates cognitive impairment, warranting evaluation by a physician. Since there are various parts of the examination, the total score may identify a cognitive deficit but does not provide information on the specific area of loss. Individualized scores of the examination sections provide a better picture of the nature of the decline. The first part of the examination measures orientation.

Serial sevens, one of the components of the MMSE, if done correctly, suggest that cognitive function is good. However, the task when failed is nonspecific, given the factors such as education or poor calculation skills that can influence the outcome. The recent memory or recall section is essential in assessment for dementia, especially in relation to functional activities. Odenheimer suggests that the one cognitive domain neglected is "executive control" or "intention," which measures stick-to-itiveness, goal setting, and flexibility.[28] Since functional independence depends on the ability to move from one task to another, it can be assessed by asking the patient to copy a figure that alternates in form or list items in a grocery store for 1 minute.

The MMSE and the Blessed Orientation-Memory-Test (BOMC)[4] are both bedside tools that have excellent test-retest reliability. They are used for identifying cognitive disabilities and in describing changes in mental status over time. Other advantages are the simplicity and clarity of the instruments, which are important because of the care-givers' minimal training in nursing homes.[42] Criticisms of these tools include limited ability to provide specific neurobehavioral descriptions as compared with more extensive tests and neglect of nonverbal functions, making them non-multidimensional.[42] Therefore, they have been reported to be vulnerable to high false-negative rates. Given these problems, the tests' wide utilization is based on the tests' ability to discriminate between different diagnostic subgroups, related to severity and course of dementia and reliability when applied in nursing home settings.

When comparing the BOMC and the MMSE, Zillmer and others found that the MMSE may be more useful since it identifies more than one mental process.[42] The study emphasized that brief mental status examination should be confined "to measuring limited dimensions of mental processes." Results of the study concluded that the BOMC and MMSE are appropriate tools if "primarily interpreted as measures of memory, attention, and limited (i.e., highly stereotyped) linguistic facility." They counseled against broader interpretation.

The cognitive deficits that the practitioner is trying to test create problems in the testing procedure, given the memory problems and impaired awareness of deficits. An informant-based scale was assessed by Koss and found to be a valid proxy of laboratory measures of memory and cognition.[20] The care-givers' perceptions of the individual's memory ability were closely related to the individual's performance on clinical measures.

Once a diagnosis is made, the interest of the rehabilitation professional lies with the functional status of the person. The Structured Assessment of Independent Living Skills (SAILS) was developed to measure the functional abilities of patients with dementia. The focus is on activities of daily living that are commonly affected in individuals with a dementia diagnosis.[24] Tasks instructions are straightforward and can be demonstrated, thereby accounting for problems encountered with batteries designed for a general population. Although the assessment identifies potential independent living skills, the question of utilization of the capabilities was not answered. The authors acknowledged the patient's motivation, care-giver availability, and environment will be influential.

THERAPEUTIC MANAGEMENT

Although the treatment goal of maximizing functional independence is consistent with the goals for patients without dementia, there are special considerations when treating an older person with a cognitive disability. Rehabilitation potential for individuals with cognitive dysfunction was considered to be minimal according to the early literature.[38] The features of dementia that most influence the rehabilitation process are memory decline and the difficulty or inability to learn new material. Since therapy is viewed as a teaching process, these features of dementia may be perceived as major obstacles to successful outcome. In addition, physical therapy reimbursement for persons with a dementing disease is often questioned based on the perceived inability to follow a treatment plan. Research now demonstrates that the presence and severity of cognitive status should not eliminate a patient from rehabilitation.[38] Therapists must modify treatment methods and goals in relation to the limitations of the cognitive disability, but therapy should not be denied based on mental dysfunction. Reassessment of progress in relation to treatment goals may be necessary on a more frequent basis, given the inconsistent pattern of mental deterioration.

The initial step in planning a therapeutic program is to determine the exact nature of the cognitive dysfunction. The screening tools discussed can be utilized for a global picture of the condition. If available, a neuropsychological assessment with consultation by a psychologist will provide additional information to delineate the deficit. The attempt is to clearly define specifics of the memory loss or other disability. Then the treatment can be modified, such as using one-step consistent commands or providing cues. The approach to teaching is to avoid criticism; use consistent, simple commands; give sensory cues: demonstrate; and allow the person to rest.[23] Learning should be approached in a simple, repetitious manner, often requiring cooperation from the family or nursing staff for consistency in the approach and directions for the individual.

The patient's physical disability may be part of the same disease that has caused the cognitive impairment, such as a cerebrovascular accident. In other cases the two components are separate, such as the patient with Alzheimer's disease who suffers a hip fracture. In either case the therapy assessment and treatment program must be modified to accommodate the mental dysfunction. A physical therapy evaluation technique such as manual muscle testing may not be valid with an individual who is inconsistent in following directions. Modification to accommodate the mental limitation may result in a generalized assessment of strength documented as "voluntary motion noted in extremities; unable to grade specifically secondary to inconsistency following directions." Muscle testing procedures are not familiar tasks to most people, which therefore necessitates learning that can be difficult for a person with dementia. While strength can be assessed and reported, the approach is modified in relation to the limitations of the mental symptoms.

The orthopedic patient with DAT and a lower extremity fracture presents an example of a need to alter the treatment program. A physician's order for gait training and partial weight-bearing with a walker is inappropriate for a person with dementia symptoms. Given the memory limitations caused by dementia, the patient will probably not be able to understand and remember the weight-bearing status nor conceptualize the mechanics of using the walker. Therefore, the physician must be consulted to change the status to either full- or non-weight–bearing status. If the dementia is severe enough, gait training may be postponed until the patient is able to walk without the use of an assistive device that may be too complicated to comprehend. Exercise for those with a cognitive deficit may be modified, with the focus on following the therapist's demonstration rather than the expectation of an independent program. Likewise, self-range of motion for a cognitively impaired person with hemiparesis is better accomplished through function rather than attempting to teach a new activity. Skills and activities that occurred daily before the onset of the mental decline such as eating, walking, or dressing can usually be relearned with a higher degree of success than introduction of a new skill.

Manipulating the patient's environment is often more successful than attempting to teach the person techniques to compensate for cognitive loss. Items and surroundings that are familiar minimize the impact of memory deficit, allowing the person to perform routine daily activities by rote without having to problem solve. The emphasis on the environment includes safety as a valid factor in the therapeutic program. Failure to recognize and react to hazards become major considerations in the person's ability to remain in an unsupervised situation. Since confusion is often an issue, protection of the patient is part of the treatment program.

Because control of the environment seems to help with the person's confusion, many facilities have developed dementia units that emphasize a structured, low-key environment with consistent staffing.[12] The focus is on safety, specially trained staff, admission criteria, physical design, and activity schedules.[30] Management is facilitated by reinforcing the environment with constant reminders to orient them to time, the place, and care-giver identity. Glickstein and Bottorf have presented suggestions for modifying the home, hospital, or day-treatment area with the goal of function at the highest level of independence.[12]

Care-Giver Issues

The health professional must address not only the patient's environment but also available support systems and family situation in order to implement an individual plan of care.[12] Education and training for the care-giver are essential since management of the patient is heavily dependent on the family support and coping resources.

Cognitive function of the care-giver, especially depression, is often related to the function of the patient and therefore a relevant issue for the therapist. A multivariate analysis by Meshefedjian showed behavioral disturbance and ADL impairment in patients to be associated with depressive symptoms in care-givers.[26] The relationship was strongest for spouse care-givers, followed by children care-givers. Further investigation of spouse involvement with Alzheimer's patients reveals wife care-givers experiencing greater degree of negative psychological well-being than husband care-givers.[34]

The therapist's awareness of the potential for care-giver mental health problems is the first step. Identification of warning signs such as care-giver denial, anger, depression, exhaustion, or health problems should be a call for action by the therapist to avoid a complex situation. Some stress can be avoided by educating the care-giver on the limitations of the patient. This should minimize unrealistic goals that are translated into demands on the patients, resulting in failure, frustration, and sometimes behavior problems. The therapist can assist in identifying patient activities that can be performed successfully without failure. Although there is no conclusive data, several studies have attempted behavioral and education interventions to decreased care-giver stress.[6] Identification of community support groups for the care-giver should be part of the treatment plan, offering an opportunity for education and emotional assistance.

Case Study

JD was an 84-year-old male living at home with his 72-year-old companion. Also living in the home was the patient's 17-year-old nephew and the nephew's pregnant 16-year-old girlfriend. According to the family, JD had been fine until he fell and fractured his left hip. After a total hip replacement, JD was placed in a nursing home for rehabilitation. Physician's orders were for physical therapy; transfer and gait training; and partial weight-bearing on the left. Upon initial evaluation the therapist found the patient to be very confused. He was unable to identify family members and was not orientated to time or place, with minimal awareness of the restrictions of his injury. Consultation with the family revealed that JD was fine before the fall, with some signs of "getting old" but much more aware than what was he was presently displaying. The therapist modified the treatment program to accommodate the cognitive status, including utilization of an adductor cushion to prevent dislocation and allowing no weight-bearing until the patient could follow partial weight-bearing limitations. The therapist considered post-surgical confusion as a possible reason for the cognitive dysfunction. When the mental function only slightly improved in the next few days, the therapist scheduled an interview with the individuals living with JD in his home.

As an introduction for the family, the therapist explained that she was interested in JD's ability to perform daily activities before the accident. She told them that "just getting old" is usually not the reason for individuals to change the way they function, that most people who experience normal aging have minimal changes in their memory, personality, or intelligence. With questioning, those interviewed recalled that JD had become more forgetful about 2 years ago. He began to get lost while driving, only to be returned by a neighbor in the small farming community. The animals were neglected, as JD either fed them five times a day or not at all for several days. When he forgot repeatedly to milk the cow, the nephew moved in to help out with the chores. In the last 6 months the family reported that they had to answer the phone, because people outside the family were unable to understand JD when he talked. JD had also become very suspicious of the neighbors, accusing them of taking down his fence. After the interview, the therapist conducted an MMSE. JD scored 15 out of 30, with low scores on the orientation and memory portion. Based on the presenting cognitive function, history as revealed by the family, and MMSE score, JD was referred to a psychologist for testing to rule out dementia of the Alzheimer type.

To maximize the therapy sessions, JD's treatment program was modified to accommodate the cognitive dysfunction. The physician was consulted regarding the difficulty of maintaining partial weight-bearing status and agreed to allow the patient to bear weight to tolerance if a wheeled walker were used. This allowed the patient to transfer with a modified standing pivot method and to begin gait training. The family was involved in therapy, as JD continued to respond to instructions when a familiar person was present. They also were instructed in simple exercises that they encouraged JD to do whenever they visited. This modification in the treatment plan compensated for JD's inability to comply with an independent exercise program. As the family was very vested in JD's returning to his prior living situation, a home assessment was conducted with resultant suggestions on safety, precautions for danger when wandering, and cues to minimize the effects of the memory loss. Family concerns were also addressed by explaining Alzheimer's disease, which had been confirmed by the consultant, and the effects on the living situation and the family members. After an extended therapy period due to the dementia, JD reached treatment goals of independent ambulation and transfers. He returned home, with supervision as a safety precaution.

SUMMARY

Within the elderly population the probability of cognitive dysfunction increases with age. While affecting only a small percentage of the population younger than 80 years, cognitive dysfunction must be considered by therapists who treat older individuals. Dementia is the most common mental dysfunction, with a varied symptomatic picture, depending on the type. With healthy aging, there are some changes in memory, intelligence, and personality. However, such variations do not interfere with daily relationships or function. Knowledge of normal aging as related to mental function allows the practitioner to recognize abnormal changes and plan an appropriate therapy program.

Memory impairment is the primary feature of dementia. Some forms of dementia are reversible. Therefore, the physical therapist must investigate the etiology to make appropriate treatment recommendations. Dementia of the Alzheimer type is the most common of the irreversible categories, with multi-infarct dementia also often diagnosed in the elderly. Depression may mimic dementia, although it is now thought that the two conditions can co-exist. Pseudodementia is an often-used term when dementia-like symptoms are eliminated with successful treatment of depression. Assessment of cognitive status can be accomplished by several brief standardized examinations. Since there are no procedures that definitively confirm dementia, clinical symptoms are often used for diagnosis. While the brief tools can be for screening purposes, referral to a psychologist or physician may be appropriate for a more comprehensive assessment.

Although the focus is the same—maximizing the individual's functional independence—the treatment for patients with a cognitive disorder is different than for patients without cognitive impairments. Teaching is an essential element of physical therapy; therefore, memory loss will influence progress and the instructional approach. Awareness of the limitations imposed by cognitive dysfunction should result in modification of the treatment program, including focus on care-giver well-being. The baseline is the therapist's understanding of the cognitive aspect of aging, both normal and abnormal. Patients with cognitive disabilities can benefit from therapy and should have the opportunity to remain as functional as possible with the intervention of knowledgeable physical therapists.

REFERENCES

1. American Psychiatric Association: *Diagnostic and Statistical Manual of Mental Disorders*, ed 4 (Revised). Washington, DC, American Psychiatric Association, 1994.
2. Baltes PB, Lindenberger U: On the range of cognitive plasticity in old age as a function of experience: 15 years of intervention research. *Behav Ther* 1988; 19:283-300.
3. Bleeker ML, et al: Age-specific norms for the Mini Mental State Exam, *Neurology* 1988; 38:1565-1568.
4. Blessed G, Tominson BE, Roth M: The association between quantitative measures of dementia and of senile change in the cerebral grey matter of elderly patients. *Br J Psychiatry* 1968; 114:797-811.
5. Buntinx F, et al: Is depression in elderly people followed by dementia? A retrospective cohort study based in general practice. *Age and Ageing* 1996; 25:231-233.
6. Burgener SC, et al: Effective caregiving approaches for patients with Alzheimer's disease. *Geriatr Nurs* 1998; 19:121-126.
7. D'Epiro NW: Alzheimer's disease: Current progress, future promise. *Patient Care* 1998; 156-168.
8. Eisdorfer C, Cohen D: Dementing illness in middle and late life, in Ebaugh FG (ed): *Geriatric Medicine*. Menlo Park, Calif, Addison-Wesley, 1981.
9. Evans DA, et al: Prevalence of Alzheimer's disease in a community population of older persons: Higher than previously reported. *JAMA* 1989; 262:2551-2556.
10. Folstein MF, Folstein SE, McHugh PR: "Mini Mental State" —a practical method for grading the cognitive state of patients for the clinician. *J Psychiatr Res* 1975; 12:189-198.
11. Forsell Y, Winblad B: Major depression in a population of demented and nondemented older people: Prevalence and correlates. *J Am Geriatr Soc* 1998; 46:27-30.
12. Glickstein JK, Bottorf S: Alzheimer's disease: Providing a meaningful existence in the absence of definitive management, in Dwyer BJ (ed): *Focus on Geriatric Care and Rehabilitation.* Frederick, Md, Aspen Publishers, 1987.
13. Grigsby J, et al: Executive cognitive abilities and functional status among community-dwelling older persons in the San Luis Valley health and aging study. *J Am Geriatr Soc* 1998; 46:590-596.
14. Haggerty JR, et al: Differential diagnosis of pseudodementia in the elderly. *Geriatrics* 1988; 43:61-74.
15. Hänninen T, et al: Prevalence of ageing-associated cognitive decline in an elderly population. *Age and Ageing* 1996; 25:201-205.
16. Hartke RJ: The aging process: Cognition, personality and coping, in Hartke RJ (ed): *Psychological Aspects of Geriatric Rehabilitation.* Frederick, Md, Aspen Publishers, 1991.
17. Hertzog C, Schaie KW: Stability and change in adult intelligence: Simultaneous analysis of longitudinal means and covariance structures. *Psychol Aging* 1988; 3:122-130.
18. Keefe FJ, Williams DA: A comparison of coping strategies in chronic pain patients in different age groups. *J Gerontol* 1990; 45:161-165.
19. Kokmen E, et al: Is the incidence of dementing illness changing? *Neurology* 1993; 43:1887-1892.
20. Koss E, et al: Memory evaluation in Alzheimer's disease: Caregivers' appraisals and objective testing. *Arch Neurol* 1993; 50:92-97.
21. Lanska DJ: Dementia mortality in the United States: Results of the 1986 national mortality followback survey. *Neurology* 1998; 50:362-367.
22. Lyketsos CG: Diagnosis and management of delirium in the elderly. *JCOM* 1998; 5(4):51-62.
23. Mace NL, Hardy SR, Rabins PV: Alzheimer's disease and the confused patient, in Jackson O (ed): *Physical Therapy of the Geriatric Patient.* New York, Churchill Livingstone, 1989.
24. Mahurin RK, et al: Structured assessment of independent living skills: Preliminary report of a performance measure of functional abilities in dementia. *J Gerontol: Psychological Sciences* 1991; 46(2):58-66.
25. McKhann GD, et al: Clinical diagnosis of Alzheimer's disease: Report of the NINCDS-ADRDA work group under the auspices of the Department of Health and Human Services Task Force on Alzheimer's disease. *Neurology* 1984; 34:939-944.
26. Meshefedjian G, et al: Factors associated with symptoms of depression among informal caregivers of demented elders in the community. *The Gerontologist* 1998; 38(2):247-253.
27. Middaugh SJ, et al: Chronic pain: Its treatment in geriatric and younger patients. *Arch Phys Med Rehabil* 1988; 69:1021-1026.
28. Odenheimer GL: Acquired cognitive disorders of the elderly. *Med Clin North Am* 1989; 73:1383-1411.
29. Pearson JL, et al: Functional status and cognitive impairment in Alzheimer's patients with and without depression. *J Am Geriatr Soc* 1989; 37:1117-1121.
30. Peppard NR: Developing a special needs dementia unit, in Glickstein JK (ed): *Focus on Geriatric Care and Rehabilitation.* Frederick, Md, Aspen Publishers, 1990.
31. Pfeiffer E: A short portable mental status questionnaire for the assessment of organic brain deficit in elderly patients. *J Am Geriatr Soc* 1975; 23:433-441.
32. Pousada L, Leipzig RM: Rapid bedside assessment of postoperative confusion in older patients. *Geriatrics* 1990; 45:59-66.
33. Rapport L, et al: Executive functioning and predictors of falls in rehabilitation setting. *Arch Phys Med Rehabil* 1998; 79:629-633.
34. Rose-Rego SK, Strauss ME, Smyth KA: Differences in the perceived well-being of wives and husbands caring for persons with Alzheimer's disease. *The Gerontologist* 1998; 38(2):224-230.
35. Stern Y, et al: Influence of education and occupation on the incidence

of Alzheimer's disease. *JAMA* 1994; 271:1004-1010.

36. Teri L, Hughes JP, Larson EB: Cognitive deterioration in Alzheimer's disease: Behavioral and health factors. *J Gerontol* 1990; 45:58-63.

37. Teri L, et al: Behavioral disturbance, cognitive dysfunction, and functional skill prevalence and relationship in Alzheimer's disease. *J Am Geriatr Soc* 1989; 37:109-116.

38. Teschendorf B: Cognitive impairment in the elderly: Delirium, depression or dementia?, in Dwyer BJ (ed): *Focus on Geriatric Care and Rehabilitation*. Frederick, Md, Aspen Publishers, 1987.

39. Tobias CR, Lippman S, Pary R: Dementia in the elderly. *Postgrad Med* 1989; 86:101-106.

40. Unverzagt FW, et al: Cognitive decline and education in mild dementia. *Neurology* 1998; 50:181-185.

41. Zarit S: *Aging and Mental Disorders: Psychological Approaches to Assessment and Treatment*. New York, Free Press, 1980.

42. Zillmer EA, et al: Comparison of two cognitive bedside screening instruments in nursing home residents: A factor analytic study. *J Gerontol* 1990; 45:69-74.

CHAPTER 10

DEPRESSION AND FUNCTION IN THE ELDERLY

ANN K. WILLIAMS, PT, PhD

INTRODUCTION

Depression is the most common psychological problem in the elderly.[15,52,63] While this is also true in other adult age-groups, depression remains a significant problem encountered by professionals working with the elderly. Although depression is commonly neglected in the elderly, it is actually quite treatable.[15,24] There are many causes of depression; however, in the elderly one factor that is commonly associated with depression is loss of health. The stress of physical illness that may be associated with physical disability, pain, and life-style changes can result in the psychological response of depression. Conversely, depression can dramatically affect the response of the elderly patient to rehabilitation. The hopelessness, apathy, and withdrawal of the depressed person make rehabilitation a challenge. While assessment and treatment of depression are the responsibility of other health professionals, they constitute a problem that physical therapists must deal with frequently. This chapter reviews the characteristics of depression, factors associated

with it, common treatment approaches, and modifications of the physical therapist's treatment plan that are appropriate for the depressed elderly patient.

CHARACTERISTICS AND ASSESSMENT OF THE DEPRESSED OLDER PERSON

Characteristics of the Depressed Person

Most people think of the predominant characteristic of depression as depressed mood, i.e., feelings of sadness, hopelessness, and loss of interest and pleasure in previously pleasurable activities. Although these emotions are a key feature of depression, experts agree that for depression to be a psychopathology or a "clinical depression," other characteristics must also be present. These include cognitive problems such as difficulty concentrating, memory complaints, slowed thinking, indecisiveness, and perceived lack of competence and control. Feelings of low self-esteem, worthlessness, decreased motivation, apathy, and excessive guilt also may be present. The depressed person has difficulties with interpersonal interactions, including withdrawal from family and friends and neglect of previously pleasurable activities. Finally, depression includes somatic symptoms such as problems with appetite, sleep, and psychomotor function. The disturbances of appetite usually involve loss of weight but may involve excessive eating. Insomnia and early morning wakening are the most common sleep disturbances, but hypersomnia may also be demonstrated. Psychomotor functioning is usually retarded but may be agitated.

To help standardize the diagnosis of depression and the terminology associated with it, the *Diagnostic and Statistical Manual of Mental Disorders,* ed. 4 (*DSM-IV*) of the American Psychiatric Association describes specific criteria for various diagnoses of mood disorders that are generally accepted.[2] The two diagnoses that are important to this discussion of depression in the elderly are Major Depressive Episode and Adjustment Disorder With Depressed Mood.

According to the *DSM-IV* the criteria for major depressive episode are either depressed mood or loss of pleasure in all activities and associated symptoms for a period of at least 2 weeks, as outlined in Box 10-1. These symptoms must be a change from previous functioning and relatively persistent. The associated symptoms include significant weight loss when not dieting or weight gain, insomnia or hypersomnia, psychomotor retardation or agitation, fatigue or loss of energy, feelings of worthlessness or excessive or inappropriate guilt, diminished ability to think or concentrate, and recurrent thoughts of death, suicide ideation, or a suicide attempt. The person must exhibit at least five of all these symptoms to be diagnosed as having a major depression. The symptoms must cause significant distress or impairment in social, occupational, or other important areas of functioning.

Adjustment disorder with depressed mood is a subcategory of adjustment disorders in the *DSM-IV*.[2] Adjustment disorders are maladaptive reactions to an identifiable psychosocial stressor that occur within 3 months of the onset of the stressor. The clinical significance of the reaction is evidenced by impairment of social or occupational functioning or by marked distress that is in excess of a normal and expected reaction. In an adjustment disorder with depressed mood the predominant symptoms are a depressed mood, tearfulness, and feelings of hopelessness. For example, a divorce may cause a person to have a depressed mood. This response would be classified as an adjustment disorder with

depressed mood if the person's social relationships or job was affected. The depression response must be considered to be excessive. If the disturbance lasts fewer than 6 months it is classified as *acute*; the term *chronic* is used if the disturbance lasts for 6 months or longer.

Physical therapists may encounter two other classifications within the *DSM-IV*: Mood Disorder Due To A Medical Disorder With Depressive Features and Dysthymic Disorder. In a mood disorder due to a medical disorder there must be a prominent and persistent disturbance in mood that causes significant distress or impairment in social, occupational, or other functioning and evidence that the disturbance is the *direct physiological* consequence of a general medical condition. An example would be a patient classified as having Mood Disorder due to Hypothyroidism, with Depressive Features. Dysthymic disorder requires a depressed mood for most of the day, for more days than not, for at least 2 years. At least two of the associated symptoms of a major depressive episode must also be present, e.g., poor appetite, insomnia, low energy, low self-esteem, poor concentration, or hopelessness.

When reading the numerous books and articles available on depression, the reader may become confused by the varied terminology that is sometimes different from that in the *DSM-IV* just outlined. For example, some authors will use the term *endogenous depression,* which is similar to a major depressive episode. Similarly, the term *reactive,* or *secondary,* depression is similar to an adjustment disorder with depressed mood. Finally, the term *dysphoria* is sometimes used to describe a milder depression characterized only by depressed mood or unhappiness. The term *depression* may be used to represent any point on this continuum from unhappiness to a clinical depression.[65]

Assessment of Depression

The various tools available for the assessment of depression are even more varied than the terms used to describe it. In the clinical setting, the diagnosis of various depressive disorders usually will be made by a health professional who is an expert in this area, e.g., a clinical psychologist or a psychiatrist. The diagnosis is based on the history, observation, and a careful interview with the patient and close family and friends.

In research studies such as those referenced in this chapter in which large numbers of persons in the community are involved, various self-report scales of depression are often used. The respondents will check off on a printed form whether they have experienced any of the symptoms of depression. Although these self-report measures depend on the honesty of the respondent to truly report symptoms, they are commonly used in the interests of conserving time and money. These self-report scales are generally accepted as good screening devices to indicate individuals who are at risk for depression and may need further professional evaluation. It is beyond the scope of this chapter to give a detailed description of all the self-report scales used for depression.

BOX 10-1
CATEGORIZATIONS OF DEPRESSION

Major Depressive Episode

1. Depressed mood*
2. Markedly diminished interest or pleasure in all, or almost all, activities
3. Weight loss or weight gain when not dieting or decrease or increase in appetite
4. Insomnia or hypersomnia
5. Psychomotor agitation or retardation
6. Fatigue or loss of energy
7. Feelings of worthlessness or excessive or inappropriate guilt
8. Diminished ability to think or concentrate or indecisiveness
9. Recurrent thoughts of death, recurrent suicidal ideation, a suicide attempt, or a specific plan for committing suicide

Adjustment Disorder with Depressed Mood

1. Emotional or behavioral symptoms in response to an identifiable stressor(s) occurring within 3 months of the onset of the stressor(s).
2. Clinically significant symptoms or behaviors as evidenced by:
   a. Marked distress that is in excess of what would be expected from exposure to the stressor
   b. Significant impairment in social or occupational functioning

*Criteria: At least five of the following symptoms present during a 2-week period and represent a change from previous functioning. One of the symptoms must be either (1) depressed mood or (2) loss of interest or pleasure. (Adapted from American Psychiatric Association: *Diagnostic and Statistical Manual of Mental Disorders*, ed. 4. Washington, DC, American Psychiatric Association, 1994.)

Some of the most commonly used scales are listed in the next paragraph with references to assist the reader who needs more information.

Four of the most commonly used depression scales are the Beck Depression Inventory, the Center for Epidemiological Studies Depression Scale (CES-D), the Geriatric Depression Scale (GDS), and the Zung Self-Rating Depression Scale (SDS).[35,83,88] Table 10-1 gives additional information about these depression scales, describing the number of items, total score, number of somatic items, and sample items. Generally, the scales make statements about feelings or situations, and the respondent indicates how frequently each item occurs.

An important issue in self-rating scales of depression is the degree of emphasis that they give to the somatic symptoms of depression.[5,24,83] Many of these symptoms, such as appetite or sleep disturbances, may be a result of aging or the many physical illnesses that are more common in the elderly. Thus a person may score high on the depression scale, not because of depression, but because of unrelated somatic symptoms. Scales that de-emphasize somatic signs of depression, such as the GDS and the CES-D, are generally considered more valid for the elderly.

Models of Depression

Numerous authors have speculated about the causes of depression, and various models have emerged. Five of the most frequently cited models are the cognitive model, the learned-helplessness model, the interpersonal model, the neurobiological model, and the social resources model. Understanding these models is important because they help to explain various treatment approaches to depression.

The *cognitive model* of depression was proposed by Aaron Beck and is based on his empirical observation of depressed patients.[30] This model emphasizes the cognitive structure underlying depression, including the negative views of the self, the environment, and the future. The depressed person uses a negative cognitive schema that influences the coding and organization of incoming stimuli. Errors of information processing occur, resulting in overestimation of negative input and underestimation of positive input. For example, a work supervisor's suggestions for improvement would be interpreted by the depressed person as an indication of unworthiness, inability to do the job, and even dislike. Loss, grief, or dysphoric feelings then trigger depression in the person with negative schemata. The perceptual bias then perpetuates the depression. In this model, the negative schemata are primary and the depressed affect is secondary.

In the *learned-helplessness model* of Seligman, uncontrollable negative events result in passive behaviors.[30] Although the research in this model was originally in animals, it has been applied to human depression. Emphasis is placed on the decreased motivation in depression and the perceptions of uncontrollability of events by the depressed person. This model may be particularly applicable to the medical patient. A series of negative health events may be perceived by the patient as uncontrollable. The sick role also promotes lack of control and passivity. The result may be excessively passive behavior, lack of motivation, and depression for the patient.

The *interpersonal model* for depression emphasizes overdependent personality traits that predispose the individual with a loss or negative life event to depression.[40] This vulnerability is often attributed to adverse childhood experiences or intrafamilial relations. This model focuses on personality rather than external causes for depression. For example, a parent's overprotectiveness might result in a child who is excessively dependent. This personality trait may then result in a depressive response to a negative life event later in life.

The *neurobiological model* of depression suggests that the somatic symptoms of depression, such as the psychomotor retardation and temporal variation, indicate a biological base for the illness.[50] Clinical observations that some drugs produced depressive symptoms, whereas other drugs re-

Table 10-1
Common Self-Report Depression Scales

Scale	No. of Items	Total Score	No. of Somatic Items	How Scored	Sample Item
Zung Self-Rating Depression Scale (SDS)	20	80	8	Scored for frequency: e.g., some of the time, most of the time, etc.	"I feel downhearted and blue."
Beck Depression Inventory	21	63	6	Subject chooses one of four choices	"I do not feel sad." "I feel sad." "I am sad all the time and can't snap out of it." "I am so sad or unhappy that I can't stand it."
Center for Epidemiological Studies Depression Scale (CES-D)	20	60	3	Scored for frequency	"I felt that I could not shake off the blues even with help from my friends and family."
Geriatric Depression Scale (GDS)	30	30	1	Scored yes/no	"Do you feel that your life is empty?"

lieved them, pointed to decreased neurotransmission or a disturbance of catecholamine transmission as the cause of depression. Deficient brain serotonergic transmission has been suggested because of the sleep disturbances that occur with depression.

In contrast to the four models just mentioned that emphasize the individual's psychological and biological response to stress, the *social resources model* emphasizes the effects of the environment on the individual.[44] Depression may result from the inability of a person to deal with certain levels of environmental stress. External factors such as income, social support, or societal resources affect the person's ability to adapt to various stressors.

Rates of Depression

Depression appears to be the most common psychopathology in all age groups.[15,52] Two age-groups appear particularly vulnerable to depression: adolescents and very elderly males.[25] When the elderly are considered as one group including all persons older than 65, their rate of depression is no different than the rest of the adult population.[25,59,63] Thus the commonly held stereotype of the elderly as lonely and depressed is not supported by research data. Selected subgroups of the elderly, such as very elderly males, show higher rates of depression in some studies, although others have not confirmed this finding. The elderly as a whole, however, have about the same rates of depression as other adult groups.

Epidemiological studies indicate a prevalence of depression in the elderly that ranges from 4% to 23%.[3,7,14,17,25,59] This wide variation of results can be due to several factors. Some studies based their rates only on patients who had sought psychiatric treatment, a research method that could underestimate rates. A wide variety of scales and classification criteria have been used across studies, making comparison difficult. Inclusion of somatic symptoms as part of the criteria for the definition of depression is problematic in the elderly because these symptoms may occur in old age or disease.[5] As described earlier, the term depression is used to describe conditions ranging anywhere from dysphoric mood to major depression. Carefully designed studies indicate a rate of depression in the elderly of around 12%.[59,76] Studies that use strict criteria for a major depression indicate lower rates, around 5%.[3] While these rates apply to all persons older than 65, certain special populations of the elderly would be expected to have higher rates of depression. These would include the institutionalized elderly[46] and, as will be discussed in detail later in this chapter, the physically ill elderly.[3] Studies of the institutionalized elderly generally indicate higher rates of severe depression—around 12%.[46] This population is especially difficult to study because of their high rates of cognitive impairment and physical illness. Not surprisingly, newly admitted residents to a nursing home are more likely to be depressed. Medical conditions that may cause depression or depression-like symptoms such as hypothyroidism, stroke, or Parkinson's disease are more common in the elderly and therefore may contribute to an increased rate of depression in older persons.[24,69]

Depression in the Elderly

An issue that is consistently debated is whether depression in the elderly is different from depression in other age-groups. A change in the characteristics of depression in the elderly is a common theme in the clinical literature.[58] Butler and Lewis suggested that feelings of guilt, self-derogation, and suicidal impulses are less common in the elderly.[9] More common in the elderly are symptoms of apathy, low motivation, low energy, sleep disturbances, and loss of appetite. Derogatis and Wise also noted increased apathy in the depressed elderly.[18] They point to an increased cognitive impairment in the depressed elderly as well as a reluctance to discuss feelings of dysphoria. Some authors believe that the elderly do not present as strongly with the somatic aspects of depression, whereas others indicate that somatization is the predominant symptom of depression in the elderly.

Unlike the clinical literature, epidemiological studies of depression generally support a picture of depression in the elderly as basically similar to depression in other age-groups.[8,22,58] Somatic symptoms are especially problematic because they may be part of a co-existing physical illness.[5,8] As will be discussed later in the chapter, this similarity of depression across the age span suggests that effective treatment strategies in younger age-groups may also be effective in the elderly.

Pseudodementia

Because the symptoms of depression may be confused with early dementia, depressed elderly persons are at risk to be diagnosed as having organic brain syndrome. This mistake is common enough to be given the name *pseudodementia*, or the *dementia syndrome of depression*, in clinical geriatric psychiatry.[70] The apathy, decreased ability to concentrate, and memory complaints of the depressed elderly person may be misinterpreted as symptoms of dementia.[17,36] Experts in geriatric psychiatry indicate that the differential diagnosis between depression and early dementia can be difficult. As guidelines for distinguishing between the two, they point out that the depressed person usually has a shorter history of illness, poorer social skills, and poorer attention to hygiene than the person with early dementia.[3,70] While the depressed older person usually has complaints of memory problems, when tested this individual shows few deficits.[3,36] Finally, symptoms of depression are usually worst in the morning and get better by the afternoon. In contrast, persons with dementia have more problems in the late afternoon.

As geriatric psychiatrists have noted, the distinction between depression and dementia is complicated by the fact that each can co-exist in the same person. If there is a clear psychosocial stressor that could lead to depression, geriatric psychiatrists recommend that treatment should be first initiated for depression. Dementia should be a diagnosis of exclusion, i.e., only given after other possible diagnoses have been eliminated. There are instruments available to measure depression in persons with high levels of cognitive deficit. These instruments are the Cornell Scale, the Demential Mood Assessment Scale, and the Depressive Signs Scale.[24] Input from family members also becomes essential when the patient has major cognitive deficits.

Factors Associated with Depression

One factor consistently associated with depression in older persons is physical illness.[4,13,23-25,37,49,65,68,78,84] This is clearly of import to health care professionals. While there are a few studies that indicate no association between physical illness and depression,[12,77] numerous studies demonstrate an increased risk of depression in physically ill persons. Various studies of patients with heart disease, rheumatoid arthritis, diabetes, cancer, and multiple sclerosis show higher rates of depression than the average in the population.[51,53,54,56,68,72,82] In addition to studies of persons with specific diseases, studies that include persons with many different diagnoses also demonstrate an increased risk for depression.

Some psychologists theorize that all persons with a physical illness will experience a "stage" of depression.[41] This traditional stage theory proposes that depression is a necessary and adaptive part of rehabilitation.[23] However, while physically ill persons have higher rates of depression, clearly not all physically ill persons develop a *clinical* depression.[23] At some point, dysphoric feelings may become excessive and maladaptive, which result in the cognitive, psychological, and somatic symptoms of a major depression. The severity and number of symptoms as well as a previous history of depression are suggestive of a major depressive episode.[10,75] Patients with an adjustment disorder with depressed mood will tend to have a decreased severity of psychological symptoms, an increased severity of stressors, and recent functioning at a higher level.[75] Studies indicate the rate of severe depression in the physically ill elderly somewhere between 20% and 35%.[23,25,37,50,68,76]

Are older persons more or less likely to respond to the stress of physical illness with depression? The few studies that have investigated age as a factor in the relationship of physical illness to depression are about equally split on both sides of the issue. Some indicate that older physically ill persons are more likely to be depressed; others indicate no relationship to age or that older persons are less likely to be depressed.[11,24,65,82] Given the high rates of physical illness in the elderly, the low overall rate of depression in this age-group suggests that older persons adapt at least as well as younger persons to the stress of physical illness.[83] Some experts have suggested that certain negative events may be more anticipated at certain times in life. Thus, older persons may expect health problems as a normal part of aging and therefore adjust better to them.[73] It remains critical to identify those whose response is maladaptive and to initiate treatment. The physical therapist may be instrumental in identifying those individuals who could benefit from referral to specialists in psychology.

Although depression in adults may be more common in women,[21,66] studies of depression in the elderly have shown variable effects of gender.[3,8,17,49] Gurland and colleagues found the highest rate of depression in very elderly males.[28] Other studies of elderly persons with a medically related de-

pression have not found gender to be a contributing factor.[7] Physical therapists might expect very elderly male patients to be at high risk for depression; however, generally, older male and female patients are equally likely to be depressed.

Higher rates of depression are linked to lower income and socioeconomic status.[17,33,59] This remains the case for depressed physically ill older persons.[83] Not surprisingly, the stress of physical illness is confounded by the stress of limited resources, and physically ill older persons with low incomes are more likely to become depressed.

One would expect that a high degree of social support from family and friends would buffer the negative effects of an illness and result in a lower risk for depression. While research has generally supported this hypothesis,[31,87] some studies have shown higher levels of anxiety and dependency in patients with more social support.[19] Perceived adequacy of social support and presence of a confident may be especially important in the ability of social support to moderate the negative effects of life's stressors.[31] Social support may only be important for persons who highly value social interaction.[86] Social support, depression, and physical illness may form a complex web of interrelationships in which persons who are ill and in pain become depressed and have difficulty mobilizing the social support that is available to them.[31,39,86] Also, older persons with chronic physical illness may require support over long periods of time. This can stress any support system, so that expected support is not available, and this may contribute to or exacerbate a depression.

The increased risk of depression in physically ill older persons makes it critical to identify factors of an illness that increase the risk for depression. Several studies have indicated higher levels of functional incapacity and disability to be associated with higher levels of depression, and one would expect higher levels of physical dependency to result in more depression.[23,37,54-56] However, very elderly persons have high rates of physical dependency without correspondingly high rates of depression.[83] The very old may have different expectations regarding disability and are therefore more likely to accept it. Research therefore indicates that the relationship of level of disability to depression is equivocable.[45]

Chronic pain patients of all ages show high rates of depression, and level of pain would be expected to be related to depression.[18,32,69,71,84] Few studies have combined physical disability and pain when assessing depression in the elderly. Williams and Schulz found that when control for other variables is added to the analysis, pain becomes a more important factor than physical disability in level of depression.[84] This strong association between pain and depression has also been shown in institutionalized elderly persons.[63,64]

The strong association of physical illness to depression would be expected to be due to many factors. In a study of elderly medical clinic outpatients, Williamson and Schulz found that health status and psychosocial factors were about equally important in explaining depression.[86] Important health variables included physician and self-rated severity of symptoms, pain medications, and activity restrictions. Key psychosocial factors included worry about transportation, need for future services, satisfaction with social support, and worry about becoming a burden and loneliness.

In summary, risk for depression is increased in physically ill persons with higher levels of pain, increased severity of symptoms, lower income and available resources, lower levels of social support (if social interaction is highly valued), and high levels of worry about future needs and life meaning.

Effects of Depression on Function in the Elderly

Because of the nature of depression, persons with depression have a reduced functional capacity.[31,52,57,81] The apathy, loss of pleasure in activities, and psychomotor retardation reduce the individual's capacity to participate in everyday activities and even perform activities of daily living. The depressed person perceives that even simple tasks require excessive amounts of energy, and these tasks become extremely difficult.[52] This decreased function is usually most evident in the morning.

For the physically ill elderly person with depression, this loss of functional capacity becomes even more problematic. The deconditioning effects of age and illness combine with depression to result in even more perceived effort required for minor everyday tasks. Long-term goals may appear unattainable. In a study of patients with hip fractures, Mossey and colleagues found increased depression to be associated with reduced functional recovery and reduced response to rehabilitation.[57] In a study of medical inpatients, Koenig and others found that after matching for age, medical condition, and functional status, depressed persons had twice the length of stay as non-depressed persons.[38] In a prospective studies, Hays and colleagues found that depression at baseline predicted increased loss of function 1 year later,[31] and Clark and others found that depression predicted increase in ADL disability over a 2-year period.[16] Depression and functional status and recovery are probably interactive, so that the depressed patient functions at a lower level, and this decreased function also reinforces the depression.

Motivation of the depressed older patient and the appropriate modifications of the rehabilitation plan will be a constant challenge to the therapist. The second part of this chapter on management of depression discusses specific suggestions for this challenge. A case history provides additional examples.

Management of Depression in the Older Person

The management of depression in the older person has many aspects. Physicians may have difficulty recognizing and treating depression in physically ill elderly persons. Two of the most common treatment approaches are pharmacotherapy and psychotherapy, each of which is discussed in this section. While psychotherapy has demonstrated positive results with older persons, it is not as frequently used with the elderly as drug treatment.[30] Reasons for this bias may include resistance to and misunderstanding of psychotherapy on the part of the elderly, bias against the elderly on the part of psychotherapists, lower cost of drug treatment, and a bias toward drug treatment in the medical community. Some experts have suggested that psychotherapy may be more effective for adjustment disorder with depressed mood, whereas drug treatment may be more effective for a major depressive episode. Nevertheless, drug treatment remains the most common approach in managing elders with depression. The use of exercise in the treatment of depression has had limited research; however, as it is of particular interest to physical therapists, it will be discussed. Finally, practical suggestions for the physical therapist working with the depressed older patient are described.

Pharmacotherapy

Pharmacological treatment is the primary therapy for major depressive episodes in the elderly.[1,80] Although there are many pharmacological treatments for depression, medications used to treat major depression can be divided into five major categories: selective serotonin reuptake inhibitors (SSRIs), tricyclic or tetracyclic antidepressants (TCAs), heterocyclic antidepressants, serotonin/norepinephrine reuptake inhibitors, and monoamine oxidase inhibitors (MAOIs).[61] Table 10-2 indicates the common drug names in these categories that the therapist might find in the medical record.

The SSRIs are the mainstay of drug treatment of depression in the elderly. They have fewer adverse side effects in the elderly, especially the lack of the anticholinergic and hypotensive effects that are characteristic of the TCAs.[61] The anticholinergic side effects of the TCAs include dizziness, tachycardia, constipation, blurred vision, urinary retention, postural hypotension, and mild tremor.[26,34,80] Of particular concern to physical therapists are the side effects of dizziness and postural hypotension. Patients taking tricyclic antidepressants may have poorer balance, particularly after moving

TABLE 10-2
Antidepressant Drug Names

Nonproprietary Name	Trade Name
Selective Serotonin Reuptake Inhibitors (SSRIs)	
Sertraline	Zoloft
Fluoxetine	Prozac
Paroxetine	Paxil
Heterocyclic Antidepressants	
Bupropion	Wellbutrin
Trazodone	Desyrel
Tricyclic or Tetracyclic Antidepressants (TCAs)	
Amitriptyline	Amitril, Elavil
Nortriptyline	Aventyl, Pamelor
Serotonin/Norepinephrine Reuptake Inhibitors	
Venlafaxine	Effexor
Monamine Oxidase Inhibitors	
Phenelzine	Nardil
Tranylcypromine	Parnate

from supine to sitting or sitting to standing. These effects are more pronounced in the period immediately after the medication is taken. While there are numerous drugs in the category of tricyclics, the differences between them are primarily in the degree of side effects produced.[1,85] These side effects are more common in the elderly and could be especially troublesome in this age-group. The serotonin/norepinephrine inhibitors have potential side-effects that are intermediate between SSRIs and TCAs.[61] The monoamine oxidase inhibitors also have major side effects similar to the tricyclics and are less commonly used in the elderly.[26,34]

The choice of an antidepressant for a particular person is dependent on many factors, including prior response, concurrent medical illnesses, and other medications used by the patient.[61] Generally the use of SSRIs and heterocyclic antidepressants is preferred in the elderly.[61]

Psychotherapy

Older patients are seldom included in studies of the effectiveness of psychotherapy.[47] Older patients may be less likely to seek psychotherapy, but also, health professionals may be biased against older persons in that they believe that elders will not benefit from psychotherapy. The few studies including older patients indicate that psychotherapy is an effective treatment for depression in the elderly.[20,29,47,79] Psychotherapy treatments for the elderly include behavioral, cognitive, and brief psychodynamic therapies. Behavioral treatments focus on modifying the behavioral components of depression, whereas cognitive approaches attempt to change the negative cognitive schemata that accompany depression. Psychodynamic therapies focus on the personality characteristics common in depression. Very few studies have compared medication and psychotherapy in the treatment of depression in the elderly, but some have indicated that psychotherapy may be at least as effective as medications in the elderly.[6,20]

Exercise

Exercise has been occasionally used as an effective treatment for depression.[27,43,60,62,67] However, the patients have usually been young or middle-aged, and the exercise was vigorous, aerobic exercise.[74] O'Connor and colleagues have completed a detailed review of the research on physical activity and depression in the elderly.[60] These authors point out the many problems with this research, including difficulties defining activity and exercise, difficulty measuring depression and activity, and inability to achieve experimental control. However, they indicated that despite these problems the research shows a clear relationship between physical inactivity and higher levels of depression in elderly persons. As expected, physical activity has little effect on mood level in nondepressed elderly persons.[60] There is little research on the effect of physical activity and exercise in physically ill or disabled elderly persons. Exercise programs that are vigorously aerobic may not be suitable for the physically ill elderly.[74] When a therapist is considering an exercise program for a depressed elderly person who is not seriously ill, the thera-

pist must consider the high rates of cardiovascular disease in this age-group. Whereas some studies indicate that heavy aerobic exercise reduces depression, others indicate that any activity, including mild recreational activity, will be associated with increases in feelings of well-being.[42,85] This improvement may be caused by time-out from periods of psychological stress, increased social interaction, or increased feelings of mastery. Some authors also hypothesize a physiological effect of increased secretion of amines that would have an antidepressant effect.[66] The exercise-induced adrenal response to stress may also affect sleep regulation and improve depressive symptoms.[60] While exercise is not a commonly accepted treatment for depression, beneficial effects of activity and exercise on well-being should be remembered by physical, occupational, and recreational therapists.

Working with the Depressed Older Patient

Suggestions for working with the depressed older patient are really little different than those for any adult who is depressed. Aerobic exercise may be a treatment modality that is less frequently used in the elderly. Also, elderly persons may be more likely to have experienced losses in their support networks, especially loss of a spouse. With a more limited support network, the stress of caring for a depressed ill person may be concentrated on a few individuals. Key support persons may also require extra assistance in dealing with the depressed patient.[31] Also depressed persons may need assistance and training to improve their interactive skills in order to maximize the effectiveness of their support networks.[23] Cognitive therapy aims at helping depressed persons redefine their self-esteem and self-perceptions.[23]

Depression can affect many aspects of physical therapy treatment. The course of therapy would be expected to be longer, because the apathy and extra energy required necessitates more time to accomplish goals. More time may need to be spent on activities of daily living, since these tasks will seem more difficult for the patient.

Physical therapists may need to modify their approach when the patient is depressed. Some professionals may believe that being overly cheerful will "jolly" the patient out of feelings of sadness and low self-esteem. Generally this is not the case, and the effect may be the opposite. The excessive cheerfulness of the therapist may only emphasize the separateness and depression of the patient and increase negative feelings. Anyone who remembers a time when he/she was quite depressed will recall that cheerfulness of others did not really decrease the depression but often only accentuated one's own sad feelings. Experts agree that a better approach to the depressed person is to be matter-of-fact and emphasize the patient's feelings of mastery rather than feelings of pleasure. Negative self-perception should be discouraged, and emphasis should be placed on achievement and appropriate perceptions of self-worth.[3] It is important to acknowledge the great degree of effort required by the depressed person to accomplish even everyday tasks. Goals should be discussed in small, easily achievable steps. The depressed person will have difficulty visualizing goals far into the future. Achievement of short-term goals will enhance the person's sense of mastery and improve motivation.

Dealing with the depressed patient may be psychologically difficult for the therapist. Research has shown that most people respond negatively and interact less with persons who exhibit depressed behaviors.[23,48] Health care professionals are not immune from these natural responses. Depressed patients are not "fun" and may appear unmotivated. It is important to remember that these people are not lazy. For them, large amounts of energy are required to accomplish even simple tasks. Working with these patients also has its rewards. Depressed persons almost always get better and will achieve therapeutic goals. Most of us have experienced depression to some extent. Remembering our own sad times can help to develop empathy for the depressed patient.

Case Study

Mr. Clark is 84 years old. Before his present hospitalization, he lived alone in his suburban home; his wife of 45 years had died 6 months previously. He has two sons, one of whom lives in the same city. He was hospitalized because he fell in his home and fractured the subcapital area of his right femur. A hemiarthroplasty was performed, and Mr. Clark was referred to physical therapy. Laboratory tests also indicated a high blood glucose level, and he is being evaluated for possible diabetes. Mr. Clark also has a history of mild congestive heart failure. The physical therapist working with Mr. Clark notes that he appears quite sad, has cried several times during treatment, and has expressed hopelessness about his future. He also has difficulty remembering the precautions regarding his hip that have been repeatedly explained to him. He is apathetic, is hard to motivate, has a poor appetite, and has difficulty sleeping. The nursing and medical staff have noted similar problems. As his son indicated that these problems had been steadily getting worse since the death of Mrs. Clark, a psychiatric consult was requested. Although Mr. Clark's memory problems could have been due to early dementia, the consult indicated that the first treatment should be for depression with later re-evaluation. Antidepressant medication and short-term therapy for depression were initiated. Mr. Clark was also prescribed insulin therapy and transferred to the rehabilitation unit.

Mr. Clark's progress in physical therapy was slower than expected, although he made steady improvement. His therapist established small short-term goals that could be accomplished in 2 to 3 days. Emphasis was placed on the mastery of these short-term goals rather than long-term goals. For example, Mr. Clark was given the goal of increasing his walking distance from 20 to 40 feet, rather than being given the long-term goal of independent ambulation. He was asked to be able to repeat one more precaution every other day, rather than learn all the precautions in 1 day. The extra effort required by Mr. Clark was acknowledged, but his negative ex-

pressions of low self-esteem and guilt were countered with more positive statements about his progress and his past and present accomplishments. The psychologist also worked with Mr. Clark to improve his personal interaction skills in order to mobilize his support network for his return home. These new skills were reinforced in physical therapy. Mr. Clark's depression gradually lifted, and he was discharged to his home. A home health agency continued his physical therapy and monitored the progress of his diabetes treatment. Antidepressant treatment was discontinued after 2 months.

SUMMARY

While depression is no more common in the elderly than in other adult age-groups, it remains the most common psychopathology of old age. The two categories of depression of greatest interest to physical therapists are major depressive episode and adjustment disorder with depressed mood. The characteristics of depression include problems with mood, cognition, self-esteem, interpersonal interactions, and somatic functions. Depression in the elderly is similar to depression in other adults, although some have suggested that the older depressed adult will show more apathy and lack of motivation. Difficulty in differentiating depression from early dementia is common enough to warrant a name: pseudodementia.

Factors that are commonly associated with depression in the elderly are the presence of physical illness, low income, and decreased social support. Among the physically ill elderly, high levels of pain, physical disability, and symptom severity may be related to depression. Depression reduces function in the physically ill elderly because of apathy, perceptions of low energy, and psychomotor retardation.

Pharmacotherapy is the primary treatment for a major depressive episode; however, psychotherapy has also been shown to be effective in the elderly. A few studies of exercise demonstrate some positive effect on depression, but the use of aerobic exercise is limited in the physically ill elderly. General physical activity is linked to increased psychological well-being.

Guidelines for working with the depressed older patient include establishing short-term goals, emphasizing achievement rather than pleasure, and avoiding excessive cheerfulness. Most depressed patients do get better with time and treatment. It is important to remember that many of us have experienced some degree of depression in our lives and can therefore be empathetic with these patients.

REFERENCES

1. Abrams WB, Berkow R: *Merck Manual of Geriatrics.* Rathway, NJ, Merck Sharp & Dome Laboratories, 1990.
2. American Psychiatric Association: *Diagnostic and Statistical Manual of Mental Disorders,* ed. 4, Washington, DC, American Psychiatric Association, 1994.
3. Baker FM: An overview of depression in the elderly: A US perspective. *J Natl Med Assoc* 1996; 88(3):178-184.

4. Ban T: Chronic disease and depression in the geriatric population. *J Clin Psychiatry* 1984, 45:18-24.

5. Berkman LF, et al: Depressive symptoms in relation to physical health and functioning in the elderly. *Am J Epidemiol* 1986; 24:372-388.

6. Beutler LE, et al: Group cognitive therapy and alprazolam in the treatment of depression in older adults. *J Consult Clin Psychol* 1987; 55: 550-556.

7. Blazer D, Williams C: Epidemiology of dysphoria and depression in an elderly population. *Am J Psychiatry* 1980; 137:439-444.

8. Bolla-Wilson K, Bleecker ML: Absence of depression in elderly adults. *J Gerontol* 1989; 44:P53-55.

9. Butler RN, Lewis M: *Aging & Mental Health.* St Louis, Mosby, 1982.

10. Cameron OG: Guidelines for diagnosis and treatment of depression in patients with medical illness. *J Clin Psychiatry* 1990; 51(suppl):32-35.

11. Cappeliez P, Blanchet D: Strategies of the elderly in coping with depressive feelings. *Can J Aging* 1986; 5:125-134.

12. Cassileth B, et al: Psychosocial status in chronic illness, a comparative analysis of six diagnostic groups. *New Engl J Med* 1984; 311:506-511.

13. Cavanaugh S: Depression in the hospitalized inpatient with various medical illnesses. *Psychother Psychosom* 1986; 45:97-104.

14. Chaisson-Stewart GM: Depression incidence: Past, present, and future, in Chaisson-Stewart GM, (ed): *Depression in the Elderly: An Interdisciplinary Approach.* New York, J Wiley & Sons, 1985.

15. Chaisson-Stewart GM: The diagnostic dilemma, in Chaisson-Stewart GM (ed): *Depression in the Elderly: An Interdisciplinary Approach.* New York, J Wiley & Sons, 1985.

16. Clark DO, Stump TE, Hui SL, Wolinsky FD: Predictors of lower body and basic ADL difficulty among adults aged 70 years and over. *The Gerontologist* 1997; 37(Special Issue 1):135.

17. Comstock G, Helsing K: Symptoms of depression in two communities. *Psychol Med* 1976; 6:551-563.

18. Derogatis LR, Wise TN: *Anxiety and Depressive Disorders in the Medical Patient.* Washington, DC, American Psychiatric Press, 1989.

19. DiMatteo M, Hays R: Social support and serious illness, in Gottlieb BH (ed): *Social Networks and Social Support.* Beverly Hills, Sage, 1981.

20. Dobson KS: A meta-analysis of the efficacy of cognitive therapy for depression. *J Consult Clin Psychol* 1989; 57:414-419.

21. Dohrenwend B: Sociocultural and social psychological factors in the genesis of mental disorders. *J Health Soc Behav* 1975; 16:365-392.

22. Downes JJ, Davies AD, Copeland JR: Organization of depressive symptoms in the elderly population: Hierarchical patterns and Guttman scales. *Psychol Aging* 1988; 3:367-374.

23. Elliott TR, et al: Previous personal experience and reactions to depression and physical disability. *Rehabilitation Psychology* 1990; 35(2): 111-116.

24. Finch EJ, Ransay R, Katona C: Depression and physical illness in the elderly. *Clin Geriatr Med* 1992; 8(2):275-287.

25. Gatz M, Hurwicz M: Are old people more depressed? Cross-sectional data on Center for Epidemiological Studies—Depression Scale. *Psychol Aging* 1990; 5:284-290.

26. Goodman AG, et al: *Goodman & Gilman's the Pharmacological Basis of Therapeutics.* New York, Macmillan, 1985.

27. Griest JH, et al: Running as a treatment for non-psychotic depression. *Behav Med* 1978; 4:19-24.

28. Gurland B, et al: *The Mind and Mood of Aging.* New York, Haworth Press, 1983.

29. Gurland BJ, Toner JA: Depression in the elderly: A review of recently published studies, in Eisdorfer C (ed): *Annual Review of Gerontology and Geriatrics.* New York, Springer, 1982.

30. Haas GL, Fitzgibbon ML: Cognitive models, in Mann JJ (ed): *Models of Depressive Disorders.* New York, Plenum Press, 1989.

31. Hays JC, et al: Social support and depression as risk factors for loss of physical function in late life. *Aging and Mental Health* 1997; 1(3): 209-220.

32. Hendler N: Depression caused by chronic pain. *J Clin Psychiatry* 1984; 45:30-38.

33. Hirschfeld R, Cross C: Epidemiology of affective disorders, psychosocial factors. *Arch Gen Psychiatry* 1982; 39:35-46.

34. Jenike MA: *Handbook of Geriatric Psychopharmacology.* Littleton, Mass, PSG, 1985.

35. Kane RA, Kane RL: *Assessing the Elderly: A Practical Guide to Measurement.* Lexington, Mass, Lexington Books, 1981.

36. Kasniak AW, Sadeh M, Stern LZ: Differentiating depression from organic brain syndromes in older age, in Chaisson-Stewart GM (ed): *Depression in the Elderly: An Interdisciplinary Approach.* New York, J Wiley & Sons, 1985.

37. Kennedy GJ, Kelman HR, Thomas C: The emergence of depressive symptoms in late life. The importance of health and increasing disability. *J Community Health* 1990; 15:93-104.

38. Koenig HG, Shelp F, Goli V: Survival and healthcare utilization in elderly medical inpatients with major depression. *J Am Geriatric Soc* 1989; 37:599-606.

39. Kessler R, Mcleod J: Social support in community samples, in Cohen S, Syme L (eds): *Social Support and Health.* San Diego, Academic Press, 1985.

40. Klerman G: The interpersonal model, in Mann JJ (ed): *Models of Depressive Disorders.* New York, Plenum Press, 1989.

41. Krueger DW: Psychological adjustment to physical trauma and disability, in Roessler R, Decker N (eds): *Emotional Disorders in Physically Ill Patients.* New York, Human Sciences Press, 1986.

42. Kugler J, et al: Hospital supervised versus home exercise in cardiac rehabilitation: Effects of aerobic fitness, anxiety, and depression. *Arch Phys Med Rehabil* 1990; 71:322-325.

43. Labbe EE: Effects of consistent aerobic exercise on the psychological functioning of women. *Percept Mot Skills* 1988; 67:919-925.

44. LaGory M, Fitzpatrick K: The effects of environmental context on elderly depression. *J Aging & Health* 1992; 4(4):459-479.

45. Langer KG: Depression & physical disability: Relationship of self-rated & observer-rated disability to depression. *Neuropsychiatr Neuropsychol Behav Neurol* 1995; 8(4):271-276.

46. Lesher EL: Validation of the Geriatric Depression Scale among nursing home residents. *Clin Gerontol* 1986; 4:21-28.

47. Levy SM, et al: Intervention with older adults and the evaluation of outcome, in Poon LW (ed): *Aging in the Eighties.* Washington DC, American Psychological Association, 1980.

48. MacNair RR, Herrick SM, Yoder B, Byrne CA: Interpersonal reactions to depression and physical disability in dyadic interactions. *J Appl Social Psychol* 1991; 21(16):1993-1302.

49. Magni G, de Leo D, Schifano F: Depression in geriatric and adult medical inpatients. *J Clin Psychol* 1985; 41:337-344.

50. Mann JJ: Neurobiologic models, in Mann JJ (ed): *Models of Depressive Disorders.* New York, Plenum Press, 1989.

51. Massei MJ, Holland JC: Depression and the cancer patient. *J Clin Psychiatry* 1990; 51(suppl):12-17.

52. Matteson M: Affective disorders, in Whanger AD, Myers AC (eds): *Mental Health Assessment and Therapeutic Intervention with Older Adults.* Rockville, Md, Aspen, 1984.

53. Mayeux R: Depression in the patient with Parkinson's disease. *J Clin Psychiatry* 1990; 51(suppl):20-23.

54. McIvor G, Riklan M, Reznikoff M: Depression in multiple sclerosis as a function of length and severity of illness, age, remissions, and perceived social support. *J Clin Psychol* 1984; 40:1028-1033.

55. Millefiorini E, et al: Depression in the early phase of MS: Influence of functional disability, cognitive impairment and brain abnormalities. *Acta Neurol Scand* 1992; 86:354-358.

56. Moos R, Solomon G: Personality factors associated with rheumatoid arthritis. *J Chronic Dis* 1964; 17:41-55.

57. Mossey JM, Knott K, Craik R: The effects of persistent depressive symptoms on hip fracture recovery. *J Gerontol* 1990; 45:M163-168.

58. Newmann JP, Engel RJ, Jansen J: Depressive symptom patterns among older women. *Psychol Aging* 1990; 5:101-118.

59. Noll G, Dubinsky M: Prevalence and predictors of depression in a suburban county. *J Community Psychol* 1985; 13:13-19.

60. O'Connor PJ, Aenchbacker III LE, Dishman RK: Physical activity and depression in the elderly. *J Aging & Physical Activity* 1993;1:34-58.

61. Omnicare, Inc: *Geriatric Pharmaceutical Care Guidelines, 1997-98 Edition.* Covington, Ky, Omnicare, Inc, 1997.

62. Palmer J, Vacc N, Epstein J: Adult inpatient alcoholics: Physical exercise as a treatment intervention. *J Stud Alcohol* 1988; 49:418-421.

63. Parmelee PA, Katz IR, Lawton MP: Depression among institutionalized aged: Assessment and prevalence estimation. *J Gerontol* 1989; 44:M22-29.

64. Parmelee PA, Katz IR, Lawton MP: The relation of pain to depression among institutionalized aged. *J Gerontol* 1991; 46:15-21.

65. Rabbitt P, et al: Unique and interactive effects of depression, age, socioeconomic advantage, and gender on cognitive performance of normal healthy older people. *Psychol & Aging* 1995; 10(3):307-313.

66. Radloff L, Rae D: Components of the sex difference in depression. *Res Community Ment Health* 1981; 2:111-137.

67. Ransford CP: A role for amines in the antidepressant effect of exercise: A review. *Med Sci Sports Exerc* 1982; 14:1-10.

68. Rodin G, Voshart K: Depression in the medically ill: An overview. *Am J Psychiatry* 1986; 143:696-703.

69. Romano J, Turner J: Chronic pain and depression: Does the evidence support a relationship? *Psychol Bull* 1985; 97:18-34.

70. Rosenberg DR, Wright B, Gershon S: Depression in the elderly. *Dementia* 1992; 3:157-173.

71. Roy R: Chronic pain and depression: A review. *Compr Psychiatry* 1984; 25:96-105.

72. Rutter B: Some psychological concomitants of chronic bronchitis. *Psychol Med* 1977; 7:459-464.

73. Schulz R, Rau M: Social support through the life course, in Cohen S, Syme L (eds): *Social Support and Health.* San Diego, Academic Press, 1985.

74. Shisslah CM, Utic J: Exercise, in Chaisson-Stewart GM (ed): *Depression in the Elderly: An Interdisciplinary Approach.* New York, J Wiley & Sons, 1985.

75. Snyder S, et al: Differentiating major depression from adjustment disorder with depressed mood in the medical setting. *Gen Hosp Psychiatry* 1990; 12:159-165.

76. Stenbach A: Depression and suicidal behavior in old age, in Birren J, Sloan RS (eds): *Handbook of Mental Health and Aging.* Englewood Cliffs, NJ, Prentice-Hall, 1980.

77. Tennant C, Wilby J, Nicholson G: Psychological correlates of myasthenia gravis: A brief report. *J Psychosom Res* 1986; 30:575-580.

78. Teuting P, Koslow SH: *Special Report on Depression Research.* National Institutes of Mental Health Science Reports. Rockville, Md, US Department of Health and Human Services, 1988.

79. Thompson LW, Gallagher E, Brechenridge JS: Comparative effectiveness of psychotherapies for depressed elders. *J Consult Clin Psychol* 1987; 55:383-390.

80. Veith RC: Depression in the elderly: Pharmacologic considerations in treatment. *J Am Geriatr Soc* 1982; 30:581-586.

81. Wade D, Legh-Smith J, Langton-Hewer R: Depressed mood after stroke: A community study of its frequency. *Br J Psychiatry* 1987; 151:200-205.

82. Westbrook M, Viney L: Psychological reactions to the onset of chronic illness. *Soc Sci Med* 1982; 16:899-905.

83. Williams A: *Physical Illness and Depression: Changes Over Time in Middle Aged and Elderly Persons* (thesis). Portland University, Portland, 1985.

84. Williams A, Schulz R: Association of pain and physical dependency with depression in physically ill middle-aged and elderly persons. *Phys Ther* 1988; 68:1226-1230.

85. Williams JM, Getty D: Effects of levels of exercise on psychological mood states, physical fitness, and plasma beta endorphin. *Percept Mot Skills* 1986; 63:1099-1105.

86. Williamson GM, Schulz R: Physical illness and symptoms of depression among elderly outpatients. *Psychol & Aging* 1992; 7(3):343-351.

87. Wortman C, Conway T: The role of social support in adaption and recovery from physical illness, in Cohen S, Syme L (eds): *Social Support and Health.* New York, Academic Press, 1985.

88. Yesavage JA, et al: Development and validation of a Geriatric Depression Scale. *J Psychiatr Res* 1983; 17:31-49.

CHAPTER 11

CLINICAL EVALUATION OF THE MEDICAL PATIENT

BARBARA ROBERGE, RNC, PhD, CS

INTRODUCTION

Clinical management and treatment of elders is often a diagnostic dilemma. How does one gather and synthesize information over an individual's lifetime into a coherent diagnostic process? Treatment decisions are based not only on physical health status but also on the interplay of psychological and social factors that comprise the patient and family unit. As in no other adult group, collaboration between health providers is paramount to success in caring for the elderly. This chapter discusses how clinicians critically analyze and prioritize complex patient issues and demonstrates how physical therapists are an integral part of that process. The health care system focuses on the delivery of quality health services. The primary value of collaboration between health providers is ensuring that the goals of providing and measuring quality care are met.

To develop and execute a rehabilitation plan, it is important that the therapist acquire the necessary skills to recognize and prioritize important symptoms. This recognition aids the process of collaboration with the health care team. In order to develop and improve the therapist's skills, this chapter discusses symptoms that therapists, due to the nature of their work, may be the first to recognize.

WELLNESS PROMOTION

Health care too often centers on what happens to an individual after a negative health event and on attempts to thwart pathological processes by medical intervention. Demographic trends are dictating new ways of analyzing the economic and health impacts of an aging society. In the early 1980s a theory evolved that garnered much interest because of its optimistic outlook. This theory, the "compression of morbidity," posited that if morbidity were postponed and life span were genetically fixed, then morbidity would be compressed into a shorter period.[19] Even though the theory itself was not confirmed in subsequent studies, it placed emphasis on health prevention and promotion activities that may delay morbidity and extend quality of life for years. Thus the goal of health promotion in geriatrics may not be focused primarily on disease prevention but on the development of wellness and the delay of functional morbidity throughout the life span. For example, effective reduction in cardiovascular mortality is related to risk factor modification and medical interventions. Most notably, cigarette smoking, inactivity, and obesity are risk factors that can be modified to improve quality of life in persons at risk for cardiovascular disease. Modifying risk factors before pathology begins should be the focus of prevention efforts with today's older adult (Box 11-1).

It is often assumed that elders are too old to change. However, modifiable risk factor reduction should be considered a worthwhile goal at any age. Research has demonstrated that modifying risk factors does affect the onset of chronic disease. However, it is important to understand that much of previous risk factor research has been done on young or middle-aged adults. Current research models focusing on elders indicate that what is known about prevention in younger populations may not always be directly applied to older persons.

Coronary heart disease (CHD) risk factors for middle-aged adults have been the focus of research for the past 40 years and have been generally incorporated into clinical

---

Box 11-1

Modifiable Cardiovascular Risk Factors for Elders

Smoking	High-fat diet
Hypertension	Hyperglycemia
Obesity	High LDL cholesterol
Sedentary life-style	Low HDL cholesterol

---

practice. Less is known about risk factor modification in elders, and the results are controversial. Studies are now examining the utility of those recommendations for elders.[8] Even though these studies are methodologically dissimilar and measure different outcomes, research demonstrates that an elder's risk factors for CHD may be different by both age and gender. Cardiac risk factors in the young old (elders aged 75 years or younger) appear similar to those of middle-aged adults, with the addition of increased left ventricular mass noted by electrocardiogram playing an important role in the incidence of CHD among all elders.[8] For those individuals in the middle-old (elders aged 76 to 84 years), or old-old (elders aged 85 years or older) age categories, total cholesterol may play a less important role in predicting CHD mortality in men. Low levels of high-density lipoprotein (HDL) cholesterol may be a more important risk factor in the incidence of CHD in these two age-groups than is total cholesterol.[38] While the role of total cholesterol as a risk factor is less clear in men, total cholesterol may play a prominent role in CHD incidence and mortality in older women.[5,8,12] Thus, elders with symptomatic CHD and a good prognosis should be encouraged to reduce modifiable risk factors.[23] It has been suggested that if an elder is healthy, and active and quality of life years may be added to the life span, then treatment of hypercholesterolemia should be undertaken. Diet modification and exercise are the recommended first line of treatment. For low-density lipoprotein cholesterol (LDL) in the 130 to 159 mg/dL range, medications to lower LDL cholesterol are best used for secondary, but not primary, prevention after diet modification is initiated for 6 months.[14] Higher LDL levels may require the consideration of low-dose "statins," e.g., lovastatin, pravastatin, simvastatin, atorvastatin, fluvastatin. Importantly, clinical recommendations in this area are changing rapidly. The elderly are more prone to drug side effects and need to be monitored carefully. It is likely that the best opportunity for reducing mortality from CHD through risk factor modification occurs at younger ages.[34] For elders in the advanced old age category or those with debilitating diseases, the benefit of no pharmacological treatment may outweigh the decision to medicate due to the increased prevalence of toxic side effects with aging. Diet and exercise should be recommended at any age because both have benefits that will improve quality of life whenever begun.

The benefits of exercise in risk factor modification in elders have been well-demonstrated. Exercise is positively associated with increased levels of HDL cholesterol, but not total cholesterol, and this positive effect has been demonstrated in very old individuals in their ninth decade.[6] Exercise also improves balance and strength and thus may prevent injury from falls.[16,26] The benefits of exercise in younger populations in reducing mortality risk have also been demonstrated in older women. Mortality in older women is inversely associated with physical activity, and the greater the intensity, the greater the benefit. Regular moderate physical activity reduced the risk of dying for women younger than 80, and the risk of dying from respiratory or cardiac disease demonstrated the greatest reduction compared with other disease states.[22] Elders are less commonly referred to cardiac rehabilitation than younger adults. Compared with that of younger adults, participation by elders in a cardiac rehabilitation program has demonstrated improvement in functional capacity and quality of life measures, with modest improvement in lipid levels,[24,25] although reduction in repeat cardiac events or/and inverse association with mortality have not been demonstrated.

While most cardiac risk factor research is performed on men, women younger than 80 have also been shown to benefit from physical activity. It may be concluded that coronary risk factor modification for young and middle-aged elders is similar to that in younger age-groups. Total cholesterol is not as strong a cardiac risk factor in elders as it is in younger age groups. Young and middle-aged elders may thus benefit from secondary prevention strategies. All elders of both genders will benefit from diet and exercise programs at all ages.

Common Presenting Signs and Symptoms

Three common symptoms may occur during the execution of a rehabilitation plan: dyspnea, dizziness, and confusion. In general, symptom analysis is physiologically based. For example, breathing successfully requires both intact oxygen transport mechanisms—i.e., lungs and heart— and an oxygen transport medium—i.e., the blood—and must meet the physiological demands of the body. Thus, analysis of the cause(s) of dyspnea must take all of these into account.

History taking helps focus the clinical examination and begins the diagnostic analysis. Symptom analysis includes knowledge of the precipitating event, symptom onset, duration, intensity, associated symptoms, timing, relieving factors, previous history, and similar episodes. After symptom analysis, a thorough physical examination adds needed information to the diagnostic process and should correlate with the history. Medications should be reviewed for any possible adverse reactions that may cause or worsen the symptom under analysis. For example, angiotensin converting enzyme (ACE) inhibitors have been known to occasionally cause dry cough, hyperkalemia, and fatigue, especially in elders.

TABLE 11-1
Common Causes of Dyspnea in Elders

System Failure	Etiology
Cardiac	Arrhythmias (atrial fibrillation)
	Myocardial infarct
	Emboli
Respiratory	Infectious lung disease
	Obstructive lung disease
Endocrine	Thyroid disease
Hematological	Hemorrhage
	Bone marrow abnormalities
Environmental	Hyperthermia

Dyspnea

Dyspnea clearly affects a person's ability to participate in a rehabilitation program, therefore the physical therapist may be the first to note this symptom. Acute dyspnea occurring at rest is an ominous sign. Focusing on a symptom analysis of the cardiac, respiratory, and circulatory systems; smoking history; work history; and self-report and observing the patient in functional activities provide insight into the severity of the problem. Any change from baseline is important and may implicate any of the causes of dyspnea outlined in Table 11-1.

Cardiac disease is the No. 1 cause of mortality in elders, a primary reason for hospitalization, and it is often first noted with dyspnea. For elders, unlike younger adults, dyspnea may be the primary and only presenting symptom signaling heart disease. The etiology of heart failure is sought among its common causes including myocardial infarct; arrhythmias; and, specifically, atrial fibrillation (see Table 11-1). Patients with paroxysmal nocturnal dyspnea (PND), orthopnea, and new onset dyspnea on exertion (DOE) are typically evaluated for heart failure, unless other etiologies are clearly evident in the history.[21] These three presentations of dyspnea, plus new onset dyspnea at rest, are important symptoms of underlying disease. More subtle symptoms, which may be first noticed by the therapist, include exercise intolerance, confusion, and nausea or abdominal pain associated with ascites and hepatic engorgement as the heart fails and fluid accumulates.

Laboratory testing includes a chest x-ray to differentiate cardiac from pulmonary disease and to evaluate heart size; however, absence of cardiomegaly (enlarged heart) does not discount heart failure. An electrocardiogram (ECG) is performed to evaluate for ischemia, arrhythmias, myocardial infarct, and conduction abnormalities. Because of the importance of data trends for accurate diagnosis, a review of serum laboratory tests allows comparison of previous results with current ones that help to identify the nature of the problem.

One important laboratory test in the evaluation of dyspnea is the complete blood count (CBC). It should be reviewed for a reduction in erythrocyte count (red blood cells, "RBCs") and the hematocrit and hemoglobin (H+H) level, which may signal anemia. The RBCs form in the bone marrow and have a life span of 120 days. A low H+H level, which is present in anemia, will aggravate heart failure because of a lack of circulating oxygen to meet the body's demands. Due to reduced reserve capacity, elders are prone to symptoms of heart failure, as cardiac output is increased in response to anemia. Hemoglobin in the RBCs combines with oxygen and carbon dioxide, forming the transport mechanism for these elements. Hemoglobin is composed of the protein portion, or globin, and an iron portion, the heme, and hence easily combines with oxygen. The hematocrit level is the ratio of packed red blood cell volume to the plasma and is expressed as a percentage. The hemoglobin and hematocrit levels are evaluated together. The hematocrit level normally measures about three times the hemoglobin level. Hematocrit levels less than 25% may mimic heart failure. Low H+H levels will affect exercise endurance, but a tolerance for low H+H levels may be demonstrated with chronic anemia. Exercise may upset this delicate balance by causing an increased demand for oxygen. New or worsening DOE may be due to an increased demand for oxygen that is not met because of poor pump performance or a filling deficit seen in heart failure or because of an inadequate delivery system resulting from anemia.

Reticulocytes are immature red blood cells released into the circulation early in response to blood cell destruction or production failure. If blood loss is suspected as a contributing factor to heart failure, a reticulocyte count may be considered. Hemorrhage results in the increased loss of cells, whereas abnormalities of the bone marrow and hemolysis result in increased destruction of the red cells. Therefore an increase in the reticulocyte count per 1000 RBCs is an indicator of hemorrhage, hemolytic anemia, or primary and secondary cancers.

In healthy elders the absolute CBC values fall within the range of normal; however, the bone marrow of elders, compared with that of younger individuals, lacks the ability to compensate in response to acute and chronic disease, putting elders at greater risk of marrow failure. This may account for the large number of anemias associated with chronic diseases seen in elderly populations.[26] Chronic anemia may be well compensated for, and, in these cases, may not be evident until severe blood loss is present. When laboratory tests are evaluated, trends in test results are as important as the actual results because of this compensation factor.

When heart failure is suspected as the cause of dyspnea, the renal laboratory tests should be reviewed, including creatinine and blood urea nitrogen (BUN) levels. Renal failure causing fluid overload will worsen heart failure, which in turn, increases fatigue levels and dyspnea. Creatinine is a measure of the products of energy metabolism excreted by the kidneys, whereas BUN is a measure of the production and excretion of urea (the end product of protein catabolism) by the kidneys. The ratio of BUN to creatinine is evaluated to determine whether renal failure is present. A ratio of 25:1 or more suggests dehydration. In patients with heart failure, a common cause of renal failure is dehydration due to the use of diuretics. A high creatinine level reveals kidney failure. It should be noted that when patients are dehydrated, the hematocrit level is falsely elevated due to the altered ratio of fluid to solids.

Laboratory tests for thyroid deficiencies are analyzed because thyroid deficiencies, common in elders, may cause or exacerbate heart failure and atrial fibrillation (AF). The thyroid-stimulating hormone (TSH) determines the level of thyroid gland activity. The level is increased in primary hypothyroidism and Hashimoto's thyroiditis.

An ECG is reviewed for ischemia, AF, or myocardial infarct. AF is more common in elders than in younger adults and may precipitate or worsen heart failure. If a diagnosis of AF is present, the potential for worsening of heart failure is present due to a reduction in cardiac output. In addition, anticoagulation therapy that is used to reduce the risk of thrombi, as blood stagnates in the atria, increases the risk of bleeding secondary to a fall.

An echocardiogram measures ejection fraction (EF), heart valve dynamics, and heart chamber size, and guides medical management of heart failure. If, for example, the ejection fraction is <40% (normal is 55% to 60%), systolic dysfunction is suspected. This is a pump problem, and treatment is directed toward improving the pumping mechanism. Coronary artery disease is a common cause of systolic dysfunction. If, however, the ejection fraction is >40% and heart failure is present, diastolic dysfunction (a filling problem) is suspected. The distinction between systolic and diastolic dysfunction is important in the management of heart failure. Older adults are more sensitive to volume changes than are younger adults. Therefore, if a filling problem is suspected, adequate filling pressure is needed to maintain cardiac output and thus heart function. The judicious use of diuretics in the treatment phase of heart failure is warranted in order to avoid volume depletion and to maintain filling pressures.[2]

It is important for the therapist to be aware of whether heart failure is present, what the etiology is, and whether anticoagulation therapy is being used. If the symptoms of DOE is worsening and syncope or chest pressure is present, close collaboration with the medical provider is important.

In the analysis of dyspnea, common elderly respiratory problems must be factored into the diagnostic equation, along with possible cardiac abnormalities. A mixed picture of cardiac and respiratory deficits is highly probable. Common elderly respiratory problems include infections and obstructive airway disease, such as asthma, bronchitis, and emphysema. Common infections include pneumonia, which may be categorized as community, long-term–care facility, or hospital-acquired pneumonia, and tuberculosis. The living situation and degree of disability must be considered because setting and disability differentiates probable pathogen type. For example, neurologically impaired individuals and those with gastrointestinal disease are at greater risk of contracting aspiration pneumonitis and aspiration pneumonia than are healthy individuals. The former is due to aspiration

of gastric contents, whereas the latter is due to aspiration of oropharyngeal contents. Cough; dyspnea; white, frothy sputum; hypotension; and agitation are hallmarks of aspiration pneumonitis. Treatment is first aimed at lowering the pH of the aspirate.

The clinical presentation of pneumonia in elders is often subtle: tachypnea may be the only presenting symptom, fever and chills may not be present, and cough and sputum production may be slight. Therefore, subtle changes in the respiratory rate noted during participation in the rehabilitation program can be a significant finding.

Pulmonary function tests help differentiate restrictive from obstructive disease. Obstructive disease is graded according to the forced expired volume in one second FEV_1. Wheezing, cough, dyspnea, and breathlessness are common in obstructive disease.[1]

Dyspnea, although not the first symptom noted, may herald dysfunction of the oxygen-carrying capacity system. In elders, upper gastrointestinal (GI) bleeding is a common cause of an insidious drop in the hematocrit and hemoglobin levels, whereas lower gastrointestinal disease often has a slower onset. Dyspnea, a late sign of blood loss, may be precipitated during exercise. Dysphagia, weight loss, and abdominal pain and discomfort are more predominant signs of gastric ulcer disease. Fatigue generally accompanies weight loss. Both gastric and duodenal ulcer disease are common causes of elderly upper GI bleeding, followed by erosive gastritis, esophagitis, esophageal varices, and neoplasm.[30] The increased use of non-steroidal anti-inflammatory drugs (NSAIDs) adds to the increased incidence of bleeding in elders. Common causes of lower tract bleeding are diverticulosis, malignancy, and colitis.

Lastly, dyspnea may be included in the constellation of symptoms present due to hyperthermia. Hyperthermia, or heat stroke, is more common in older than in younger adults due to a decrease in the thirst mechanism accompanying aging and a decline in cognition and functional levels, requiring assistance to procure food and fluids. Hyperthermia increases mortality risk in cardiac patients.[41] Early symptoms may include dizziness, delirium, nausea, headache, and dyspnea.

Dizziness

Dizziness is a common complaint encountered by the physical therapist and is an important identifier of increased risk of hip fracture.[40] For ease of diagnosis, dizziness is categorized as vertigo or a spinning sensation, disequilibrium or imbalance sensation, near-syncope or light-headedness, or non-specific dizziness.[29,39] The evaluation of dizziness presents a plethora of diagnostic possibilities, including vestibular, cardiac, neurological, visual, and psychiatric disorders. However, it has been demonstrated that physical examination, provocation studies, and psychological assessment are more helpful diagnostically than expensive radiological, electrophysiological, and laboratory testing.[11] Therefore, it is important to obtain a careful history of dizziness, ascertaining a clear picture of the symptoms and precipitating events.

The patient with vertigo is more likely to suffer from vestibular problems than from other problems. Spinning, which occurs 15 to 20 seconds after head and neck movement, is often associated with labyrinthine disease. Balance is dependent on sensory cues and vestibular function, both central and peripheral. Therefore, inner ear problems and gait disturbance affect balance and increase the risk of falls.

Near-syncope, or fainting, is often related to cardiovascular disease rather than to a peripheral or central nervous system disorder. If syncope is present, a search for a cardiac etiology should be initiated. An ECG and a loop ambulatory cardiac monitor are obtained to evaluate for rhythm disturbances. Syncope also requires a careful physical examination and echocardiogram for blood flow abnormalities. Faintness during standing or bowel movements may relate to orthostatic hypotension or to a Valsalva maneuver, respectively.

Inability to describe symptoms may be related to dementia or psychiatric disorders. Individuals with dementia may be trying to describe the confusion they experience and not true dizziness. An evaluation for depression, anxiety, and dementia may be included in the differential diagnosis, if symptoms are difficult to describe. Finally, iatrogenic postural hypotension that causes positional dizziness is more common in elders than in younger adults due to the increased prevalence of polypharmacy in elders. Medications are always implicated initially as causative agents, until proven otherwise. These include antihypertensives, diuretics, and drugs that cause sedation.

Confusion

Confusion is a common and complex symptom, often first noted yet often overlooked by the providers most familiar with the elder exhibiting the symptom. Especially difficult is the differential diagnosis of acute confusion (delirium) in a demented individual. The assessment of confusion starts with differentiating symptom onset and course.

Because delirium is reversible, the evaluation centers on a hunt for metabolic, infectious, or neurological disturbances, including alcohol and drug withdrawal. An example of the latter is the abrupt withdrawal of benzodiazepines and antipsychotic medications. The hallmark of delirium is an acute onset with a fluctuating course. Knowing the baseline cognitive functional level of the patient is key to the evaluation. Altered levels of consciousness with inattention are common. These patients often will be able to participate in a rehabilitation plan at one time during the day, but be lethargic or unable to follow instructions at another. Cognitive impairment and memory disturbance may be present and not related to any previous diagnosis of dementia. Fluctuating psychotic symptoms include visual and tactile hallucinations and delusions. Increased agitation and confusion, starting in the late afternoon (sundowning), is more commonly diagnosed in institutional residents than community-dwelling

residents and is associated with dementia and related to sleep disturbance. The treatment aim in these cases is improvement of the individual's sleeping patterns and remediation of the behavior disturbance.

Common causes of delirium in the ambulatory setting include infections, especially of the urinary tract and the respiratory system; blood loss; new cardiac abnormalities; and adverse medication reactions. Laboratory analysis is an important part of the delirium evaluation. Metabolic, hematologic, and infectious abnormalities appear in laboratory test results. The laboratory analysis of a suspected infectious etiology begins with an analysis of the CBC—specifically, the leukocytes or white blood cells (WBCs). Leukocytosis, or a rise in the WBCs, is due to an increase of one of the many types of white blood cells in response to inflammation. A rise may result from infections, steroid use, malignant disease, leukemia, drugs, or the release of toxins into the system. A reduction in the total WBCs, known as leukopenia, may result from viral infections or bone marrow disorders. Leukopenia is analyzed as a problem characterized by reduced production or increased destruction of cells.

The five subtypes of WBCs are presented in Table 11-2 and together are called the differential count. The differential count gives information regarding the type of inflammatory response present. The differential count is always interpreted in relation to the total leukocyte count. During normal conditions, each subtype falls in a normal range and is expressed as a percent of the total white blood cell count and the absolute value.

Neutrophils are the most numerous of the white blood cells and their increase indicates the severity of an infection, whereas the total white blood cell count indicates the patient's ability to mount an infectious response. Neutrophils are the primary response to invading microorganisms and work by phagocytosis. Considering neutrophils linearly, specific inflammatory responses cause different percents of immature or mature neutrophils to rise and shift the most frequent percentage (mode) of these cells to the left or right on an imaginary line. This information is referred to as a *shift-to-the-left* if an increase in immature cells is present, indicating a regenerative process, or as a *shift-to-the-right* if mature neutrophils predominate. The shift is diagnostically significant and evaluated in response to the total leukocyte count. In those with a weakened immune response—frail elders, those with overwhelming infections or AIDS, or chemotherapy patients—there may be a shift-to-the-left without an increase in the overall white blood cell count. Conversely, an increase in immature neutrophils with a proportional rise in the total leukocyte count indicates an infection with a good immune response.

Lymphocytes provide cellular immunity by the production of immunoglobulins. They respond to antigens and are the chief cells of the lymph nodes. Monocytes also respond to infection by phagocytosis, but occur later than neutrophils. They are the body's second line of defense against invading organisms. Eosinophils are involved in allergic and

Table 11-2
Differential White Blood Cell Count

White Blood Cells	Relative Value as a % of total	Absolute Value per cu mm	Etiology -(increase)	Etiology-(decrease)
Neutrophils	60%-70%	3000-7000	Bacterial infections Exercise Burns Infarction Chronic inflammation Hemolysis	Viral infections Leukemia Aplastic anemia Pernicious anemia Overwhelming infection
Lymphocytes	20%-40%	1000-4000	Chronic lymphocytic leukemia Mononucleosis Infectious hepatitis Tuberculosis	Acute illness stress Sepsis Hodgkin's disease Chemotherapy Heart failure
Monocytes	2%-6%	100-600	Leukemia Infections (viral/bacterial) Sarcoidosis Rheumatoid arthritis	No specific disease
Eosinophils	1%-4%	50-400	Allergies Parasites Chronic skin infections Endocrine disease Malignant neoplasm Steroids mask eosinophilia	Mononucleosis Adrenal disorders Drugs
Basophils	0.5%-1%	25-100	Allergic reactions Leukemia Chronic inflammation	Prolonged steroids Acute allergic reactions Acute illness stress

immune responses. Basophils, the smallest proportion of the WBCs, are involved in acute allergic responses.

Common Syndromes Affecting Rehabilitation

Syndromes are multi-causal entities. Syndromes, due to their inherent complexity, present diagnostic and management dilemmas. Three syndromes common to elders are discussed: failure to thrive, dehydration, and malnutrition. All of these syndromes require modification of current rehabilitation plans or the development of innovative methods of delivering rehabilitation to older adults.

Failure to Thrive
Failure to thrive (FTT) is described as a progressive loss of function and general deterioration greater than expected when compared to a matched age group. It is a term used for our most vulnerable populations at both ends of the age spectrum. Patients present with weight, functional, and muscle loss. Weight loss, the hallmark of FTT, is often gradual. It may be accompanied by weakness, self-care deficits, dizziness, memory loss, or depression. These symptoms should not be mistaken for the natural aging process, but be recognized as abnormal findings and markers for disease. It is theorized that FTT may be a hallmark of mortality or alternatively have a reversible etiology. The diagnostic evaluation seeks to differentiate between reversible and irreversible etiologies of the syn-

drome, and therefore the health history focuses on the evaluation of four domains: physical functioning, malnutrition, depression, and dementia.[33] Symptoms of worsening chronic diseases; the onset of new acute illnesses; and risk factors for malignancy, gastrointestinal malabsorption, and depression are important considerations.

Malnutrition
Malnutrition is defined as deficient or excess consumption of calories or nutrients.[10] This section focuses on nutritional inadequacies and underweight states. It is important to note that nutritional inadequacies include the spectrum of both overweight and underweight states. Overweight is not synonymous with adequate nutritional intake. One study of community dwelling elders found that 42% of elders were overweight.[15]

Because of the important correlation between caloric intake and energy expenditure, a nutritional assessment should be part of any physical therapist's examination. Successful rehabilitation and adequate nutrition are synergistic. Nutritional excess and deficiency are common problems in elders and have enormous policy and individual implications for an aging society.[3] At the societal level, malnutrition is associated with longer hospitalization, higher mean hospital cost per hospitalization, and greater use of community services once hospital discharge occurs.[9] At the individual level, muscle wasting and weight loss or excess negatively affect the individual's ability to perform basic functions, heal injured tissue, and fight infections.

TABLE 11-3
QUICK NUTRITION EVALUATION FOR ELDERS*

DOMAINS	ASSESSMENT AREAS	INTERVENTION/OUTCOME
Caloric/ Vitamin Intake	No. of meals per day Weight loss > 10 lbs past 6 months Use of vitamin supplements	Adequate caloric intake Weight gain
Dentition and Swallow	Chewing and swallow food consistency	Referral to dentist Swallow evaluation
Environmental	Food availability Able to procure food	Referral to social service Meals on Wheels
Functional	Self-feed ability Functional dependency	Maximize independence
Financial	Able to afford food	Referral to social service
Health Behaviors	Smoking Excessive alcohol	Stop smoking Reduce alcohol intake
Polypharmacy	Appetite suppressant Taste change Nausea Dry mouth	Minimize medications
Physiological Normal vs. Disease	Advanced age Organ function change	Adequate nutritional intake
Psychological	Depression Motivation Dementia	Depression treatment Feeding groups Assist with feeding Family involvement Family support

*A 10-item evaluation covering some of these domains has been developed and distributed by the Nutrition Screening Initiative of the American Academy of Family Physicians, The American Dietetic Association, and the National Council on the Aging Inc.

Nutritional risk screening has become widely publicized since the advent of the Nutrition Screening Initiative (NSI).[15] Although a popular 10-item weighted response survey developed by this initiative has not been validated as a direct indicator of malnutrition, it is a useful educational tool identifying potential risk of poor nutritional intake.[32] The NSI provides in-depth assessment for those initially identified as being at risk.

Risk factors for malnutrition are advanced age, poor dentition, low income, and tobacco use.[30] Weight loss of greater than 10 pounds in 6 months and low serum cholesterol and low albumin levels are all indicators of malnutrition and signs of a poor prognosis.

The common domains of a nutritional risk assessment are outlined in Table 11-3. Vitamin intake and supplements; percent and variety of meals eaten; and the ability to self-feed, chew, and swallow are important assessment factors. It should be recognized that the evaluation of life-long eating patterns is mandatory. A life-long history of anorexia, due to

body image concerns, has been reported in the literature.[28] Anorexia in elders, related to body image, is often undetected and poorly understood. The availability of and financial ability to purchase food should be assessed. Physiological and psychological factors are key elements of a nutritional assessment. With advancing age and disease come changes in taste; salivary gland function; reduced secretion of digestive enzymes; changes in hepatic catabolism; alteration in intestinal mobility; and reduced ability to synthesize vitamin D, which may affect nutritional intake. In addition, depression and dementia may have profound effects on adequate nutritional intake.

Dietary guidelines are based on the Food Guide Pyramid, which provides sound nutritional recommendations, though not specific to older populations.[35] Bread, cereals, rice, and pasta are the basis from which a healthy diet is constructed, followed by vegetables and fruits, with limited use of meat, poultry, and fish. Two to three servings of low-fat milk, yogurt, and cheese are recommended. However, it could be argued that recommendations in this category, especially low-fat fortified milk, need to be increased due to the high incidence of osteoporosis and the lack of adequate vitamin D intake and absorption in elders. Limited use of fats, oils, and sweets is recommended and thus tops the pyramid.

The need for or abuse of vitamin supplements is an issue about which elders often ask. A balanced diet is the best source of an adequate vitamin intake and probably safer than supplementation. However, elders may need supplements of vitamins D and B_{12}. Sources of vitamin D are meat, fish, and fortified milk. Vitamin D, especially important in slowing the rate of bone loss, is often inadequate in elders. Vitamin D recommendations for those aged 51 to 70 are 400 IU (International Units) daily, which increases to 600 IU after age 70.[20] The incidence of atrophic gastritis is greater in elders than in younger adults. This condition prevents the absorption of B_{12} from dietary sources, but allows for the absorption of crystalline B_{12} normally. Therefore, elders may benefit from a supplement of B_{12}, at least at the recommended daily allowance (RDA) of 2.4 g/day.[7] In general, the use of multivitamin supplements is not associated with lower morbidity and mortality.

The search within each domain of nutritional risk focuses on modifiable causes of the syndrome. The patient and family should be actively involved in the decision to evaluate, treat, and manage FTT. If unmodifiable factors are not evident or if treatment is not desired, end of life support and comfort may be reasonable approaches after the initial evaluation.

Dehydration

Dehydration is a common problem in elders and directly increases rates of morbidity and mortality. Dehydration is a costly societal, as well as individual, problem. In 1991, the cost to Medicare for dehydration, not including long-term–care costs, was $446 million. At the individual level, 47% of hospitalized elders with a primary diagnosis of dehydration died within 1 year of the indexed hospitalization.[36]

Incidence has a linear association to aging, and thus there is a great likelihood that a physical therapist working with adults will encounter this problem.

Elders are more susceptible to dehydration because of blunting of homeostatic mechanisms that prevent hypovolemia. Changes in the homeostatic mechanism controlling volume and osmolality of extracellular fluid result in reduced reserve capacity when the system is stressed by changes in physical, psychological, or environmental conditions governing the system. First, thirst response, stimulated by dehydration, is diminished, resulting in an increased solute to water ratio. Second, decreased renal plasma flow may be responsible for a decline in urine concentration ability, which prevents the body from retaining enough fluid to avert dehydration. Finally, vasopressin release, stimulated by low fluid volume, is diminished.[18]

Presenting symptoms of dehydration may include confusion, lethargy, rapid weight loss, and functional decline, all of which will interfere with rehabilitation goals. Therefore, the physical therapist is in a good position to alert the medical team to the emergence of this syndrome. The most common causes of dehydration are poor fluid intake, iatrogenesis induced by medications, gastrointestinal fluid loss, and preparation for procedures.

The most significant laboratory abnormality is sodium imbalance, and this should be carefully monitored. Because of this association, dehydration is categorized by the relationship between free water and sodium. In one kind of dehydration, known as *isotonic dehydration,* there is a balanced loss of water and sodium. Equal loss of both water and sodium is often seen in vomiting and diarrhea. A second type of dehydration, *hypertonic* or *hypernatremic dehydration,* occurs when water loss is greater than sodium loss. Examples of hypertonic dehydration are febrile states and poor fluid intake. Finally, hypotonic dehydration occurs when sodium loss is greater than water loss, resulting in hyponatremia. Inappropriate use of diuretics causes hypotonic dehydration with low sodium.[13]

A common clinical finding in hyponatremia of older adults, which can often be misdiagnosed, is the inability to excrete free water. The kidneys conserve water because of an increase in vasopressin release. Thus the ratio of free water to sodium solute is increased. This clinical syndrome is termed *inappropriate secretion of antidiuretic hormone (SIADH).* Urine osmolality is greater than 300 mOsm/kg in the individual with a low serum sodium level. Treatment is aimed at restricting free water.

Laboratory Values

The evaluation of laboratory tests is an important part of the evaluation of older adults. While laboratory values for elders are often within the same numerical range as those for younger adults, the probability of an imbalance is greater in elders because of polypharmacy, the increased number of diseases per individual compared with younger adults, and

TABLE 11-4
Reference Ranges for Laboratory Tests*

Laboratory Test	Reference Range
Complete blood count	
Hematocrit	Male 47 ± 5%
	Female 42 ± 5%
Hemoglobin	Male 16.2 ± 2 g/dL
	Female 14 ± 2 g/dL
White blood count	7.8 ± 3 × 10⁹
Platelet count	140-400 × 10⁹
Biochemical tests	
Sodium	135-148 mEq/dL
Chloride	98-106 mmol/dL
Carbon dioxide	23-30 mmol/dL
BUN	7-18 mg/dL
Creatinine	0.6-1.2 mg/dL
Potassium	3.6-5.1 mEq/dL
Calcium	9.0-10.5 mEq/dL
Magnesium	1.2-2.3 mg/dL
Glucose	67-109 mg/dL
Alkaline phosphatase	45-126 IU/L
Total protein	6.3-8.3 g/dL
Albumin	3.4-4.8 g/dL
T_4	5.0-12.5 mcg/dL
T_3 resin uptake	25%-35%
TSH	0.4-4.8 mc$_{IU}$/mL

*Reference ranges may vary according to laboratory.
T_4 = thyroxine; T_3 = triiodothyronine; TSH = thyroid-stimulating hormone.

physiological changes that occur with aging (Table 11-4). Important laboratory tests with implications for a rehabilitation plan include the electrolyte panel, liver function test (LFT), and thyroid function test (TFT). The albumin and total protein levels reveal important nutritional information. A urinalysis is a simple urine test that imparts a wealth of knowledge about aging kidneys. Finally, the importance of the electrocardiogram must be noted.

The electrolyte panel ("lytes") consists of basic electrolytes, sodium, potassium, chloride, and carbon dioxide. It is often combined with BUN, creatinine, and glucose to form the basic metabolic panel referred to as the "chemistry seven," or "chem. 7." Basic electrolyte levels do not change with aging. Under standard conditions, the aging body is able to adapt to usual conditions for maintaining fluid volume. Under extreme conditions of stress, physiological reserve is diminished, resulting in an increased probability of electrolyte abnormalities. Three classes of drugs often administered to elders are common causes of hyperkalemia or increased potassium levels.[4] The drug classes are (1) potassium-sparing diuretics—e.g., spironolactone and triamterene—which interfere with potassium excretion; (2) NSAIDs; and (3) ACE inhibitors—e.g., quinapril, captopril, lisinopril, and enalapril.

Serum creatinine concentration, a measure of kidney function, does not change with normal aging. In the elderly, the most common cause of a rise in the creatinine and BUN levels is due to acute renal failure caused by the syndrome of prerenal azotemia secondary to dehydration.

Liver function tests are a measure of hepatic destruction and function. A basic hepatic laboratory panel may consist of measurement of albumin, total protein, globulin, bilirubin, alkaline phosphatase (ALP), alanine aminotransferase (ALT) or serum glutamate pyruvate transaminase (SGPT), and aspartate transaminase (AST) or serum glutamic-oxaloacetic transaminase (SGOT).

Albumin, globulin, and total protein levels are used to measure hepatic function. Formed in the liver, they control the normal distribution of body water by the forces of colloidal osmotic pressure. Proteins also help in the transport of hormones, fatty acids, enzymes, and some drugs.[17] Hypoalbuminemia is often associated with edema and poor drug distribution, leading to toxic levels of drugs in the body. Malnutrition, liver disease, malabsorption syndromes, and increased loss of albumin are some of the causes of low albumin and total protein levels.

The other liver function tests measure enzymes released into the circulation during cell destruction. These enzymes occur in varying amounts in liver and other organ tissues. For example, elevated levels of AST or SGOT occur during a myocardial infarct or with liver disease. ALT or SGPT is more specific to liver destruction than is AST. Finally, alkaline phosphatase (ALP) is a marker of liver and certain bone disease.

Thyroid disease is more common in elders than in younger adults. The effects of aging on thyroid function laboratory tests are minimal. However, illness and medications may have a marked effect on tests of thyroid function. Hypothyroidism may contribute to fatigue, constipation, cold intolerance, and muscle stiffness, often observed with the aging process and therefore often misdiagnosed as due to old age. First-line testing to distinguish primary hypothyroidism is the TSH test. TSH is released into the blood by a feedback mechanism between the anterior pituitary, which releases TSH in response to low levels of circulating thyroid hormone. When hypothyroidism occurs, TSH secretion increases. Alternatively, elders with hyperthyroidism often describe feelings such as fatigue, restlessness, weight loss, and "not feeling well." Weight loss occurs and may be accompanied by nausea and diarrhea. Cardiac manifestations of hyperthyroidism include AF, congestive heart failure, and angina pectoris and occur more frequently in the elderly than in younger adults.

The urinalysis is a simple test of basic kidney function. The physiological changes that occur in the aging kidney include decreased renal blood flow and glomerular filtration rate (GFR), with accompanying smaller kidney size. Under disease-free circumstances the normal aging kidney, even with the physiological changes described, is able to maintain fluid homeostasis but is at greater risk of imbalance under conditions of stress. Renal drug clearance is affected by the depressed GFR of aging and is one cause of the greater incidence of drug toxicity seen in elders. The dipstick is a small, easily portable strip that is impregnated with chemicals that detect urine compounds. Color changes occur in the presence of abnormalities. The dipstick detects the presence of abnormal amounts of glucose, protein, blood, leukocytes, and nitrates in the urine. The presence of leukocytes may signal a urinary tract infection, and a urine culture may be warranted. The presence of nitrates, however, may be a sign of kidney dysfunction.

The ECG records electrical impulses that stimulate the heart to contract. Heart cells produce a wave of electricity that depolarizes or positively charges the inside of the heart cell, causing it to contract. As this wave passes through the heart from the atria to the ventricles, the electrical charge is recorded on the electrocardiogram. The cell recovers its negative or resting charge during repolarization. Both depolarization and repolarization are recorded on the ECG. Six limb and six chest leads compose the standard ECG.

The electrical impulse starts in the posterior wall of the right atrium at the sinoatrial (SA) node, which is also called the *pacemaker* because it controls heart rate. As the atria contract, the positive electrical impulse of depolarization spreads across the atria to produce the P wave on the ECG. Blood is forced through the mitral and tricuspid valves after which the electrical impulse travels down to the atrioventricular (AV) node. From the AV node the impulse travels down the right and left bundle branches that comprise the ventricular conduction system. This ventricular depolarization appears on the ECG as the second impulse and is described at the QRS complex. The first negative deflection of the complex is the Q wave. The R wave is the first positive impulse of the complex and reflects ventricular repolarization, and the S wave is the negative deflection after the R wave. The complex is completed by ventricular repolarization, which allows the heart cells to regain a negative charge and is noted on the ECG as the T wave. The low-voltage U wave sometimes follows the T wave and represents repolarization of the intraventricular conduction system (Fig. 11-1). The ECG paper contains a grid that allows measurement of the height, length, and duration of the cardiac cycle. Abnormalities of measurement occur during cardiac dysfunction and allow the diagnosis of diseases, such as ischemia, infarction, arrhythmia, hypertrophy, and conduction delays.

Two cardiac abnormalities more common in elders than in younger adults are AF and angina pectoris. AF occurs when many atrial foci fire at one time. It appears on the ECG as an irregular baseline without a P wave. The QRS complex is irregular, and the atria do not empty efficiently or completely. Patients are at risk for thromboembolic events and are treated with warfarin. Even though the risk of falls is a consideration for frail elders, older adults are candidates for anticoagulation therapy but are often undertreated. It is important for the physical therapist to know whether a patient is receiving this type of treatment, due to the increased risk of bleeding. Warfarin is potentiated by numerous classes of drugs, including the infrequent use of acetaminophen, and thus careful monitoring of the prothrombin time and international normalization ratio (INR) and knowledge of the patient's medication regimen are mandatory.

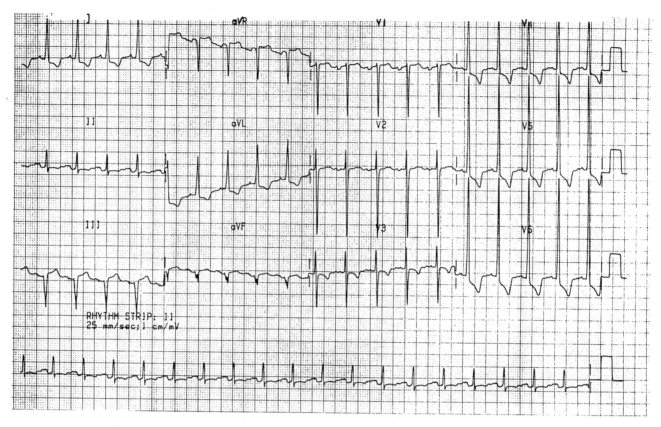

FIG. 11-1   Left ventricular hypertrophy with strain. This pattern is characterized by very tall R waves and deeply inverted T waves.

Angina pectoris results from transient myocardial ischemia. In elders, dyspnea—not chest pain—may be the presenting symptom. T-wave inversion in the chest leads characterizes ischemia, or reduced blood supply, on the ECG. If ischemia progresses to injury, the ST segment that follows the QRS complex is elevated (see Fig. 11-1). In ischemic disease, elders' ECGs may demonstrate nonspecific changes, especially when associated with the commonly seen increased QRS voltage of left ventricular hypertrophy.[37]

SUMMARY

Clinical management of elders is complex. Treating illness while promoting optimal health is the common goal of all professional practitioners in geriatric health care. A critical shift in geriatric health care has occurred, moving from an illness paradigm to a wellness one. Wellness, for older adults, focuses on health promotion and management of chronic illness with an emphasis on quality of life. Research findings consistently demonstrate the value of risk factor reduction, including positive benefits of exercise, even in very old individuals. Symptom analysis is foremost in the diagnosis and management of illness, including symptoms commonly encountered by physical therapists: dyspnea, dizziness, and delirium. Syndromes such as malnutrition, failure to thrive,

and dehydration, also require innovative methods of care delivery involving physical therapists as key members of the geriatric health care team.

REFERENCES

1. Adair N: Chronic airflow obstruction and respiratory failure, in Hazard WR, et al (eds): *Principles of Geriatric Medicine and Gerontology.* New York, McGraw-Hill, 1994.
2. Aronow WS: Treatment of congestive heart failure in older persons. *J Am Geriatr Soc* 1997; 45:1252-1258.
3. Barents Group: *The Clinical Cost Effectiveness of Medical Nutrition Therapy: Evidence and Estimates of Potential Medicare Savings from the Use of Selected Nutritional Interventions.* (Summary Report for *The Nutrition Screening Initiative.*) Washington, DC, 1996.
4. Beck LH: Aging changes in renal function, in Hazard WR, et al (eds): *Principles of Geriatrric Medicine and Gerontology.* New York, McGraw-Hill, 1994.
5. Benfante R, Reed D: Is elevated serum cholesterol level a risk factor for coronary heart disease in the elderly? *JAMA* 1990; 263:393-396.
6. Bijnen FC, et al: Physical activity and cardiovascular risk factors among elderly men in Finland, Italy, and Netherlands. *Am J Epidemiol* 1996; 143:553-561.
7. Carmel R: Cobalmin, the stomach, and aging. *Am J Clin Nutr* 1997; 66:750
8. Castelli WP, Wilson P, Levy D, Anderson K: Cardiovascular risk factors in the elderly. *Am J Cardiol* 1989; 63:12H-19H.
9. Chima CS, et al: Relationship of nutritional status to length of stay, hospital cost, and discharge status of patients hospitalized in the medicine service. *J Am Diet Assoc* 1997; 97:975-978.

10. Codispoti CL, Bartlett BJ: Food and Nutrition for Life: Malnutrition and Older Americans. *Report by the Assistant Secretary for Aging Administration on Aging.* Department of Health and Human Services, Washington, DC, 1994.

11. Colledge NR, et al: Evaluation of investigations to diagnose the cause of dizziness in elderly people: A community based controlled study. *BMJ* 1996; 313(28):788-792.

12. Corti M, et al: HDL cholesterol predicts coronary heart disease mortality in older adults. *JAMA* 1995; 274:539-544.

13. Davis KM, Minaker KL: Disorders of fluid balance: Dehydration and hyponatremia, in Hazard WR, et al (eds): *Principles of Geriatric Medicine and Gerontology.* New York, McGraw-Hill, 1994.

14. Denke MA, Grundy SM: Hypercholesterolemia in elderly persons: Resolving the treatment dilemma. *Ann Intern Med* 1990; 112:780-792.

15. Dwyer J: *Nutrition Screening Manual for Professionals Caring for Older Americans.* Washington, DC, Nutrition Screening Initiative, 1991.

16. Fiatarone MA, O'Neil EF, Doyle N: Exercise training and nutritional supplements for physical frailty in very elderly people. *New Engl J Med* 1994; 330:1769-1775.

17. Fischback, F: *A Manual of Laboratory and Diagnostic Tests.* Philadelphia, JB Lippincott, 1994.

18. Fish LC, Davis KM, Minaker KL: Dehydration, in Morris J, Lipsitz L, Murphy K, Belleville-Taylor P, (eds): *Quality Care in the Nursing Home.* St Louis, Mosby, 1997.

19. Fries JF: Aging, natural death and the compression of morbidity. *New Engl J Med* 1980; 303:130-134.

20. Hansten PD, Steigbigel NH: Vitamin supplements, in Abramowicz M (ed): *The Medical Letter* 1998: 1032(40):75-77.

21. Konstam M, Dracup K, Baker D: Heart Failure: Management of Patients with Left Ventricular Systolic Dysfunction, *Clinical Practice Guideline, Publication No. 94-0612,* Agency for Health Care Policy and Research, Washington, DC, 1994.

22. Kushi LH, et al: Physical activity and mortality in postmenopausal women. *JAMA* 1997; 277:1287-1292.

23. LaRosa JC, et al: Cholesterol lowering in the elderly. Results of the cholesterol reduction in seniors program (CRISP) pilot study. *Arch Intern Med* 1994; 154:529-539.

24. Lavie CJ, Milani RV: Benefits of cardiac rehabilitation and exercise training in elderly women. *Am J Cardiol* 1997; 79:664-666.

25. Lavie CJ, Milani RV: Effects of cardiac rehabilitation programs on exercise capacity, coronary risk factors, behavioral characteristics, and quality of life in a large elderly cohort. *Am J Cardiol* 1995; 76:177-179.

26. Lipsitz L: Aging of the hematopoietic system, in Hazard WR, et al (eds): *Principles of Geriatric Medicine and Gerontology.* New York, McGraw-Hill, 1994.

27. McCarthy N, Hicks A, Martin J, Webber C: A longitudinal trial of weight training in the elderly: Continued improvement in 2 years. *J Gerontol* 1996; 51A:B425.

28. Miller DK, Morley JE, Rubenstein LZ, Pietruska FM: Abnormal eating attitudes and body image in older undernourished individuals. *J Am Geriatr Soc* 1991; 39:462-466.

29. Palmi JV, Lipsitz LA: Dizziness and syncope, in Hazzard WR, et al (eds): *Principles of Geriatric Medicine and Gerontology.* New York, McGraw-Hill, 1994.

30. Posner BM, et al: Nutritional risk in New England elders. *J Gerontol* 1994; 49:M123-M132.

31. Reuben DB, Yoshikawa TT, Besdine RW: *Geriatrics Review Syllabus.* Dubuque, Iowa, Kendall/Hunt Publishing Co, 1996.

32. Rush D: Evaluating the Nutrition Screening Initiative. *Am J Public Health* 1993; 83:944-945.

33. Sarkisian CA, Lachs MS: Failure to thrive in older adults. *Ann Intern Med* 1996; 124:1072-1078.

34. Shipley MJ, Pocock SJ, Marmot MG: Does plasma cholesterol concentration predict mortality from coronary heart disease in elderly people? 18 year follow up in Whitehall study. *BMJ* 1991; 303:89-92.

35. U.S. Department of Agriculture: *Food Guide Pyramid.* Washington, DC, US Government Printing Office, 1990.

36. Warren JL, et al: The burdens and outcome associated with dehydration among US elderly, 1991. *Am J Public Health* 1994; 84:1265-1269.

37. Wei JY: Disorders of the heart, in Hazard WR, et al (eds): *Principles of Geriatric Medicine and Gerontology.* New York, McGraw-Hill, 1994.

38. Weijenberg MP, Feskens E, Kromhout D: Total and high density lipoprotein cholesterol as risk factors for coronary heart disease in elderly men during 5 years of follow-up. *Am J Epidemiol* 1996; 143: 151-158.

39. Weinstein BE, Devons CA: The dizzy patient: Stepwise workup of a common complaint. *Geriatrics* 1995; 50:42-46.

40. Wolinski FD, Fitzgerald JF: Subsequent hip fracture among older adults. *Am J Public Health* 1994; 84:1316-1318.

41. Wongsurawat N: Thermoregulatory failure in the elderly. *JAMA* 1990; 38:899-903

CHAPTER 12

GERIATRIC PHARMACOLOGY

CHARLES D. CICCONE, PT, PhD

INTRODUCTION

Physical therapists working with any patient population must be aware of the drug regimen used in each patient. Therapists must have a basic understanding of the beneficial and adverse effects of each medication and must be cognizant of how specific drugs can interact with various rehabilitation procedures. This idea seems especially true for geriatric patients receiving physical therapy. The elderly are generally more sensitive to the adverse effects of drug therapy, and many adverse drug reactions impede the patient's progress and ability to participate in rehabilitation procedures. An adequate understanding of the patient's drug regimen, however, can help physical therapists recognize and deal with these adverse effects as well as capitalize on the beneficial effects of drug therapy in their geriatric patients.

The purpose of this chapter is to discuss some of the pertinent aspects of geriatric pharmacology with specific emphasis on how drug therapy can affect older individuals receiving physical therapy. This chapter begins by describing the pharmacological profile of the geriatric patient, with emphasis on why adverse drug reactions tend to occur more commonly in the elderly. Specific adverse drug reactions that commonly occur in the elderly are then discussed. Finally, the beneficial and adverse effects of specific medications are examined, along with how these medications can have an impact on the rehabilitation of the older adult.

PHARMACOLOGICAL PROFILE OF THE GERIATRIC PATIENT

In general, the elderly are two to three times more likely than younger adults to experience an adverse drug reaction.[160] The increased incidence of adverse drug effects in the elderly is influenced by two principal factors: the pattern of drug use that occurs in a geriatric population and the altered response to drug therapy in the elderly.[56,245] A number of other contributing factors such as multiple disease states, lack of proper drug testing, and problems with drug education and compliance also increase the likelihood of adverse effects in older adults. The influence of each of these factors on drug response in the elderly is discussed briefly here.

Pattern of Drug Use in the Elderly: Problems of Polypharmacy

The elderly consume a disproportionately large amount of drugs relative to younger people.[148,191,232] For example, adults older than 65 currently compose about 12% of the U.S. population, but they consume 33% of all prescription drugs.[216] By the year 2030, it is predicted that the elderly will account for 21% of the population and consume 40% of all drugs.[3]

A logical explanation for this disproportionate drug use is that the elderly take more drugs because they suffer more illnesses. Indeed, upward of 80% of individuals older than 65 suffer from one or more chronic conditions, and drug therapy is often the primary method used to treat these conditions.[212] For example, consumption of two or more different medications each day is common in the general population of people older than 65.[36,191,223] Drug use in certain elderly subpopulations is even higher, with nursing home residents receiving an average of five to eight prescription medications each day.[148] Use of nonprescription (over-the-counter) products is also an important factor in geriatric pharmacology, especially in the community dwelling elderly who have greater access to these products.[121]

The elderly therefore rely heavily on various prescription and nonprescription products, and medications are often essential in helping resolve or alleviate some of the illnesses and other medical complications that commonly occur in the elderly. A distinction must be made, however, between the reasonable and appropriate use of drugs and the phenomenon of polypharmacy. Polypharmacy occurs whenever the patient's drug regimen includes one or more unnecessary medications.[43] Owing to the extensive use of medications in this population, the elderly are often at high risk for polypharmacy.[13,30,88]

Polypharmacy can be distinguished from a more reasonable drug regimen by the criteria listed in Table 12-1. Of these criteria, the use of drugs to treat adverse drug reactions is especially important. The administration of drugs to treat drug-related reactions often creates a vicious cycle in which additional drugs are used to treat adverse drug reactions, thus creating more adverse effects, thereby initiating the use of more drugs, and so on (Fig. 12-1).[101] This cycle can rapidly accelerate until the patient is receiving a dozen or more medications.

In addition to the risk of creating the vicious cycle seen in Fig. 12-1, there are several other obvious drawbacks to polypharmacy in the elderly. Because each drug will in-

TABLE 12-1

CHARACTERISTICS OF POLYPHARMACY IN THE ELDERLY[*]

CHARACTERISTIC	EXAMPLE
Use of medications for no apparent reason	Digoxin use in patients who do not exhibit heart failure
Use of duplicate medications	Simultaneous use of two or three laxatives
Concurrent use of interacting medications	Simultaneous use of a laxative and an antidiarrheal agent
Use of contraindicated medications	Use of aspirin in bleeding ulcers
Use of inappropriate dosage	Failure to use a lower dose of a benzodiazepine sedative-hypnotic
Use of drug therapy to treat adverse drug reactions	Use of antacids to treat aspirin-induced gastric irritation
Patient improves when medications are discontinued	Withdrawal of a sedative-hypnotic results in clearer sensorium

[*]Adapted from Simonson W: *Medications and the Elderly: A Guide for Promoting Proper Use.* Rockville, Md, Aspen Publications, 1984.

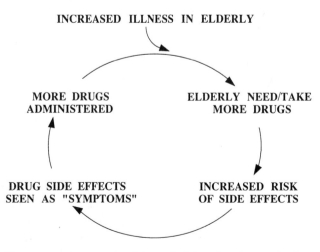

FIG. 12-1 Vicious cycle of drug administration that can lead to polypharmacy in the elderly.

evitably produce some side effects when used alone, the number of side effects will begin to accumulate when several agents are used concurrently.[12] More importantly, the interaction of one drug with another (drug-drug interaction) increases the risk of an untoward reaction because of the ability of one agent to modify the effects and metabolism of another drug. If many drugs are administered simultaneously, the risk of adverse drug reactions increases exponentially.[12,28] Other negative aspects of polypharmacy are the risk of decreased patient compliance with the drug regimen[196] and the increased financial burden of using large numbers of unnecessary drugs.[30,88]

Polypharmacy can occur in the elderly for a number of reasons. In particular, physicians may rely on drug therapy to accomplish goals that could be achieved through non-pharmacological methods, i.e., it is often relatively easy to prescribe a medication to resolve a problem in the older adult even though other methods that do not require drugs could be used. For instance, the patient who naps throughout the day will probably not be sleepy at bedtime. It is much easier to administer a sedative-hypnotic agent at bedtime rather than institute activities that keep the patient awake during the day and allow nocturnal sleep to occur naturally.

In some cases, the patient may also play a contributing role toward polypharmacy. Patients may obtain prescriptions from several different practitioners, thus accumulating a formidable list of prescription medications. Elderly individuals may receive medications from friends and family members who want to "share" the benefits of their prescription drugs. Some older adults may also use over-the-counter and self-help remedies to such an extent that these agents interact with one another and with their prescription medications.

Polypharmacy can be prevented if the patient's drug regimen is reviewed periodically and any unnecessary or harmful drugs are discontinued.[4,13,88,90] Also, new medications should only be administered if a thorough patient evaluation indicates that the drug is truly needed in that patient.[30] When several physicians are dealing with the same patient, these practitioners should make sure that they communicate with one another regarding the patient's drug regimen.[86] Physical therapists can play a role in preventing polypharmacy by recognizing any changes in the patient's response to drug therapy and helping to correctly identify these changes as drug reactions rather than disease "symptoms." In this way, therapists may help prevent the formation of the vicious cycle illustrated in Fig. 12-1.

Altered Response to Drugs

There is little doubt that the response to many drugs is affected by age and that the therapeutic and toxic effects of any medication will be different in an older adult than in a younger individual. Alterations in drug response in the elderly can be attributed to differences in the way the body handles the drug (pharmacokinetic changes) as well as differences in the way the drug affects the body (pharmacody-

namic changes).[245] The effects of aging on drug pharmacokinetics and pharmacodynamics are discussed briefly here.

Pharmacokinetic Changes

Pharmacokinetics is the study of how the body handles a drug, including how the drug is absorbed, distributed, metabolized, and excreted. Several changes in physiological function occur as a result of aging that alter pharmacokinetic parameters in the elderly. The principal pharmacokinetic changes associated with aging are summarized in Fig. 12-2 and are discussed briefly here. The effects of aging on pharmacokinetics has been the subject of fairly extensive research, and the reader is referred to several excellent reviews for more information on this topic.[42,54,170,244,245]

Drug Absorption

Several well-documented changes occur in gastrointestinal (GI) function in the older adult that could potentially affect the way drugs are absorbed from the GI tract. Such changes include decreased gastric acid production, decreased gastric emptying, decreased GI blood flow, diminished area of the absorptive surface, and decreased intestinal motility.[42,62,244] The effect of these changes on drug absorption, however, is often inconsistent, i.e., aging does not appear to significantly alter the absorption of most orally administered drugs. This may be due in part to the fact that the aforementioned

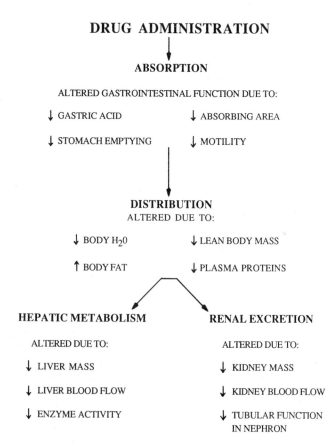

FIG. 12-2 Summary of the physiological effects of aging that may alter pharmacokinetics in the elderly.

changes may offset one another. For instance, factors that tend to decrease absorption (e.g., decreased GI blood flow, decreased absorptive surface area) could be counterbalanced by factors that allow the drug to remain in the gut for longer periods (decreased GI motility), thus allowing more time for absorption. Hence, altered drug absorption does not appear to be a major factor in determining pharmacokinetic changes in the elderly.

Drug Distribution

After a drug is absorbed into the body, it undergoes distribution to various tissues and body fluid compartments (e.g., vascular system, intracellular fluid, and so forth). Drug distribution may be altered in the elderly due to several physiological changes such as decreased total body water, decreased lean body mass, increased percent body fat, and decreased plasma protein concentrations.[170,244] Depending on the specific drug, these changes can affect how the drug is distributed in the body, thus potentially changing the response to the drug. For instance, drugs that bind to plasma proteins (e.g., aspirin, warfarin) may produce a greater response because there will be less drug bound to plasma proteins and more of the drug will be free to reach the target tissue. Drugs that are soluble in water (e.g., alcohol, morphine) will be relatively more concentrated in the body since there is less body water in which to dissolve the drug. Increased percentages of body fat can act as a reservoir for lipid-soluble drugs, and problems related to drug storage may occur with these agents. Hence, these potential problems in drug distribution must be anticipated, and dosages must be adjusted accordingly in elderly individuals.

Drug Metabolism

The principal role of drug metabolism (biotransformation) is to inactivate drugs and create water-soluble by-products (metabolites) that can be excreted by the kidneys. Although some degree of drug metabolism can occur in tissues throughout the body, the liver is the primary site for metabolism of most medications. Several distinct changes in liver function occur with aging that affect hepatic drug metabolism. The total drug-metabolizing capacity of the liver decreases with age because of a reduction in liver mass, a decline in hepatic blood flow, and decreased activity of drug-metabolizing enzymes.[130,135,170,264,265] As a result, drugs that undergo inactivation in the liver will remain active for longer periods because of the general decrease in the hepatic-metabolizing capacity seen in older adults.

Drug Excretion

The kidneys are the primary routes for drug excretion from the body. Drugs reach the kidney in either their active form or as a drug metabolite after biotransformation in the liver. In either case, it is the kidney's responsibility to filter the drug from the circulation and excrete it from the body via the urine. With aging, declines in renal blood flow, renal mass, and function of renal tubules result in a reduced ability of the kidneys to excrete drugs and their metabolites.[54,131,152,244] These changes in renal function tend to be one of the most important factors affecting drug pharmacokinetics in the elderly, and reduced renal function should be taken into account whenever drugs are prescribed to these individuals.[19,152]

The cumulative effect of the pharmacokinetic changes associated with aging is that drugs and drug metabolites often remain active for longer periods, thus prolonging drug effects and increasing the risk for toxic side effects. This is evidenced by the fact that drug half-life (the time required to eliminate 50% of the drug remaining in the body) is often substantially longer in an older individual versus a younger adult.[28,32] For example, the half-life of certain medications such as the benzodiazepines (e.g., diazepam [Valium], chlordiazepoxide [Librium]) can be increased as much as fourfold in the elderly.[83] Obviously, this represents a dramatic change in the way the elderly body deals with certain pharmacological agents. Altered pharmacokinetics in the elderly must be anticipated by evaluating changes in body composition (e.g., decreased body water, increased percentages of body fat) and monitoring changes in organ function (e.g., decreased hepatic and renal function) so that drug dosages can be adjusted and adverse drug reactions minimized in elderly individuals.[149,152,170,177]

Finally, it should be noted that the age-related pharmacokinetic changes described here vary considerably from person to person within the geriatric population.[177] These changes are, however, considered part of the "normal" aging process. Any disease or illness that affects drug distribution, metabolism, or excretion will cause an additional change in pharmacokinetic variables, thus further increasing the risk of adverse drug reactions in the elderly.[32,82,177]

Pharmacodynamic Changes

Pharmacodynamics is the study of how drugs affect the body, including systemic drug effects as well as cellular and biochemical mechanisms of drug action. Changes in the control of different physiological systems can influence the systemic response to various drugs in the elderly.[229,244] For instance, deficits in the homeostatic control of circulation (e.g., decreased baroreceptor sensitivity, decreased vascular compliance) may change the response of the elderly patient to cardiovascular medications. Other age-related changes, such as impaired postural control, decreased visceral muscle function, altered thermoregulatory responses, and declines in cognitive ability, can alter the pharmacotherapeutic response as well as the potential side effects that may occur when various agents are administered to the older adult.[229] The degree to which systemic drug response is altered will vary depending on the magnitude of these physiological changes in each individual.

In addition to these systemic changes, the way a drug affects tissues on a cellular level may be different in the older adult. Most drugs exert their effects by first binding to a receptor that is located on or within the specific target cells that are influenced by each type of drug. This receptor is usually coupled in some way to the biochemical "machinery" of the target cell, so that when the drug binds to the receptor, a biochemical event occurs that changes cell function in a predictable way (Fig. 12-3). For instance, binding of epinephrine (adrenaline) to beta-1-receptors on myocardial cells causes an increase in the activity of certain intracellular enzymes, which in turn causes an increase in heart rate and contractile force. Similar mechanisms can be described for other drugs and their respective cellular receptors. The altered response to certain drugs seen in the elderly may be caused by one or more of the cellular changes depicted in Fig. 12-3. For instance, alterations in the drug-receptor attraction (affinity) could help explain an increase or decrease in the sensitivity of the older adult to various medications.[14,198,229] Likewise, changes in the way the receptor is linked or coupled to the cell's internal biochemistry have been noted in certain tissues as a function of aging.[85,163] Finally, the actual biochemical response within the cell may be blunted because of changes in cellular structure and function that occur with aging.[110,229]

Consequently, pharmacodynamics may be altered in the elderly due to systemic physiological changes acting in combination with changes in drug responsiveness that occur on a cellular or even subcellular level. These pharmacodynamic changes along with the pharmacokinetic changes discussed earlier help explain why the response of a geriatric individual to drug therapy often differs from the analogous response in a younger individual.

Other Factors That Increase the Risk of Adverse Drug Reactions in the Elderly

In addition to the pattern of drug use and the altered response to drugs seen in the elderly, several other factors may also contribute to the increased incidence of adverse drug reactions seen in these individuals. Several of these additional factors are presented here.

Presence of Multiple Disease States

The fact that elderly people often suffer from several chronic conditions greatly increases the risk of adverse drug reactions.[32] The presence of more than one disease (comorbidity) often necessitates the use of several drugs, thus increasing the risk of drug-drug interactions. Even more important is the fact that various diseases and illnesses usually alter the pharmacokinetic and pharmacodynamic variables discussed earlier. For instance, the age-related changes in hepatic metabolism and renal excretion of drugs are affected to an even greater extent if liver or kidney disease is present. Many elderly patients suffer from diseases that further decrease function in both of these organs as well as cause diminished function in other physiological systems. The involvement of several organ systems, combined with the presence of several different drugs, makes the chance of an adverse drug reaction almost inevitable in the elderly patient with multiple disease states.

Lack of Proper Drug Testing and Regulation

The Food and Drug Administration (FDA) is responsible for monitoring the safety and efficacy of all drugs marketed in the United States. The FDA requires all drugs to undergo extensive preclinical (animal) and clinical (human) trials before they receive approval. With regard to the elderly, some question has been raised about the evaluation of drugs in geriatric individuals prior to FDA approval. It has been recognized that an adequate number of patients older than 65 should be included at various stages of the clinical testing, especially for drugs that are targeted for problems that occur in the elderly (e.g., Parkinson's disease and dementia).[3] It is unclear, however, whether efforts to increase drug testing in geriatric subjects have been successful in providing improved information about drug safety in older adults.[1] Additional efforts on the part of the FDA and the drug manufacturing companies may be necessary to help reduce the risk of adverse side effects through better drug testing.

There also has been concern that many drugs are overprescribed and misused in older adults. This concern seems especially true for certain classes of psychotropic agents (e.g., antipsychotics, sedative-hypnotic agents).[178,220] Fortunately, efforts have been made to institute government regulations and guidelines that limit the use of these medications.[140,220,267] Enforcement of existing regulations and development of guidelines for other types of drugs will hopefully reduce the incidence of inappropriate drug use in older adults.

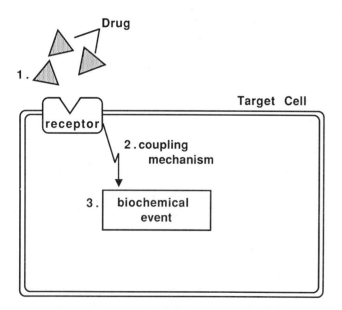

Fig. 12-3   Potential sites for altered cellular responses in the elderly. Changes may occur (1) in drug-receptor affinity, (2) in the coupling of the receptor to an intracellular biochemical event, and (3) in the cell's ability to generate a specific biochemical response.

Problems with Patient Education and Self-Adherence to Drug Therapy

Even the most appropriate and well-planned drug regimen will be useless if the drugs are not taken as directed. Patients may experience an increase in adverse side effects, especially if drugs are taken in excessive doses or for the wrong reason.[196] Conversely, elderly patients may stop taking their medications, resulting in a lack of therapeutic effects and a possible increase in disease symptoms. The fact that older patients often neglect to take their medications is one of the most common types of drug noncompliance.[196]

Many factors can disrupt the older individual's self-adherence (compliance) to drug therapy. A decline in cognitive function, for example, may impair the older person's ability to understand instructions given by the physician, nurse practitioner, or pharmacist. This can hamper the ability of the geriatric patient to take drugs according to the proper dosing schedule, especially if several different medications are being administered, with a different dosing schedule for each medication.[196,232] Other factors such as poor eyesight may limit the older person's ability to distinguish one pill from another, and arthritic changes may make it difficult to open certain "childproof" containers.

The older adult may also stop taking a medication because of an annoying but unavoidable side effect.[196] For instance, the elderly patient with hypertension may refuse to take a diuretic because this particular medication increases urinary output and may necessitate several trips to the bathroom in the middle of the night. To encourage patient self-adherence, it must be realized that these annoying side effects are not trivial and can represent a major source of concern to the patient. Hence, health care professionals should not dismiss these complaints but should make an extra effort to help the patient understand the importance of adhering to the drug regimen whenever such unavoidable side effects are present.

Additional Factors

Other factors, including poor diet, excessive use of over-the-counter products, cigarette smoking, and consumption of various other substances (e.g., caffeine, alcohol), may help contribute to the increased risk of adverse drug effects in the elderly.[9,31,195] These factors must be taken into consideration when a prescription drug program is implemented for the elderly individual. For instance, it must be realized that the older adult with a protein-deficient diet may have extremely low plasma protein levels, thus further altering drug pharmacokinetics and increasing the risk of an adverse drug effect. It is therefore important to consider all aspects of the life-style and environment of the older adult that may affect drug therapy in these individuals.

COMMON ADVERSE DRUG REACTIONS IN THE ELDERLY

An adverse drug reaction (ADR) is any unwanted and potentially harmful effect caused by a drug when the drug is given at the recommended dosage.[212] Listed here are some of the more common ADRs that may occur in older adults. Of course, this is not a complete list of all the potential ADRs,

but these are some of the responses that physical therapists should be aware of when dealing with geriatric patients in a rehabilitation setting.

Gastrointestinal Symptoms

GI problems such as nausea, vomiting, and diarrhea are among the most commonly occurring adverse drug reactions in the elderly.[12,89] These reactions can occur with virtually any medication, and GI symptoms are especially prevalent with certain medications such as the opioid (narcotic) and non-opioid (non-steroidal anti-inflammatory drugs) (NSAIDs) analgesics. Although these symptoms are sometimes mild and transient in younger patients, elderly individuals often require adjustments in the type and dosage of specific medications that cause gastrointestinal problems.

Sedation

The elderly seem especially susceptible to drowsiness and sleepiness as a side effect of many medications. In particular, drugs that produce sedation as a primary effect (e.g., sedative-hypnotics) as well as drugs with sedative side effects (e.g., opioid analgesics, antipsychotics) will often produce excessive drowsiness in older adults.

Confusion

Various degrees of confusion ranging from mild disorientation to delirium may occur with a number of medications, such as antidepressants, narcotic analgesics, and drugs with anticholinergic activity.[192] Confusion can also indicate that certain drugs, such as lithium and digoxin, are accumulating and reaching toxic levels in the body. Elderly individuals who are already somewhat confused may be more susceptible to drugs that tend to further increase confusion.

Depression

Symptoms of depression (e.g., intense sadness and apathy, as described elsewhere in this text) may be induced in older adults by certain medications. Drugs such as barbiturates, antipsychotics, alcohol, and several antihypertensive agents (e.g., clonidine, reserpine, propranolol) have been implicated in producing depression as an ADR in the elderly.[22]

Orthostatic Hypotension

Orthostatic (postural) hypotension is typically described as a 20 mm Hg or greater decline in systolic blood pressure or a 10 mm Hg or greater decline in diastolic blood pressure that occurs when an individual assumes a more upright posture (e.g., moving from lying to sitting or from sitting to standing).[226] Owing to the fact that many older adults are relatively sedentary and have diminished cardiovascular function, these individuals tend to be more susceptible to episodes of orthostatic hypotension, even without the influence of drug therapy.[48,112] A number of medications, however, augment the incidence and severity of this blood pressure decline.[48,251] In particular, drugs that tend to lower blood pressure (e.g., antihypertensives, antianginal medications) are a common cause of orthostatic hypotension in older adults. Orthostatic hypotension often leads to dizziness and syncope because blood pressure is too low to provide adequate cerebral perfusion and oxygen delivery to the brain. Hence, orthostatic hypotension may precipitate falls and subsequent injury (e.g., hip fractures, other trauma) in elderly individuals.[171] Since elderly patients are especially susceptible to episodes of orthostatic hypotension during certain rehabilitation procedures (e.g., gait training, functional activities), physical therapists should be especially alert for this ADR.

Fatigue and Weakness

Strength loss and muscular weakness may occur for a number of reasons in response to drug therapy. Some agents, such as the skeletal muscle relaxants, may directly decrease muscle contraction strength, whereas other drugs, such as the diuretics, may affect muscle strength by altering fluid and electrolyte balance. Elderly individuals who are already debilitated will be more susceptible to strength loss as an ADR.

Dizziness and Falls

Drug-induced dizziness can be especially detrimental in older adults because of the increased risk of loss of balance and falling. Problems with dizziness result from drugs that produce sedation or from agents that directly affect vestibular function. Examples of such agents include sedatives, antipsychotics, opioid analgesics, and antihistamine drugs.[141,154,184,236,239] Dizziness may also occur secondary to drugs that cause orthostatic hypotension (see previous discussion). Drug-induced dizziness and increased risk of falling may be especially prevalent in older adults who already exhibit balance problems, and physical therapists should be especially alert for these ADRs in these individuals.

Anticholinergic Effects

Acetylcholine is an important neurotransmitter that controls function in the central nervous system and also affects peripheral organs such as the heart, lungs, and GI tract. A number of drugs exhibit anticholinergic side effects, meaning that these agents tend to diminish the response of various tissues to acetylcholine. In particular, antihistamines, antidepressants, and certain antipsychotics tend to exhibit anticholinergic side effects. Acetylcholine affects several diverse physiological systems throughout the body, and drugs with anticholinergic effects are therefore associated with a wide range of ADRs. Drugs with anticholinergic effects may produce central nervous system effects such as confusion, nervousness, drowsiness, and dizziness. Peripheral anticholinergic effects include dry mouth, constipation, urinary retention, tachycardia, and blurred vision. The elderly seem to be more sensitive to anticholinergic effects, possibly due to the fact that acetylcholine influence has already started to diminish as a result of the aging process. In any event, physical therapists should be aware that a rather diverse array of potentially serious ADRs may arise from drugs with anticholinergic properties.

Extrapyramidal Symptoms

Drugs that produce side effects that mimic extrapyramidal tract lesions are said to exhibit extrapyramidal symptoms. Such symptoms include tardive dyskinesia, pseudoparkinsonism, akathisia, and other dystonias. Antipsychotic medications are commonly associated with an increased risk of extrapyramidal symptoms. The problem of extrapyramidal symptoms as an antipsychotic ADR is presented in more detail later in this chapter.

DRUG CLASSES COMMONLY USED IN THE ELDERLY: IMPACT ON PHYSICAL THERAPY

This section provides a brief overview of drug therapy in the elderly. Included are some of the more common groups of drugs that are prescribed to older adults. For each group, the principal clinical indication or indications are listed, along with a brief description of the mechanism of action of each type of drug. The primary adverse effects and any specific concerns for physical therapy in elderly patients receiving these drugs are also discussed. Examples of typical drugs found in each of the major groups are indicated in several tables in this section. For additional information about specific agents listed here, the reader can refer to one of the sources listed at the end of this chapter.[39,91,176]

Psychotropic Medications

Psychotropic drugs include a variety of agents that affect mood, behavior, and other aspects of mental function. As a group, the elderly exhibit a high incidence of psychiatric disorders.[106,237] Psychotropic drugs are therefore commonly used in elderly individuals and are also associated with a high incidence of adverse effects that can have an impact on rehabilitation.[155,219] The major groups of psychotropic drugs are listed in Table 12-2, and pertinent aspects of each group are discussed here.

Sedative-Hypnotic and Antianxiety Agents

Sedative-hypnotic drugs are used to relax the patient and promote a relatively normal state of sleep. Antianxiety drugs are intended to decrease anxiety without producing excessive sedation. Insomnia and disordered sleep may occur in elderly individuals concomitant to normal aging or in response to medical problems and life-style changes that occur with advanced age.[80,132,153] Likewise, medical illness, depression, and other aspects of aging may result in increased feelings of fear and apprehension in older adults.[16,65,100,203,224,256,261] Hence, use of sedative-hypnotic and antianxiety drugs is commonly encountered in the elderly.

The primary group of agents used to promote sleep and decrease anxiety in the elderly is the benzodiazepines (see Table 12-2).[16,132,224] Benzodiazepines are typically regarded as

TABLE 12-2
PSYCHOTROPIC DRUG GROUPS

	COMMON EXAMPLES	
GROUP	GENERIC NAME	TRADE NAME
Sedative-Hypnotic Agents		
Benzodiazepines	Flurazepam	Dalmane
	Temazepam	Restoril
	Triazolam	Halcion
Barbiturates	Pentobarbital	Nembutal
	Secobarbital	Seconal Sodium
Antianxiety Agents		
Benzodiazepines	Chlordiazepoxide	Librium
	Diazepam	Valium
	Lorazepam	Ativan
Azapirones	Buspirone	BuSpar
Antidepressants		
Tricyclics	Amitryptyline	Elavil, Endep
	Imipramine	Tofranil, Tripramine
MAO* inhibitors	Isocarboxazid	Marplan
	Phenelzine	Nardil
Second-generation agents	Bupropion	Wellbutrin
	Maprotiline	Ludiomil
	Fluoxetine	Prozac
Antipsychotics		
Phenothiazines	Chlorpromazine	Thorazine
	Thioridazine	Mellaril
Thioxanthenes	Chlorprothixene	Taractan
	Thiothixene	Navane
Butyrophenones	Haloperidol	Haldol

*MAO = monoamine oxidase.

the principal sedative-hypnotic and antianxiety drugs because they are somewhat safer and more effective than other agents, such as the barbiturates and meprobamate (Miltown).[107] Benzodiazepines exert their beneficial effects by increasing the central inhibitory effect of the neurotransmitter gamma-aminobutyric acid (GABA).[231] This increase in GABA-mediated inhibition seems to account for the decreased anxiety and increased sleepiness associated with these drugs.

Despite the relative safety of currently used agents, several problems still occur when benzodiazepines are used to treat insomnia in the elderly. For instance, residual or "hangover" effects may occur, producing drowsiness and sluggishness the morning after a sedative-hypnotic is used. These effects seem especially prevalent if a relatively long-acting benzodiazepine, such as chlordiazepoxide, diazepam, or flurazepam, is administered to an older patient.[81] Physical therapists should be especially aware of the possibility of residual effects of sedative-hypnotic drugs when scheduling elderly patients for rehabilitation first thing in the morning. Other potential adverse effects include "anterograde amnesia," in which patients have lapses in short-term memory for the period immediately preceding drug administration and "rebound insomnia," in which sleeplessness increases when the drug is discontinued.[132]

Use of benzodiazepines to treat sleep disorders can also result in problems associated with addiction if these drugs are used indiscriminately for prolonged periods (4 weeks or longer).[132] These problems include the need to progressively increase dosage to achieve beneficial effects (tolerance) and the onset of withdrawal symptoms when the drug is discontinued (physical dependence). Clearly, benzodiazepines can help the older patient cope with occasional sleep disturbances, but these drugs should be used at the lowest possible dose and for only short periods while trying to find nonpharmacological methods (e.g., counseling and decreased caffeine use) to deal with the patient's insomnia.[25,132,153]

Benzodiazepines are also associated with specific adverse responses when used to treat anxiety in older adults. As previously described, these agents can cause tolerance and physical dependence when used for prolonged periods. Likewise, sedation and cognitive impairment are possible side effects when benzodiazepines are used to treat anxiety in the elderly.[222] Physical therapists should therefore realize that the use of benzodiazepines in elderly patients is a two-edged sword. Decreased anxiety may enable the patient to be more relaxed and cooperative during rehabilitation, but any benefits will be negated if the patient experiences significant psychomotor slowing and is unable to remain alert during the therapy session.

In order to treat anxiety more effectively in the elderly, newer agents known as the azapirones (e.g., buspirone) have been developed.[27,222] These agents appear to decrease anxiety by directly stimulating serotonin receptors in certain parts of the brain (dorsal raphe nucleus) rather than by increasing GABA-mediated inhibition like the benzodiazepines.[27] More importantly, azapirones such as buspirone do not cause sedation, do not impair cognition and psychomotor function, and appear to have a much lower potential for the patient developing tolerance and physical dependence than traditional agents such as the benzodiazepines.[27,172] Azapirones are therefore much better tolerated in older adults and are used increasingly in the treatment of various forms of anxiety in the elderly.[27,172] It will be interesting to see whether buspirone and similar azapirones continue to gain favor as drugs of choice in treating anxiety in older adults.

Antidepressants

Depression is the most common form of mental illness in the general population as well as the most commonly observed mental disorder in the elderly.[190] Feelings of intense sadness, hopelessness, and other symptoms may occur in the elderly after a specific event (e.g., loss of a spouse, acute illness) or in response to the gradual decline in health and functional status often associated with aging. Drug therapy may be instituted to help resolve these symptoms, along with other nonpharmacological methods, such as counseling and behavioral therapy.

There are several distinct groups of antidepressant medications: tricyclics, monoamine oxidase (MAO) inhibitors, and the newer "second-generation" drugs (see Table 12-2).

All antidepressant drugs share a common goal—to increase synaptic transmission in central neural pathways that use amine neurotransmitters such as norepinephrine, dopamine, or 5-hydroxytryptamine (serotonin). The rationale is that symptoms of depression are due to hypersensitivity of central amine receptors, and drugs that bring about overstimulation of these receptors will cause a compensatory decrease (downregulation) in the number of functioning receptors.[102] As receptor sensitivity stabilizes, the clinical symptoms of depression appear to be resolved.

A primary focus in treating depression in the elderly has been identifying which agents produce the best effects with the least side effects.[243] In the past, tricyclic antidepressants were often the drugs of choice, even though these drugs tend to produce anticholinergic and other side effects (see the following discussion). Certain second-generation drugs, however, appear to be as effective as the tricyclics but may be better tolerated in older adults. In particular, agents such as fluoxetine (Prozac), sertraline (Zoloft), and paroxetine (Paxil) have been advocated as drugs of choice in the elderly because they generally have fewer severe side effects than other antidepressants.[60,63,92,168,214] These agents are known collectively as selective serotonin reuptake inhibitors (SSRIs) because they tend to preferentially affect CNS synapses that use serotonin as a neurotransmitter rather than affect synapses using other amine transmitters, such as norepinephrine or dopamine. Considerable debate still exists, however, and optimal use of SSRIs and other antidepressants in the elderly remains under investigation.[206,243]

Antidepressants produce various side effects, depending on the particular type of drug. As indicated earlier, tricyclic antidepressants produce anticholinergic effects and may cause dry mouth, constipation, urinary retention, and central nervous system (CNS) symptoms such as confusion, cognitive impairment, and delirium. Tricyclics also cause sedation and orthostatic hypotension, and these drugs can produce serious cardiotoxic effects after overdose.[214] Monoamine oxidase inhibitors also produce orthostatic hypotension and tend to cause insomnia. Side effects associated with the second-generation drugs vary depending on the specific agent. As previously noted, certain effects that are particularly troublesome in the elderly (i.e., sedation, anticholinergic effects, orthostatic hypotension) tend to occur less frequently with the SSRIs. SSRIs, however, have a greater tendency to cause other bothersome effects, such as GI distress.[92]

Physical therapists should be aware that antidepressants may help improve the patient's mood and increase the patient's interest in physical therapy. Certain side effects, however, such as sedation and confusion may impair the patient's cognitive ability and make it difficult for some elderly patients to participate actively in rehabilitation procedures. Hence, selection of drugs that minimize these effects may be especially helpful. Therapists should also be aware that it may take 6 or more weeks from the onset of drug therapy until an improvement occurs in the depressive symptoms. This substantial time lag is critical because the patient may actually become more depressed before mood begins to improve. Therapists should therefore look for signs that depression is worsening, especially during the first few weeks of antidepressant drug therapy. A suspected increase in depressive symptoms should be brought to the attention of the appropriate member of the health care team (e.g., physician or psychologist).

Manic-Depression: Lithium Treatment

As the name implies, manic-depression is a form of mental illness characterized by mood swings from an excited, hyperactive state (mania) to periods of apathy and dysphoria (depression). Although the cause of manic-depression is unknown, this condition responds fairly well to the drug lithium. It is not exactly clear how lithium prevents episodes of manic-depression, but this drug may prevent the excitable, or manic, phase of this disorder, thus stabilizing disposition and preventing the mood swings characteristic of this disease.[210]

It is important to be aware of the use of lithium for the treatment of manic-depression in elderly patients since this drug can rapidly accumulate to toxic levels in these individuals.[117] Lithium is an element and cannot be degraded in the body to an inactive form. The body must therefore rely solely on renal excretion to eliminate this drug. Because renal function is reduced in the elderly, the elimination of this drug is often impaired. Accumulation of lithium beyond a certain level results in lithium toxicity.[117] Symptoms of mild lithium toxicity include a metallic taste in the mouth, fine hand tremor, nausea, and muscular weakness and fatigue. These symptoms increase as toxicity reaches moderate levels, and other CNS signs such as blurred vision and incoordination may appear. Severe lithium toxicity may cause irreversible cerebellar damage,[117] and prolonged lithium neurotoxicity can lead to coma and even death.

Hence, physical therapists working with elderly patients who are taking lithium must continually be alert for any signs of lithium toxicity. This idea is especially important if there is any change in the patient's health or activity level that might cause an additional compromise in lithium excretion.

Antipsychotics

Antipsychotic medications are often used to help normalize behavior in older adults. *Psychosis* is the term used to describe the more severe forms of mental illness that are characterized by marked thought disturbances and altered perceptions of reality.[118] Aggressive, disordered behavior may also accompany symptoms of psychosis. In the elderly, psychotic-like behavior may occur because of actual psychotic syndromes (e.g., schizophrenia, severe paranoid disorders) or may be associated with various forms of dementia.[119,238,258] In any event, antipsychotic drugs may be helpful in improving behavior and compliance in elderly patients.

There are several major chemical classifications of antipsychotic drugs (see Table 12-2). These drugs all share a common mechanism in that they impair synaptic transmission in central dopamine pathways.[70,267] It is theorized that psychosis may be due to increased central dopamine influence. Antipsychotic drugs are believed to reduce this dopaminergic influence, thus helping to decrease psychotic-like behavior.

Antipsychotic drugs are associated with several annoying but fairly minor side effects, such as sedation and anticholinergic effects (e.g., dry mouth, constipation). Orthostatic hypotension may also occur, especially within the first few days after drug treatment is initiated. A more serious concern with antipsychotic drugs is the possibility of extrapyramidal side effects.[109,242] As discussed earlier in this chapter, motor symptoms that mimic lesions in the extrapyramidal tracts are a common ADR associated with these medications, especially in the elderly.[109] For instance, patients may exhibit involuntary movements of the face, jaw, and extremities (tardive dyskinesia), symptoms that resemble Parkinson's disease (pseudoparkinsonism), extreme restlessness (akathisia), or other problems with involuntary muscle movements (dystonias).[75,124,193] Early recognition of these extrapyramidal signs is important since they may persist long after the antipsychotic drug is discontinued, or these signs may even remain permanently. This fact seems especially true for drug-induced tardive dyskinesia, which may be irreversible if antipsychotic drug therapy is not altered when these symptoms first appear.[124]

The use of antipsychotic drugs may have beneficial effects on rehabilitation outcomes since patients may become more cooperative and less agitated during physical therapy. Therapists should be especially alert for the onset of any extrapyramidal symptoms because of the potential that these symptoms may result in long-term or permanent motor side effects. Therapists should realize, however, that antipsychotics have often been used inappropriately in older adults.[178,219,220] These medications are approved to help control certain psychotic-related symptoms, including behavioral problems such as aggression and severe agitation. These drugs, however, should not be used indiscriminately as "tranquilizers" to control all unwanted behaviors in the elderly. As indicated earlier, government regulations have been instituted to help decrease the inappropriate and unnecessary use of these medications in older adults.[227,267]

Treatment of Dementia

Dementia is a term used to describe a fairly global decline in intellectual function, with marked impairments in cognition, speech, personality, and other skills.[47] Some forms of dementia may be due to specific factors such as an infection, metabolic disorder, or an adverse reaction to drugs that have psychoactive side effects.[192,258] These so-called reversible dementias are often resolved if the precipitating factor is identified and corrected. Irreversible dementia is typically associated with progressive degenerative changes in cortical structure and function such as those occurring in Alzheimer's disease. Drug treatment of irreversible dementia follows two primary strategies: improving cognitive function and treating behavioral symptoms. These strategies are discussed briefly here.

In the past, attempts to improve cognitive function using various medications resulted in only limited success in persons with irreversible dementia. Recent drug development, however, has focused on the use of agents that increase acetylcholine function in the brain. It is known that acetylcholine influence in the brain begins to diminish because of the neuronal degeneration inherent to Alzheimer's disease. Therefore, drugs that increase cholinergic activity may help improve intellectual and cognitive function in persons with Alzheimer-type dementia. As a result, agents such as tacrine (Cognex) and donepezil (Aricept) have been developed to specifically improve cognition and behavioral function in persons with Alzheimer's disease.[53,235] These drugs inhibit the acetylcholinesterase enzyme, thus decreasing acetylcholine breakdown and prolonging the activity of this neurotransmitter in the brain.

Regrettably, cholinergic stimulants provide only moderate benefits in patients who are in the relatively early stages of this disease,[250] i.e., these drugs may help patients retain more cognitive and intellectual function during the mild to moderate stages of Alzheimer's disease, but these benefits are eventually lost as the disease progresses. Likewise, these drugs do not appear to delay the neurodegenerative changes that underlie this disease, and side effects such as GI distress and liver toxicity may limit the use of these drugs in some patients.[6,250] Still, these agents may help sustain cognitive function during the early course of Alzheimer's disease, thus enabling patients to continue to participate in various activities, including physical therapy. Other pharmacological strategies that enhance cognition or delay the degenerative changes in Alzheimer's disease are currently being explored, and these strategies may help provide more long-lasting effects in the future.[161,203]

Consequently, there do not appear to be any drugs at present that conclusively improve or maintain intellectual function in patients with advanced cases of irreversible dementia. However, some of the other drugs already discussed in this chapter may be used to help normalize and control behavior in patients with Alzheimer's disease and other forms of dementia. In particular, antipsychotic drugs may help improve certain aspects of behavior, such as decreased hallucinations and diminished feelings of hostility and suspiciousness.[57,215,227] Response to these drugs, however, is highly variable, and side effects are quite common when these drugs are given to older people.[47]

As noted earlier, efforts are also being made to decrease the indiscriminate use of antipsychotics in persons with Alzheimer's disease. For example, nonpharmacological interventions such as therapeutic activities, environmental modification, and care-giver support/education should be considered before resorting to drug therapy.[64,182,204,227,234] If drug therapy is required, choice of a specific medication should be based on the specific symptoms exhibited by each patient.[204] For example, the severely anxious patient may respond better to an antianxiety drug, the depressed patient may respond to an antidepressant, and so on.[234] The idea that antipsychotics are not a panacea for all dementia-like symptoms is certainly worth considering, and the use of alternative interventions may decrease the incidence of polypharmacy and antipsychotic-related side effects.

Neurological Agents

In addition to the drugs that affect mood and behavior, there are specific agents that are important in controlling certain neurological conditions in the elderly. Drug treatment of two of these conditions, Parkinson's disease and seizure disorders, is discussed here.

Drugs Used for Parkinson's Disease

Parkinson's disease is one of the more prevalent disorders in the elderly, with more than 1% of the population older than 60 years of age being afflicted. This disease is caused by the degeneration of dopamine-secreting neurons located in the basal ganglia.[50] Loss of dopaminergic influence initiates an imbalance in other neurotransmitters, including an increase in acetylcholine influence. This disruption in transmitter activity ultimately results in the typical parkinsonian motor symptoms of rigidity, bradykinesia, resting tremor, and postural instability.[50]

Drug treatment of Parkinson's disease usually focuses on restoring the balance of neurotransmitters in the basal ganglia.[50,188] The most common way of achieving this is to administer 3,4-dihydroxyphenylalanine (dopa), which is the immediate precursor to dopamine. Dopamine itself will not cross the blood-brain barrier, meaning that dopamine will not move from the bloodstream into the brain, where it is ultimately needed. However, levodopa (the L-isomer of dopa) will pass easily from the bloodstream into the brain, where it can then be transformed into dopamine and help restore the influence of this neurotransmitter in the basal ganglia.

Levodopa is often administered orally with a drug known as carbidopa. Carbidopa inhibits the enzyme that transforms levodopa to dopamine in the peripheral circulation, thus allowing levodopa to cross into the brain before it is finally converted to dopamine. If levodopa is converted to dopamine before reaching the brain, the dopamine will be useless in Parkinson's disease because it becomes trapped in the peripheral circulation. The simultaneous use of carbidopa and levodopa allows smaller doses of levodopa to be administered, because less of the levodopa will be wasted due to premature conversion to dopamine in the periphery.

Levodopa therapy often produces dramatic beneficial effects, especially during the mild to moderate stages of Parkinson's disease. Nonetheless, levodopa is associated with several troublesome side effects.[50] In particular, levodopa may cause GI distress (e.g., nausea, vomiting) and cardiovascular problems (e.g., arrhythmias, orthostatic hypotension), especially for the first few days after drug therapy is initiated. Neuropsychiatric problems (e.g., confusion, depression, anxiety, hallucinations) and problems with involuntary movements (e.g., dyskinesia) have also been noted in patients on levodopa therapy.[103] Perhaps the most frustrating problem, however, is the tendency for the effectiveness of

levodopa to diminish after 4 or 5 years of continuous use.[136] The reason for this diminished response is not fully understood but may be related to the fact that levodopa replacement simply cannot adequately restore neurotransmitter dysfunction in the final stages of this disease, i.e., levodopa therapy may help supplement endogenous dopamine production in early to moderate Parkinson's disease, but this effect is eventually lost when the substantia nigra neurons degenerate beyond a certain point. Other fluctuations in the response to levodopa have been noted with long-term use.[136] These fluctuations include a spontaneous decrease in levodopa effectiveness in the middle of a dose interval (on-off phenomenon) or loss of drug effects toward the end of a dose cycle (end-of-dose akinesia). The reasons for these fluctuations are poorly understood but may be related to problems in the absorption and metabolism of levodopa in the later stages of Parkinson's disease.

Fortunately, several other agents are currently available to help alleviate the motor symptoms associated with Parkinson's disease (Table 12-3).[50] Drugs such as bromocriptine (Parlodel) and pergolide (Permax) mimic the effects of dopamine and can be used to replace the deficient neurotransmitter. Anticholinergic drugs (e.g., biperiden, ethopropazine) act to decrease acetylcholine influence in the brain and can attenuate the increased effects of acetylcholine that occur when dopamine influence is diminished. Amantadine (Symmetrel) is actually an antiviral drug that also exerts antiparkinson effects, presumably by facilitating the release of dopamine from storage sites in the basal ganglia.

TABLE 12-3
Drugs Used in Neurological Disorders

	Generic Name	Trade Name
Drugs Used in Parkinson's Disease		
Dopamine precursors	Levodopa	Sinemet*
Dopamine agonists	Bromocriptine	Parlodel
	Pergolide	Permax
Anticholinergic drugs	Benztropine	Cogentin
	Biperiden	Akineton
	Ethopropazine	Parsidol
	Procyclidine	Kemadrin
Others	Amantadine	Symadine, Symmetrel
	Selegiline	Eldepryl
Drugs Used in Seizure Disorders		
Barbiturates	Mephobarbital	Mebaral
	Phenobarbital	Solfoton
Benzodiazepines	Clonazepam	Klonopin
	Clorazepate	Tranxene
Hydantoins	Ethotoin	Peganone
	Mephenytoin	Mesantoin
	Phenytoin	Dilantin
Succinimides	Ethosuximide	Zarontin
	Methsuximide	Celontin
Others	Carbamazepine	Tegretol
	Valproic acid	Depakene

*Indicates trade name for levodopa combined with carbidopa, a peripheral decarboxylase inhibitor.

Selegiline (Eldepryl) inhibits the enzyme that degrades dopamine, thus prolonging the effects of any dopamine that exists in the basal ganglia.

Consequently, levodopa therapy is still the cornerstone of treatment in persons with Parkinson's disease, but several other agents are now available that can be used in combination with or instead of levodopa to create an optimal drug regimen for each patient.[8,95,254] Nonetheless, current pharmacotherapy of Parkinson's disease has some considerable shortcomings, and treatment of patients is often limited by inadequate effects or toxic side effects, especially during the advanced stages of this disease. Additional drug treatments are being considered that may actually help delay the neurodegenerative changes inherent to Parkinson's disease.[37,87] If proven effective, these treatments would offer substantial benefits because they would help slow the progression of this disease rather than merely treat the parkinsonian symptoms.

Physical therapists working with patients with Parkinson's disease should attempt to coordinate rehabilitation sessions with the peak effects of drug therapy whenever possible. For instance, scheduling physical therapy when levodopa and other antiparkinson drugs reach peak effects (usually 1 hour after oral administration) will often maximize the patient's ability to actively participate in exercise programs and functional training. Therapists should also be cognizant of the potential side effects of levodopa, including the tendency for responses to fluctuate or diminish with prolonged use. Physical therapists may also play an important role in documenting any decline or alteration in drug effectiveness while working closely with patients with Parkinson's disease.

Drugs Used to Control Seizures

Seizure disorders such as epilepsy are characterized by the sudden, uncontrolled firing of a group of cerebral neurons.[200] This uncontrolled neuronal excitation is manifested in various ways, depending on the location and extent of the neuronal involvement, and seizures are classified according to the motor and sensory symptoms that occur during a seizure. In the general population, the exact cause of the seizure disorder is often unknown. In the elderly, however, seizure activity may be attributed to a fairly well-defined cause such as a previous CNS injury (e.g., stroke, trauma), tumor, or degenerative brain disease.[133] If the cause cannot be treated by surgical or other means, pharmacological management remains the primary method of preventing recurrent seizures.

The primary goal of antiseizure drugs is to normalize the excitation threshold in the group of hyperexcitable neurons that initiate the seizure.[199] Ideally this can be accomplished without suppressing the general excitation level within the brain. Several groups of chemically distinct antiseizure drugs are currently in use, and each group uses a different biochemical mechanism to selectively decrease excitability in the seizure-prone neurons (see Table 12-3). The selection of a particular antiseizure drug depends primarily on the type of seizure present in each patient.[137,199]

Sedation is the most common side effect that physical therapists should be aware of when working with elderly patients who are taking seizure medications. Other annoying side effects include GI distress, headache, dizziness, incoordination, and dermatological reactions (e.g., rashes). More serious problems, such as liver toxicity and blood dyscrasias (aplastic anemia), may occur in some patients. In addition to monitoring these side effects, physical therapists can play an important role in helping assess the effectiveness of the antiseizure medications by observing and documenting any seizures that may occur during the rehabilitation session.

Treatment of Pain and Inflammation

Pharmacological treatment of pain and inflammation is used in the elderly to help resolve symptoms of chronic conditions (e.g., rheumatoid arthritis and osteoarthritis) as well as acute problems resulting from trauma and surgery.[55,61] Drugs used for analgesic and anti-inflammatory purposes include the opioid analgesics, non-opioid analgesics, and glucocorticoids (Table 12-4). These are discussed briefly here.

TABLE 12-4
DRUGS USED TO TREAT PAIN AND INFLAMMATION

	COMMON EXAMPLES	
CATEGORY	**GENERIC NAME**	**TRADE NAME**
Opioid Analgesics	Codeine	Many trade names
	Meperidine	Demerol
	Morphine	Many trade names
	Oxycodone	Roxicodone
	Propoxyphene	Darvon, others
Non-opioid Analgesics		
NSAIDs	Aspirin	Many trade names
	Ibuprofen	Advil, Motrin, others
	Ketoprofen	Orudis
	Naproxen	Naprosyn, Anaprox
	Piroxicam	Feldene
	Sulindac	Clinoril
Acetaminophen	—	Tylenol, Panadol
Corticosteroids	Betamethasone	Celestone
	Cortisone	Cortone Acetate
	Hydrocortisone	Cortef, Hydrocortone, others
	Prednisone	Deltasone, others
Disease-Modifying Drugs*		
Gold compounds	Auranofin	Ridaura
	Aurothioglucose	Solganal
	Gold sodium thiomalate	Myochrysine
Antimalarials	Chloroquine	Aralen HCl
	Hydroxy-chloroquine	Plaquenil Sulfate
Others	Penicillamine	Cuprimine, Depen
	Methotrexate	Rheumatrex Dose Pack, others
	Azathioprine	Imuran

*Drugs used to slow the progression of rheumatoid arthritis.
NSAIDs = nonsteroidal anti-inflammatory drugs.

Opioid Analgesics

Opioid analgesics compose the group of drugs used to treat relatively severe, constant pain. These agents, also known as *narcotics,* are commonly used to reduce pain in elderly patients after surgery or trauma, or in more chronic situations such as cancer.[67] Opioids vary in terms of their relative analgesic strength, with drugs such as morphine and meperidine (Demerol) having strong analgesic properties, and drugs such as codeine having a more moderate ability to decrease pain. These drugs exert their beneficial effects by binding to opioid receptors in the brain and spinal cord, thereby impairing synaptic transmission in pain-mediating pathways.[59,266] Opioid analgesics are often characterized by their ability to alter pain perception rather than completely eliminating painful sensations. This effect allows the patient to focus on other things rather than being continually preoccupied by the painful stimuli.

Physical therapists should be aware that the analgesic effects of opioid drugs tend to be accompanied by many side effects that can influence the patient's participation in rehabilitation.[67] Adverse side effects such as sedation, mood changes (e.g., euphoria or dysphoria), and GI problems (e.g., nausea, vomiting, constipation) are quite common. Orthostatic hypotension and respiratory depression are also common side effects, especially for the first few days after opioid analgesic therapy is started. Confusion may be a problem, particularly in older adults. Finally, aspects of drug addiction, including tolerance and physical dependence, are always a concern when opioid analgesics are used for prolonged periods.

Non-Opioid Analgesics

Treatment of mild to moderate pain is often accomplished by the use of two types of non-opioid agents: NSAIDs and acetaminophen. NSAIDs compose a group of drugs that are therapeutically similar to aspirin (see Table 12-4). These aspirin-like drugs produce four therapeutic effects: analgesia, decreased inflammation, decreased fever (antipyresis), and decreased platelet aggregation (anticoagulant effects). Acetaminophen appears to have analgesic and antipyretic properties similar to the NSAIDs, but acetaminophen lacks any significant anti-inflammatory or anticoagulation effects. NSAIDs and acetaminophen exert most, if not all, of their beneficial effects by inhibiting the synthesis of a group of compounds known as the *prostaglandins.* Prostaglandins are produced locally by many cells and are involved in mediating certain aspects of pain and inflammation.[51,123] Aspirin and other NSAIDs inhibit the enzyme that synthesizes prostaglandins in the central nervous system as well as peripheral tissues, thus diminishing the painful and inflammatory effects of these compounds throughout the body.[189,246] Acetaminophen also inhibits prostaglandin biosynthesis, but this inhibition may only occur in the central nervous system, thus accounting for the differences in acetaminophen and NSAID effects.[66]

NSAID use in elderly patients tends to be fairly safe when these drugs are used in moderate doses for short periods.[162,174,194] The most common side effect is gastrointestinal irritation, and problems ranging from minor stomach upset to serious gastric ulceration can occur in older adults.[99,213] Renal and hepatic toxicity may also occur, especially if higher doses are used for prolonged periods or in patients with pre-existing kidney or liver disease.[7,233] Other problems that may occur in elderly patients include allergic reactions (e.g., skin rashes) and possible CNS toxicity (e.g., confusion, hearing problems). In particular, tinnitus (a ringing or buzzing sound in the ears) may develop with prolonged aspirin use, and this side effect may be especially annoying and distressing to older adults.

Acetaminophen does not produce any appreciable gastric irritation and may be taken preferentially by elderly patients for that reason. It should be noted, however, that acetaminophen lacks anti-inflammatory effects and may be inferior to NSAIDs if pain and inflammation are present. Acetaminophen may also be more hepatotoxic than the NSAIDs in cases of overdose or in persons who are dehydrated, consume excessive amounts of alcohol, and so forth.

Glucocorticoids

Glucocorticoids are steroids produced by the adrenal cortex that have a number of physiological effects, including a potent ability to decrease inflammation.[202] Synthetic derivatives of endogenously produced glucocorticoids can be administered pharmacologically to capitalize on the powerful anti-inflammatory effects of these compounds. These agents are used to treat rheumatoid arthritis and a variety of other disorders that have an inflammatory component. Glucocorticoids exert their anti-inflammatory effects through several mechanisms, including the ability to suppress leukocyte function and to inhibit the production of pro-inflammatory substances, such as prostaglandins and leukotrienes, at the site of inflammation.[126,189,202]

The powerful anti-inflammatory effects of glucocorticoids must be balanced against the risk of several serious adverse effects. In particular, physical therapists should be aware that these drugs produce a general catabolic effect on supporting tissues throughout the body.[96,122] Breakdown of bones, ligaments, tendons, skin, and muscle can occur after prolonged systemic administration of glucocorticoids. This breakdown can be especially devastating in the elderly patient who already has some degree of osteoporosis or muscle wasting.[96] Glucocorticoids also produce other serious adverse effects, including hypertension, peptic ulcer, aggravation of diabetes mellitus, glaucoma, increased risk of infection, and suppression of normal corticosteroid production by the adrenal cortex. Adrenocortical suppression can have devastating or even fatal results if the exogenous (drug) form of the glucocorticoid is suddenly withdrawn because the body is temporarily incapable of synthesizing adequate amounts of these important compounds. Finally, it should be realized that glucocorticoids often treat a disease manifestation (inflammation) without resolving the underlying cause of the disease. For instance, the elderly patient with rheumatoid arthritis may appear quite healthy due to this "masking" effect of glucocorticoids, whereas other sequelae of this disease (e.g., bone erosion, joint destruction) continue to worsen.

Other Drugs Used in Inflammatory Disease: Disease-Modifying Agents

Because NSAIDs and other anti-inflammatory drugs do not usually slow the disease process in rheumatoid arthritis, efforts have been made to develop drugs that try to curb the progression of this disease.[147] These so-called disease-modifying antirheumatic drugs (DMARDs) include an assortment of agents with different chemical and pharmacodynamic properties (see Table 12-4).[46,73] In general, these agents have immunosuppressive effects that blunt the autoimmune response that is believed to underlie rheumatic joint disease.[23,49,73,128,201,249] The use and effectiveness of various drugs in this category remain under investigation, but it seems that certain agents such as the gold compounds and methotrexate have been successful in arresting or even reversing some of the arthritic changes in certain patients

with this disease.[77,98,111,164,183] Hence, a current trend is to use DMARDs fairly early in the course of rheumatoid arthritis so that these drugs can help prevent some of the severe joint destruction associated with this disease.[21,105,114,179,248] Regrettably, use of these DMARDs is limited in many patients because of toxic effects such as GI distress and renal impairment.[45,73,263] Future studies should provide more information about the optimal use of DMARDs and other innovative treatments for rheumatoid arthritis.[35,71,143,201]

Cardiovascular Drugs

Cardiovascular disease is one of the leading causes of morbidity and mortality in elderly individuals. Various drugs are therefore used to prevent and treat cardiovascular problems in older adults, and many of these medications can directly affect rehabilitation of the elderly. Some of the more common cardiovascular drugs are listed in Table 12-5 and are discussed briefly here.

Beta-Adrenergic Blockers

Beta-adrenergic antagonists, or "beta-blockers," are so named because they bind to beta-1-receptors on the heart and block the effects of catecholamines (epinephrine, norep-

TABLE 12-5
CARDIOVASCULAR DRUGS

DRUG GROUP	PRIMARY INDICATIONS	COMMON EXAMPLES	
		GENERIC NAME	TRADE NAME
Alpha-blockers	Hypertension	Phenoxybenzamine	Dibenzyline
		Prazosin	Minipress
Angiotensin-converting enzyme inhibitors	Hypertension, CHF	Captopril	Capoten
		Enalapril	Vasotec
Anticoagulants	Overactive clotting	Heparin	Liquaemin Sodium
		Warfarin	Coumadin
Beta-blockers	Hypertension	Atenolol	Tenormin
	Angina	Metoprolol	Lopressor
	Arrhythmias	Nadolol	Corgard
		Propranolol	Inderal
Calcium channel blockers	Hypertension	Diltiazem	Cardizem
	Angina	Nifedipine	Adalat, Procardia
	Arrhythmias	Verapamil	Calan, Isoptin SR
Centrally acting sympatholytics	Hypertension	Clonidine	Catapres
		Methyldopa	Aldomet
Digitalis glycosides	CHF	Digoxin	Lanoxin
Diuretics	Hypertension, CHF	Chlorothiazide	Diuril
		Furosemide	Lasix
		Spironolactone	Aldactone
Drugs that prolong repolarization	Arrhythmias	Amiodarone	Cordarone
		Bretylium	Bretylol
Organic nitrates	Angina	Nitroglycerin	Nitrostat, others
Presynaptic adrenergic depletors	Hypertension	Guanethidine	Ismelin
		Reserpine	Serpalan
Sodium channel blockers	Arrhythmias	Quinidine	Cin-Quin, others
		Lidocaine	Xylocaine, others
Vasodilators	Hypertension	Hydralazine	Apresoline
		Minoxidil	Loniten

CHF = congestive heart failure.

inephrine) on myocardial tissues. Catecholamines normally accelerate cardiac function, and beta-blockers negate this effect thus causing decreased heart rate (negative chronotropic effect) and decreased myocardial contraction force (negative inotropic effect). Owing to their ability to slow heart rate and contractile force, these drugs have become a mainstay in managing a number of cardiovascular problems such as hypertension, angina pectoris, and cardiac arrhythmias.[38,74] The ability of beta-blockers to reduce cardiac workload also enables these drugs to reduce mortality and enhance recovery after myocardial infarction[10,78] as well as to help treat certain types of heart failure.[41,94]

Beta-blockers are therefore used extensively to treat a number of common cardiovascular problems. These drugs are also used extensively because they tend to be fairly well-tolerated and have a relatively low incidence of serious adverse effects. Elderly individuals, however, tend to be more susceptible to certain side effects of these agents, such as depression, lethargy, and sleep disorders.[116] Other problems with beta-blockers occur because of the tendency of these drugs to attenuate cardiac pumping ability. For instance, heart rate will be lower at any given exercise workload in a patient taking beta-blockers.[173] Orthostatic hypotension may occur due to the decreased ability of the heart to redistribute vascular fluid after a change in posture. Naturally, these cardiac effects will be exaggerated in the elderly patient with pre-existing cardiovascular problems or decreased cardiac function secondary to prolonged inactivity. Physical therapists working with the elderly should recall that beta-blockers will limit the cardiac response to exercise and postural changes, and some rehabilitation procedures (e.g., ambulation activities, various exercise regimens) may have to be changed accordingly.

Diuretics

Diuretics act on the kidneys to increase the excretion of water and sodium.[38] This action decreases the amount of fluid in the vascular system, thus decreasing cardiac workload, i.e., the heart does not have to work as hard since there is less fluid to pump. Diuretics are classified according to their chemical structure (thiazides) or according to their mechanism of action (loop and potassium-sparing agents). Diuretic agents are used primarily in the treatment of hypertension and congestive heart failure.[38,113]

The primary problems with diuretics are associated with the tendency of these drugs to cause fluid volume depletion and electrolyte imbalances, such as low blood sodium (hyponatremia) and low blood potassium (hypokalemia).[26,69] These effects can be particularly harmful in the older patient with pre-existing volume depletion or hypokalemia due to poor diet.[158] Problems with fluid and electrolyte balance are often manifested through central symptoms (e.g., confusion, mood change) and peripheral problems involving skeletal muscle (e.g., weakness, fatigue). Orthostatic hypotension may also result due to an inadequate amount of intravascular fluid being available for redistribution on standing. Physical therapists working with the elderly can play an impor-

tant role in recognizing these drug-related changes in function and alerting the medical staff of a potential problem in diuretic therapy.

Organic Nitrates

Organic nitrates such as nitroglycerin are used to prevent episodes of angina pectoris.[38] Angina typically occurs when myocardial oxygen demand exceeds myocardial oxygen supply. Nitroglycerin decreases myocardial oxygen demand by vasodilating the peripheral vasculature.[169] Peripheral vasodilation causes a decrease in the amount of blood returning to the heart (cardiac preload) as well as the amount of pressure in the vascular system that the heart must pump against (cardiac afterload). Consequently, cardiac workload and oxygen demand are temporarily reduced, thus allowing the anginal attack to subside.

Nitrates can be administered at the onset of an anginal attack by placing the drug under the tongue (sublingually). These drugs can also be administered transdermally using drug-impregnated patches that allow slow, steady absorption of nitrate into the bloodstream. The use of nitrate patches has gained favor because the continuous administration of small amounts of drug may help prevent the onset or reduce the severity of anginal attacks.[93,253]

The primary adverse effects that may affect physical therapy are related to the peripheral vasodilating effects of the nitrates. Blood pressure may decrease in patients taking nitroglycerin, and dizziness due to hypotension is a common problem. Likewise, orthostatic hypotension may occur if the patient stands suddenly. Headache may also occur due to vasodilation of meningeal vessels. These side effects are most common immediately after the patient takes a rapid-acting sublingual dose. Hence, therapists should be especially concerned about hypotensive effects from the first minutes to 1 hour after a patient self-administers a sublingual dose of nitrates. Finally, patients who take nitrates sublingually must be sure to bring their medications with them to physical therapy so that the patient can self-administer the nitrate if anginal symptoms occur during the rehabilitation session.

Antiarrhythmic Drugs

Disturbances in cardiac rhythm—i.e., a heart rate that is too slow, too fast, or irregular—may occur in the elderly for various reasons.[247] A variety of different drugs can be used to stabilize heart rate and normalize cardiac rhythm, and these agents are typically grouped into four categories.[156,207] Sodium channel blockers (lidocaine, quinidine) control myocardial excitability by stabilizing the opening and closing of membrane sodium channels. Beta-blockers (metoprolol, propranolol) normalize heart rate by blocking the effects of cardioacceleratory substances such as norepinephrine and epinephrine. Drugs that prolong cardiac repolarization (bretylium) stabilize heart rate by prolonging the refractory period of cardiac action potentials. Calcium channel blockers (diltiazem, verapamil) decrease myocardial excitability and conduction of action potentials by limiting the entry of calcium into cardiac muscle cells. Although different antiarrhythmic drugs have various side effects, the most common adverse reaction is an increased risk of cardiac arrhythmias,[252] i.e., drugs used to treat one type of arrhythmia may inadvertently cause a different type of rhythm disturbance. Physical therapists should be alert for changes in cardiac rhythm by monitoring heart rate in elderly patients who are taking antiarrhythmic drugs.

Drugs Used in Geriatric Hypertension

An increase in blood pressure is commonly observed in the elderly, and this increase is believed to be due to changes in cardiovascular function (e.g., decreased compliance of vascular tissues, decreased baroreceptor sensitivity) and diminished renal function (e.g., decreased ability to excrete water and sodium) that normally occur with aging.[2] A mild increase in blood pressure may not necessarily be harmful in the older adult and may in fact have a protective effect in maintaining adequate blood flow to the brain and other organs.[217] However, blood pressure values above certain levels (systolic and diastolic values greater than 180 mm Hg and 100 mm Hg, respectively) are treated in elderly patients in order to reduce the risk of mortality and morbidity due to cardiovascular complications.[165,166,180,181,221] The goal of antihypertensive therapy is not to reduce blood pressure in the older adult to levels equivalent to those seen in normotensive young adults who have systolic and diastolic values of 120 mm Hg and 80 mm Hg, respectively. Rather, target values of 160 mm Hg systolic and 90 mm Hg diastolic are recommended as much more realistic and safer goals in treating geriatric hypertension.[180]

Fortunately, a large and diverse array of antihypertensive agents is available for treating geriatric patients with hypertension (see Table 12-5). Diuretic agents (discussed earlier) reduce blood pressure by diminishing the volume of fluid in the vascular system. Sympatholytic agents (e.g., beta-blockers, alpha-blockers) work in various ways to interrupt sympathetic stimulation of the heart and peripheral vasculature. Vasodilators reduce peripheral vascular resistance by directly relaxing vascular smooth muscle. Angiotensin-converting enzyme (ACE) inhibitors block the formation of angiotensin II, a potent vasoconstrictor that also produces adverse structural changes in vascular tissues. Finally, calcium channel blockers inhibit the entry of calcium into cardiac muscle cells and vascular smooth muscle cells, thus reducing contractility in these tissues.

Which antihypertensive agent or agents will be used in a given geriatric patient depends on several factors, such as the magnitude of the hypertension and any other medical problems existing in that patient. Often, a "stepped-care" approach is used, in which one drug is used initially, and other drugs are added sequentially until blood pressure is adequately reduced.[138] For example, diuretics and beta-blockers are often used initially to control hypertension in the older adult.[125,186,255] Other drugs such as ACE inhibitors and calcium channel blockers can be added or substituted based on

the individual needs of each patient.[127,209,240] Regardless of which agent is used initially, a successful antihypertensive drug regimen should be designed specifically for each patient and should incorporate the "low-and-slow" philosophy of starting with low doses of each drug and slowly increasing dosages as needed.

The various drugs that could be used to manage hypertension are all associated with specific side effects. A common concern, however, is that blood pressure will be reduced pharmacologically to the point where symptoms of hypotension become a problem. Therapists should always be aware that dizziness and syncope may occur due to low blood pressure when the patient is stationary and especially when the patient stands (orthostatic hypotension). Also, any physical therapy intervention that causes an additional decrease in blood pressure should be used very cautiously in geriatric patients who are taking antihypertensive drugs. Treatments such as systemic heat (e.g., large whirlpool, Hubbard tank) and exercise using large muscle groups may cause peripheral vasodilation that acts synergistically with the antihypertensive drugs to produce a profound and potentially serious decrease in blood pressure.

Drugs Used in Congestive Heart Failure

Congestive heart failure is a common disorder in older adults and is characterized by a progressive decline in cardiac pumping ability.[139,187,208] As the pumping ability of the heart diminishes, fluid often collects in the lungs and extremities (hence the term congestive heart failure). Treatment of this disorder typically consists of using drugs that improve myocardial pumping ability (e.g., digitalis glycosides, beta-blockers) combined with drugs that reduce fluid volume and vascular resistance (e.g., diuretics, ACE inhibitors, vasodilators).[11,38,139] Digitalis glycosides such as digoxin cause an increase in myocardial pumping ability by a complex biochemical mechanism that increases the calcium concentration in myocardial cells. Beta-blockers reduce excessive sympathetic stimulation of the heart, thus stabilizing heart rate and allowing more normal ventricular function in certain types of heart failure. Diuretics are used to increase renal excretion of water and sodium, thus decreasing some of the excess fluid in the lungs and body tissues. ACE inhibitors and vasodilators, such as the organic nitrates, reduce peripheral vascular tone, thus decreasing the pressure the heart must pump against.

The adverse effects of beta-blockers, diuretics, and nitrates were discussed earlier in this chapter. These agents are relatively safe when used to treat heart failure in the elderly. Likewise, ACE inhibitors are tolerated fairly well in older adults, although hypotension and orthostatic hypotension may occur when these drugs are first administered to elderly individuals.[241] Digoxin and similar drugs, however, are often associated with some common and potentially serious side effects. These agents can accumulate rapidly in the bloodstream of an elderly patient, resulting in digitalis toxicity.[79] Digitalis toxicity is characterized by gastrointestinal symptoms (e.g., nausea, vomiting, diarrhea), CNS disturbances (e.g., confusion, blurred vision, sedation), and cardiac arrhythmias. Arrhythmias can be quite severe and may result in cardiac fatalities if digitalis toxicity is not quickly rectified. Physical therapists should be alert for signs of digitalis toxicity because early recognition is essential in preventing the more serious and potentially fatal side effects of these drugs.

Drugs Used in Coagulation Disorders

Excessive hemostasis, or a tendency for the blood to clot too rapidly, is a common and serious problem in the older adult.[225] Formation of blood clots may result in thrombophlebitis and thromboembolism. These problems are especially important in the older patient after surgery and prolonged bed rest.[5,18] The use of two anticoagulants, heparin and warfarin, is a mainstay in preventing excessive hemostasis.[5] These agents work by different mechanisms to prolong and normalize the clotting time of the blood.[20,167] Heparin is usually administered parenterally via intravenous or subcutaneous injection, whereas warfarin can be taken orally. Typically, heparin is used initially to achieve a rapid decrease in blood clotting, followed by long-term management of excessive coagulation through oral warfarin administration.

The most common problem with anticoagulant drug therapy is an increased tendency for hemorrhage.[68,257] Use of heparin and warfarin can result in too much of a delay in blood clotting, so that excessive bleeding occurs. Physical therapists should be cautious when dealing with open wounds or procedures that potentially induce tissue trauma (e.g., chest percussion, vigorous massage) because of the increased risk for hemorrhage.

Respiratory and Gastrointestinal Drugs
Drugs Used in Respiratory Disorders

Older adults may take drugs to treat fairly simple respiratory conditions associated with the common cold and seasonal allergies. Such drugs include cough medications (antitussives), decongestants, antihistamines, and drugs that help loosen and raise respiratory secretions (mucolytics and expectorants). Drugs may also be taken for more chronic, serious problems such as chronic obstructive pulmonary disease (COPD) and bronchial asthma.[185] Drug therapy for asthma and COPD includes bronchodilators such as beta-adrenergic agonists (albuterol, epinephrine), xanthine derivatives (aminophylline theophylline), and anticholinergic drugs (ipratropium). Corticosteroids may also be given to treat inflammation in the respiratory tracts that is often present in these chronic respiratory problems.

These respiratory drugs are associated with various side effects that may affect physical therapy of the older adult. In particular, the elderly may be more susceptible to sedative side effects of drugs such as antihistamines and cough suppressants. For some of the prescription medications, side effects are often reduced if the medication can be applied directly to the respiratory tissues by inhalation.[58,230] For instance, even corticosteroids can be used fairly safely in the elderly if these drugs are inhaled rather than administered orally and distributed into the systemic circulation. If medications are administered systemically, however, lower doses of the prescription bronchodilators may be necessary in older adults. This fact is especially true in the elderly patient with reduced liver or kidney function, since metabolism and elimination of the active form of the drug will be impaired. Finally, some elderly patients may use excessive amounts of certain over-the-counter products. Physical therapists should question the extent to which their geriatric patients routinely take large doses of cough suppressants, antihistamines, and other over-the-counter respiratory drugs.

Drugs Used in Gastrointestinal Disorders

Gastrointestinal drugs such as antacids and laxatives are among the most commonly used medications in the elderly.[211,228] Antacids typically consist of a base that neutralizes hydrochloric acid, thus helping to alleviate stomach discomfort caused by excess gastric acid secretion. Other drugs that decrease gastric acid secretion include the H_2 blockers (e.g., cimetidine, ranitidine), which work by blocking certain histamine receptors (H_2 receptors) that are located in the gastric mucosa. Laxatives stimulate bowel evacuation and defecation by a number of different methods depending on the drug used. Drugs used to treat diarrhea are also commonly taken by elderly patients. These drugs consist of agents such as opioids (diphenoxylate, loperamide) that help decrease GI motility and products such as the adsorbents (e.g., kaolin, pectin) that help sequester toxins and irritants in the GI tract that may cause diarrhea.

The major concern for GI drug use in the elderly is the potential for inappropriate and excessive use of these agents.[211] Most of these drugs are readily available as over-the-counter products. Elderly individuals may self-administer these agents to the extent that normal GI activity is compromised. For instance, the older person who relies on daily laxative use (or possibly even several laxatives each day) may experience a decline in the normal regulation of bowel evacuation. Drugs may also be used as a substitute for proper eating habits. Antacids, for example, may be taken routinely to disguise the irritant effects of certain foods that are not tolerated well by the older adult. Physical therapists can often advise their geriatric patients that most GI drugs are meant to be used for only brief episodes of GI discomfort. Therapists can discourage the long-term use of such agents and advise their patients that proper nutrition and eating habits are a much safer and healthier alternative than prolonged use of GI drugs.

Hormonal Agents
General Strategy: Use of Hormones as Replacement Therapy

The endocrine glands synthesize and release hormones that travel through the blood to regulate the physiological function of various tissues and organs. If hormonal production is interrupted, natural or synthetic versions of these hormones can be administered pharmacologically to restore and maintain normal endocrine function. This replacement therapy is commonly used in the elderly when endocrine function is diminished because of age-related factors (e.g., loss of ovarian hormones after menopause) or if endocrine function is lost after disease or surgery.[120,260] Some of the more common hormonal agents used in the elderly are listed in Table 12-6 and are discussed here.

Estrogen Replacement

The primary female hormones—estrogen and progesterone—are normally produced by the ovaries from puberty until approximately the fifth or sixth decade when menopause occurs. Loss of these hormones is associated with a number of problems, including vasomotor symptoms (hot flashes), atrophic vaginitis, and atrophic dystrophy of the vulva. Replacement of the ovarian hormones, especially estrogen, can help resolve all these symptoms.[262] In addition, estrogen replacement can substantially reduce the risk of osteoporosis and cardiovascular disease in postmenopausal women.[104,262] Preliminary evidence also suggests that estrogen may improve cognition and mood in older adults and that estrogen replacement may delay the neurodegenerative changes associated with Alzheimer's disease.[17,205]

Although estrogen replacement is clearly associated with certain beneficial effects, there is concern that estrogen therapy may increase the risk of some forms of cancer, including breast and endometrial cancer.[29,72,104,262] However, the exact relationship between estrogen replacement and the risk of cancer remains uncertain.[104,262] At the present time, it appears that the benefits of estrogen replacement outweigh the potential problems, especially in women who are at high risk for developing osteoporosis or cardiovascular disease.[104,144,218] Likewise, newer estrogen-like compounds such as raloxifene are currently being studied because these agents may produce beneficial effects on bone and cardiovascular function without causing carcinogenic side effects.[44,146] The development of effective and safer hormonal strategies will certainly be a welcome addition to the drug regimen for older women who require estrogen replacement.

Diabetes Mellitus

Insulin is normally synthesized by pancreatic beta cells, and this hormone regulates the metabolism of glucose and other energy substrates. Diabetes mellitus is a complex metabolic disorder caused by inadequate insulin production, decreased peripheral effects of insulin, or a combination of inadequate insulin production and decreased insulin effects. Diabetes mellitus consists of two principal types: type I (insulin-dependent diabetes mellitus) and type II (non-insulin-dependent diabetes mellitus). Type I diabetes mellitus is commonly associated with younger individuals, whereas type II diabetes mellitus occurs quite commonly in the elderly.[145] As many as 10% to 20% of Americans older than 60 may be diagnosed with type II mellitus.[129] If diabetes mellitus is not managed appropriately, acute effects (e.g., impaired glucose metabolism, ketoacidosis) and chronic effects (e.g., neuropathy, renal disease, blindness) may occur.

In contrast to the younger type I diabetic, the older adult with type II diabetes mellitus may not require exogenous insulin to manage this disease. The principal methods of managing type II diabetes mellitus in the elderly are diet, exercise, and maintenance of proper body weight.[129] When drug therapy is required in the older type II diabetic, it is usually in the form of oral hypoglycemic drugs (see Table 12-6).[108,150] These agents are taken orally to lower blood glucose levels, hence the term *oral hypoglycemic*. Depending on the exact agent, these drugs help improve glucose metabolism by enhancing the release of insulin from the pancreas, increasing the sensitivity of peripheral tissues to insulin, stabilizing hepatic glucose output, or delaying absorption of glucose from the GI tract.[24]

TABLE 12-6
DRUGS USED IN ENDOCRINE DISORDERS

CATEGORY	INDICATION	COMMON EXAMPLES	
		GENERIC NAME	TRADE NAME
Estrogens	Osteoporosis	Conjugated estrogens	Premarin, others
	Severe postmenopausal symptoms	Estradiol	Estrace, others
	Some cancers		
Insulin	Diabetes mellitus	—	Iletin, Humulin, Velosulin, others
Oral hypoglycemic agents	Diabetes mellitus	Acarbose	Precose
		Chlorpropamide	Diabinese
		Glipizide	Glucotrol
		Metformin	Glucophage
		Tolbutamide	Orinase
Antithyroid agents	Hyperthyroidism	Methimazole	Tapazole
		Propylthiouracil	Propyl-Thyracil
Thyroid hormones	Hypothyroidism	Levothyroxine (T_4)	Synthroid, others
		Liothyronine (T_3)	Cytomel

The principal problem associated with drug therapy in elderly diabetic patients is that the blood glucose level may be reduced too much, resulting in symptoms of hypoglycemia. Physical therapists should be alert for signs of a low blood glucose level, such as headache, dizziness, confusion, fatigue, nausea, and sweating.

Thyroid Disorders

The thyroid gland normally produces two hormones: thyroxine and triiodothyronine. These hormones affect a wide variety of tissues and are primarily responsible for regulating basal metabolic rate and other aspects of systemic metabolism. Thyroid dysfunction is quite common in the elderly and can be manifested as either increased or decreased production of thyroid hormones.[34] Excess thyroid hormone production (hyperthyroidism, thyrotoxicosis) produces symptoms such as nervousness, weight loss, muscle wasting, and tachycardia. Inadequate production of the thyroid hormones (hypothyroidism) is characterized by weight gain, lethargy, sleepiness, bradycardia, and other features consistent with a slow body metabolism.

Hyperthyroidism can be managed with drugs that inhibit thyroid hormone biosynthesis, such as propylthiouracil, methimazole, or high doses of iodide.[97] The primary problems associated with these drugs are transient allergic reactions (e.g., skin rashes) and blood dyscrasias, such as aplastic anemia and agranulocytosis. A more permanent treatment of hyperthyroidism can be accomplished by administering radioactive iodine.[97] The radioactive iodine is taken up by the thyroid gland, where it selectively destroys the overactive thyroid tissues.

Hypothyroidism is usually managed quite successfully by replacement therapy using natural and synthetic versions of one or both of the thyroid hormones. The most significant problem associated with thyroid hormone replacement in older patients is that the elderly require smaller doses of these hormones than younger individuals.[52,197] Replacement doses that are too high evoke symptoms of hyperthyroidism, such as nervousness, weight loss, and tachycardia. Physical therapists should be alert for these symptoms when working with elderly patients who are receiving thyroid hormone replacement therapy.

Treatment of Infections

Various microorganisms such as bacteria, viruses, fungi, and protozoa can invade and proliferate in the elderly individual. Often the immune system is able to combat these microorganisms successfully, thus preventing infection. Occasionally, however, drugs must be used to supplement the body's normal immune response in combating infection caused by pathogenic microorganisms. The elderly are often susceptible to such infections, especially if their immune system has already been compromised by previous illness or a general state of debilitation. Two of the more common types of infections, bacterial and viral, are presented along with a brief description of the related drug therapy.

Antibacterial Drugs

Although some bacteria exist in the body in a helpful or symbiotic state, infiltration of pathogenic bacteria may result in infection. If the immune system is unable to contain or destroy these bacteria, antibacterial drugs must be administered. Some of the principal groups of antibacterial drugs are shown in Table 12-7. These agents are often grouped according to how they inhibit or kill bacterial cells. For instance, certain drugs (e.g., penicillins, cephalosporins) act by inhibiting bacterial-cell–wall synthesis. Other drugs (e.g., aminoglycosides, tetracyclines) specifically inhibit the synthesis of bacterial proteins. Drugs such as the fluoroquinolones (e.g., ciprofloxacin) and sulfonamides (e.g., sulfadiazine) work by selectively inhibiting the synthesis and function of bacterial deoxyribonucleic acid (DNA) and ribonucleic acid (RNA). The selection of a specific agent from one of these groups is based primarily on the type of bacterial infection present in each patient.

Table 12-7
Treatment of Infection

	Common Examples	
	Generic Name	Trade Name
Antibacterial Drugs		
Major Groups		
Aminoglycosides	Gentamicin	Garamycin; others
	Streptomycin	—
Cephalosporins	Cefaclor	Ceclor
	Cephalexin	Keflex; others
Erythromycins	Erythromycin	Many trade names
Fluoroquinolones	Ciprofloxacin	Cipro
	Norfloxacin	Noroxin
Penicillins	Penicillin G	Bicillin, many others
	Penicillin V	V-Cillin K, many others
	Amoxicillin	Amoxil, many others
	Ampicillin	Polycillin, many others
Sulfonamides	Sulfadiazine	Silvadene
	Sulfisoxazole	Gantrisin
Tetracyclines	Doxycycline	Vibramycin, others
	Tetracycline	Sumycin, others
Antiviral Drugs		
Principle Indication		
Herpes viruses	Acyclovir	Zovirax
	Vidarabine	Vira-A
Cytomegalovirus	Foscarnet	Foscavir
	Ganciclovir	Cytovene
Influenza A	Amantadine	Symadine, Symmetrel
Human immunodeficiency virus (HIV)	Zidovudine (AZT)	Retrovir
	Didanosine	Videx
	Zalcitabine	HIVID
	Ritonavir	Norvir
	Saquinavir	Invirase

The side effects that tend to occur with these agents vary from drug to drug, and it is not possible in this limited space to discuss all the potential antibacterial ADRs. With regard to their use in elderly patients, many of the precautions discussed earlier tend to apply. For instance, adverse drug reactions tend to occur more frequently because of the decreased renal clearance of antibacterial drugs in older adults.[76,142] Hence, physical therapists should be alert for any suspicious reactions in elderly patients who are taking antibacterial drugs, especially if renal function is already somewhat compromised. Resistance to antibacterial drugs is also a major concern in all age-groups, including the elderly.[134] Overuse and improper use of these agents have enabled certain bacterial strains to develop anti-drug mechanisms, thus rendering these drugs ineffective against these bacteria. Physical therapists should be aware of the need to prevent the spread of bacterial infections through the use of frequent handwashing and other universal precautions.

Antiviral Drugs

Viruses are small microorganisms that can invade human (host) cells and use the biochemical machinery of the host cell to produce more viruses. As a result, the virus often disrupts or destroys the function of the host cell, causing specific symptoms that are indicative of viral infection. Viral infections can cause disease syndromes ranging from the common cold to serious conditions such as acquired immunodeficiency syndrome (AIDS). Because the viral invader usually functions and co-exists within the host cell, it is often difficult to administer a drug that will kill the virus without simultaneously destroying the host cell. The number of antiviral agents is therefore limited (see Table 12-7), and these drugs often attenuate viral replication rather than actually destroy a virus that already exists in the body.

Due to the relatively limited number of effective antiviral agents, pharmacological management of viral disease often focuses on preventing viral infection through the use of vaccines. Vaccines are usually a modified, inactive form of the virus that stimulates the patient's immune system to produce specific antiviral antibodies. When exposed to an active form of the virus, these antibodies help destroy the viral invader before an infection is established.

Physical therapists should realize that the antiviral agents shown in Table 12-7 are often poorly tolerated and produce a number of adverse side effects, especially in elderly or debilitated patients.[159] Hence, prevention of viral infection through the use of vaccines is especially important in the elderly. For instance, influenza vaccines are often advocated for elderly individuals before seasonal outbreaks of the "flu."[151,157] Of course, some vaccines are not always completely effective in preventing viral infections, and an appropriate vaccine has yet to be developed for certain viral diseases such as AIDS. Still, vaccines represent the most effective method of dealing with viral infections in elderly individuals.

Cancer Chemotherapy

Cancer is the term used to describe diseases that are characterized by a rapid, uncontrolled cell proliferation and conversion of these cells to a more primitive and less functional state. Cancer is often treated aggressively through the use of a combination of several different techniques, such as surgery, radiation, and one or more cancer chemotherapeutic agents.

The elderly represent the majority of patients who will ultimately require some form of anticancer medication.[40,115,175] In general, the cancer chemotherapy regimens in older adults are similar to those used in younger individuals, with the exception that dosages are adjusted according to changes in liver and kidney function or other changes that affect drug pharmacokinetics. The results of cancer chemotherapy in the older patient also parallel those seen in the younger individual, with the possible exception that some hematological malignancies (certain leukemias) do not appear to respond as well to drug therapy in the elderly.[175] The principal chemotherapeutic strategies and types of anticancer agents are presented here.

Basic Strategy of Cancer Chemotherapy

Most anticancer drugs work by inhibiting the synthesis and function of DNA and RNA. This impairs the proliferation of cancer cells because they must rely on the rapid replication of genetic material in order to synthesize new cancer cells. Of course, DNA and RNA function is also impaired to some extent in healthy noncancerous cells, and this accounts for the many severe side effects and high level of toxicity associated with cancer chemotherapeutic agents. Cancer cells, however, should suffer to a relatively greater degree because these cells typically have a greater need to replicate their genetic material in order to sustain a high rate of cell reproduction. Still, most of the common adverse effects discussed here occur because of the nonselective effect of many anticancer drugs on normal cell function.

Types of Anticancer Drugs

Anticancer medications are classified according to their biochemical characteristics and mechanism of action (Table 12-8).[33] For example, alkylating agents form strong bonds between nucleic acids in the DNA double helix so that the DNA strands within the helix are unable to unwind and allow replication of the cell's genetic code. Antimetabolites impair the normal biosynthesis of nucleic acids and other important cellular metabolic components necessary for cell function. Antimitotic agents directly inhibit the mitotic apparatus that is responsible for controlling the actual division of one cell into two identical cells (mitosis). Certain antibiotics are effective as anticancer agents because they become inserted (intercalated) directly into the DNA double helix and either inhibit DNA function or cause the helix to break at the point where the drug is inserted. Hormones and drugs that block hormonal effects (antiestrogens, antiandrogens) are often used to attenuate the growth of hormone-sensitive

Table 12-8
Cancer Chemotherapeutic Agents

	Common Examples	
Major Groups	Generic Name	Trade Name
Alkylating Agents	Busulfan	Myleran
	Carmustine	BCNU, BiCNU
	Cyclophosphamide	Cytoxan, Neosar
	Mechlorethamine	Mustargen
	Uracil mustard	—
Antimetabolites	Cytarabine	Cytosar-U
	Floxuridine	FUDR
	Fluorouracil	Adrucil
	Methotrexate	Mexate
Antimitotics	Paclitaxel	Taxol
	Vinblastine	Velban
	Vincristine	Oncovin, Vincasar
Antineoplastic antibiotics	Daunorubicin	Cerubidine
	Doxorubicin	Adriamycin
	Idarubicin	Idamycin
Hormones		
Estrogens	Conjugated estrogens	Premarin, others
	Estradiol	Estrace, others
Antiestrogens	Tamoxifen	Nolvadex
Androgens	Testosterone	Many trade names
Antiandrogens	Flutamide	Eulexin
Interferons	Interferon alfa-2a	Roferon-A
	Interferon alfa-2b	Intron A

tumors such as breast cancer and prostate cancer. Interferons inhibit genes in the cancerous cell (oncogenes) that cause excessive proliferation of cancerous tissues, and interferons may also enhance the immune system's ability to destroy cancerous cells.

Anticancer drugs therefore inhibit replication and function of the cancer cell through one of the mechanisms just described. Likewise, several different drugs are often used simultaneously to achieve a synergistic effect between the antiproliferative actions of each drug.

Adverse Effects and Concerns for Rehabilitation

As mentioned, patients receiving cancer chemotherapy typically experience a number of severe adverse drug effects. Side effects such as GI distress (e.g., anorexia, vomiting), skin reactions (e.g., hair loss, rashes), and toxicity of various organs are extremely common. Elderly patients receiving cancer chemotherapy are especially prone to certain adverse effects such as cardiotoxicity, neurotoxicity, and blood disorders (e.g., anemia, thrombocytopenia).[15,115] Unfortunately, these adverse effects must be tolerated because of the serious nature of cancer and the fact that death will ensue if these drugs are not used. In terms of rehabilitation of elderly patients, physical therapists must recognize that these adverse effects will inevitably interfere with rehabilitation procedures. There will be some days that the patient is simply unable to participate in any aspect of physical therapy. Still, the

therapist can provide valuable and timely support for the elderly patient receiving cancer chemotherapy and reassure the patient that these drug-related effects are often unavoidable because of the cytotoxic nature of the drugs.

General Strategies for Coordinating Physical Therapy with Drug Treament in the Elderly

Based on the preceding discussion, it is clear that various medications can produce beneficial and adverse effects that may affect physical therapy of the elderly in many different ways. There are, however, some basic strategies that therapists can use to help maximize the beneficial aspects of drug therapy and minimize the detrimental drug effects when working with geriatric individuals. These general strategies are summarized here.

Distinguishing Drug Effects from Symptoms

When evaluating a geriatric patient, therapists must try to account for the subjective and objective findings that may be due to ADRs rather than true disease sequelae and the effects of aging. For instance, the patient who appears confused and disoriented during the initial physical therapy evaluation may actually be experiencing an adverse reaction to a psychotropic drug, cardiovascular medication, or some other agent. The correct distinction of true symptoms from ADRs allows better treatment planning and clinical decision making.

As discussed earlier, therapists can also take steps to prevent inappropriate drug use and polypharmacy by helping distinguish ADRs from true disease symptoms. Distinguishing drug-related signs from true patient symptoms may require careful observation and consultation with family members or other health professionals to see whether these signs tend to increase after each dosage. Periodic re-evaluation should also take into account any changes in drug therapy, especially if new medications are added to the patient's regimen. Finally, the medical staff should be alerted to any change in the patient's response that may indicate an ADR.

Scheduling Physical Therapy Sessions Around Dosage Schedule

Physical therapy should be coordinated with peak drug effects if the patient's active participation will be enhanced by drug treatment. For instance, drugs that improve motor performance (e.g., antiparkinson agents), improve mood and behavior (e.g., antidepressants, antipsychotics), and decrease pain (e.g., analgesics) may increase the older patient's ability to take part in various rehabilitation procedures. Conversely, physical therapy should be scheduled when drug effects are at a minimum for elderly patients receiving drugs that produce excessive sedation, dizziness, or other adverse effects that may impair the patient's cognitive or motor abilities. Unfortunately, there is often a tradeoff between desirable effects and adverse effects with the same drug, such as the opioid analgesic that also produces sedation. In these cases, it may take some trial and error in each patient to find a treatment time that capitalizes on the drug's benefits with minimum interference from the adverse effects.

Promoting Synergistic Effects of Physical Therapy Procedures with Drug Therapy

One must not lose sight of the fact that many of the rehabilitation procedures used with geriatric clients may augment drug therapy. For instance, the patient with Parkinson's disease may experience an optimal improvement in motor function through a combination of physical therapy and antiparkinson drugs. In some cases, drug therapy may be reduced through the contribution of physical therapy procedures (e.g., reduction of pain medications through the simultaneous use of TENS, physical agents, and so forth). This synergistic relationship between drug therapy and physical therapy can help achieve better results than if either intervention is used alone.

Avoiding Potentially Harmful Interactions Between Physical Therapy Procedures and Drug Effects

Some physical therapy interventions used in the elderly could potentially have a negative interaction with some medications. For instance, the use of rehabilitation procedures that cause extensive peripheral vasodilation (e.g., large whirlpool, some exercises) may produce severe hypotension in the patient receiving certain antihypertensive medications. These negative interactions must be anticipated and avoided when working with geriatric patients.

Improving Education and Compliance with Drug Therapy in the Elderly

Proper adherence to drug therapy is one area in which physical therapists can have a direct impact. Therapists can reinforce the need for adhering to the prescribed regimen, and therapists can help monitor whether drugs have been taken as directed. Therapists can also help educate their geriatric patients and their families as to why specific drugs are indicated and what side effects should be expected and tolerated as opposed to side effects that may indicate drug toxicity.

Case Studies

Case 1: Parkinson's Disease

Brief History

A 71-year-old male patient was diagnosed with Parkinson's disease 15 years ago. Drug therapy was initiated in the form of the dopamine agonist bromocriptine (Parlodel). Levodopa therapy was added to the drug regimen approximately 5 years ago when symptoms became incapacitating. Levodopa dosage was progressively increased over the next few years as the patient's condition gradually worsened. Recently, symptoms of bradykinesia and rigidity increased to the point that the patient's spouse was no longer able to care

for him, and he was admitted to a nursing home. At the time of admission, the patient was receiving 500 mg of levodopa given in combination with 50 mg of carbidopa 3 times per day. Dosages were administered at mealtimes to decrease stomach irritation caused by these drugs. Upon admission, the patient began receiving daily physical therapy to help maintain mobility and joint range of motion.

Problem/Influence of Medication

The therapist began seeing the patient each morning in the physical therapy clinic at the nursing home. Although symptoms of rigidity and bradykinesia were fairly marked, the therapist found that the patient was able to actively participate to some extent in range-of-motion exercises and some ambulation activities. During the second session, however, the patient suddenly became extremely rigid and exhibited a complete loss of all voluntary movement. The therapist found this surprising since the patient had started the physical therapy session with a reasonable amount of voluntary motor activity. The patient had also completed the entire session on the preceding day without any such akinetic episodes. Upon further consideration, the therapist realized that the patient was seen later in the morning on the second day and that the akinetic episode occurred about 1 hour before the patient's next dose of levodopa.

Decision/Solution

The therapist realized that the patient was exhibiting end-of-dose akinesia. Patients who have been on levodopa therapy for several years often exhibit this phenomenon, in which the effectiveness of levodopa appears to wear off before the next dose. To prevent a recurrence of this problem, the therapist made a point of scheduling this patient about 1 hour after his initial (breakfast) dose of antiparkinson medications. This at least allowed the patient to participate as much as possible in his daily exercise regimen. The therapist also notified the patient's physician of the end-of-dose akinesia. This problem was ultimately resolved by increasing the levodopa dosage so that a sufficient amount of drug was available to maintain motor function throughout each dosing cycle.

Case 2: Lithium Toxicity

Brief History

A 76-year-old woman living at home fell and fractured her right hip. She was admitted to the hospital, where she underwent total hip arthroplasty. The patient had been in relatively good health before her fall but had been receiving treatment for bipolar syndrome (manic-depression) for several years. At the time of admission, she was maintained on a dosage of 300 mg of lithium taken 3 times daily. The patient began receiving physical therapy in the hospital on the day after her hip surgery and was ambulating independently with a walker within 1 week after admission to the hospital. She was discharged to her home, but physical therapy was recommended at home to ensure continued progress and full recovery.

Problem/Influence of Medication

The physical therapist visiting this patient at home initially found her to be alert and enthusiastic about resuming her rehabilitation. By the second visit, however, the therapist noticed some confusion and slurred speech in this patient. Upon closer inspection, the therapist also observed symptoms such as hand tremors and muscle weakness. When ambulating, the patient exhibited some incoordination and became fatigued very easily.

Decision/Solution

The therapist became concerned of the potential for lithium toxicity in this patient. Apparently the hip surgery and subsequent change in activity level in this patient had altered renal excretion of lithium to the extent that this drug was slowly accumulating in the patient's body. The therapist immediately notified the patient's physician. Laboratory tests revealed a serum concentration of 2.1 mEq/L, indicating moderate levels of lithium toxicity. The patient's dosage of lithium was decreased until serum levels returned to values that were within the therapeutic range. The patient continued to receive physical therapy at home and completed her recovery from hip surgery without any further incidents.

Summary

Drug intervention in geriatric individuals can be regarded as a two-edged sword: the beneficial and therapeutic effects of any given medication must be balanced against the risk that the older adult will experience an adverse reaction to that drug. There is no doubt that many illnesses and afflictions that typically occur in a geriatric population can be alleviated through appropriate pharmacological measures. However, the risk of adverse drug reactions is increased in the elderly due to factors such as disproportionate drug use and an altered response to many medications. The potential for beneficial drug effects therefore co-exists with an increased chance for serious adverse effects in the older adult.

Physical therapists must be aware of the drug regimen used in their geriatric patients and how the beneficial and adverse effects of each medication can affect rehabilitation of these individuals. Physical therapists can also play an important role in recognizing adverse drug reactions in the elderly. Finally, therapists can help encourage proper compliance with drug therapy and discourage the excessive and inappropriate use of unnecessary medications in their geriatric patients.

References

1. Abernethy DR, Azarnoff DL: Pharmacokinetic investigations in elderly patients: Clinical and ethical considerations. *Clin Pharmacokinet* 1990; 19:82-93.
2. Abrams WB: Pathophysiology of hypertension in older patients. *Am J Med* 1988; 85(suppl 3b):7-13.
3. Abrams WB: Introduction: The concept of geriatric clinical pharmacology. *Clin Pharmacol Ther* 1987; 42:659-662.
4. Ackermann RJ, Meyer von Bremen GB: Reducing polypharmacy in the nursing home: An activist approach. *J Am Board Fam Pract* 1995; 8: 195-205.
5. Agnelli G, Sonaglia F: Prevention of venous thromboembolism in high risk patients. *Haematologica* 1997; 82:496-502.
6. Ahlin A, Junthe T, Hassan M, Nyback H: One year of tacrine (THA): Clinical and biochemical effects in patients with dementia of the Alzheimer type. *Int Psychogeriatr* 1995; 7:75-83.
7. Ailabouni W, Eknoyan G: Nonsteroidal anti-inflammatory drugs and acute renal failure in the elderly. A risk-benefit ratio. *Drugs Aging* 1996; 9:341-351.
8. Albanese A: Emerging treatments in Parkinson's disease. *Eur Neurol* 1997; 38:175-183.
9. Anderson KE: Influence of diet and nutrition on clinical pharmacokinetics. *Clin Pharmacokinet* 1988; 14:325-346.
10. Aronow WS: Postinfarction use of beta-blockers in elderly patients. *Drugs Aging* 1997; 11:424-432.
11. Aronow WS: Therapy of congestive heart failure in elderly persons. *Compr Ther* 1997; 23:639-647.
12. Atkin PA, Shenfield GM: Medication-related adverse reactions and the elderly: A literature review. *Adverse Drug React Toxicol Rev* 1995;14: 175-191.
13. Avorn J, Gurwitz JH: Drug use in the nursing home. *Ann Intern Med* 1995; 123:195-204.
14. Baker SP, et al: Age-related changes in cardiac muscarinic receptors: Decreased ability of the receptor to form a high affinity agonist binding state. *J Gerontol* 1985; 40:141-146.
15. Balducci L, Extermann M: Cancer chemotherapy in the older patient: What the medical oncologist needs to know. *Cancer* 1997; 80: 1317-1322.
16. Banazak DA: Anxiety disorders in elderly patients. *J Am Board Fam Pract* 1997; 10:280-289.
17. Beckmann CR: Alzheimer's disease: An estrogen link? *Curr Opin Obstet Gynecol* 1997; 9:295-299.
18. Bergqvist D, et al: Low-molecular-weight heparin (enoxaparin) as prophylaxis against venous thromboembolism after total hip replacement. *N Engl J Med* 1996; 335:696-700.
19. Bernus I, Dickinson RG, Hooper WD, Eadie MJ: Anticonvulsant therapy in aged patients. Clinical pharmacokinetic considerations. *Drugs Aging* 1997; 10:278-289.
20. Bjork I, Lindahl U: Mechanism of the anticoagulant action of heparin. *Mol Cell Biochem* 1982; 48:161-182.
21. Blackburn WD: Management of osteoarthritis and rheumatoid arthritis: Prospects and possibilities. *Am J Med* 1996; 100(suppl 2a):24s-30s.
22. Blumenthal MD: Depressive illness in old age: Getting behind the mask. *Geriatrics* 1980; 35:34-43.
23. Bondeson J: The mechanisms of action of disease-modifying antirheumatic drugs: A review with emphasis on macrophage signal transduction and the induction of proinflammatory cytokines. *Gen Pharmacol* 1997; 29:127-150.
24. Bressler R, Johnson DG: Oral antidiabetic drug therapy in the elderly. *Drugs Aging* 1996; 9:418-437.
25. Brown SL, et al: Occult caffeine as a source of sleep problems in an older adult population. *J Am Geriatr Soc* 1995; 43:860-864.
26. Byatt CM, Millard PH, Levin GE: Diuretics and electrolyte disturbances in 1000 consecutive geriatric admissions. *J R Soc Med* 1990; 83:704-708.
27. Cadieux RJ: Azapirones: An alternative to benzodiazepines for anxiety. *Am Fam Physician* 1996; 53:2349-2353.
28. Cadieux RJ: Drug interactions in the elderly: How multiple drug use increases risk exponentially. *Postgrad Med* 1989; 86:179-186.
29. Cahn MD, Tran T, Theur CP, Butler JA: Hormone replacement therapy and the risk of breast lesions that predispose to cancer. *Am Surg* 1997; 63:858-860.
30. Carlson JE: Perils of polypharmacy: 10 steps to prudent prescribing. *Geriatrics* 1996; 51:26-30.
31. Cartwright A: Medicine taking by people aged 65 or more. *Br Med Bull* 1990; 46:63-76.
32. Catterson ML, Preskorn SH, Martin RL: Pharmacodynamic and pharmacokinetic considerations in geriatric psychopharmacology. *Psychiatr Clin North Am* 1997; 20:205-218.

33. Chabner BA, Allegra CJ, Curt GA, Calabresi P: Antineoplastic agents, in Hardman JG, Gilman AG, Limbird LE (eds): *The Pharmacological Basis of Therapeutics,* ed 9. New York, McGraw-Hill, 1996.

34. Chiovato L, Mariotti S, Pinchera A: Thyroid diseases in the elderly. *Ballieres Clin Endocrinol Metab* 1997; 11:251-270.

35. Choy EH, Scott DL: Drug treatment and rheumatic diseases in the 1990s. Achievements and future developments. *Drugs* 1997; 53: 337-348.

36. Chutka DS, Evans JM, Fleming KC, Mikkelson KG: Symposium on geriatrics—Part I: Drug prescribing for elderly patients. *Mayo Clin Proc* 1995; 70:685-693.

37. Ciccone CD: Update: Free radical toxicity and antioxidant medications in Parkinson's disease. *Phys Ther* 1998; 78:313-319.

38. Ciccone CD: Current trends in cardiovascular pharmacology. *Phys Ther* 1996; 76:481-497.

39. Ciccone CD: *Pharmacology in Rehabilitation,* ed 2. Philadelphia, FA Davis, 1996.

40. Cleary JF, Carbone PP: Palliative medicine in the elderly. *Cancer* 1997; 80:1335-1347.

41. Cleland JG, et al: Beta-blocking agents in heart failure. Should they be used and how? *Eur Heart J* 1996; 17:1629-1639.

42. Cohen JL: Pharmacokinetic changes in aging. *Am J Med* 1986; 80(suppl 5a):31-38.

43. Colley CA, Lucas LM: Polypharmacy: The cure becomes the disease. *J Gen Intern Med* 1993; 8:278-283.

44. Compston JE: Hormone replacement therapy. *Ballieres Clin Rheumatol* 1997; 11:583-596.

45. Conaghan PG, Brooks P: Disease-modifying antirheumatic drugs, including methotrexate, gold, sulfasalazine, antimalarials, and D-penicillamine. *Curr Opin Rheumatol* 1996; 8:176-182.

46. Conaghan PG, Lehmann T, Brooks P: Disease-modifying antirheumatic drugs. *Curr Opin Rheumatol* 1997; 9:183-190.

47. Corey-Bloom J, Galasko D: Adjunctive therapy in patients with Alzheimer's disease. A practical approach. *Drugs Aging* 1995; 7:79-87.

48. Craig GM: Clinical presentation of orthostatic hypotension in the elderly. *Postgrad Med J* 1994; 70:638-642.

49. Cronstein BN: The mechanism of action of methotrexate. *Rheum Dis Clin North Am* 1997; 23:739-755.

50. Cutson TM, Laub KC, Schenkman M: Pharmacological and nonpharmacological interventions in the treatment of Parkinson's disease. *Phys Ther* 1995; 75:363-373.

51. Davies P, Bailey PJ, Goldenberg MM: The role of arachidonic acid oxygenation products in pain and inflammation. *Annu Rev Immunol* 1984; 2:335-357.

52. Davis FB, et al: Estimation of a physiologic replacement dose of levothyroxine in elderly patients with hypothyroidism. *Arch Intern Med* 1984; 144:1752-1754.

53. Davis KL, et al: A double-blind, placebo-controlled multicenter study of tacrine for Alzheimer's disease. The Tacrine Collaborative Study Group. *N Engl J Med* 1992; 327:1253-1259.

54. Dawling S, Crome P: Clinical pharmacokinetic considerations in the elderly. An update. *Clin Pharmacokinet* 1989; 17:236-263.

55. Dellasega C, Keiser CL: Pharmacological approaches to chronic pain in the older adult. *Nurse Pract* 1997; 22:20-24.

56. Denham MJ: Adverse drug reactions. *Br Med Bull* 1990; 46:53-62.

57. Devanand DP, Levy SR: Neuroleptic treatment of agitation and psychosis in dementia. *J Geriatr Psychiatry Neurol* 1995; 8(suppl 1): s18-s27.

58. Dow L, Holgate ST: Assessment and treatment of obstructive airway disease in the elderly. *Br Med Bull* 1990; 46:230-245.

59. Duggan AW, North RA: Electrophysiology of the opioids. *Pharmacol Rev* 1983; 35:219-281.

60. Dunner DL: Therapeutic considerations in treating depression in the elderly. *J Clin Psychiatry* 1994; 55(suppl):48-58.

61. Egbert AM: Postoperative pain management in the frail elderly. *Clin Geriatr Med* 1996; 12:583-599.

62. Evans MA, et al: Gastric emptying rate in the elderly: Implications for drug therapy. *J Am Geriat Soc* 1981; 29:201-205.

63. Finkel SI: Efficacy and tolerability of antidepressant therapy in the old-old. *J Clin Psychiatry* 1996; 57(suppl 5):23-28.

64. Fleming KC, Evans JM: Pharmacological therapies in dementia. *Mayo Clin Proc* 1995; 70:1116-1123.

65. Flint AJ: Epidemiology and comorbidity of anxiety disorders in later life: Implications for treatment. *Clin Neurosci* 1997; 4:31-36.

66. Flower RJ, Vane JR: Inhibition of prostaglandin synthetase in brain explains the antipyretic action of paracetamol (4-acetamidophenol). *Nature* 1972; 240:410-411.

67. Forman WB: Opioid analgesic drugs in the elderly. *Clin Geriatr Med* 1996; 12:489-500.

68. Francis CW, et al: Comparison of two warfarin regimens in the prevention of venous thrombosis following total knee replacement. *Thromb Haemost* 1996; 75:706-711.

69. Freis ED: The cardiovascular risks of thiazide diuretics. *Clin Pharmacol Ther* 1986; 39:239-244.

70. Friedhoff AJ: A strategy for developing novel drugs for the treatment of schizophrenia. *Schizophr Bull* 1983; 9:504-527.

71. Furst DE: Clinical pharmacology of combination DMARD therapy in rheumatoid arthritis. *J Rheumatol Suppl* 1996; 44:86-90.

72. Gambrell RD: Estrogen-progesterone replacement and cancer risk. *Hosp Pract* 1990; 25:81-91.

73. Gardner G, Furst DE: Disease-modifying antirheumatic drugs. Potential effects in older patients. *Drugs Aging* 1995; 7:420-437.

74. Gerber JG, Nies AS: Beta-adrenergic blocking drugs. *Annu Rev Med* 1985; 36:145-164.

75. Gershanik OS: Drug-induced parkinsonism in the aged. Recognition and prevention. *Drugs Aging* 1994; 5:127-132.

76. Gleckman RA, Czachor JS: Reviewing the safe use of antibiotics in the elderly. *Geriatrics* 1989; 44:33-39.

77. Glennas A, et al: Auranofin is safe and superior to placebo in elderly-onset arthritis. *Br J Rheumatol* 1997; 36:870-877.

78. Goldstein S: Beta-blocking drugs and coronary heart disease. *Cardiovasc Drugs Ther* 1997; 11(suppl 1):219-225.

79. Gosselink AT, van Veldhuisen DJ, Crijns HJ: When, and when not, to use digoxin in the elderly. *Drugs Aging* 1997; 10:411-420.

80. Gottlieb GL: Sleep disorders and their management: Special considerations in the elderly. *Am J Med* 1990; 88(suppl 3a):29-33.

81. Grad RM: Benzodiazepines for insomnia in community-dwelling elderly: A review of benefit and risk. *J Fam Pract* 1995; 41:473-481.

82. Greenblatt DJ: Basic pharmacokinetic principles and their application to psychotropic drugs. *J Clin Psychiatry* 1993; 54(suppl):8-13.

83. Greenblatt DJ, Shader RI, Harmatz JS: Implications of altered drug disposition in the elderly: Studies of benzodiazepines. *J Clin Pharmacol* 1989; 29:866-872.

84. Grierson DJ: Hydroxychloroquine and visual screening in a rheumatology outpatient clinic. *Ann Rheum Dis* 1997; 56:188-190.

85. Guarnieri T, et al: Contractile and biochemical correlates of beta-adrenergic stimulation of the aged heart. *Am J Physiol* 1980; 239:H501-H508.

86. Gupta S, Rappaport HM, Bennett LT: Polypharmacy among nursing home geriatric Medicaid recipients. *Ann Pharmacother* 1996; 30: 946-950.

87. Hagan JJ, Middlemiss DN, Sharpe PC, Poste GH: Parkinson's disease: Prospects for improved drug therapy. *Trends Pharmacol Sci* 1997; 18:156-163.

88. Hamdy RC, et al: Reducing polypharmacy in extended care. *South Med J* 1995; 88:534-538.

89. Hanlon JT, et al: Adverse drug events in high risk outpatients. *J Am Geriatr Soc* 1997; 45:945-948.

90. Hanlon JT, et al: A randomized, controlled trial of a clinical pharmacist intervention to improve inappropriate prescribing in elderly outpatients with polypharmacy. *Am J Med* 1996; 100:428-437.

91. Hardman JG, Gilman AG, Limbird LE (eds): *The Pharmacologicalal Basis of Therapeutics,* ed 9. New York, McGraw-Hill, 1996.

92. Harris MG, Benfield P: Fluoxetine. A review of its pharmacodynamic and pharmacokinetic properties, and therapeutic use in older patients with depressive illness. *Drugs Aging* 1995; 6:64-84.

93. Hayashi H, et al: The utility of Nitroderm TTS in angina pectoris: Long-term treatment after switching from long-acting oral isosorbide dinitrate. *Clin Cardiol* 1994; 17:31-36.

94. Heidenreich PA, Lee TT, Massie BM: Effect of beta-blockade on mortality in patients with heart failure: A meta-analysis of randomized clinical trials. *J Am Coll Cardiol* 1997; 30:27-34.

95. Hely MA, Morris JG: Controversies in the treatment of Parkinson's disease. *Curr Opin Neurol* 1996; 9:308-313.

96. Henderson NK, Sambrook PN: Relationship between osteoporosis and arthritis and effect of corticosteroids and other drugs on bone. *Curr Opin Rheumatol* 1996; 8:365-369.

97. Hennessey JV: Diagnosis and management of thyrotoxicosis. *Am Fam Physician* 1996; 54:1315-1324.

98. Hillson JL, Furst DE: Pharmacology and pharmacokinetics of methotrexate in rheumatic disease. Practical issues in treatment and design. *Rheum Dis Clin North Am* 1997; 23:757-778.

99. Hirschowitz BI: Nonsteroidal anti-inflammatory drugs and the gut. *South Med J* 1996; 89:259-263.

100. Hocking LB, Koenig HG: Anxiety in medically ill older patients: A review and update. *Int J Psychiatry Med* 1995; 25:221-238.

101. Hogan DB: Revisiting the O complex: Urinary incontinence, delirium and polypharmacy in elderly patients. *Can Med Assoc J* 19XX; 157:1071-1077.

102. Hollister LE: Current antidepressants. *Annu Rev Pharmacol Toxicol* 1986; 26:23-37.

103. Hughes AJ: Drug treatment of Parkinson's disease in the 1990s. Achievements and future possibilities. *Drugs* 1997; 53:195-205.

104. Jacobs S, Hillard TC: Hormone replacement therapy in the aged. A state of the art review. *Drugs Aging* 1996; 8:193-213.

105. Jain R, Lipsky PE: Treatment of rheumatoid arthritis. *Med Clin North Am* 1997; 81:57-84.

106. Jenike MA: Psychiatric illnesses in the elderly: A review. *J Geriatr Psychiatry Neurol* 1996; 9:57-82.

107. Jenike MA: Psychoactive drugs in the elderly: Antipsychotics and anxiolytics. *Geriatrics* 1988; 43:53-65.

108. Jennings PE: Oral antihyperglycemics. Considerations in older patients with non-insulin-dependent diabetes mellitus. *Drugs Aging* 1997; 10:323-331.

109. Jeste DV, et al: Management of late-life psychosis. *J Clin Psychiatry* 1996; 57(suppl 3):39-45.

110. Johnson JE: *Aging and Cell Structure,* 2 vols. New York, Plenum Press, 1984.

111. Jones G, Brooks PM: Injectable gold compounds: An overview. *Br J Rheumatol* 1996; 35:1145-1158.

112. Jonsson PV, Lipsitz LA: Cardiovascular factors contributing to falls in the older adult. *Top Geriatr Rehabil* 1990; 5:21-33.

113. Kaplan NM: Diuretics: Cornerstone of antihypertensive therapy. *Am J Cardiol* 1996; 77:3b-5b.

114. Khraishi MM, Singh G: The role of anti-malarials in rheumatoid arthritis—the American experience. *Lupus* 1996; 5(suppl 1):s41-s44.

115. Kimmick GG, Fleming R, Muss HB, Balducci L: Cancer chemotherapy in older adults. A tolerability perspective. *Drugs Aging* 1997; 10:34-49.

116. Koella WP: CNS-related (side) effects of beta-blockers with special reference to mechanism of action. *Eur J Clin Pharmacol* 1985; 28 (suppl 1):55-63.

117. Kores B, Lader MH: Irreversible lithium toxicity: An overview. *Clin Neuropharmacol* 1997; 20:283-299.

118. Lacro JP, Jeste DV: Geriatric psychosis. *Psychiatr Q* 1997; 68:247-260.

119. Lake JT, Rahman AH, Grossberg GT: Diagnosis and treatment of psychotic symptoms in elderly patients. *Drugs Aging* 1997; 11:170-177.

120. Lamberts SW, van den Beld AW, van der Lely AJ: The endocrinology of aging. *Science* 1997; 278:419-424.

121. Lamy PP: Nonprescription drugs and the elderly. *Am Fam Physician* 1989; 39:175-179.

122. LaPier TK: Glucocorticoid-induced muscle atrophy. The role of exercise in treatment and prevention. *J Cardiopulm Rehabil* 1997; 17:76-84.

123. Larsen GL, Henson PM: Mediators of inflammation. *Annu Rev Immunol* 1983; 1:335-359.

124. Latimer PR: Tardive dyskinesia: A review. *Can J Psychiatry* 1995; 40(suppl):s49-s54.

125. Lever AF, Ramsay LE: Treatment of hypertension in the elderly. *J Hypertens* 1995; 13:571-579.

126. Lewis GD, Campbell WB, Johnson AR: Inhibition of prostaglandin synthesis of glucocorticoids in human endothelial cells. *Endocrinology* 1986; 119:62-69.

127. Lindholm LH: Antihypertensive treatment in the elderly. *Clin Exp Hypertens* 1996; 18:435-447.

128. Lipsky PE: Remission-inducing therapy in rheumatoid arthritis. *Am J Med* 1983; 75(suppl 4b):40-49.

129. Lipson LG: Diabetes in the elderly: Diagnosis, pathogenesis, and therapy. *Am J Med* 1986; 80(suppl 5a):10-21.

130. Loi C-M, Vestal RE: Drug metabolism in the elderly. *Pharmacol Ther* 1988; 36:131-149.

131. Lonergan ET: Aging and the kidney: Adjusting treatment to physiologic change. *Geriatrics* 1988; 43:27-33.

132. Maczaj M: Pharmacological treatment of insomnia. *Drugs* 1993; 45:44-55.

133. Mahler ME: Seizures: Common causes and treatment in the elderly. *Geriatrics* 1987; 42:73-78.

134. Mao CA, Siegler EL, Abrutyn E: Antimicrobial resistance patterns in long term geriatric care. Implications for drug therapy. *Drugs Aging* 1996; 8:162-170.

135. Marchesini G, et al: Galactose elimination capacity and liver volume in aging man. *Hepatology* 1988; 8:1079-1083.

136. Marsden CD: Problems with long-term levodopa therapy for Parkinson's disease. *Clin Neuropharmacol* 1994; 17(suppl 2):s32-s44.

137. Mattson RH: Efficacy and adverse effects of established and new antiepileptic drugs. *Epilepsia* 1995; 36(suppl 2):s13-s26.

138. McDonald RH: The evolution of current hypertension therapy. *Am J Med* 1988; 85(suppl 3b):14-18.

139. McMurray L, McDevitt DG: Treatment of heart failure in the elderly. *Br Med Bull* 1990; 46:202-229.

140. McNutt LA, et al: Impact of regulation on benzodiazepine prescribing to a low income elderly population, New York State. *J Clin Epidemiol* 1994; 47:613-625.

141. Mendelson B: The use of sedative/hypnotic medication and its correlation with falling down in the hospital. *Sleep* 1996; 19:698-701.

142. Meyers BR, Wilkinson P: Clinical pharmacokinetics of antibacterial drugs in the elderly: Implications for selection and dosage. *Clin Pharmacokinet* 1989; 17:385-395.

143. Michet CJ, et al: Common rheumatologic diseases in elderly patients. *Mayo Clin Proc* 1995; 70:1205-1214.

144. Miller KL: Hormone replacement therapy in the elderly. *Clin Obstet Gynecol* 1996; 39:912-932.

145. Miller M: Type II diabetes: A treatment approach for the older patient. *Geriatrics* 1996; 51:43-44.

146. Mitlak BH, Cohen FJ: In search of optimal long-term female hormone replacement: The potential of selective estrogen replacement modulators. *Horm Res* 1997; 48:155-163.

147. Moncur C, Williams HJ: Rheumatoid arthritis: Status of drug therapies. *Phys Ther* 1995; 75:511-525.

148. Monette J, Gurwitz JH, Avorn J: Epidemiology of adverse drug events in the nursing home setting. *Drugs Aging* 1995; 7:203-211.

149. Montamat SC, Cusack BJ, Vestal RE: Management of drug therapy in the elderly. *N Engl J Med* 1989; 321:303-309.

150. Mooradian AD: Drug therapy of non-insulin-dependent diabetes mellitus in the elderly. *Drugs* 1996; 51:931-941.

151. Morgan R, King D: Influenza vaccination in the elderly. *Postgrad Med J* 1996; 72:339-342.

152. Morike K, Schwab M, Klotz U: Use of aminoglycosides in elderly patients. Pharmacokinetic and clinical considerations. *Drugs Aging* 1997; 10:259-277.

153. Mullen E, Katona C, Bellew M: Patterns of sleep disorders and sedative hypnotic use in seniors. *Drugs Aging* 1994; 5:49-58.

154. Mustard CA, Mayer T: Case-control study of exposure to medication and the risk of injurious falls requiring hospitalization among nursing home residents. *Am J Epidemiol* 1997; 145:738-745.

155. Naranjo CA, Herrmann N, Mittmann N, Bremner KE: Recent advances in geriatric psychopharmacology. *Drugs Aging* 1995; 7:184-202.

156. Nattel S: Comparative mechanisms of action of antiarrhythmic drugs. *Am J Cardiol* 1993; 72:13f-17f.

157. Nichol KL, Margolis KL, Wouremna J, von Sternberg T: Effectiveness of influenza vaccine. *Gerontology* 1996; 42:274-279.

158. Nicholls MG: Age-related effects of diuretics in hypertensive subjects. *J Cardiovasc Pharmacol* 1988; 12(suppl 8):51-59.

159. Nicholson KG: Use of antivirals in influenza in the elderly: Prophylaxis and therapy. *Gerontology* 1996; 42:280-289.

160. Nolan L, O'Malley K: Prescribing for the elderly. Part I: Sensitivity of the elderly to adverse drug reactions. *J Am Geriatr Soc* 1988; 36:142-149.

161. Nordberg A: Pharmacological treatment of cognitive dysfunction in dementia disorders. *Acta Neurol Scand Suppl* 1996; 168:87-92.

162. Nuki G: Pain control and the use of nonsteroidal analgesic anti-inflammatory drugs. *Br Med Bull* 1990; 46:262-278.

163. O'Connor SW, Scarpace PJ, Abrass IB: Age-associated decrease of adenylate cyclase activity in rat myocardium. *Mech Ageing Dev* 1981; 16:91-95.

164. O'Dell JR: Methotrexate use in rheumatoid arthritis. *Rheum Dis Clin North Am* 1997; 23:779-796.

165. Ooi HH, Coleman PL, Duggan J, O'Meara YM: Treatment of hypertension in the elderly. *Curr Opin Nephrol Hypertens* 1997; 6:504-509.

166. Oparil S: Introduction: Treating the older hypertensive patient—an overview. *Am J Med* 1988; 85(suppl 3b):1.

167. O'Reilly RA: Vitamin K and the oral anticoagulant drugs. *Annu Rev Med* 1976; 27:245-261.

168. Oxman TE: Antidepressants and cognitive impairment in the elderly. *J Clin Psychiatry* 1996; 57(suppl 5):38-44.

169. Paratt JR: Nitroglycerin—the first one hundred years: New facts about an old friend. *J Pharm Pharmacol* 1979; 31:801-809.

170. Parker BM, Cusack BJ, Vestal RE: Pharmacokinetic optimization of drug therapy in elderly patients. *Drugs Aging* 1995; 7:10-18.

171. Passant U, Warkentin S, Gustafson L: Orthostatic hypotension and low blood pressure in organic dementia: A study of prevalence and related clinical characteristics. *Int J Geriatr Psychiatry* 1997; 12:395-403.

172. Pecknold JC: A risk-benefit assessment of buspirone in the treatment of anxiety disorders. *Drug Saf* 1997; 16:118-132.

173. Peel C, Mossberg KA: Effects of cardiovascular medications on exercise responses. *Phys Ther* 1995; 75:387-396.

174. Phillips AC, Polisson RP, Simon LS: NSAIDs and the elderly. Toxicity and economic implications. *Drugs Aging* 1997; 10:119-130.

175. Phister JE, Jue SG, Cusack BJ: Problems in the use of anticancer drugs in the elderly. *Drugs* 1989; 37:551-565.

176. *Physician's Desk Reference*, ed. 52. Montvale, NJ, Medical Economics Co, 1998.

177. Planchock NY, Slay LE: Pharmacokinetic and pharmacodynamic monitoring of the elderly in critical care. *Crit Care Nurs Clin North Am* 1996; 8:79-89.

178. Pollock BG, Mulsant BH: Antipsychotics in older patients. A safety perspective. *Drugs Aging* 1995; 6:312-323.

179. Pope RM: Rheumatoid arthritis: Pathogenesis and early recognition. *Am J Med* 1996; 100(suppl 2a):3s-9s.

180. Potter JF, Haigh RA: Benefits of antihypertensive therapy in the elderly. *Br Med Bull* 1990; 46:77-93.

181. Prince MJ: The treatment of hypertension in older people and its effect on cognitive function. *Biomed Pharmacother* 1997; 51:208-212.

182. PV: Developing treatment guidelines for Alzheimer's disease and other dementias. *J Clin Psychiatry* 1996; 57(suppl 14):37-38.

183. Rau R, Schleusser B, Herborn G, Karger T: Long-term treatment of destructive rheumatoid arthritis with methotrexate. *J Rheumatol* 1997; 24:1881-1889.

184. WA, Griffin MR: Prescribed medications and the risk of falling. *Top Geriatr Rehabil* 1990; 5:12-20.

185. Renwick DS, Connolly MJ: Prevalence and treatment of chronic airways obstruction in adults over the age of 45. *Thorax* 1996; 51:164-168.

186. Reynolds E, Baron RB: Hypertension in women and the elderly. Some puzzling and some unexpected findings of treatment studies. *Postgrad Med* 1996; 100:58-63.

187. Rich MW: Epidemiology, pathophysiology, and etiology of congestive heart failure in older adults. *J Am Geriatr Soc* 1997; 45:968-974.

188. Robertson DRC, George CF: Drug therapy for Parkinson's disease in the elderly. *Br Med Bull* 1990; 46:124-146.

189. Robinson DR: Prostaglandins and the mechanism of action of anti-inflammatory drugs. *Am J Med* 1983; 75(suppl 4b):26-31.

190. Rothschild AJ: The diagnosis and treatment of late-life depression. *J Clin Psychiatry* 1996; 57(suppl 5):5-11.

191. Rumble RH, Morgan K: Longitudinal trends in prescribing for elderly patients: Two surveys four years apart. *Br J Gen Pract* 1994; 44: 571-575.

192. Rummans TA, Evans JM, Krahn LE, Fleming KC: Delirium in elderly patients: Evaluation and management. *Mayo Clin Proc* 1995; 70:989-998.

193. Sachdev P: The epidemiology of drug-induced akathisia: Part II. Chronic, tardive, and withdrawal akathisia. *Schizophr Bull* 1995; 21:451-461.

194. Sack KE: Update on NSAID's in the elderly. *Geriatrics* 1989; 44:71-90.

195. Salerno E: Psychopharmacology and the elderly. *Top Geriatr Rehabil* 1986; 1:35-45.

196. Salzman C: Medication compliance in the elderly. *J Clin Psychiatry* 1995; 56(suppl 1):18-22.

197. Sawin CT, et al: Aging and the thyroid: Decreased requirement for thyroid hormone in older hypothyroid patients. *Am J Med* 1983; 75: 206-209.

198. Scarpace PJ, Abrass IB: Decreased beta-adrenergic agonist affinity and adenylate cyclase activity in senescent rat lung. *J Gerontol* 1983; 38:143-147.

199. Schachter SC: Review of the mechanisms of antiepileptic drugs. *CNS Drugs* 1995; 4:469-477.

200. Scheuer ML, Pedley TA: Current concepts: The evaluation and treatment of seizures. *N Engl J Med* 1990; 323:1468-1471.

201. Schiff M: Emerging treatments for rheumatoid arthritis. *Am J Med* 1997; 102(suppl 1a):11s-15s.

202. Schimmer BP, Parker KL: Adrenocorticotropic hormone; adrenocortical steroids and their synthetic analogs; inhibitors of the synthesis and action of adrenocortical hormones, in Hardman JG, Gilman AG, Limbird LE (eds.): *The Pharmacologicalal Basis of Therapeutics*, ed 9. New York, McGraw-Hill, 1996.

203. Schneider LS: New therapeutic approaches to Alzheimer's disease. *J Clin Psychiatry* 1996; 57(suppl 14):30-36.

204. Schneider LS: Efficacy of treatment for geropsychiatric patients with severe mental illness. *Psychopharmacol Bull* 1993; 29:501-524.

205. Schneider LS, Finch CE: Can estrogens prevent neurodegeneration? *Drugs Aging* 1997; 11:87-95.

206. Schneider LS, Olin JT: Efficacy of acute treatment for geriatric depression. *Int Psychogeriatr* 1995; 7(suppl):7-25.

207. Scholz H: Classification and mechanism of action of antiarrhythmic drugs. *Fundam Clin Pharmacol* 1994; 8:385-390.

208. Senni M, Redfield MM: Congestive heart failure in elderly patients. *Mayo Clin Proc* 1997; 72:453-460.

209. Shammas E, Dickstein K: Drug selection for optimal treatment of hypertension in the elderly. *Drugs Aging* 1997; 11:19-26.

210. Sheard MH: The biological effects of lithium. *Trends Neurosci* 1986; 3:85-86.

211. Sihvo S, Hemminki E: Self-medication of dyspepsia: How appropriate is it? *Scand J Gastroenterol* 1997; 32:855-861.

212. Simonson W: *Medications and the Elderly: A Guide for Promoting Proper Use*. Rockville, Md, Aspen Publications, 1984.

213. Singh G, et al: Gastrointestinal tract complications of nonsteroidal anti-inflammatory drug treatment in rheumatoid arthritis. A prospective observational cohort study. *Arch Intern Med* 1996; 156:1530-1536.

214. Skerritt U, Evans R, Montgomery SA: Selective serotonin reuptake inhibitors in older patients. A tolerability perspective. *Drugs Aging* 1997; 10:209-218.

215. Sky AJ, Grossberg GT: The use of psychotropic medication in the management of problem behaviors in the patient with Alzheimer's disease. *Med Clin North Am* 1994; 78:811-822.

216. Sloan RW: Principles of drug therapy in geriatric patients. *Am Fam Physician* 1992; 45:2709-2718.

217. Smith WF: Epidemiology of hypertension in older patients. *Am J Med* 1988; 85(suppl 3b):2-6.

218. Speroff L: Postmenopausal hormone therapy into the 21st century. *Int J Gynaecol Obstet* 1997; 59(suppl 1):s3-s10.

219. Spore D, et al: Psychotropic use among older residents of board and care facilities. *J Am Geriatr Soc* 1995; 43:1403-1409.

220. Spore D, et al: Regulatory environment and psychotropic use in board-and-care facilities: Results of a 10-state study. *J Gerontol A Biolog Sci Med Sci* 1996; 51:M131-M141.

221. Staessen J, et al: Antihypertensive drug treatment in elderly hypertensive subjects: Evidence of protection. *J Cardiovasc Pharmacol* 1988; 12(suppl 18):33-38.

222. Steinberg JR: Anxiety in elderly patients. A comparison of azapirones and benzodiazepines. *Drugs Aging* 1994; 5:335-345.

223. Stewart RB, Cooper JW: Polypharmacy in the aged. Practical solutions. *Drugs Aging* 1994; 4:449-461.

224. Stoudemire A: Epidemiology and psychopharmacology of anxiety in medical patients. *J Clin Psychiatry* 1996; 57(suppl 7):64-72.

225. Stults BM, Dere WH, Caine TH: Long-term anticoagulation: Indications and management. *West J Med* 1989; 151:414-429.

226. Stumpf JL, Mitrzyk B: Management of orthostatic hypotension. *Am J Hosp Pharm* 1994; 51:648-698.

227. Sunderland T: Treatment of the elderly suffering from psychosis and dementia. *J Clin Psychiatry* 1996; 57(suppl 9):53-56.

228. Sweeney M: Constipation. Diagnosis and treatment. *Home Care Provid* 1997; 2:250-255.

229. Swift CG: Pharmacodynamics: Changes in homeostatic mechanisms, receptor and target organ sensitivity in the elderly. *Br Med Bull* 1990; 46:36-52.

230. Taburet AM, Schmit B: Pharmacokinetic optimization of asthma treatment. *Clin Pharmacokinet* 1994; 26:396-418.

231. Tallman JF, Gallager DW: The GABA-ergic system: A locus of benzodiazepine action. *Annu Rev Neurosci* 1985; 8:21-44.

232. Tamblyn R: Medication use in seniors: Challenges and solutions. *Therapie* 1996; 51:269-282.

233. Tannenbaum H, et al: An evidence-based approach to prescribing NSAIDs in musculoskeletal disease: A Canadian consensus. *Can Med Assoc J* 1996; 155:77-88.

234. Tariot PN: Treatment strategies for agitation and psychosis in dementia. *J Clin Psychiatry* 1996; 57(suppl 14):21-29.

235. Tariot PN, Schneider L, Porsteinsson AP: Treating Alzheimer's disease. Pharmacological options now and in the near future. *Postgrad Med J* 1997; 101:73-76.

236. Thapa PB, Gideon P, Fought RL, Ray WA: Psychotropic drugs and risk of recurrent falls in ambulatory nursing home residents. *Am J Epidemiol* 1995; 142:202-211.

237. Thompson TL, Moran MG, Nies AS: Psychotropic drug use in the elderly. *N Engl J Med* 1983; 308:134-138, 194-199.

238. Thorpe L: The treatment of psychotic disorders in late life. *Can J Psychiatry* 1997; 42(suppl 1):19s-27s.

239. Tinetti ME, Speechley M, Ginter SF: Risk factors for falls among elderly persons living in the community. *N Engl J Med* 1988; 319:1701-1707.

240. Tomlinson B: New insights into the treatment of hypertension. *Clin Exp Pharmacol Physiol* 1997; 24:978-981.

241. Tomlinson B: Optimal dosage of ACE inhibitors in older patients. *Drugs Aging* 1996; 9:262-273.

242. Tonda ME, Guthrie SK: Treatment of acute neuroleptic-induced movement disorders. *Pharmacotherapy* 1994; 14:543-560.

243. Tourigny-Rivard MF: Pharmacotherapy of affective disorders in old age. *Can J Psychiatry* 1997; 42(suppl 1):10s-18s.

244. Tregaskis BF, Stevenson LH: Pharmacokinetics in old age. *Br Med Bull* 1990; 46:9-21.

245. Tsujimoto G, Hashimoto K, Hoffman BB: Pharmacokinetic and pharmacodynamic principles of drug therapy in old age: Part 1. *Int J Clin Pharmacol Ther Toxicol* 1989; 27:13-26.

246. Vane JR: Inhibition of prostaglandin synthesis as a mechanism of action for aspirin-like drugs. *Nature* 1971; 231:232-235.

247. Van Gelder IC, Brugemann J, Crijns HJ: Pharmacological management of arrhythmias in the elderly. *Drugs Aging* 1997; 11:96-110.

248. van Gestel AM, Haagsma CJ, Furst DE, van Piel PL: Treatment of early rheumatoid arthritis patients with slow-acting antirheumatic drugs (SAARDs). *Ballieres Clin Rheumatol* 1997; 11:65-82.

249. van Noort JM, Amor S: Cell biology of autoimmune diseases. *Int Rev Cytol* 1998; 178:127-206.

250. van Reekum R, Black SE, Conn D, Clarke D: Cognition-enhancing drugs in dementia: A guide to the near future. *Can J Psychiatry* 1997; 42(suppl 1):35s-50s.

251. Verhaeverbeke I, Mets T: Drug-induced orthostatic hypotension in the elderly: Avoiding its onset. *Drug Saf* 1997; 17:105-118.

252. Vigreux P, et al: Antiarrhythmic drug-induced side effects: A prospective survey of 300 patients. *Therapie* 1995; 50:413-418.

253. Wainwright RJ, et al: The long-term safety and tolerability of transdermal glyceryl trinitrate, when used with a patch-free interval in patients with stable angina. *Br J Clin Pract* 1993; 47:178-182.

254. Watts RL: The role of dopamine agonists in early Parkinson's disease. *Neurology* 1997; 49(suppl 1):s34-s48.

255. Weir MR, Flack JM, Applegate WB: Tolerability, safety, and quality of life and hypertensive therapy: The case for low-dose diuretics. *Am J Med* 1996; 101(suppl 3a):83s-92s.

256. Weiss KJ: Management of anxiety and depression syndromes in the elderly. *J Clin Psychiatry* 1994; 55(suppl):5-12.

257. Wester JP, et al: Risk factors for bleeding during treatment of acute venous thromboembolism. *Thromb Haemost* 1996; 76:682-688.

258. Whalley LJ, Bradnock J: Treatment of the classical manifestations of dementia and confusion. *Br Med Bull* 1990; 46:169-180.

259. Wilske KR: Approaches to the management of rheumatoid arthritis: Rationale for early combination therapy. *Br J Rheumatol* 1993; 32(suppl 1):24-27.

260. Winger JM, Hornick T: Age-associated changes in the endocrine system. *Nurs Clin North Am* 1996; 31:827-844.

261. Wise MG, Griffies WS: A combined treatment approach to anxiety in the medically ill. *J Clin Psychiatry* 1995; 56(suppl 2):14-19.

262. Witt DM, Lousberg TR: Controversies surrounding estrogen use in postmenopausal women. *Ann Pharmacother* 1997; 31:745-755.

263. Wolfe F: Adverse drug reactions of DMARDs and DC-ARTs in rheumatoid arthritis. *Clin Exp Rheumatol* 1997; 15(suppl 17):s75-s81.

264. Woodhouse KW, James OF: Hepatic drug metabolism and aging. *Br Med Bull* 1990; 46:22-35.

265. Wynne HA, et al: The effect of age upon liver volume and apparent liver blood flow in healthy men. *Hepatology* 1989; 9:297-301.

266. Yaksh TL, Noueihed R: The physiology and pharmacology of spinal opiates. *Annu Rev Pharmacol Toxicol* 1985; 25:433-462.

267. Zaleon CR, Guthrie SK: Antipsychotic drug use in older adults. *Am J Hosp Pharm* 1994; 51:2917-2943.

PART III

PROBLEMS AND PROCEDURES

CHAPTER 13

FUNCTIONAL TRAINING

MICHAEL MORAN, PT, ScD AND EDMUND M. KOSMAHL, PT, EdD

OUTLINE

INTRODUCTION

Living at home and interacting with the community can be challenging for the older adult. Often, a delicate balance must exist between functional capability, adaptation of the environment, and reliance upon support services. The purposes of this chapter are to present some of the challenges that confront the older adult living at home and to offer some strategies for minimizing their impact.

GENERAL CONSIDERATIONS

Challenges for the Older Adult to Remain in the Community

To live independently, people must be able to safely perform a complement of self-care and home management activities. The specific nature of the activities required by any given individual depends on many variables. Still, one can identify two broad groups of activities and tasks that are usually necessary for independent living—*activities of daily living (ADLs)* and *instrumental activities of daily living (IADLs)*.

People perform ADLs to manage basic personal hygiene and survival needs. Functional activities that may be in-

cluded in this category are bed mobility, getting in and out of a bed or chair, bathing, toileting, dressing, grooming, eating, and ambulating. These activities are sometimes called *personal* activities of daily living.[94]

IADLs are more complex functional abilities that are also required for independent community living. These include activities such as preparing meals, laundering clothes, doing housework, using the telephone, traveling (using public transportation or driving), shopping, taking medications, and managing money.[53]

Dependence (requiring the assistance of another person) for ADLs and IADLs increases the risk of institutionalization and mortality.[94] The capacity to perform IADLs independently is strongly associated with velocity of gait, balance, grip strength, and chair rise time.[43] Researchers have shown that exercise can improve strength, balance, and velocity of gait for older persons.[17,26,42,44] Assistive devices can be used to facilitate independent performance of ADLs and IADLs, e.g., using a shower seat to facilitate bathing or a motorized scooter to facilitate shopping. Clearly, appropriate use of therapeutic exercise, functional training, and prescription and application of assistive devices can promote independence for community-dwelling elders.

Team Approach to Challenges

Regardless of the setting in which an older individual may reside, multiple challenges may arise, especially those affecting function. Those challenges are often best dealt with by a team or multidisciplinary approach. Incorporating the expertise and perspectives of several professionals facilitates differentiation of problems and enhances holistic care for individual patients.[20] Team approach treatment strategies have been reported as likely to be successful in terms of compliance and effectiveness.[112] In addition, a team approach encourages patients and care-givers to be active participants in developing and carrying out an overall management plan.[15]

Many of the functional challenges experienced by older individuals have been successfully met in a variety of settings using a team approach. For instance, the rehabilitation of patients with hip fractures can include an interdisciplinary approach.[97] Similarly, team decision making may aid the recovery of a patient who has sustained a cerebrovascular accident (CVA).[40] Sensory problems such as low vision can complicate the performance of daily activities, but a team approach can enhance patient independence. For example, an ophthalmologist can assess visual acuity, whereas a therapist can determine how a patient may use remaining vision to perform ADLs.[107] In addition, chronic pain management[84] and foot care[21] are facilitated by the application of a multidisciplinary program.

Interdisciplinary care of elders can occur in a number of settings and offers many benefits. For patients at home, comprehensive assessments can delay the development of disability and reduce nursing home stays.[95] Older individuals in a nursing home benefit in terms of improved quality of life,[3] whereas hospitalized patients may return home more quickly because of reduced lengths of stay.[101]

RETURNING TO HOME
Multiple Service Sites

There are a variety of reasons why a community-dwelling older individual may require services from or placement in a health-care facility. An aged individual may be treated for minor injuries or illnesses in a hospital emergency department and discharged to home. Serious injuries, such as hip fracture or CVA, may precipitate admission to an acute-care facility with possible subsequent short- or long-term rehabilitation after the acute episode. Other hospital admissions may be necessary to manage one or more chronic problems, such as congestive heart failure or pain. The course of care will depend on the needs of the patient, with some individuals returning directly home from the hospital. Others may require care from another facility, such as a skilled nursing facility or rehabilitation center, before returning home.

Given the managed health-care environment, patient intervention outcomes need to emphasize function and a return to home as soon as possible. If an elder is treated as an outpatient in an emergency department, follow-up care (possibly including physical therapy) in the home may be required for the patient to deal with new dependency and support needs.[87] Necessary physical therapy interventions may include strengthening, transfer training, gait training, an environmental assessment, or other strategies to increase the likelihood of returning the individual to an independent life-style.

Factors That Affect Acute Hospital-Based Interventions

If a person is admitted to a hospital, medical/surgical management may require that individual to be dependent on others and immobile for a period of time. It is important that physical therapists perform comprehensive examinations[50] and assist patients to regain their independence and mobility in preparation for returning home. A team approach, including physical therapist patient management, has been found effective to improve ADL performance, such as autonomy in bed mobility, transfer, locomotion, eating, and personal hygiene. In addition, patients receiving a combined rehabilitation approach in a study were more likely to return home than matched control patients.[50] Such a combined approach may occur more frequently if the hospital has a specialized geriatric unit.

A number of physical therapy interventions may be used to help older patients return home from a hospital. Selecting an appropriate mobility aid[73] can promote early mobilization and reduce clinical complications.[89] Practice in ADLs[30] and dressing skills[96] can improve patient performance and independence. Frequency of physical therapy interventions is also important. It has been found that patients who received physical therapy more than once a day had a greater likelihood of returning directly home.[33] Further, patient satisfaction has also been related to the amount of therapy services received.[72]

Factors That Affect Short-Term Rehabilitation Interventions

After a hospital stay, a geriatric individual may require additional time and therapy before being able to return home. Such subacute care may occur at another unit of the hospital, a skilled nursing facility, or possibly a transitional-care center.[106] Overall, the highest rates of discharge to home for the older population occur from subacute care that focuses on geriatric principles and rehabilitation.[106] For example, the goals for a patient with impaired aerobic capacity and endurance secondary to deconditioning associated with systemic disorders (*Guide to Physical Therapist Practice*, pp 1461-1471)[33a] should be based on the expected demands of the patient's home environment,[8] and intervention should emphasize specific functional activities, such as transfers and ambulation.

Varying lengths of time will be required to prepare different patients to return home. During that time, sensitivity to cultural factors will facilitate the patient-therapist relationship. The process of inquiry—asking questions to determine cultural factors—has been offered as a helpful mechanism in judging a patient's cultural status, rather than making assumptions or generalizing.[36] While time is a factor in rehabilitation, intensity of care is also an important consideration. Intensive physical therapy has been associated with enhanced rates of recovery in patients who sustained a CVA.[51] Further, Medicare (and other third-party payers) may mandate that a patient receive a minimum number of hours of rehabilitation services to qualify for reimbursement.[8]

The number of staff and staffing patterns has also been found to affect patient outcomes. Nursing interventions may decrease urinary incontinence and urinary retention,[78] enhancing discharge to home. Also, facilities that employ their own therapists (rather than contract for them) report having more patients receiving daily services, which is positively correlated with patient discharges.[47]

Specialized geriatric units may provide short-term rehabilitation that emphasizes comprehensive geriatric pathways.[22] The reported outcomes of such services have been significant, and some evidence links those outcomes to the use of quality assurance tools.[27] Some units may offer specialized services for patients with common disorders such as a hip fracture and CVA, whereas others may focus on a more narrow patient population such as geriatric patients after amputation.[25] These specialized facilities have demonstrated the potential for successful problem resolution in the older population. For example, older individuals have shown as great an improvement as individuals in other age-groups in a majority of measures after pain-center treatment.[18]

Factors That Affect Long-Term Rehabilitation Interventions

Some older patients may require extended periods of time to recover from disease or disability. The presence of multiple chronic conditions such as arthritis, vascular insufficiency, and pain may be superimposed on a primary problem such as a hip fracture. A greater number of clinical considerations can complicate rehabilitation efforts.

Some patients may benefit from prolonged rehabilitation because the additional time permits more elaborate examination and evaluation. One example of more extensive testing includes using an obstacle course to assess balance and mobility in elders. Research indicated the course was valid and useful to evaluate older persons with balance and mobility impairments.[63]

Long-term rehabilitation has also been studied in terms of the effectiveness of interventions aimed at functional performance of older individuals. Researchers have reported that interactions of amount of therapy time and factors such as medication, practice, or motivation appeared to contribute to the overall improved functional status of a group of cognitively impaired older persons.[12]

The site of rehabilitation may also play a role in the functional recovery of some older patients, depending on the precipitating illness. Patients with a hip fracture admitted to rehabilitation hospitals did not differ from patients admitted to nursing homes in returning to the community. However, patients who sustained a CVA and were admitted to nursing homes were less likely to return home than patients who received care in a rehabilitation hospital.[49]

INTERVENTIONS THAT KEEP PEOPLE LIVING AT HOME

Probably the single most important aspect of keeping older people living at home is injury prevention. Unfortunately, common ailments associated with aging, such as knee osteoarthritis, have a relationship to loss of balance.[111] Falls are common in elders and can result in severe injuries, causing reduced mobility and dependence.[2] In terms of costs, the total direct cost of fall injuries in 1994 among persons aged 65 and older was $20.2 billion.[24]

Various strategies have been developed to help prevent falls in the older population. Home-barrier assessments to eliminate environmental hazards are a start, but issues such as medications, nutrition, and illness must also be considered.[23] The importance of a comprehensive approach to fall prevention cannot be overstated. Physical therapists must keep normal age-related changes in mind and differentiate those changes from other factors such as polypharmacy, inadequate food intake, and inactivity.

Typical problems for the older adult living at home include difficulty getting in and out of the bathtub or shower, using a toilet, turning faucet handles and doorknobs, and negotiating steps. A therapist can reduce or eliminate all of those problems by recommending adaptive equipment such as grab bars, transfer benches, elevated toilet seats, handle extensions, and railings. Further, ensuring that appropriate footwear is used and that eyeglass prescriptions are up-to-date will also help older adults remain functional in their home.

Home assessments can reveal common problems such as poor lighting, loose carpets or slippery surfaces, and clutter. While these assessments (in and outside of the home) can be easily performed, implementing changes based on them are not always successful. A possible service therapists could provide is fall-prevention educational programs.[90] Although shown to be in an unsafe home, many older people will nevertheless resist making recommended changes.[23] This response to professional recommendations is unfortunate since the risk of falling can be lowered by more than one-half by incorporating simple modifications to the home.[99] Therapists should note that a favorable attitude toward home modifications is a strong predictor of adaptation.[31] Even if prevention measures are taken, a fall may still occur. Therefore, it is important for therapists to teach elders how to cope after a fall.[76]

Two additional types of interventions may assist an older adult to remain at home: program assistance and technology. Program assistance includes services from home health agencies, private aides or certified nursing assistants,[13,32] hospice organizations,[19,108] Meals on Wheels,[9,55] and chore services.[67,92] Technology includes devices and equipment[68] that allow aged people to perform tasks for themselves or call for assistance if required.[64,85]

A local (perhaps county) bureau of aging is a good initial contact point to identify the types of program assistance available in a given community. It is wise to consider multiple sources of assistance over the course of an illness, as, for example, the length of time a home health agency can provide reimbursable services is quite limited. Private assistance for ADLs and IADLs may be required, and an individual is likely to have to pay out-of-pocket expenses for this kind of help. Community groups and religious organizations oftentimes maintain a list of volunteers to assist older adults to remain in their homes.

Program assistance such as Meals on Wheels can help an older adult maintain adequate nutrition. Nutrition is an important factor in remaining healthy, especially as elders are often taking a variety of medications. Chore services can perform home modifications such as enlarging bathrooms and building ramps.

Hospice is a special type of care, designed to assist those in the final stage of life to remain comfortable and at home. While certainly not limited to hospice patients, technology is often the reason why a terminally ill individual may remain at home rather than being institutionalized. Devices such as infusion pumps,[80] portable oxygen equipment, and bedside nebulizers permit continuous treatment to occur in the home setting.

Technology also includes using the telephone as part of a support program for older adults.[98] Friends and relatives can place "safety check" calls to help monitor another's safety.[110] Telephones also can be used to provide reassurance to patients recently discharged to home from a hospital.[93] The use of computers by older adults has been investigated,[45,66,81] and using computers and computer networks can help to maintain contact with others, thereby promoting socialization.

Staying at Home with a Care-Giver

Many older individuals are able to remain at home because a care-giver is available. The actual availability of a care-giver can vary depending on whether that person is a volunteer, e.g., relative or friend, or paid employee. Depending on individual circumstances, the need for a care-giver will range from brief visits to care lasting 24 hours a day.

It is important that care-givers receive adequate training.[37] This is especially important in the area of normal aging changes so that care-givers can distinguish between such normal changes and pathology. They should understand the proper use of any relevant assistive equipment[7] as well as appropriate positioning, transfer, and guarding techniques. Care-givers must use correct body mechanics while assisting. Further, if the older individual uses a wheelchair for assisted mobility, the care-giver must take things like rugs and thick carpets into consideration.

If an older individual requires care at home, the role of care-giver is often assumed by female family members.[6,36] The role of care-giver, in addition to demands such as job, children, and homemaking, may create excessive stress for the individual.[35] For continuity of care, the health and safety of the care-giver are as important as for the person receiving care.[62] This is especially true if the care-giver also is older.[10]

Care-giver stress can adversely affect that person's health.[61] Relief from care-giving responsibilities (respite) is often a primary concern of care-givers[86] and may be related to fatigue.[79] If possible, care-givers should seek regular relief of duties and try to share responsibilities with others.

Even with a care-giver, some older individuals will be more functional if the home environment is modified to accommodate their limitations and those of the care-giver. For instance, using a ramp and wheelchair may be far easier for both patient and care-giver than having a care-giver attempt to help the patient walk up and down steps. Transfers will be facilitated by raised toilet seats and an adjustable height bed and chair. If custom features are needed, physical therapists are ideally suited to recommend home adaptations.

Staying at Home without a Care-Giver

Many older individuals chose to remain alone in their own homes. That decision may be made for several reasons: economic necessity, i.e., avoid institutional care; a desire to remain independent; not wanting to leave familiar surroundings; and others. Living alone may offer benefits but also requires planning for expected changes and problem solving.

Reliable assistance when needed is paramount for an older individual to live alone. Friends, family, and neighbors may be available in times of need, but their absence must be anticipated. Community resources, e.g. companions and Meals on Wheels, should be investigated. Research has shown that age and chronic illness are strongly related to the use of community services.[9] Difficulty in cleaning the house was found to be a strong predictor of using home help.[75] Further, transportation accessibility was identified as a major obstacle, especially for rural elders.[91] The use of professional home-care by elders has been studied, and it was found that the greatest users were more often female, older, and not married.[29]

In addition to community resources, professional help may be needed for an older individual to remain home. A home assessment by a physical therapist may be required to recommend adaptive equipment or environmental changes.

The home environment can be modified to permit a person with functional limitations to live alone. Telephones can be adapted, increasing the ability of someone living alone to stay in contact with others.[56] While furniture and televisions are considered cherished objects by elders,[16] they can be rearranged to enhance functional mobility and safety. Loose throw rugs should be secured and thresholds identified by contrasting colors. Other indoor modifications include installing grab bars, hand rails, adapted sink faucets, wall socket or light switch adapters, ramps, and lever-type door handles.[102] The outdoor environment must also be considered because steps, irregular surfaces, and inclement weather may predispose an older person to injuries and falls.

In addition to home modifications, assistive equipment can be used to enhance safety and function. Many devices are available in categories such as mobility, personal care, and positioning aids. Examples for those categories are walkers, bath benches, and orthotics, respectively. It is important that physical therapists match individuals with the appropriate device since research indicates that some older individuals consider mobility aids a visible symbol for stigmatization and a reminder of diminishing capabilities.[88] One possible way to encourage an older person to use an assistive device is to include that person in the selection process. Other strategies are to have a therapist who has visited the home (rather than one who has not) recommend the assistive equipment and conduct training in its use.[109]

In a national data-based study[109] of individuals older than 65, including a substantial number who lived alone, more than 23% reported using assistive devices. Persons living alone reportedly had a greater need for numerous devices compared with those living with someone. This finding is not surprising because a number of devices may be required if a person is to perform ADLs and IADLs independently.

The most commonly used type of assistive device is a mobility aid. Canes and walkers are the top two mobility aids in terms of number of users.[57] A wide variety of designs and features are available.[57,58] For example, four-wheeled walkers give more stability on carpets and hard surfaces than do two-wheeled walkers. However, the four-wheeled walker is less stable for transfer support.[100]

While allowing many older individuals to ambulate independently, walkers have several disadvantages. They can encourage a flexed trunk posture, become tangled in cords and clutter, prevent individuals from carrying items along with them, and cause upper extremity pain from weight bearing and lifting. Solutions to these problems may include selecting a walker of appropriate height, eliminating clutter, using a waist pack or attaching a basket to the walker, and using a wheeled walker with padded or molded handles.

Advantages of walkers may be perceived in the functional mobility of the person using them. Walkers can include seats, brakes, baskets, and carry bags, and they can fold for easier storage. Skis/sleds can be placed on the rear legs of a roller-walker, easing the user's effort to move the walker, especially on carpets.

Canes also present advantages and disadvantages. They can support up to 25% of an individual's weight[71] and are used primarily for support and balance. Canes may incorporate a variety of handles and be made of wood or other materials. Very light-weight canes made from carbon-fiber[71] may be preferred over wood canes by some users. Canes may also be distinguished by the number of legs and width of their bases.

Some disadvantages of canes are that they offer limited support; may be too wide for some activities, e.g., a wide-base cane may be too wide for use on steps; and handles may aggravate arthritic hands. Furthermore, like walkers, they are useless if not used: 42% of older people eventually abandon their canes.[71]

Mobility in the Community

Pedestrian

Older pedestrians are at greater risk of traffic-related fatality than individuals of any other age-group. The National Highway Traffic Safety Administration reports that 1011 (19%) of 5472 pedestrian fatalities in 1994 were persons aged 70 and older. The age-group with the next highest level of pedestrian fatalities (ages 35 to 39) accounted for only 479 (9%) fatalities.[104] What are some of the reasons for the high number of fatalities among elders, and what can be done to reduce this number?

Traffic safety engineers use detailed guidelines to design pedestrian and traffic control devices.[59] Issues such as signal timing, curb height, wheelchair curb cuts, pedestrian intervals, and green-light intervals are specified in the guidelines. Generally, a pedestrian walking speed of 1.22 meters per second (4.0 feet per second) and a curb height of 20.32 centimeters (8 inches) are assumed. In areas where a significant number of older persons are likely to use pedestrian crosswalks, a walking speed of 0.92 meters per second (3.0 feet per second) is recommended.

Existing pedestrian and traffic control devices do not accommodate elders. Hoxie and Rubenstein observed pedestrians crossing an intersection in Los Angeles.[39] Twenty-seven percent of older pedestrians were unable to cross the intersection before the signal changed. Data from the Established Populations for Epidemiologic Studies of the Elderly show that 11% of New Haven, Conn., older residents (aged 72 or older) reported having difficulty crossing intersections.[52] The New York City Police Department discovered that many older pedestrians attempting to cross Queens Boulevard were unable to cross in the time allowed by the signals. In addition, elders experienced a disproportionately higher number of injuries and fatalities.[74]

Inadequate walking speed accounts for most of the difficulty that older persons experience when crossing intersections. The older pedestrians observed by Hoxie and Rubenstein had a mean walking speed of 0.86 meters per second (2.8 feet per second).[39] Data from the Established Populations for Epidemiologic Studies of the Elderly show that fewer than 1% of older pedestrians had a normal walking speed of at least 1.22 meters per second (4.0 feet per second). Only 7% had an average walking speed of 0.92 meters per second (3.0 feet per second).[52] Clearly, the typical older pedestrian cannot walk fast enough to cross intersections within the time intervals recommended by established guidelines.[59]

Older independent community dwellers use walking as their major means of transportation. Trips to the supermarket and bank are the most common reasons for ambulation outside of the home.[77] Other important destinations are the post office, physician's office, department store, and pharmacy.[54] To use these facilities, distances of approximately 300 meters (984 feet) must be ambulated, and curb heights of 18 to 20 centimeters (7.1 to 7.9 inches) must be negotiated.[14,54,83]

A host of interventions by a physical therapist can assist older pedestrians. Generally speaking, physical therapists should train their pedestrian patients to meet functional benchmarks required for community ambulation (Table 13-1). Therapists should measure distances, curb heights, crosswalk timings, and other potential barriers that the patient will encounter in the normal pedestrian area. Locations such as the supermarket, bank, post office, physician's office, pharmacy, and department store should be evaluated. Therapists should use specific data obtained from these measurements to establish criteria for treatment outcomes. Assistive devices such as powered scooters may offer an alternative for patients who are unable to meet measured criteria.

Table 13-1
Functional Benchmarks for Pedestrians

Parameter	Benchmark
Walking speed	1.22 m/s[a] (4.0 f/s[b])
Walking distance	300 m (984 f)
Curb height	20.32 cm (8 in)

[a] meters per second, [b] feet per second

Traffic safety interventions can also help the older pedestrian. Some traffic safety interventions that can improve safety for older pedestrians include installing pedestrian signals at intersections, assistive technology such as audible signals, median areas in the middle of crosswalks, curb cuts at intersections, minimizing curb corner radius to decrease the speed of turning motorists, eliminating right turns on red, and eliminating visual obstructions in the crosswalk area.[38] Although physical therapists do not have a direct role in the implementation of traffic safety interventions, they can express these concerns to local municipalities as advocates of public health and safety.

Transportation

The Americans with Disabilities Act (ADA) of 1990 specifies that public transportation systems must provide accessible services to individuals with disabilities.[5] By virtue of the ADA definition of "disability," many older persons may qualify for consideration with regard to public transportation.

"The term 'disability' means, with respect to an individual - (A) a physical or mental impairment that substantially limits one or more of the major life activities of such individual; . . ."[5]

The ADA mandates that any new vehicle purchased for use in a public transportation system must be readily accessible to persons with disabilities, including people who use wheelchairs. Essentially, this mandate specifies that public transportation vehicles must be equipped with a wheelchair-lift device that can also be used by standees who cannot manage stairs. This includes persons using crutches or a walker. There are no specifications for bus stair riser height or tread depth because vehicle undercarriage, width, and right-of-way considerations prevent buses from complying with architectural building stair requirements.[103] Interestingly, automobiles that are used as taxis need not meet ADA accessibility requirements, although other vehicle types used by taxi services, e.g., vans, must be compliant.[1]

Paratransit is another transportation option for older persons with disabilities. *Paratransit* means comparable transportation service required by the ADA for individuals with disabilities who are unable to use fixed-route transportation systems.[1] Persons who cannot use a lift-equipped bus because they require assistance (other than that provided by the lift operator) are eligible for paratransit services. Generally, paratransit provides door-to-door, on-demand service. Vehicles are usually small, specially-equipped vans with wheelchair lifts and trained operators. Typically, 24-hour advance notice is required, and service is usually on a first-come, first-served basis. The cost for paratransit service is generally minimal. Contact the local public transportation authority to inquire about the availability of service in a particular area.

Driving

Driving an automobile is an important way to maintain community independence. Society places a high value on the ability to drive. Cessation of driving is associated with an increase in depressive symptoms among older individuals.[60]

The risk of traffic-related injury increases substantially for people older than 70 years.[11] In one review, 61.5% of trauma victims older than 65 admitted to the Milwaukee County Medical Complex between July 1991 and October 1992 were involved in motor vehicle crashes—more than falls or auto-pedestrian injuries. The mortality rate for these individuals was high (29.2%).[105] Older people are more susceptible to medical complications following injuries, which accounts for higher mortality rates.[65]

What factors can help to identify older drivers who are at risk of injury and should discontinue driving? One factor that seems to be associated with increased risk is reduced cognitive function, or dementia.[28,41,82] Johansson and colleagues found that even mild cognitive impairment contributed to losing a driver's license because of automotive accidents.[41] Beyond this, there is little agreement about which factors can be used to identify older drivers who should discontinue driving. Some other factors that may be related to the decline of driving ability in older persons are visual acuity, useful field of vision, visual-spatial attention, diabetes, coronary heart disease, back pain, and use of non-steroidal anti-inflammatory drugs.[28,41,48,69]

When surveyed as to why they stopped driving, elders offered the following reasons: health problem other than eyesight or hearing impairment (30%); trouble with eyesight (29%); and being uncomfortable with driving (27%). The average age at which these former drivers stopped driving was 60 years, and only 4% reported having their driver's license revoked.[46] An interesting finding of a study by Kington and co-workers is that elders who lived in households with more adults were less likely to drive. This fact suggests that elders are likely to relinquish driving privileges when assistance is available.

Perhaps because of the multiplicity of variables that have been associated with increased risk of injury for older drivers, there are no standardized guidelines available to identify older drivers who are at increased risk of injury. There is some evidence that age-related medical screening of older drivers does not improve traffic safety.[34] Wiseman and Souder have offered a detailed checklist of risk factors that may be used to identify older persons with driving problems.[113] Their checklist includes items such as motor vehicle safety record; episodes of confusion; family observations of person's poor driving ability; alcohol abuse; use of sedating drugs; neurological or musculoskeletal conditions that may slow reaction time; compromised cognitive or visual function; poor decision-making ability; and inappropriate behaviors, such as impulsivity.

Several resources are available to assist the older driver. At least two national organizations (American Automobile Association and American Association of Retired Persons) offer educational programs for mature drivers. Persons who successfully complete these programs may receive a discount on their automobile insurance premium. Many driver rehabilitation programs exist in which driving skills can be evaluated and adaptations can be suggested. The Association of Driver Educators for the Disabled certifies Driver Rehabilitation Specialists. This association can also provide information about the local availability of certified specialists and driver rehabilitation programs. A comprehensive resource guide for driver rehabilitation has been published by the American Occupational Therapy Association.[4] This resource guide lists many useful sources of help for older drivers and clinicians who assist them.

What can physical therapists do to help the older driver? The first step is to speak to the patient about the issue. Amazingly, in a focus group study of older ex-drivers, only 32% of physicians and only 9% of nurses or therapists had raised the topic of driving with their patients.[70] At the very least, therapists should conduct a screening examination of cognitive function, visual acuity, and reaction time. If the screening reveals potential deficits that are beyond the scope of physical therapy, then a referral to the appropriate health care practitioner is necessary. If neuromuscular deficits seem to contribute to unsafe driving abilities and if there is a reasonable expectation that these deficits can be mediated by exercise, functional training, or assistive and adaptive devices, these interventions should be implemented. Finally, if cessation of driving becomes necessary, therapists should advise their patients to take advantage of community resources such as family and friends and public transportation, paratransit, or ambulance services. Although these accommodations may be inconvenient, the safety of all concerned should take precedence.

Case Studies

Case 1: Impaired Joint Mobility, Motor Function, Muscle Performance, and Range of Motion Associated with Joint Arthroplasty

Mr. CS is a 76-year-old male who received a total knee joint arthroplasty of the right knee on June 6, 1997. Mr. CS has a long history of degenerative joint disease of the right knee. He experienced a gradual increase of pain in the knee and a gradual decline of ambulation ability over a 2-year period. Before onset of significant pain 2 years ago, Mr. CS had been an active out-of-doors ambulator with no significant con-

TABLE 13-2

FUNCTIONAL MEASURES FOR MR. CS UPON DISCHARGE FROM REHABILITATION HOSPITAL

PARAMETER	MEASUREMENT
Passive range of motion: Right knee (all other ranges within normal limits for 76-year-old male)	Extension minus 5° Flexion 100°
Strength: Right knee (all other strengths within normal limits for 76-year-old male)	Extensors 3+/5 (10° quad lag noted, i.e., active range of extension limited to minus 15°) Flexors 3+/5
Ambulation	61 meters (200 feet) with walker, allowed weight bearing as tolerated on right
Stairs	Up and down 12 stairs with railing
Transfers	Independent to and from bed, chair, toilet

comitant medical problems. When pain with ambulation could no longer be controlled by conservative measures and ambulation became limited to within the home only, Mr. CS's physician recommended surgery.

The postoperative recovery was uneventful. After an acute-care hospitalization of 5 days, the patient was transferred to a rehabilitation hospital. Since Mr. CS lived alone, the therapists at the rehabilitation hospital concentrated on independence with ADLs as functional outcomes. Table 13-2 lists Mr. CS's functional measures at the time of discharge from the rehabilitation hospital.

The home-care physical therapist visited Mr. CS for the first time on the 14th postoperative day (second day after discharge from the rehabilitation hospital). The patient reported that he was managing well in the home with support services (Meals on Wheels, home health aide). He was able to negotiate the one flight of stairs to the second-floor bedroom and bathroom using the railing and folded walker. The home-care nurse had removed surgical staples on the previous day, and a light dressing was in place for protection of the healing wound. The nurse's note indicated that the wound was not draining and there was no sign of infection. When asked about his long-range goals, Mr. CS stated that he would like to walk to the small shopping center down the street and be able to drive his automobile (something he was able to do up until the day of his surgery).

The physical therapist began the evaluation by confirming that the patient could safely ambulate throughout the home, negotiate the stairs, and perform all necessary transfers. The therapist and patient noted that there were four stair steps leading to the front door of the home, and these steps did not have a railing. Range-of-motion and strength measures were similar to the measurements taken upon discharge from the rehabilitation hospital (see Table 13-2). The therapist measured the patient's walking speed by marking a 7.62-meter (25-foot) runway in the patient's living room and hallway. The patient was able to walk this length in 10 seconds—a walking speed of 0.762 meters per second (2.5 feet per second). This walking speed was well short of the benchmark required for community ambulation (see Table 13-1).

The community evaluation revealed that the shopping center was two blocks away (a distance of 183 meters, or 600 feet). There were four curbs of 20 centimeters (about 8 inches) on the way to the shopping center. There was a traffic light with pedestrian signals at the intersection where the shopping center was located. The timing of the pedestrian signal required a walking speed of 1.22 meters per second (4.0 feet per second). Mr. CS's automobile was kept in his garage that was easily accessible once the four stair steps in front of the home had been negotiated. Based on all available information, the therapist developed several goals and a treatment plan (Table 13-3).

The therapist began the treatment program by teaching open- and closed-chain active terminal knee extension exercises. The patient was instructed to perform 15 repetitions 3 times daily. The patient was advised that he might experience a stretching sensation or mild discomfort while performing exercises. He was told that he should stop exercises and alert the therapist if he experienced significant pain that lasted more than a half hour after exercising.

OPEN-CHAIN: The patient was instructed to sit on the bed with the thighs supported and legs dangling over the edge. The patient slowly straightened the right knee, held the maximal achievable extension range for a count of five, then slowly returned to the starting position.

CLOSED-CHAIN #1: The patient was instructed to lie supine with a towel roll placed under the right ankle. The patient tightened the knee extensor muscles while pushing the posterior aspect of the knee down toward the bed. The patient held the maximal achievable extension range for a count of five, then slowly returned to the starting position.

CLOSED-CHAIN #2: The patient was instructed to stand with his back toward a wall. The posterior aspects of the heels, buttocks, and shoulders touched the wall. The patient tightened the knee extensor muscles while pushing the posterior aspect of the knee back toward the wall. The patient held the maximal achievable extension range for a count of five, then slowly returned to the starting position.

After completing closed-chain exercise #2, the patient was instructed to modify that exercise to add self-assisted range of motion. The patient was told to cross the left thigh over the right thigh and to gently push down on the right thigh with the left thigh while actively straightening the right knee. The patient was told to hold the maximum achievable extension range for a count of five, then return to the starting position.

The patient was given the following advice for self-assisted flexion range-of-motion exercise: sit in a sturdy wooden chair placed on a non-carpeted floor; place the right foot on a towel on the floor; cross the left foot in front of the right; slide both feet back until you feel a stretching sensation at the right knee; hold this position for a count of five, then return to the starting position.

To accomplish endurance ambulation training, the therapist used the 7.62-meter (25-foot) runway that had been marked in the patient's living room and hallway. The therapist observed the patient while he walked at a moderate pace to ensure safety of technique. The therapist instructed the patient to walk nine runway lengths (68.58 meters, or 225 feet) on the first day of training. This distance was 7.62 meters (25 feet) longer than the patient's capability on discharge from the rehabilitation hospital. The patient was told to increase the distance by one runway length each day. After completing

TABLE 13-3
FUNCTIONAL PROBLEMS, GOALS, AND TREATMENT PLAN FOR MR. CS AT FIRST HOME-CARE VISIT

FUNCTIONAL PROBLEM	GOAL	PLAN
10° quad lag	Eliminate quad lag (4 weeks postoperative)	Active terminal knee extension exercises
Passive range of motion limited to minus 5° extension and 100° flexion	Increase passive range to full extension and 110° flexion (6 weeks postoperative)	Active and self-assisted range of motion exercises
Unable to negotiate stairs without railing in front of home	Install railing (3 weeks postoperative)	Have local chore service install railing
Walker encumbers ambulation	Ambulate with cane (3 weeks postoperative)	Advance to cane ambulation (check with surgeon first)
Unable to walk to shopping center	Ambulate 300 meters (984 feet) (6 weeks postoperative)	Endurance ambulation training
Unable to walk quickly enough to cross intersection at shopping center	Ambulate at a rate of 1.22 meters per second (4.0 feet per second) (6 weeks postoperative)	Speed ambulation training
Unable to drive automobile	Return to driving (8-10 weeks postoperative)	Refer for driver evaluation (when surgeon agrees)

the endurance walk, the patient was instructed to rest for 3 minutes, then repeat the endurance walk. This cycle could be repeated three or four times. The patient was taught to monitor his heart rate. He was told to stop walking if his heart rate exceeded 122 beats per minute (85% of age-predicted maximum heart rate) or if he felt "very hard" exertion. Once the railing for the entrance-way stairs had been installed and the surgeon authorized advancement to a single-tipped cane, endurance ambulation was often conducted outdoors.

The therapist also used the 7.62-meter (25-foot) runway that had been marked in the patient's living room and hallway for ambulation speed training. To walk at a speed of 1.22 meters per second (4.0 feet per second) the patient needed to walk the length of the runway in 6.25 seconds. A clock with a large face and second hand was placed at the end of the hallway. The patient was instructed to time himself while he walked one length of the runway a little faster (but always mindful of safety) each day. This training activity could be repeated as often as the patient wished each day. The patient was advised to rest for at least 1 minute between each speed-training walk.

Mr. CS made steady progress toward all functional goals. He was advanced from walker to cane during the third postoperative week. The quad lag was eliminated by the end of the fourth postoperative week, and strength and range-of-motion measures steadily improved. During the fourth through the sixth postoperative weeks, the therapist conducted all ambulation endurance and speed training outdoors. The patient was able to safely ambulate to the shopping center by the beginning of the seventh postoperative week. Since all home-care physical therapy goals had been met, the patient was given instructions for exercises to maintain strength, range of motion, and endurance. Home-care physical therapy was discontinued at that point. When Mr. CS visited the surgeon for a 6-week postoperative follow up, the surgeon authorized referral to the rehabilitation center for driver evaluation. This evaluation was accomplished during the eighth postoperative week. Mr. CS was cleared for driving at that point in time.

Case 2: Impaired Gait, Locomotion, and Balance Secondary to Lower Extremity Amputation

The patient is a 71-year-old male who underwent surgical above-knee amputations secondary to diabetes mellitus. He was initially placed in a long-term–care facility for preprosthetic care and returned home 2 months after surgery. The home environment was a two-story single-family dwelling. At that time the patient was using a wheelchair for mobility, and home modifications included adapting the bathroom for a wheelchair user (Fig. 13-1, *A* and *B*). The shower area was designed with transfers in mind, as was the toilet. In this case, curtains rather than doors permitted easy entry and use. In addition, other important elements of the modifications included the adjustable shower head and floor drain. The toilet bars were made from PVC pipe and were

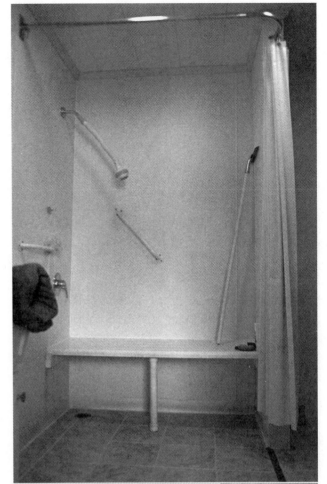

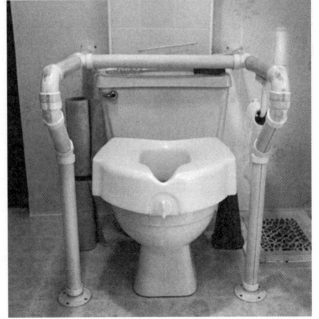

FIG. 13-1 Shower area, **A,** and toilet, **B,** designed for a wheelchair user.

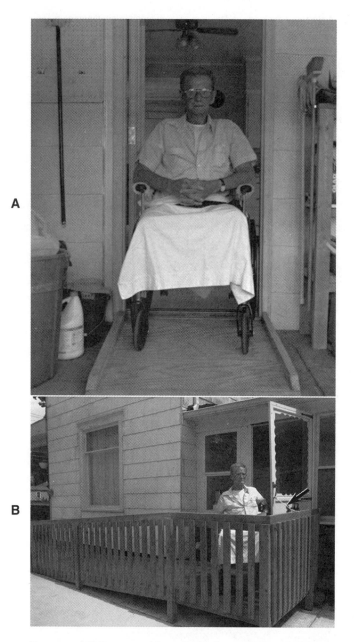

FIG. 13-2 **A,** Ramps enable a wheelchair user to enter and exit the home without negotiating difficult stairs. **B,** A piece of rope *(arrow)* secures a screen door in the open position, and concrete surrounds the front of the home to facilitate mobility.

custom designed. After an inpatient stay, the patient returned home using a walker with platform attachments and two above-knee prostheses to ambulate short distances. The energy cost of ambulation was high, and the patient sometimes preferred to use the wheelchair. As steps were difficult for the patient to negotiate, a ramp was constructed to enter and exit the home (Fig. 13-2, *A* and *B*), and a simple piece of rope secured a screen door in the open position. Concrete was continued around the front of the home, facilitating mobility.

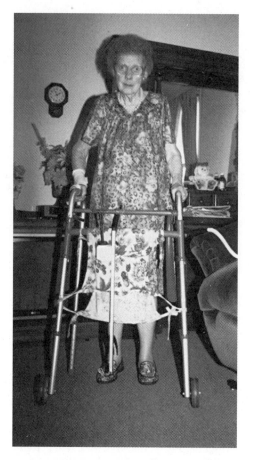

FIG. 13-3 A wheeled walker can be substituted when the patient experiences pain lifting a pickup walker.

Case 3: Impaired Joint Mobility, Motor Function, Muscle Performance, and Range of Motion Associated with Localized Inflammation

The patient is an 82-year-old female guest at a personal care home. Her history included carpal tunnel syndrome (right wrist) and rheumatoid arthritis. She declined surgery for the syndrome, preferring to use a wrist support for pain relief. The carpal tunnel syndrome and rheumatoid arthritis were challenges to this patient's mobility. Lifting a walker worsened her wrist pain, but hip and knee pain prevented her from ambulating without the device. To accommodate her needs, a wheeled walker was substituted for a pickup walker (Fig. 13-3). Fortunately, the home environment included low pile carpeting and wood floors. Those surfaces offered very little resistance to the wheeled walker. The addition of a lift chair (Fig. 13-4) enabled the woman to transfer sit-stand without assistance and have independent mobility in her room. An electric hospital bed was used in a fashion similar to the lift chair to maintain independence in bed transfers. Using grab bars and a raised toilet seat, the patient was independent in toilet transfers.

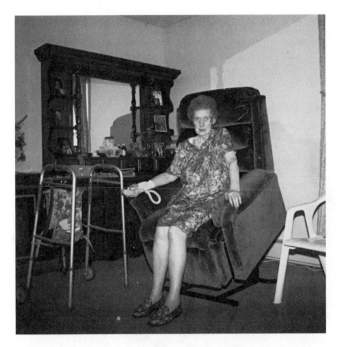

FIG. 13-4   A lift chair adds ease to the sit-stand transition.

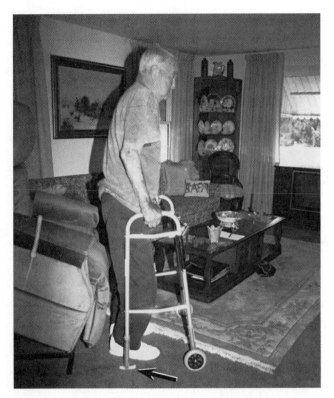

FIG. 13-6   Posterior skis on the wheeled walker *(arrow)* reduce the energy expended when moving about the house.

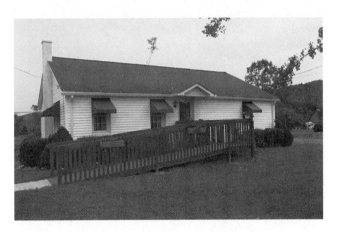

FIG. 13-5   A ramp on the exterior of the home allows for frequent trips and independence for the wheelchair patient.

Case 4: Impaired Aerobic Capacity and Endurance Associated with Cardiovascular Pump Dysfunction

The patient was an 80-year-old man with a history including renal failure, congestive heart failure, gouty arthritis, and syncope. He returned home after a hospital stay to begin dialysis. The home environment was modified with a ramp (Fig. 13-5) to allow for frequent trips (via wheelchair and an adapted van) for outpatient dialysis. An "L" shape design was used to allow for a 1-inch rise for every foot of ramp. Indoors, the patient's home contained very thick pile carpeting. He used a wheeled walker to ambulate, but the back legs of the walker dragged on the carpeting, causing him to

overexert himself. Posterior skis (Fig. 13-6) significantly reduced the energy cost of ambulation and permitted him to ambulate freely about his home.

Case 5: Impaired Aerobic Capacity and Endurance Secondary to Deconditioning Associated with Systemic Disorders

The patient was a 73-year-old male who underwent surgical resection of a malignant lung tumor. A course of chemotherapy and radiation followed the surgery, leaving the patient weak. The weakness hampered functional mobility, including bed transfers. The problem was that the bed was too high. Rather than cutting the bedposts to reduce the bed height, a box (Fig. 13-7, *A*) was fabricated to assist in bed transfers. Another difficulty the patient encountered was using the toilet. An elevated toilet seat and tub-mounted grab bar made it possible for the patient to remain independent in toilet transfers (Fig. 13-7, *B*). Stair climbing was aided by the installation of suitable railings. To ascend and descend stairs, angled railings were used. The angled railings allowed the patient to self determine the height of his hand grip. Readers should note the level railing at the stairs' landing (Fig. 13-7, *C*). The use of level railings on a flat surface was easier for the patient rather than angled ones. The level railings allowed the patient to weight bear in a fashion similar to the walker he was using at the time.

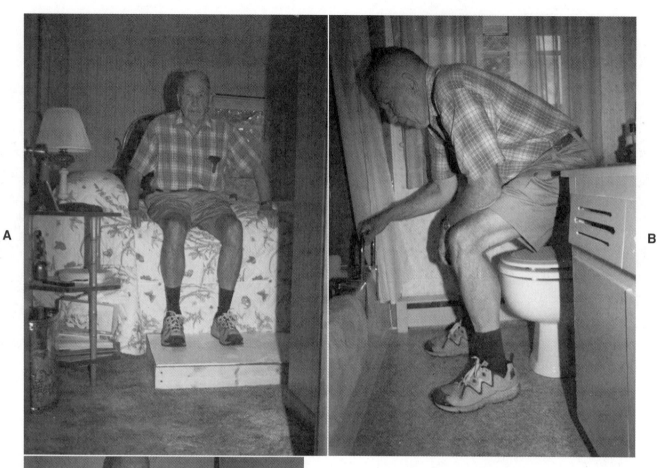

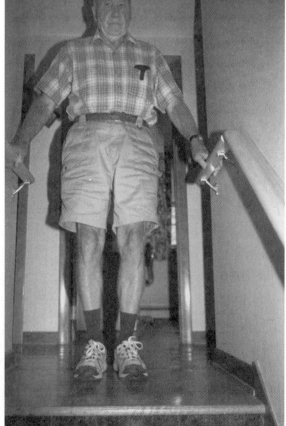

FIG. 13-7   **A,** A box can allow for easy transitions into and out of the bed. **B,** Elevated toilet seats and tub-mounted grab bars make it possible for toilet transfers to remain an independent task. **C,** Level railings on a flat surface allow weight bearing in a fashion similar to a walker.

Summary

Remaining at home can be difficult for the older adult. Adequate and appropriate physical therapy interventions can improve the odds for living successfully at home. Adaptation of the environment, especially in the context of the community, often requires the cooperation of many interested parties. Sometimes, the functional abilities and support resources needed for independent living are not achievable. An accurate and thorough examination and evaluation of the patient and the environment should provide the data needed to make a judgment about living at home.

References

1. *ADA Regulations, 49 CFR part 37*. United States Department of Transportation, Washington, DC, 1990.
2. Alexander BH, Rivara FP, Wolfe ME: The cost and frequency of hospitalization for fall-related injuries in older adults. *Am J Pub Health* 1992; 82(7):1020-1023.
3. Alt-White AC, Romano EL: An interdisciplinary approach to improving the quality of life for nursing home residents. *Nsg Connect* 1993; 6(4):51-59.
4. American Occupational Therapy Association, Inc: *Driver Rehabilitation Resource Guide*. Bethesda, MD, 1995.
5. Americans With Disabilities Act of 1990. *Public Law 101-336*.
6. Baharestani MM: The lived experience of wives caring for their frail, homebound, elderly husbands with pressure ulcers. *Adv Wound Care* 1994; 7(3):40-42, 44-46, 50.
7. Ballinger C: Mobility aides for daily tasks. *Pract Nurse* 1996; 11(7):473, 475-476.
8. Bonder BR, Wagner MB: *Functional Performance in Older Adults*. Philadelphia, 1994, FA Davis.
9. Boniface DR, Denham MJ: Factors influencing the use of community health and social services by those aged 65 and over. *Health Soc Care Community* 1997; 5(1):48-54.
10. Brown S, Zamprogna A: Focus in quality. Balancing act. . . who will care for and support these aging caregivers? *Can Nurse* 1996; 92(3):53-54.
11. Burke M: Motor vehicle injury prevention for older adults. *Nurse Pract* 1994; 19(2):26-28.
12. Cartwright DL, Madill HM, Dennis S: Cognitive impairment and functional performance of patients admitted to a geriatric assessment and rehabilitation centre. *Phys Occup Ther Geriatr* 1996; 14(3):1-21.
13. Cervantes E, Heid-Grubman J, Schuerman CK: Prevention: The effect of medication on older adults. *Caring* 1996; 15(3):58-63.
14. Cohn JJ, et al: Establishing criteria for community ambulation. *Top Geriatr Rehabil* 1987; 3:71-77.
15. Collier P, Early A: A team approach to geriatric case management. *J Case Manage* 1995; 4(2):66-70.
16. Cookman CA: Older people and attachment to things, places, pets, and ideas. Image. *J Nurs Scholar* 1996; 28(3):227-231.
17. Cress ME, et al: Effects of training on VO$_2$ max, thigh strength, and muscle morphology in septuagenarian women. *Med Sci Sports Exerc* 1991; 23:752-758.
18. Cutler RB, et al: Outcomes in treatment of pain in geriatric and younger age groups. *Arch Phys Med Rehabil* 1994; 75(4):457-464.
19. Delong MF: Caring for the elderly, part 5: Managing end of life issues. *Nurseweek* 1995; 8(9):8-9, 11.
20. Dubin S: Geriatric assessment. *Am J Nurs* 1996; 96(5):49-50.
21. Echevarria KH, et al: A team approach to foot care. *Geriatr Nurs* 1988; 9(6):338-340.
22. Editor: Skilled nursing facility comprehensive geriatric pathway. *Focus Geriatr Care Rehabil* 1996; 9(10):insert 4p.
23. El-Faizy M, Reinsch S: Home safety intervention for the prevention of falls. *Phys Occup Ther Geriatr* 1994; 12(3):33-49.
24. Englander F, Hodson TJ, Terregrossa RA: Economic dimensions of slip and fall injuries. *J Foren Sci* 1996; 41(5):733-746.
25. Esquenazi A: Geriatric amputee rehabilitation. *Clin Geriatr Med* 1993; 9(4):731-743.
26. Fiatrone MA, et al: Exercise training and nutritional supplementation for physical frailty in very elderly people. *N Engl J Med* 1994; 330:1769-1775.
27. Flemming P: Improving outcomes in hip fracture patients: Using qa tools in a skilled nursing facility physical therapy clinic. *J Healthc Qual* 1993; 15(4):21-25.
28. Foley DJ, Wallace RB, Eberhard J: Risk factors for motor vehicle crashes among older drivers in a rural community. *J Am Geriatr Soc* 1995; 43(7):776-781.
29. Frederiks CMA, et al: Why do elderly people seek professional home care? Methodologies compared. *J Community Health* 1992; 17(3):131-141.
30. Gladman JRF, et al: Survey of a domiciliary stroke rehabilitation service. *Clin Rehabil* 1995; 9(3):245-249.
31. Gosselin C, et al: Factors predicting the implementation of home modifications among elderly people with loss of independence. *Phys Occup Ther Geriatr* 1993; 12(1):15-27.
32. Guariglia W: Sensitizing home care aides to the needs of the elderly. *Home Health Nurse* 1996; 14(8):618-623.
33. Guccione AA, Fagerson TL, Anderson JJ: Regaining functional independence in the acute care setting following hip fracture. *Phys Ther* 1996; 76(8):818-826.
33a. Guide to physical therapist practice. *Phys Ther* 1997; 1163-1650.
34. Hakamies-Blomqvist L, Johansson K, Lundberg C: Medical screening of older drivers as a traffic safety measure—a comparative Finnish-Swedish evaluation study. *J Am Geriatr Soc* 1996; 44(6):650-653.
35. Hawkins B: Daughters and caregiving, taking care of our own. *AAOHN J* 1996; 44(9):433-437.
36. Henderson JN, Whaley M: Cultural factors in geriatric rehabilitation: Ethnic-specific generational cultures. *Top Geriatr Rehabil* 1997; 12(3):1-9.
37. Hilling L: AARC clinical practice guideline: Providing patient and caregiver training. *Respir Care* 1996; 41(7):658-663.
38. Hoxie RE, Rubenstein LZ, Hoenig H, Gallagher BR: The older pedestrian. *J Am Geriatr Soc* 1994; 42:444-450.
39. Hoxie RE, Rubenstein LZ: Are older pedestrians allowed enough time to cross intersections safely? *J Am Geriatr Soc* 1994; 42(3):241-244.
40. Hubschen S: The course of stroke rehabilitation—interdisciplinary teamwork as practiced in a geriatric acute care clinic. *Rehab Stuttgart* 1996; 35(1):49-53.
41. Johansson K, et al: Can a physician recognize an older driver with increased crash risk potential? *J Am Geriatr Soc* 1996; 44(10):1198-1204.
42. Judge JO, et al: Balance improvements in older women: Effects of exercise training. *Phys Ther* 1993; 73:254-265.
43. Judge JO, Schechtman K, Cress E, FICSIT Group: The relationship between physical performance measures and independence in instrumental activities of daily living. *J Am Geriatr Soc* 1996; 44:1332-1341.
44. Judge JO, Underwood M, Gennosa T: Exercise to improve gait velocity in older persons. *Arch Phys Med Rehabil* 1993; 74:400-406.
45. Kautzmann LN: Introducing computers to the elderly. *Phys Occup Ther Geriatr* 1990; 9(1):27-36.
46. Kington R, Reuben D, Rogowski J, Lillard L: Sociodemographic and health factors in driving patterns after 50 years of age. *Am J Public Health* 1994; 84(8):1327-1329.
47. Kochersberger G, Hielema F, Westlund R: Rehabilitation in the nursing home: How much, why and with what results. *Pub Health Rep* 1994; 109(3):372-376.
48. Koepsell TD, et al: Medical conditions and motor vehicle collision injuries in older adults. *J Am Geriatr Soc* 1994; 42(7):695-700.
49. Kramer AM, et al: Outcomes and costs after hip fracture and stroke, a comparison of rehabilitation settings. *JAMA* 1997; 277(5):396-404.
50. Landi F, et al: Physiotherapy and occupational therapy: A geriatric experience in the acute care hospital. *Am J Phys Med Rehabil* 1997; 76(1):38-42.
51. Langhorne P, Wagenaar R, Partridge C: Physiotherapy after stroke: More is better? *Physio Res Int* 1996; 1(2):75-88.
52. Langlois JA, et al: Characteristics of older pedestrians who have difficulty crossing the street. *Am J Pub Health* 1997; 87(3):393-397.

53. Lawton MP, Brody EM: Assessment of older people: Self-maintaining and instrumental activities of daily living. *Gerontologist* 1969; 9:179-185.

54. Lerner-Frankiel MB, et al: Functional community ambulation: What are your criteria? *Clin Manage* 1986; 6(2):12-15.

55. Lewis CK: The Relationship of Health Status, Population Characteristics, and Specific Chronic Health Conditions of the Frail Rural Elderly to the Availability/Utilization of Community-Based Services With Implications for Future Policy. *Dissertation.* George Mason University, 1993.

56. Mann WC, et al: The use of phones by elders with disabilities: Problems, interventions, costs. *Assist Technol* 1996; 8(1):23-33.

57. Mann WC, et al: An analysis of problems with walkers encountered by elderly persons. *Phys Occup Ther Geriatr* 1995; 13(1/2):1-23.

58. Mann WC, et al: An analysis of problems with canes encountered by elderly persons. *Phys Occup Ther Geriatr* 1995; 13(1/2):25-49.

59. *Manual on Uniform Traffic Control Devices for Streets and Highways.* Washington, DC, United States Department of Transportation, Federal Highway Administration, 1988.

60. Marottoli RA, et al: Driving cessation and increased depressive symptoms: Prospective evidence from the New Haven EPESE. Established Populations for Epidemiologic Studies of the Elderly. *J Am Geriatr Soc* 1997; 45(2):202-206.

61. Mastrian KG, Ritter C, Deimling GT: Predictors of caregiver health strain. *Home Healthc Nurse* 1996; 14(3):209-217.

62. McKibbon J, Genereux L, Seguin-Roberge G: Who cares for the caregivers? *Can Nurse* 1996; 92(3):38-41.

63. Means KM, Rodell DE, O'Sullivan PS: Use of an obstacle course to assess balance and mobility in the elderly: A validation study. *Am J Phys Med Rehabil* 1996; 75(2):88-95.

64. Montgomery C: Personal response systems in the United States. *Home Health Care Serv Q* 1992; 13(3/4):201-222.

65. National Center for Prevention and Control: *Fact Sheet: Motor Vehicle Deaths in Older Americans.* National Center for Injury Prevention and Control, Division of Unintentional Injury Prevention, Atlanta, 1997.

66. O'Leary S, Mann C, Perkash I: Access to computers for older adults: Problems and solutions. *Am J Occup Ther* 1991; 45(7):636-642.

67. Osterkamp LB, Chapin RK: Community-based volunteer home repair and home maintenance programs for elders: An effective service paradigm? *J Geron Soc Work* 1995; 24(1/2):55-75.

68. Parker MG, Thorslund M: The use of technical aids among community-based elderly. *Am J Occup Ther* 1991; 45(8):712-718.

69. Perryman KM, Fitten LJ: Effects of normal aging on the performance of motor-vehicle operational skills. *J Geriatr Psychiatry Neurol* 1996; 9(3):136-141.

70. Persson D: The elderly driver: Deciding when to stop. *Gerontologist* 1993; 33(1):88-91.

71. Phillips B: Technology abandonment from the consumer point of view. *Naric Q* 1993; 3(2):1-10.

72. Pound P, Gompertz P, Ebrahim S: Patients' satisfaction with stroke services. *Clin Rehabil* 1994; 8(1):7-17.

73. Prajapati C, et al: The s test—a preliminary study of an instrument for selecting the most appropriate mobility aid. *Clin Rehabil* 1996; 10(4):314-318.

74. Queens Boulevard Pedestrian Safety Project—New York City. *MMWR* 1989; 38:61-64.

75. Ranhoff AH: Activities of daily living, cognitive impairment and other psychological symptoms among elderly recipients of home help. *Health Soc Care Community* 1997; 5(3):147-152.

76. Reece AC, Simpson JM: Preparing older people to cope after a fall, *Physiotherapy* 1996; 82(4):227-237.

77. Regnier V, Gordan G, Murakami E: How Neighborhood characteristics affect travel patterns, in *Transportation for the Elderly and Handicapped: Programs and Problems II.* Washington, DC, US Department of Transportation, 1980.

78. Resnick B, Slocum D, Ra L, Moffett P: Geriatric rehabilitation: Nursing interventions and outcomes focusing on urinary function and knowledge of medications. *Rehabil Nurs* 1996; 21(3):142-147.

79. Riccio PA: Perceived quality of sleep and levels of daytime sleepiness among elderly women caregivers of Alzheimer's disease patients. *Home Health Care Manage Pract* 1996; 8(6):52-57.

80. Richardson RJ: A look at home infusion therapy. *Computertalk Homecare Providers* 1994; 2:46-47.

81. Riviere CN, Thakor NV: Effects of age and disability on tracking tasks with a computer mouse: Accuracy and linearity. *J Rehabil Res Dev* 1996; 33(1):6-15.

82. Rizzo M, et al: Simulated car crashes and crash predictors in drivers with Alzheimer Disease. *Arch Neurol* 1997; 54:545-551.

83. Robinett CS, Vondran MA: Functional ambulation velocity and distance requirements in rural and urban communities. *Phys Ther* 1988; 68:1371-1373.

84. Rook JL: Managing chronic pain: The evolution of geriatric pain management will require a team approach part 1. *Rehab Manage* 1994; 7(6):41-45.

85. Roush RE, et al: Impact of a personal emergency response system on hospital utilization by community-residing elders. *South Med J* 1995; 88:917-922.

86. Rudin DJ: Caregiver attitudes regarding utilization and usefulness of respite services for people with Alzheimer's disease. *J Gerontol Soc Work* 1994; 23(1/2):85-107.

87. Runciman P, et al: Discharge of elderly people from an accident and emergency department: Evaluation of health visitor follow-up. *J Adv Nurs* 1996; 24:711-718.

88. Rush KL, Ouellet LL: Mobility aids and the elderly client. *J Geron Nurs* 1997; 23(1):7-15.

89. Rush S: Rehabilitation following orif of the hip. *Top Geriatr Rehabil* 1996; 12(1):38-45.

90. Ryan JW, Spellbring AM: Implementing strategies to decrease risk of falls in older women. *J Geron Nurs* 1996; 22(12):25-31.

91. Schultz AA: Identification of needs of and utilization of resources by rural and urban elders after hospital discharge to the home. *Pub Health Nurs* 1997; 14(1):28-36.

92. Seifert S, Suther M: Breaking home care tradition with home repairs and other services. *Caring* 1994; 13(6):60-63.

93. Shu E, Mirmina Z, Nystrom K: A telephone reassurance program for elderly home care clients after discharge. *Home Healthc Nurse* 1996; 14(3):154-161.

94. Sonn U, Grimby G, Svanborg A: Activities of daily living studied longitudinally between 70 and 76 years of age. *Disabil Rehabil* 1996; 18(2):91-100.

95. Stuck AE, et al: A trial of annual in-home comprehensive geriatric assessments for elderly people living in the community. *N Engl J Med* 1995; 333:1184-1189.

96. Thomas KS, Hicks JJ, Johnson OA: A pilot project for group cognitive retraining with elderly stroke patients . . . learning of new motor skill patterns used in upper extremity dressing. *Phys Occup Ther Geriatr* 1994; 12(4):51-66.

97. Thomas RL: Management of hip fracture in the geriatric patient: A team approach in the institutional setting. *Top Geriatr Rehabil* 1996; 12(1):59-69.

98. Thomas T: A telephone group support program for the visually impaired elderly. *Clin Gerontol* 1993; 13(2):61-71.

99. Thompson PG: Preventing falls in the elderly at home: A community based program, *Med J Aust* 1996; 164(9):530-532.

100. Tideiksaar R: Comparison of a two-wheeled walker and a four-wheeled walker in a geriatric population, *Proceedings of the Annual Meeting of the American Geriatrics Society (psa32).* New Orleans, 1993.

101. Trella RS: A multidisciplinary approach to case management of frail, hospitalized older adults. *J Nurs Adm* 1993; 23(2):20-26.

102. Trickey F, et al: Adapting older person's homes to promote independence. *Phys Occup Ther Geriatr* 1993; 12(1):1-14.

103. US Architectural and Transportation Barriers Compliance Board: *Accessibility Guidelines for Transportation Vehicles.* Access Board, Washington, DC, 1990.

104. US Department of Transportation National Highway Traffic Safety Administration. *Traffic Safety Facts 1994.* National Center for Statistics and Analysis, Washington DC 1994.

105. Valley VT, et al: A profile of geriatric trauma in southeastern Wisconsin. *Wis Med J* 1994; 93(4):165-168.

106. Von Sternberg T, et al: Post-hospital subacute care: An example of a managed care model, *JAGS* 1997; 45(1):87-91.

107. Warren M: Providing low vision rehabilitation services with occupational therapy and ophthalmology: A program description. *Am J Occup Ther* 1995; 49(9):877-883.

108. Watt K: Hospice medicine. Hospice and the elderly: A changing perspective. *Am J Hosp Palliat Care* 1996; 13(6):47-48.

109. Watts JH, et al: Assistive device use among the elderly: A national data-based study. *Phys Occup Ther Geriatr* 1996; 14(1):1-18.

110. Weber J, et al: Safety at home: A practical home injury control program for independent seniors. *Caring* 1996; 15(6):62-66.

111. Wegener L, Kisner C, Nichols D: Static and dynamic balance responses in persons with bilateral knee osteoarthritis. *JOSPT* 1997; 25(1):13-18.

112. Wells NL, Balducci L: Geriatric oncology: Medical and psychosocial perspectives. *Cancer Pract* 1997; 5(2):87-91.

113. Wiseman EJ, Souder E: The older driver: A handy tool to assess competence behind the wheel. *Geriatrics* 1996; 51(7):36-45.

CHAPTER 14

IMPAIRED VENTILATION AND RESPIRATION IN THE OLDER ADULT

MARY C. BOURGEOIS, PT, MS, CCS AND CYNTHIA C. ZADAI, PT, MS, CCS

OUTLINE

INTRODUCTION

One of the many challenges facing health care providers who manage pathology and impairment in older adults is the question: Are the patient's presenting signs, symptoms, and complaints during the latter decades of life a sign of specific pathology or merely the manifestation of advancing age?

Formulating an accurate diagnosis that discriminates between the two requires careful assessment across all body systems and the ability to integrate the findings. It also relies on the examiner having a strong working knowledge of the expected anatomical and physiological changes associated with normal aging and how those changes differ from or contribute to common pathologies.

Anatomical and physiological aging have many inherent characteristics. Most notably, aging is an inevitable and predictable progression of tissue and system decline. All living cells have a predetermined life span whether in an organism or a species, yet variability exists among and within each organism or species.[17] Gilchrest and Rowe have described human aging as "an irreversible process that begins or accelerates at maturity, and results [over time] in an increasing number and range of deviations from the ideal state."[17] They comment that although the average human life expectancy has increased over time, the expected maximum life span of the species has not, implying inevitable anatomical and physiological decline. Furthermore, people die of physiological processes rather than pathological processes.

As medical science advances to more effectively manage pathology, the clinical consequences of human aging that physical therapists face in the 21st century may be different than those therapists faced in the previous century. The focus may soon evolve to become management of physiological aging, with management goals directed exclusively toward wellness and prevention strategies rather than the consequences of pathology. The population of elders today, however, probably sits closer to the pathology end of the wellness / pathology continuum. Today's demographics include a rapidly increasing number of older men and women who currently have many existing pathologies and impairments that drive a variety of health-care needs. The ability of medical practitioners to treat pathology as well as the ability of physical therapists and others to promote functional independence over the life span have created a progressively larger demand for services related to impairment and disability. Consequently, the development of physical therapy science requires attention across the complete spectrum of physical ability through to disability to meet the needs of today's and tomorrow's patients.

The purpose of this chapter is to provide a detailed overview of the anatomical and physiological functions of ventilation and respiration and to describe the tissue and pulmonary system changes that occur with normal aging as well as the subsequent impact these changes have on function. The differences between the consequences of normal aging and the impairments produced by cellular and system pathology are examined. Special attention is afforded to the investigation of dyspnea in the older adult, with emphasis on the role that symptom evaluation plays in differential diagnosis. The scope of therapeutic interventions based on examination findings is presented with consideration of specific tests for and diagnosis of impairments of the pulmonary system. The chapter concludes with suggestions for optimizing function and preventing pulmonary dysfunction in the older adult.

VENTILATORY PUMP AND RESPIRATORY DEVELOPMENT

Growth is characterized by the proliferation of cells, tissues, and organs with new structures or functions, whereas senescence is characterized by the loss of adaptation ability and greater vulnerability to disease.[29] Growth and full development are therefore requirements for achieving maximum functional capacity and for the development of an adequate ventilatory and gas exchange *reserve capacity*. While at rest the adult individual uses approximately 10% of the pulmonary system's vital capacity (VC) to uptake adequate volume for oxygen extraction. The remaining 90% of VC can be considered the reserve capacity available for responding to increased oxygen demands, such as exercise or the metabolic demands of disease. Consequently, any injury, disease, or impairment that occurs during maturation can significantly affect the potential for full development of the reserve capacity and therefore have a subsequent impact on pulmonary system function in the long term.

Ventilatory Pump Development

The neonate's thorax is comprised of 12 pairs of ribs arranged in parallel fashion and consisting of predominantly cartilage cells.[11] At birth the ribs are nearly horizontal, and their motion is essentially en bloc. The initial thoracic pressure change required for ventilation is produced by the diaphragm, relying on its piston action to compress the abdominal contents and displace the compliant chest wall. The ventilatory muscles are skeletal muscles comprised of a mix of white and red, fast- and slow-twitch fibers. The diaphragm includes all these fiber types and is the primary muscle of ventilation. At birth, the diaphragm's arching curve is located high in the thorax, resulting in a smaller ra-

dius of curvature than in the adult. From this position the muscle is able to generate an efficient inspiratory force. The diaphragm at this time also has limited ventilatory reserve capacity as little *endurance conditioning* occurs intrautero, and the neonate has a lower preponderance of type I and a larger number of type IIa fibers than do adults. This combination leaves the neonate at risk for, and prone to, diaphragmatic fatigue.

The work of breathing (WOB) at birth is produced by diaphragmatic and chest wall muscle contraction, which displace the abdominal contents against a relatively weak abdominal wall and pull on the compliant thorax.[12] The minute ventilation ($[\dot{V}e]$ = respiratory rate [RR] × tidal volume $[V_t]$) is produced by a rapid respiratory rate and small tidal volume at birth. As the lungs become more compliant with the reabsorption of amniotic fluid, volume increases and rate decreases. Ventilatory muscles of neonates initially gain in strength and endurance with resulting increase in ventilatory capacity simply by performing the continued WOB independently.

As the child develops in height and lays down osteophytes to replace the cartilage in the ribs, a more rigid elliptically shaped ventilatory pump develops.[11,12] The progressive nature of growth and development allows for gradual strengthening and increased endurance of the muscles as the child conditions the muscles by participating in functional activities and exercise throughout adolescence. By age 20, the maximum force capacity, or strength of the ventilatory muscles, is 7 to 10 times that needed to create inspiratory flow, and nearly twice the maximum inspiratory force of an individual is available to generate the expiratory flows essential for coughing and airway clearance.[36]

Respiratory System Development

Murray describes the basic formation of the 23 generations of cartilaginous conducting airways that are completed by birth, with no additional division occurring after delivery.[29] However, some additional structural changes occur during growth and development that continue to affect the morphology of the airway. A decrease in the total number of generations in the conducting airways takes place through a process called *alveolarization*. Non-respiratory bronchioles are converted to respiratory bronchioles in the alveolarization process, which progressively increases the gas-exchange capacity of the lung. The conversion occurs continuously from birth through approximately 3 years of age, after which the total number of conducting airways remains constant throughout life.

The growth of each segment of the conducting airways continues throughout adolescence and ceases with the completion of growth of the thorax. Among individuals there remains great variability in the number of bronchial divisions within the lung. Each individual's surface area for conducting and exchanging gas depends on the conduction length of the pathways from the pharynx to the segmental bronchi and from the segmental bronchi to the gas exchange units.

Then, the number of terminal units, including the actual amount of bronchiole and alveolar surface area, completes the surface area for gas exchange.

Neonatal alveoli are less complex than those in adults but still serve in the function of gas exchange. They increase in number from approximately 25 million at birth to approximately 300 million when the lung is fully grown.[1,29] Two processes contribute to this increase. The first process is a multiplication of old alveoli whereby a single alveolar unit replaces itself. The precise period for completion of multiplication is not known, is probably variable, and does stop before growth of the thorax is complete. The second process, alveolarization, stops by approximately age 3, although growth of the individual's lung continues to maturity. During this time the alveoli increase in size and complexity to eventually provide a larger amount of surface area for gas exchange at any given lung volume. The total alveolar surface area of a normal adult has been reported to be approximately 80 m², and 85% to 95% of that surface is covered with pulmonary capillaries.[29]

The end result of ventilatory pump and lung development for a 20-year-old without disease or injury of the pulmonary structures is a gas-exchanging system with a contact area between the body and the external environment that is 40 times greater than that of the skin.[29] This lung development combined with ventilatory pump development contribute to the tremendous reserve capacity available for the functions of ventilation and respiration in the adult. Tidal volume is easily achieved at rest by ventilatory muscles generating force at less than 10% of maximum capacity and using less than 2% of the body's total oxygen uptake ($\dot{V}O_2$) to perform the WOB. The 70 square meters of lung/capillary interface provide more than adequate surface area to achieve the oxygen uptake required either at rest or with exercise and contribute to the significant reserve capacity of the pulmonary system required for gas exchange over the course of a lifetime.

VENTILATORY PUMP, AIRWAY, AND LUNG ALTERATIONS WITH AGING

The *physiological function of ventilation* can be described as the activity performed by the biomechanical action of the ventilatory muscles on the anatomically elliptical thoracic cage to achieve the intrathoracic pressure changes required for gas flow. The *WOB* is the work performed by the ventilatory muscles, and the *integrated musculoskeletal activity of ventilation* is described as the physiological work of the ventilatory pump.

Ventilatory Muscles

Tolep and Kelsen have studied the specific effects of aging on ventilatory muscles.[46] In general, both the strength and endurance of skeletal muscles have been found to decline with age. The ventilatory muscles are a mix of type I slow-twitch and type II fast-twitch muscle fibers, which is similar to other skeletal muscles. The mixture allows the composition

TABLE 14-1

TYPICAL VALUES FOR STATIC RESPIRATORY PRESSURES

PRESSURE* (CM H₂O)	LUNG VOLUME		
	RV	FRC	TLC
PEmax	0	200	240
PImax	-130	-115	0
Prs	-30	0	30
Pmus exp	30	200	210
Pmus insp	-100	-115	-30

*Maximal static respiratory pressures at the mouth = PEmax, PImax; Respiratory system recoil = Prs; Respiratory muscle pressures = Pmus exp (PEmax – Prs) and Pmus insp (PImax – Prs).
RV = residual volume; *FRC* = functional residual capacity; *TLC* = total lung capacity. From Rochester DF: Respiratory muscles: Function in health and disease. *Clin Chest Med* 1988; 9:250.

of the muscle to be specifically responsive to the pattern of activity and the functional role the muscle has in the body.

During normal resting breathing, the slow-twitch motor units of respiratory muscles are active. These fiber types generate tension more slowly but are resistant to fatigue. The fast-twitch motor units are recruited, and the fibers respond quickly during more strenuous breathing efforts, but they are also more susceptible to fatigue. All motor unit types appear to be recruitable in the setting of a maximal inspiratory effort or during forceful exhalations, such as coughing. The function of the motor units remains intact over the course of a lifetime.

Ventilatory muscle strength can be tested indirectly by measuring static inspiratory and expiratory pressures at the airway opening during occluded ventilatory efforts. The actual force values achieved are dependent not only on muscle strength but also on the subject's motivation and coordination. The measured values reflect the mechanical action of the entire inspiratory and expiratory muscles contracting in aggregate. The force generated is also a function of lung volume, making measures of pulmonary function and ventilatory mechanics interdependent. Pulmonary function and inspiratory/expiratory force values can reflect the elastic recoil properties of the lungs and chest wall (Table 14-1), both of which are altered in aging, and by measuring strength at volumes other than functional residual capacity (FRC) (Fig. 14-1).[46]

Physiological Measures of Ventilation

There are several physiological parameters that can be measured over time as indicators of a given individual's maintenance of ventilatory muscle strength and volume, or capacity. These include pulmonary function test measures of volume, flow and lung compliance, and ventilatory mechanical tests of muscle strength and endurance. To understand how aging of the lung in combination with the associated musculoskeletal and chest wall changes impact these measures of physiological function, large population studies have been performed to specifically document the change in males versus females and during specific decades of life.

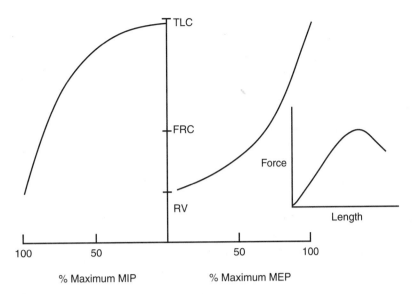

FIG. 14-1 Effect of lung volume on maximum inspiratory and maximum expiratory pressures as a function of the force-length relationship of the muscles (*MIP* = maximal inspiratory pressure; *MEP* = maximum expiratory pressure; *TLC* = total lung capacity; *FRC* = functional residual capacity; *RV* = residual volume). (Redrawn from Clanton TL, Diaz PT: Clinical assessment of the respiratory muscles. *Phys Ther* 1995; 75:11.)

Lung volumes such as total lung capacity (TLC), vital capacity (VC), and residual volume (RV) increase in value from birth through the completion of growth, which usually occurs in the late teens. Adolescent lung volumes are well-correlated with increasing body height and increase in the size of the musculoskeletal frame as well as with the increases in intrathoracic space and lung tissue surface area.[29] Normal values for lung volumes can therefore be determined by using prediction nomograms that correlate to gender, height, and age. Consequently, as height progressively declines over the course of a lifetime, the size of the thoracic container and its volume capacity are reduced (Fig. 14-2).

Tolep and Kelsen analyzed the work of Black and Hyatt and others who examined and compared changes in ventilatory muscle strength with age.[46] All investigators noted that maximal static respiratory pressures declined 15% to 20% over the age span from 20 to 70 years. The decline, however, did not become significant statistically until age 55. Tolep and Kelsen also assessed diaphragm strength by measuring it transdiaphragmatically. They found a 20% to 25% reduction in diaphragmatic strength, specifically when comparing older adult values with those of young adults. The authors stated that the differences did not appear to be the result of either level of fitness or nutritional status. Additional conclusions described WOB as increased with age, and requiring greater muscle oxygen consumption at any workload since both respiratory muscle strength and endurance are decreased.

Given the aforementioned findings, the older individual is at greater risk for developing respiratory muscle fatigue and subsequent failure when subjected to injury or disease that affects ventilatory mechanics or inspiratory muscle

strength and endurance.[46] Muscle fatigue can be assessed by measuring the amount of time a particular ventilatory load, or $\dot{V}e$, can be sustained or by looking at the maximum level of ventilation that can be sustained for a predetermined amount of time, i.e., the maximum sustained ventilatory capacity (MSVC) or the maximum voluntary ventilation (MVV).[46]

Airway/Lung Alterations

Wright has described normal lung tissue at full maturation as having a network of elastic fibers that provides a supporting framework for the primary lobule, including the terminal bronchiole, respiratory bronchiole, alveolar ducts, and alveoli.[49] In the large bronchus the elastic fibers are longitudinally arranged in a layer in the mucosa. Occasional small fibers may be circumferential and intermeshed with the thick longitudinal fibers. Circular fibers are abundant in the bronchioles. In total, there is an elaborate continuous framework of elastic fibers that unifies the various pulmonary structures into an elastic unit. Microscopic examination of healthy lung tissue extracted from a wide range of adults showed alterations in elastic tissue that were most distinct in those older than 80 but present in those older than 50. The alterations in configuration were confined primarily to the alveolar ducts and alveoli and showed a generalized and uniform reduction in the number of elastic fibers. The ducts and alveolar openings were also slightly dilated.

Other tissue changes described during Wright's examination included localized deposits of granular black pigment.[49] These deposits were noted mostly in the walls of respiratory

Lung Volume

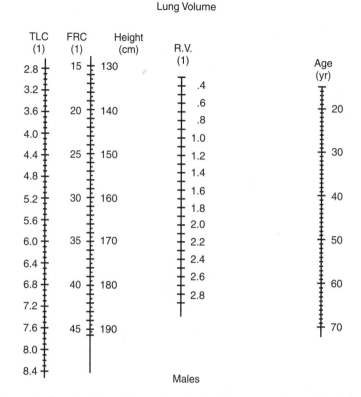

FIG. 14-2   Nomogram for calculation of lung volume in healthy non-smoking adults. (From Cherniack R: *Pulmonary Function Testing.* Philadelphia, WB Saunders, 1977.)

bronchioles and alveolar ducts. Immediately surrounding these pigmented areas, the elastic tissue was more fragmented and in some instances absent. The collective tissue changes described were postulated by the author to be responsible for the loss of elastic recoil in the lungs of older adults that leads to the progressive retention of volume, which has been documented as associated with aging. Turner and co-workers also investigated pulmonary changes associated with aging and found reduction in static recoil pressures, which are the physiological corroboration of the fragmenting of elastic fibers.[47] Turner and colleagues also attributed the resultant increase in residual lung volume to the changes in lung elasticity and compliance.

Thoracic Pump Alterations

Although the alteration of the elastic fibers in the lung tissue produces a more compliant, or "floppier," lung, there are summary anatomical changes in the thoracic skeleton that result in a more rigid chest wall frame. The mobility reduction in the thoracic rib cage is suggested to result from two primary tissue alterations. The first is an increase in the cross-linking of collagen fibers both in the ribs and in the connecting sternal cartilage.[52] The second is primarily a vertebral column change whereby the intervertebral annulus fibrosis becomes stiffer due to water loss, causing a subsequent reduction in the cushioning distance between the intervertebral disks. The composite result is a shorter, more

rigid thorax that is resistant to deformation and therefore requires greater ventilatory muscle force to achieve a change in the intrathoracic pressure (Table 14-2).

Campbell and Lefrak[4] and Shepard[39] have researched and reported measurable changes associated with increasing lung compliance and decreasing chest wall compliance over time.

They noted that the combination of a rigid thorax, reduced ventilatory muscle strength, and loss of elastic recoil in older individuals combines to produce physiological alterations in both the ventilation and gas exchange functions of the respiratory system. As noted, the primary system for measurement of ventilatory capacity is pulmonary function testing or ventilatory mechanics, which assess muscle strength, ventilatory volume, and expiratory flow.

Testing of lung volume over decades demonstrates that TLC is not increased despite the increasing lung compliance associated with breakdown of alveolar ducts and alveoli. The stiffer chest wall and concomitant reduction in ventilatory muscle strength probably prevents further increase in the maximum volume that might be achievable with the more compliant lung. Residual volume and FRC are however increased with the loss of elastic recoil and increased stiffness of the chest wall. Additionally, distal airway closure during expiration, or closing volume (CV), increases with loss of the lung's supporting network, resulting in collapse of distal lung segments and gas trapping in the lungs.[4] Since VC is the

TABLE 14-2
PULMONARY ANATOMICAL AND PHYSIOLOGIC AL CHANGES WITH AGING

AGING ALTERATION	PHYSIOLOGICAL CHANGE	MEASURABLE CONSEQUENCES
• Rearrangement and fragmentation of elastic fibers	• Decreased elastic recoil • Increased compliance of lung tissue	• Progressive retention of alveolar volume • Increased closing volume/ airtrapping
• Stiffened cartilage • Water loss from annulus fibrosis	• Increased rigidity of thorax • Reduction in inter-vertebral cushioning	• Decreased chest wall compliance • Increased work of breathing • Shortened thoracic cage
• Decreased ventilatory muscle strength and endurance	• Decreased MVV decreased MSVC • Increased muscle fatigue at lower workloads	• Decreased inspiratory force • Decreased efficacy of cough • Decreased exercise tolerance
• Increased closing volume	• Increased V/Q mismatch	• Decreased resting PaO_2

TABLE 14–3
CHANGE IN PHYSIOLOGICAL MEASURES OF LUNG FUNCTION WITH AGING

PULMONARY FUNCTION TEST	TEST DESCRIPTOR	CHANGE WITH AGE
Total lung capacity (TLC)[38]	The amount of gas in the lungs at maximal inspiration	No change
Functional residual capacity (FRC)[38]	The volume of gas remaining in the lungs at the end of a resting exhalation	Increased
Residual volume (RV)[38]	The volume of gas that remains in the lungs after a maximal exhalation	Increased
Vital capacity (VC)[38]	The total volume of gas that can be exhaled after a maximal inspiration	Decreased
Forced vital capacity (FVC)[38]	The largest volume of gas that can be forcefully exhaled after deepest inspiration	Decreased
Forced expiratory volume in 1 second (FEV_1)[38]	The largest volume of gas that can be exhaled in 1 second after deepest inspiration	Decreased
Maximal inspiratory pressure (MIP)[50]	The maximum inspiratory force that can be generated at the mouth, usually performed at RV	Decreased
Maximum expiratory pressure (MEP)[50]	The maximum expiratory force that can be generated at the mouth, usually performed at TLC	Decreased
Maximal voluntary ventilation (MVV)[38]	The largest volume of gas that can be breathed per minute, with voluntary effort	Decreased
Compliance lung/thorax	The volume change per unit of pressure change	Increased/Decreased

difference between TLC and RV, there is a proportional decline in VC as the RV increases (Table 14-3).

Ventilatory Work of Breathing
The structural cellular and system changes just described have distinct clinical implications for physical therapists working with older adults. Essentially, the musculoskeletal ventilatory pump has to carry out its function at a progressively increasing mechanical disadvantage over the course of time.[52]

A portion of the increased ventilatory work and decreased mechanical advantage results from the increase in RV and FRC. The retained volume at the end of a resting exhalation (FRC) means that the chest wall is actually held in a position of partial inspiration. This altered position serves to shorten the inspiratory muscles' resting length and primarily flattens the diaphragm. The position change alters both the muscle's length tension curve and zone of apposition while it reduces the muscle's potential contractile force. The increasingly stiff chest wall is also more difficult to displace, so a greater muscle force is needed to achieve a change in intrathoracic pressure or volume. Simultaneously, the disruption in the elastic framework of the lung at the alveolar level results in increased lung compliance with loss of elastic recoil. The summary effect on ventilatory work is a higher oxygen cost for the WOB at any given tidal volume or an overall decrease in the efficiency of ventilation.

Aging-induced change in the elastic fiber support of the conducting tubules (which become more rigid over time) produces a less distensible airway and increases flow resistance while narrowing the tubules' radius. The thickened mucosal layer associated with aging narrows the collective conducting tubule radius even further. Both changes increase the flow resistive WOB during the same time period that the chest wall changes are occurring and increasing the elastic WOB.

In the early decades of adult life, the ventilatory muscles require less than 1% of the total $\dot{V}O_2$ to accomplish WOB at rest. In contrast, up to 10% of the total $\dot{V}O_2$ can be required by the ventilatory muscles to perform the WOB at extremes of exercise.[20] This physiological range allows the ventilatory system to perform efficiently over a wide range of functions, from activities of daily living (ADL) and instrumental activities of daily living (IADL) to sports and work activities. With aging, the anatomical changes that inevitably increase the WOB at rest automatically result in a rise in the oxygen cost of ventilation for any level of activity or exercise. The same progressive aging changes that decrease efficiency of ventilation at rest also produce a reduction in the pump's maximum capacity and decrease the ventilatory reserve capacity available to meet the oxygen demands of activity or the onset of pathology.

OXYGEN UPTAKE AND DELIVERY ALTERATIONS WITH AGING

Examining the impact of aging on the function of external and internal respiration focuses the discussion on the physiological functions of gas exchange, diffusion and oxygen uptake, and delivery. Murray has offered that the pattern of increase in arterial PO_2 from birth to adulthood followed by an age-related decline is similar to the course of change in elastic recoil between birth and advanced age.[29] He also comments that the two variables are related because of the interrelated impact of elastic recoil on airway caliber and the distribution of ventilation. Weiss concurs that the distribution of ventilation and perfusion determines the potential for gas exchange and oxygen uptake.[48]

Ventilation/Perfusion Matching

Regional differences in the ratio of ventilation to perfusion exist in the normal adult, and they are significantly related to body position at rest. In the upright position there is a greater degree of both ventilation and blood flow at the base versus the apex of the lung. Gravity is responsible for the large volume of blood flow at the lung bases, which increases the interstitial pressure on alveolar structures and keeps them relatively collapsed when compared with alveoli in the lung apices. The larger number of alveoli at the base, however, compensates for their small size when compared with the overdistended alveoli at the apex. The end result is an overall alveolar ventilation perfusion ratio ($\dot{V}/\dot{Q}$) of 0.8 for the whole lung.

Factors contributing to mild mismatching of ventilation and perfusion at rest include the mixing of venous blood with arterialized blood in the pulmonary veins and the physiological dead space that results from low pulmonary artery perfusion pressure in areas that are less well-ventilated. Regional $\dot{V}/\dot{Q}$ differences are easily overcome in the normal adult lung

with simple physical activity. Increase in oxygen demand at the peripheral muscle produces an increase in all the physiological components of gas exchange. Increased cardiac output and systolic blood pressure with exercise result in an increased pulmonary artery perfusion pressure and flow with more even distribution of circulation throughout the lung. Simultaneous increase in tidal volume more evenly distributes ventilation throughout the lung. Use of both the ventilatory and circulatory reserves during activity overcomes regional differences in both ventilation and perfusion and improves $\dot{V}/\dot{Q}$ relationships and the *respiration*, or gas exchange, function across the lung.

Gas Exchange Alteration with Aging

Multiple authors have described the steady decline in resting arterial PO_2 with aging.[4,29,39,49,52] The reported decline in PaO_2 can be calculated with the regression equation: $PaO_2 = 100.1 - 0.323$ (age).[29] This formula is predicated on the progressive anatomical changes described earlier. As the supporting framework for the alveolar structures breaks down, the resultant lung collapse produces both uneven ventilation and uneven circulation or greater potential for $\dot{V}/\dot{Q}$ mismatch. The progressive airway closure and alveolar breakdown that occur at the lung bases with aging indicate that the inspired gas, traveling in the path of least resistance, preferentially distributes to the lung apices, thereby creating more $\dot{V}/\dot{Q}$ mismatching as blood flow continues to be greater at the bases.

Arterial carbon dioxide (CO_2) levels are not subject to the same physiological changes as is oxygen. The diffusing capacity of CO_2 allows continued elimination throughout life despite the progressive increase in $\dot{V}/\dot{Q}$ mismatching. The intrauterine-to-extrauterine change in the PCO_2 during the neonatal period (which decreases from 76 mm Hg at birth to approximately 33 mm Hg by 24 hours of life followed by the gradual rise in PCO_2 back to 40 mm Hg) is literally the only age-related change in PCO_2 that occurs over the lifetime. CO_2 then remains at the normative value of 40 mm Hg throughout adulthood, assuming the absence of pathology.

Diffusion

Diffusion is another factor that potentially impacts arterial blood gas values. Multiple factors may influence the rate of diffusion of a given gas and therefore the percentage of gas in the alveoli or in the blood stream. Diffusion is enhanced with a greater membrane surface area and a reduced membrane thickness.[18] Additionally, the larger the pressure gradient and the lower the molecular weight of a gas, the more rapid the diffusion rate. In normal development, the diffusing capacity of the newborn is approximately half of that of the adult, but by 5 to 6 years of age, diffusing capacity values in the child are comparable with adult values.[29] Throughout the rest of the normal growth period, diffusing capacity increases in close proportion to height. An increase in diffusing surface area corresponds to an increase in body mass and is associated with an increase in the reserve gas exchange capacity of the lung. With advancing age, the progressive breakdown of alveolar and capillary walls and consequential reduction in alveolar capillary surface area results in reduced diffusing capacity.[29] The decrease in diffusing capacity is not considered pathological nor is it cited as a reason for the change in the resting value of PaO_2. The decline in arterial PO_2 is thought to be the result of ventilation-perfusion imbalances, or mismatching.

Oxygen Delivery

The cardiac and pulmonary systems work in a complimentary manner to accomplish the systemic functions of oxygen uptake and delivery. The ventilatory pump is responsible for moving gas from the atmosphere into the alveoli. Alveolar oxygen moves into the pulmonary capillaries by the process of diffusion. Oxygen then combines with blood-borne hemoglobin and travels to the left atrium in preparation for left ventricular pumping and delivery to the body tissues. The cardiac pump receives the oxygenated blood from the pulmonary system and delivers it to the tissues via pumping through the arterial system. Maximum oxygen consumption ($\dot{V}O_2$max) is the measure of an individual's level of cardiopulmonary fitness and is the product of cardiac output ($\dot{Q}$) and arteriovenous oxygen tension difference (a-$\bar{v}O_2$) and is calculated by the formula: $\dot{V}O_2$max $= \dot{Q} \times$ (a-$\bar{v}O_2$ difference).[52] Alteration or change in any one aspect of the oxygen uptake and delivery system will certainly have a potential impact on all aspects of the system.

Beginning with the pulmonary aging changes described, any rise in WOB or oxygen cost of breathing increases total body oxygen demand and potentially diminishes oxygen available to limb muscles and other organs, particularly during exercise. An increased demand for oxygen results in an increase in $\dot{V}e$.[20] The increased ventilatory muscle effort associated with an increase in Ve has an associated oxygen cost. Ventilatory muscle work during resting minute ventilation generally requires little of the total body $\dot{V}O_2$, whereas high levels of exercise may require up to 10% or more of the total $\dot{V}O_2$. The process of aging and pathology can significantly affect those values.

Pardy and co-workers summarized and applied work by Otis in their research and reported that by calculating the $\dot{V}O_2$ of the ventilatory muscles and the total WOB, it is possible to project that at minute ventilations greater than 140 L/min in patients with impaired gas exchange, all additional increases in $\dot{V}O_2$ that could be achieved would be used by the ventilatory muscles.[30,32] This projection was based on actual measurement of $\dot{V}O_2$ and calculated blood flow to the ventilatory muscles to demonstrate the impact of increased WOB in individuals with pulmonary impairment. These authors further commented that if a large portion of $\dot{V}O_2$ is directly consumed by the ventilatory muscles, then a significant portion of the cardiac output is delivered to the ventilatory muscles, thereby reducing O_2 availability to other skeletal muscles. These proportional changes affect the amount of

$\dot{V}O_2$ required to perform an activity and the $\dot{V}O_2$max achievable by an individual.

Cardiac output (CO)—the product of stroke volume (SV) and heart rate (HR)—is also influenced by aging, predominantly as a result of the progressive decline in maximal HR.[40] Shepard has noted that except for in the extremes of old age, SV is relatively well-preserved.[39] This physiological phenomenon would explain the lack of change in resting HR values throughout the lifetime. SV values that are smaller during the adult years are primarily a result of pathology or the poorer conditioning level of less-fit individuals. However, at very high levels of work, SV may be less in the older adult because of a variety of additional influencing factors, including poorer myocardial contractility, decreased diastolic filling, and increased afterload—which are all associated with aging.[39,52] Thus, an increase in the load on the cardiovascular system potentially decreases CO and in turn influences $\dot{V}O_2$.

Concomitantly, older individuals are also more at risk for the presence and progression of coronary artery disease. Any previous infarction of cardiac muscle reduces pump function, limits distensibility, and potentially decreases the maximum and reserve capacity of the cardiovascular pump. Systemic demands for increased oxygen delivery require both an increased CO and oxygen supply to the myocardium. Any blockage of coronary arteries that produces cardiac ischemia secondary to inadequate blood flow results in a stiffer left ventricle with elevated end-diastolic pressures. Both conditions further reduce myocardial blood flow and produce potential for cardiac pump failure and inability to meet systemic oxygen demands. In this case, exercise capacity may be greatly reduced and the individual may likely experience the symptoms of angina and dyspnea.

Cellular Oxygen Uptake

Examination of a-$\bar{v}O_2$ difference caused Shepard to state that there are several factors that may influence both the amount of oxygen available at the tissue level and the tissue's ability to extract oxygen in older individuals. The oxygen carrying capacity of the blood is certainly one factor to be considered. However, anemia is not commonly thought to be much of a concern in the general elder population.[40] Decline in pulmonary function and $\dot{V}/\dot{Q}$ matching could certainly diminish the amount of available oxygen in the capillaries; however, the impact on PaO_2 is relatively small. Therefore, the impact on a-$\bar{v}O_2$ difference has also not been reported as substantial.

Shepard has indicated that through study of multiple organ systems, the factor most responsible for the reduction in a-$\bar{v}O_2$ difference with aging is the relatively large blood flow that continues to regions where oxygen extraction is limited.[40] Areas of declining perfusion with age include the skin, kidneys, and other viscera, while the blood flow to exercising muscles may also be relatively decreased. The young adult has a demonstrated effective oxygen extraction in the working muscles due to the dense capillary beds and high levels of aerobic enzymes in skeletal muscles. The older individual who has decreasing muscle density and potentially obstructed arteries combined with the reduced capillary/muscle fiber ratio may have a poor overall oxygen extraction ability that results in a lower maximum a-$\overline{v}O_2$ difference.

Integration of Cardiovascular and Pulmonary Response to Increased Oxygen Demand

Examination of ventilatory and respiratory physiological function reveals similarities between the cardiovascular and pulmonary systems when responding to an increased oxygen demand. The ventilatory and cardiac pumps simultaneously increase their rate of contraction and volume of gas or blood output when responding to an increase in systemic stress or oxygen demand.[52] Both V_t and SV steadily increase in response to a progressive O_2 demand up to approximately 50% of the $\dot{V}O_2$max. Both pumps rely on smaller increases in rate and larger increases in volume to meet increased output demand when they function efficiently. Beyond that volume midpoint, each system relies on RR and HR increases, respectively, to produce greater $\dot{V}e$ and CO while V_t and SV level off. The ability of each system to either uptake or output the greater volume needed to meet O_2 demand is dependent on the intact physiological components of each system ($\dot{V}e = RR \times V_t$ and $CO = HR \times SV$) performing the work and a significant reserve capacity.

Steady state is achieved by each system once oxygen supply meets the demand. This is measured by a steady respiratory and heart rate at a given workload. Consequently, it is the *efficiency* (work performed/oxygen used) of the cardiovascular and pulmonary systems' response to an increased oxygen demand that progressively declines with age due to the progressive decline of the working components and the slowed responses of advancing age.[52] Work or exercise at a given intensity level potentially demands relatively larger $\dot{V}e$ and CO to achieve the same oxygen uptake and delivery in an older individual. The simultaneous overall reduction in efficiency and maximum capacity in both systems means that the older individual reaches 50% of maximum $\dot{V}O_2$ at a lower workload level than a younger individual in similar physiological condition. This can be measured clinically through assessment of HR and RR while the individual is performing exercise at objectively measured workloads. The systems of older individuals will potentially take longer to achieve a steady state and concomitantly may take longer to return to resting level values. These clinical changes are not unlike those seen in the presence of pathology.

From a functional perspective, loss of ventilatory muscle function, gas exchange, and cardiovascular oxygen delivery capacity with age contributes to a reduced maximum functional capacity for older individuals. The combination of inevitable physiological aging and loss of fitness, or deconditioning, can result in a functionally significant reduction in both the ventilatory and cardiovascular reserve capacity available to meet $\dot{V}O_2$ demands during activity.[52] According to data regarding exercise capacity in the normal adult (age 20 to 60 years), it is common for most individuals to perform functional activity or ambulation at approximately 40% or less of their maximum $\dot{V}O_2$.[3] Additionally, when adults are at greater than 60% $\dot{V}O_2$max, they experience dyspnea.[52] Consequently, most individuals function between 10% and 40% of $\dot{V}O_2$max to perform ADL. Thus, as $\dot{V}O_2$max declines with aging, an individual may modify activity performance, i.e., slow down, to keep oxygen consumption at or less than 40% of max. If situations arise that require the individual to exceed 50% to 60% $\dot{V}O_2$max, anaerobic metabolism and dyspnea are experienced and the individual will generally self-limit the activity. The challenge then for most clinicians is to differentiate whether the symptoms of dyspnea on exertion in older adults are the result of the level of exercise compared to the level of conditioning, the impact of aging, or the development of pathology.

PATHOLOGY THAT PRODUCES IMPAIRMENT AND IMPACTS FUNCTION
Physiological Effects of Pathology

There are many pathological processes—both acute and chronic—that can result in impaired oxygen uptake or delivery in the older adult. Any pathology that affects the chest wall, ventilatory muscle strength and endurance, gas exchange surface area, or oxygen transport and delivery essentially interferes with the metabolic kinetic chain. Commonly, older adults have multiple comorbidities that concurrently affect several of the physiological component functions and thereby impair both the resting and exercise $\dot{V}O_2$ and $\dot{V}O_2$max.

Chronic alterations in the bony thorax of the ventilatory pump such as those seen in scoliosis, kyphosis, or ankylosing spondylitis can result in reduced chest wall compliance and increased WOB secondary to both the increased load and the mechanical disadvantage during diaphragmatic descent and accessory muscle rib cage lift. Acute pathology such as rib fracture, surgical incision, or pleuritic pain associated with chest wall inflammation creates a similar set of physiological circumstances, again restricting V_t and necessitating an increase in RR to meet the demands of ventilation. With limitation in chest wall expansion, the increases in $\dot{V}e$ needed for gas exchange probably result from increase in RR rather than an increase in V_t. Consequently, some activities may be selectively eliminated by older individuals due to the discomfort associated with an increased RR. Increased frequency of respiration also affects the force/frequency curve of the ventilatory muscles by reducing the maximum force of contraction and increasing the oxygen cost of ventilation, serving as another potential limit to exercise.

The muscles associated with ventilatory pump motion can also undergo acute and chronic changes due to pathological processes, which can translate into functional impairments. Acutely, a hemidiaphragm paralysis, whether due to idiopathic cause or one associated with a surgical procedure, can greatly reduce ventilatory muscle strength and endurance. This too will result in dyspnea on exertion (DOE) or again elimination of activities that produce or are associated with uncomfortable symptoms. Perhaps more chronic in impact is the progressive muscle weakness associated with some neurological diseases or the immediate reduction in force that results from spinal cord trauma, reducing VC and the ability to successfully maintain or increase V̇e.

The airways and lung parenchyma are also at risk for pathological compromise. Acute processes such as asthma exacerbation that cause airway edema and inflammation create resistance to airflow by narrowing the diameter of the airways. Similarly, hypertrophy of the mucous glands produces excessive mucus in the airway that is thicker and more difficult to mobilize. Edema and secretions, in combination with the impaired mucociliary transport often associated with bronchitis and airway inflammation, will increase airway resistance and WOB. This set of conditions may be acute, chronic, or acute superimposed on a chronic condition.

Atelectasis may also result from many of these pathological circumstances, which effectively reduce V̇e and contribute to gas exchange impairment with an alteration in ventilation/perfusion matching. A greater intrathoracic pressure change will be required (increased WOB) to achieve re-expansion of collapsed lung areas when compared with the WOB associated with tidal ventilation in partially inflated or compliant parenchyma.

All of these examples of acute and chronic pathology serve to describe some of the physiological mechanisms that can affect or permanently alter the WOB and reduce gas exchange capacity. Chronic conditions that continually and progressively impair or eliminate the ventilatory and gas exchange reserve capacity often produce greater decline over time than those associated with acute pathology. Although the initial functional change at the individual level may present as a simple slowing down in the performance of work or community activity, the incremental, progressive loss in combination with physiological aging may lead to eventual reduction in or elimination of independence and function in ADL.

Identification and Impact of Common Pathologies

Acute lung pathology is important to identify in its early stages because it can have significant and long-lasting ventilatory and respiratory consequences in the older adult. Ability to fight infection is a significant issue for the aging population whether the individual is healthy or already compromised. Meyer and colleagues studied whether increasing age would be a factor in the presence of immune dysregulation and inflammation in the lungs of clinically normal older persons.[26] Their results indicated that altered inflammatory cell profiles and low-grade inflammation of the lower respiratory tract were more prominent in the older age-groups that they studied.

Gyetko and Loews studied the ability of older individuals to fight infection.[19] Upper airway protection can be compromised by the change in elastic recoil and the rigidity of the chest wall as well as the progressive impairment of cough re-

sponse associated with aging. These changes occur in the absence of other neuromuscular and musculoskeletal pathology. Alterations in the defense mechanisms of the lower respiratory tract of elders may increase their vulnerability to infection. The cells involved in specific immune responses have been reported to be the most affected by aging in terms of both slowed response and a decrease in the magnitude of response.

Pneumonia

The diminished respiratory reserve and declining immunity associated with the aging process increase the risk of contracting and experiencing severe consequences from community-acquired pneumonia.[6] The prevalence and severity of pneumonia in older populations has been linked to the extensive use of immunosuppressive drugs for treatment of a variety of disorders. Micro-aspiration has also been identified as a significant cause for bacterial pneumonia in this population, though in many cases no causative agent is ever conclusively identified.[6]

Atypical presentation of pneumonia symptoms in elders may often delay diagnosis and subsequent treatment. Chan and Welsh discussed the difficulties associated with geriatric respiratory medicine.[6] They summarized that many patients presented with functional decline, confusion, falls, angina, exacerbation of chronic obstructive pulmonary disease (COPD), or metabolic abnormalities instead of the typical respiratory symptoms common to pneumonia in a younger population. They added that the delayed or missed diagnosis of pneumonia may contribute to the increased mortality rate associated with this disease in elders. This has clinical significance for many physical therapy providers in a variety of practice settings who may be the first to observe or identify the change in behavior or atypical symptoms. Standardized physical examination and review of systems in this population are essential to identify all signs and symptoms of abnormality and to accurately identify acute impairment in its earliest state. The slowed physiological responses and decreased reserve capacity in advancing age decreases the margin for error and increases the risk associated with any pathology.

Asthma

Fanta has reported on the difficulty of diagnosing asthma in elders.[14] He noted that it may be extremely challenging to distinguish between the presentation of chronic obstructive lung disease and asthma, especially in older individuals who are smokers. It is entirely possible that the individual with fixed airway obstruction secondary to chronic lung disease may additionally develop a reversible obstructive component that responds to bronchodilators and corticosteroid therapy. He offers that asthmatic bronchitis may be a better descriptor for reactive airways disease in these patients. He emphasizes that advancing age does not mandate irreversible airway obstruction. Consequently, those patients who would benefit from use of a bronchodilator to reduce WOB and improve functional performance should be identified.

Again, the presence of potential comorbidities makes differential diagnosis in the setting of wheezing quite difficult. It is important to rule out other acute processes such as lung lesions, pulmonary emboli, or other chronic system problems such as congestive heart failure and recurrent aspiration. Examination of standardized test values and the response to therapies can assist in the diagnosis.

Tuberculosis (TB)

Couser and Glassroth have noted that except for patients with human immunodeficiency virus (HIV), the elderly have the greatest incidence of tuberculosis.[9] They postulate that factors determining whether an infected elder develops active disease may be related to the presence of an associated underlying illness, use of immunosuppressive drugs, baseline nutritional status, and the degree of immunocompromise in a particular individual. They note that a diagnosis may be delayed or missed secondary to older patients who are poor historians; have cognitive impairments; or simply have masked symptoms such as cough, dyspnea, fatigue, night sweats, or weight loss that can be attributed to aging or another comorbidity. Symptoms may also vary from those of younger patients, and radiographic findings may also be unusual as skeletal, lung tissue, and aging changes can confound the picture. Careful testing and monitoring can often lead to previously missed diagnoses such as TB in older individuals. Certainly, the lack of an accurate diagnosis in this instance could have dire consequences, particularly with residents of health institutions.

Lung Cancer

The increased incidence of lung cancer in the elderly is another significant cause of mortality and morbidity. Older adults are predisposed to development of lung cancer because of their longer lifetime exposure to cigarette smoking and other environmental irritants.[24] Symptoms common to many of the diseases discussed earlier are often the presenting features here as well, i.e., chest pain, dyspnea, weight loss, and cough or hoarseness. Physical therapists may become involved in one of the many case management phases for these patients, from participating in the diagnostic process by collecting sputum samples for diagnostic testing to preoperative rehabilitation that includes reconditioning through acute postoperative airway clearance management and eventual reconditioning. Examination and evaluation at every phase with careful testing can identify specific emerging and resolving impairments. Consideration of the individual's prognosis and objective measures of improvement or decline are the key factors for assuring the accuracy of the impairment diagnosis at every stage.

Chronic Obstructive Pulmonary Disease

Chronic lung diseases are prevalent in this country, and the onset is generally in the fifth (chronic bronchitis) through the seventh (emphysema) decades of life. They are commonly confused with the onset and impact of aging due to their physiological similarities. Emphysema is characterized by extensive destruction of the elastic network in the lung parenchyma, causing a loss of alveolar surface area and capillaries.[44] The resultant impaired gas exchange, which may or may not be present at rest, is readily identified during exercise tests that monitor ventilation and blood gases or pulse oximetry. Limitations in an individual's ability to increase $\dot{V}e$ secondary to increased flow resistance with collapsible airways and/or weak, fatiguing ventilatory muscles result in the clinical signs and symptoms of dyspnea; decreasing levels of blood oxygen; change in ventilatory pattern; and the likely termination of exercise at low maximum voluntary ventilation (MVV), or achievement of predicted MVV at low workloads.

Individuals with chronic bronchitis or bronchiectasis have obstruction to airflow and a greater WOB due to the reduced airway diameter associated with smooth muscle contraction and excess secretions. Concomitantly, they are at risk for and frequently have airway inflammation as a result of immobile and retained secretions. Many individuals experience a combination of pathologies, whereby components of both chronic bronchitis and emphysema co-exist, probably because cigarette smoking is the most predominant etiology in both pathologies. Air trapping in the lungs due to the parenchymal disintegration associated with aging is of far greater consequence in the older adult with obstructive lung disease than in the aging adult without underlying lung pathology. The increased WOB and loss of gas exchange capacity impair physical function at lower workloads and often steadily progress to loss of independence in unassisted physical functional activity.

The anatomical and physiological aging changes that reduce the pulmonary reserve capacity of seniors work in concert with COPD pathology to exaggerate the pulmonary symptoms associated with aging.[52] The normal individual's ventilatory strategy for meeting increased oxygen demand includes increasing V_t and shortening and equaling the inspiratory/expiratory phases of breathing while increasing respiratory rate and breathing at a higher lung volume.[20] The ability to move a larger volume of gas at a faster rate and with a shorter expiratory phase depends on many factors: an effective muscle mechanical response to stretch, force frequency and length tension, and the ability to improve the muscle force response to load to take advantage of the maximal flow rates achievable at high lung volumes. Older individuals with COPD are often unable to take advantage of these physiological mechanisms as a result of the progression of aging and disease.

The difficulty associated with the ventilatory response to increased work demand in these patients is a result of the compounding effects of aging and pathology. The overdistended floppy lung increases its residual volume over time and shortens the resting position of the ventilatory muscles. Increasing ventilatory volume from this resting position requires the muscles to shorten even further, which significantly reduces the force generation potential of the ventilatory pump. This force reduction occurs in a setting where the stiffer thoracic cage increases the elastic WOB and the narrowed obstructed airways increase the flow resistive WOB. Similarly, increasing respiratory rate to improve gas exchange will also reduce force generation potential based on the force frequency curve of muscle. Reducing the expiratory phase time and increasing the expiratory force and pressure will promote more airway collapse and trapping in this population, further compounding the problem.

Consequently, the exact strategies that improve the ventilatory mechanics for normal individuals are costly in terms of WOB and oxygen consumption for older patients with COPD. These breathing strategies are thereby self-limiting since they are being performed by muscles with decreased strength and endurance capacity working against progressively increasing loads at a greater mechanical disadvantage.[32] The ability to sustain exercise in this patient population will eventually be severely limited and can potentially progress to early onset of DOE and ventilatory muscle fatigue or even onset of dyspnea and fatigue at rest.

Osteoporosis

The onset of osteoporosis with aging can also have a significant impact on ventilatory function and cardiovascular fitness. While osteoporosis is not inevitable with aging, measures must be taken to delay or defer its onset.[16] Some persons are genetically at greater risk for the development of osteoporosis, but diets low in calcium, sedentary life-styles, and the postmenopausal state all contribute to the development of osteoporosis. Restrictive lung disease may develop as the thoracic spine becomes more kyphotic and the chest wall becomes more rigid. Pain associated with decline in bone mass diminishes ventilation or ventilatory efforts and has a negative effect on the desire to participate in activity/exercise. The diminished ventilatory capacity associated with restrictive disease necessitates an increase in respiratory rate to meet the demand for increased minute ventilation and precipitates dyspnea at an earlier onset during activity. Maintenance of an active life-style through the aging process is associated with improved cardiovascular fitness and increased bone and muscle mass.

EXAMINATION AND EVALUATION TO DISCRIMINATE BETWEEN AGING AND PATHOLOGY

Examination

The consistent combined symptom presentation in older adults that includes dyspnea, early onset fatigue, and slowed activity rate challenges clinicians to be careful and thorough during examination and evaluation to ensure accuracy of diagnosis and appropriateness of prognosis and treatment plan. The overlapping signs and symptoms of aging, deconditioning, and cardiovascular or pulmonary pathology present an excellent rationale for performing a standardized examination and evaluation with every patient. A complete history, review of systems, and use of standardized tests and measures provide a baseline set of information and test values that can be compared with known normative values for identification and classification of actual pathology, impairment, and functional limitation.

History and Systems Review

Past medical and surgical history, history of the current condition, and symptom description for rest and activity are essential beginning components of the examination. The patient's description of his/her current functional level and whether that has been consistent for years or recently developed gives the provider a picture of the patient's perception of himself/herself and his/her function compared with others. Standardized tests such as the Functional Status Questionnaire (FSQ) and the Klein Bell Activities Scale can be used to establish a functional baseline and to compare the patient with others or himself/herself over the course of therapy.[21,22,37]

The work and environmental living history will also contribute to the patient composite picture. Each of these data sets allows the clinician a view of how patients perceive themselves compared with their baseline, describe their function in terms of their current life-style, and set out their expectations for the future. A sedentary individual may not perceive slight shortness of breath at rest as a problem, whereas a lifetime tennis player may perceive the inability to play multiple sets as a disaster. The patient history and expectations present the context for the next steps in the process: review of systems and test/measures.

Review of systems serves to screen each system for pathology to indicate whether additional objective testing is required. Any abnormality in baseline values such as heart rate, blood pressure, or respiratory rate at rest will indicate whether further tests, such as monitoring vital signs with activity, are necessary. Normative values obtained for any system may also allow the clinician to rule out certain pathologies or impairments and eliminate the need for any further testing.

Tests and Measures

Tests that document cardiovascular and pulmonary function at rest and with activity are the essential components of this examination. Observation and documentation of the thoracic cage shape, mobility, and muscle function are the initial steps. Physical examination steps including palpation, percussion, and auscultation are performed initially and repeatedly over the course of care since these tests may illustrate change fairly rapidly in response to changing conditions.

Tests and measures of ventilatory function, such as pulmonary function tests (PFTs) and ventilatory mechanics, and tests and measures of gas exchange, such as arterial blood gases (ABGs), oximetry, and capnometry, are essential to compare the objective values with the subject's description of symptoms or information presented during the interview. These standardized, reliable, and valid tests are invaluable to the clinician making the initial diagnosis and measuring progress over time.

Investigators have questioned whether older individuals with slowed processes or mild cognitive impairments would be able to adequately perform compliance-dependent tests, such as PFTs.[41] Sherman and colleagues found that overall, seniors can perform PFTs in compliance with the acceptability and reproductibility standards of the American Thoracic Society. Although most subjects were unable to meet the exact standards for achieving a plateau in the flow/volume curve or reproductibility standards for multiple performance, the diagnostic utility was still deemed useful. Despite the fact that objective testing of the population is standardized, one of the most difficult things to measure accurately and repeatedly is symptoms. Quantification of symptoms is essential in older adults because one symptom, such as dyspnea, could represent multiple pathologies or impairments.

Silvestri and Mahler have discussed the problem of dyspnea in the elderly and do not feel it is a normal consequence of aging.[42] Most persons who experience dyspnea tend to seek medical attention when the symptom interferes with functional activities. An unfortunate consequence of dyspnea is that individuals tend to reduce their physical activity in response to symptom onset, which leads to progressive deconditioning, which in turn leads to dyspnea onset at lower levels of physical exertion. It is therefore essential to determine the source of an individual's dyspnea to appropriately address the impairment and resolve the issue precipitating the problem.

Quantification of dyspnea by standardized methods is strongly suggested. Acute dyspnea that is characterized by rapid onset is more likely due to an acute pathological problem such as pneumonia, pulmonary embolus, or pleural effusion.[25] Slow insidious dyspnea onset that is commonly attributed to the "aging process" can often be traced to the simultaneous progression of chronic disease and deconditioning. Consequently, exercise testing or walk testing that documents and measures the onset and severity of symptoms and then compares the results with standardized values is an effective way to objectively document and classify the symptoms.[20]

Measures of lung volume and flow, maximal inspiratory and expiratory pressures and gas exchange and qualification of symptoms at rest are often not enough to get a complete picture of the patient or to make an accurate diagnosis of impairment, functional limitation, and disability. Monitored exercise tolerance tests that track signs and symptoms at measured workloads make an essential contribution to identifying and discriminating among the signs and symptoms of pathology versus aging.[42]

A cardiopulmonary exercise test is designed to stress the oxygen transport system. Metabolic, cardiac, ventilatory, respiratory, and subjective data are all examined and compared with predicted normative values for gender, age, and level of training. Interpretation of the data generally indicates whether a ventilatory, respiratory, cardiovascular, or symp-

tomatic limitation to exercise exists. Ventilatory limits or impairments are identified when the $\dot{V}$emax is greater than or equal to 85% of the predicted MVV. A gas exchange limit or impairment is diagnosed by a decrease in partial pressure or saturation of oxygen with increasing activity level. Neither of these changes is associated with normal aging. A cardiac pump impairment is identified by a flat or falling systolic blood pressure in response to increasing levels of work. Additionally, the $\dot{V}O_2$ may fail to increase early in exercise, demonstrating the pump's inability to increase SV with increased oxygen demand, or the $\dot{V}O_2$ may level off quickly and before maximum exercise, denoting a limitation in cardiac reserve and indicating abnormality rather than aging.

Deconditioning is common among older adults and is represented in exercise testing by a low $\dot{V}O_2$max and low anaerobic threshold. Changes in signs and symptoms, such as angina onset with change in electrocardiogram configuration (ECG change), are identified as ischemia and not deconditioning. Consequently, when the patient describes onset of chest tightness or dyspnea during exercise that is associated with rales and falling blood pressure, the clinician can rule out deconditioning as the impairment. Similarly, DOE can certainly be associated with deconditioning but a decline in oxygen saturation or onset of paradoxical breathing pattern of ventilation cannot be. Deconditioned individuals most often complain of leg fatigue or discomfort at the termination of exercise in addition to the symptoms of general fatigue and dyspnea.[42] Physiological abnormalities associated with increasing workloads are measured and recorded to serve as the basis for identifying and classifying impairments to be managed in physical therapy or patients who need to be referred for medical evaluation.

Evaluation, Diagnosis, Prognosis

The final step in evaluation is the clinical judgment process. The clinician considers all the findings from the examination to determine what impairments are amenable to physical therapy intervention, what diagnostic pattern best describes the patient, and what are reasonable outcomes and prognosis for the course of care. Patients who have localized problems such as muscle performance or the systemic problems associated with deconditioning may be well-managed in a short treatment course and quickly achieve an improved functional performance. Older individuals with serious and significant impairment of ventilatory pump function or gas exchange mechanisms may require more complex interventions and a longer course of care and may never achieve a return to full functional capacity. The goals and expected outcomes for seniors should consider the slowed healing process, the decreased maximum capacity of the system, and a realistic functional potential.

THERAPEUTIC INTERVENTION

Design of an accurate and effective treatment program is dependent on the previously described processes of examination and evaluation. Identification of the existence and severity of each impairment allows the therapist to prioritize interventions and direct the care provided to maximize the probable improvement any patient can achieve. Individuals with reduced ventilatory pump capacity will receive programs that effectively reduce the work of breathing or improve the strength and endurance of ventilatory muscles. Reduction in the WOB is often accomplished through change in body position to reduce the biomechanical load, e.g., upright sitting reduces abdominal resistance. Muscle length and stretch are often affected by variables that can be manipulated, such as intrathoracic lung volume; body position (supine vs upright); and degree of external compression, e.g., abdominal binder. Therapeutic intervention is directed at the balance between minimizing load and maximizing efficiency. Other strategies to reduce WOB include those that lower flow resistance, e.g., use of bronchodilators; use of medications, e.g., steroids to reduce inflammation; and control of breathing pattern to improve flow rate and muscle contraction.

Breathing Strategies

From a physical therapy perspective there are strategies that can be used to decrease the work of breathing for patients with an increase in both the elastic and the flow resistive work of breathing. Diaphragmatic breathing, pursed lip breathing, and paced breathing with exercise are techniques that are designed to reduce the WOB, decrease the oxygen cost of ventilation, and improve the efficiency of ventilatory pump function.[23] Diaphragmatic breathing as a technique focuses on reduction of the RR to improve efficiency of alveolar ventilation; recruitment of the abdominal muscles to facilitate use of the diaphragm to its best advantage on its length tension curve; and finally, reduction of $\dot{V}O_2$ per unit of work by decreasing the repetitive contraction of the accessory muscles.[27]

Reduction of the RR improves alveolar ventilation in multiple ways. A lower rate reduces the $\dot{V}/\dot{Q}$ mismatch by decreasing inefficient ventilation of the anatomical dead space. It also slows the velocity of diaphragmatic contraction, which facilitates recruitment of intercostal and other accessory muscles. Finally, it increases the overall strength of each muscle contraction by potentiating the force frequency curve and allowing time for motor unit recruitment.[5,31]

Improving the strength and efficiency of each breath potentially lengthens the time before the onset of fatigue in an impaired individual. Tactile facilitation of efficient and effective diaphragmatic contraction assists with expiration through muscle cueing. Abdominal pressure in the subxiphoid region generates a quick stretch before the next inspiratory effort, improving inspiratory contraction. Selecting the appropriate technique for each patient is based on the previous examination or re-examination.[23]

Pursed lip breathing is a strategy used to diminish the symptom of dyspnea. It is spontaneously adopted by some individuals with obstructive lung disease. A summary of the findings of multiple investigators offers a variety of ratio-

nales to describe the mechanism for its success. The proposed reasons include: facilitation of increased inspiratory tidal volume by increasing the volume exhaled with each breath, decreased respiratory rate by slowing and prolonging expiratory flow, decrease peak and mean expiratory flow rates that potentially decrease turbulent flow and airway collapse, and finally improved alveolar ventilation.[28,45] The technique can be taught to patients by using visual aids such as a mirror and careful tactile and vocal facilitation of the therapist.

Paced breathing is another technique that is expected to reduce the work of breathing and diminish the symptom of dyspnea during activity.[23] Varying ratios of inspiratory time to expiratory time have been tested with multiple functional activities in an effort to find a ratio that provides subjective comfort during activity performance. Practice or repetition of maneuvers during basic activities of daily living (BADL) may enhance the process of integrating the behaviors into daily living. Change at that level improves the likelihood the patterns will become ingrained behaviors and improve the patient's ability to participate in social and work activities, enhancing overall quality of life.

The most severely limited patients may need to implement a program that incorporates most or all of the aforementioned strategies. Exhale with effort is a technique that attempts to break down an activity into one or more breaths per task, with the intent of decreasing the rate of activity performance and reducing the overall or maximum metabolic demand.[23] Applying expiratory control throughout the breathing cycle allows the inspiratory ventilatory muscles to be active during inspiration, and the abdominal and some parasternal muscles to be active during expiration. This shortens the active cycle for each group, allows them to potentiate function for one another, and again prolongs the onset of fatigue.[23] Silvestri and Mahler support the use of breathing strategies, with the additional expectation that patients will be able to gain control of their breathing and stave off the usual panic that accompanies the onset of dyspnea.[42]

Strength and Endurance Conditioning of Ventilatory Muscles

Once the patient has begun to master some of the strategies or techniques for reducing the work of breathing and improving the efficiency of the pattern of breathing, there may be an opportunity to address strength and endurance needs of the ventilatory muscles. Inherent in this process is the need to have measured and documented any impairment. It is appropriate that strength is measured through the assessment of the maximum inspiratory and expiratory pressures (MIP and MEP) and the comparison of values with normative data. Assessment of MVV or that which can be sustained for 15 minutes or longer (MSVC) measures endurance.[36] Other tests are not as practical for clinical use.

The same principles that accomplish skeletal muscle strength training apply to training the ventilatory muscles. To achieve a change in muscle fiber size or response to load, an acceptable level of intensity must be applied using the overload principle. Specificity is important in that improved performance for an outcome is achieved by training using a like activity.[2] Finally, the principle of reversibility applies, meaning that cessation of the training activity will result in a decline in the positive benefit previously achieved.[33]

While there are multiple ways of training the ventilatory muscles, threshold training has been suggested to achieve both strength and endurance goals.[34,35] In this method, a calibrated load is applied during inspiration, and no load or resistance exists during expiration. Reid and Samrai reviewed the results of studies by multiple authors and reported improvements with this method of training in a variety of populations (asymptomatic persons and those with COPD, asthma, and cystic fibrosis).[35] An alternative method for addressing the strength and endurance needs of the ventilatory muscles is to have the individual perform exercise, as the WOB itself presents the overload training stimulus. With this method it is possible to apply the principles of overload, specificity, and reversibility and have a patient participate in an activity that can be reproduced during day-to-day function. From a clinical perspective, there may be improved compliance on the part of the patient if he/she is not obliged to perform multiple forms of therapeutic activity throughout the day for the same end result.

Airway Clearance

Excessive secretions in the airways can obstruct airflow and increase the flow resistive work of breathing. Manual techniques of percussion, shaking, and vibration in appropriate segmental drainage positions can enhance the mobilization of secretions.[43] Clearance of secretions by cough, huff, forced expiratory techniques, or suctioning removes the obstruction to airflow—at least on a temporary basis—and reduces the work of breathing. There are conditions of excessive mucus production (chronic bronchitis, bronchiectasis) or impaired mucociliary transport (immotile cilia syndrome) that may require secretion clearance measures on a chronic or long-term basis to assist in managing airway obstruction and in maintaining a tolerable work of breathing. Many of these techniques can be effectively performed by the patient in chronic situations, which promotes self-care and independence.

Endurance Conditioning

The last intervention to be discussed is exercise training or conditioning. The exercise program for any individual is based on reducing or eliminating impairments and is therefore prescribed using the exercise test results.[51] Healthy older adults may have required a routine standardized exercise test protocol during examination to elicit symptoms and document maximum capacity or exercise limitation.[52] Individuals who have been sedentary or who have been diagnosed with significant pulmonary disease likely will have undergone a modified exercise test protocol or a timed walk test to objectively elicit their exercise limitation and allow for measure-

ment of clinical signs and symptoms. Severity of pre-existing cardiopulmonary disease may have warranted additional data collection that included 12-lead ECG monitoring, analysis of expired gases, or assessment of heart sounds to accurately identify system impairment during exercise.[52]

An exercise program should be designed based on the documented impairment, the patient's functional goals, and the prognosis for outcome. Often the most significant key to the success of an exercise program is a patient-selected reasonable mode of exercise. *Reasonable* is defined in terms of ease of access, simplicity of performance, and patient comfort. The physiologically successful prescription has to combine the elements of intensity, duration, and frequency that best address the type and severity of impairment, e.g., strength training/intensity for strength deficits.[15] Accommodations that are often necessary for older patients include an initially low intensity of exercise, an intermittent workload, and a goal that focuses on prolonged duration. An initial approach that is too aggressive may result in an excessive respiratory rate, early onset of symptoms, and rapid patient discomfort, which could lead to early termination of the activity. Programs that result in early successes and goal achievement will often increase the confidence of the participant and enhance his/her willingness to continue.

Physiological training principles should focus on low-intensity loads until the duration of exercise achieves a reasonable endurance level, e.g., 30 minutes. Once the patient can ambulate or bike for 30 continuous minutes, the load can be increased to address functional strength goals. Specificity of program design relates to the task to be accomplished, e.g., quad strengthening for stair climbing. Incorporating the patient's goals for improvement in performance of any basic or instrumental activities of daily living will undoubtedly improve compliance with the exercise program. Giving the patient suggestions for modifying all daily activities to an intensity that does not provoke an unacceptable subjective rating of dyspnea may enhance his/her compliance with the exercise program until overall functional capacity improves.

Wellness/Prevention Techniques

Given that aging is inevitable and the consequences of aging are not preventable, the question arises, how can the risks of ventilatory and respiratory dysfunction be minimized for the older adult? Clearly many individuals lead a normal life without excessive adaptations for performance of functional activities, and not all forms of pathology produce dysfunction. However, many individuals may increase the risk of developing impairment as a result of unhealthy behaviors, particularly in the setting of other environmental factors.

Smoking Cessation

Cigarette smoking is a major health concern for everyone; however, there are special problems that are unique to the older adult. Most older smokers have a higher nicotine addiction, making it more difficult to quit. Additionally they have smoked longer and are consequently at greater risk for more smoking-related problems.[10] Cox has reported that " . . . quitting smoking at any age will increase both the quality and quantity of life . . . . "[10] Clinicians who understand this will not have an attitude of "age prejudice" toward their patients by deciding that it is too late to refer older individuals to smoking cessation programs.

Nutrition

Nutrition is an important consideration for good health at any age. In examining dyspnea in the elderly, Silvestri and Mahler commented that one third of patients with COPD were underweight.[42] They projected a host of consequences that were related to weight loss and poor nutrition, including shorter survival, decreased ventilatory muscle strength, and greater risk of infection. There is obvious concern that reduced ventilatory muscle strength may contribute to increased breathlessness and a greater WOB. A recent study by Dow examined whether dietary antioxidant intake in elderly persons was related to lung function.[13] While vitamin C had no association with FEV_1 or FVC, vitamin E was positively associated with both. Implications were that further study should investigate the value of dietary supplementation and the effect that may have on reducing the decline in lung function longitudinally.

Immunizations

Vaccinations are another means of reducing pathology risk in older adults, especially in terms of common pulmonary disorders that compromise function. Seniors should avail themselves of the publicly circulated vaccines for influenza and pneumococcal pneumonia. While illness is not prevented in 100% of cases, severity is reported to be much less in vaccinated individuals—a significant benefit to persons with diminished reserve capacity.[10]

Stress Management

Management of stress needs consideration as well. Both the immune and cardiovascular systems are influenced negatively by stress.[16] Additionally, stress and anxiety have a detrimental effect on an individual's ability to cope with shortness of breath or dyspnea.

Case Studies

BJ

BJ is a 73-year-old English speaking white male who was admitted to the hospital 1 day ago after a medical evaluation in the emergency unit. He is undergoing an examination by a physical therapist in the acute medical service. One week before admission he noted a fever of 102°F associated with cough and sputum production and was prescribed an antibiotic by his primary care physician. Yesterday, he complained of increasing shortness of breath, increased cough with yellow sputum, and decreased activity tolerance. He was transported to the emergency unit by ambulance.

History

Pertinent social history includes that he is married and lives with his wife. He has seven children and many grandchildren who are his primary interest and socialization, though many live out of state. He is a retired high school principal and currently is not involved in any community activities. BJ lives in a two-story home that he owns. There are eight steps into the house from the front walk, which has railings on both sides. His bedroom is on the second floor, but there are bathrooms on both levels. He describes himself as independent in self-care, but says that "everything takes a long time" and his wife will assist as needed. He does not participate in any IADL, except for driving. He had to give up his hobby of gardening 2 years ago. Medications on admission include albuterol, ipratropium and fluticasone inhalers, glyburide, levofloxacin, verapamil, digoxin, and supplemental O_2.

The most recent laboratory tests show a slightly elevated white blood cell count, normal hematocrit value, and normal platelet count. The chest radiograph reveals a calcified nodule in the right hilum and infiltrates in the left upper lobe, lingula, and left lower lobe. The sputum specimen shows gram positive cocci. An arterial blood gas on 5 L O_2 via nasal prongs revealed significant hypoxemia with a compensated respiratory acidosis. The most recent measures of spirometry from 1 month ago demonstrate an FVC of 1.94 L (50% predicted) and an FEV_1 of 0.39 L (15% predicted). BJ had been hospitalized for a right lower lobe pneumonia within the last month and before admission was receiving home nursing and physical therapy services. Past medical history is significant for COPD; frequent pneumonias, including respiratory failure requiring prolonged mechanical ventilation 3 years ago; type II diabetes; hypertension; supraventricular tachycardia; and a remote history of an appendectomy.

Social habits include an 80-pack per year smoking history and no alcohol use. The patient admits that he continues to "sneak" cigarettes, and his wife smokes at home.

Systems Review

A review of systems reveals a resting respiratory rate of 28, a heart rate of 102, and blood pressure of 152/60 mm Hg. The skin is warm, dry, and intact with no evidence of clubbing. There are no active musculoskeletal or neuromuscular problems that would limit the patient. He is alert and oriented, communicates well, and understands instructions.

Tests and Measures

Appropriate tests and measures to conclude the examination included the following:
- Aerobic capacity and endurance: Able to ambulate 300 feet with a rolling walker with two rest periods of 1 to 2 minutes; on 3 L of oxygen (baseline at home) his saturation dropped from 93% to 86%; activity was rated as "very heavy"
- Anthropometric characteristics: Height = 66 inches, weight = 160 pounds

- Arousal, attention, cognition: Fully alert, oriented, and communicative
- Muscle performance: All extremities within functional limitations
- Posture: Rounded shoulders, forward head, forearm leaning position at rest
- Self-care and home management: Independent in bed mobility, moves supine to sit to stand, ambulates with a rolling walker (assist needed for wheeling O_2)
- Ventilation and respiration: Breath sounds markedly diminished bilaterally; bronchial over left upper lobe, rhonchi over left lower lobe laterally; cough effective, wet, and clearing moderate amounts of thick green sputum; poor chest wall mobility and barrel chest evident; at rest HR 102, BP 152/60 mm Hg, RR 28, SpO_2 93% on 3 L O_2.

After objective information was collected, the evaluation was formulated. A list of pertinent impairments included the following:
- Impaired ventilation
- Impaired gas exchange
- Impaired airway clearance
- Impaired ADL/IADL performance
- Impaired aerobic capacity

Based on the examination findings an appropriate physical therapy diagnostic classification for this patient was impaired ventilation, respiration, and aerobic capacity associated with airway clearance dysfunction.

The clinical impression was that this elderly gentleman had been experiencing an acute pulmonary process superimposed on a chronic condition. He was not able to maintain baseline status in this setting and required PT intervention to assist with secretion clearance, to improve gas exchange, and to prevent further deconditioning. He would require further short-term rehabilitation before returning home. Prognostically, it was anticipated that he should return to his baseline status of independent secretion clearance with 6 visits over 4 days. However, he might not return to his baseline status with regard to gas exchange for 2 to 3 weeks. By the time he returns home, the physical therapist expects no evidence of acute infiltrate by chest x-ray. BJ also should experience less dyspnea on exertion with basic ADL and should be able to resume driving.

Appropriate interventions for this patient included supplemental O_2 with titration to keep saturation at least 92%; BJ required teaching to ensure appropriate use. Positioning and manual techniques to enhance secretion clearance were instituted to reduce the WOB and to improve gas exchange. A progressive walking program was implemented to improve exercise tolerance, while instruction in energy conservation and pacing improved his ability to perform self-care at home. Although the focus of therapy is remediating impairments in the acute setting, the intent is to achieve meaningful outcomes for any patient. Reasonable outcomes for this patient included the following:
- Return to optimal level of daily function
- Return to ability to socialize with friends and family
- Improved health related quality of life
- Safe performance of basic and instrumental ADL

- Understanding of strategies to prevent further functional limitations and disabilities
- Patient satisfaction with health care interventions

This case demonstrates the examination and evaluation processes for a patient with an acute on chronic process and offers strategies for a return to functional independence with PT intervention.

CE

CE is a 60-year-old white male with emphysema and chronic bronchitis who was referred to outpatient physical therapy secondary to progressive DOE. His chief complaint is an inability to walk more than 100 feet without resting. He has noticed a significant decrease in activity tolerance since his last hospital admission for pneumonia 4 months ago.

History

Pertinent social history includes that he is a widower and lives with his son and daughter-in-law in their two-story home. There are two steps to enter the house, and the patient stays on the first floor. He is retired from maintenance work secondary to his health, and has been on disability for 8 months. Functionally, he is independent in basic ADL, but it takes him a longer time to shower and dress. Additionally, showering precipitates increased cough and shortness of breath. With regard to instrumental ADL, CE is quite limited. Most cooking, cleaning, and laundry is done by his family. He drives and does light marketing and minimal cooking. He uses no assistive devices. He has no hobbies. Medications include salmeterol, albuterol, ipratropium and budesonide metered-dose inhalers, prednisone, theophylline, and trazodone. There are no laboratory tests available except spirometry, which demonstrates an FVC of 2.01 L (46% predicted) and FEV_1 of 0.85 L (27% predicted).

The past medical history is unremarkable, except for pulmonary issues. He was diagnosed with emphysema 4 years ago by his report. He has had multiple pneumonias, requiring hospitalization four times in the last year. Social habits include a 120-pack per year smoking history, currently 3 to 4 cigarettes/day. He admits to occasional ETOH use (alcohol consumption).

Systems Review

The review of systems showed a resting regular HR at 108, BP of 140/80 mm Hg, RR of 24, SpO_2 of 91% on room air. No clubbing or lower-extremity edema were noted. No apparent limitations related to musculoskeletal or neuromuscular problems were identified. The patient admitted that he feels discouraged by his current limitations.

Tests and Measures

Appropriate tests and measures to conclude the examination included:
- Aerobic capacity: 6-minute walk test, covering 850 feet, requiring 3 brief rests; small but appropriate elevations in HR, BP; RR increased to 32; SpO_2 dropped to 86%; perceived exertion was "very heavy"

- Anthropometric characteristics: Weight = 131 pounds, with 10-pound weight loss in last 6 months; height = 70 inches
- Arousal, attention, cognition: Alert and oriented, good historian, appears motivated to improve health status
- Gait, locomotion, balance: No abnormalities noted
- Muscle performance: Proximal muscles 3+ to 4/5 in all extremities, otherwise normal; maximal inspiratory pressure −30 cm H_2O from RV, maximal expiratory pressure in normal range
- Posture: Forward head, rounded shoulders, elevated clavicles, significant thoracic kyphosis
- Ventilation and respiration: Breath sounds are decreased throughout with low-pitched wheezes at bases; synchronous pattern of breathing at rest with significant recruitment of accessory muscles with ambulation; poor chest wall mobility and diaphragmatic excursion; cough is effective, dry now, but frequently productive of tan secretions throughout the day

Based on the examination findings, the evaluation was formulated and a list of pertinent impairments included the following:

- Impaired ventilation with increased work of breathing, inefficient pattern, and low MIP
- Impaired gas exchange
- Impaired muscle performance
- Impaired aerobic capacity
- Impaired knowledge regarding use of O_2, medications, self-monitoring, and exercise progression
- Impaired ability to engage in IADLs and socialization
- Inability to climb stairs in a functional manner

The examination findings supported a diagnostic classification of impaired ventilation, respiration and aerobic capacity, and endurance associated with ventilatory pump dysfunction.

This patient had one significant comorbidity that could impede his progress—his nutritional status. He could require dietary supplements or might benefit from a referral to a nutritionist. He was motivated to make gains and already reduced his smoking to 3 to 4 cigarettes per day. He understood that another exacerbation of bronchitis would negatively affect his progress and that it is imperative that he achieve full cessation of smoking. It should take approximately 6 to 8 weeks for him to meet his goals and experience functional gains.

The anticipated goals and expected outcomes for this patient included:

- Increased proximal muscle strength to 4 to 4+/5 in 6 to 8 weeks
- Decreased sense of dyspnea with ambulation on level surfaces and stairs in 6 weeks
- Appropriate use of supplemental O_2 within 2 weeks
- Appropriate use of metered-dose inhalers within 2 to 3 weeks
- Adherence to home exercise program within 2 weeks
- Ability to self-monitor exercise/symptom response in 8 weeks

- Ability to ambulate for 30 minutes with increased distance in 8 weeks
- Improved participation in basic and instrumental ADL in 8 weeks with decreased sense of dyspnea

Intervention was scheduled for 2 to 3 times per week during the next 6 to 8 weeks. The focus in weeks 1 and 2 was on breathing retraining to improve efficiency and to minimize the work of breathing. Given the history of recurrent infections, it was worthwhile to ensure that the patient adequately cleared secretions without bronchopulmonary hygiene (manual techniques). Additionally, education was provided regarding appropriate use of supplemental oxygen and metered-dose inhalers as well as symptom identification. Inspiratory muscle training was introduced at this time as well as peripheral muscle strengthening. The focus in weeks 2 to 6 was on an exercise assessment and creating an exercise prescription that led to a conditioning program.

Given the severe functional limitations, ĊE initially walked in an interval format using short walk segments (e.g., 2 minutes) alternating with rests (30 seconds), attempting to complete at least 20 minutes of exercise. By week 6 he was performing 20 to 30 minutes of continuous walking with only one rest period. It was expected that he would carry out a walking program at home and use an exercise log as an effective tool for monitoring his success and adherence. While all aspects of the program were monitored and modified throughout the course of physical therapist intervention, the focus in weeks 6 to 8 was on finalizing all aspects of the exercise prescription and ensuring independence in performance. It was important to re-examine all objective tests and measures to determine improvement over the course of intervention as well as to obtain the patient's subjective view. Re-examination in 4 to 6 weeks was the ideal time for further modification of the exercise prescription and assessment of patient compliance.

SUMMARY

The ventilatory and respiratory functions of older adults undergo a process of change related to aging that begins in early adulthood. In the absence of other pulmonary insults or illness, these changes do not usually result in a severe enough decline to affect resting function or performance of activities that require a moderate level of $\dot{V}O_2$. However, the impact of disease in conjunction with environmental factors or high-risk behaviors can be significant. Disease processes can easily be accelerated and result in functional limitations if not addressed early in their course or treated adequately.

The physical therapist practicing in a geriatric setting needs to be knowledgeable about the normal consequences of aging to be able to identify the origin of and differences between impairments of aging or pathology. The ability to measure and discriminate between the process of aging and the sequelae of pathology are essential to appropriate management of impairment and prevention of functional decline. Interpretation of the results of varied testing procedures in addition to the thorough interview and examination allow the therapist to perform the differential diagnostic process and proceed with an appropriate plan for intervention. Interventions are directed at patient-identified goals, when appropriate, and the success of any program is based on improvement in the quality of life and prevention of functional decline.

REFERENCES

1. Angus GE, Thurlbeck WM: Number of alveoli in the human lung. *J Appl Physiol* 1972; 32:483-485.
2. Belman MJ, Gaesser GA: Ventilatory muscle training in the elderly. *J Appl Physiol* 1988; 64(3):899-905.
3. Blessey RL, et al: Metabolic energy cost of unrestrained walking. *Phys Ther* 1976; 56(9):1019-1024.
4. Campbell EJ, Lefrak SS: How aging affects the structure and function of the respiratory system. *Geriatrics* 1978; June:68-74.
5. Casciari RJ, et al: Effects of breathing retraining in patients with chronic obstructive pulmonary disease. *Chest* 1981; 79(4):393-398.
6. Chan ED, Welsh CH: Geriatric respiratory medicine. *Chest* 1998; 114:1704-1733.
7. Cherniak RM: *Pulmonary Function Testing.* Philadelphia, WB Saunders, 1977.
8. Clanton TL, Diaz PT: Clinical assessment of the respiratory muscles. *Phys Ther* 1995; 75:983-995.
9. Couser JI, Glassroth J: Tuberculosis, an epidemic in older adults. *Clin Chest Med* 1993; 14(3):491-498.
10. Cox EJ: Smoking cessation in the elderly patient. *Clin Chest Med* 1993; 14(3):423-428.
11. Crane LD: Functional anatomy and physiology of ventilation, in Zadai CC (ed): *Pulmonary Management in Physical Therapy.* New York, Churchill Livingstone, 1992.
12. Davis GM, Bureau MA: Pulmonary and chest wall mechanics in the control of respiration in the newborn. *Clin Perinatol* 1987; 14:551.
13. Dow L, et al: Does dietary intake of vitamins C and E influence lung function in older people. *Am J Respir Crit Care Med* 1996; 154: 1401-1404.
14. Fanta CH: Asthma in the elderly. *J Asthma* 1989; 26(2):87-97.
15. Fiatarone MA, et al: High intensity strength training in nonagenarians. *JAMA* 1990; 263(22):3029-3034.
16. Gambert SR, Gupta KL: Preventative care: What it's worth in geriatrics. *Geriatrics* 1989; 44(8):61-67.
17. Gilchrest BA, Rowe JW: The biology of aging, in Rowe JW, Besdine RW (eds): *Health and Disease in Old Age.* Boston, Little, Brown, 1982.
18. Grippi MA: Gas exchange in the lung, in Grippi MA (ed): *Pulmonary Pathophysiology.* Philadelphia, JB Lippincott, 1995.
18a. Guide to physical therapy practice. *Phys Ther* 1997; 77:1163-1650.
19. Gyetko MR, Loews GB: Immunology of the aging lung. *Clin Chest Med* 1993; 14(3):379-391.
20. Irwin S, Zadai CC: Cardiopulmonary response to exercise, in Zadai CC (ed): *Pulmonary Management in Physical Therapy.* New York, Churchill Livingstone, 1992.
21. Jette AM, et al: The Functional Status Questionnaire. *J General Intern Med* 1986; 1:143-149.
22. Klein RM, Bell B: Self-care skills: Behavioral measurement with Klein Bell ADL Scale. *Arch Phys Med Rehabil* 1982; 63:335-338.
23. Levenson CR: Breathing exercises, in Zadai CC (ed): *Pulmonary Management in Physical Therapy.* New York, Churchill Livingstone, 1992.
24. Lee-Chiong TL, Matthay R: Lung cancer in the elderly patient. *Clin Chest Med* 1993; 14(3):453-478.
25. Lillington GA: Dyspnea in the elderly: Old age or disease? *Geriatrics* 1984; 39(11):47-52.
26. Meyer KC, et al: Immune dysregulation in the aging human lung. *Am J Respir Crit Care Med* 1996; 153:1072-1079.
27. Miller WF: A physiologic evaluation of the effects of diaphragmatic breathing training in patients with chronic pulmonary emphysema. *Am J Med* 1954; 17:471-477.
28. Mueller RE, Petty TL, Filley GF: Ventilation and arterial blood gas changes induced by pursed lips breathing. *J Appl Physiol* 1970; 28: 784-789.
29. Murray JF: *The Normal Lung.* Philadelphia, WB Saunders, 1976.
30. Otis AB: The work of breathing. *Physiol Rev* 1954; 34:449.
31. Paul G, et al: Some effects of slowing respiration rate in chronic emphysema and bronchitis. *J Appl Physiol* 1966; 21:877-882.
32. Pardy RL, Hussain SN, Macklem PT: The ventilatory pump in exercise. *Clin Chest Med* 1984; 5(1):35-49.
33. Pardy RL, Reid WD, Belman MJ: Respiratory muscle training. *Clin Chest Med* 1988; 9(2):287-296.
34. Reid WD, Dechman G: Considerations when testing and training the respiratory muscles. *Phys Ther* 1995; 75(11):971-982.
35. Reid WD, Samrai B: Respiratory muscle training for patients with chronic obstructive pulmonary disease. *Phys Ther* 1995; 75(11):996-1005.
36. Rochester DF: Tests of respiratory muscle function. *Clin Chest Med* 1988; 9(2):249-261.
37. Rubenstein LV, et al: Health status assessment for elderly patients. *JAGS* 1988; 37:562-569.
38. Ruppel G: *Manual of Pulmonary Function Testing.* St Louis, Mosby, 1979.
39. Shepard RJ: *Physical Activity and Aging.* Rockville, Md, Aspen, 1987.
40. Shepard RJ: The cardiovascular benefits of exercise in the elderly. *Top Geriatr Rehabilitation* 1985; 1(1):1-10.
41. Sherman CB, et al: Cognitive function and spirometry performance in the elderly. *Am Rev Respir Dis* 1993; 148:123-126.
42. Silvestri GA, Mahler DA: Evaluation of dyspnea in the elderly patient. *Clin Chest Med* 1993; 14(3):393-404.
43. Starr JA: Manual techniques of chest physical therapy and airway clearance techniques, in Zadai CC (ed): *Pulmonary Management in Physical Therapy.* New York, Churchill Livingstone, 1992.
44. Tecklin JS: Common pulmonary diseases, in Irwin S, Tecklin JS (ed): *Cardiopulmonary Physical Therapy,* 3rd ed. St Louis, Mosby, 1995.
45. Toman RL, Stolar GL, Ross JC: The efficacy of pursed lips breathing in patients with chronic obstructive pulmonary disease. *Am Rev Respir Dis* 1966; 93:100-106.
46. Tolep K, Kelsen SG: Effect of aging in respiratory skeletal muscles. *Clin Chest Med* 1993; 14(3):363-378.
47. Turner JM, Mead J, Wohl ME: Elasticity of human lungs in relation to age. *J Appl Physiol* 1968; 25(6):664-671.
48. Weiss ST: Pulmonary system, in Rowe JW, Besdine RW (eds): *Health and Disease in Old Age.* Boston, Little, Brown, 1982.
49. Wright RR: Elastic tissue of normal and emphysematous lungs. *Am J Pathology* 1961; 39(3): 355-367.
50. Zadai CC: Comprehensive physical therapy evaluation: Identifying potential pulmonary limitations, in Zadai CC (ed): *Pulmonary Management in Physical Therapy.* New York, Churchill Livingstone, 1992.
51. Zadai CC: Cardiopulmonary aging and exercise, in Pryor JA (ed): *Respiratory Care.* New York, Churchill Livingstone, 1991.
52. Zadai CC, Irwin SC: Cardiopulmonary rehabilitation of the geriatric patient, in Lewis CB (ed): *Aging, The Health Care Challenge,* 3rd ed. Philadelphia, FA Davis, 1990.
53. Zadai CC: Pulmonary physiology of aging: The role of rehabilitation. *Top Geriatr Rehabilitation* 1985; 1(1):49-57.

CHAPTER 15

ENDURANCE TRAINING OF THE OLDER ADULT

WENDY M. KOHRT, PHD AND MARYBETH BROWN, PT, PHD

INTRODUCTION

A decline in cardiovascular functional capacity occurs with aging, regardless of life-style. However, the sedentary life-style that is typical of older adults in the United States accelerates the decline in functional capacity and increases the risk for losing independence at a relatively young age. Some older adults, particularly women, are so debilitated that they use nearly 100% of their cardiovascular functional capacity just to perform instrumental activities of daily living (IADL). Habitual exercise training slows the rate of decline in cardiovascular function, thereby delaying the onset of frailty.

Even though cardiovascular fitness declines with aging, most older adults have the potential to improve fitness markedly through endurance exercise training. Although the primary benefit of endurance training is an improvement in maximal cardiovascular functional capacity, there are secondary benefits that are of significant practical importance. For example, an activity that demands 100% of functional capacity before training may require only 80% of functional capacity after training, thereby reducing the fatigue and discomfort associated with the activity. Other potential health benefits of endurance exercise training translate into an improved quality of life by reducing the risk of developing age-related diseases, such as atherosclerosis, hypertension, non-insulin–dependent diabetes, and osteoporosis.

The best index of cardiovascular functional capacity is maximal oxygen uptake, or $\dot{V}O_2max$. Briefly, $\dot{V}O_2max$ is the maximal rate at which the body can utilize oxygen (O_2) or, in other words, the maximal rate at which energy can be produced through aerobic mechanisms. Usually, $\dot{V}O_2max$ is expressed as the volume of O_2 consumed (mL) relative to time (per minute) and body weight (per kg)—or mL/min/kg. To provide a degree of perspective, a world-class male endurance athlete may have a $\dot{V}O_2max$ of 80 mL/min/kg, whereas it is not uncommon for a frail 80-year-old woman to have a $\dot{V}O_2max$ of 14 mL/min/kg. For additional perspective, the energy cost of walking 3 mph is approximately 12 mL/min/kg. Thus, walking 3 mph would require only 15% of the elite endurance athlete's $\dot{V}O_2max$, but 86% of the 80-year-old's $\dot{V}O_2max$. Because the degree of fatigue and discomfort experienced during an activity depends on the intensity of the exercise relative to an individual's $\dot{V}O_2max$, walking 3 mph would be perceived as very easy by the elite athlete but as very difficult by the frail woman. Thus, the higher a person's $\dot{V}O_2max$, the greater the opportunity for that person to enjoy a variety of physical activities without undue fatigue.

CHANGES IN CARDIOVASCULAR FUNCTION WITH AGING

The rate of O_2 consumption ($\dot{V}O_2$) increases linearly as exercise intensity increases and is a function of the rate at which O_2 is delivered to (cardiac output, or $\dot{Q}$) and extracted by the tissues (arteriovenous oxygen content difference, or a-$\overline{v}O_2$ difference). The $\dot{V}O_2max$ an individual can reach is influenced by factors such as heredity, gender, age, body composition, and endurance exercise training.[5] In most individuals, $\dot{V}O_2$max is limited by $\dot{Q}$, which is the product of heart rate (HR) and stroke volume (SV). For this reason, $\dot{V}O_2$max is considered the best available index of cardiovascular fitness. It is usually measured during a treadmill or cycle ergometer test, during which exercise intensity is progressively increased. The objective determination of $\dot{V}O_2$max is a failure to increase $\dot{V}O_2$ with an increase in exercise intensity, i.e., a plateau in $\dot{V}O_2$. Because this criterion is often difficult to attain, particularly in the elderly, other indices of a near-maximal effort include a respiratory exchange ratio greater than 1.10, a HR within 10 beats per minute of the age-predicted maximal HR, or a blood lactate level greater than 8 mmol/L.[5,76] Using these criteria, it has been shown that healthy older men and women up to 80 years of age reach $\dot{V}O_2$max values during treadmill exercise that are reproducible.[52] When $\dot{V}O_2$max is measured during cycle ergometer exercise, however, individuals are often limited by muscular fatigue and attain peak $\dot{V}O_2$ values that are approximately 10% less than the treadmill value.[58] This deficit may be exaggerated in the elderly due to declining quadriceps muscle mass and/or strength.

Average $\dot{V}O_2$max values in healthy, sedentary 25-year-old men and women are 46 to 48 mL/min/kg and 34 to 36 mL/min/kg, respectively.[46,64,76] The effect of aging, per se, on the decline in $\dot{V}O_2$max is difficult to determine due to the increase in body fat content[37,77] and decline in physical activity[125] that also typically occur with advancing age; both will accelerate the decline in $\dot{V}O_2$max. Cross-sectional and longitudinal studies indicate that $\dot{V}O_2$max decreases about 4 to 5.5 mL/min/kg/decade in men and 2 to 3.5 mL/min/kg/decade in women, or approximately 12% to 13% per decade.[61] This probably reflects the rate of decline due to the combined effects of age, increasing adiposity, and a sedentary life-style. In men and women who remain relatively lean, the estimated rate of decline in $\dot{V}O_2$max is about 9% per decade,[57,76] and in master athletes, who remain lean and maintain a vigorous level of physical activity, the estimated rate of decline is only about 5% per decade.[46,57,108]

It has been suggested that the age-related decline in $\dot{V}O_2$max in sedentary persons is due in large part to the loss of muscle mass that occurs with aging.[46] This seems unlikely, however, as muscle mass is essentially maintained to age 50 but $\dot{V}O_2$max is not.[61] The decline of $\dot{V}O_2$max in well-trained athletes also does not appear to be linked to changes in body composition but rather to a decline in maximal HR.[51,57,108]

DETERMINANTS OF $\dot{V}O_2$MAX

Heart Rate
Maximal HR (HRmax) is determined primarily by age, as evidenced by the following equation recommended for its estimation.[5]

$$HRmax = 220 - age$$

However, a number of studies of exercise capacity of the elderly have found that HRmax is actually greater than predicted.[51,52,76,123] For example, among groups of healthy people whose age averaged 58 years,[51] 65 years,[76] and 72 years,[52] HRmax averaged 176, 165, and 157 beats per minute (bpm), respectively, or approximately 10 bpm higher than the age-predicted values. HRmax is not different between older men and women[59,76] and is not markedly altered by endurance exercise training.[7,36,52,54,76,123]

To determine the effect of age, per se, on cardiovascular responses to exercise, researchers have studied master athletes, who remain lean and maintain a high level of physical activity. These studies[51,57,102,108] indicate that HRmax plays a major role in the age-related decline of $\dot{V}O_2$max. Rivera and colleagues found that HRmax, SV, and a-$\bar{v}O_2$ difference were all lower in older compared with young distance runners.[108] However, others[51,56] have found that O_2 pulse (defined as $\dot{V}O_2$max divided by HRmax), SV, and a-$\bar{v}O_2$ difference were similar in young and older athletes, indicating that a slower HR was responsible for the lower $\dot{V}O_2$max in older athletes. In comparisons of master athletes and age-matched sedentary controls,[51,56] HRmax was similar but $\dot{V}O_2$max values were 40% to 50% lower in the untrained men due to reductions in both SV and a-$\bar{v}O_2$ difference. Thus, the age-related decline in $\dot{V}O_2$max is due primarily to the decline in HRmax but, at any age, differences among individuals in $\dot{V}O_2$max reflect differences in the capacity of the heart to deliver O_2 and the muscles to utilize O_2.

The cause of the age-related decline in maximal HR is not fully understood. Sympathetic drive may be attenuated, since catecholamine levels, i.e., epinephrine, norepinephrine, have been observed to be lower in older than in young persons in response to exercise at the same relative intensity.[80] Furthermore, with aging there appears to be a decreased sensitivity[67,117,140] and responsiveness[46,97,139] to the effects of catecholamines. Thus, the chronotropic response, i.e., increase in HR, to a given plasma catecholamine concentration is reduced with aging.

Stroke Volume
SV is the difference between end-diastolic and end-systolic volumes. Maximal SV may be maintained or actually increased with aging to help offset the decline in maximal $\dot{Q}$ (cardiac output) due to the reduction in HRmax. From studies of men and women aged 20 to 75 years,[59,64] it has been determined that there is no relationship between age and stroke index (SV per m² body surface area). These studies reported significant declines in $\dot{V}O_2$max with aging due to the decline in maximal $\dot{Q}$ that occurred as a result of a lower HRmax. It is possible, however, that this apparent decline in cardiac function was complicated by the high prevalence of occult coronary artery disease.[86,110] Indeed, when subjects were rigorously screened to eliminate those with cardiovascular disease,[119] the older subjects had a greater increase in SV during vigorous exercise than did the younger subjects. This was accomplished by an increase in end-diastolic volume rather than a reduction in end-systolic volume. Endurance exercise training has been shown to result in an increase in maximal $\dot{Q}$ due to an increase in SV in older

men[124,132,133,135] but not women,[132-134] suggesting that sex hormones may play an important role in the adaptive response.

Although end-diastolic volume may increase with age in healthy people, end-systolic volume apparently also increases and ejection fraction is reduced.[40,119] The decline with aging in ejection fraction at peak exercise has been attributed to an increase in aortic stiffness[47,66] and/or peripheral vascular resistance,[30,54] both of which may be related to altered autonomic modulation.

Arteriovenous Oxygen Content Difference

The extraction of O_2 across a working muscle is expressed as the difference in the arterial and venous O_2 content measured in mL of O_2 per 100 mL of blood. At rest, O_2 content in arterial and venous blood is approximately 20 and 15 mL/100 mL, and the a-$\bar{v}O_2$ difference is 5 mL/100 mL. During maximal exercise, the a-$\bar{v}O_2$ difference increases to 16 to 17 mL/100 mL in both young and master athletes.[51,95,110] Therefore age, per se, does not seem to alter the ability of skeletal muscle to extract O_2. However, in sedentary people there is a decline in a-$\bar{v}O_2$ difference with advancing age.[30,54,95]

The decrease in O_2 extraction that has been reported to occur with aging does not appear to be due to a reduction in O_2 carrying capacity of arterial blood[30,63] or to a decline in the metabolic potential of skeletal muscle.[4,26,48] There is, however, a decreased capillary/fiber ratio in aged muscle[26,99] as well as a reduction in maximal peripheral blood flow[87] that could contribute to the decrease in a-$\bar{v}O_2$ difference in sedentary older people.

BENEFITS OF ENDURANCE EXERCISE TRAINING

Cardiovascular Fitness

Early studies of the effect of endurance exercise training on aerobic power in the elderly led to equivocal results. On one hand there was a report[10] that older men and women increased $\dot{V}O_2$max by 38% with training, a large increase in comparison with the 15% to 25% improvement that typically occurs in young people.[6,25] On the other hand, there were studies[1,11,35] showing little or no increase in $\dot{V}O_2$max in older people in response to training. More recent studies indicate that the relative increase in aerobic power with training is not age dependent, at least through the eighth decade.[52,76,80,123,133] The lack of a marked training response in the aforementioned studies may have been the result of an insufficient training stimulus, i.e., training duration, intensity, or both. Conversely, the 38% improvement in $\dot{V}O_2$max reported by Barry and colleagues was probably an overestimation of the adaptability of older people, since maximal heart rate, respiratory exchange ratio, and blood lactate concentration were all markedly higher after training than before, indicating that a true $\dot{V}O_2$max had not been attained in the initial assessments.[10]

It is now accepted that older people can increase $\dot{V}O_2$max with endurance exercise training to the same relative degree as young people, i.e., 15% to 25%. While no significant gender differences in the increases in $\dot{V}O_2$max in response to training have been reported, a tendency toward less improvement in women was noted by Blumenthal and colleagues[16] (9% in women versus 14% in men) and by Seals and co-workers[122] (19% in women versus 27% in men). It is not known whether the exercise training prescriptions were similar for men and women in these studies. However, a report by Kohrt and colleagues indicated that the increases in $\dot{V}O_2$max in older men (26%) and women (23%) were not significantly different when the exercise stimulus was of similar frequency (4 days per week), duration (45 minutes per day), and relative intensity (80% HRmax).[76] In that study, the individual improvements in $\dot{V}O_2$max for the 53 men and 57 women who completed the exercise program varied markedly, ranging from 0% to 54%. Earlier studies suggested that the degree to which $\dot{V}O_2$max could be improved was dependent on the intensity of the exercise, i.e., higher intensity of exercise resulted in larger improvements,[53,122,137] and on the initial level of fitness, i.e., patients with lower fitness showed larger improvements.[28,118,137] However, Kohrt and co-workers have found that the magnitude of improvement in $\dot{V}O_2$max with training was not related to any specific component of the exercise prescription—i.e., frequency, duration, or intensity—nor was it related to the initial fitness level of the participant.[76] Thus, it seems likely that most older men and women, whether they lead very sedentary or fairly active lives, can improve cardiovascular fitness through regular endurance exercise training. The level of cardiovascular function that the average 65-year-old man or woman can attain through vigorous exercise is equivalent to that of someone 15 to 20 years younger.[76]

Metabolic Fitness

In addition to improvements in cardiovascular function, endurance exercise training can provide a number of other health benefits for older men and women. It has been estimated that people who are sedentary are twice as likely to develop coronary artery disease (CAD) as people who exercise regularly.[84,90,96] Part of this protective nature of exercise is due to its effects on coronary risk factors. Risk factors for CAD that can be improved through exercise include hypercholesterolemia,[14,123,138] hypertension,[53] hyperinsulinemia,[56,62] glucose intolerance,[62,112,113] and obesity.[78,120] Exercise is also one of the few interventions that can successfully increase plasma high-density lipoprotein (HDL) cholesterol, which is negatively correlated with CAD.[112,138]

Aging is often associated with a decline in glucose tolerance that may progress to non-insulin–dependent diabetes mellitus, or type 2 diabetes. This deterioration is not due to insulin deficiency, as in insulin-dependent diabetes mellitus, but rather to the resistance of peripheral tissues (primarily skeletal muscle) to the actions of insulin.[32,106] Thus, as insulin resistance develops, there is typically an excess of insulin secreted to try to maintain glucose homeostasis. Insulin resistance and hyperinsulinemia are very common in older people, particularly in those who accumulate fat in the abdominal region, i.e., apple-shaped, as opposed to the gluteal-femoral region, i.e., pear-shaped. There is evidence that hyperinsulinemia is associated with the development of not only type 2 diabetes but also hypertension[45,106] and CAD.[8,100] Exercise can be very effective in reducing hyperinsulinemia. Even a single bout of exercise can make skeletal muscle more sensitive to the glucoregulatory actions of insulin, thereby reducing insulin requirements.[70,71,89,111,113] Thus, through its effects on insulin action, regular exercise can play a major role in both the treatment and prevention of type 2 diabetes, CAD, and hypertension.

Body Composition

Many of the beneficial effects of exercise are only short lived. For example, the increased sensitivity of muscle to the action of insulin persists for only 48 to 72 hours after a bout of exercise.[60,71] Longer-lasting benefits of exercise are probably mediated primarily through the reduction in body fat levels, particularly in the abdominal region. Although obesity is a potent risk factor for the development of CAD, type 2 diabetes, and hypertension, it has become apparent that it is abdominal obesity that is particularly detrimental.[15,33,75] The accumulation of intraabdominal fat appears to begin in young- to middle-aged men and progresses with advancing age. The majority of women, on the other hand, appear to be protected against this until menopause, at which time they, too, accumulate visceral fat.[18,33,41,126] Furthermore, although premenopausal women are at far lower risk for developing CAD than age-matched men, the risk profile of postmenopausal women who are not receiving sex hormone replacement therapy becomes more like that of their male counterparts, and the incidence of CAD increases dramatically.[9,21,23] It is currently not known to what extent the accumulation of intraabdominal fat mediates the increased risk for CAD in postmenopausal women.

There is evidence that endurance exercise training results in a preferential loss of fat from the central,[78] and possibly the visceral,[34,120] regions of the body. There is also evidence that a reduction in intraabdominal fat is predictive of improvements in plasma insulin and cholesterol concentrations.[34] Habitual exercise training seems to prevent much of the accumulation of abdominal fat that typically occurs with advancing age. Master athletes are much leaner than age-matched nonathletes, with the greatest differences in fat deposition being in central regions of the body.[54,77,103,121]

It is important to recognize that endurance exercise training does not usually bring about increases in lean body mass, even when sedentary older people engage in vigorous aerobic exercise.[76] Small increases in lean mass may occur when the endurance training program incorporates exercises that have modest resistance components, such as stair climbing or rowing.[20] Thus, if one of the goals of an exercise program is to increase muscle mass and strength, the program should include progressive resistance exercise training, i.e., weight lifting.

Bone Health

Another potential benefit of exercise training of particular importance for older women is the reduction in risk for osteoporosis. The effect of physical inactivity on bone is profound. When loading forces on the skeleton are markedly reduced, such as during bedrest[83] or space flight,[27] there is a rapid loss of bone mineral. The finding that exercise performed during space flight does not fully prevent the loss of calcium has been taken as evidence that exercise must be weight bearing in nature to have beneficial effects on the skeleton. However, it is unlikely that relatively short-duration exercise sessions in space could fully compensate for the drastic reduction in gravitational and load-bearing forces that is inevitable in a microgravity environment.

Although it is widely accepted that exercise is an important factor in maintaining skeletal integrity, the type of exercise that will optimize bone mass remains poorly defined. Studies using animal models have yielded important information regarding adaptive responses of the skeleton to mechanical loading forces. Using an avian model, Lanyon and colleagues demonstrated that the osteogenic response is maximized by just a few loading cycles when the loading forces are of high magnitude, applied at a fast rate, and represent a unique stimulus to the bone.[94,114-116] It is likely that the magnitude of the peak loading forces acting on specific regions of the skeleton is the major determinant of whether that region will undergo remodeling in response to an exercise program. Telemetry data from patients fitted with instrumented hip prostheses indicate that peak joint forces are 2.8 to 4.8 times body weight during walking at slow to moderate speeds (0.5 to 3 mph). Fast walking, jogging, and going up and down stairs all generate higher peak hip joint forces, with the upper limit being approximately 6 times body weight.[12,13,31,82] Although telemetry data are not available from patients performing resistance types of exercises, it has been estimated that compressive forces at the knee during a squat exercise can be as high as 6 times body weight.[55] Thus, it appears that both endurance, e.g., jogging, stair climbing, and resistance, e.g., weight lifting, types of exercises can introduce forces to the skeleton that are of relatively high magnitude.

Several studies have now shown that bone mass can be increased, even in older postmenopausal women, in response to exercise training. Increases of 1% to 5% in total body, lumbar spine, and proximal femur bone mineral density (BMD) have been reported in older women and men.[69,74,79,85,88,91,105] While this magnitude of increase may seem small, it must be considered in the context that the usual rate of bone mineral loss is ~0.5% to 1% per year. Endurance-exercise, e.g., walking, jogging, stair stepping, and resistance-exercise, e.g., weight lifting, training programs have been shown to induce similar increases in BMD of the total body and lumbar spine.[74,128] Weight-bearing–endurance exercise training, but not resistance training,[69,74,85] has also been shown to be effective in increasing bone mineral content of the neck region of the proximal femur, which is a clinically important site because of the morbidity and mortality associated with hip fractures. While this finding might suggest that weight-bearing exercise is more effective in preventing osteoporotic fractures, some adaptations that are specific to resistance training, namely the increase in muscle mass and strength, may be important not only in preventing osteoporotic fractures by reducing the risk for falls,[91] but also in preventing the muscle atrophy that contributes to the decline in functional independence and overall health with advancing age.[42]

It should be noted that not all studies have found beneficial effects of exercise on bone mass. In fact, some have shown that the rate of bone mineral loss is the same, or even greater, in exercisers as compared with nonexercisers.[24,109] In general, studies that have demonstrated favorable effects of exercise on bone have used exercises that exert loading forces on the skeleton that are of relatively high magnitude. The importance of the magnitude of the loading forces was demonstrated in humans by Kerr and colleagues, who found that bone mass increased in older women in response to high intensity, but not moderate intensity, resistance training.[69] Importantly, even though moderate intensity exercise may not induce increases in bone mass, it does appear that a physically active life-style, in combination with appropriate nutrition, may help to at least slow the rate of bone loss.[131,136]

Estrogen deficiency in postmenopausal women causes an acceleration in the rate of bone mineral loss. Currently, there is no evidence that even vigorous exercise can prevent the menopause-related decline in bone mass in women. Indeed, the importance of the role of female sex hormones in protecting the skeleton is apparent even in young women. Amenorrheic female athletes typically have lower bone mineral density than their eumenorrheic counterparts, even at skeletal sites subjected to high-impact loading during exercise.[129,130] In postmenopausal women, it has been demonstrated that there are independent and additive effects of estrogen and exercise on bone mineral density at some clinically relevant skeletal sites.[73,79,93] Importantly, estrogen also appears to preserve exercise-induced increases in bone mass when exercise is reduced or discontinued.[29,73]

ENDURANCE EXERCISE FOR OLDER ADULTS

Exercise prescription for older adults is challenging because often there are factors that may limit activity or narrow the range of possibilities for exercise. Factors to consider include, but are not limited to, heart disease, medications that alter heart rate or blood pressure responses to exercise, severe osteoarthritis, lung disease, osteoporosis, postural deformity, diabetes, obesity, painful or insensitive feet, claudication, and incontinence. Taking all these factors into consideration and designing a program that is adequately vigorous yet enjoyable, or at least tolerable, can be very challenging.

By definition, endurance exercise will stress the cardiovascular system, resulting in an increase in HR and blood pressure (BP). Selecting the activities appropriate for an individual is based in large measure on initial fitness level and orthopedic limitations. For those who are unfit, with low $\dot{V}O_2$max values, e.g., less than 18 mL/min/kg, even slow walking may raise HR to near maximal levels. Men and women with higher $\dot{V}O_2$max values, without musculoskeletal or other impairments, may be able to walk briskly, bicycle, or even jog.

For developing and maintaining cardiovascular fitness, the American College of Sports Medicine (ACSM) recommends that healthy adults exercise 3 to 5 days/week, for 20 to 60 minutes/day, at an intensity of 50% to 85% of $\dot{V}O_2$max (Table 15-1[104]).[2] If HR is used to monitor exercise intensity, the corresponding levels would be either 50% to 85% of HR reserve or 60% to 90% of maximal HR. Because the estimation of maximal HR may not closely approximate an individual's true maximal HR, the Borg scale (Table 15-2[17]) should be used as an adjunct to determine the appropriateness of the exercise intensity.[92] This instrument is a simple way of having someone provide a rating of perceived exertion (RPE) during exercise. Exercise that requires 50% to 85% of $\dot{V}O_2$max is typically associated with a score of 12 to 16 on the RPE scale.

For all components of the exercise prescription, a range of values is provided to accommodate people of varying fitness levels. Thus, someone who is deconditioned should start with the low end of the recommended ranges for frequency, duration, and intensity of exercise. To reduce the likelihood

TABLE 15-1
RELATIONSHIPS AMONG METHODS OF QUANTIFYING EXERCISE INTENSITY DURING ENDURANCE EXERCISE

RELATIVE INTENSITY (%)				
HRMAX	$\dot{V}O_2$MAX	HR RESERVE	RATING OF PERCEIVED EXERTION	CLASSIFICATION OF INTENSITY
<35%	<30%	<30%	<10	Very light
35%-59%	30%-49%	30%-49%	10-11	Light
60%-79%	50%-74%	50%-74%	12-13	Somewhat hard
80%-89%	75%-84%	75%-84%	14-16	Hard
>89%	>84%	>84%	>16	Very hard

Adapted from Pollock ML, Wilmore JH: *Exercise in Health and Disease: Evaluation and Prescription for Prevention and Rehabilitation*, 2nd ed. Philadelphia, WB Saunders, 1990.

TABLE 15-2

ORIGINAL AND REVISED SCALES FOR RATINGS
OF PERCEIVED EXERTION (RPE)

ORIGINAL SCALE		REVISED SCALE	
6		0	Nothing at all
7	Very, very light	0.5	Very, very weak
8		1	Very weak
9	Very light	2	Weak
10		3	Moderate
11	Fairly light	4	Somewhat strong
12		5	Strong
13	Somewhat hard	6	
14		7	Very strong
15	Hard	8	
16		9	Very, very strong
17	Very hard	10	
18		>10	Maximal
19	Very, very hard		
20			

From Borg GAV: Psychophysical bases of perceived exertion. *Med Sci Sports* 1982; 14:377-381.

of injury or orthopedic discomfort, it is recommended that increases in exercise volume be made initially by increasing frequency and/or duration.[68] When predetermined goals for frequency and duration, e.g., 45 min/day, 5 days/week, are reached, intensity of exercise can be gradually increased. Perhaps the greatest difference in prescribing exercise for older people, as compared with young people, is that it takes longer for adaptations to occur. Whereas a 20-year-old may increase $\dot{V}O_2$max by 25% after 12 weeks of endurance exercise training, a 60-year-old may require 36 weeks of training to achieve a 25% gain.

The ACSM guidelines for prescribing exercise intensity are not age-specific. However, it has been shown that using the HR reserve method to prescribe exercise intensity in 60- to 75-year-old women and men will result in the exercise being performed at a higher-than-expected percentage of $\dot{V}O_2$max.[81,98] It is therefore recommended that target HR during exercise be prescribed as a percentage of maximal HR and that RPE values be used to verify the appropriateness of the exercise intensity.[81]

The mode of exercise that is appropriate for an endurance exercise training program is any activity that uses large muscle groups, can be maintained continuously, and is rhythmical and aerobic in nature. Such activities include walking, bicycling, hiking, dancing, running, rowing, stair climbing, cross-country skiing, swimming, and skating. For older adults in particular, an activity program with multiple forms of endurance exercise is less likely to cause muscle and joint overuse and fatigue than a program that features only one activity, particularly when exercise is being performed 5 or more times per week (M. Brown and colleagues, unpublished observations). Also, warm-up and cool-down periods seem to be important to keep muscle strain to a minimum and to maintain flexibility. One exercise session of 60 minutes duration may include a warm-up, brisk walking, riding a stationary cycle ergometer, and rowing at an appropriate HR and RPE for each activity, and a cool-down.

Alternating days of reduced or less-intense activity with days of rigorous activity may also decrease the risk of injury and allow an adequate recovery.[101] For example, a 45-minute run may be performed Monday, Wednesday, and Friday, with swimming or walking performed on Tuesday and Thursday. All exercisers, regardless of age, need adequate rest cycles, which should be incorporated into a fitness program. In general, the older the individual, the longer the period of recovery from an intense exercise bout.

Walking is a popular form of exercise for women and men of all ages, particularly older adults. If this form of activity is prescribed, attention to proper footwear is important. Name-brand walking shoes may provide adequate comfort for most people, but if feet are unusually wide, if foot deformities are present, or if the plantar fat pad is diminished in thickness, a running shoe may be more comfortable. There is more impact absorption built into a running shoe than a walking shoe. For the runner, a proper running shoe is imperative. A physical therapy evaluation of the foot can help determine whether the individual should look for specific features in a shoe, such as a straight, semi-curved, or curved last, or rigid hindfoot control.

An examination and evaluation by a physical therapist are also highly recommended to identify postural abnormalities or orthopedic conditions that might predispose a person toward injury or pain. For example, if a long history of knee arthritis is present and there is obvious joint impairment, a program of swimming or other form of activity that minimizes stress on the knees should be suggested. Components of the examination and evaluation are covered elsewhere in this text. Many of these evaluation tools should be used for determining the mode of activity and the duration and frequency of exercise that are appropriate for the individual.

Another consideration in prescribing exercise for older adults, particularly women, is that they may experience urinary stress incontinence during some forms of exercise. If stress incontinence is present, appropriate strengthening exercises may help. Prescribing endurance exercise that does not exacerbate the problem will likely enhance adherence to the exercise program. Generally, non-weight–bearing exercise such as bicycling, rowing, and swimming will be more successful than loading activities, e.g., jogging, aerobics, that may cause fear of an accident.

Heart disease is not a contraindication to exercise in most instances, as exercise is a treatment for ischemic heart disease. Stress testing will reveal the presence of heart disease and provide guidelines on the degree to which the cardiovascular system can be stressed. Physician input is imperative, providing information on target HR or BP responses that are safe yet adequately challenging. Patients with heart disease must be fully informed of the danger signs—e.g., shortness of breath, profuse sweating, lightheadedness—and be able to monitor their HR. If the exercise program is of high intensity or the patient is considered high risk, it may be recommended that a physician be present or nearby and on call.

Unless a physician feels endurance training is unsafe, patients with heart disease generally can exercise rigorously, and they often improve cardiovascular fitness significantly.[38,39]

Age, per se, is not a contraindication to endurance exercise. Advancing age will limit the choices for endurance training, given the decline in $\dot{V}O_2$max that occurs with each successive decade. A wide range of possibilities, e.g., jogging, dancing, cycling, cross-country skiing, and hiking, exist for the healthy "young-old" adult. Musculoskeletal complaints become more commonplace with advancing age, and fewer individuals are capable of activities as rigorous as jogging. Age, however, is but one factor that determines the choice of endurance exercise.

To summarize, selection of an exercise program to enhance aerobic capacity is based primarily on level of fitness as determined by a treadmill or other test to determine $\dot{V}O_2$max. Other factors such as strength, flexibility, postural deviations, painful joints, and stress incontinence, as revealed by evaluation, also must be considered in the design of an exercise program. Finally, the patient's desire for a particular form of activity needs to be considered carefully and seriously. It should be borne in mind that women and men aged 90 years or older have scaled some of the major mountains in the world and completed marathons, and that desire can result in remarkable achievements at any age. The program chosen should be challenging yet prudent, reasonable, and, above all, safe.

ENDURANCE EXERCISE FOR THE VERY OLD

It is commonly believed that, in the absence of disease, the physical frailty of very old age is due in large measure to the loss of muscle mass and strength, a condition that has been referred to as *sarcopenia*.[42] Perhaps it is for this reason that studies of the physiological adaptations to exercise in the very old have focused on resistance exercise.[43,44] Low aerobic power is not typically thought of as a determinant of frailty. Yet maximal attainable $\dot{V}O_2$ values for women in their 80s average approximately 14 mL/min/kg.[65] For these women, walking fast enough to cross a street before the traffic light turns red—i.e., 3 mph or, 80 m/min—is extremely demanding, requiring about 85% of their maximal aerobic capacity. In elderly women and men, objective measures of functional capacity[49,107] are inversely related to maximal attainable $\dot{V}O_2$, suggesting that low-aerobic power is either a cause or a consequence of physical frailty (W. Kohrt and colleagues, unpublished observations). In either case, exercise programs for the very old should incorporate both endurance and resistance components, as both are likely to have beneficial effects on the performance of instrumental and advanced activities of daily living.

SAFETY CONSIDERATIONS

Before exercise can be prescribed for an older adult, it must be determined that the person can exercise safely. Although endurance exercise training is a form of treatment for ischemic heart disease and hypertension, prescribing exercise without prior knowledge of the presence or extent of a disease can result in tragic outcomes. The American College of Sports Medicine provides recommendations for determining when a diagnostic medical examination and exercise test should be performed before an exercise program is begun and when a physician should be present for the exercise test (Table 15-3).[3] The need for a stress test is based on the gender and age of the patient, whether he/she will be performing

TABLE 15-3
AMERICAN COLLEGE OF SPORTS MEDICINE'S EXERCISE TESTING AND PRESCRIPTION GUIDELINES

Medical Examination and Clinical Exercise Test Recommended Before:

	APPARENTLY HEALTHY		INCREASED RISK[a]		KNOWN DISEASE[b]
	YOUNGER[c]	OLDER	NO SYMPTOMS	SYMPTOMS	
Moderate exercise[d]	No[e]	No	No	Yes	Yes
Vigorous exercise[f]	No	Yes[g]	Yes	Yes	Yes

Physician Supervision Recommended During Exercise Test:

	APPARENTLY HEALTHY		INCREASED RISK[a]		KNOWN DISEASE[b]
	YOUNGER[c]	OLDER	NO SYMPTOMS	SYMPTOMS	
Submaximal testing	No[e]	No	No	Yes	Yes
Maximal testing	No	Yes[g]	Yes	Yes	Yes

[a] Persons with two or more risk factors or one or more signs or symptoms.
[b] Persons with known cardiac, pulmonary, or metabolic disease.
[c] Younger implies ≤40 years for men, ≤50 years for women.
[d] Moderate exercise as defined by an intensity of 40% to 60% $\dot{V}O_2$max; if intensity is uncertain, moderate exercise intensity may alternately be defined as an intensity well within the individual's current capacity, one which can be comfortably sustained for a prolonged period of time, i.e., 60 minutes, which has a gradual initiation and progression, and is generally noncompetitive.
[e] A "No" response means that an item is deemed "not necessary."
The "No" response does **not** mean that the item should not be done.
[f] Vigorous exercise is defined by an exercise intensity >60% $\dot{V}O_2$max; if intensity is uncertain, vigorous exercise may alternately be defined as exercise intense enough to represent a substantial cardiorespiratory challenge or if it results in fatigue within 20 minutes.
[g] A "Yes" response means that an item is recommended. For physician supervision, this suggests that a physician is in close proximity and readily available should there be an emergent need.
From American College of Sports Medicine: *Guidelines for Exercise Testing and Prescription,* ed 5. Baltimore, Williams & Wilkins, 1995.

TABLE 15-4
RISK FACTORS FOR CORONARY ARTERY DISEASE

POSITIVE RISK FACTORS	CRITERIA
Age	Men >45 yr; women >55 yr or premature menopause without estrogen replacement therapy
Family history	Myocardial infarction or sudden death before 55 yr of age in father or other male first-degree relative or before 65 yr of age in mother or other first-degree female relative
Current cigarette smoking	
Hypertension	Blood pressure ≥140/90 mm Hg, confirmed by measurements on at least 2 separate occasions; or person is taking anti-hypertensive medication
Hypercholesterolemia	Total serum cholesterol >200 mg/dL (5.2 mmol/L) or HDL cholesterol
Diabetes mellitus	Persons with insulin-dependent diabetes mellitus (IDDM) who are >30 yr of age or have had IDDM for >15 yr; persons with non-insulin–dependent diabetes mellitus who are >35 yr of age should be classified as patients with disease
Physical inactivity	Persons comprising the least active 25% of the population, as defined by the combination of sedentary jobs involving sitting for a large part of the day and no regular exercise or active recreational pursuits
NEGATIVE RISK FACTOR	**CRITERIA**
High serum HDL cholesterol	>60 mg/dL (1.6 mmol/L)

NOTE: It is common to sum risk factors in making clinical judgements. If HDL is high, subtract one risk factor from the sum of positive risk factors, since high HDL decreases CAD risk.
From American College of Sports Medicine: *Guidelines for Exercise Testing and Prescription,* ed 5. Baltimore, Williams & Wilkins, 1995.

moderate or vigorous exercise, and the risk for or presence of heart disease. The purposes of a stress exercise test are to (1) evaluate risk level, (2) obtain HR and BP (and $\dot{V}O_2$, if available) data for prescribing exercise, and (3) provide baseline and follow-up data that facilitate evaluation of progress.

If moderate intensity exercise, defined as 40% to 60% of $\dot{V}O_2$max, is to be performed, it is not necessary for women and men to undergo a stress exercise test unless they have been diagnosed with cardiac, pulmonary, or metabolic disease or unless they have signs or symptoms of disease (Table 15-4). If vigorous exercise, defined as greater than 60% of $\dot{V}O_2$max, is to be performed, stress tests should be conducted before an exercise program is initiated in apparently healthy women older than 50 years and men older than 40 years and in women and men of any age who have two or more risk factors (Box 15-1) or signs or symptoms of disease. A physician should be present during a stress exercise test whenever the patient has known disease or signs or symptoms of disease and when maximal tests to exhaustion are performed in people with two or more risk factors and in apparently healthy older women (older than 50 years) and men (older than 40 years) (see Table 15-3). In all cases, the personnel administering an exercise test must be fully aware of absolute and relative contraindications to exercise testing and the absolute and relative indications for stopping an exercise test.[3]

Whether an exercise test should be maximal or submaximal depends on factors such as the reason for the test, the health status of the patient, and the availability of equipment and trained personnel. Maximal tests with the assessment of $\dot{V}O_2$max are typically performed only in certain research or clinical settings. For patients who do not require a stress test with monitoring of the electrocardiogram for diagnostic purposes, a submaximal test with assessment of HR and BP can provide very useful information for prescribing exercise intensity. Such a test typically consists of three submaximal ex-

---

BOX 15-1
MAJOR SYMPTOMS OR SIGNS SUGGESTIVE OF CARDIOPULMONARY DISEASE

1. Pain, discomfort (or other anginal equivalent) in the chest, neck, jaws, or other areas that may be ischemic in nature
2. Shortness of breath at rest or with mild exertion
3. Dizziness or syncope
4. Orthopnea or paroxysmal nocturnal dyspnea
5. Ankle edema
6. Palpitations or tachycardia
7. Intermittent claudication
8. Known heart murmur
9. Unusual fatigue or shortness of breath with usual activities

From American College of Sports Medicine: *Guidelines for Exercise Testing and Prescription,* ed 5. Baltimore, Williams & Wilkins, 1995.

ercise stages of progressively increasing intensity, e.g., walking at 2, 3, and 4 mph or cycling at 50, 75, and 100 W, with each stage lasting at least 3 min in duration, and with HR and BP assessed at the end of each stage. As shown in Fig. 15-1, the HR data are plotted against exercise intensity, or estimated $\dot{V}O_2$; the line can be extrapolated out to the age-predicted maximal HR to derive an estimate of $\dot{V}O_2$max. Equations are available to predict the energy cost, i.e., $\dot{V}O_2$, during submaximal walking, running, cycling, and stepping.[3]

Although the treadmill is the modality of choice for exercise stress tests, some older adults may not be able to walk on a treadmill because they are limited by musculoskeletal impairments, balance problems, fear, incoordination, lightheadedness, or pain. An alternative modality for testing for these individuals is the cycle ergometer, which has the advantages of being weight supporting while allowing the subject to hold on to the handlebars. There is also a greater sense

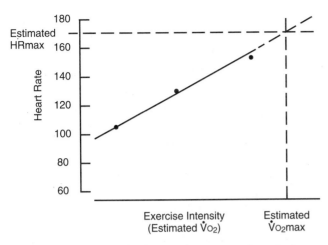

FIG. 15-1 The relationship between heart rate and exercise intensity measured during submaximal exercise bouts. Exercise intensity can be expressed in units specific to the activity (e.g., walking speed or cycling resistance) or as an estimate of the energy cost of the exercise (i.e., V̇O₂).

_____

of safety knowing that the test can be terminated by the participant, rather than the examiner. Cycle ergometer testing is not indicated if a person has quadriceps weakness or suffers from leg pain, particularly with exertion.

If exercise equipment is not available, an alternative method of evaluating fitness is the One-Mile Walk Test.[72] The patient walks continuously at a self-chosen brisk pace that is perceived as appropriate for the distance required. For the final quarter of a mile, the time required to cover this distance and the heart rate at the end are recorded. V̇O₂max is estimated using the following equation:

$$\dot{V}O_2max = 6.9652 + (0.0091 \times wt) - (0.0257 \times age) + (0.5955 \times gender) - (0.2240 \times T1) - (0.0115 \times HR)^*$$

Advantages of this form of testing include lack of need for equipment, performing an activity most people can do, and ease of administration. Disadvantages are that not many old-old adults can walk that far, people with dizziness or impaired balance may be at risk for falling, and fatigue may overcome the participant before the end of the test.

The 6-minute walk test[22,50] is another inexpensive and easy-to-perform evaluative procedure, originally developed for patients with pulmonary disease, that can be done with just a stopwatch and a walkway of reasonable length. A resting HR is obtained before administration of the test. The stopwatch is started as the patient begins to walk at the fastest self-selected pace that can be maintained for 6 minutes. If a patient needs to slow down or rest during the 6-minute test, he/she is permitted to do so, as this will be reflected in less distance being covered. HR is measured again immediately after the test, the distance walked is recorded,

and patients are asked to rate their level of perceived exertion (see Table 15-2). The 6-minute walk test is a simple way to assess functional capacity and changes in functional capacity in response to therapy, but it does not provide quantitative information about aerobic power.

The chair step test[127] was developed to accommodate the older, frail adult who has limited muscle strength and very low V̇O₂max (less than 10 mL/kg/min) and may be unsafe on a treadmill. A chair, metronome, stopwatch, and adjustable bar are all that are required for the test. Subjects are positioned comfortably in a chair and, to the beat of a metronome, are asked to place a foot on the bar, which is positioned 6 inches above the ground. Alternate stepping at a rate of one step/second is performed for 3 minutes, at which time the bar is raised to 12 inches and the test is repeated for another 3 minutes. The third stage is alternate "stepping" to a bar raised to 18 inches. The fourth stage is a repeat of the third stage, except the arms are raised overhead each time a foot is raised to the bar. HR is recorded at the end of each exercise stage.

Safety of the participant must be the first and foremost concern in conducting an exercise test and in prescribing exercise for the older adult. If appropriate precautions are taken, even very old women and men can engage in endurance exercise training that can lead to improvements in health status, functional capacity, and quality of life.

EXERCISE AND INJURY

When older women and men who have been relatively sedentary for many years start a low-intensity exercise program, as many as 20% may develop some form of orthopedic discomfort.[19] Conservative measures—cessation of the activity for a day or two, icing, elastic wrapping, modification of the activity, nonsteroidal anti-inflammatory drugs—are usually successful in alleviating the discomfort. High-intensity training, on the other hand, is likely to induce a painful episode in the majority of participants, perhaps as many as 75%.[19] The majority of painful episodes involve nonspecific joint pain, probably of osteoarthritic origin, typically at the knee or foot-ankle complex. Again, conservative measures can be used to successfully manage the majority of the problems. Some form of musculoskeletal discomfort should be expected when older adults initiate endurance training. Informing patients of the likelihood that they may experience such discomforts may help to alleviate their concern and promote adherence to exercise. Additionally, if physical therapy intervention is provided immediately, fears are allayed and small, painful episodes do not progress to serious injuries. Thus, older adults should understand that endurance training will probably result in some form of musculoskeletal discomfort and that it should not be ignored when it occurs.

Should the high incidence of musculoskeletal discomfort in older adults be a contraindication to endurance exercise training? Absolutely not, since the numerous potential ben-

_____

*wt = body weight in pounds; age is measured in years; gender = 0 for women, 1 for men; T1 = the time in minutes to complete the final 0.25 miles; HR = the heart rate measured at the end of the test.

efits to health and functional capacity far outweigh the risks associated with the incidental and usually transient problems associated with increased activity. Exercise should be part of the daily routine for all adults, regardless of age.

Case Studies

The following three case studies detail the exercise regimens of individuals from the seventh, eighth, and ninth decades of life. This large age span was chosen to highlight some of the considerations and activities that tend to change with advancing age. Probably the most important consideration is the decline in $\dot{V}O_2$max normally seen with advancing age, i.e., activities that have a modest impact on the cardiovascular system at 70 years of age may represent a significant cardiovascular challenge at the age of 90 years. For example, given the decline in $\dot{V}O_2$max that occurs with aging, the rate of energy expenditure during walking 3 mph on a level surface would be approximately 45% of $\dot{V}O_2$max for a 60-year-old woman but 85% of $\dot{V}O_2$max for an 80-year-old woman. Instrumental and advanced activities of daily living may be a sufficient aerobic stimulus for very deconditioned elderly people, particularly women.

Celeste C (age, 63 years)

This young older woman had a history of not engaging in regular exercise but had been physically active as a result of rearing 12 children. Motivation to exercise consisted of "knowing that she should" and fear of becoming like her 83-year-old mother who was now in a nursing home. After physician clearance for aerobic exercise, Celeste came in for a physical therapy evaluation, which consisted of assessments of lower-extremity strength, range of motion, posture, balance, and $\dot{V}O_2$max. Testing revealed the following: adequate strength and range with the exception of hip flexor tightness (10 degrees bilaterally), ankle dorsiflexion range (0 degrees left, 5 degrees right), minimal balance trouble, and no functional ADL or IADL compromise. Problems identified that needed to be considered in exercise design were the presence of stress incontinence and significant genu varum. $\dot{V}O_2$max was 22 mL/min/kg, and maximal HR was 156 bpm.

Celeste expressed interest in a walking program but admitted that her knees hurt when she walked for extended periods. A walking program was developed with the caveat that if her knees became painful with exercise, an alternate exercise method would be necessary. Initially, exercise was prescribed at a HR of 101 to 117 bpm—i.e., 65% to 75% of maximal HR—with the intent of Celeste progressing gradually to performing exercise at a HR of 125 to 133 bpm—i.e., 80% to 85% of maximal HR. Celeste began a walking exercise program that initially consisted of a 30-minute walk at a speed that brought her HR into the desired range. Her neighborhood was hilly and it was not difficult for her to

reach this HR goal, even at a preferred walking pace. Celeste found, however, that after 0.5 miles, her knees were aching and that the ache would persist for several hours after cessation of exercise. After 1 month of walking, knee pain had not improved and an alternative strategy for exercise was discussed. Exercise equipment in the home consisted of a treadmill and exercise cycle. Celeste initially tried the exercise cycle and found this mode of activity boring after 10 minutes, but a reasonable HR response was possible. Treadmill walking at 3 mph was well-tolerated, but an adequate HR response was possible only if the incline was increased to 5%. Again, Celeste found the treadmill uninspiring but was able to perform ~45 total minutes of activity if warm-up exercises were performed initially and the aerobic portion of activity alternated between cycling and treadmill walking. Self-discipline was enhanced when the stationary cycle was set up to permit reading while cycling and a television was placed in front of the treadmill.

Once a training effect began to take place, it was necessary to raise the treadmill grade. The steeper incline resulted in a shorter stride length, which markedly reduced exercise-related knee pain. These forms of activity also reduced the potential for exercise-induced incontinence, which further enhanced compliance, and weather was no longer a consideration. The final program consisted of warm-up stretching exercises, 10 minutes of cycling at 400 kgm/min, 10 minutes of treadmill walking up a 10-degree incline, another 10 minutes each of cycling and walking, and a series of cool-down stretches. On alternate days, the aerobic component of the exercise program consisted of 10 minutes of walking, 10 minutes of cycling, and 10 minutes of walking.

Mabel E (age, 71 years)

This retired bookkeeper was interested in joining some of her friends who gathered three mornings a week at a local indoor shopping center to walk. The social nature of the activity was probably the most powerful motivator, as breakfast usually followed the mall walking. An additional motivation for exercise, in conjunction with the social stimulation, was that Mabel's spouse had died and she was living alone. Mabel had noticed that she became breathless rather quickly and thought that walking might improve her "wind" and ability to accomplish her chores. She was cleared for exercise by her physician, and physical therapy examination did not reveal any musculoskeletal abnormalities or other physical problems that were a source of concern.

A graded treadmill exercise test revealed that Mabel had an estimated $\dot{V}O_2$max of 17 mL/min/kg, a value somewhat lower than expected for her age (about 20 mL/min/kg), suggesting that she was quite deconditioned. Her training HR range was determined to be between 92 and 124 bpm, and a mall walking program was designed to elicit a HR that was within this range. During week 1, for example, Mabel was instructed to walk at a "normal," or preferred, gait speed from one department store to another particular store (0.25 mile), at a faster speed from that store to another department store (slightly less than 0.25 mile), and at an even faster speed for the remaining 0.25 mile. HR checks were performed at specified locations along the way. An exercise sheet was provided for Mabel to record her HR responses and subjective perceived exertion. Any orthopedic discomfort was also noted. At the end of the week, the results were discussed with the physical therapist and the prescription changed to accommodate fatigue, HR responses, and any musculoskeletal trouble or other observations. By the end of 2 months (program changed nearly weekly), Mabel could walk from one end of the mall to the other four times (3 miles) at an average pace of 3 mph. HR averaged 112 bpm, and no rest stops were required.

Before the walking program was instituted, Mabel was instructed on what to look for in a decent pair of walking shoes. Her feet were flat, bony, and very narrow, which diminished her options for brand-name selections. After shoe purchase, shoe modifications (molefoam or moleskin) were made by the physical therapist to further raise the arch of the shoe, provide additional cushion, and to keep the heel from pistoning. In addition, Mabel was taught some simple stretching exercises to maintain flexibility. She was also taught how to take her own pulse, how to use the perceived exertion scale, instructed on possible discomforts that might occur, and how to record distances and times on her exercise sheet. The physical therapist made weekly phone calls to check on Mabel's progress, to troubleshoot as able, and to answer questions. During the first 3 months, Mabel made two additional clinic visits to permit a more detailed examination of progress, especially a HR and BP check at actual walking velocities. These visits also included a discussion of walking distances and times, perceived exertion, a range-of-motion check at the hip (hip-flexor tightness) and ankle (dorsiflexion range), and examination of shoes. Independence in exercise was achieved, but Mabel was made aware that she could receive assistance at any time, if required.

Liz F (age, 83 years)

This patient had a long history of osteoarthritis of the knees and hips, hypertension, asthma, glaucoma, and falling. She lived alone in a large apartment complex in which the majority of occupants were pensioners. Liz wanted an exercise program that would improve her walking. She was fearful that a fall would result in injury. She could not cross the street quickly enough to beat the stoplight, and she was exhausted by the time she reached the church where she did volunteer work. Liz had fallen several times on her way to the church and had sustained fractures of the wrist and coccyx.

Treadmill testing (symptom limited) revealed a maximal attainable $\dot{V}O_2$ of 12 mL/min/kg. Dizziness and fatigue were encountered during the stress test, where HR reached 108 bpm and BP rose to 165/95 mm Hg. The patient also felt quite breathless for about 5 minutes after the test.

Physical therapy evaluation revealed lower extremity strength of F+ to good, with deficiencies primarily in the muscles of weight bearing: plantar flexors, quadriceps, and hip abductors and extensors. Standing balance was diminished. Liz could accomplish only two of six stages on the sharpened Romberg, was completely unable to stand on one leg, and required assistance with weight-shifting activities. Liz used a cane for all walking activities outside and inside the home. Range of motion was within normal limits with the exception of knee flexion, which was 110 degrees, and ankle dorsiflexion, which was 0. The patient was able to dress herself and take care of the easier day-to-day chores. She had help with grocery shopping, cleaning, and laundry. She could not get out of the tub, get up off the floor, step up more than a 6-inch stair, or descend/ascend steps without a railing.

For the first 3 weeks, training consisted of relatively easy chair exercises to enhance strength and challenge balance while sitting or while standing and holding on to the arm of the chair. A walking program was initiated that started with a distance of 25 feet. Liz stood from a chair, walked 25 feet, rested a few seconds, and then returned to the chair while walking at a faster-than-normal pace. Walking was done next to a wall in the apartment complex so that Liz could hold her cane with one hand and use the wall for balance as necessary. For the first few weeks, chair exercise for 20 minutes and three to four repetitions of the 50-foot walk were all that she could tolerate. After 1 month, she could walk 50 feet without resting and at a slightly faster pace four times. After 2 months, Liz walked 75 feet briskly, then normally, and then again briskly. Ultimately the patient progressed to walking briskly around the entire apartment complex, a distance of 220 feet, without resting and at a faster-than-normal pace. Walking on carpeted surfaces and up and down stairs would be added to the program in time. Liz was able to walk further without undue fatigue a little more quickly, with better balance, but still could not get across the street before the light turns green—the ultimate goal of the program.

These case histories exemplify typical real-life situations in which patients are interested in exercise but do not know how to begin a safe and effective program, have some physical difficulties to accommodate, and have varying levels of ability. Exercise prescription was successful for each of these individuals because programs were tailored to their needs, physical capabilities, and desires. All these individuals made significant gains in fitness, and the improvements resulted in enhanced functional capacity.

All three of the case histories presented were those of women because women are more likely than men to exhibit functional decline and, thus the need for exercise. Using examples from the same gender also permitted illustration of the decline in $\dot{V}O_2$max values that is typical for deconditioned women in this age range. Physical activities that are traditionally regarded as aerobic exercises were appropriate for the first patient since she had an adequate aerobic capacity. The last patient was so deconditioned that many activities of daily living represented aerobic exercise. Tailoring exercises appropriate to level of fitness is an important consideration in endurance training.

Summary

Although cardiovascular functional capacity declines with aging, even in people who remain physically active, a sedentary life-style markedly accelerates the rate of decline. Additionally, sedentary behavior promotes undesirable changes in body composition, particularly increased abdominal adiposity, that further compromise functional capacity and health. Ideally, age-related changes in fitness and functional capacity are minimized if a person remains physically active over the course of a lifetime.

Importantly, however, even older adults who have been sedentary for many years retain the ability to improve their functional capacity through endurance exercise training. Yet many older people are hesitant to start exercising because they don't know what type or how much exercise they should do or whether it is safe for them. Exercise can raise concern or even fear in the older person who has led a sedentary life, because he/she may be unaccustomed to the "usual discomforts" of exercise—shortness of breath, increased heart rate, sweating—that might be perceived as, and sometimes are, indicators of cardiovascular problems. Thus, it is important that people in a position to prescribe exercise for older adults, such as physical therapists, understand the benefits to be gained from endurance exercise training and how to prescribe a safe, yet effective, training program to help the older adult realize those benefits.

Acknowledgments

Unpublished data cited in this chapter were from research by the authors and their colleagues (J.O. Holloszy, A.E. Ehsani, R.J. Spina, E.B. Binder, D.R. Sinacore) at the Washington University Older Americans Independence Center supported by the National Institute on Aging (AG13629).

References

1. Adams GM, DeVries HA: Physiological effects of an exercise training regimen upon women aged 52 to 79. *J Gerontol* 1973; 28:50-55.
2. American College of Sports Medicine: The recommended quantity and quality of exercise for developing and maintaining cardiorespiratory and muscular fitness in healthy adults. *Med Sci Sports Exerc* 1990; 22:265-274.
3. American College of Sports Medicine: *Guidelines for Exercise Testing and Prescription*, ed 5. Baltimore, Williams & Wilkins, 1995.
4. Aniansson A, et al: Muscle morphology, enzymatic activity, and muscle strength in elderly men: A follow-up study. *Muscle Nerve* 1986; 9: 585-591.
5. Astrand P-O, Rodahl K: *Textbook of Work Physiology: Physiological Bases of Exercise.* New York, McGraw-Hill, 1986.
6. Åstrand I: Aerobic work capacity in men and women with special reference to age. *Acta Physiol Scand* 1960; 49(Suppl 169):92.
7. Badenhop DT, et al: Physiological adjustments to higher- and lower-intensity exercise in elders. *Med Sci Sports Exerc* 1983; 15:496-502.
8. Barnard RJ, et al: Role of diet and exercise in the management of hyperinsulinemia and associated atherosclerotic risk factors. *Am J Cardiol* 1992; 69:440-444.
9. Barrett-Connor E, Wingard DL, Criqui MH: Postmenopausal estrogen use and heart disease risk factors in the 1980s. *JAMA* 1989; 261:2095-2100.
10. Barry AJ, et al: The effects of physical conditioning on older individuals. I. Work capacity, circulatory-respiratory function, and work electrocardiogram. *J Gerontol* 1966; 21:182-191.
11. Benestad AM: Trainability of old men. *Acta Med Scand* 1965; 178:321-327.
12. Bergmann G, Graichen F, Rohlmann A: Hip joint loading during walking and running, measured in two patients. *J Biomechanics* 1993; 26:969-990.
13. Bergmann G, Graichen F, Rohlmann A: Is staircase walking a risk for the fixation of hip implants? *J Biomech* 1995; 28:535-553.
14. Binder EF, Birge SJ, Kohrt WM: Effects of endurance exercise and hormone replacement therapy on serum lipids in older women. *J Am Geriatr Soc* 1996; 44:231-236.
15. Björntorp P: Body fat distribution, insulin resistance, and metabolic diseases. *Nutrition* 1997; 13:795-803.
16. Blumenthal JA, et al: Cardiovascular and behavioral effects of aerobic exercise training in healthy older men and women. *J Gerontol* 1989; 44:M147-157.
17. Borg GAV: Psychophysical bases of perceived exertion. *Med Sci Sports* 1982; 14:377-381.
18. Borkan GA, et al: Age changes in body composition revealed by computed tomography. *J Gerontol* 1983; 38:673-677.
19. Brown M: Physical and orthopaedic limitations to exercise in the elderly, in Buckwalter JA, Goldberg VM, Woo SLY (eds): *Musculoskeletal Soft-Tissue Aging: Impact on Mobility.* Rosemont, IL, American Academy of Orthopaedic Surgeons,1992.
20. Brown M, Birge SJ Jr, Kohrt WM: Hormone replacement therapy does not augment gains in muscle strength or fat-free mass in response to weight-bearing exercise. *J Gerontol: Biol Sci* 1997; 52A:B166-B170.
21. Bush TL, et al: Cardiovascular mortality and noncontraceptive use of estrogen in women: Results from the Lipid Research Clinics Program Follow-up Study. *Circulation* 1987; 75:1102-1109.
22. Butland RJ, et al: Two-, six-, and 12-minute walking tests in respiratory disease. *Br Med J* 1982; 284:1607-1608.
23. Campos H, Wilson PWF, Jiménez D et al: Differences in apolipoproteins and low-density lipoprotein subfractions in postmenopausal women on and off estrogen therapy: Results from the Framingham Offspring Study. *Metabolism* 1990; 39:1033-1038.
24. Cavanaugh DJ, Cann CE: Brisk walking does not stop bone loss in postmenopausal women. *Bone* 1988; 9:201-204.
25. Coggan AR, et al: Endurance training decreases plasma glucose turnover and oxidation during moderate-intensity exercise in men. *J Appl Physiol* 1990; 68:990-996.
26. Coggan AR, et al: Skeletal muscle adaptations to endurance training in 60- to 70-year-old men and women. *J Appl Physiol* 1991; 72:1780-1786.
27. Collet P, et al: Effects of 1- and 6-month spaceflight on bone mass and biochemistry in two humans. *Bone* 1997; 20:547-551.
28. Cunningham DA, et al: Exercise training of men at retirement: A clinical trial. *J Gerontol* 1987; 42:17-23.
29. Dalsky GP, et al: Weight-bearing exercise training and lumbar bone mineral content in postmenopausal women. *Ann Int Med* 1988; 108:824-828.
30. Davies CTM: The oxygen transporting system in relation to age. *Clin Sci* 1972; 42:1-13.
31. Davy DT, et al: Telemetric force measurements across the hip after total arthroplasty. *J Bone Joint Surg* 1988; 70:45-50.
32. DeFronzo RA: Glucose intolerance and aging: Evidence for tissue insensitivity to insulin. *Diabetes* 1979; 28:1095-1101.
33. Després J-P, et al: Regional distribution of body fat, plasma lipoproteins, and cardiovascular disease. *Arteriosclerosis* 1990; 10:497-511.
34. Després J-P, et al: Loss of abdominal fat and metabolic response to exercise training in obese women. *Am J Physiol* 1991; 24:E159-E167.
35. DeVries HA: Physiological effects of an exercise training regimen upon men aged 52 to 88. *J Gerontol* 1970; 25:325-336.
36. Drinkwater BL, Horvath SM, Wells CL: Aerobic power in females, ages 10 to 68. *J Gerontol* 1975; 30:385-394.
37. Durnin JV, Womersley J: Body fat assessed from total body density and its estimation from skinfold thickness; measurements on 481 men and women aged from 16 to 72 years. *Br J Nutr* 1974; 32:77-97.

38. Ehsani AA, et al: The effect of left ventricular systolic function on maximal aerobic exercise capacity in asymptomatic patients with coronary artery disease. *Circulation* 1984; 70:552-560.

39. Ehsani AA, et al: Effects of twelve months of intense exercise training on ischemic ST-segment depression in patients with coronary artery disease. *Circulation* 1981; 64:1116-1124.

40. Ehsani AA, et al: Exercise training improves left ventricular systolic function in older men. *Circulation* 1991; 83:96-103.

41. Enzi G, et al: Subcutaneous and visceral fat distribution according to sex, age, and overweight, evaluated by computed tomography. *Am J Clin Nutr* 1986; 44:739-746.

42. Evans WJ: What is sarcopenia? *J Gerontol* 1995; 50A:5-8.

43. Fiatarone MA, et al: High-intensity strength training in nonagenarians. Effects on skeletal muscle. *JAMA* 1990; 263:3029-3034.

44. Fiatarone MA, et al: Exercise training and nutritional supplementation for physical frailty in very elderly people. *N Engl J Med* 1994; 330:1769-1775.

45. Flack JM, Sowers JR: Epidemiologic and clinical aspects of insulin resistance and hyperinsulinemia. *Am J Med* 1991; 91(Suppl 1A):11S-21S.

46. Fleg JL, Lakatta EG: Role of muscle loss in the age-associated reduction in VO$_2$max. *J Appl Physiol* 1988; 65:1147-1151.

47. Gerstenblith G, Lakatta EG, Weisfeldt ML: Age changes in myocardial function and exercise response. *Prog Cardiovasc Dis* 1976; 19:1-21.

48. Grimby G, et al: Morphology and enzymatic capacity in arm and leg muscles in 78-81 year-old men and women. *Acta Physiol Scand* 1982; 115:125-134.

49. Guralnik JM, et al: A short physical performance battery assessing lower extremity function: Association with self-reported disability and prediction of mortality and nursing home admission. *J Gerontol* 1994; 49:M85-M94.

50. Guyatt GH, et al: The 6-minute walk: A new measure of exercise capacity in patients with chronic heart failure. *Can Med Assoc J* 1985; 132:923.

51. Hagberg JM, et al: A hemodynamic comparison of young and older endurance athletes during exercise. *J Appl Physiol* 1985; 58:2041-2046.

52. Hagberg JM, et al: Cardiovascular responses of 70- to 79-yr-old men and women to exercise training. *J Appl Physiol* 1989; 66:2589-2594.

53. Hagberg JM, et al: Effect of exercise training in 60- to 69-year-old persons with essential hypertension. *Am J Cardiol* 1991; 64:348-353.

54. Hagberg JM, et al: Metabolic responses to exercise in young and older athletes and sedentary men. *J Appl Physiol* 1988; 65:900-908.

55. Hattin HC, Pierrynowski MR, Ball KA: Effect of load, cadence, and fatigue on tibio-femoral joint force during a half squat. *Med Sci Sports Exerc* 1989; 21:613-618.

56. Heath GW, et al: Effects of exercise and lack of exercise on glucose tolerance and insulin sensitivity. *J Appl Physiol* 1983; 55:512-517.

57. Heath GW, et al: A physiological comparison of young and older endurance athletes. *J Appl Physiol* 1981; 51:634-640.

58. Hermansen L, Saltin B: Oxygen uptake during maximal treadmill and bicycle exercise. *J Appl Physiol* 1969; 26:31-37.

59. Higginbotham MB, et al: Physiologic basis for the age-related decline in aerobic work capacity. *Am J Cardiol* 1986; 57:1374-1379.

60. Higuchi M, et al: Superoxide dismutase and catalase in skeletal muscle: Adaptive response to exercise. *J Gerontol* 1985; 40:281-286.

61. Holloszy JO, Kohrt WM: Exercise, in Masoro EJ, (ed): *Handbook of Physiology-Aging*, Oxford, University Press, 1995.

62. Holloszy JO, et al: Effects of exercise on glucose tolerance and insulin resistance. *Acta Med Scand Suppl* 1986; 711:55-65.

63. Horvath SM, Borgia JF: Cardiopulmonary gas transport and aging. *Am Rev Respir Dis* 1984; 129(2 Pt 2):S68-S71.

64. Hossack KF, Bruce RA: Maximal cardiac function in sedentary normal men and women: Comparison of age-related changes. *J Appl Physiol* 1982; 53:799-804.

65. Host HH, et al: Indicators of mild to moderate physical frailty in older adults. *Phys Ther* 1996; 76:518.

66. Julius S, et al: Influence of age on the hemodynamic response to exercise. *Circulation* 1967; 36:222-230.

67. Kaijser L, Sachs C: Autonomic cardiovascular responses in old age. *Clin Physiol* 1985; 5:347-357.

68. Kallinen M, Markku A: Aging, physical activity and sports injuries. An overview of common sports injuries in the elderly. *Sports Med* 1995; 20:41-52.

69. Kerr D, et al: Exercise effects on bone mass in postmenopausal women are site-specific and load-dependent. *J Bone Miner Res* 1996; 11: 218-225.

70. King DS, et al: Effects of exercise and lack of exercise on insulin secretion and action in trained subjects. *Am J Physiol* 1988; 254:E537-E542.

71. King DS, et al: Effects of exercise and lack of exercise on insulin sensitivity and responsiveness. *J Appl Physiol* 1988; 64:1942-1946.

72. Kline GM, et al: Estimation of VO$_2$max from a one-mile track walk, gender, age, and body weight. *Med Sci Sports Exerc* 1987; 19:253-259.

73. Kohrt WM, Ehsani AA, Birge SJ Jr: HRT preserves increases in bone mineral density and reductions in body fat after a supervised exercise program. *J Appl Physiol* 1998; 84:1506-1512.

74. Kohrt WM, Ehsani AA, Birge SJ Jr: Effects of exercise involving predominantly either joint-reaction or ground-reaction forces on bone mineral density in older women. *J Bone Miner Res* 12:1253-1261, 1997.

75. Kohrt WM, et al: Insulin resistance in aging is related to abdominal obesity. *Diabetes* 1993; 42:273-281.

76. Kohrt WM, et al: Effects of gender, age, and fitness level on the response of VO$_2$max to training in 60- to 71-year-olds. *J Appl Physiol* 1991; 71:2004-2011.

77. Kohrt WM, et al: Body composition of healthy sedentary and trained, young and older men and women. *Med Sci Sports Exerc* 1992; 24:832-837.

78. Kohrt WM, Obert KA, Holloszy JO: Exercise training improves fat distribution patterns in 60- to 70-yr-old men and women. *J Gerontol* 1992; 47:M99-M105.

79. Kohrt WM, et al: Additive effects of weight-bearing exercise and estrogen on bone mineral density in older women. *J Bone Miner Res* 1995; 10:1303-1311.

80. Kohrt WM, et al: Effects of age, adiposity, and fitness level on plasma catecholamine responses to standing and exercise. *J Appl Physiol* 1993; 75:1828-1835.

81. Kohrt WM, et al: Prescribing exercise intensity for older women. *J Am Geriatr Soc* 1998; 46:1-5.

82. Kotzar GM, et al: Telemeterized in vivo hip joint force data: A report on two patients after total hip surgery. *J Orthop Res* 1991; 9:621-633.

83. LeBlanc AD, et al: Bone mineral loss and recovery after 17 weeks of bed rest. *J Bone Miner Res* 1990; 5:843-850.

84. Leon AS, et al: Leisure-time physical activity levels and risk of coronary heart disease and death. *JAMA* 1987; 258:2388-2395.

85. Lohman T, et al: Effects of resistance training on regional and total bone mineral density in premenopausal women: A randomized prospective study. *J Bone Miner Res* 1995; 10:1015-1024.

86. Mann DL, et al: Effects of age on ventricular performance during graded supine exercise. *Am Heart J* 1986; 111:108-115.

87. Martin WH III, et al: Exercise training enhances leg vasodilatory capacity of 65-year-old men and women. *J Appl Physiol* 1990; 69: 1804-1809.

88. Menkes A, et al: Strength training increases regional bone mineral density and bone remodeling in middle-aged and older men. *J Appl Physiol* 1993; 74:2478-2484.

89. Mikines KJ, et al: Effect of physical exercise on sensitivity and responsiveness to insulin in humans. *Am J Physiol* 1988; 254:E248-E259.

90. Morris JN, et al: Vigorous exercise in leisure-time: Protection against coronary heart disease. *Lancet* 1980; 2:1207-1210.

91. Nelson ME, et al: Effects of high-intensity strength training on multiple risk factors for osteoporotic fractures: A randomized controlled trial. *JAMA* 1994; 272:1909-1914.

92. Noble BJ, et al: A category-ratio perceived exercise scale: Relationship to blood and muscle lactates and heart rate. *Med Sci Sports Exerc* 1983; 15:523-528.

93. Notelovitz M, et al: Estrogen therapy and variable-resistance weight training increase bone mineral in surgically menopausal women. *J Bone Miner Res* 1991; 6:583-590.

94. O'Connor JA, Lanyon LE, MacFie H: The influence of strain rate on adaptive bone remodeling. *J Biomechanics* 1982; 15:767-781.

95. Ogawa T, et al: Effects of aging, sex, and physical training on cardiovascular responses to exercise. *Circulation* 1992; 86:494-503.

96. Paffenbarger RSJ, et al: Physical activity, all-cause mortality and longevity of college alumni. *N Engl J Med* 1986; 314:605-613.

97. Palmer GJ, Ziegler MG, Lake CR: Response of norepinephrine and blood pressure to stress increases with age. *J Gerontol* 1978; 33:482-487.

98. Panton LB, et al: Relative heart rate, heart rate reserve, and V_{O_2} during submaximal exercise in the elderly. *J Gerontol: Biol Sci* 1996; 51A: M165-M171.

99. Parizkova J, et al: Body composition, aerobic capacity, and density of muscle capillaries in young and old men. *J Appl Physiol* 1971; 31:323-325.

100. Peiris AN, et al: Adiposity, fat distribution, and cardiovascular risk. *Ann Int Med* 1989; 110:867-872.

101. Pollock ML, et al: Injuries and adherence to walk/jog and resistance training programs in the elderly. *Med Sci Sports Exerc* 1991; 23:1194-1200.

102. Pollock ML, et al: Effect of age and training on aerobic capacity and body composition of master athletes. *J Appl Physiol* 1987; 62:725-731.

103. Pollock ML, et al: Twenty-year follow-up of aerobic power and body composition of older track athletes. *J Appl Physiol* 1997; 82:1508-1516.

104. Pollock ML, Wilmore JH: *Exercise in Health and Disease: Evaluation and Prescription for Prevention and Rehabilitation,* ed 2. Philadelphia, WB Saunders, 1990.

105. Pruitt LA, Taaffe DR, Marcus R: Effects of a one-year high-intensity versus low-intensity resistance training program on bone mineral density in older women. *J Bone Miner Res* 1995; 10:1788-1795.

106. Reaven GM: Insulin resistance, hyperinsulinemia, and hypertriglyceridemia in the etiology and clinical course of hypertension. *Am J Med* 90(Suppl 2A):7S-12S, 1991.

107. Reuben DB, Siu AL: An objective measure of physical function of elderly outpatients. *J Am Geriatr Soc* 1990; 38:1105-1112.

108. Rivera AM, et al: Physiological factors associated with the lower maximal oxygen consumption of master runners. *J Appl Physiol* 1989; 66:949-954.

109. Rockwell JC, et al: Weight training decreases vertebral bone density in premenopausal women: A prospective study. *J Clin Endocrinol Metab* 1990; 71:988-993.

110. Rodeheffer RJ, et al: Exercise cardiac output is maintained with advancing age in healthy human subjects: Cardiac dilatation and increased stroke volume compensate for diminished heart rate. *Circulation* 1984; 69:203-213.

111. Rogers MA, et al: Effect of 10 days of inactivity on glucose tolerance in master athletes. *J Appl Physiol* 1990; 68:1833-1837.

112. Rogers MA, et al: The effect of 7 years of intense exercise training on patients with coronary artery disease. *J Am Coll Cardiol* 1987;10:321-326.

113. Rogers MA, et al: Improvement in glucose tolerance after one week of exercise in patients with mild NIDDM. *Diabetes Care* 1988; 11:613-618.

114. Rubin CT, Lanyon LE: Regulation of bone formation by applied dynamic loads. *J Bone Joint Surg* 1984; 66-A:397-402.

115. Rubin CT, Lanyon LE: Regulation of bone mass by mechanical strain magnitude. *Calcif Tissue Int* 1985; 37:411-417.

116. Rubin CT, Lanyon LE: Osteoregulatory nature of mechanical stimuli: Function as a determinant for adaptive remodeling in bone. *J Orthop Res* 1987; 5:300-310.

117. Rubin PC, et al: Noradrenaline release and clearance in relation to age and blood pressure in man. *Eur J Clin Invest* 1982; 12:121-125.

118. Saltin B, et al: Physical training in sedentary middle-aged and older men. *Scand J Clin Lab Invest* 1969; 24:323-334.

119. Schocken DD, et al: Physical conditioning and left ventricular performance in the elderly: Assessment by radionuclide angiocardiography. *Am J Cardiol* 1983; 52:359-364.

120. Schwartz RS, et al: The effect of intensive endurance exercise training on body fat distribution in young and older men. *Metabolism* 1991; 40:545-551.

121. Seals DR, et al: Glucose tolerance in young and older athletes and sedentary men. *J Appl Physiol* 1984; 56:1521-1525.

122. Seals DR, et al: Effects of endurance training on glucose tolerance and plasma lipids in older men and women. *JAMA* 1984; 252:645-649.

123. Seals DR, et al: Endurance training in older men and women. I. Cardiovascular response to exercise. *J Appl Physiol* 1984; 57:1024-1029.

124. Seals DR, et al: Enhanced left ventricular performance in endurance trained older men. *Circulation* 1994; 89:198-205.

125. Shephard RJ: Assessment of physical activity and energy needs. *Am J Clin Nutr* 1989; 50(Suppl):1195-1200.

126. Shimokata H, et al: Studies in the distribution of body fat: I. Effects of age, sex, and obesity. *J Gerontol* 1989; 44:M66-M73.

127. Smith EL, Gilligan C: Physical activity prescription for the elderly. *Phys Sports Med* 1983; 11:91-101.

128. Snow-Harter C, et al: Effects of resistance and endurance exercise on bone mineral status of young women: A randomized exercise intervention trial. *J Bone Miner Res* 1992; 7:761-769.

129. Snow-Harter CM: Bone health and prevention of osteoporosis in active and athletic women. *Clin Sports Med* 1994; 13:389-404.

130. Sowers MF, et al: Joint influence of fat and lean body composition compartments on femoral bone mineral density in premenopausal women. *Am J Epidemiol* 1992; 136:257-265.

131. Specker BL: Evidence for an interaction between calcium intake and physical activity on changes in bone mineral density. *J Bone Miner Res* 1996; 11:1539-1544.

132. Spina RJ, et al: Gender-related differences in left ventricular filling dynamics in older subjects after endurance exercise training. *J Gerontol: Biol Sci* 1996; 51:B232-B237.

133. Spina RJ, et al: Differences in cardiovascular adaptations to endurance exercise training between older men and women. *J Appl Physiol* 1993; 75:849-855.

134. Spina RJ, et al: Effect of exercise training on left ventricular performance in older women free of cardiopulmonary disease. *Am J Cardiol* 1993; 71:99-104.

135. Spina RJ, Turner MJ, Ehsani AA: Exercise training enhances cardiac function in response to an afterload stress in older men. *Am J Physiol* 1997; 272(2 Pt 2):H995-H1000.

136. Suleiman S, et al: Effect of calcium intake and physical activity level on bone mass and turnover in healthy, white, postmenopausal women. *Am J Clin Nutr* 1997; 66:937-943.

137. Thomas SG, et al: Determinants of the training response in elderly men. *Med Sci Sports Exerc* 1985; 17:667-672.

138. Wood PD, et al: The effects on plasma lipoproteins of a prudent weight-reducing diet, with or without exercise, in overweight men and women. *N Engl J Med* 1991; 325:461-466.

139. Young JB, et al: Enhanced plasma norepinephrine response to upright posture and oral glucose administration in elderly human subjects. *Metabolism* 1980; 29:532-539.

140. Ziegler MG, Lake CR, Kopin IJ: Plasma noradrenaline increases with age. *Nature* 1976; 261:333-335.

CHAPTER 16

MUSCLE FATIGUE AND IMPAIRED MUSCLE ENDURANCE IN OLDER ADULTS

MARYBETH BROWN, PT, PhD

OUTLINE

INTRODUCTION

Muscle fatigue is such a common complaint from the older deconditioned patient that it causes no surprise when brought to the attention of a physical therapist. Frequently, after a few repetitions of an activity, fatigue is apparent, as evidenced by inability to move the body part through the same range of motion, actual muscle quivering, or shaking of the entire extremity. Therapists commonly indicate "improve endurance" as a goal of intervention, and yet there is not a universally accepted definition of what this goal means. Some therapists who attempt to enhance physical performance through the improvement of muscular endurance often have developed their own approaches to testing and treating fatigue and deficiencies in endurance. Oddly, there has been very little sharing of information in the literature regarding examination, evaluation, and intervention for this ubiquitous problem. Thus, the primary purpose of this chapter is to bring attention to the problem of poor muscular endurance and fatigue in the older adult. It is hoped that this chapter will stimulate clinical research into the development of tests for muscle fatigue and poor endurance and stimulate therapists to examine strategies to treat fatigue and limited muscular endurance.

The terms *endurance* and *fatigue* are often used synonymously, yet from a investigative standpoint, they are not viewed as interchangeable. In this chapter, fatigue is defined as a reduced ability to achieve the same level of force output. An example of fatigue is illustrated by a patient who performs a series of contractions and generates 100% of maximum during the first contraction, 90% of maximum the second contraction, 80% of maximum during the third contraction and so on, to the point of inability to move. Endurance is the ability to sustain a selected force output (usually 50%) for as long a time as possible. Hand grip endurance, for example, is often measured as the duration that 50% of a one-repetition maximum can be maintained. Grip endurance typically lasts 1 to 2 minutes, whereas fatigue may occur within a matter of seconds. Since fatigue is the phenomenon we tend to observe most commonly, the remainder of this discussion is directed primarily toward this problem.

What are the causes of fatigue? In general, fatigue can be the consequence of failure at a number of sites, both central and peripheral. Briefly, fatigue can result from failure in motor unit recruitment and impulse transmission at multiple sites: brain, spinal cord, peripheral nerve. Fatigue can also be the consequence of failure in transmission at the neuromuscular junction or through the transverse tubular system. The excitation process can be diminished substantially by the sarcoplasmic reticulum failing to release adequate calcium. Altered excitation-contraction coupling and energy substrate depletion may play a role, affecting the binding of adenosine triphosphate (ATP) and the attachment of the cross-bridge. Because there are so many potential sites for failure to occur, it is not surprising that fatigue is difficult to characterize, as detailed in the reviews on fatigue by MacLaren and colleagues[12] and Fitts.[4] Regardless of the etiology or site of fatigue, the more important clinical consideration is the recognition and characterization of this frequently encountered phenomenon.

Muscular endurance is related in large measure to the aerobic capacity of muscle, the volume of mitochondria (and hence, aerobic enzymes such as citrate synthase), and fiber type. The higher the proportion of type I fibers, the better the endurance capacity of that muscle. Clearly, the more aerobically trained an individual, the more endurant are those muscles involved in the activity. Thus, a jogger has more endurant quadriceps than a sedentary adult, because training has resulted in increases in mitochondrial volume and aerobic enzyme capacity. Jogging probably has also caused a shift in fiber type distribution (more type IIa fibers than type IIb fibers) toward a more aerobic profile.[1,3,7,9] Muscles involved in endurance or aerobic exercise activity perform better (longer) on endurance tests.

SUSCEPTIBILITY OF OLDER ADULTS TO FATIGUE

Although there are not many studies of fatigue in older adults, particularly those beyond the seventh decade, there is little evidence to suggest that older adults are more susceptible to fatigue than young adults. Lindstrom and colleagues, for example, asked healthy older men and women to perform 100 repeated maximum dynamic knee extensions at 90°/s (degrees/second) using a Cybex II dynamometer.[11] Peak torque was recorded for each contraction. Although maximum voluntary contraction (MVC) was significantly lower in the older men and women, there was no discernible difference in relative muscle force production or fatigue rate between young and old individuals. Similar data have been collected in the laboratory and are presented in Fig. 16-1. These data were collected for 65 men and women between the ages of 60 and 72 years and 25 younger individuals between the ages of 20 and 29 years. The test was done on a Cybex dynamometer at 180°/s. One maximum contraction was performed each second for a total of 60 contractions. The slope of the line in the illustration indicates fatigue and is essentially the same for the young and older adults. "Fatigue" in both instances was approximately 50%. If the concept of "work" is introduced into the equation, clearly older adults are not able to produce as much work (i.e., the area under the curve [see Fig. 16-1]) as young adults. Nonetheless, for the same relative work load, there does not seem to be an age-related penalty.

In one of the few investigations of older adults who were not healthy/normal, fatigue was found to occur more readily. Schwendner and colleagues studied 27 normal older women and 26 women with a history of falling.[17] They had subjects perform maximal concentric knee extensions until the force output fell below 50% of MVC. Time to fatigue was significantly faster in the women with a history of falls as compared with the women of similar age with no history of falls. As observed in other studies, however, the women with a history of no falls did not tire any more quickly than the 29 young women examined whose mean age was 22 years.[13] Strength values were not reported, so it is not known whether the women with a history of falls fatigued more readily because of poorer strength values.

DIFFERENCES IN MUSCLE ENDURANCE BETWEEN YOUNGER AND OLDER ADULTS

Curiously, the evidence to support a decrease in muscular endurance with age is not that strong. A number of studies have been performed that ask subjects to maintain a certain force level (from 5% to 80% of maximum voluntary force) for as long as possible. These studies involve a variety of muscle groups, including the back extensors,[10] finger flexors,[8] and quadriceps.[18] In general, force levels less than approximately 15% of maximum can be maintained indefinitely. As the amount of force required is increased, endurance time decreases rapidly, regardless of the muscle group being tested.[10]

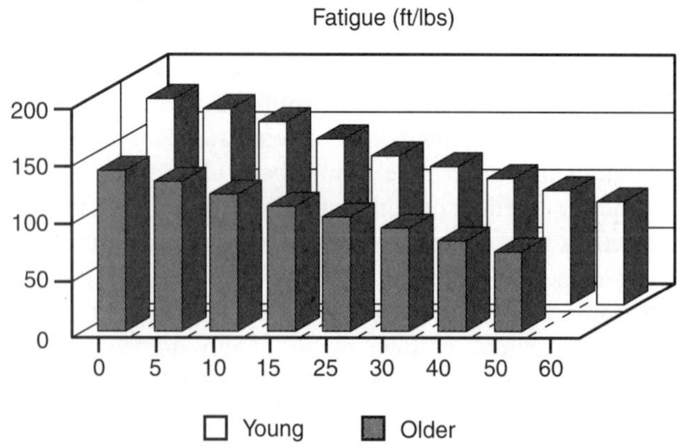

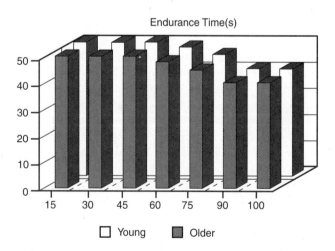

FIG. 16-1   Decline in maximum force (*Y axis*) with 60 contractions (*X axis*). A ~50% decline in quadriceps force generating ability occurred for young and older adults during the 60-second contraction period. The slope of the decline is identical for young and older men and women, suggesting a comparable rate of fatigue.

FIG. 16-2   Grip strength endurance for young and older adults. The decline in grip force does not differ with age. On the *Y axis* is percent grip force, whereas on the *X axis* is time in seconds.

Studies of endurance that have included elders as subjects seem to indicate that the initial starting value for strength is the only likely difference between young and old. When young and older adults are asked to maintain a 50% grip (half of maximum grip strength) for as long as possible, older subjects do as well or even better than young subjects.[8] The ability to maintain 50% of maximum grip strength is depicted in Fig. 16-2. Differences between young and older adults is not apparent. However, the initial starting value for grip strength is not reflected, which is 90 pounds for young adults (men and women combined) and 60 pounds for older adults (60 to 75 years).

FACTORS THAT INFLUENCE FATIGUE

Muscle Strength

Clearly, lack of muscle strength is a major factor contributing to fatigue, and thus the stronger the patient becomes with exercise, the less likely he or she is to experience fatigue. For example, if six dinner plates weigh 10 pounds and an individual is capable of lifting 10 pounds, then 100% of available strength is being used to accomplish the task of lifting those plates. Under these circumstances, the task can be repeated only once before fatigue limits performance. If a patient has the capability of lifting 20 pounds, then placing 10 pounds of plates into a cupboard represents only a 50% challenge. Given such a modest challenge, the lifting task can be repeated multiple times before fatigue becomes a problem. The strategy of reducing the amount of weight to permit multiple repetitions of a task is routinely used in the industry.

Intuitively, humans embrace behaviors that reduce the amount of force required for a particular task, i.e., reduce the potential for fatigue. If strength is limited, a person places less clothing into a suitcase before embarking on a trip. With advancing age, it is not uncommon to see older adults pack more bags of groceries with fewer items, thus reducing the weight of each bag to facilitate placement of the bags into the car. Obviously, lower forces can be sustained longer than high forces, and individuals with little ability to generate force, i.e., those who become easily fatigued, are likely to become patients of physical therapists.

From a rehabilitation standpoint, increasing strength to the highest levels possible will have a positive effect on fatigue. The greater the available strength, the smaller the percentage demand on each muscle group. An interesting example of this is the case of an 82-year-old man who had been weight-lifting for more than 60 years who was tested in the laboratory. Although the amount of weight he could lift had decreased over the years by more than 50%, his lifting capability still was vastly superior to that of men in younger age categories. This man could not comprehend why his peers were having difficulty with fatigue. Even though his strength was diminished, he had far more capability than needed to perform the basic repetitive tasks, e.g., walking and lifting, associated with activities of daily living with ease.

If initial strength values are so low that all tasks become too difficult, fatigue will overwhelm the individual and there is a threat of lost independence. There is a clear association between the loss of lean muscle mass and inability to accomplish routine activities of daily living.[2,15] Thus, increasing strength will have a positive effect on muscle mass and function and will result in the reduction of fatigue. It cannot be overemphasized that the initial starting value for strength is a major determinant in fatigue.

Strength enters into the clinical equation in another capacity as well. Consider that a muscle contraction greater than approximately 15% of maximum constricts the muscle sufficiently to diminish circulation to that muscle.[14] In other words, the muscle becomes anoxic when contractions exceed a certain threshold level, leading to the build-up of waste products that limit performance. Anoxia also impedes the delivery of oxygen and nutrients to a working muscle. Thus, the greater the strength capacity of the muscle, the higher the likelihood of avoiding the constriction of vessels leading to anoxia in a contracting muscle. If a patient's maximum force output of a muscle is 10 pounds and blood vessels are compressed with lifting a 1.5-pound (15% of maximum) load, then this patient is likely to experience fatigue secondary to circulatory constriction—just lifting a large glass of water.

Aerobic Conditioning

Another factor that influences fatigue is the state of aerobic conditioning. Men and women who are conditioned to aerobic exercise fatigue to a lesser extent and recover more quickly than those who are deconditioned. In the laboratory, men and women between the ages of 55 and 84 years participated in a fatigue test. Subjects included 24 master athletes and 24 age-matched controls who were relatively sedentary but healthy individuals. Master athletes typically were runners and cyclists, many of them world class, who participated in the Senior Olympics. The test required each subject to exert 60 maximum contractions of the quadriceps repetitively during 60 seconds. Subjects were seated on a Cybex machine, which was set at a speed of 180°/s, and then were asked to extend the knee maximally each second to the beat of a metronome. Once the fatiguing protocol (which is not a recommended protocol for most older adults) was over, subjects rested for 30 seconds and then were asked to produce a maximum contraction. After 1 minute of rest, subjects were asked to generate another maximum contraction and so forth, until full recovery was obtained (maximum of 5 minutes). Results for these two groups are presented in Table 16-1. Note in particular the athletes' higher starting point, i.e., greater strength values; smaller drop in force with the fatiguing protocol; and rapid rate of recovery. Some of the sedentary subjects had not recovered 100% of initial torque after 5 minutes, which was the end of the test, whereas most of the athletes had full recovery of maximum torque at the end of 1 minute. The percent decline and rapid recovery are reflective of resistance to fatigue and good endurance.

TABLE 16-1
INITIAL AND FINAL QUADRICEPS TORQUE OF ATHLETES AND AGE-MATCHED SEDENTARY CONTROLS[*]

	ATHLETES	SEDENTARY CONTROLS
Initial Torque (ft/lbs)	78±19	69±20[†]
End Torque	52±10	35±8[†]
% Decline	33%	49%[†]
30s recovery	88±11%	79±17%[†]
60s recovery	94±9%	87±15%[†]

[*] Values (means±sd) at 180°/s after a 60-second fatigue protocol.
[†] p<0.05 indicating values for athletes are significantly higher than those for age-matched sedentary controls.

One additional factor that likely influences fatigue is inactivity. Men and women who are sedentary may lose the ability to fully activate their muscles.[5] It is possible that the shakiness observed in a patient who has been on bed rest, for example, reflects disuse rather than fatigue, per se. Regardless, to the patient, it feels as though the arm or leg weighs 6 tons, and the perception of fatigue is very real to that individual.

Lastly, the issue of motivation is outside the scope of this discussion, but very real nonetheless. If a patient is simply unwilling to perform to the best of his/her ability, the lack of motivation may appear as fatigue.

FACTORS THAT INFLUENCE MUSCLE ENDURANCE

In reality, the factors that influence muscle fatigue also affect muscular endurance. Thus, the separation of fatigue and endurance represents a somewhat artificial partition. Muscle strength and aerobic condition are major determinants of endurance as well. Men and women, regardless of age, who are in excellent physical shape, with optimal strength and aerobic capacity, have excellent muscle endurance, as mitochondrial volume, aerobic enzyme activity, and capillary supply are higher than in sedentary individuals. ATP can be generated more quickly in "fit" individuals.[16] Conversely, those who are unfit, deconditioned, or inactive because of bed rest are likely to show signs of poor muscle endurance.[6]

It was noted previously that a task requiring 15% or less of maximum strength can be maintained indefinitely.[8] This finding once again underscores the importance of muscle mass and strength as key determinants of muscular endurance. Obviously, the stronger the individual, the greater the array of tasks to choose from without a reduction in muscular endurance. If walking requires 10% of an individual's strength capability, that individual probably can walk all day. If walking requires 25% of an individual's capacity, then walking endurance will be limited considerably. Obviously, potential cardiovascular and pulmonary limitations are not being taken into consideration in this discussion, but they are discussed elsewhere in this text.

TESTS AND MEASURES FOR FATIGUE AND ENDURANCE

Tests for the assessment of fatigue are limited and not readily applicable to the clinical setting or the geriatric population. The most commonly used test, 50 to 60 maximal knee extensions on an isokinetic device, requires equipment that is not likely to be on site in many facilities. Many older adults are not able to grasp the isokinetic nature of the test, and it can be risky for those with significant cardiac compromise. In many clinical situations the patient is fatigued by the time four to six repetitions are completed, so a test requiring a multitude of contractions is not helpful. However, because fatigue is a common patient complaint and is commonly observed, some means for assessing the magnitude of the problem is needed. One suggested method is to select a cuff weight that is reasonable (based on clinical judgment), strap it onto the extremity of interest, and then choose a functional task that is pertinent. For example, a patient's functional limitation could be measured by placing a cuff on the patient's upper extremity, having the patient reach up along a yardstick to the highest point possible, and then determining how many times the patient reached the set goal. This measure provides a distance that is reproducible and quantifies the number of repetitions achieved. Improvement in fatigue would be noted as an increase in number of repetitions achieved, a greater distance reached, and the more weight lifted. A similar protocol could be developed for the lower extremity, e.g., putting a cuff weight around the patient's ankle and then having the patient bring the knee to a certain height forward to a line to challenge the hip flexors or the knee extensors. These suggestions are provided to encourage the reader to develop better protocols. An acceptable fatigue protocol must be reliable, valid, easy to use, understandable to most patients and third party payers, and require little or no equipment.

When the goal of "improve endurance" is written, the likely intent of the therapist is to reduce fatigue. Endurance tests, such as holding a contraction for as long as possible, are probably not indicative of the patient's compromise as a test for fatigue. Regardless, some type of test that underscores the need to "improve endurance" is sorely needed for clinical practice. Those in the geriatric community of care are the most capable of developing such a tool.

Case Study

Rita M (age, 72 years)

This sprightly, trim woman had a primary diagnosis of rheumatoid arthritis of long-standing duration (more than 30 years). Rita has had both knees and hips replaced and has had numerous other surgeries on her hands and feet to reduce deformity. Nonetheless, she was an independent community ambulator (no cane) and could perform all her activities of daily living with the use of assistive devices, e.g., button hook. Even though Rita could accomplish the fundamental tasks of dressing, food preparation, house management, etc., she was exhausted at the end of the day. Trips to the grocery store, physician's office, and theater were a chore, resulting in "muscle fatigue." In addition to fatigue, Rita's only other complaint was inability to pick up her grandchildren. Thus, the patient's goals were to make chores a little easier to perform (decrease fatigue) and lift up and hold her 2- and 4-year-old grandchildren (improve strength).

Tests to identify deficits in strength, fatigue, and endurance were performed at initial evaluation. These tests consisted of (1) determining maximum isometric strength of the major muscle groups of the upper extremities and hip extensors and abductors, using a hand-held dynamometer; (2) determining how many repetitions of upper extremity lift could be performed using a weight that was 50% of maximum; (3) having Rita perform an isoki-

netic test for the quadriceps and hamstrings at 0, 60, 180, and 300°/s and plantar and dorsiflexors at 0, 60 and 180°/s; and (4) having the patient perform an isokinetic endurance test (50 maximum contractions at 180°/s). In addition, tests of function were performed and consisted of preferred gait speed, book-lift test, and chair rise. Initial examination findings are displayed in Table 16-2.

Isokinetic testing of the knee extensors and flexors revealed that Rita could not move the arm of the dynamometer faster than 180°/s. In other words, torque output at 300°/s was zero. The endurance test was highly remarkable as there was no decline in torque over the 1-minute test period (Fig. 16-3). The 18-foot/pound output (a very low value) was maintained throughout the entire test. Functional testing indicated that preferred gait speed was 45 m/min, a total of 8 pounds could be lifted overhead three times before the onset of fatigue, and that Rita could not get up from a chair without using her arms to assist.

Exercise intervention was initiated and consisted of the following:

1. General body strengthening using primarily body weight and the weight of the body part, such as supine straight leg raising while maintaining abdominal control and wall slides
2. Walking with a weight belt around the waist to load the hips, in particular
3. Stationary cycling with no resistance to reduce swelling of the knees and reduce perceived lower extremity joint stiffness

As progress was made, exercises with resistive elastic were added to the regimen. Rita's hand function was so poor that it was difficult for her to hold traditional weights, and cuff weights resulted in enough joint traction to cause discomfort. Resistive elastic strips that could be looped around up-

TABLE 16-2
SELECTED STRENGTH VALUES FOR ISOMETRIC/ISOKINETIC TESTS BEFORE AND AFTER INTERVENTION

	INITIAL EXAMINATION	3 MONTHS
Shoulder flexion	7 lbs	10 lbs
Elbow flexion	18 lbs	25 lbs
Grip	18 lbs	18 lbs
Hip extension	20 lbs	28 lbs
Hip abduction	32 lbs	38 lbs
Knee extension	28 ft/lbs	48 ft/lbs
Knee flexion	18 ft/lbs	32 ft/lbs
Plantar flexion	28 ft/lbs	36 ft/lbs

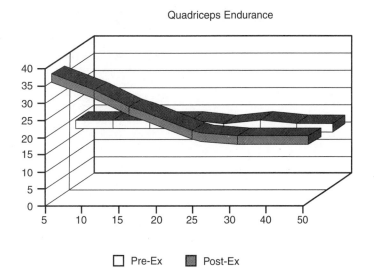

Quadriceps Endurance

□ Pre-Ex ■ Post-Ex

FIG. 16-3 Quadriceps endurance before and after 3 months of physical therapy exercise. On the *X axis* is torque output in ft/lbs, and on the *Y axis* are the number of contractions performed. A metronome was set to elicit 50 contractions for 1 minute, and the dynamometer was set at 180°/s.

per and lower extremities proved to be the most comfortable resistance exercise. At the end of 3 months of exercise that was done on site under supervision 3 times week, a re-examination was performed. Substantial progress was made, as indicated in Table 16-2.

With regard to muscle fatigue (Fig. 16-3), torque values were so low that there was no decline in torque during the fatigue test before exercise intervention. Torque output doubled after 3 months of intervention and declined to the original starting value of 18 feet/pounds with the endurance test. Interpretation of this type of test is challenging since, as the slope of the curve suggests (see Fig. 16-3), there was no compromise in endurance before exercise and a 50% decline in endurance capacity after exercise. It is easy to misconstrue this finding as an indication of a worsening of endurance. Another way of looking at the data is that the amount of work (area under the curve in Fig. 16-3) performed increased by about 30%, suggesting an important improvement in endurance (and strength) capacity.

With regard to the book-lift task, Rita could complete eight repetitions of 10 pounds after physical therapy intervention, which was a marked improvement. More importantly, she could hold (but not lift) her grandchildren after exercise and spend more time in the community without undue fatigue. Her preferred gait speed increased 5 m/min, and she could now get up from a chair without using her arms.

This case study demonstrates that it is possible to identify fatigue and endurance compromise, but it also shows the need for better tests to illustrate deficits, particularly to third party payers. This case study also shows that it is possible to influence strength, fatigue, and endurance with standard treatment principles. Improvements in strength likely contributed to the reduction in fatigue and improvement in endurance. The combined effect of all of the positive changes was enhanced physical function. However, it must also be noted that the investment required to achieve this outcome was more than 30 patient visits in 3 months, highlighting the importance of excellent documentation to demonstrate the value of physical therapy intervention.

SUMMARY

Older adults commonly exhibit signs of fatigue and poor muscular endurance. The identification of fatigue and impaired endurance should be routine components of physical therapists' examination, just as the inclusion of exercises to reduce fatigue and poor endurance should become standard interventions to improve the physical function and quality of life of older adults.

REFERENCES

1. Alway SE, et al: Functional and structural adaptations in skeletal muscle of trained athletes. *J Appl Physiol* 1988; 64:1114-1120.
2. Buchner D, Wagner EH: Preventing frail health. *Clin Geriatr Med* 1992; 8:1-17.
3. Costill DL, et al: Skeletal muscle enzymes and fiber composition in male and female track athletes. *J Appl Physiol* 1976; 40:149-154.
4. Fitts RH: Cellular mechanisms of fatigue. *Physiol Rev* 1994; 74:49-94.
5. Häkkinen K, Komi PV: Electromyographic changes during strength training and detraining. *Med Sci Sports Exerc* 1983;15:455-460.
6. Henriksson J, Reitman J: Time course changes in human skeletal muscle succinate dehydrogenase and cytochrome oxidase activities and maximal oxygen uptake with physical activity and inactivity. *Acta Physiologica Scand* 1977; 99:91-97.
7. Ingjer F: Capillary supply and mitochondrial content of different skeletal muscle fiber types in untrained and endurance-trained men. A histochemical and ultrastructural study. *Eur J Appl Physiol* 1979; 40:197-209.
8. Laforest S, St-Pierre DM, Cyr J, Gayton D: Effects of age and regular exercise on muscle strength and endurance. *Eur J Appl Physiol* 1990; 60:104-111.
9. Larsson L, Ansved T: Effects of long-term physical training and detraining on enzyme histochemical and functional skeletal muscle characteristics in man. *Muscle Nerve* 1985; 8:714-722.
10. Lennmarken C, Bergman T, Larsson J, Larsson LE: Skeletal muscle function in man: Force, relaxation rate, endurance and contraction-time dependence on sex and age. *Clin Physiol* 1985; 5:243-255.
11. Lindstrom B, Lexell J, Gerdle B, Downham D: Skeletal muscle fatigue and endurance in young and old men and women. *J Gerontol* 1997; 52:B59-66.
12. MacLaren DPM, Gibson H, Parry-Billings M, Edwards RHT: A review of metabolic and physiological factors in fatigue. *Exerc Sport Sci Rev* 1989;17:29-66.
13. Merton PA: Voluntary strength and fatigue. *J Physiol* 1954; 123:553-564.
14. Naamani R, Hussain SNA, Magder S: The mechanical effects of contractions on blood flow to the muscle. *Eur J Physiol* 1995; 71:102-112.
15. Ringsberg K, Gerdhem P, Johansson J, Obrant KJ: Is there a relationship between balance, gait performance and muscular strength in 75-year-old women? *Age Ageing* 1999; 28:289-293.
16. Rogers MA, et al: Decline in VO_{2max} with aging in master athletes and sedentary men. *J Appl Physiol* 1984; 57:1024-1029.
17. Schwendner KI, et al: Differences in muscle endurance and recovery between fallers and nonfallers and between young and older women. *J Gerontol* 1997; 52:M155-160.
18. Viitasalo JT, Komi PV: Rate of force development, muscle structure and fatigue. *Biomechanics* 1981; 136-141.

CHAPTER 17

POSTURE IN THE OLDER ADULT

Carolee Moncur, PT, PhD

INTRODUCTION

When one is asked to imagine a picture of the posture of an elderly person, too often the image is that of a bent or stooped individual who, more often than not, is of the female gender and has a high risk of falling (Fig. 17-1). Often, previous experience as a student or clinician has created a picture of the posture of only those elderly persons who are confined to nursing homes or similar circumstances.

Posture can be a statement about an individual. It may be an outward demonstration of wellness, illness, self-esteem (or the lack thereof), the vicissitudes of life, or simply the processes of development or aging. As physical therapists, it is important to decipher between the circumstances to be expected as a result of aging and those conditions extraneous to growing old, thereby altering upright posture.

The purpose of this chapter is to review these parameters and to demonstrate the process of designing and implementing a physical therapy plan of care for common postural problems seen in the elderly person. It is imperative that posture be evaluated on an individual basis as, in the case of other human characteristics, the upright position has great variability among this population of people.

POSTURE THROUGH THE LIFE SPAN
Development of Upright Posture

During fetal life, childhood, and adolescence, increase in the number of cells is of prime importance to growth of the body systems responsible for the development of posture. The central nervous system matures concurrent with the continuous changes occurring in the musculoskeletal system. Martin suggests that children develop postural control in various stages corresponding with their ability to integrate sensory information.[65] In the early years, vision is the primary source used to reinforce upright orientation, with the proprioceptive systems being of secondary importance. In order to effectively develop proprioception as a mode of input, the child must continue to practice motor skills to perfect the system.

Aging of the child, as well as increased use of the somatosensory and vestibular systems, enhances the adaptation of the individual to the upright position. The somatosensory systems continue to be the primary sources used by both children and adults to achieve postural stability.[36] It is important to appreciate that, notwithstanding the importance of the nervous system, other factors must develop parallel with the development of movement, such as strength and endurance against gravity. This of course requires the appropriate integration of healthy cardiopulmonary, musculoskeletal, and neuromuscular systems. In essence, posture is derived from the relationship of body parts to one another as well as the maturation and interaction of a number of body systems.[56,104,105] Once postural control has been established, the child can begin coordinated, sequential movements about the environment.[65]

A brief description of the development of posture would not be complete if some comment were not made regarding the influence of psychosocial factors on the upright position. In the pre-school age youngster, parental and sibling influences affect the mobility of the child and can give rise to the intensity, duration, and selection of activity in which the child participates. When boys and girls enter school, obvious differences begin to appear with respect to motor behavior, as demon-

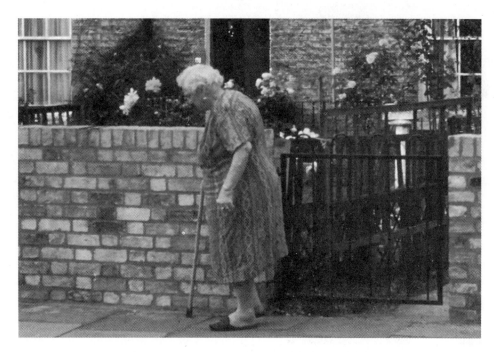

Fig. 17-1   Traditional perception of elderly posture.

strated by Hayes and co-workers.[45] Physical growth during adolescence, as well as other changes associated with that time period, can have an important effect on the individual's belief in oneself. Fears of being different from peers may interfere with self-image and be reflected in the youth's posture.[45]

Since it is outside the scope of this chapter to elaborate on the theories of aging, we will assume for our purposes that growth, development, and differentiation of the human continues throughout life and does not stop at young adulthood.[98] Furthermore, it will be assumed that the elderly are those who have had long lives with varied experiences that demonstrate great differentiation. How the elder person maintains the capacity to adapt to the growth and changes of life will decide how the individual will master the tasks of later maturity and old age, including optimizing upright posture.[16]

Factors Influencing Postural Changes During Senescence

It is clear that one person who is elderly is not the same as another person who is elderly. *Variability* is the important word to keep in mind as postural changes characteristic of aging are discussed. The description here will be of what one might find to be typical or reflective of the aging process; however, it should be recognized that the posture of the individual may be altered or changed by disease, medication, trauma, state of mind, or the setting and time of day when the patient is evaluated.

Musculoskeletal Changes

Some authors draw a fine line between decreases occurring in the density of long bones and the vertebral column due to aging changes in bone mineral balance and decreases that result

in osteopenic or more severe osteoporotic bone. Results of scientific studies have demonstrated that a decrease of height or stature can generally be expected due to senescence.[25,96]

Age-related changes in bone density differ from site to site. Bone mineral at peripheral sites (such as the radius) remains relatively stable until menopause, but bone loss of the spine and neck of the femur occurs 5 to 10 years earlier, respectively. Simply stated, changes in bone during aging occur earlier in the spine than in the limbs.[69] Bone loss in men occurs at a rate of about 0.4% per year, beginning at age 50, and does not characteristically become problematic until the male is in his 80s.[68,69] In both men and women between the ages of 60 and 80 years, the average rate of decrease in height is about 2 cm per decade and may be as much as a total of 12 cm in extreme cases of bone loss.[24]

These changes commence around age 40 and are more noticeable in women than in men, likely due to the increased vulnerability for women to lose bone mass. In aging women, bone loss begins at 0.75% to 1% per year beginning at age 30 to 35 years. A higher rate (2% to 3%) of bone mineral loss occurs after menopause. A greater loss occurs in the spine the first 5 years after menopause than during the subsequent 15 years of the woman's life.[41] At this rate, women may lose 30% of bone mineral mass of the spine by 70 years of age. Interestingly, bone mineral loss does not occur as readily in overweight women.[86] Longcope and colleagues suggested that this is a consequence of peripheral estrogen production by adipose tissue.[62]

Since the upright posture of an individual is reflected dramatically in the spine and related structures, the following discussion concentrates on the life span changes in the musculoskeletal properties of these structures. The focus is limited to the intervertebral disks, spine ligaments, vertebrae, ribs, articular cartilage, entheses, muscles, and related biomechanics.

Age-related change in the intervertebral disk is a well-known phenomenon occurring throughout the life span, beginning about 30 years of age.[77,113] Briefly, the intervertebral disks are composed of fibroblasts, collagen, elastin, and a polysaccharide ground substance consisting of hyaluronic acid and proteoglycans. While serving various functions, the individual disk is subjected to considerable forces and moments throughout the life span. In concert with the facet joints, it is responsible for responding to the compressive loads placed on the trunk.[46,85] Nachemson and colleagues[74,76,113] have described these forces, stating that the forces on a disk are greater during the standing anatomical position than the weight of the portion of the body above it. The sitting position is another matter. When it comes to the forces on the lumbar disks, the summation of forces on the lumbar spine during sitting is greater than three times the weight of the trunk.[74,76] Dynamic loads such as jumping or running will obviously increase the forces to perhaps twice as high as those in standing or sitting positions.[10] Not only are intervertebral disks subjected to compressive stresses,[17,30,46,47,64,87,109] they must also endure tensile stress[17,39,113] and axial rotation of the trunk, which results in shear stresses.[17,30,31,47,52,64]

Anatomically, the intervertebral disk constitutes 20% to 30% of the cumulative height of the spinal column.[113] The disk is composed of a nucleus pulposus, an annulus fibrosus, and the cartilaginous end plates. Centrally located, the nucleus pulposus is composed of a loose, translucent network of fibers that lie in a mucoprotein gel containing a variety of mucopolysaccharides. The water content of the nucleus ranges from 70% to 90%, being highest at birth and diminishing in amount with age. The relative size of the nucleus to the total disk area depends on where it is located in the bony column, with the nuclei of the lumbar spine being 30% to 50% of the disk area.

The annulus fibrosus is composed of fibroelastic tissue arranged in concentrically laminated bands that are arranged in a helicoid fashion. Any two adjacent bands demonstrate fibers that run in opposite directions from each other such that the fibers of two bands are oriented at 120 degrees to each other (Fig. 17-2). The annulus fibers are attached to the cartilaginous end plates on the inner zone of the vertebral body, while peripherally they are attached by Sharpey's fibers to the edges of the body. The cartilaginous end plate is composed of hyaline cartilage and separates the nucleus and annulus from the vertebral body.[113]

In general, aging alters both the properties and the relative proportion of the connective tissue elements of the disk. Specifically, there is an increase in the stability and density of collagen with the exception of some tissues, such as the skin.[67] With aging, elastin becomes less distensible and can undergo fragmentation. Collagen molecules that form elastin may change either by degradation or by incorrect synthesis, resulting in an intermediate form of elastin called *pseudoelastin*.[96] This departure from normal collagen fibers

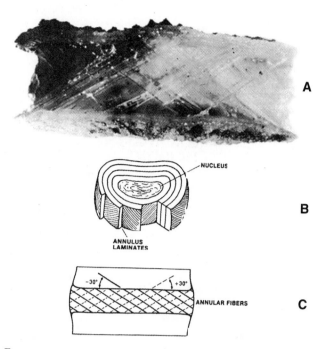

FIG. 17-2 Components of the intervertebral disk. **A,** Photograph of a disk showing the annular fibers and their orientation. **B,** Drawing of the lamellar configuration of the annular fibers. **C,** Orientation of fibers at about 30 degrees with respect to placement of the disk. (From White AA, Panjabi MM: *Clinical Biomechanics of the Spine,* ed 2. Philadelphia, JB Lippincott, 1990. Used by permission.)

is predominantly found in the exposed dermis of the neck of the elderly person.

The nucleus pulposus contains considerable water and mucopolysaccharides that coalesce as a gelatinous mass up to about age 25 to 30. This anatomical feature is significant in protecting the spinal elements when the vertebrae are subjected to stress and loads. Alterations of these constituents found in the disk may cause it to collapse, thus diminishing the height of the individual as well as decreasing the soft, yellow core of pulpy elastic material that forms the nucleus pulposus.[76]

The *ligaments of the spine* are depicted in Fig. 17-3. Ligaments surrounding any anatomical structure act much like guy wires and/or rubber bands with respect to their function. In the spine, one might conceptualize that the ligaments respond to tensile forces by becoming taut. The reverse is true when the spine is subjected to compressive loads; namely, the collagen fibers in ligaments buckle and become slack. Ligaments allow mobility in the spine while maintaining fixed postural relationships between vertebrae. Additionally, they need to do this with the least amount of effort. This suggests that as long as the spinal column is healthy, properly aligned, and supported by strong musculature and ligaments, upright posture will be sustained. However, should the ligaments be maintained in a slackened position, changes will occur in postural patterns. The tensile ability of the ligaments of the spine degenerates with age. In an extensive study on 484 samples, Tkaczuk determined that the tensile characteristics of both

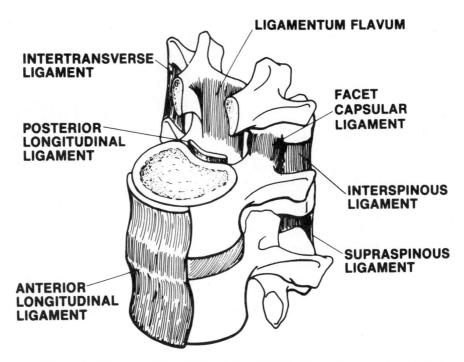

FIG. 17-3   Ligaments of the spine. (From White AA, Panjabi MM: *Clinical Biomechanics of the Spine,* ed 2. Philadelphia, JB Lippincott, 1990. Used by permission.)

the anterior and posterior ligaments of the lumbar spine decreased with age.[106] This was particularly true of the ligaments' ability to respond to shock absorption. Likewise, Nachemson and Evans determined that the ligamentum flavum declines in its ability to perform "resting" tension upon the spine. This duty is important in lending to the stability of the spine.[75] Without the tensile strength in ligaments and resultant laxity, it seems apparent that these changes might contribute to the flexed forward posture of the elderly person.

Studies of the strength characteristics of the *human vertebra* began more than 100 years ago and have received considerable attention since that time.[1,8,72,84,110] It has been observed that the vertebra decreases in strength with age, particularly beyond age 40. Fig. 17-4 depicts the results of an investigation by Bell and associates that demonstrates a definite relationship between the strength (stress of failure) and relative ash content (osseous tissue) of the vertebra.[8] These data indicate that vertebral strength is lost with age and is directly related to the decrease in the amount of bone. Furthermore, a small loss of osseous tissue produces considerable decrease in vertebral bone strength. As seen in Fig. 17-4, a 25% loss in osseous tissue results in a greater than 50% decrease of strength of a vertebra.[8]

The separate components of the vertebra—including the body,[8,83,110] cortical shell,[7,8,88,110] cancellous core,[61,88] end plates,[84,89] neural arch,[57,90,111] and facets[30,32,54,74,81,112,114]—have been investigated to determine the response of each to compressive loads on the spine. To summarize this literature, it has been determined that cancellous bone contributes 25% to 55% of the strength to the lumbar vertebrae. In a person younger than 40 years, 55% of the load is carried by the cancellous core, and in a person older than 40 years, this share decreases to about 35%.[66] Failure patterns in the end plates of vertebrae can be central or peripheral or involve the entire end plate.[84,89] Strength in the neural arch decreases with age and when loaded with compressive forces, the arch is most likely to fail through the pedicles.[57] The facet joints appear to carry about 18% of the total compressive load borne by a motion segment.[74] However, King and colleagues determined that the share of the load carried by the facets could be from 33% to 0%, depending on the spinal postures.[54]

Atkinson and co-workers[6,26] evaluated the vertebral trabecular bone to determine age-related patterns. The earliest changes seen were related to the orientation of the trabeculae from horizontal to vertical structures. The horizontal trabeculae were decreased first; however, there was a concomitant thickening of some of the vertical trabeculae. Therefore, there was no appreciable loss of osseous tissue on the whole until age 50 but rather a decrease in the mechanical strength of the vertebral body due to the loss of the horizontal trabeculae.

Not only did a loss in the horizontal trabeculae occur, the loss was in the central region of the vertebral body, whereas the peripheral trabeculae were largely unaltered. The implication is that the loss of strength with age is preferential to the center of the vertebrae. Microcollapse of the vertebral body, not sufficient to be diagnosed as osteoporosis, may contribute to the reduction in height that an elderly person experiences. Extensive collapse correlates well with the clinical findings of central collapse of the body in individuals who have developed osteoporosis.[68,69]

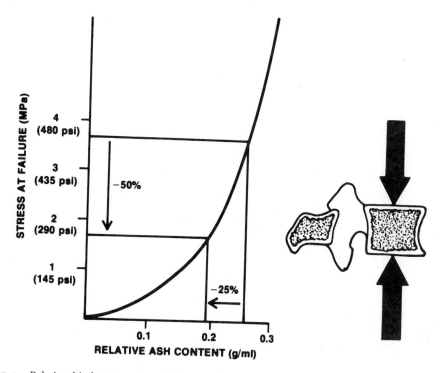

FIG. 17-4   Relationship between osseous tissue and vertebral strength. (From Bell GH, et al: *Calcif Tissue Res* 1967; 1:75-86. Adapted from White AA, Panjabi MM: *Clinical Biomechanics of the Spine*, ed 2. Philadelphia, JB Lippincott, 1990. Used by permission.)

It is difficult to determine the contribution of the *rib cage* or its components to the inherent stability of the spine. The individual components of the rib cage may be quite flexible. However, using mathematical modeling on a computer, Andriacchi and colleagues studied a variety of simulations to determine the effects of the rib cage on the stiffness properties of the normal spine, on the stability of the normal spine under axial compression, and on the scoliotic spine subjected to traction.[3] Essentially, the results demonstrated that the stiffness properties of the spine were found to be greatly increased by the presence of the rib cage during various spinal motions. The rib cage was also found to increase the mechanical stability of the spine by 4 times when a compression load was placed on it. Finally, while traction increased axial stiffness in the normal spine 40% due to the presence of a rib cage, this was not the case in a scoliotic spine. Flexibility in the scoliotic spine with a rib cage was found to be 2½ times greater, which might be attributed to the abnormal geometric curvature found in scoliosis.[3] One might conjecture that changes occurring in the geometric relationship of the ribs and the spinal column due to aging could reduce its stiffness and ability to maintain an upright position.

Articular cartilage, with similar components found in other connective tissues, likewise undergoes change. Healthy cartilage in fresh cadavers is translucent, glistening, and pearl-like, whereas the cartilage of older cadavers is opaque and yellow and may have undergone some decrease in thickness. So a reduction in the thickness of the articular cartilage of the lower extremities in particular will contribute to the decrease of upright height. Degenerative joint disease may be present in some specimens but should not be equated with age-related changes in the cartilage. Rather, while there are age-related changes in the structure of the collagen—including a loss of resilience, decreases in the content and aggregation of the hydrophilic proteoglycans (chondroitin and keratin sulfate side chains), and a reduction in the length of the chondroitin chains in articular cartilage[11]—this does not mean that joint disease will occur. It does mean that there is an increased possibility that the articular cartilage could sustain microfractures or damage[19] from forces such as overuse, obesity, trauma, metabolic disease, or hereditary factors.

It is not uncommon for physical therapists to see older individuals who have participated in a physical activity that has caused a sprain, strain, or rupture of a muscle or tendon. Age-related changes modify not only the tendon but also the *entheses.* These changes unfortunately make the older person more vulnerable to injury of tendons by reducing the distensibility of the collagen and elastic fiber when pressed to complete vigorous activity. Indirectly, the tendinous age-related changes may contribute to the alterations in upright posture.

Lastly and extremely important are the aging changes that occur in *muscular tissue.* It has been demonstrated for quite some time by various authors[2,4,5,35,42,58,60,107] that muscle strength peaks at about 30 years of age and remains constant to about 50 years, whereupon it begins to show an accelerating loss somewhat parallel to the decline of lean body tissue (Fig. 17-5). It has been demonstrated that there is a reduction of myosin adenosine triphosphatase (ATPase) activity

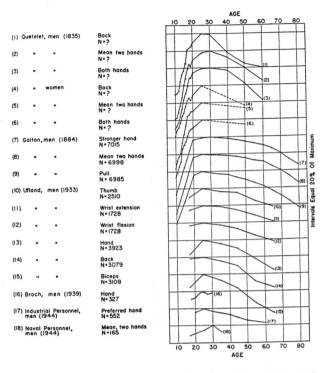

	AGE
(1) Quetelet, men (1835)	Back N=?
(2) " "	Mean two hands N=?
(3) " "	Both hands N=?
(4) " women	Back N=?
(5) " "	Mean two hands N=?
(6) " "	Both hands N=?
(7) Galton, men (1884)	Stronger hand N=7015
(8) " "	Mean two hands N=6998
(9) " "	Pull N=6985
(10) Ufland, men (1933)	Thumb N=2510
(11) " "	Wrist extension N=1728
(12) " "	Wrist flexion N=1728
(13) " "	Hand N=3923
(14) " "	Back N=3079
(15) " "	Biceps N=3108
(16) Broch, men (1939)	Hand N=327
(17) Industrial Personnel, men (1944)	Preferred hand N=552
(18) Naval Personnel, men (1944)	Mean, two hands N=165

FIG. 17-5   Relationship of strength to age. (From Fisher MB, Birren JE: J *Appl Psychol* 1947; 31:628-630. Used by permission.)

as well as a selective decrease in the number of fast-twitch, type II muscle fibers as one ages. This tends to explain why there is a lengthening of the time to peak tension, a decrease in peak tension of muscle, and a lengthening of the half-relaxation time. The functional consequences of the prevertebral and postvertebral muscle becoming atrophied could result in some of the postural and biomechanical changes seen in some older persons.

Neurological Changes

Distinguishing between uncomplicated aging of the nervous system and comorbid factors such as cerebrovascular disease is sometimes difficult to accomplish. Aging of the nervous system does not affect all neural structures in the same fashion.* Of particular importance is the contribution that degeneration of the nigrostriatal pathways makes to decreasing motor performance and posture in the elderly. Extensive degeneration of these same monoaminergic neuronal systems occurs in Parkinson's disease,[59,78,108] leading to flexed posture, muscular rigidity, tremor, and slow movement.

While the clinical appearance of some elderly individuals bears a remarkable similarity to Parkinson's disease, one should not presume that all elderly persons have the disease.[103] Minor extrapyramidal signs may be present in the elderly and are often overlooked as a result of the aging process. Pyramidal tract and cerebellar signs are less common in the younger elderly. The significance of the age-related imbal-

ances between the motor systems that may occur in aging are not clearly understood. It is possible that when one observes the older person who is flexed forward, has a slight tremor, weak voice, and shuffling gait, it could be related to the aging process occurring in the basal ganglia and associated nuclei.[103] Postural tremor that occurs in the elderly[29,94] and impairment of balance may be caused by cerebellar degeneration[23] or any of its connections.[103] Therefore, neurological causes of postural change should also be examined.

Decreases in voluntary movement control and reaction time occur in the elderly.[22,50,91,101,102,115] It has been reported that the effects of age are more marked when the individual is asked to accomplish complex reaction time tasks,[35,80,97,116] complicated motor responses,[90] or sudden postural adjustments.[50,115] Muscular atrophy of the postural muscles in the elderly has been discussed previously in this chapter and elsewhere.[14,90]

Although the foregoing events occur with aging, it appears that some of the decline in motor performance, including postural control, may be more related to a decrease in physical activity on the part of the elder. Various authors have demonstrated that individuals who are physically active and continue to maintain maximal oxygen uptake during senescence enjoy the benefits derived from an improved heart rate, cardiac output, blood pressure,[4,9,21,27,37,43,95] joint mobility,[20] and increased flexibility.

Psychosocial Factors

The impact of psychosocial factors on the posture of elderly individuals has not been well-documented; therefore, this discussion is mostly anecdotal from observations made by the author, who is also a physical therapist for elderly individuals with arthritis and associated psychosocial concerns. It is beyond the scope of this chapter to address the multiple psychosocial problems that could affect posture. Three of the more common phenomena seen in a physical therapy practice are depression,[13,15] delirium (acute confusional state),[92] and dementia[40,48,49,55,73] and are covered in detail in other chapters.

Depression is the single most common problem of mental health occurring in the elderly and is the most treatable.[12] The following case study demonstrates how depression altered both posture and general affect.

Mrs. VJ is a 73-year-old woman who lives with her husband, a recently retired obstetrician, in an affluent high-rise condominium. She has a 25-year history of osteoarthritis of the lumbar spine including both the disks and the facet joints of L1 to L5. On x-ray the L4-5 segment has collapsed and fused, and there are large osteophytes protruding into the intervertebral foramina. The facet joints of these segments are fused.

Mrs. VJ is overweight by 50 pounds. About 8 months ago (about the same time her husband completely retired from his practice), she developed intolerable low back pain. She responded initially to a nonsteroidal anti-inflammatory drug and a carefully planned therapeutic exercise and walking pro-

*References 3, 16, 18, 44, 63, 71, 79, 82, 105

gram. She was seen weekly for 1 month, then once a month thereafter. Each time she returned for her monthly appointment, it was noted that her complaints of fatigue and lack of sleep increased. She also seemed apathetic about her appearance and about 4 months ago began to wear the same workout clothes for treatment along with her fur coat. Her complaints about her low back pain increased as did the complaints of fatigue and low endurance, and she began to sleep for 2 to 4 hours during the day. She walked lethargically and with a more stooped, bent-forward posture. She claimed to be compliant at home with her home program of exercises.

When confronted with the question as to whether she was depressed, she openly admitted she was and burst into tears. Multiple problems were bothering her, including unresolved feelings and beliefs about a daughter who had died 20 years ago, resentment that her husband was home "under my feet all day," and a feeling that she had no freedom. She was referred to a psychiatrist who prescribed an antidepressant and counseling for her. Although she was seeing a psychiatrist, the physical therapist continued to follow her case monthly to monitor her exercise program as well as to provide support during her initial counseling sessions. In 1 month her entire demeanor, depression, countenance, and posture improved. She continued with counseling and her exercise program and has been discharged from physical therapy to be followed *ad libitum.*

Pharmaceutical Factors

Many drug groups may change posture. Pepper and Robbins have suggested that the major mechanisms by which drugs impair mobility and alter posture are sedation (decreased motivation); postural instability (imbalance that contributes to falls and fear of falling that causes elders to limit activity); sensory or psychomotor impairment (altered visual, proprioceptive, or vestibular compensatory mechanisms necessary for balance); and postural hypotension (syncope, dizziness, weakness).[83] Learning what drugs the patient is taking can be valuable information before making any final evaluative decisions regarding the posture of the elder.

Comorbidity Factors

Comorbidity factors that may alter the posture and postural control of the elderly person might be tinnitus, visual impairment, deafness, headaches, hypertension, or hypotension. Control of the posture is governed by the vestibular system in the inner ear, by the visual system, and by proprioceptive information from the peripheral nervous system. Degenerative changes or other insult to these mechanisms could impair postural control. Alterations in the cerebroregulatory function probably contribute an important part in postural disturbances in old people.[99] The list of comorbid factors could be lengthy, and to explain each is outside the scope of this chapter. The physical therapist must be cognizant of any comorbid factors that may be present in the elder, no matter how subtle or unimportant they appear when an initial history is taken.

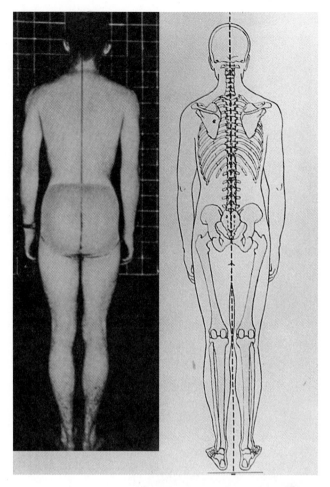

Fig. 17-6 Posture in the standing position viewed from the posterior. (From Kendall EP, McCreary EK: *Muscles: Testing and Function.* Baltimore, Williams & Wilkins, 1993. Used by permission.)

Evaluation of Posture and Postural Changes

Before beginning a discussion on the evaluation process, a precautionary note should be emphasized again. The model for correct postural alignment is a young, healthy individual who has a well-integrated neuromusculoskeletal system and postural control, as reflected in Figs. 17-6 and 17-7.[53] While this information is important in general, it may not be specific to the elder person. Figs. 17-8 and 17-9 are more reflective of the postural changes particular to the elderly.[51] As can be seen, with advancing age the head moves forward, the thoracic spine is more kyphotic, and there is a loss of the normal lumbar lordosis. One should remember, however, that postural alignment in elderly persons can be highly individualized in appearance.

Alignment

To assess the total body alignment, visual inspection should occur in the sagittal, coronal, and horizontal planes as well as from anterior, posterior, and lateral views. Typically, one uses a plumb line or a posture grid to determine a reference point

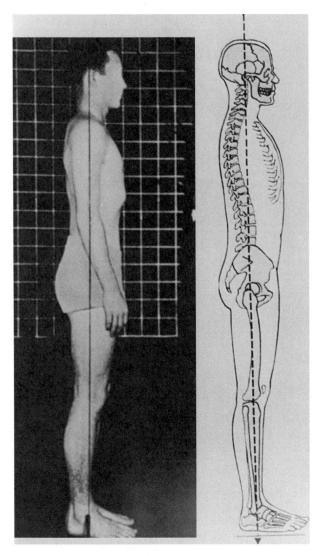

FIG. 17-7 Posture in the standing position viewed from the side. (From Kendall EP, McCreary EK: *Muscles: Testing and Function.* Baltimore, Williams & Wilkins, 1993. Used by permission.)

for inspection from each view. Although the proximal fixation points for the plumb line are (1) mental protuberance of the mandible for the anterior view, (2) anterior margin of the mastoid process of the temporal bone for the lateral view, and (3) the external occipital protuberance on the occipital bone for the posterior view as in the young adult, deviations from what is expected in younger persons should be anticipated.

For example, Friedenburg and Miller identified that 70% of their subjects had appreciable degenerative changes in the cervical spine by the seventh decade of life.[38] Likewise, Brain reported that spondylosis of the cervical spine was present in 80% of subjects in his study of persons older than 55.[11] These cervical changes can restrict motion in the cervical spine and contribute to the forward head posture seen in older persons. Furthermore, it might be observed that the pelvis tends to tilt posteriorly more often than is seen in

younger patients. This might be due to prolonged sitting postures and hypokinesis of the postural muscles. Deviations of the posture in the posterior and lateral views can be seen in Figs. 17-10 and 17-11.[70]

While assessing the alignment of the body, it is also important to determine the extent to which the person is able to maintain the posture (posture holding) or position of the body without extraneous movements (equilibrium or postural sway). Maintaining postural control in a static position decreases with age and is potentially problematic for the elder, as the loss of postural control increases the risk of falling.[10,33,34] Sample tests for determining disturbances in posture are depicted in Box 17-1. Suggested tests for assessing equilibrium coordination are outlined in Box 17-2.[93] Assessment of postural sway may be as simple as observation by the therapist or as complex as objective data that may be generated from a computer-assisted force plate as the subject stands on it.

It should be noted that elders with significant sensory losses of vision and proprioception may have difficulty maintaining a stable posture.[10,28] It is an important component of assessment to view posture as a total integration of multiple systems. Hence, while static positions are important to assess, it is equally important to assess posture in terms of dynamic balance and coordination by asking the subject to execute a sit-to-stand movement, establish immediate standing balance, react to a nudge by the examiner when standing, turn in a circle, perform a one-legged stance, and sit down.

The "get-up-and-go" test was described by Mathias and colleagues.[66] The purpose is to have the person complete a series of postural adjustments in sequence, including sitting in a chair, standing up, maintaining static bipedal stance, walking a distance, turning around without touching any object for support, walking back to the chair, and turning around and sitting down in the chair. The subject's performance is scored using a five-point Likert scale, with 1 being normal and 5 being a severely abnormal performance.

Joint alignment, joint stability, and range-of-motion examinations are generic tests used in physical therapy but applied with consideration given for age-related changes previously mentioned. Soft tissue changes, stiffness, and stretch weakness of muscles are common in the elder person.

Respiratory Function

While the primary goal of a postural assessment is not necessarily to determine how the respiratory apparatus is functioning, it is an opportunity to determine whether the posture of the individual has the potential of compromising how one breathes. Speads and Leong suggest that while some disturbances in breathing are quite obvious, others will require close observation to determine whether posture is impairing the airflow of the patient.[100] For example, these authors suggest that the observer should watch the patient in the supine position and observe whether the patient experi-

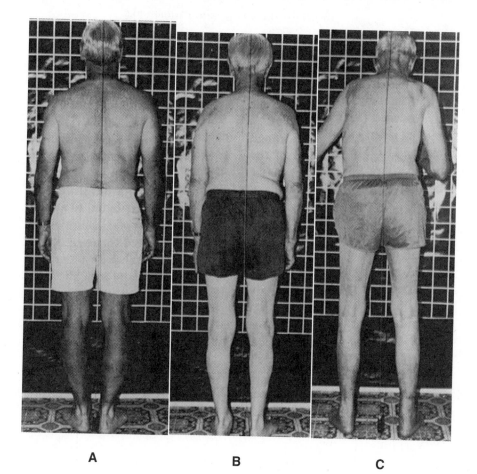

FIG. 17-8 Posterior posture of (**A**) a 60-year-old man, (**B**) a 78-year-old man, and (**C**) a 93-year-old man (From Kauffman T: *Top Geriatr Rehabil* 1987; 2(4):13-28. Used by permission.)

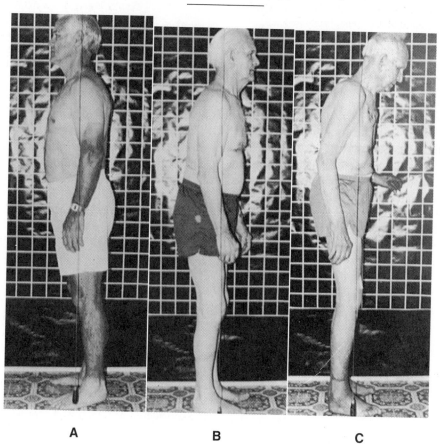

FIG. 17-9 Lateral posture of (**A**) a 60-year-old man, (**B**) a 78-year-old man, and (**C**) a 93-year-old man. (From Kauffman T: *Top Geriatr Rehabil* 1987; 2(4):13-28. Used by permission.)

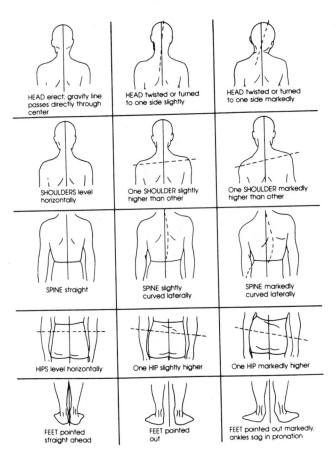

FIG. 17-10   Postural deviation from the posterior view. (Redrawn from McGee DJ: Assessment of posture, in McGee DJ (ed): *Orthopedic Physical Assessment*, ed 3. Philadelphia, WB Saunders, 1997. Used by permission.)

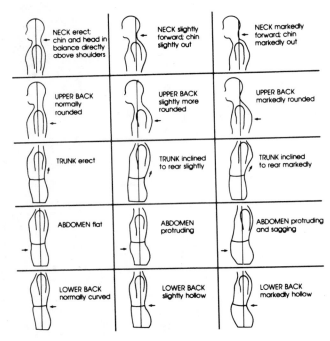

FIG. 17-11   Postural deviations from the lateral view. (Redrawn from McGee DJ: Assessment of posture, in McGee DJ (ed): *Orthopedic Physical Assessment*, ed 3. Philadelphia, WB Saunders, 1997. Used by permission.)

BOX 17-1
TESTS FOR DISTURBANCES OF POSTURE

1. Fixation or position holding (upper and lower extremities).
2. Displace balance unexpectedly in sitting or standing positions.
3. Standing, alter base of support.
4. Standing, one foot directly in front of the other.
5. Standing on one foot.

From Schmitz TJ: Coordination assessment, in Sullivan SB, Schmitz TJ (eds): *Physical Rehabilitation: Assessment and Treatment*, ed 2. Philadelphia, FA Davis, 1988.

ences difficulty breathing or is able to lie comfortably. Sitting postures will also reveal whether the thorax is able to move air appropriately. If the person bends forward while sitting, this may compress the contents of the abdomen against the diaphragm, causing breathing to be restricted. Observations should be made of the rhythm of breathing as well as the movement of the whole thorax. Is the rhythm regular? Is the movement of the thorax too fast or too slow? Does the patient sigh more often than is necessary? Does the person execute Valsalva's maneuver when changing positions or when doing a task? It is important that the air is moving freely, without strain and without interference.[100]

It is useful also to watch for signs of fatigue or lack of endurance as the patient changes positions or completes the posture examination. Casual and routine questions such as "Do you sleep well at night?" and "How long could you walk outdoors before you would have to sit down because you were tired?" may be interspersed into a conversation with the patient during the examination. Answers to these questions can provide direction for further endurance and fatigue testing.

Muscle Strength

Given the variability in changes of the muscular tissue in the elderly person, traditional manual muscle testing may be both spurious and disinclined to provide a true picture of what the person is able to accomplish. Performance-based assessment is much more useful as a global indicator of what the person can accomplish, whereas isolated manual muscle testing or isokinetic testing may be used when there are questions about specific muscle groups.

Coping with Postural Change

Having assessed the person's posture and having determined that there are some noticeable variations from what would be considered normal posture for an elderly person, several

---

BOX 17-2
EQUILIBRIUM COORDINATION TESTS

1. Standing in a normal, comfortable posture.
2. Standing, feet together (narrow base of support).
3. Standing, with one foot directly in front of the other (toe of one foot touching heel of opposite foot).
4. Standing on one foot.
5. Arm position may be altered in each of the above postures (i.e., arms at side, over head, hands on waist, etc.).
6. Displace balance unexpectedly (while carefully guarding patient).
7. Standing, alternate between forward trunk flexion and return to neutral.
8. Standing, laterally flex trunk to each side.
9. Walking, placing the heel of one foot directly in front of the toe of the opposite foot.
10. Walk along a straight line drawn or taped to the floor; or place feet on floor markers while walking.
11. Walk sideways and backward.
12. March in place.
13. Alter speed of ambulatory activities (increased speed will exaggerate coordination deficits).
14. Stop and start abruptly while walking.
15. Walk in a circle, alternate directions.
16. Walk on heels or toes.
17. Normal standing posture. Observe patient both with patient's eyes open and with patient's eyes closed (or vision occluded). If patient is able to maintain balance with eyes open but not with vision occluded, it is indicative of a proprioceptive loss. This inability to maintain an upright posture without visual input is referred to as a positive *Romberg's sign*.

From Schmitz TJ: Coordination assessment, in Sullivan SB, Schmitz TJ (eds): *Physical Rehabilitation: Assessment and Treatment,* ed 2. Philadelphia, FA Davis, 1988.

---

questions need to be answered before a plan of care for the patient can be formulated. Some questions are:

1. Does the patient agree that there is a problem with his/her posture?
2. Are the postural deformities flexible or fixed in nature?
3. Is the patient suffering from comorbidity? What effect would correcting the posture problem have on the comorbidity? Which is more important to the person: the comorbidity or the posture problem?
4. What is the extent of the person's ability to care for himself/herself at home?
5. What are the home conditions of the patient?
6. What occupational or recreational activities does the person enjoy? Would a correction in posture result in the individual's ability to enjoy them more?

Once you have determined that the answers to these questions reflect that the person is motivated, willing to commit to taking charge of the plan of care (with supervision as necessary from a physical therapist), and believes that he/she can succeed for the most part, it is appropriate to develop the plan of care.

THE PLAN OF CARE

Four different postural disorders of primarily musculoskeletal origin (commonly seen by this author in elderly persons) will be used to illustrate how to develop and implement a physical therapy plan of care. The postural disorders to be discussed are those that occur in hypokinetics, osteoporosis, cervical spine dysfunction, and degenerative joint disease. As these types of patients are typically seen in an outpatient setting in a tertiary care hospital, they rarely present with a simple clinical problem but rather have several comorbid conditions.

Case Studies

Hypokinesis

Hypokinesis is a decrease in activity that results in an accentuation of the age-related changes that may be seen in the elder person, such as increased flexed posture, decreased flexibility, decreased muscle strength, decreased endurance, and decreased functional ability. Hypokinesis may occur separately or with comorbidity. Mr. HS is an 85-year-old white male who was first seen in physical therapy for lower extremity strengthening and aerobic and balance exercises in July 1986. His past medical history was remarkable for hypertension, tinnitus, and occasional bouts with syncope. He was able to execute the "get-up-and-go" test, with mild difficulty getting up and down out of a chair. He exhibited decreased one-legged stance balance on each leg but did not exhibit rigidity, cerebellar signs, or tremor. His home exercise routine consisted of walking with his wife through his neighborhood and caring for a very large flower garden. His chief complaint in 1986 was the difficulty he was experiencing with getting up from a chair or the toilet and up and down stairs. He was retired and financially secure and lived with his wife who was 4 years his senior in age.

In November 1990, he reported to his physician that he was falling more often, had "the shakes" when he ate his food, and was easily fatigued with just walking from his home to the garage to get into his car. His wife had died suddenly in 1988, and in 1989, he remarried. During the past year he has not been able to do any kind of air travel, which he previously could do, nor can he play golf. He complained of being house-bound because he had become so weak and shaky. He was not able to complete the "get-up-and-go" test and demonstrated a positive Romberg's sign. He walked with a shuffling flat-footed gait, taking short steps. Although he was now using a cane for balance, he tended to walk in a flexed position reminiscent of an individual with Parkinson's. His physician referred him to a neurologist for a complete work-up, which was only remarkable for symptoms compatible with 85 years of age.

In this particular case, he was described as having hypokinesis and referred to physical therapy for a "tune-up" on his exercise program. Since it was thought that he might also be depressed, he was referred to a physical therapist who worked in a sports physical therapy setting, was also trained with a gerontologic background, and worked with elder exercisers. Mr. HS joined with the group of elders and young athletes doing exercise in the clinic. While his improvement physically is slow, his increase in morale has given him some zest to be more active.

What is important to note here is that the aging process, along with inactivity and depression, can accentuate the elder person's decreased functional ability and loss of freedom to move around. In this case, Mr. HS was carefully matched in an environment for physical therapy where he might experience success in his physical functioning, however modest. Since he loved athletics as a young person, he greatly enjoyed interacting with the young and elder athletes.

Osteoporosis

Mrs. TB is a 68-year-old white female who is widowed and has a 35-year history of rheumatoid arthritis. Considering her numerous upper extremity joint deformities, particularly the instability of the right shoulder and the left elbow, she does very well functionally. During the past 10 years she has developed severe scoliosis of the spine with a right thoracic and left lumbar curvature. Associated with these changes, she has degenerative joint disease of the lumbosacral spine involving both the facet joints and the intervertebral disks. Her current medical problems are degenerative joint disease, osteoporosis, rheumatoid arthritis, scleritis, and hypertension. Her medications list includes azathioprine (Imuran), dexamethasone (Decadron), estrogens (Premarin), medroxyprogesterone (Provera), acetaminophen (Tylenol 3), enalapril (Vasotec), and ranitidine (Zantac). She has been using some form of corticosteroid in various dosages for more than 30 years. Her current dosage is 5 mg orally per day, which is considered a maintenance dose.

Her risk factors for osteoporosis are postmenopausal female, white, light skeletal mass, and steroid dependence for more 30 years. She presented herself to the physical therapy clinic because of a long-standing patient-therapist association. Her chief complaint was of localized back pain that seemed to start at her spine and follow around her rib cage. She also felt that she was twisting more and was having great difficulty getting up and down from the bed, chairs, and toilet. Asked when the symptoms began, she reported that they had been ongoing for about 2 weeks. The only activity she could attribute it to was straining to close the door on her car, which had become caught on a grassy curb.

Anterolateral assessment of her back revealed the dramatic scoliotic curvature of her spine. Upon visual inspection it could not be determined whether the scoliotic curves were increasing; however, she did complain of greater difficulty breathing, sometimes having sharp, stabbing pain on forced inhalation and upon coughing. Palpation of her spine revealed point tenderness at the level of the 12th thoracic vertebra toward the right side of the spine within the mass of the sacrospinalis muscles. The pain followed the dermatome out to approximately the midaxillary line on the right side. Mrs. TB was unable to bend the trunk to the right or rotate the trunk to either side because of pain. She demonstrated a positive straight leg test (Lasegue's sign) on the right.

Given the results of Mrs. TB's evaluation and her history of steroid dependency, she was referred to her rheumatologist for a medical work-up, which revealed that she had sustained a compression fracture of the 11th thoracic vertebra on the 12th. She was prescribed bedrest for 3 weeks, with subsequent home visits from the physical therapist to instruct her in deep-breathing and bed mobility exercises and to help her put on a soft spinal corset. Owing to the instability and deformities of her upper extremities, she was unable to care for herself and hence stayed with a daughter. She was gradually progressed to weight-bearing exercises and returned to independence.

The significance of this case is that Mrs. TB had more than one diagnosis that could have caused her back pain. Because of her osteoporosis, risk factors, the type of event that could have elicited her pain, as well as the distribution of the pain, a vertebral compression fracture is a strong alternative diagnosis that requires confirmation before an appropriate physical therapy plan of care can be devised or implemented.

Cervical Spine Dysfunction

Mr. MJ is a 63-year-old custodian who was referred to physical therapy with a diagnosis of cervical spondylosis and radiculopathy to the right upper extremity. Cervical spine x-rays demonstrated moderate degenerative changes in C5 and C6, with anterior osteophytes from the margins of the vertebral bodies. There was narrowing of the cartilage space of the facet joints, with sclerosis and osteophytes encroaching the right neuroforamina of C5 and C6.

Upon physical examination of the cervical spine, it was noted that rotation to the right was limited to 45 degrees. Forward flexion was within the normal limits; however, hyperextension was limited to 20 degrees, with the presence of pain and crepitus. Rotation to the left was 50 degrees, with crepitus. Palpation revealed point tenderness over the coracoid process and tendon of the supraspinatus on the right. Postural examination of the cervical spine revealed a forward head posture. Mr. MJ reported that he had a history of migraine headaches and has become addicted to triazolam (Halcion) and propoxyphene napsylate (Darvocet). His addiction is currently being medically managed to get him off these drugs.

When asked about his job and work style, Mr. MJ described himself as a workaholic and a perfectionist. He claimed to exercise his neck every day to strengthen the muscles. When asked to demonstrate the exercises, he executed rapid rotatory motions of the neck as well as rapid flexion and extension exercises. His upper extremity exercises were demonstrated at the same velocity.

Given his diagnosis, forward head, work style, drug addiction, and methods of exercise, the treatment plan centered around his taking the responsibility to modify the way he was working, standing, and exercising. He was instructed to do long, slow stretching motions of the neck; to perform shoulder shrug exercises at a slow pace; to assess his workplace; and to pace himself so that he did not mechanically aggravate his neck. At night he was to use a cervical pillow, and during the day he was to use a cervical traction unit at home at least once a day. The traction was attached to his bed, which allowed him to lie down to do his treatment. Furthermore, he agreed to begin a swimming program of aerobic work to help his arthritis and to reduce stress.

In this particular case, the forward head posture could not be substantially reversed. Mr. MJ was, however, able to realize the value of gentle exercise on sore joints, relaxation techniques, life-style modifications, and aerobic conditioning. Too often, cervical exercises are performed incorrectly by the elder person, resulting in greater pain and immobility. Careful attention to avoid "overkill" in performing the exercise program can reap significant pain relief.

Degenerative Joint Disease of the Lumbosacral Spine

Mrs. HJ is a 78-year-old widow who was referred to the clinic with a diagnosis of degenerative joint and disk disease of the lumbosacral spine. She also has degenerative disease of the distal interphalangeal joints of both hands (Heberden's nodes), the carpometacarpal joint of the right thumb, the right hip, and both knees. Her x-ray findings of the lumbosacral spine revealed that she also had diffuse osteoporosis, discogenic sclerosis between T11 and T12 and L1 through S1 disk spaces, abundant osteophyte formation, spondylolisthesis of L4 on L5, and sacralization of L5—all of which are consistent with degenerative joint disease of the spine. Her right knee x-ray demonstrated degenerative changes in the patellofemoral compartment with cartilage loss in both the lateral and medial compartments of the knee. The left knee x-rays revealed mild osteophyte formation and subchondral sclerosis of the medial compartment of the knee.

Examination of the back revealed a kyphosis of the lumbar spine, decreased mobility in all active ranges of motion, bilateral positive straight leg raise signs, pain on palpation of the central low back region, and pain when asked to hyperextend the back. Assessment of her functional status revealed Mrs. HJ to be a very active 78-year-old person, particularly when one observed her x-rays. She noted that sitting or standing too long exacerbated her symptoms; however, if she intermingled rest with activity, she was able to get many things accomplished during the day. Mrs. HJ is highly active in managing her arthritis on a personal level. She is a positive individual with many hobbies, including having sung for 20 years with an internationally acclaimed religious choir.

Evaluation of her posture demonstrated that she had a slight forward head without any concurrent thoracic kyphosis, no scoliosis, and a lumbar kyphosis. She had a leg length difference of $1/2$ inch, which was easily corrected by an insole she wore in her right shoe. She commented that when she did not wear her orthosis, she noticed that her back would become more painful. She has been advised to have surgery in the past but has chosen to use exercise and other means of conservative treatment rather than take the risk of a surgical failure.

Her treatment in the clinic included applying heat, performing gentle flexion exercises (since hyperextension aggravates her symptoms), riding a stationary bike, and instruction in the use of a home transcutaneous electrical nerve stimulation (TENS) unit for pain control. Because of the arthritis in her knees and back, the stationary bicycle had to be adjusted so that she did not bend forward over the handlebars. The seat also had to be raised so that her knees were extended as much as possible when she peddled the bike. She was instructed to avoid flexion of the knee to 90 degrees.

Mrs. HJ's case is instructive because a hasty conclusion, based only on her x-rays, would project a life of severe disability. This serves to point out that all patients have a different level of self-efficacy and handle low back pain quite differently. Because of her mental and emotional outlook and careful incorporation of energy-conserving techniques in her daily life-style, Mrs. HJ was able to increase her quality of life, which could have been quite different if she had a lesser sense of mastery over the impact of arthritis on her life or if she had avoided consulting physical therapy at the appropriate time.

Summary

This chapter has reviewed the posture and postural changes found in elderly persons. Evaluation and treatment of posture are accomplished by using the generic skills of physical therapy and adapting them to the elderly patient. What is most important for the physical therapist to consider and remember is that not all elderly persons are alike—not all are stooped forward, and not all are unmotivated to change their posture. With professional guidance, they can make changes in their posture that will enhance the positive process of getting older.

References

1. Amstutz HC, Sisson HA: The structure of the vertebral spongiosa. *J Bone Joint Surg* 1969; 51B:540-550.
2. Amussen E, Freunsgaard K, Norgaard S: A follow-up longitudinal study of selected physiologic functions in former physical education students: After forty years. *J Am Geriatr Soc* 1975; 23:442-450.
3. Andriacchi TP, et al: A model for studies of mechanical interactions between the human spine & rib cage. *J Biomech* 1974; 7:497-507.
4. Anianson A, et al: Muscle function in 75-year-old men and women: A longitudinal study. *Scand J Rehabil Med Suppl* 1983; 90:92-102.
5. Anianson A, Grimby G: Muscle strength and endurance in elderly people with special reference to muscle morphology, in Amussen E, Jorgensen R (eds): *Biomechanics VI-A.* Baltimore, University Park Press, 1977.
6. Atkinson PJ: Variation in trabecular structure of vertebrae with age. *Calcif Tissue Res* 1967; 1:24-32.

7. Bartley MH, et al: The relationship of bone strength and bone quantity in health, disease and aging. *J Gerontol* 1966; 21:517-521.

8. Bell GH, et al: Variation in strength of vertebrae with age and their relation to osteoporosis. *Calcif Tissue Res* 1967; 1:75-86.

9. Benestad AM: Trainability of older men. *Acta Med Scand* 1965; 178:321-327.

10. Bohannon RW, et al: Decrease in timed balance test scores with aging. *Phys Ther* 1984; 64:1067-1070.

11. Brain L: Some unsolved problems of cervical spondylosis. *Br Med J* 1963; 1:771-777.

12. Brandt K, Palmoski M: Organization of ground substance proteoglycans in normal and osteoarthritic knee cartilage. *Arthritis Rheum* 1976; 19:209-215.

13. Bressler R: Treating geriatric depression: Current options. *Drug Ther* 1984; 9:129-144.

14. Briggs RC, et al: Balance performance among noninstitutionalized elderly women. *Phys Ther* 1989; 69:748-756.

15. Brody EM: Aging and family personality: A developmental view. *Fam Process* 1974; 13:23-39.

16. Brody H: An examination of cerebral cortex and brainstem aging, in Terry RD, Gershon S (eds): *Neurobiology of Aging.* New York, Raven Press, 1976.

17. Brown T, Hanson RJ, Yorra AJ: Some mechanical tests on the lumbosacral spine with particular reference to the intervertebral discs: A preliminary report. *J Bone Joint Surg* 1957; 39A:1135-1164.

18. Bugiani O, et al: Nerve cell loss with aging in the putamen. *Eur Neurol* 1978; 17:286-291.

19. Calkins E, Challa HR: Disorders of the joints and connective tissue, in Andres R, Bierman EL, Hazzard WR (eds): *Principles of Geriatric Medicine.* New York, McGraw-Hill, 1985.

20. Chapman EA, DeVries HA, Swezey R: Joint stiffness: Effects of exercise on young and old men. *J Gerontol* 1972; 27:218-221.

21. Choquette G, Ferguson RJ: Blood pressure reduction in "borderline" hypertensives following physical training. *Can Med Assoc J* 1973; 108:699-703.

22. Clarkson PM: The effect of age and activity level on simple and choice fractionated response time. *Eur J Appl Physiol* 1978; 40:17-25.

23. Corsellis JAN: Some observations on the Purkinje cell population and on brain volume in human aging, in Terry RD, Gershon S (eds): *Neurobiology of Aging.* New York, Raven Press, 1976.

24. Courpron P, Meunier PJ: Osteopenie et pathologie osseuse, in Bourliere F (ed): *Gerontologie.* Biologie et clinique. Paris, Flammarion, 1982.

25. Damon A, et al: Age and physique in healthy white veterans at Boston. *J Gerontol* 1972; 27:202-208.

26. Dunhill MS, Anderson JA, Whitehead R: Quantitative histological studies on age changes in bone. *J Pathol Bacteriol* 1967; 94:275.

27. Ekblom B: Effects of physical training on oxygen transport in man. *Acta Physiol Scand Suppl* 1969; 328:9.

28. Era T, Heikkinen E: Postural sway during standing and unexpected disturbance of balance in random sample of men of different ages. *J Gerontol* 1985; 40:287-295.

29. Fahn S: Differential diagnosis of tremors. *Med Clin North Am* 1972; 56:1363-1375.

30. Farfan HF: *Mechanical Disorders of the Low Back.* Philadelphia, Lea & Febiger, 1973.

31. Farfan HF, et al: The effects of torsion on the lumbar intervertebral joints, the role of torsion in the production of disc degeneration. *J Bone Joint Surg* 1970; 52A:468-497.

32. Farfan HF, Sullivan JD: The relationship of facet orientation to intervertebral disc failure. *Can J Surg* 1967; 10:179-185.

33. Fernie G, et al: The relationship of postural sway in standing to the incidence of falls in geriatric subjects. *Age Ageing* 1982; 11:11-16.

34. Ferris S, et al: Reaction time as a diagnostic measure in senility. *J Am Geriatr Soc* 1976; 24:529-533.

35. Fisher MB, Birren JE: Age and strength. *J Appl Psychol* 1947; 31:628-630.

36. Forssberg H, Nashner LM: Ontogenic development of postural control in man: Adaptation to altered support and visual conditions during stance. *J Neurosci* 1982; 2:545-552.

37. Frick MH, Konttinen A, Sarajas HSS: Effects of physical training at rest and during exercise. *Am J Cardiol* 1963; 12:142-147.

38. Friedenburg ZB, Miller WT: Degenerative disc disease of the cervical spine. *J Bone Joint Surg* 1963; 43A:1171-1178.

39. Galante JO: Tensile properties of the human lumbar annulus fibrosus. *Acta Orthop Scand* 1967; (Suppl 100):1-91.

40. Galasko D, et al: Neurological findings in Alzheimer's disease and normal aging. *Arch Neurol* 1990; 47:625-627.

41. Gallagher JC, Goldgar D, Moy A: Total bone calcium in normal women: Effect of age and menopausal status. *J Bone Miner Res* 1987; 2:491-496.

42. Grimby G, et al: Morphology and enzymatic capacity in arm and leg muscles in 78-81 year old men and women. *Acta Physiol Scand* 1982; 115:125.

43. Hartley LH, et al: Physical training in sedentary middle-aged and older men. III. Cardiac output and gas exchange at submaximal and maximal exercise. *Scand J Clin Lab Invest* 1969; 24:335-344.

44. Hassler R: Extrapyramidal control of the speed of behavior and its change by primary age processes, in Welford AT, Birren JE (eds): *Behaviour, Aging and the Nervous System.* Springfield, Ill, Charles C Thomas, 1965.

45. Hayes SC, et al: The development of the display and knowledge of sex-related motor behavior in children. *Child Behav Ther* 1981; 3:1.

46. Hirsch C: The reaction of intervertebral discs to compressive forces. *J Bone Joint Surg* 1955; 37A:1188-1196.

47. Hirsch C, Nachemson A: New observations on the mechanical behavior of lumbar discs. *Acta Orthop Scand* 1954; 23:254-283.

48. Huff FJ, et al: The neurologic examination in patients with probable Alzheimer's disease. *Arch Neurol* 1987; 44:929-932.

49. Huff FJ, Growdon JH: Neurological abnormalities associated with severity of dementia in Alzheimer's disease. *Can J Neurol Sci* 1986; 21:403-405.

50. Inglin B, Woollacott M: Age-related changes in anticipatory postural adjustments associated with arm movements. *J Gerontol* 1988; 43: 105-113.

51. Kauffman T: Posture and age. *Top Geriatr Rehabil* 1987; 2(4):13-28.

52. Kazarian LE: Creep characteristics of the human spinal column. *Orthop Clin North Am* 1975; 6:3-18.

53. Kendall EP, McCreary EK: *Muscles: Testing and Function.* Baltimore, Williams & Wilkins, 1993.

54. King AI, Prasad P, Ewing CL: Mechanism of spinal injury due to caudocephalad acceleration. *Orthop Clin North Am* 1975; 6:19-31.

55. Koller WC, et al: Motor signs are infrequent in dementia of the Alzheimer's type. *Ann Neurol* 1984; 16:514-515.

56. Kugler PN, Turvey MT: *Information, Natural Law and the Self Assembly of Rhythmic Movement.* Hillsdale, NJ, Erlbaum, 1987.

57. Lamy C, et al: The strength of the neural arch and the etiology of spondylolysis. *Orthop Clin North Am* 1975; 6:215-231.

58. Larsson L, Grimby G, Karlsson J: Muscle strength and speed of movement in relation to age and muscle morphology. *J Appl Physiol* 1979; 46:451-456.

59. Lewis PD: Parkinsonism-neuropathology. *Br Med J* 1971; 3:690-692.

60. Lexell JK, Henriksson-Larsson E, Sjostrom M: Distribution of different fiber types in human skeletal muscles. A study of cross-sections of whole muscle vastus lateralis. *Acta Physiol Scand* 1983; 117:115-122.

61. Lindahl O: Mechanical properties of dried defatted spongy bone. *Acta Orthop Scand* 1976; 47:11-19.

62. Longcope C, et al: Aromatization of androgens by muscle and adipose tissue in vivo. *J Clin Endocrinol Metab* 1978; 46:146-152.

63. Mann DMA, Yates PO: The effects of aging on the pigmented nerve cells of the human locus caeruleus and substantia nigra. *Acta Neuropathol (Berl)* 1979; 47:93-97.

64. Markolf KL, Morris JM: The structural components of the intervertebral disc. *J Bone Joint Surg* 1974; 56A:675-687.

65. Martin T: Normal development of movement and function: Neonate, infant and toddler, in Scully RM, Barnes MR (eds): *Physical Therapy.* Philadelphia, JB Lippincott, 1989.

66. Mathias S, Nayak U, Isaacs B: Balance and elderly patients: The "get up and go" test. *Arch Phys Med Rehabil* 1986; 67:387-389.

67. Maurel E, et al: Age dependent biochemical changes in dermal connective tissue. Relationship to histological and ultrastructural observations. *Connect Tissue Res* 1980; 8:33-39.

68. Mazess RB: Measurement of skeletal status by noninvasive methods. *Calcif Tissue Int* 1979; 28:89-92.

69. Mazess RB: Bone densiometry in osteoporosis. *Intern Med Specialist* 1987; 8:133.

70. McGee DJ: Assessment of posture, in McGee DJ (ed): *Orthopedic Physical Assessment.* Philadelphia, WB Saunders, 1997.

71. McGeer PL, McGeer EG, Suzuki JS: Aging and extrapyramidal function. *Arch Neurol* 1977; 34:33-35.

72. Messerer O: *Uber Elasticitat und Festigkeit Meuschlichen Knochen.* Stuttgart, JG Cottaschen Buchhandling, 1880.

73. Molsa PK, Marttila RJ, Rinne UK: Extrapyramidal signs in Alzheimer's disease. *Neurology* 1985; 34:1114-1116.

74. Nachemson A: The influence of spinal movements on the lumbar intradiscal pressure and on the tensile strength in the annulus fibrosus. *Acta Orthop Scand* 1963; 33:183-207.

75. Nachemson AL, Evans JH: Biomechanical study of human lumbar ligamentum flavum. *J Anat* 1969; 105:188-189.

76. Nachemson A, Morris JM: In vivo measurements of intradiscal pressure. Discometry, a method for determination of pressure in the lower lumbar discs. *J Bone Joint Surg* 1964; 46A:1077-1092.

77. Naylor A, Happy F, MacRae T: Changes in the human intervertebral disc with age: A biophysical study. *J Am Geriatr Soc* 1955; 3:964-973.

78. Ohama E, Ikuta F: Parkinson's disease: Distribution of Lewy bodies and monoaminergic neuron system. *Acta Neuropathol (Berl)* 1976; 34: 311-319.

79. Pakkenberg H, Brody H: The number of nerve cells in the substantia nigra in paralysis agitans. *Acta Neuropathol (Berl)* 1965; 5:320-324.

80. Panek PE: Age differences in perceptual style, selective attention and perceptual-motor reaction time. *Exp Aging Res* 1978; 4:377-387.

81. Panjabi MM, White AA, Johnson RM: Cervical spine mechanics as a function of transection components. *J Biomech* 1975; 8:327-336.

82. Peng MT, Lee LR: Regional differences of neuron loss of rat brain in old age. *Gerontology* 1979; 25:205-211.

83. Pepper GA, Robbins LJ: Improving geriatric drug therapy. *Generations* 1987; 12:57-61.

84. Perry O: Fracture of the vertebral end-plate in the lumbar spine. *Acta Orthop Scand* 1957; 25(suppl):1.

85. Prasud P, King AI, Ewing CL: The role of the articular facets and +Gz acceleration. *J Appl Mech* 1974; 41:321.

86. Ribot C, et al: Obesity and postmenopausal bone loss: The influence on vertebral density and bone turnover in postmenopausal women. *Bone* 1988; 8:327-331.

87. Roaf R: A study of the mechanics of spinal injuries. *J Bone Joint Surg* 1960; 42B:810-823.

88. Rockoff SD, Sweet E, Bleustein J: The relative contribution of trabecular and cortical bone to the strength of human lumbar vertebrae. *Calcif Tissue Res* 1969; 3:163-175.

89. Rolander SD, Blair WE: Deformation and fracture of the lumbar vertebrae end-plate. *Orthop Clin North Am* 1975; 6:75-81.

90. Rothschild BM: Age-related changes in skeletal muscle. *Geriatr Med Today* 1986; 5:87-95.

91. Salthouse TA: Speed and age: Multiple rates of age decline. *Exp Aging Res* 1976; 2:349-359.

92. Saylor C: Stigma, in Lubkin IM (ed): *Chronic Illness: Impact and Intervention.* Boston, Jones and Bartlett, 1990.

93. Schmitz TJ: Coordination assessment, in Sullivan SB, Schmitz TJ (eds): *Physical Rehabilitation: Assessment and Treatment,* ed 2. Philadelphia, FA Davis, 1994.

94. Scott TR, Netsky MG: The pathology of Parkinson's syndrome: A critical review. *Int J Neurol* 1961; 2:51-60.

95. Shepherd RJ: *Fitness of a Nation—The Canada Fitness Survey.* Basel, Karger, 1986.

96. Shephard RJ: Gross changes of form and function, in Shephard RJ (ed): *Physical Activity and Aging,* ed 2. Rockville, Md, Aspen, 1987.

97. Simon JR, Pouraghabagher AR: The effect of aging on the stages of processing in a choice reaction time task. *J Gerontol* 1978; 33:553-561.

98. Sinclair D: *Human Growth After Birth.* London, Oxford University Press, 1973.

99. Sixt E, Landahl S: Postural disturbances in a 75-year-old population: I. Prevalence and functional consequences. *Age Ageing* 1987; 16:393-398.

100. Speads CH, Leong MJ: Breathing: An approach for facilitating movement, in Jackson OL (ed): *Therapeutic Considerations for the Elderly.* New York, Churchill Livingstone, 1987.

101. Stelmach GE, Diewert GL: Aging information processing and fitness, in Borg G (ed): *Physical Work and Effort.* Oxford, Pergamon Press, 1977.

102. Surwillo WW, Titus TG: Reaction time and the psychological refractory period in children and adults. *Dev Psychobiol* 1976; 9:517-527.

103. Teravainen H, Calne DB: Motor system and normal aging, in Katzman R, Terry RD (eds): *The Neurology of Aging.* Philadelphia, FA Davis, 1983.

104. Thelen E, Kelso JAS, Fogel A: Self organizing systems and infant motor development. *Dev Rev* 1987; 7:39-65.

105. Thelen E, Ulrich B, Jenson J: The developmental origins of locomotion, in Woollacott MH, Shumway-Cook A (eds): *The Development of Posture and Gait Across the Lifespan.* Columbia, University of South Carolina Press, 1989.

106. Tkaczuk H: Tensile properties of human lumbar longitudinal ligaments. *Acta Orthop Scand Suppl* 1968; 115:1.

107. Viitsala JJ, et al: Muscular strength profiles and anthropometry in random samples of men aged 31-35, 51-55 and 71-75 years. *Ergonomics* 1985; 28:1563-1574.

108. Vijayashankar N, Brody H: A quantitative study of the pigmented neurons in the nuclei locus coeruleus and subcoeruleus in man as related to aging. *J Neuropathol Exp Neurol* 1979; 38:490.

109. Virgin W: Experimental investigations into physical properties of the intervertebral disc. *J Bone Joint Surg* 1951; 33B:607-611.

110. Weaver JK, Chalmers K: Cancellous bone: Its strength and changes with aging and an evaluation of some methods for measuring mineral content. *J Bone Joint Surg* 1966; 48A:289-298.

111. Weiss EB: Stress at the lumbosacral junction. *Orthop Clin North Am* 1975; 6:83-103.

112. White AA, Hirsch C: The significance of the vertebral posterior elements in the mechanics of the thoracic spine. *Clin Orthop* 1971; 81: 2-14.

113. White AA, Panjabi MM: *Clinical Biomechanics of the Spine.* Philadelphia, JB Lippincott, 1990.

114. White AA, et al: Biomechanical analysis of clinical stability in the cervical spine. *Clin Orthop* 1975; 109:85-96.

115. Woollacott M, Inglin B, Manchester D: Response and posture control: Neuromuscular changes in the older adult. *Ann N Y Acad Sci* 1988; 515:42-53.

116. Wright GR, Shephard RJ: Brake reaction time-effects of age, sex, and carbon monoxide. *Arch Environ Health* 1978; 33:141-150.

CHAPTER 18

BALANCE AND FALLS IN THE ELDERLY: ISSUES IN EVALUATION AND TREATMENT

JULIE M. CHANDLER, PT, PhD

INTRODUCTION

Everybody falls. Regardless of age, falling is a ubiquitous event experienced by all throughout life. Most falls, especially in children and young adults, are of minor consequence, are readily forgotten, and have no impact on subsequent function. Falls in the elderly, by contrast, are a major cause of morbidity and mortality—the consequences often extending far beyond minor injury to significant loss of functional independence and even death. The reason that falling becomes a major health hazard in persons older than 65 is a result of the complex and poorly understood interaction of biomedical, physiological, psychosocial, and environmental factors.

The overall objective of this chapter is to provide the reader with an understanding of the complex issues in the evaluation and treatment of the older person with instability. To meet this objective, we will follow a five-step process.

First, we will define the problem of falls in the elderly from an epidemiological perspective. Then we will delineate the multiple interacting factors in falls. Because the contribution of physiological impairment to falls is particularly important for the therapist to assess, we will review the role of postural control in instability. Based on the aforementioned information, we will present a strategy for the comprehensive assessment of the older faller, and finally, we will discuss the principles of intervention.

DEFINING THE PROBLEM OF FALLS

Falls are a major cause of morbidity and mortality in persons older than 65. They are the leading cause of death from injury, a rate that increases with advancing age. In persons older than 85, approximately two thirds of injury-related deaths are due to falls.[1] It is estimated that 30% of community-dwelling elders older than 65, 40% of those older than 80 years, and 66% of institutionalized elders fall each year. There is a greater-than-linear increase in the rate of falls between the ages of 60 to 65 and 80 to 85.[46] Because most falls do not result in injury requiring medical attention, it is likely that many falls go unreported and that fall rates are grossly underestimated.[44]

Major morbidity from falls includes hip and other fractures and serious soft tissue injuries that require immobilization or hospitalization. The majority of falls in the elderly, however, result in minor or no injury.[70] Regardless of injury severity, sequelae from even a benign fall can be devastating. A single fall often results in a fear of falling, which leads to a loss of confidence in one's ability to perform routine tasks, restriction in activities, social isolation, and increased dependence on others.[69] The ensuing deconditioning, joint stiffness, and muscle weakness that result from immobility can lead to more falls and further mobility restriction.[35,44] Fear of falling can also affect those with impaired mobility who have not fallen, leading to similar sequelae of restricted activity, social isolation, and increasingly greater dependence.[9,68]

Risk Factors

Seriousness of the consequences of falls coupled with the recognition of falling as an escalating problem in an aging population has prompted many investigators in the field of geriatrics to examine risk factors associated with falls. The U.S. Public Health Service estimates that two thirds of falls by the elderly are potentially preventable.

Identification of significant risk factors is an important step toward fall prevention. Risk factors associated with falls can be classified as either intrinsic (host) or extrinsic (environmental).[49] Host factors include symptoms such as dizziness, weakness, difficulty walking, or confusion, whereas environmental factors include conditions such as a slippery surface, loose rug, poor lighting, and obstacles. Tinetti and colleagues found that intrinsic factors such as sedative use, cognitive impairment, lower extremity disability, palmomental reflex, and foot problems increase the likelihood of falling in community-dwelling elders older than 75.[67] Not surprisingly, the likelihood of falling increases as risk factors accumulate. Overwhelming medical or environmental events such as stroke, syncope, or slipping on the ice account for a very small percentage of falls in the elderly and are usually eliminated from falls rate and risk factor analysis. Lach and co-workers found that intrinsic factors such as dizziness, weakness, difficulty walking, and confusion accounted for 45% of falls in community-dwelling elders, whereas slippery surfaces, loose rugs, loose objects, or poor lighting accounted for 39% of falls.[29] For most falls in the elderly, however, it is difficult to distinguish between those that are intrinsically and extrinsically precipitated. It is likely that most falls are a result of the complex interaction of host and environmental factors.[30,64,65] Multisystem failure can lower one's threshold for environmentally precipitated falls. In the 80-year-old diabetic person with severe osteoarthritis of the hip, peripheral neuropathy, and failing vision, the likelihood of tripping over a carpet edge or raised threshold increases dramatically.

Aging Theory: Concepts Pertinent to Falls in the Elderly

While it is useful to identify potential markers of physical frailty that may contribute to falls risk, one must be careful not to simply treat a "laundry list" of host and environmental conditions with the hope that falls risk will diminish. The reason for this is that the process of aging itself is a complex event; several important axioms in gerontology should be considered in the comprehensive evaluation and treatment of the frail older person.[61]

The first of these axioms is the notion of functional reserve. *Functional reserve* refers to the excess or redundant function that is present in virtually all physiological systems such that a significant degree of physiological function can be lost long before clinical symptoms appear. In the older adult, functional reserve is markedly diminished, and the threshold for clinically observable loss of function is lowered. For the older faller, it may be that redundant functions within the postural control system are lost gradually. As losses accumulate, a critical threshold is reached, and clinical signs and symptoms such as falling and instability are observed.

The second important axiom is that aging is heterogeneous. Variability between individuals increases with age, and the discrepancy between biological age and chronological age widens. It is therefore difficult to examine the effect of age on any one physiological system because individuals have different combinations of subtle and interacting pathologies.

Third, an elderly person's function may represent more or less than the sum of losses in his/her physiological systems. Function is likely to be maintained when only one sensory component is compromised.[15] When additional subtle losses occur across other domains, e.g., central processing or effector, compensatory capacity may become compromised and function lost. In other words, function is the outcome produced by the integration of the system's physiological components. When a single component is lost, function can be maintained by compensatory mechanisms through other components. When multiple subtle losses accumulate across other components, compensatory capacity may become compromised. It is therefore critical when interpreting diagnostic and physiological information to examine integrated measures of functional performance to understand the functional consequences of physiological losses.

Finally, the consequences of impaired mobility and poor balance in the older person may vary depending on his/her social, emotional, and behavioral resources. A strong social support network and sound judgment in risk-taking behavior may mitigate the effect of poor balance control and reduce falls risk.

MULTIFACETED APPROACH TO THE FALLS PROBLEM

Falls themselves are a heterogeneous phenomenon. Falls represent a failure of the body to remain upright but do not necessarily signal a disruption in the integrity of the postural control system. For some, a fall or series of falls may be a marker of an acute illness or other overwhelming medical event. For others, a fall or falls can occur in the presence of extreme environmental conditions or unusual activity. In most cases, however, falls represent the failure of the person with impaired functional capacity to meet the intrinsic and extrinsic demands of mobility within specific environments.[44] In general, as one ages, falls risk shifts from being spread out over many diverse activities, situations, and environments to being focused on basic movements required for routine daily activities.[46,48]

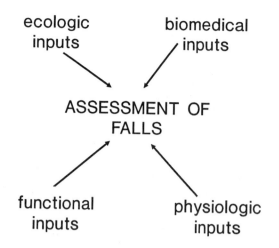

FIG. 18-1   Four approaches to the assessment of falls. (Adapted from Studenski S: Falls, in Calkins E (ed): *The Practice of Geriatrics*, ed 2. Philadelphia, WB Saunders, 1992.)

Because of the complexity of falls themselves and of interpreting falls risk, a multifaceted approach to examining the falls phenomenon in the geriatric patient is useful. Studenski suggests four approaches to assessing the falling syndrome in the geriatric patient: ecological, biomedical, physiological, and functional (Fig. 18-1).[58] The ecological approach focuses on the extrinsic components of a fall event, i.e., the interaction between the organism and the environment. A fall can occur in the presence of an unusual environment, e.g., icy surface, in a person with minimal impairment. A fall can also occur in a mildly impaired person attempting to negotiate a gravel pathway in unfamiliar territory. Or a severely impaired person may fall while walking in his home. Such an approach allows the examiner to assess the contribution and potential modification of environmental factors in fall events.

The biomedical component of the assessment focuses on medical events that are potentially contributory to falls. It is important for the practitioner to identify acute and chronic diseases that result in instability. For example, acute illnesses and conditions such as electrolyte abnormalities, infections, drug side effects, dehydration, orthostatic hypotension, blood loss, and hypoxemia can all cause weakness, lightheadedness, and falls. The possibility of an acute process in the chronic faller can be signaled by a sudden, unexplained change in fall frequency. Diseases that cause falls can be classified by organ system. For example, cardiovascular conditions include arrhythmias, aortic stenosis, and carotid sinus sensitivity. Neuromuscular diseases such as cerebrovascular accidents (CVAs), seizures, Parkinson's disease, myelopathies, cerebellar disease, normal pressure hydrocephalus, brain tumors, myopathies, peripheral neuropathies, and vestibular disease can also cause instability and falling. While it is relatively rare for a single diagnosis to account wholly for falls in the geriatric patient (with the exception of Parkinson's disease), this approach is useful for identifying treatable disease components of the falls syndrome.

The pathophysiological component of geriatric falls assessment allows for identification of deficits in postural control that contribute to instability. Components of the postural control system that are assessed include sensory; effector (strength, range of motion, biomechanical alignment, flexibility); and central processing. Current postural control theory as outlined in the next section of this chapter forms the conceptual basis for the physical therapist's assessment and treatment of the geriatric faller.

Finally, the functional components of the assessment allow the examiner to identify important routine movements with which the patient has difficulty. These movements represent the integrated function of the postural control system and signal how the "output" of the system is affected by deficits in its components.

POSTURAL CONTROL THEORY
Physiology of Balance
Adequate postural control requires keeping the center of gravity over the base of support during both static and dynamic situations. The body must be able to respond to translations of the center of gravity voluntarily imposed, e.g., intentional movement, and involuntarily or unexpectedly imposed, e.g., slip, trip.

Physiologically speaking, how does the body maintain balance? First, a person must continually acquire information about the body's position and trajectory in space. This is done through the sensory system. Second, the body must determine, in advance, an effective and timely response (central processing). And third, the body must carry out that response via the effector system (strength, range of motion, flexibility, endurance).

Sensory data critical to balance are provided primarily from visual, vestibular, and somatosensory systems. Vision helps to orient the body in space by referencing vertical and horizontal axes of objects around them. In standing, vision helps to detect slight postural shifts by providing information to the central nervous system (CNS) about the position and movements of the body parts in relation to each other and the external environment.

Components of vision that are clinically important to consider include (1) acuity, (2) contrast sensitivity, (3) peripheral vision, and (4) depth perception. *Acuity* refers to the ability to detect subtle differences in shapes and letters, whereas *contrast sensitivity* is the ability to detect subtle differences in shading and patterns, e.g., the ability to discriminate steps covered with a heavily patterned carpet. *Peripheral vision* is the ability to see from the side while looking straight ahead, and *depth perception* is the ability to distinguish distances.

The vestibular system also provides key sensory data for balance control. This system provides the CNS with information (via the otoliths and semicircular canals) regarding head movement and position. Vestibular input is used to generate compensatory eye movements and postural responses during head movements and helps to resolve conflicting information from visual images and actual movement. Information from sensory receptors in the vestibular apparatus interacts with visual and somatosensory information to produce proper body alignment and postural control.

Somatosensation is the third important input to the sensory system for balance control. Proprioceptive input provided to the CNS by joint, tendon, and muscle receptors gives information regarding the motion of the body with respect to the support surface and motion of the body segments with respect to each other.

Sensory information provided from visual, vestibular, and somatosensory systems is somewhat redundant in balance control. Blind people can stand and walk without losing balance. Nevertheless, it is well-documented that in the absence of diagnosable disease, visual (especially contrast sensitivity),[18] vibratory, and proprioceptive input are commonly diminished in the older adult.[31,37] Specifically, Lord and colleagues found that clinical loss of contrast sensitivity was associated with a higher incidence of falls in older adults.[32] Thus, redundancy in sensory input may be compromised either as a result of aging alone or as a result of subclinical disease processes to which older adults are particularly prone.[23,76]

Central processing is the second major physiological component of balance control. It can be regarded as the process of "setting up" the postural response. Horak and Nashner's systems approach to balance control proposes that the central nervous system maps the location of the center of gravity and adaptively organizes its response to disequilibrium by preprogramming postural sensorimotor strategies. The preprogrammed strategies are based on the body's biomechanical constraints, available sensory information, the environmental context, and prior experience.[22]

In simpler terms, the CNS receives sensory information provided by the visual, vestibular, and somatosensory systems; processes it in the context of previously learned responses; and executes a corrective automatic postural response that is guided by or expressed through the mechanical structure in which it sits. Automatic postural responses are sometimes referred to as *long loop reflexes* that occur at latencies of approximately 100 to 120 msec in normal young adults. They are distinguished from stretch (monosynaptic) reflexes, which occur rapidly (at about 50 msec) in a very stereotypical pattern, and voluntary movement that is not stereotypical and occurs at latencies of at least 150 msec. Automatic postural responses are elicited in both feedback and feedforward situations. *Feedback* refers to situations in which the body is perturbed by an external event, such as slipping on a rug, tripping, or being pushed. The center of gravity is displaced, and the CNS, based on the sensory information it has received, sets up a postural response to bring the center of gravity back over the base of support. Responses can be either protective or corrective. *Feedforward* describes a situation in which the CNS sets up a postural response in anticipation of a disturbance of the center of gravity, such as catching a ball or simply raising the arms. The movement of reaching to catch a ball is a voluntary displacement of the center of gravity, but the automatic postural responses must precede the voluntary movement in order to stabilize the center of gravity and allow the movement to take place.

Research in automatic postural responses has focused on neurophysiological responses to postural perturbations in feedback paradigms. Movable platforms have been used to create perturbations (forward, backward, or rotatory) as the patient stands in his/her normal stance. In this paradigm, the base of support is displaced, and a postural response to restore normal upright alignment is elicited. Using electromyography (EMG), muscle responses to such perturbations have been identified. The primary variables examined are latency (time to muscle response) and sequence (the order in which muscles respond). Based on his original work in this area, Nashner has proposed a model to interpret postural responses using this paradigm.[40-43] Though recent research in this area suggests that postural response mechanisms are more complex than originally proposed by this model, it does provide a framework from which to understand postural responses better. Nashner describes three basic strategies as "normal" responses to unexpected postural perturbations:

1. An ankle strategy is used with relatively small disturbances of the base of support. The center of gravity is perturbed backward or forward, and the body moves as a relatively rigid mass about the ankle joints, like an inverted pendulum, to bring the center of gravity back over the base of support. The latency is approximately 100 to 120 msec for healthy young adults, and the typical muscle sequence follows a distal-to-proximal pattern of lower extremity activation. For example, a forward movement of the platform induces a posterior displacement of the center of gravity, similar to a slip on a rug. Because this perturbation is relatively mild on a wide stable base of support, the response is subtle, and corrective movement occurs primarily around the ankle joint. In a typical healthy young adult, the tibialis anterior would be activated first (about 100 msec), followed by a quadriceps response as the center of gravity is pulled back over the base of support. A perturbation in the opposite direction (induced forward sway) would stimulate a gastrocnemius-hamstring response.

2. For more forceful perturbations or for perturbations that occur while a person is standing on a narrow or unstable base of support, a hip strategy is typically seen. In this response, primary movement occurs at the hip (flexion or extension) as the center of gravity moves rapidly back and forth over a relatively short distance. Instead of distal-to-proximal sequencing, the reverse is typically seen, i.e., a proximal-to-distal pattern.

3. The third major classification is the stepping strategy, which occurs in situations in which the center of gravity is displaced beyond the limits of the base of support. A stepping or stumbling strategy is necessary to regain equilibrium because neither the ankle nor hip strategy is sufficient to move the center of gravity back over the base of support.

Investigation in this area has expanded immensely during the past decade. Recent studies stress the importance of medial-lateral stability in addition to anteroposterior stability. Impairment of responses to mediolateral perturbation may be more strongly related to falls than anteroposterior response abnormalities in older adults. McIlroy and Maki have shown that older adults tend to take multiple steps to recover from unexpected perturbations, with the later steps usually directed toward recovering lateral stability.[39] In addition, kinematic analysis of postural responses and of actual falls demonstrate that arm movements are critical components of the postural response. Arm movements can contribute to stability by altering the center of mass (compensatory movement), grasping, or protecting against injury.[36,50]

Examination of EMG responses along the axial skeleton to the neck during postural perturbation show that normal postural control mechanisms as evaluated electromyographically are more complex and variable than originally postulated in the Nashner model.[27] Keshner found that response patterns do not always ascend in a distal-to-proximal sequence, even to subtle perturbations.[26] She postulates that sequences vary because muscles are activated either by a combination of inputs from different sensory components (vestibular, visual, neck proprioceptors) activated by the perturbation or by proprioceptive inputs at each joint. It appears that people have distinct muscle response patterns but that response patterns are variable among individuals. Her work suggests that the CNS should provide multiple alternatives for attaining the goal of postural stability. The key to success in maintaining balance is to develop adaptable and flexible strategies that will meet the demands of a complex and constantly changing environment. Many investigators have examined the effects of age on postural responses.[24,33,34,37,55,77,79] While distal-to-proximal sequencing in response to platform perturbation appears to be the predominant pattern, a higher incidence of proximal-to-distal sequencing in the older adult has been observed. A higher incidence of co-contraction in antagonist muscle groups has also been observed. Such altered sequencing may indicate compromised postural control in the older adult.[78] Other studies have shown similar variability in response patterns in healthy older adults and older fallers alike.[59] It is thus not clear exactly what significance EMG sequence has in the postural response of the aging adult.

Findings from studies of response latencies have consistently demonstrated delays of approximately 20 to 30 msec in the healthy older adult.[56,59,77,78] It has been postulated that specific timing, if delayed sufficiently, may significantly affect one's ability to produce an effective response. Thus, inability to fire fast enough, regardless of activation sequence, may be a significant factor in the patient who presents with instability. Studenski and colleagues reported evidence of delayed latency in older fallers when compared with age-matched nonfallers. Latencies are not only delayed in the healthy older adult but are even further delayed in the older person with a history of unexplained falls.[59]

In summary, the variables of sequence and latency are used to describe central-processing mechanisms in both feedback and feedforward paradigms. The relationship between responses to artificially imposed perturbations and responses to balance disturbances in everyday life is not known. Nevertheless, it would appear that a patient with significantly delayed latencies or a patient who demonstrates co-contraction instead of an organized distal-to-proximal or proximal-to-distal response to a platform perturbation is likely to also respond ineffectively to mild or moderate center of gravity displacements during functional activities. The CNS should be able to provide multiple alternatives for attaining the single goal of postural stability.[26] The key to successful balance control is to develop adaptable strategies that will meet the demands presented in a complex environment.

The third major physiological component of balance is the effector component, which constitutes the biomechanical apparatus through which the centrally programmed response must be expressed. Factors such as range of motion, muscle torque and power, postural alignment, and endurance can all affect the capacity for a person to effectively respond to a disturbance of balance. Studenski determined that elderly fallers produce significantly weaker distal lower extremity torque than healthy older adults.[59] Similarly, Whipple and colleagues found that nursing home residents with a history of recurrent falls demonstrated diminished torque production of both the ankle and knee.[72] The ability to generate ankle torque rapidly is also a key factor in balance recovery and can be diminished in the older adult.[63] Thus, sufficient muscle power of the lower extremity muscles is a key element in effective balance control.

Less is known about the influence of joint limitations on righting reactions and falls. Back extension and neck range of motion may be reduced and arthritis more common in elderly fallers.[67] Intuitively, sufficient flexibility in the mechanical structure is needed for effective execution of the balance response. Loss of flexibility may lead to a less efficient or ineffective response strategy.[51]

Summary: Influence of Age on Postural Control

The aging process affects all components of postural control—sensory, effector, and central processing. In the sensory system, visual acuity, contrast sensitivity, and depth perception worsen with age. Changes in the vestibular-ocular reflex are consistent with age-related peripheral anatomical changes in the vestibular system. Mild proprioceptive and vibratory sense loss have also been demonstrated in older adults. In the effector system, joint stiffness and loss of range of motion occur as a result of age-related degenerative changes in the joints themselves. Declines in muscle strength with age are associated with decreases in the size and number of muscle fibers. Increased stiffness in connective tissues in general likely contributes to age-related losses in joint range of motion and flexibility. In the central processing component, general slowing of sensory information processing coupled with slowing of nerve conduction velocity may contribute to the observed 20 to 30 msec delay in onset (latency) of automatic postural responses. Other manifestations of age-related changes in central processing include increased incidence of proximal-to-distal sequencing, increased incidence of co-contraction of antagonist muscle groups, increased static sway, and increases in the number of steps required to recover balance after perturbation. In the aging adult, it is difficult to distinguish pure age effects from effects of the subtle subclinical diseases and life-style changes that accompany the aging process. Nevertheless, it is important to understand that subtle changes in any single component of the postural control system are not likely to be sufficient to cause postural instability. Redundancy in the system can guard against subtle losses in any single component. Accumulation of mild deficits across multiple components of postural control, however, may diminish the compensatory capacity of the system, leading to a lowered threshold for instability.

Relationship Between Postural Control and Falls: A Model

It is clear from the previous discussion that the issue of balance impairment and falls is a complex and multifaceted problem in the aging adult. With the exception of overwhelming medical or environmental events, falls in the elderly usually occur in those with physical impairment.[6,25,54] Yet the relationship between physical impairment and falls is not linear. Factors outside of physical function—psychosocial, cognitive, environmental—can modify the risk of falling in persons with severely impaired mobility.[62] Thus, physical impairment may be a necessary but not sufficient condition for falling.[61]

At the highest levels of physical mobility and balance control, falls risk is very low. At very low levels of physical mobility and balance control, falls risk is also low because the person is unable to displace his/her center of gravity. The relationship between falls risk and physical impairment between those two extremes is not clear. In a person with moderately impaired mobility, the risk of falling may be modified if he/she has social support to help with risky tasks. A person's risk-taking behavior can also affect his/her falls risk. If a person recognizes that he/she is at risk for falling in a particular situation and modifies his/her behavior, falls risk will be minimized. If, on the other hand, he/she recognizes the risk of falling but prefers to take the risk by performing the task, the risk of falling is heightened. Another important consideration is that improved physical function may not necessarily reduce falls risk but may simply alter the types of activities during which falls occur. Finally, cognitive impairment can include a loss of judgment in risk-taking behavior and has been strongly associated with falls risk.[67]

Comprehensive assessment of the older faller must include not only evaluation of physiological impairments and physical performance deficits but also an assessment of cognitive, behavioral, environmental, and social factors.

EXAMINATION AND EVALUATION

Comprehensive assessment of the older faller requires a multidisciplinary team effort, of which the physical therapist is an integral part. Other members include a physician, a social worker, a nurse, and possibly a psychologist or counselor. Medical screening crucial to the evaluation process includes (1) examination of the patient's current and past medications for potential interactions and side effects (hypnotics, sedatives, tricyclic antidepressants, tranquilizers, and antihypertensive drugs have all been associated with falls and instability)[5,7,49,67] and (2) identification of medical conditions that may contribute to unsteadiness (focal neurological lesion, cardiovascular conditions, orthostasis); diseases manifesting with balance disorders; and metabolic causes of instability. The social worker or psychologist can gather information from the patient and family about social and financial resources, depression, cognitive function, and family dynamics. The physical therapist gathers information about impairments in the postural control system and about functional performance deficits that contribute to the person's disability. Successful management of the geriatric faller, then, is based on input from all sources of the evaluation.

How should you approach the older patient referred for instability and falls? Because of the complex nature of the problem, a systematic approach to the evaluation procedure is useful (Box 18-1).

Box 18-1

ELEMENTS IN THE ASSESSMENT OF INSTABILITY IN THE OLDER FALLER

I. Falls history
   A. Onset—sudden vs. gradual, frequency
   B. Environmental factors
   C. Activities at time of fall
   D. Presence of dizziness, vertigo, lightheadedness
   E. Current medications, past medications
   F. Direction of falls
II. Etiological assessment
   A. Sensory
      1. Vision
      2. Proprioception, vibration
      3. Vestibular
   B. Effector
      1. Strength
      2. Range of motion, flexibility
      3. Endurance
   C. Central processing
      1. Feedback
      2. Feedforward
      3. Response to changing conditions
III. Functional assessment
   A. Standing reach
   B. Mobility skills
   C. Varied conditions of performance
IV. Environmental assessment
   A. Functional home assessment—interaction of patient and home

History

It is useful to have a clear idea of the patient's perception of his/her unsteadiness problem before gathering other relevant historical information. Knowing how the unsteadiness is primarily affecting the patient or family member provides a useful framework from which to proceed with the evaluation. It is important to gather specific information regarding the patient's falls, such as onset of falls, environmental conditions, activities at the time of falls, direction of falls, and medications. For example, it is useful to know whether the onset of falls is sudden (acute medical condition) or gradual (slowly deteriorating compensatory mechanisms). In addition, it is important to know what environmental conditions are associated with falls. Was the fall inside the home (consider factors such as lighting, chair height, steps) or outside the home (review factors such as unfamiliar territory, uneven surfaces, more vigorous activities)? Finding out about the activity at the time of the fall can give insight into how much the postural control system was being stressed. The presence of vertigo or dizziness at the time of the fall can signal a circulatory or vestibular function problem. Information regarding the direction of falls (forward, backward, to the side) is useful because reproducible circumstances of falls may signal specific postural control deficits. Finally, the patient's current and past medications should be noted for their possible contribution to unsteadiness, e.g., antidepressants, sedatives, tranquilizers, and antihypertensives.

Etiological Assessment

The etiological assessment allows identification of deficits in the sensory, effector, and central-processing systems that may contribute to the falls problem.

Sensory

Sensory examination should include vision, vestibular, and somatosensory systems. Important aspects of vision to consider include acuity, contrast sensitivity (ability to discriminate fine details in a cluttered environment), peripheral fields, and depth perception.

Acuity, peripheral fields, and depth perception can be easily screened in the clinic. For acuity, having the patient read a pocket-size Snellen chart (Fig. 18-2) can give a quick gross estimate of his/her ability to discriminate fine detail. A score of 20/200 may signal that vision is contributing to the patient's instability. For peripheral fields, the examiner brings his/her fingers from behind the patient's head at eye level while the patient stares straight ahead. The patient identifies when he/she first notices the examiner's finger in his/her side view. A significant field cut unilaterally or bilaterally would be noteworthy. For depth perception, the examiner holds his/her index fingers parallel and pointing upward in front of the patient at eye level. As the examiner moves his/her fingers apart (one forward, one back), the patient identifies when the fingers are back together (parallel). If the patient is off by 3 inches or more, then depth perception may be a problem. Examination of existing lenses may also be useful.

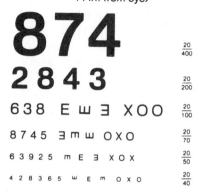

Fig. 18-2   Pocket-sized Snellen chart for gross visual acuity screening.

Bifocals magnify objects and can be very disorienting during activities such as stair climbing and descent.

Vestibular function should also be assessed. Vestibuloocular and vestibulospinal reflexes are critical in balance control. Vestibulospinal input is particularly important for maintaining upright body position during movement. Because of the complexity of the pathway, few good clinical tests of vestibulospinal function exist. Vestibuloocular tests are therefore used more frequently to assess vestibular function. Vestibuloocular function can be tested by having the patient maintain gaze on a fixed object, e.g., examiner's finger, while he/she turns his/her head rapidly to the right or left. Normally, a person should be able to maintain gaze without difficulty. In the presence of vestibular dysfunction the patient's eyes will move off target and will make a corrective saccade to regain fixation. Other clinical tests of dynamic stability that grossly assess integrated vestibular function include (1) reading a book while walking or (2) marching in place with eyes closed. In the first test, the patient should be able to read while walking without losing balance. The patient with vestibular dysfunction will be unable to maintain visual fixation on the reading material and move at the same time. Marching in place with the eyes closed is also difficult for the patient with a vestibular lesion. When asked to perform this test, he/she will deviate markedly from his/her initial position.[21]

Somatosensory examination includes proprioception and vibration. Both should be assessed in a distal-to-proximal sequence. A patient with normal proprioception should be able to detect very subtle motion of the great toe (less than 5 mm). Vibratory sense can be assessed by placing a tuning fork at the first metatarsal head. If vibratory sense and proprioception are present distally, there is no need to proceed proximally.

The Sensory Integration Test (SIT) developed by Shumway-Cook and Horak can also be used clinically to assess the influence of vision, somatosensation, and vestibular function on standing balance.[53] The SIT includes a series of six tests under varying sensory conditions during which the patient is timed and standing balance is assessed. Visual, proprioceptive, and vestibular inputs are manipulated in various combinations to provide six different sensory conditions. It is important to note that as sensory conditions change, the expected response also changes. That is, under conditions of diminished sensory input, increased sway is anticipated. The patient with severe joint motion loss or weakness may be unable to maintain his/her balance under the conditions of increased sway. This patient may not have a problem with sensory integration but rather with a faulty effector system that is unable to execute a sufficient motor response to maintain stability under those conditions. While the SIT cannot identify specific causes of balance dysfunction, it can be useful in identifying conditions under which the patient may have difficulty. Technologically sophisticated versions of the sensory integration test, referred to generically as *dynamic posturography,* are available commercially and provide information about balance performance under different sensory conditions.

Effector

Effector components that should be evaluated are strength, range of motion, and endurance.

Strength. Traditional methods of manual muscle testing may not provide the most useful information with regard to balance control. This is especially true in muscle groups for which large displacements and fast, forceful movements are required, i.e., quadriceps, hamstrings. Isokinetic testing of the quadriceps, hamstrings, dorsiflexors, and plantarflexors at both slow and moderate speeds gives a more accurate picture of the patient's torque-generating capacity under different conditions. A patient who can produce sufficient torque at very slow speeds but has difficulty generating torque at faster speeds may have difficulty generating torque quickly enough to produce an effective postural response.[63] In the more proximal hip and trunk muscles, whose primary function is stabilization, an isometric muscle test may be more appropriate.

Range of Motion. Measurement of range of motion and flexibility using standard goniometric methods is an important component of the etiological evaluation. Important musculoskeletal regions to be assessed include ankle, knee, hip, trunk, and cervical spine. While it is not known to what extent limited flexibility contributes to instability in the frail older adult, it is clear that a patient with severe limitation of trunk, neck, or lower extremity motion will be constrained by the biomechanical apparatus through which his/her postural response must be expressed. The variety of postural response strategies that are required to function in a complex environment may be restricted as a result of a stiff body segment.

Endurance. Another effector component to consider in overall stability and function is endurance. A patient may be able to generate adequate force during a few repeated contractions but may have difficulty during tasks that require continued efforts. One useful quantitative test for assessing endurance in frail older adults is the 6-minute walk. In this test, the patient walks up and down a premeasured walkway, e.g., a hospital corridor, at his/her normal pace for 6 minutes, resting as needed. The distance covered after 6 minutes is recorded.[11,19]

Central Processing

Central processing can be grossly assessed in both feedforward and feedback situations. The examiner looks for (1) the effectiveness of the patient's response to induced, unexpected perturbations (feedback) and (2) the ability of the patient to maintain stability during movements that intentionally displace the center of gravity (feedforward). It is important to note, however, that responses to such tests represent integrated function of the postural control system and not just central processing. Because responses are ultimately expressed through the effector system, an ineffective response to a perturbation may be the result of weakness or stiffness rather than faulty central processing.

A simple semiquantitative method of testing responses to induced posterior perturbation is the Postural Stress Test (PST).[75] In this test, motor responses to postural perturbations of varying degrees are measured during normal standing using a simple pulley-weight system that displaces the center of gravity behind the base of support. The PST measures an individual's ability to withstand a series of destabilizing forces applied at the level of the subject's waist. Scoring of the postural responses is based on a nine-point ordinal scale, in which a score of 9 represents the most efficient postural response, and a score of 0 represents complete failure to remain upright. Mild perturbations should require minimal response (corresponding to a score of 8 or 9), whereas larger perturbations may require a stepping strategy (corresponding to a score of 4, 5, or 6). Studies have shown that healthy elders demonstrate effective balance responses during this test but that elderly fallers are likely to show ineffective responses (corresponding to scores of 0, 1, or 2).[8] The test is useful in grossly assessing the patient's capacity to withstand mild, unexpected perturbations. An alternative to the PST is a simple manual test that can be performed in any clinic setting. In this test, the therapist stands behind the patient and pulls him/her backward at waist level several times with varying degrees of force (mild to moderate). The therapist looks for the appropriateness of the patient's responses to a given level of perturbation. For example, the patient should be able to maintain upright stance using minimal postural response (ankle dorsiflexion only) when the pull backward is very mild. With a more forceful pull backward, the patient should be able to recover his/her balance using a hip or stepping strategy. The patient who cannot execute an effective response will require intervention by the therapist to keep from falling. Similarly, the patient who requires multiple steps to recover balance when given a very mild perturbation will likely lose his/her balance with more forceful balance disturbances.

Feedforward postural responses can be assessed by having the patient perform voluntary movements that require mild to moderate displacements of his/her center of gravity. For example, in his/her normal standing position, asking the patient to raise his/her arms in front of him/her requires subtle postural stabilization by the lower extremity and trunk muscles in preparation for mild displacement of the center of gravity caused by arm raising. Varying the speed of the task can give further information regarding the patient's ability to organize his/her preparatory postural responses in a timely fashion. Catching a ball thrown slightly off center, slowly, then faster, is an example of a higher-level feedforward task that further stresses the postural control system.

Reaction time is another element of central processing that may be useful to assess. Tests involving simple lower or upper extremity movements in response to a light cue are examples of reaction time tests and may be abnormally slowed in the older faller.[45, 57] Patla and colleagues developed a lower extremity reaction time test in which the subject takes a step forward, backward, or to the side in response to the appropriate light cue.[47] This task may be particularly relevant in the older faller because it requires movements that are initiated to avoid collision and potential falls and requires weight transfer to the other limb before the initiation of movement. Total reaction time in this test reflects the process of stimulus detection, response selection, and planning and movement execution.

Functional Assessment

While identification of defective components of the postural control system can help to guide specific treatment planning, more critical is the assessment of the patient's functional performance. It is during this part of the evaluation that the therapist must determine how specific deficits in the system affect the patient's overall function. Given a significant level of hip abductor and hip extensor weakness, for example, one would expect the patient to demonstrate instability during activities such as walking, stair climbing, or rising from a chair. If the patient's balance problems are not manifested during those activities but rather during simple reaching tasks or when turning to change direction, then hip weakness may not be a key component of the patient's instability and may not need to be addressed in treatment. A series of progressively challenging mobility tasks can be used to screen for functional balance deficits. The progressive mobility skills protocol takes the patient through a series of increasingly complex tasks from sitting unsupported to stair climbing (Table 18-1).[60] Failure to perform a task at any point during the test theoretically precludes further testing. Overall performance can be scored and used as baseline information against which to measure change. Performance on individual tasks in the protocol can be used to identify specific functional deficits that can be addressed in treatment. Other quantitative performance-oriented scales such as the Balance Scale,[2,3] the "get-up and go" test,[38] the Performance Oriented Mobility Assessment (POMA)[66], and the Physical Disability Index[17] have also been developed for use in both clinic and research settings. Choice of the appropriate scale depends on the mobility level of the patient. Some scales were developed in relatively healthy older adults (mobility skills, POMA), whereas others were developed for use in more frail populations (Balance Scale, Physical Disability Index). Another quantitative and informative measure of functional performance is the functional reach measure.[13] During this test the patient is asked to reach forward as far as possible from a comfortable standing posture. The excursion of the arm from start to finish is measured via a yardstick affixed to the wall (Fig. 18-3). This measure tests the ability and willingness of the patient to move to the margins of his/her base of support voluntarily. Duncan and colleagues have shown that frail persons with reaches less than 6 inches have 4 times the likelihood of falling than persons with a reach greater than 10 inches.[14] An excellent critical review of validated functional performance measures has been published recently.[4]

While quantitative tests are useful for measurement and documentation purposes, qualitative description and observation are also important. During the functional assessment

Table 18-1
Progressive Mobility Skills Assessment Task

Task	Performance (scoring)
Sitting balance	Subjects sit in firm-surfaced chair with arms crossed, unsupported
Sitting reach	Subjects grasp ruler held at shoulder level 12 inches from outstretched arm
Chair rise	Subjects rise from standard straight chair with arms folded
Standing balance	Subjects stand steadily, without support, for 60 seconds
Pick up object	Subjects pick up ruler placed on the floor 2 ft in front of them without holding on for support
Walking	Subjects walk 10 ft with a safe, stable gait without assistive device
Abrupt stop	Subjects walk as fast as they can for several steps and then, on command, stop abruptly without stumbling or grabbing for support
Turning	Subjects walk at normal pace, then turn around with smooth, continuous steps
Obstacle	Subjects step over shoebox in walking path without hesitating or stumbling over box
Standing reach	Subjects grasp ruler held at shoulder level 12 inches beyond outstretched arm without taking a step
Stairs	Subjects ascend and descend stairs, step over step, without support

Adapted from Studenski S, et al: *Progressive mobility skills.* Presented at the American Geriatrics Society Annual Meeting. Boston, Massachusetts, May 12, 1989.

process, the therapist should vary the conditions under which the patient performs the tasks. For example, it is useful to see how the patient responds to changes in gait speed and direction, negotiates obstacles, and handles changing surfaces and other environmental distractions and conditions.

Environmental Assessment

Another aspect of functional performance that is important to consider is how the patient functions at home. Often, decisions are made to modify a person's environment based on performance deficits that may have been observed during evaluation in a hospital room or clinic. Not surprisingly, the unstable patient is often able to maneuver around his/her own home much more steadily and safely than he/she can in an unfamiliar hospital or clinic environment. Chandler and co-workers have developed an instrument that allows the therapist to assess performance-based environmental risk (Table 18-2).[7] Ideally, home modifications or other interventions should be designed based on the patient's performance during routine activities within his/her home. The therapist can perform the assessment by asking the patient to show him/her how he/she maneuvers around his/her home on a typical day. Getting in and out of a favorite chair; turning on the television; opening high and low cabinets and the refrigerator; getting on and off the commode, in and out of the shower or bath, and in and out of bed are examples of typical activities that should be assessed. Access to lighting and illumination is important to assess. It is unnecessary to suggest bathroom modification if the patient has no difficulty with such transfers. Obstacles, cords, and clutter become particularly relevant in the patient with serious visual deficits or gait abnormality but need to be addressed only to the extent that they pose a threat to the patient's safe function. Using this instrument, environmental risk can be quantified by evaluating both the degree of environmental hazard and the frequency with which it is encountered.

Psychosocial Assessment

Factors outside of physical performance that should be covered in the comprehensive evaluation of the geriatric faller include social support and behavioral/cognitive function. While other members of the interdisciplinary team are better equipped to identify specific problems in these areas, the therapist should be aware of how these factors may influence falls risk. The presence of a strong social support network may minimize falls risk because other people may be available to perform the "risky" activities for the patient. The patient who is no longer able to climb ladders or do yardwork safely must first recognize that these activities are no longer safe. Then one must decide the willingness to restrict activities or whether to take the risk of falling. Patients with severe cognitive loss are generally unable to recognize risk and consequently do not make sound judgments regarding safe activity.

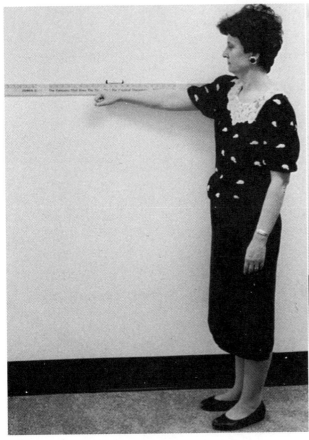

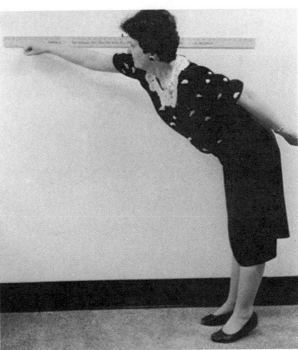

A

B

FIG. 18-3   Functional reach. **A,** Starting position. **B,** Ending position.

TABLE 18-2
FUNCTIONAL HOME ASSESSMENT PROFILE

PATHWAYS	POTENTIAL RISK ITEMS	FREQUENCY		HAZARD		SUM
1. Entrance into home	Access (railing)	_____	×	_____	=	_____
	Door	_____	×	_____	=	_____
	Threshold	_____	×	_____	=	_____
	Other	_____	×	_____	=	_____
				Total	=	_____
2. Living room	Lighting	_____	×	_____	=	_____
3. Kitchen	Floor	_____	×	_____	=	_____
4. Bedroom	Storage	_____	×	_____	=	_____
5. Bathroom	Furniture	_____	×	_____	=	_____
	Other	_____	×	_____	=	_____
				Total*	=	_____
6. Other (hallway)	Floor	_____	×	_____	=	_____
	Lighting	_____	×	_____	=	_____
	Other	_____	×	_____	=	_____
				Total	=	_____

VARIABLES (FOR EACH POTENTIAL RISK ITEM)

Hazard
0 = No risk
1 = Low-to-moderate risk (patient would likely have difficulty 10% to 40% of time hazard is encountered)
2 = Moderate-to-high risk (patient would likely have difficulty 50% to 100% of time hazard is encountered)
Frequency (frequency of encounter)
0 = Never
1 = < 1× / month
2 = < 1× / week
3 = 2-3× / week
4 = 1-2× / day
5 = > 2× / day
Total = Sum (frequency × hazard)

Adapted in part from Chandler JM, Prescott BL, Duncan PW, Studenski SA: Reliability of a new instrument: The Functional Environmental Assessment. *Phys Ther* 1991; 71(suppl):586.
*The sum (frequency × hazard) should be totaled for each of the rooms: living room, kitchen, bedroom, and bathroom.

INTERVENTION

Comprehensive multidisciplinary examination and evaluation should guide the management of the geriatric patient with instability. The universal goal of intervention is to maximize independence in mobility and function. Within the limits of safety, it is always preferable to improve mobility and function than to restrict activity. Indeed, the consequences of immobilization and restricted activity can be more devastating than the instability itself. The typical sequelae of restricted activity include decreased life space, fear of movement, deconditioning, depression, and often a high financial and emotional cost to family and society. The goal of maximum functional independence can be achieved by using the following principles to guide treatment planning:
- Identify and treat modifiable deficits
- Identify and compensate for fixed deficits

Based on the evaluation, the therapist should first be able to identify possible etiological components of the patient's instability. For example, major visual dysfunction is a fixed deficit but can be potentially treated by altering eyewear. Glasses with prisms can compensate for peripheral-field deficits, tinted glasses can increase contrast sensitivity, and different glasses for near and far vision can reduce problems caused by bifocals. A referral to a geriatric optometrist can be extremely useful.

Loss of proprioception is also a fixed deficit and may be a potential contributor to the patient's instability. Because the probability of reversing proprioceptive loss is low, training the patient to compensate with increased visual input may be the most effective strategy. Patients with vestibular lesions can be potentially treated with specific exercises to improve vestibular function or can be taught compensatory techniques using vision.[20,21]

When irreversible neurological disease is the basis for instability, it is necessary to address the treatable aspects of the condition in order to improve or maintain mobility within the limits of safety. In the patient with Parkinson's disease, emphasis on flexibility and range of motion, particularly of the axial skeleton, may help to provide a more supple biomechanical apparatus through which an effective balance strategy might be better expressed.[52] Teaching the patient with Parkinson's disease to keep his/her weight forward in both standing and sitting situations can facilitate walking and rising from a chair, respectively. A rolling walker may be a useful tool to facilitate this movement strategy and provide additional safety.

To the extent that strength, range of motion, and endurance are contributing to the patient's instability, they need to be addressed in treatment. Research has indicated that lower extremity weakness, especially at the ankle and knee, is significantly associated with recurrent falls in the elderly.[59,72] It has also been well-established that strength gains can be made in all age-groups, even in nonagenarians, by applying the physiological exercise principles of overload and specificity.[10,16]

No treatment will be effective without specifically addressing the patient's functional deficits. Just as in treating the young orthopedic patient, vigorous strength training will not improve function unless specific functional training is incorporated into the exercise program. The functional assessment allows the therapist to identify specific functional limitations, so treatment should focus on similar activities. If, for example, reaching is limited, the therapist might incorporate functional activities that stress the patient's margin of stability, such as reaching for a glass, leaning forward, reaching behind self (as if to put arm in coat sleeve), and catching a ball off center. Weakness of the hip musculature can be effectively addressed by incorporating rising from a chair and climbing stairs into the exercise program. Similarly, teaching the most biomechanically efficient chair-rise strategy can lead to immediate functional improvement.[71]

For the patient who demonstrates poor balance responses to either feedforward or feedback displacements of the center of mass, it may be useful to practice effective balance responses, such as weight-shifting techniques. However, there is little evidence that balance training carries over to improved functional performance.[12] Evidence does suggest that balance is highly task specific and that muscles respond differently to different center-of-mass displacements. Interventions for balance deficits should therefore be functionally driven and task specific. Recent studies have shown that the ancient Chinese martial art form of Tai Chi Quan is effective in reducing falls in older adults.[73] This exercise, which involves slow rhythmical movement, weight transfer, and concentration, is thought to sufficiently enhance physical and mental control to reduce falls even though physiological measures of postural stability (postural sway) may not improve.[28,74]

Compensatory treatment strategies must be applied when balance deficits cannot be changed. Such strategies must include environmental modification—e.g., grab bars, railings, improved lighting, altered chair heights—assistive devices, and increased external support—e.g., home health aide.

SUMMARY

Falls in the elderly are a multifaceted and heterogeneous problem. The most effective management strategy requires a multidisciplinary approach in which pathophysiological, functional, and environmental issues can be thoroughly

evaluated and treated. The goal of intervention should always be to maximize functional independence within the margins of safety.

REFERENCES

1. Baker SP, Harvey AH: Fall injuries in the elderly. *Clin Geriatr Med* 1985; 1(3):501-512.
2. Berg K, et al: Measuring balance in the elderly: Validation of an instrument. *Can J Public Health* 1992; 83(suppl 2):s7-s11.
3. Berg K, Wood-Dauphinee S, Williams JI: The Balance Scale: Reliability assessment for elderly residents and patients with acute stroke. *Scand J Rehabil Med* 1995; 27:27-36.
4. Berg K, Norman KE: Functional assessment of balance and gait. *Clin Geriatr Med* 1996; 12:705-723.
5. Blake AJ, et al: Falls by elderly people at home: Prevalence and associated factors. *Age Ageing* 1988; 17:365-372.
6. Campbell JA, Borrie MJ, Spears GF: Risk factors for falls in a community-based prospective study of people 70 years and older. *J Gerontol* 1989; 44:M112-M117.
7. Chandler JM, Prescott BL, Duncan PW, Studenski SA: Reliability of a new instrument: The Functional Environmental Assessment. *Phys Ther* 1991; 71(suppl):586.
8. Chandler JM, Duncan PW, Studenski SA: Comparison of postural responses in young adults, healthy elderly and fallers using postural stress test. *Phys Ther* 1990; 70:410-415.
9. Chandler JM, Duncan PW, Studenski SA: The fear of falling syndrome: Relationship to falls, physical performance and activities of daily living in frail elders. *Top Geriatr Rehabil* 1996; 11:55-63.
10. Chandler JM, Duncan PW, Kochersberger G, Studenski SA: Is lower extremity strength gain associated with improvement in physical performance and disability in frail, community dwelling elderly? *Arch Phys Med Rehabil* 1998; 79:24-30.
11. Cooper KH: A means of assessing maximal oxygen intake: Correlation between field and treadmill testing. *JAMA* 1968; 203:201-204.
12. Daleiden S: Weight shifting as a treatment for balance deficits: A literature review. *Physiother Can* 1990; 42:81-87.
13. Duncan PW, et al: Functional reach: A new measure of balance. *J Gerontol* 1990; 45:M192-197.
14. Duncan PW, Studenski SA, Chandler JM: Functional reach: Predictive validity. *J Gerontol* 1992; 47(3):M93-98.
15. Duncan PW, et al: How do physiologic components of balance affect function in elders? *Arch Phys Med Rehabil* 1993; 74:1343-1349.
16. Fiatarone MA, et al: High intensity strength training on nonagenarians. *JAMA* 1990; 263:3029-3034.
17. Gerety MB, et al: Development and validation of a physical performance instrument for the functionally impaired elderly: The Physical Disability Index (PDI). *J Gerontol* 1993; 48:M33-38.
18. Greene HH, Madden DJ: Adult age difference in visual acuity, stereopsis and contrast sensitivity. *Am J Optom Physiol Opt* 1986; 63:724-732.
19. Guyatt G, Thompson PJ: How should we measure function in patients with chronic heart and lung diseases? *J Chronic Dis* 1985; 38:517-524.
20. Herdman SJ: Exercise strategies in vestibular disorders. *Ear Nose Throat J* 1989; 68:961-964.
21. Herdman SJ: Assessment and treatment of balance disorders in the vestibular deficient patient, in Duncan P (ed): Balance. *Proceedings of the American Physical Therapy Association Forum.* Alexandria, Va, APTA Publications, 1990.
22. Horak FB, Nashner LM: Central programming of postural movements: Adaptations to altered support-surface configurations. *J Neurophysiol* 1986; 55:1369-1381.
23. Horak FB, Shupert CL, Mirka A: Components of postural dyscontrol in the elderly: A review. *Neurobiol Aging* 1989; 10:727-738.
24. Inglin B, Woollacott M: Age-related changes in anticipatory postural adjustments associated with arm movements. *J Gerontol* 1988; 43:M105-M113.
25. Kauffman T: Impact of aging-related musculoskeletal and postural changes on falls. *Top Geriatr Rehabil* 1990; 5(2):34-43.
26. Keshner EA: Reflex, voluntary, and mechanical process in postural stabilization, in Duncan PW (ed): Balance. *Proceedings of the American Physical Therapy Association Forum.* Alexandria, Va, APTA Publications, 1990.

27. Keshner EA, Allum JHJ, Pfaltz CR: Postural coactivation and adaptation in the sway stabilizing responses of normals and patients with bilateral peripheral vestibular deficit. *Exp Brain Res* 1987; 69:66-72.

28. Kutner NG, et al: Self-report benefits of Tai Chi practice by older adults. *J Gerontol* 1997; 52:P242-6.

29. Lach HW, et al: Falls in the elderly: Reliability of a classification system. *J Am Geriatr Soc* 1991; 39:197-202.

30. Lipsitz LA, et al: Causes and correlates of recurrent falls in ambulatory frail elderly. *J Gerontol* 1991; 46:M114-M122.

31. Lord SR, Clark RD, Webster IW: Postural stability and associated physiological factors in a population of aged persons. *J Gerontol* 1991; 46:M69-M76.

32. Lord SR, Clark RD, Webster IW: Visual acuity and contrast sensitivity in relation to falls in an elderly population. *Age Ageing* 1991; 20:175-181.

33. Lord SR, Ward JA, Williams P, Anstey KJ: Physiological factors associated with falls in older community dwelling women. *J Am Geriatr Soc* 1994; 42:1110-1117.

34. Lord SR, Lloyd DG, Li SK: Sensorimotor function, gait patterns and falls in community dwelling women. *Age Ageing* 1996; 25:292-299

35. Maki BE, Holliday PJ, Topper AK: Fear of falling and postural performance in the elderly. *J Gerontol* 1991; 46:M123-M131.

36. Maki BE, McIlroy WE: The role of limb movements in maintaining upright stance: The 'change in support' strategy. *Phys Ther* 1997; 77:488-507.

37. Manchester D, et al: Visual, vestibular and somatosensory contributions to balance control in the older adult. *J Gerontol* 1989; 44:M118-M127.

38. Mathias S, Nayak USL, Isaacs B: Balance in elderly patients: The "get-up and go" test. *Arch Phys Med Rehabil* 1986; 67:387-389.

39. McIlroy WE, Maki BE: Age-related changes in compensatory stepping in response to unpredictable perturbations. *J Gerontol* 1996; 51:M289-296.

40. Nashner LM: Fixed patterns of rapid postural responses among leg muscles during stance. *Exp Brain Res* 1977; 30:13-24.

41. Nashner LM, McCollum G: The organization of human postural movement: A formal basis and experimental synthesis. *Behav Brain Sci* 1985; 8:135-172.

42. Nashner LM, Woollacott MH: The organization of rapid postural adjustments of standing humans: An experimental-conceptual model, in Talbott RE, Humphrey DR (eds): *Posture and Movement.* New York, Raven Press, 1979.

43. Nashner LM, Woollacott M, Tuma G: Organization of rapid response to postural and locomotor-like perturbation of standing man. *Exp Brain Res* 1979; 36:463-476.

44. Nevitt MC: Falls in older persons; Risk factors and prevention, in Berg RL, Cassells JF (eds): *The Second Fifty Years: Promoting Health and Preventing Disability.* Washington DC, Institute of Medicine National Academy Press, 1990.

45. Nevitt MC, et al: Risk factors for recurrent nonsyncopal falls: A prospective study. *JAMA* 1989; 261:2663-2668.

46. Nickens H: Intrinsic factors in falling among the elderly. *Arch Intern Med* 1985; 145:1089-1093.

47. Patla A, et al: Identification of age-related changes in the balance control system, in Duncan PW (ed): Balance. *Proceedings of the American Physical Therapy Association Forum.* Alexandria, Va, APTA Publications, 1990.

48. Prudham D, Evans J: Factors associated with falls in the elderly: A community study. *Age Ageing* 1981; 10:141-146.

49. Robbins AS, et al: Predictors of falls among elderly people: Results of two population-based studies. *Arch Intern Med* 1989; 149:1628-1633.

50. Romick-Allen R, Schultz AB: Biomechanics of reactions to impending falls. *J Biomech* 1998; 21:591-600.

51. Schenkman M: Interrelationship of neurological and mechanical factors in balance control, in Duncan PW (ed): Balance. *Proceedings of the American Physical Therapy Association Forum.* Alexandria, Va, APTA Publications, 1990.

52. Schenkman M, et al: Exercise to improve axial flexibility and function for people with Parkinson's disease—a randomized controlled trial. *J Am Geriatr Soc* 1998; 46(10)1207-1216.

53. Shumway-Cook A, Horak F: Assessing the influence of sensory interaction on balance. *Phys Ther* 1986; 66:1548-1550.

54. Speechley M, Tinetti M: Assessment of risk and prevention of falls among elderly persons: Role of the physiotherapist. *Physiother Can* 1990; 42:75-79.

55. Stelmach GE, et al: Age, functional postural reflexes and voluntary sway. *J Gerontol* 1989; 44:B100-106.

56. Stelmach GE, et al: Age related decline in postural control mechanisms. *Int J Aging Hum Dev* 1989; 23:205-223.

57. Stelmach GE, Worringham CJ: Sensorimotor deficits related to postural stability: Implication for falling in elderly. *Clin Geriatr Med* 1985; 1(3):679-694.

58. Studenski S: Falls, in Calkins E (ed): *The Practice of Geriatrics,* ed 2. Philadelphia, WB Saunders, 1992.

59. Studenski SA, Duncan PW, Chandler JM: Postural responses and effector factors in persons with unexplained falls: Results and methodologic issues. *J Am Geriatr Soc* 1991; 39:229-234.

60. Studenski S, et al: *Progressive mobility skills.* Presented at the American Geriatric Society Annual Meeting, May 12, 1989.

61. Studenski S, et al: The role of instability in falls among older persons, in Duncan PW (ed): Balance. *Proceedings of the American Physical Therapy Association Forum.* Alexandria, Va, APTA Publications, 1990.

62. Studenski SA, et al: Predicting falls: The role of mobility and nonphysical factors. *J Am Geriatr Soc* 1994; 42:297-302.

63. Thelen DG, Schultz AB, Alexander NB, Ashton-Miller JA: Effects of age on rapid ankle torque development. *J Gerontol* 1996; 51:M226-232.

64. Tideiksaar R: Geriatric falls in the home. *Home Health Nurse* 1986; 4:14-23.

65. Tideiksaar R: Geriatric falls: Assessing the cause, preventing recurrence. *Geriatrics* 1989; 44:57-64.

66. Tinetti ME: Performance oriented assessment of mobility problems on elderly patients. *J Am Geriatr Soc* 1986; 34:119-126.

67. Tinetti ME, Speechley M, Ginter SF: Risk factors for falls among elderly persons living in the community. *N Engl J Med* 1988; 319:1701-1707.

68. Tinetti ME, Mendes-de-Leon CF, Doucette JT, Baker DI: Fear of falling and fall-related efficacy in relationship to functioning among community-living elders. *J Gerontol* 1994; 49: M140-147.

69. Vellas BJ, et al: Fear of falling and restriction of mobility in elderly fallers. *Age Aging* 1997; 26:189-193.

70. Waller JA: Falls among the elderly—human and environmental factors. *Accid Anal Prev* 1978; 10:21-33.

71. Weiner DK, et al: When older adults face the chair rise challenge. A study of chair height availability and height-modified chair-rise performance in the elderly. *J Am Geriatr Soc* 1993; 41:6-10.

72. Whipple RH, Wolfson LI, Amerman P: The relationship of knee and ankle weakness to falls in nursing home residents: An isokinetic study. *J Am Geriatr Soc* 1987; 35:13-20.

73. Wolf SL, et al: Reducing frailty and falls in older persons: An investigation of Tai Chi and computerized balance training. *J Am Geriatr Soc* 1996; 44:489-497.

74. Wolf Sl, Barnhart HX, Ellison GL, Coogler CE: The effect of Tai Chi Quan and computerized balance training on postural stability in older subjects. Atlanta FICSIT Group. *Phys Ther* 1997; 77:371-381.

75. Wolfson LI, Whipple R: Stressing the postural response. *J Am Geriatr Soc* 1986; 34:845-850.

76. Wolfson LI, et al: Gait and balance in the elderly. *Clin Geriatr Med* 1985; 1(3):649-659.

77. Woollacott MH: Changes in posture and voluntary control in the elderly: Research findings and rehabilitation. *Top Geriatr Rehabil* 1990; 5(2):1-11.

78. Woollacott MH, Shumway-Cook A, Nashner L: Aging and posture control: Changes in sensory organs and muscular coordination. *Int J Aging Hum Dev* 1986; 23:97-114.

79. Woollacott MH, Shumway-Cook A, Nashner L: Postural reflexes and aging, in Mortimer J, Rororzzolo F, Maletta G (eds): *The Aging Nervous System.* New York, Praeger Publishers, 1989.

CHAPTER 19

AMBULATION: A FRAMEWORK OF PRACTICE APPLIED TO A FUNCTIONAL OUTCOME

PATRICIA E. SULLIVAN, PT, PhD AND PRUDENCE D. MARKOS PT, MS

INTRODUCTION

One of the primary purposes of physical therapy is to enhance the individual's physical ability to interact within the environment and to function in the community. Particularly important with the elderly is to improve, restore, or maintain the functional outcome of ambulation. Independent ambulation and walking at a functional speed are two of the most important factors in maintaining a self-reliant life-style for older individuals.[78] The ability to walk without undue fatigue at a functionally adequate speed for a reasonable time contributes to a comfortable and independent life.[7]

This chapter describes an examination, evaluation, and intervention strategy focusing on the functional outcome of ambulation for elderly persons. The Framework of Clinical Practice is used to guide the clinical decision-making process as the functional limitations and impairments of this specific problem are assessed and as intervention programs are developed (Fig. 19-1). Impairments related to postural control and falling also are discussed because of their importance in the elderly population and their relationship to ambulation. Although there is no differentiation among the sub-groups of elders by age or activity level in this chapter, age and activity level need to be considered in the clinic so that the therapist can identify appropriate outcomes and implement the most effective intervention program for each patient.

Walking velocity can be used as a marker of disability and dependency in older persons.[26,32] Ambulation is important for its implication related to community independence and also as an exercise in and of itself. Rakowski and Mor reported on the association of physical activity, particularly ambulation, with mortality in the elderly. In a sample of 5901 persons, ages 70 and older, a higher mortality was associated with walking less than 1 mile once a week or never, as was not getting enough exercise or not having a regular exercise routine, particularly for the women in the sample. It is not clear from these results what the specific effect walking may have on cardiopulmonary-vascular health, on psychological health, or on the maintenance of postural control and strength. However, the strong association for women

FRAMEWORK OF CLINICAL PRACTICE

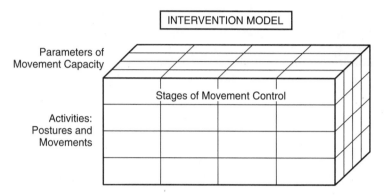

Functional Abilities

Functional Limitations

Environmental/Social/
   Cultural Factors
Medical/Psychological Factors
Physical Factors

INTERVENTION MODEL

Parameters of
Movement Capacity

Stages of Movement Control

Activities:
Postures and
Movements

FIG. 19-1   Framework of Clinical Practice, including the Evaluation and Intervention Models.

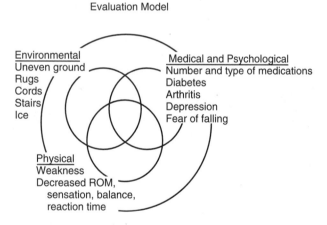

FIG. 19-2   Application of the Evaluation Model to factors that contribute to falls in the elderly.

between walking 1 mile more than once a week and improved longevity seems clear.[66] For many elderly, walking is the most common form of physical activity.[25]

To better match the individual's ambulatory capability to the demands of the community, walking speed standards, or norms, have been established and vary from a speed of 1.07 to 1.4 meters/second (m/sec). However, in many studies, elderly subjects or those following hip fracture have not been able to achieve these walking speeds.[24,52] A speed of 0.82 m/sec in patients who have had hip fracture has been reported. Interestingly, most of the hip fracture subjects achieved the desired walking speed after an exercise rehabilitation program.[24]

Ambulatory ability also is related to other markers. For example, dependent ambulation and reduced safety during gait activities are common reasons for admission to nursing homes or other residential facilities.[32] A large percentage of falls occur in elderly individuals while they are walking and may be attributed to various factors (Fig. 19-2). Some falls result in injury. Estimates suggest that as many as 25% of those who enter a hospital because of a hip fracture will die within 1 year. There is a societal need to decrease the number of falls, to reduce the need for nursing home placement, and to improve or maintain functional independence in the elderly.[2,44] Thus, the examination and evaluation of ambulation and intervention to preserve or restore walking ability are critical.

A sedentary life-style for elderly persons is not uncommon. It has been estimated that only 45% to 66% of older persons participate in regular exercise, even though activity seems to be critical to maintaining mental and physical health.[71] Physical therapists must continue to analyze and implement intervention programs to prevent and counteract many of the impairment changes found in older persons and to improve their functional ambulatory ability and general overall health.

The focus of this chapter is to analyze the function of ambulation and the common changes that occur in the component physical characteristics in the aging population. This information will serve as a basis for the physical therapy evaluation and intervention. The chapter is based on the following principles:

1. *An individual's functional capability* is an interaction between environmental demands or restrictions and the individual's abilities. Both the person who enters the therapeutic situation and the environment in which that person functions must be considered during the examination, evaluation, and intervention.[31]

2. *Functional outcomes* can be attained by a combination of intervention strategies. These include rehabilitating the individual, if change is possible or appropriate, and providing adaptive and assistive devices and aids as well as instruction and education in their use and modification of the environment. This principle also includes prevention of impairments and functional limitations so that intervention can promote an individual's abilities most effectively.

3. *Intervention* is designed to remedy both the primary and secondary impairments that limit function through a program that enhances movement control and capacity by proceeding through a logical sequence of procedures. Intervention encompasses the promotion of wellness, the improvement or maintenance of functional abilities, the prevention of limitations, as well as rehabilitation if impairments are present.[38,75]

Examination

The examination is used to subjectively and objectively assess the patient's capability to perform functional activities. The therapist compiles these data to design the most effective and efficient intervention strategies to achieve anticipated functional outcomes. In this section the commonly observed gait characteristics in the older individual are discussed, followed by a presentation of other potentially relevant findings within their physical and physiological systems. In addition to these factors, the environmental, social, psychological, and medical factors relative to the elderly require consideration. These factors are discussed as they are relevant to the function of ambulation and possible intervention strategies.

Environmental Factors

Environmental factors that may influence ambulatory ability include architectural barriers or the lack of aides that may provide needed assistance. Examples of barriers are stairs without banisters, elevations without ramps, and curbs without cutouts. Modifications of the environment or the use of adaptive and assistive devices and aides may be effective means of achieving the goal of maintaining community ambulatory status. The following recommendations should be considered: cross walks with the option of slower pedestrian crossing signals, elimination of highly polished floors in public buildings, walkways without bricks or cobble-

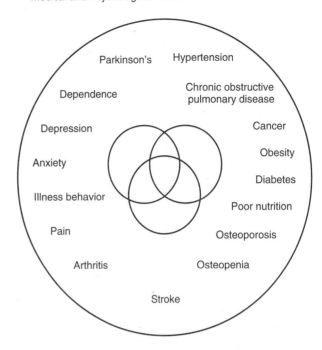

Fig. 19-3 Medical and psychological factors that affect functional abilities.

stones, adequate cleaning of icy or snowy sidewalks, rest benches in shopping areas, and the installation of stall bars next to curbs at commonly used intersections. Also, curb and stair-stepheights should be restricted to 150 mm in locations frequented by adults older than 80 for easier access.[12a] Modifying environmental challenges may be an efficient and effective intervention strategy in achieving functional outcomes.

Psychological/Medical Factors

Acute or chronic psychological and medical conditions and altered nutrition compound the physical impairments that accompany aging and diminished activity (Fig. 19-3).[22] Although depression is a common finding in the elderly,[7] mood status seems to change with disability. Barbisoni investigated the influence of physical therapy on a number of factors, including depression, and found that depressive symptoms, when marked on admission, had substantially improved after a course of physical therapy and that smaller improvements were seen in patients with less initial symptomatology.[5] Patients with improved walking speed after an exercise program have reported more social interactions and more community involvement.[24] The fear of falling may lead to apprehension and postural instability in some patients,[53] whereas others may fear falling due to postural instability. Both groups may limit community involvement. A more positive attitude toward life has been demonstrated in persons who walk at least 30 minutes a day compared with those who do not.[25] In contrast, poor self-perceived health is included in a group of risk factors for falls.[37]

When assessing the elderly with a falling complaint or who have improved ambulation as a functional outcome, the therapist must be aware that the elderly commonly have multiple medical problems whose symptoms or pharmacological management may contribute to physical dysfunction. Comorbidities found in a group of elderly with a mean age of 77 included visual deficits (71%), hypertension (47%), coronary artery disease (23%), and other cardiac involvement (23%).[28] The strength and sensory deficits, particularly proprioceptive loss in the lower extremities associated with diabetes, need to be considered with many elderly.

Ambulatory Characteristics

General changes in ambulation that are associated with aging are slower velocity and decreased stride length. Mean comfortable gait speed has been recorded as 1.27 m/sec for women in their 70s. A range for the mean maximum gait speed for elderly women has been reported, including 1.32 m/sec,[33] 1.5 m/sec,[17] and 1.74 m/sec.[9] Maximum gait speed in the elderly declines more steeply than does the speed of walking at a comfortable pace. An elderly group was reported to ambulate 28% faster during maximum speed of walking compared with self-paced speed, whereas a younger age group could walk 43% faster during maximum effort compared with self-paced walking. This loss of reserve, indicated as a narrowing between what an individual actually does compared with the capacity for doing, may be critical in the elderly as they attempt to physically cope with additional strains. For those in nursing homes, gait velocity has been found to be even slower. Those with a history of falls walked at 0.37 m/sec and those without a falling history walked at speeds of 0.64 m/sec.[84]

Slower gait speed in the elderly has been related to pathophysiological findings. For example, walking speed can help

identify those who are at greater risk for medical complications, such as an increased risk of hip fracture.[18] In addition, the time an individual ambulates per day or the distance walked has implications: those who walk 30 minutes or more a day have better exercise capacity, higher bone mineral content, and lower blood triglycerides.[25] Reduced visual acuity has also been implicated in determining walking speed.[18]

Related Movement Control Characteristics

Although some characteristics vary with different reports, the following are common ambulatory findings. During the stance phase of gait, elderly persons generally use a wider base of support (BoS) and exhibit a shorter step length, thereby spending a longer time in double support. Decreased dorsiflexion is common during the early swing phase and may be compensated for by use of greater hip and knee flexion to accomplish toe clearance. At late swing, when the compensatory increase in knee flexion seen in early swing becomes impossible, toe clearance is minimized. The decreased ankle range of motion (ROM) found during gait may be associated with the slower walking speeds.[33] Also, there seems to be less deceleration control at late swing and early stance.[83] Within the trunk and the proximal joints, there is less pelvic rotation and trunk counter-rotation, increased shoulder extension and elbow flexion, increased hip abduction, greater toeing out, and less vertical projection of the trunk and pelvis at toe-off.[7,12,34,59,82] In addition to measuring velocity during free walking, examining the initiation of gait has proved fruitful.[14] Older persons initiate stepping with a longer reaction time and longer weight transfer time than do younger subjects.[82]

The association between changes during walking and various physical impairments can be evaluated from multiple perspectives, including the elder's attempts to improve stabilization as well as the consequence of physical change (Box 19-1). The older individual's attempts to improve stabilization during ambulation may result in decreased trunk counter-rotation, decreased pelvic forward rotation, shorter step length, wider BoS, and decreased vertical projection at heel-off.[83]

The effects of decreased range in the trunk, hips, and ankles; decreased force production in the postural extensors and plantar flexors; and diminished proprioceptive awareness may result in diminished velocity. Similarly, the altered speed of walking, especially during stair climbing, may be due to a decrease in the number of type II muscle fibers, a reduction in the ability to perform unilateral stance, or a decreased aerobic capacity. Other possible reasons that the elderly may walk slower include slower reaction time and decreased strength, particularly of the knee extensors. Walking velocity was found to relate to strength of hip abduction when walking at comfortable speeds and knee extension when walking at maximum speed.[9] The increased shoulder extension noted during gait may be a mechanism to counterbalance the increased kyphosis and flexed hips that move the center of mass anteriorly. Substantiation of the second perspective was provided by Judge, who found that gait ve-

---

BOX 19-1
IMPAIRMENTS ASSOCIATED WITH COMMON FINDINGS OF GAIT ANALYSIS IN THE ELDERLY

Gait Examination Results	*Physical Impairments*
Slower velocity	Reduced aerobic capacity
Decreased stride length	Muscle and joint tightness
Decreased initial swing height	Decreased strength
Decreased control terminal swing	anterior tibialis,
Longer double support time	quadriceps, and
Toeing out	gluteus medius
Wider BOS	Decreased hamstring control
	Altered postural alignment
	Decreased balance control
	Decreased proprioception

locity was enhanced after an exercise program to improve strength and balance.[42]

Stair-climbing characteristics also deserve a brief mention. Speed and quality of stair-climbing pattern are associated with age, unilateral balance time, and active hip flexibility.[12a] The ankle dorsiflexion range that is required during stair climbing may not be found in many elderly.

Dizziness related to vestibular function needs to be considered. Patients with disequilibrium have been found to have gait and balance abnormalities and tend to veer from side to side, particularly with rapid turning, but do not seem to have a greater frequency of reported falls.[23] When vestibular dysfunction is coupled with either visual or peripheral sensory involvement, the redundant sensory postural mechanisms are challenged. When vestibular involvement leads to ambulatory changes, a compromised musculoskeletal system may not be able to meet the demand.

Related Movement Capacity Characteristics

Characteristic changes in the capacity to sustain movement for a given speed of ambulation, as measured by oxygen consumption, become more pronounced with advancing age. Energy expenditure in ambulation over level ground and during stair climbing is similar for many elderly and younger persons because the elderly seemingly regulate their energy consumption by walking more slowly.[7] However, even when stair climbing is performed more slowly, the energy cost can exceed the ability of some elderly persons. Oxygen consumption for walking at a self-paced speed does not differ with age. However, free speed gait requires approximately 32% of $\dot{V}O_2$max in younger individuals and nearly 48% in older persons. Even healthy elderly have progressively smaller aerobic reserves due to the decline in $\dot{V}O_2$max.[17] This decline in aerobic reserves makes it more difficult for an elderly person to accommodate to the energy demand of a gait disorder or the need for faster speed. The elderly tend to walk slower when attempting fast speed to stay below the anaerobic threshold. In a study of more than 200 elderly subjects aged 79 years old, 18% of the women and 26% of the men had cardiovascular involvement, implying limitations in those systems.[52]

The preferred walking speed of active elderly at 1.43 m/sec is similar to the speed of young sedentary individuals at 1.41 m/sec. Sedentary elderly subjects walked 15% slower than active elderly, whereas sedentary young subjects walked only 6% slower than active young subjects.[55] Sedentary lifestyle in the elderly seems to have more of a deleterious effect than in younger populations.

Variations in ambulation related to gender differences in the elderly have also been reported. Women take shorter steps than men. To increase their speed, women take more steps, whereas men increase step length.[7,36] It is not clear whether these gender differences are related to variations in leg length, flexibility, strength, general physical condition, or some combination of these factors. In a group of 79-year-old subjects, walking aids were used by 27% of women and by 25% of men.[52]

Measurement Considerations

The method and procedure of measuring gait characteristics affect the interpretation of the findings. For example, some measures are primarily temporal distance tools, such as the 10 meter gait test.[48,61] Other measures, such as the Tinetti, focus on the quality and symmetry of movement.[79] Still other measures such as the "Up&Go" and the timed "Up&Go" combine ambulation with a sit-to-stand-to-sit maneuver.[64] When a longer distance or duration is used, e.g., the 6-minute walk test,[55] gait speed in populations with cardiac or pulmonary dysfunction is related to cardiovascular-pulmonary (CVP) measures. In elders without overt CVP pathology, lower extremity strength is predictive of distance. When a shorter distance is measured, strength, balance, and proprioceptive variables are related to gait speed. If gait speed is determined by calculating from the first step as compared to calculating after gait has been initiated, variations also will be seen.[61] No standardized distance has been used, with distances varying between 7.62 meters (25 feet)[9] to 10 meters.[48,61] Walking over and around obstacles also has been investigated to simulate the environmental conditions that may lead to trips and slips.[15]

As previously mentioned, many falls occur during ambulation. At least two different relationships have been investigated. One is concerned with differentiating physical characteristics of those who fall compared with those who do not in an attempt to develop risk factors for falling; the other is to examine and differentiate possible reasons for falling. Risk factors for falls and factors that differentiate fallers and nonfallers have included gait disturbances, such as shorter stride length and slow gait velocity; balance as measured by one-foot stance; body sway; and backward walking.[80] Also implicated are strength of the hip, knee, and ankle extensors; complaints of dizziness; poor self-perceived health; difficulties with activities of daily living (ADL); and non-practice of "morning walk."[27,29,36,37,45] Additional factors related to falling include reaction time, tactile sensitivity, cognitive impairment, psychoactive drug use, and age.[51] Because many falls are a result of tripping, understanding the mechanisms of controlling movement when stepping over objects is an important line of investigation in the elderly. Chen and colleagues measured the reaction time in young and older subjects. The older group was regularly active in walking. The reaction time in the older females was 29 to 54 msec slower than in young females. The older subjects had more difficulty avoiding obstacles. When attention was divided, scores decreased for both young and old. The older subjects avoided obstacles in fewer than 50% of trials, whereas the younger subjects avoided the obstacles in 75% of trials. Older adults seemingly have more difficulty because of the dual nature of the task. They performed poorer on each individual task and poorer still on the combined task. They had more difficulty attending to multiple tasks simultaneously.[15] Even with the adoption of a slower speed and shorter stride length, the results suggest that normal aging requires that a greater proportion of attentional resources be allocated to the balance demands of postural tasks.[46] However, the elderly may not attend to the balance aspect of the task and may tend to fall more than younger persons who may maintain balance and disregard other aspects of the task.[87] Reaction time has also been measured during the initiation of stepping with a decrease of 36% seen during this complex, but common lower extremity movement, which also requires a transition from static to dynamic postural stabilization.[62]

Because of the many complaints of tripping and slipping during walking, Winter conducted a multifaceted assessment of gait and determined that primary contributing factors included poor deceleration of the foot in late swing and early stance associated with reduced hamstring control.[83] Preventative programs for recurrent fallers may focus on improvements in balance, reaction and response time in specific muscle groups, leg extension strength, walking speed, and ability to negotiate obstacles. Patients who have attentional dysfunction may need to be reminded to focus on the walking task and not to attempt to perform more than one activity at a time.

Physical Systems Review: Impairment Changes Related to Ambulation

Because each physical system can contribute to motor performance, the therapist examines each physical system and its overlapping physiological areas to determine the cause of the impairment. For example, the abnormal performance of the dorsiflexors exhibited during gait may be a problem of movement control that is demonstrated as abnormal timing and sequencing of the response; the deficit could be within the musculoskeletal system, which may be seen as decreased

torque generation regardless of position or time; or it could be abnormal movement capacity noted as an inability to perform repetitive movement.

The nervous (N), musculoskeletal (MS), and cardiovascular-pulmonary (CVP) systems are three physical systems of primary concern to physical therapy and as illustrated in Fig. 19-4 should be regarded as interrelated systems. The anatomical structure of each system is depicted in the unique area; the physiological nature of the systems is represented in the overlap between the systems. The physiological capacity for movement is represented in the area between the CVP and MS systems, the neurophysiological control of movement is depicted in the area between the N and MS systems, and neural perfusion is represented in the area between the CVP and N systems. Common to all are the physiological functions of the autonomic nervous system (ANS) and the immune system.[75]

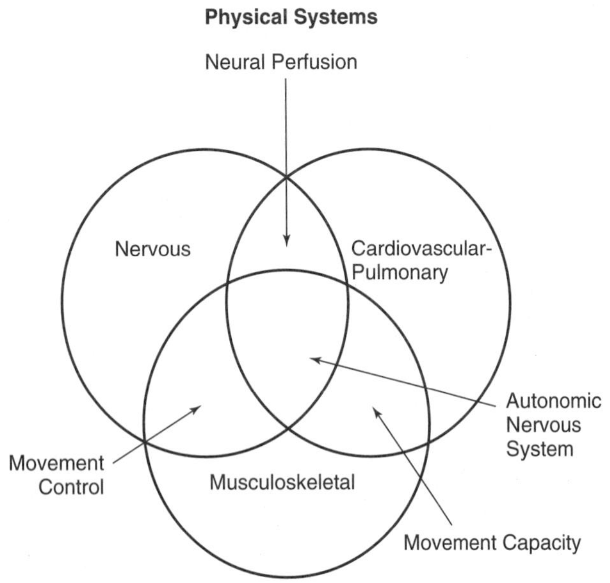

Nervous System

For the elderly, changes in the nervous system may contribute to alterations in ambulation (Fig. 19-5). These changes include reduced sensory input from proprioceptive, visual, and vestibular mechanisms that may be related to a longer latency and a higher threshold from cutaneous and proprioceptive receptors.[54,70,72,73,87,88] Because proprioception is diminished, the elderly may demonstrate abnormalities in postural control, measured as increased sway while standing with the eyes closed and during ambulation.[16,39] Impaired proprioception has been related to decreased gait speed, lower scores relative to the quality of gait,[78] and poorer functional balance scores as measured by the Berg Balance Scale.[8,61]

Other neurological changes that may affect ambulation in the elderly include presence of fewer dendrites, reduced nerve conduction velocity, greater monosynaptic latency, decreased excitability at the myoneural junction, decreased numbers of functional motor units, decreased reaction time, and a higher threshold for the H-reflex. These neural changes slow the generation of automatic motor programs, increase the time required for peripheral feedback to be received centrally, and delay the transmission of efferent responses.[47,68]

Physical Systems

Neural Perfusion

Nervous

Cardiovascular-Pulmonary

Autonomic Nervous System

Movement Control

Musculoskeletal

Movement Capacity

FIG. 19-4 Integration of physical systems pertinent to physical therapist examination.

Nervous System

Decreased orientation
Decreased ability to follow
    commands
Reduced number of synapses
Diminished sensory input
    (visual, vestibular, proprioceptive)
Increased receptor threshold

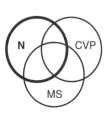

FIG. 19-5 Changes in the nervous system that may contribute to problems with ambulation in the elderly.

Musculoskeletal System

Many changes in the musculoskeletal system occur with aging that are relevant to ambulation. These include less tightly packed muscle fibers, an increase in fat content between muscle fibers, an increase in fibrin deposits, a decrease in the number of type II fibers and functional motor units, and loss of bone density (Fig. 19-6).[76] Clinically, a predominant finding in the elderly is a reduction in general flexibility. Any of these findings, as well as the changes that occur in the cartilage and joint surfaces, may lead to postural alterations.[43]

Gibbs reported that joint impairments in the elderly were 70% in the spine, 54% in the feet, 35% in the knees, 19% in the hips, and 19% in the ankles.[28] If degeneration is accompanied by inflammation, pain may result and alter the individual's gait pattern.

Cardiovascular-Pulmonary System

Elderly persons commonly exhibit an increased prevalence of coronary artery disease and hypertension (Fig. 19-7). Cardiac pathophysiology may be demonstrated by an increase in blood pressure; decreases in stroke volume, maximum heart rate, and coronary artery circulation; and a narrowing of the coronary vessels and stenosis of the cardiac valves.[63]

The pulmonary system often shows altered compliance of the bony thorax and the lung tissue with a resultant decrease in diffusing capacity and efficiency in breathing. In the peripheral vasculature, there is an increase in the resistance to peripheral blood flow and a decrease in the elasticity of vessels and the number of capillary beds in the muscles. In addition to the aforementioned impairments, patients taking cardiac medication may be at more risk for falls; digitalis and calcium blockers have been reported as risk factors.[45]

Movement Control and Capacity

The quality and quantity of ambulation are related to impairments leading to alterations in control and capacity for movement. Control alterations in the programming, planning, or execution of movement can be depicted as impairments in the area overlapping the nervous and musculoskeletal systems. Impairments in the area overlapping the cardiovascular-pulmonary and musculoskeletal systems can limit the individual's capacity to sustain movement, including ambulation. In the following paragraphs, the effects of control and capacity impairments are discussed.

Movement Control

The control of movement, postural responses, and ambulation is the result of complex interactions between the nervous and musculoskeletal systems (Fig. 19-8). Automatic, reflexive, and volitional levels of control may be influenced.[50,69] The automatic level of control relies on central mechanisms to interpret the position of body segments; implement common movements; judge disturbances accurately; and respond with the appropriate timing, sequencing, and force.[88]

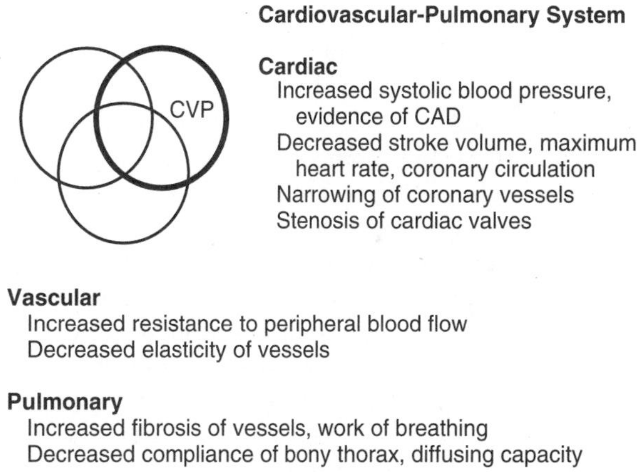

Cardiovascular-Pulmonary System

Cardiac
Increased systolic blood pressure, evidence of CAD
Decreased stroke volume, maximum heart rate, coronary circulation
Narrowing of coronary vessels
Stenosis of cardiac valves

Vascular
Increased resistance to peripheral blood flow
Decreased elasticity of vessels

Pulmonary
Increased fibrosis of vessels, work of breathing
Decreased compliance of bony thorax, diffusing capacity

FIG. 19-7 Changes in the cardiovascular-pulmonary system that may contribute to problems with ambulation in the elderly.

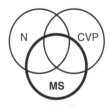

Musculoskeletal System

Less tightly packed muscle fibers
Increased fat content, increased fibrin
Decreased number of type II muscle fibers
Decreased bone density
Increased stiffness
Decreased extensibility in the trunk, shoulder, and ankle
Changed postural alignment

FIG. 19-6 Changes in the musculoskeletal system that may contribute to problems with ambulation in the elderly.

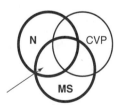

Movement Control
Decline in:
Proximal dynamic stability
BoS-CoG adaptability
Abnormal timing and sequencing of movements
Reduced redundancy in balance control
Decreased lower extremity strength

FIG. 19-8 Interaction of nervous and musculoskeletal systems that affects problems with ambulation in the elderly.

These mechanisms are needed to maintain a posture and to respond to minor or previously encountered changes in the external environment. Automatic ambulatory patterns are generated from central feedforward mechanisms and result in responses to known situations. These automatic programs may not be adequate in some elderly individuals because the total system for the control of movement may be slowed. Abnormalities also may exist and interfere with correct observation and interpretation of environmental conditions, as well as with adequate strength and timing of motor responses. Any novelty in environmental conditions may exaggerate the impairment. The reflexive level of control involves peripheral sensorimotor links that consist of proprioceptive and stretch receptor mechanisms and the vestibulo-ocular reflex.[3,50,54,86] Volitional control requires conscious attention to the activity. Such attention is more important if the environmental conditions are unusual, such as walking in the dark, or if the ability to monitor these conditions has been altered internally, as can occur with diminished distal sensation. Conscious effort usually results in a reduction of speed and an increase in energy cost. The decreased sensory inputs that occur with aging, coupled with the inability to vary motor strategies, reduce the overlapping of sensory input and the adaptability of motor responses.[86]

Some of the motor control problems found in the elderly during ambulation can be analyzed by examining three conditions inherent in purposeful movement: the position of the body must be known, the target position or goal to be achieved must be identified, and the correct combination of muscle forces in the correct sequence must be generated to move from the starting position to the goal position.

The combination of feedforward and feedback mechanisms and the sensory input contributing to movement control normally allow movement to occur from the existing body position toward a subsequent target position in a coordinated fashion. Programs within the central nervous system (CNS) underlying the automatic nature of ambulation are altered with aging through changes in both peripheral and central inputs. Visual, vestibular, and proprioceptive mechanisms that monitor conditions internal to the body, such as limb position, muscle length-tension relations, and the ability to monitor environmental conditions external to the individual also change with aging.[86] If the sensitivity of any or all of these modalities is reduced, integration of the necessary afferent information into a motor plan can be difficult.

The speed of walking is influenced by the intensity of lower extremity muscle activation.[11] The ability to generate sufficient motor force in the proper sequence is diminished in the elderly.[58] Thus, the decreased walking speed of elderly individuals may be an accommodation to the decreased ability to generate sufficient force in the required time.[81] The decrease in muscle activation may be due to delayed nerve conduction velocity, diminished sensory awareness, disuse atrophy, or a combination of all these factors. Any of these can create a cycle in which reduced ambulation leads to disuse weakness, which in turn further limits ambulation. In addition to the effect these impairments have on the function of ambulation, they also have been associated with abnormalities in static and dynamic postural control.

Movement Capacity

In addition to changes in movement control, functional limitations in ambulation can be due to changes in the capacity for movement—the physiological overlap between the cardiovascular-pulmonary and musculoskeletal systems (Fig. 19-9). Clinically, CVP changes may be manifested in the elderly as lowered aerobic capacity, diminished exercise tolerance, and positional hypotension. A decline in cardiac output, decreased maximum heart rate, reduced vital capacity, increased residual volume, decreased oxygen saturation, increased resistance to peripheral blood flow, diminished blood flow to the muscles, and decreased ability to extract oxygen from the blood[4] can all adversely affect the interdependent relationship between the cardiovascular-pulmonary and musculoskeletal systems. All of these changes can lead to a reduced ability to respond to the aerobic demand of functional activities and thus promote further decline in aerobic capacity.[1] Elderly individuals with CVP system impairments may be forced to decrease the speed of walking and stair climbing due to an inability to sustain the output of energy required by the increased metabolic cost of these activities. The loss of speed, in turn, leads to an overall decrease in endurance for functional activities. For this reason, the 6-minute walk test, which measures the distance walked in the designated time, is a common tool used to assess endurance.[56] In general, the ability of elderly persons declines with advancing years, but the individual results seem more related to activity level rather than to age. However, even healthy elderly individuals have progressively smaller aerobic reserves due to the decline in $\dot{V}O_2$max. This decline in aerobic reserve makes it more difficult for elderly to accommodate the energy demand of a gait disorder or the need for faster speed. Cunningham and Martin examined the influence of age and sedentary life-style on walking speed by measuring the metabolic cost of walking at preferred speeds and at speeds

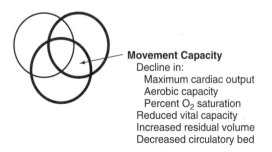

Movement Capacity
Decline in:
   Maximum cardiac output
   Aerobic capacity
   Percent O_2 saturation
Reduced vital capacity
Increased residual volume
Decreased circulatory bed

FIG. 19-9   Interaction of cardiovascular-pulmonary and musculoskeletal systems that affect problems with ambulation in the elderly.

across a spectrum. Findings in this study indicated that there was a 10% decline in walking speed in sedentary individuals by age. The metabolic cost exceeded the difference in speed, which may indicate an altered efficiency in the speed of muscle contraction and of muscle fiber recruitment patterns.[17,55]

Interrelationship of Control and Capacity

Improving an individual's capacity for exercise seems to influence his/her movement control. Baylor and Spirduso investigated the relationship between aerobic exercise and components of reaction time in older women. They found that in older women regular aerobic exercise was an important factor in influencing the speed of reactions to simple and discriminatory stimuli and also was associated with enhanced speed of reaction-type responses both in the central and peripheral components. It was speculated that exercise may affect the oxidative capacity of the brain and of the central nervous system function in general. In the group of elderly who did not exercise, contraction times were slower.[6]

EVALUATION

Interpretation of Findings Related to Intervention Strategies

One purpose for examining the physical systems is to identify impairments that contribute to the limitations found during the gait analysis. During the evaluation the therapist clusters these findings to determine the proportional contribution of the impairments to the functional limitation, and to the extent possible, determines the most effective and efficient means of remediating both the functional deficits and the impairments through the implementation of a comprehensive intervention program. For example, decreased toe-off and limited dorsiflexion during swing may be clinical findings of the gait analysis. Before an effective intervention can be designed, the therapist must determine whether these findings are due to a loss of ROM at the ankle, weak plantarflexors and dorsiflexors, diminished proprioception, poor motor control, limited capacity for repetitive movement, or any combination of these factors. In addition to treatment of specific impairments, conscious changes in the gait pattern also may be an effective means to enhance voluntary control of the task. If the problem has been long standing, changes in the patient may occur slowly, if at all; therefore supportive devices, such as an ankle foot orthosis (AFO), need to be considered. In addition, the individual may need education regarding elimination of any obstacles that may increase the chance of "catching his/her toe" and may need to be cautioned about walking on uneven surfaces.

Clinical Impression: Relating Impairments to Possible Functional Changes

It is difficult to differentiate impairments that result from aging from those that are due to diseases, such as diabetes, or to a sedentary life-style.[43] For example, persons who fall and those who are sedentary tend to be weaker than those who do not fall or who are active.[81] However, it is not always clear which of these problems has occurred first: the falling, the sedentary behavior, or the weakness. What is evident is that if a fall occurs, many elderly persons, even those who have been quite active, may reduce their activity level because of anxiety or fear of falling and thus put themselves at further ambulatory risk, e.g., sedentary individuals are more at risk for hip fracture.[18,20,30]

In the evaluation process, the therapist considers examination findings in each of the physical systems, determines the proportional contribution of these to the patient's functional limitation, assesses the patient's potential for change, and determines the availability of intervention strategy options.[75] For example, the inability to climb stairs after a hip fracture may be related to decreased aerobic capacity, diminished lower extremity strength, and abnormal balance responses (Fig. 19-10). The poor balance may be the result of decreased ROM, proprioception, and stability in the ankles and diminished strength and proprioception at the hip. All of these contribute to the functional limitation, with strength involved in both ambulation and balance dysfunction. The patient in this example had been sedentary before the hip fracture so the therapist determines that aerobic deconditioning is a large contributor to the short ambulatory distance. Because aerobic conditioning and strengthening exercises may take a few weeks before functional changes may be noted the therapist includes assistive and environmental changes in the total intervention plan. Other considerations that are factored into the treatment plan include the length of time the patient has had the functional limitation and impairments, the course of the disability, and the environmental constraints.

In this example, the mix of the most effective and efficient modes of intervention to remedy the impairments and maximize functional capability has not yet been determined, most probably because a range of strengthening, flexibility, aerobic, and balance exercises needs to be coupled with education, adaptive and assistive devices and aides, and environmental modifications. At this point, the clinical question can be framed as "to what extent, in what combination, and when should intervention focus on changing the individual, on providing adaptive or assistive devices or aides, or on modifying the environment?" Therapists can target interventions more specifically on the underlying cause when the relationships between pathology, impairments, functional limitation, and disability are better known[31,75] as well as the influence of an active or sedentary life-style. The therapist's decision making will improve when more is known about the reversibility of the deficits and the ability of the individual to respond to the intervention in a realistic time period.

In addition to assisting individuals in changing, the therapist can help to modify the environment. Environmental modifications may be a more efficient way to effect change and reach the functional outcomes when a number of individuals share common impairments, such as reduced speed of ambulation, decreased extremity ROM, and decreased postural stability. Interventions may include decreasing step height, varying chair height, raising the height of toilet seats, removing area rugs, prolonging the walk time at crossing lights, installing stall showers with grab bars and night-lights in bathrooms, and altering the size or shape of doorknobs.[77]

INTERVENTION

The physical therapist's intervention is directed toward functional outcomes desired by both the patient and the physical therapist. The outcome emphasized in this chapter is ambulation with sufficient control and capacity to be safe at a speed that allows independence with or without an assistive device on a variety of surfaces. Although the focus of this chapter is toward improved ambulation, the individual's ability to perform ADL and to communicate effectively also would be included in the complete physical therapy program.

Intervention has been shown to be effective in altering the changes that accompany aging and that may result from a sedentary existence. Therapeutic exercise programs administered to a wide range of elderly persons have resulted in improvements in their strength, flexibility, and exercise capacity.[1,22,42] Lord investigated whether a program of regular exercise improved gait patterns in older women and whether any such improvement in gait is mediated by increased lower-limb muscle strength. A 22-week trial of exercise was conducted with 160 women between the ages of 60 to 83, with a mean age of 71.1 years. The exercise subjects showed improved strength in five lower-limb muscle groups and increased walking speed, cadence, and stride length and shortened their stride times. Increased cadence was associated with improved ankle dorsiflexion strength, and increases in stride length were related to improved hip extension strength. Exercise subjects with a lower initial walking speed showed greater changes in velocity, stride length, ca-

dence, and stance duration than those with a faster initial walking speed.[49] Finlay demonstrated that exercise in patients with hip fracture or total hip replacement could improve walking speed from 0.82 m/sec to 1.13 m/sec—an improvement of 82%. These patients had standard postoperative treatment but had not participated in follow-up exercise interventions after the acute stay.[24]

Chandler and Hadley, in reviewing the impact of exercise in elderly men and women, reported that the musculoskeletal and cardiovascular systems, regardless of age, can respond to both resistance and aerobic training as measured by impairments, such as diminished strength and maximum oxygen uptake. The magnitude of physiological effect may be dampened in frailer individuals in response to lower-intensity exercise stimuli. In the most impaired elders, exercise may help to forestall further decline in physiological reserve rather than produce significant gains. The extent to which exercise programs affect performance and disability is less clear. Exercise programs in frailer individuals appear to have greater effect on gait speed and chair rise time than similar programs in healthier individuals. The impact of exercise on measures of disability has not been widely reported. Studies reviewed by Chandler and Hadley suggest that exercise training in elders is a potential means of reducing the burden of impairments and ultimately improving function.[13]

Myers identified 52 studies that examined risk factors for falls and nine intervention studies. Intervention studies that were directed at nursing home populations did not result in prevention of falls but had other statistically and clinically significant outcomes. Studies among the community dwelling that targeted potential or current risk factors and included an exercise component reported a significant reduction in falls, prevention of the onset of new disabilities, and reduction of baseline risk factors.[60]

A functional outcome can be characterized as being performed either with control or with compensatory strategies. Normal control assumes a standard timing and sequencing of movement with an amount of force appropriate to perform the task; normal movement is efficient and requires the least amount of energy. When normal control is not possible because of unalterable impairments, compensatory strategies are indicated. However, compensatory movements commonly require more energy. Age-appropriate comparison movements must be kept in mind when determining functional outcomes and treatment goals for elderly patients. Changes in the pattern and speed of gait, in sensory inputs, and in the strength and timing of muscle responses all occur with aging. Thus, "normal" standards both at the functional and impairment level are age dependent.

As previously stated, the patient's functional capability, the impairments related to the limitations in ambulation, and the patient's potential for change are all determined during the evaluation. The next step in the clinical decision-making process is to translate these examination findings into an intervention plan. To do so, the impairments that limit function should be clustered into the classifications de-

Functional Limitation: Stair Climbing

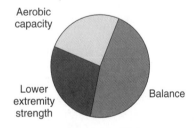

Balance impairment further related to:
   Decreased ROM trunk, hips, and ankles
   Strength and proprioception in ankles
   Strength and proprioception in hips

FIG. 19-10   Analysis of impairments that contribute to functional limitations in stair climbing.

scribed in the intervention model (see the following section). Realistic treatment goals can be prioritized according to the assessments of which changes are possible for the individual and which changes most probably will have the greatest influence on improving the outcome of ambulation. The general goals could include increasing ROM, increasing the time that standing can be maintained without assistance, and improving the ability to repeatedly assume standing from sitting. The goals also can include the teaching of compensatory movements and modification of the environment.

Intervention Model

The intervention model is a three-dimensional matrix that classifies physical characteristics associated with functional ability (Fig. 19-11). The classifications encompass the control of and capacity for posture and movement. The model describes a general intervention strategy designed to achieve functional outcomes by sequencing the difficulty of movements. Anatomical and biomechanical principles and theories of motor control, motor learning, and exercise physiology are integral to this strategy and formulate the basis for the principles of physical therapist intervention. The model and principles guide the therapist in designing effective and efficient treatment strategies to achieve the functional outcome. The impact of impairments can be decreased by combining the four strategies of intervention: remediating the patient's deficits, providing adaptive and assistive devices and aides, providing education and modifying the environment.

The following is a list of impairments associated with gait changes that will be the focus of intervention to be discussed:

- Lowered sensory acuity—proprioception, vision, vestibular
- Decreased ROM
- Altered postural alignment
- Decreased strength overall, but particularly in the hip and knee extensors and knee and ankle flexors
- Altered static and dynamic balance
- Decreased reaction time, especially when attention is shared
- Decreased muscle endurance and general aerobic capacity

The postures and movements included in the treatment are termed *activities* and are sequenced along the model's vertical axis. Movement control, delineated into stages that progress the complexity of motor tasks,[74] constitutes the horizontal axis. Movement control is enhanced with the use of various treatment *techniques* that are used in conjunction with the specific activities. The third axis describes *parameters* of capacity that correspond to the stress imposed on the patient by the movement. The actual values of these parameters are determined by the patient's level of healing, physiological requirements, and cognitive status. By classifying the patient's impairments within the components of the model, the therapist may be able to better analyze the relationship between impairments and function, prioritize and sequence intervention procedures, and determine the most appropriate intervention strategies.[75]

The patient's impairments associated with the functional limitation are classified in the intervention model, and the

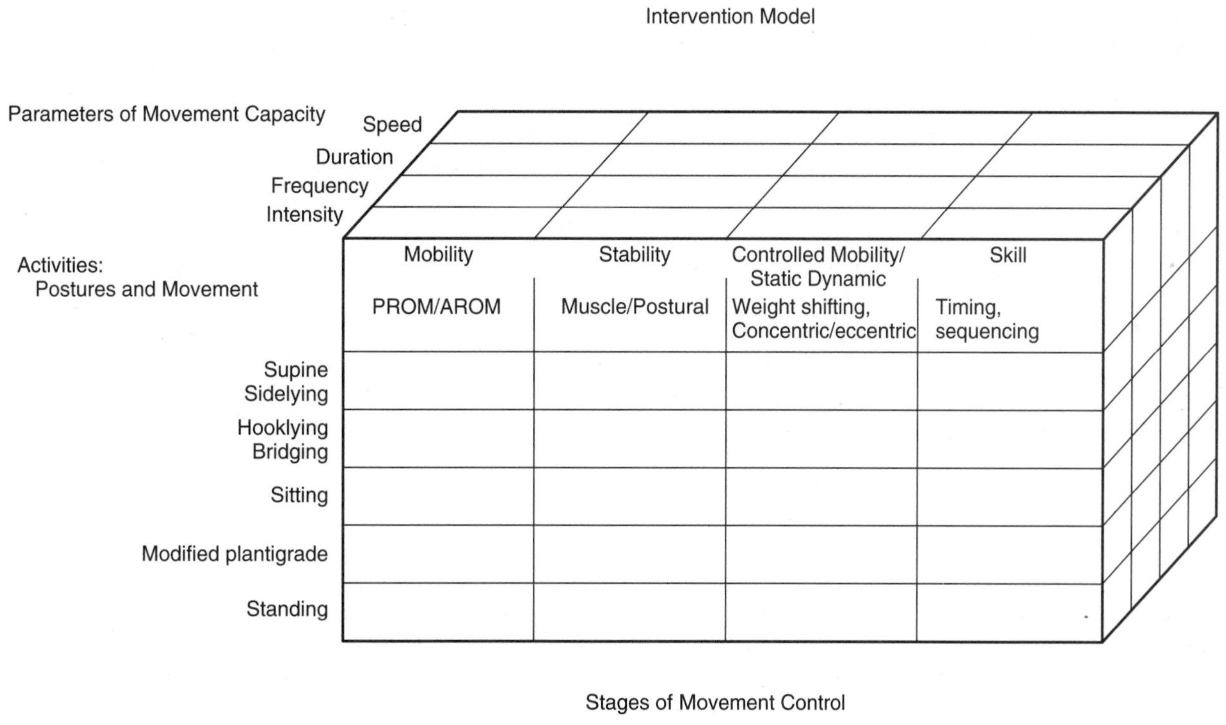

Intervention Model

FIG. 19-11 The intervention model classifies stages of movement control and parameters of movement capacity in relationship to postures and movements.

decision-making process is continued. A patient may demonstrate limitations in walking and climbing stairs associated with impairments of decreased ankle ROM, knee and hip extensor strength, dynamic balance, and generalized decreased muscle endurance. These impairments correspond to movement classifications described by the stages of control and parameters of capacity. The impairments that the therapist determines can be changed are translated into treatment goals. For this patient, the anticipated goals might include the achievement of sufficient ankle ROM to ambulate and descend stairs by sustaining isometric contractions of the trunk, hip, and knee extensors for at least 30 seconds; increasing eccentric strength of the hip and knee extensors; and maintaining unilateral weight bearing in standing for 10 seconds. These treatment goals are designed to achieve the functional outcomes of ambulation for 1/4 mile and stair descent at a functional pace. The treatment procedures are developed, sequenced, implemented, and progressed to achieve the treatment goals and demonstrate functional outcomes. The treatment goals reflect both improvements in movement control, e.g., improved ROM and muscle stability, and movement capacity, e.g., holding a moderate intensity contraction up to 30 seconds. For example, passive range of motion (PROM) around the ankle may first be developed with moderate intensity of hold relax and joint oscillations, and muscle stability in the lower limb may be promoted with low-intensity isometric contractions. If the patient has difficulty learning the movement, the frequency of the task may be altered and verbal or visual feedback may be varied. The progression of the home exercise program, patient-related instruction regarding adaptive and assistive devices and aides, and modification of the environment are ongoing throughout the rehabilitation program. Initial improvements found in strength and capacity measures may actually be displayed by learning and neural control modifications. Actual changes in strength and capacity may require up to 6 weeks to achieve. The therapist needs to educate the patient regarding the indicators that can be monitored to adjust the difficulty of the procedure. For example, the Borg rating of perceived exertion (RPE) can be used when an individual performs independent or home exercises.[10] If the patient has a cardiac or diabetic condition that may affect his/her strength, balance, or capacity, then additional treatments with the therapist may be needed to ensure adequate understanding of the exercise monitors.

The objective and subjective changes in the impairments and functional abilities are continually noted so that appropriate modifications to the general strategy and specific procedures can be made. The patient's subjective report of functional change does not always parallel the objective findings. The therapist needs to monitor both types of outcome measures to adequately determine treatment effectiveness and the need for further intervention. Easy-to-use, reliable, valid, and sensitive measures need to be chosen.[65] The impairments that cannot be changed by any of the physical therapy strategies are determined, and appropriate referrals are made.

Units of the Procedure

Intervention procedures combine the three components of treatment: the activities, the techniques, and the parameters. Procedures, designed to achieve one or more treatment goals, always begin with exercises the patient can perform and progress toward achieving the functional outcome.[75]

Activities

Activities are postures and movement patterns incorporated in the intervention to achieve the treatment goals and functional outcomes. The postures associated with ambulation include those that occur during the assumption of standing and those in which specific motor abilities can be practiced and achieved. The sequence of postures, which includes supine, sidelying, sitting, and standing, can aid in the assumption and control of standing. The control of the lower trunk and lower extremities required for the assumption of standing and for ambulation can be further enhanced in hooklying, bridging, and modified plantigrade. These postures are included in treatment to improve ambulatory control, as well as to increase weight-bearing stress. Weight-bearing stress in the upper extremity can also be achieved in quadruped. However, quadruped may be too difficult for many elderly persons and is therefore not included in the program.

Techniques

Techniques are sensory inputs and types of muscle contractions used to enhance the stages of movement control. The treatment techniques used may include those that increase passive or active ROM (mobility), improve the ability to sustain an isometric contraction and to maintain a posture (stability), enhance the ability to move within or between postures (controlled mobility and static-dynamic control), and improve the timing and sequencing of movement (skill).

Parameters

The exercise parameters are the frequency, duration, intensity, and speed of each of the treatment procedures. These parameters are varied according to the patient's learning ability, cardiovascular-pulmonary status, or the acuteness of the dysfunction.

For those patients who demonstrate difficulty with learning due to attention-span deficits or decreased sensory-motor integration, the parameters can be altered to affect the practice schedule and the internal and external feedback. The duration of each treatment can be reduced and the frequency increased to distribute the repetition of the task, and the intensity of patient effort can be altered to increase feedback and enhance the response of various peripheral receptors.[19,54,86]

Patients who are limited by exercise capacity deficits and involvement of the cardiovascular-pulmonary system may

require modifications in the exercise parameters so that appropriate physiological stress occurs during the procedures. Heart rate, blood pressure, and perceived exertion[10] during the intervention program should be monitored in such circumstances.

If the patient is recovering from a musculoskeletal injury or surgery, exercise parameters should be adjusted according to the tissue's reactivity[35] or ability to respond to varying amounts of intensity or frequency of exercise. Elderly patients may recover more slowly, manifest different responses to internal and external stress, and be more affected by the deleterious results of bedrest.

Various intensities of exercise have been used to improve strength. In a group of very elderly persons, high-intensity exercise was used to counteract muscle weakness in the hip and knee extensors. These muscle performance changes were associated with an improvement in walking speed.[23] Strengthening exercise is a generic phrase requiring more definition before treatment effectiveness can be determined. Some patients' functional limitations reflect the need for muscle aerobic training, therefore increased repetitions at low to moderate intensity may improve the distance walked. Some may not be able to generate the muscle force to climb stairs or assume standing from sitting. In such cases fewer repetitions but at a greater intensity would seem indicated. Others seem to have a general fatigue impairment that limits the distance walked or the number of stairs climbed, indicating the need for general aerobic training of progressive intensity with increased repetitions and frequency of a total body exercise program, such as that provided by a stationery bicycle, treadmill, or walking program. Not uncommon is the need for a combination of all three "strengthening" exercise protocols.

Impairments Classified According to the Stages of Control

Examples of impairments related to the control of movement are classified within the model along the horizontal axis. From these classifications, treatment goals and appropriate treatment techniques can be determined. For example, a patient receiving treatment may be limited in weight shifting forward during the transition from sitting to standing as a result of impairments that include tightness of the hip capsule and of the hip extensor muscle. Limited range is classified within the mobility stage. To determine the treatment goal, the therapist considers the patient's range in comparison to that required for moving from sitting to standing,[41] the type of tissue involved (capsule and muscle), and the duration of involvement. If the limitation is in soft tissue and is of short duration, the assumption can be made that change can occur. If the impairment is chronic or if bone limits ROM, soft tissue changes are unlikely, necessitating physical therapy treatment aimed at compensation that might include raising seat height and adding rails to the toilet; referral for surgical intervention might also be considered.

Mobility—Passive Range of Motion

Impairment. PROM deficits that impede ambulation, assumption of standing, or stair climbing can be due to shortening or stiffness of the skin; connective tissue; muscle; ligament; and capsule in the trunk, hip, knee, or ankle.

Functional Implications. During the stance and swing phases of gait, impairments of range in the trunk, hip, and ankle may limit trunk counter-rotation, pelvic rotation, step length, the ability to maintain an erect posture, and tibial translation over the talus.[59] For example, decreased range into lumbar extension combined with tight hip flexors and plantar flexors may reduce terminal stance and step length. Patients with decreased range in the trunk and lower extremity may have difficulty moving from sitting to standing[16,41] and may be restricted to climbing stairs one step at a time. The first phase of assuming standing normally requires upper body and hip flexion and flexion of the knees and ankles as the feet move or are positioned under the front of the chair. If these joints or surrounding tissues are stiff, these initial flexion movements will be restricted. Another common finding—difficulty with erect standing following prolonged sitting—may result from impairments that include stiffness in the flexor muscles and decreased joint flexibility. Abnormal range in the thoracic and cervical spine also can influence posture and gait. Typically, an elderly person will demonstrate thoracic and cervical changes that anteriorly translate the upper body's center of gravity. To offset this change, the individual may alter muscular activity or position the upper extremities posteriorly to control postural responses in sitting and standing and while walking.

Treatment Goals. These include improvement of trunk and limb ROM by decreasing tissue stiffness and improving muscle and soft tissue length. The measure of effectiveness could be joint ROM, muscle length, the stiffness or resistance to passive movement, and the achievement of the range that commonly occurs during functional activities. For example, during the assumption of standing from sitting or during stair descent the position or movement of the lower leg is an indication of the functional ankle ROM.

Treatment Techniques. If specific joint motions are limited by capsular or ligamentous tightness or by chronic joint effusion, joint mobilization and measures to reduce edema should be incorporated. The therapist must note that edema around the ankle may be associated with cardiac disease—requiring special examination procedures—and stiffness may be related to diabetic tissue changes. If muscle tightness is noted, hold relax (HR) to increase contractile tissue extensibility is indicated. Active warm-up activities or heat may be useful before ROM procedures. Self-stretching has an advantage in that it can be performed independently, although it is not as specific to any one tissue. During self-stretching, the movements and instructions should be sufficiently specific to limit the stretch to the involved area. Whether individual or group exercise is performed, care must be taken with persons who have osteoporosis or whose bones are osteopenic.

ROM exercises can be performed in any position in which the involved joint is non-weight bearing. To ensure relaxation, supine, side-lying, or sitting postures are common.

Mobility—Initiation of Active Movement

Impairment. The ability to initiate active movement is decreased and the speed with which movement is initiated may be delayed. The weakness that reduces the initiation of movement may be due to a combination of fewer type II fibers, resistance from stiff antagonistic tissues, and a sedentary life-style. Peripheral neural involvement, as occurs with diabetes or central involvement from Parkinson's disease or hemiplegia, also may affect movement initiation.

Functional Implications. When initiation of movement is too slow or weak, postural reactions and automatic movements in standing or during ambulation may not occur with sufficient speed to respond to environmental demands or to allow for an adequate rate of walking. For example, activation of the dorsiflexors or everters may be delayed if the tissues around the ankle are stiff. Weakened muscle may have difficulty overcoming internal tissue resistance impeding movements during postural disturbances,[3,81] ambulation, and stair climbing. Decreased sensory input from proprioceptive, visual, and vestibular receptors also can lead to diminished movement initiation as can cognitive inattention. The therapist, if possible, needs to differentiate a sensory input from a motor output impairment and also differentiate these from a deficit in cognitive functioning so that the appropriate intervention can be implemented.

Treatment Goals. Goals are to improve initiation of active movement, including the "strength" and the speed of the motion. Treatment measures may include testing the speed or delay in movement initiation, the range through which movement occurs, and the strength of the response.

Treatment Techniques. If the patient has difficulty initiating movement in the presence of increased tone, e.g., an individual with Parkinson's disease, rhythmic initiation (RI) is chosen to facilitate active movement. Because of the repetitive motion, RI also is appropriate for patients experiencing difficulty in learning movements. If the patient has difficulty initiating contractions in the postural extensors associated with muscle weakness, hold relax active motion (HRAM) is performed to improve the holding ability in shortened ranges and the ability to initiate movement from the lengthened range. If weakness is primarily in the flexor muscles, the technique of repeated contractions (RC) may promote increased motor unit activation by superimposing a stretch response onto a voluntary contraction. By stimulating muscle spindle activity, these techniques also may enhance peripheral proprioceptive input. Electrical stimulation may augment voluntary contractions if the problem is localized, e.g., in the anterior tibialis muscle.

As with the exercises to improve PROM, when promoting the initiation of movement, postures are chosen in which the involved segment is non-weight bearing. For example, if the goal is to improve the initiation of ankle dorsiflexion, sitting with the knee in a comfortable amount of extension may be appropriate.

Stability

Muscle Stability

Muscle stability is the ability of postural muscles to hold for at least 10 seconds in their shortened ranges. Holding in the shortened range requires co-activation of the alpha and gamma motor units to contract the extrafusal and intrafusal muscle fibers. Thus, stretch sensitivity of the muscle spindle is indirectly assessed as the patient holds the contraction in the shortened range.

Impairment. The postural extensor muscles are weak, with decreased ability to sustain isometric contractions in the shortened range against gravitational or manual resistance. Diminished proprioception associated with poor position or movement sense, in other than extreme ranges, also is related to decreased muscle spindle responses.[70]

Functional Implications. Maintenance of a contraction with resistance and approximately 40% effort is performed primarily by type I muscle fibers. In elderly patients with decreased strength and a decreased circulatory muscle bed, attempts at holding may require proportionally more effort and muscular contractions may become anaerobic more rapidly. Another factor that may contribute to their weakness is a sedentary life-style, in particular prolonged sitting, that results in maintained lengthened ranges of the trunk and lower extremity postural extensors. Although in elderly patients the loss of type II motor units appears to predominate, many clinical findings suggest a decreased holding ability or loss of type I motor unit functioning. These findings include fatigue; reduced aerobic capacity; poor postural stability; and the decreased ability to maintain erect, upright postures. Promoting muscle stability provides the prerequisite control in the postural muscles of the trunk, hips, knees, and ankles to more adequately maintain body weight in upright positions. The improved postural awareness that may accompany improved muscle spindle feedback may enhance the learning of gait patterns and "correct" posture.

Treatment Goals. The goal is to improve isometric "strength," endurance, or duration of low- to moderate-intensity muscle contractions. Treatment measures include tests of isometric strength in the shortened range for a longer duration, the reduction of an active lag, improvement in proprioceptive awareness, and improved muscle endurance. Functionally, muscle stability improvement may be observed as the patient stands more erect for a longer duration because the hip and lower trunk extensors can hold in the shortened range.

Treatment Techniques. The technique of a shortened held resisted contraction (SHRC) can be used to facilitate an isometric contraction of the trunk, hip, knee, and ankle extensors in their shortened ranges. With this technique, the patient maintains an isometric contraction in or near the shortened range of the extensor muscles for approximately 10 seconds, then progresses to greater duration. Increasing the duration of the contraction is the initial means of progressing the challenge and is essential to reducing muscle fatigue. The type and amount of resistive force can be altered among gravity or manual or mechanical forces. The contractions should be graded to approximately 40% of maximum effort to foster contraction of primarily slow-twitch fibers. The duration of the contraction is gradually increased while the patient maintains this intensity level. The individual should be able to breathe comfortably during the exercise, which assists in ensuring that the response remains aerobic. Heart rate and blood pressure may need to be monitored, particularly if the patient has cardiac dysfunction. In these cases the intensity of response may need to be decreased. The duration of the contraction can be progressed by counting the number of breaths the patient takes while maintaining the contraction rather than by counting the number of seconds. For example, "hold the position for three breaths and progress to holding for five breaths." After increasing the duration, the number of repetitions, or frequency, of the exercise is increased. The patient should be encouraged to hold in progressively shorter and shorter ranges until holding in the shortened range can be achieved.

The supine position is initially chosen when the goal is to improve muscle stability in the extensors of the lower trunk, hip, and knee to decrease the resistive effects of gravity. A pillow is placed under the knees, and the patient instructed to "push the knees down into the pillow and lift the hips and lower body." Upper body muscle stability also can be performed in supine by instructing the patient to "push the elbows into the bed, pinch the shoulder blades together, and lift the chest up toward the ceiling." This upper body exercise also can be performed in the sitting position using elastic-band or pulley resistance.

Postural Stability

Postural stability is the ability to maintain weight-bearing postures for the amount of time needed by the patient to perform functional tasks. This stage is also termed *static postural control, static balance,* and *static stability.*

Impairment. The decreased ability to maintain midline or weight-bearing postures may be the result of diminished ROM, sensory awareness, speed or strength of muscular responses, ability to alter contraction between antagonists in midranges, or ability to grade the strength or timing of the response. ROM is addressed in the mobility stage and sensory awareness in the muscle stability level of control.

Functional Implications. A posture must be maintained either by external supports or by muscular forces before functional activities can be performed in that posture. Maintaining the upright posture of standing—important for many ADL functions—is prerequisite to ambulation for most individuals. However, standing and walking differ in their muscular activity and kinetics due to their varied static and dynamic nature.

Some patients who have impairments commonly associated with poor balance, such as diminished proprioception and strength, seem to abnormally stiffen while attempting to maintain a static position. They demonstrate less than the usual amount of sway and may have great difficulty progressing onto dynamic stability. The underlying muscle and postural stability impairments that have necessitated the stiffening compensation need to be addressed with appropriate intervention.

Treatment Goals. The goal is to increase the length of time the patient is able to maintain postures such as sitting and standing. At the muscle level, measures can be improvement in the "strength" of the isometric response; in the timing of the response, i.e., reducing the time lag between the application of resistance and the muscle's response; and in position or movement sense. The clinical measures also can include the duration that the posture is maintained, the correctness and awareness of postural alignment, and the amount of sway that occurs while the position is maintained. Postural stability, particularly in the lower body extensors, can be promoted in less-demanding positions, such as bridging and modified plantigrade, as well as in standing.

Treatment Techniques. Alternating isometrics (AI) and rhythmic stabilization (RS) are techniques that can be applied to the shoulders or hips with the patient in upright postures. A minimal to moderate amount of resistance is applied slowly, consistent with the patient's ability. The speed of resistance can be gradually increased, coupled with a reduced intensity to improve the patient's response time. Initially, resistance may be performed in a rhythmic manner, allowing the patient to anticipate the changes to assist in learning the responses. The timing and intensity of the resistance progresses to an irregular pattern to promote the anticipatory responses needed during dynamic functional activities. As these parameters are gradually altered, sensory stimuli also are diminished by having the patient maintain postures and balance without vision or to stand on foam. During these more difficult conditions, to improve awareness of peripheral input, the patient may be cued to focus on foot and ankle sensations as the techniques are applied. Resistance can be applied with free weights, pulleys, or elastic, and the patient can isometrically "disturb" his/her own balance by pushing or pulling against an immovable object. In other postures, e.g., bridging or modified plantigrade, AI and RS can be applied to promote specific hip or knee control, or the patient can attempt to maintain the postures without external resistance for longer periods to improve muscle endurance. If the patient seems to have difficulty with stability at the ankle, noted either by an excessive ankle strategy or a compensatory hip strategy, AI and RS can be applied with the patient sitting, placement of the limb in a non–weight-bearing position, and with a manual contact above and below the ankle to enhance the muscle and sensory responses.

Controlled Mobility

The concentric-eccentric muscle contractions in weight-bearing postures that occur at this stage are also termed *dynamic stability, weight shifting,* and *eccentric control* in the posture.

Impairments. Many of the impairments classified at this stage can result from deficits in the mobility and stability stages. However, studies have noted that during weight shifting within a posture, older persons have less ability to control the outer limits of sway, even though they may be able to maintain a static posture.[86] It is not clear whether this weight-shifting difficulty is related to the range required during movement, to the decreased sensory awareness, or to the diminished motor ability to modify and increase force production as the center of mass moves.[85] Eccentric contractions, although requiring less capacity and force, may require more control than concentric contractions and are essential to self-controlled weight-shifting activities. In addition to promoting more advanced movement control, weight shifting over a limb increases the muscular and weight-bearing forces on bones—a consideration for those with osteoporosis. Within the trunk, this stage is addressed during rolling movements by controlling a log-rolling movement.

Functional Implications. Pelvic rotation during gait is commonly limited in the elderly. However, analysis of trunk motion has not differentiated between the available passive movement and the active ability to control that movement. Functionally, older persons tend to rotate the body less and have difficulty isolating neck rotation. In addition, weight transference time has been shown to be delayed in the elderly during gait initiation.[62] As weight shifting improves, the speed of the movement also should increase, which may be demonstrated as improved gait initiation and weight exchange. A deficit in eccentric control in the quadriceps and gluteals may be evaluated during the functional activities of descending stairs and moving from standing to sitting.

Treatment Goals. Goals can include increased excursion of sway, greater control of sway at the ankles rather than at more cephalo areas, and improved timing of gait initiation. Clinical monitors can include the distance that movement can be controlled, termed *dynamic balance,* or the limit of stability. Sitting and standing reaching tests in different planes of movement can standardize the measure.[21] Anticipatory responses to changes in the body's center of mass can be observed, e.g., as the patient sways in standing or moves an upper extremity while standing. The therapist also may monitor concentric-eccentric movement through increasing range at this stage. Because muscle control through range is needed, measures can be concentric-eccentric "strength and endurance," including determining movement of knee extension in the sitting posture, testing the amount of weight lifted and lowered by the quadriceps, and counting the number of repetitions performed with a consistent amount of weight.

Treatment Techniques. Weight shifting can be performed either as a concentric-eccentric reversal of one muscle group, *termed agonistic reversal (AR),* or as a reversal of antagonists, termed *slow reversal hold (SRH)* or *slow reversal (SR).* In either condition, resistance can be applied manually or with weights. Progression is achieved by (1) increasing the range of movement, which in turn requires an increase in the ability to control the excursion of the center of gravity; (2) moving the center of gravity over a fixed base of support, then moving the base of support under the center of mass; (3) performing movements on a stable surface, then on an unstable base; and (4) altering the sensory conditions. For example, in standing, weight shifting or swaying over the feet is performed before raising on the toes or heels, which decreases the size of the base. On a balance board a similar sequence is to maintain the position, then shift the position of the board. In both conditions, the weight-shifting motion is encouraged at the ankle to promote a more normal ankle strategy.[86] The sensory conditions can be altered to challenge vestibular and proprioceptive mechanisms: vision can be obscured or the individual can stand on foam.

The technique of AR can promote eccentric control of the quadriceps in the modified plantigrade position and of the gluteals in bridging. AR can also be applied to limb movements such as knee extension to improve the "strength" of the quadriceps. The patient can be sitting and lifting a weight, which makes the exercise non-weight bearing, or the patient may be in modified plantigrade with an elastic band secured to a table to resist knee extension, which would be a weight-bearing exercise. Proprioceptive feedback and motor unit activity are enhanced during these procedures as body weight or additional resistance is added.

Static-Dynamic

The static-dynamic level is a transition between controlled mobility and skill. In weight-bearing postures it encompasses activities in which the base of support is reduced, e.g., unilateral standing. Within the trunk, segmental upper- and lower-body movements occur at this level. In total body activities, this level is represented by movements between postures or transitional movements, e.g., moving from sitting to standing back to sitting.

Impairment. Diminished stability in a posture in which the base of support has been reduced is not an uncommon finding. An example is the difference in the length of time that bilateral compared with unilateral standing can be maintained. With the reduced base there is a greater amount of body weight supported by the remaining limbs, a more limited possible excursion of the center of pressure, and a greater compression through the weight-bearing joints. Impairments that can contribute to static-dynamic limitations include diminished dynamic balance from motor or sensory loss, decreased strength, limited PROM, or pain with increased weight bearing. These impairments can also limit control of trunk segmental movements.

Functional Implications. Unilateral stance is important for many functional activities, such as climbing stairs and dressing. The time that unilateral standing can be maintained has been shown to be related to the time and quality of stair climbing.[12a,15] Elderly persons have a great deal of difficulty with both unilateral weight bearing in standing and transitional movements. However, the functional implications of these findings have been controversial. Winter and colleagues, in their assessment of ambulation in elite elderly, described a poor relationship between static balance in unilateral standing and ambulation. They found that during the unilateral stance phase of gait, the center of pressure stayed more central and did not shift laterally as much as occurred when the person maintained unilateral standing.[82] In younger persons and in the fit elderly, the muscular responses that control the mass of the upper body during ambulation occur primarily in the hip and back extensors and hip abductors. In contrast to the findings with elite elderly patients, the gait pattern of less active elderly subjects demonstrates a slower ambulatory speed, longer stance time, and increased lateral sway in the upper body.[36,59] These conditions may alter the center of mass–BoS relationship and the needed muscular responses to support the biomechanical requirements of ambulation. In some elderly persons the wider BoS that occurs during ambulation may alter the amount of abductor muscle activity required and increase the similarity between unilateral standing and gait. During ambulation, trunk counter-rotation occurs. At this static-dynamic level, segmental trunk movements are encouraged in anticipation of the progression to counter-rotation.

Another difference between unilateral standing and gait is the distribution of forces at the ankle and hip. Unilateral standing requires sufficient range; position sense; and muscular control in the subtalar and hip joints, primarily in the medial-lateral direction. Gait on a flat, smooth surface—the most commonly measured—is controlled more in an anterior-posterior plane. However, walking on uneven surfaces also challenges medial-lateral control. Because of the difficulty in obtaining objective measures of sensation and motor control in these regions, deficits are not commonly documented in elderly populations.

Many older people are reported to fall during transitional movements from supine to sitting and from sitting to standing,[67] which may be due to decreased range weakness in the quadriceps and gluteals, postural hypotension, and dizziness. To determine whether hypotension is the problem, heart rate and blood pressure should be measured before and after positional change. In anticipation of hypotension, elderly patients should be encouraged to maintain the new position for a few seconds before continuing with an activity.

Treatment Goals. The ability to maintain unilateral stance and perform transitional movements between postures is the focus at this stage. Dynamic stability required for unilateral stance; the simulation of one step of the gait cycle; segmental trunk rotation; and the ability to perform transitional movements between postures, such as from supine to sidelying, then to sitting, and standing are included at this stage.

Treatment Techniques. The patient can independently maintain a variety of weight-bearing positions with a reduced base of support, with or without resistance. AI and RS can be used to enhance stability control of the supporting segments; active movement, SRH, and SR can be added to improve dynamic control. A home exercise program can easily include unilateral limb movements in modified plantigrade that progress to contralateral movements. Within the trunk, segmental upper and lower trunk motions can be emphasized in a variety of postures. For example, while sitting, trunk segmental movements can first be performed with the upper body moving on a fixed lower trunk; this is followed by lower trunk movement under a stabilized upper body. Both of these movements are needed to assist the patient in scooting forward in a chair.

Skill

Locomotion and Manipulation

The skill stage encompasses the functional activities the patient performs. These ambulatory activities and ADL can be performed with age-adjusted normal control, or functionally with abnormal timing, incoordination, or bilateral inequality. Most commonly, when performed with normal control the activity is less energy consuming. However, the outcome of intervention is improved function. The therapist needs to consider all types of intervention strategies beyond remediation, including compensatory movements, adaptive and assistive devices and aides, and environmental modifications, to achieve the outcome.

Impairment. The impairments at this skill stage include deficits in the normal distal-to-proximal timing of movement and the sequencing and speed of the functional task.

Functional Implications. The therapist needs to differentiate between ambulation with normal control and functional ambulation, which may be slower and performed with assistive devices. Some patients appear to have no control impairments yet have difficulty ambulating within their environment. In these cases the deficit may be due to decreased automatic movement, difficulty learning and transferring functional abilities to other environmental conditions, or reduced exercise capacity for movement. For example, some elderly patients with primarily cognitive deficits may have difficulty walking in a new environment, particularly if they cannot remember directions.[19] The problem may be one of motor learning, of adapting to the environment, or of understanding the task—rather than of deficits of motor control or exercise capacity. Difficulty with execution that is not related to range, strength, or control may be due to deficits in memory and cognitive function, necessitating particular learning strategies, including increasing practice repetitions or modifying the environmental demands. Some patients who fear falling may have increased anxiety during ambulation, which can alter the movement quality.

Treatment Goals. When setting goals the therapist must keep in mind the age-appropriate standard for each patient. At this stage the normal timing and sequencing of movement are promoted to achieve a more normal quality and velocity of ambulation. To improve gait velocity, McIntosh investigated the addition of rhythmic auditory stimulation in persons with Parkinson's disease and healthy elderly. Auditory input set at 10% faster speed than the person's baseline gait pattern produced greater gait velocity, cadence, and stride length in all groups.[57] Goals also include ambulation on a variety of surfaces, including uneven ground, ramps and stairs. These additional ambulatory challenges may be limited by impairments at earlier stages. For example, walking on uneven ground may be limited by impaired ankle stability, and ascending ramps may be problematic due to decreased ankle PROM (the mobility stage). Even when the patient is functionally ambulatory, impairments at earlier stages need to be considered when determining the most effective intervention procedures. As has been described, many of these procedures can be performed in group or home exercise programs.

Treatment Techniques. Practicing the functional task—whether it be walking, dressing, or feeding—under a variety of environmental conditions is emphasized at this skill stage. When the patient has difficulty performing the functional movement, the therapist determines the underlying impairments and develops a program to rectify those components, as has been described. The techniques at the skill stage promote the timing and sequencing of responses. Resisted progression (RP) is used to improve the sequencing of body segments during gait. Manual contacts are commonly positioned on the pelvis to guide and direct the proper progression. Additional support may be provided by parallel bars, an assistive device, or having the patient hold the therapist's shoulders. If the patient has difficulty activating the distal musculature at the initiation of movement, the technique of normal timing (NT) may be indicated. For example, at the beginning of the swing phase, a patient may have difficulty initiating dorsiflexion, even though there is sufficient strength at other points in the range. At the initiation of the limb movement, the speed of dorsiflexion is facilitated by repeated stretches added to the voluntary attempt. For patients who have more difficulty with the timing and control of proximal segments, the techniques of SR, SRH, and AR are used in less challenging postures, such as modified plantigrade.

Strength and Endurance

Impairment. Power and endurance of responses commonly are decreased. Strengthening is an inherent aspect of each stage of control and capacity. Strength impairments may be a result of delayed or improper neural messages leading to activation of an insufficient number of motor units in an inappropriate sequence, a reduction in the actual number of motor units, or an inadequate actin-myosin bond. Reduced aerobic capacity can be a result of decreased circulatory bed in the muscle, poor nutrients to the muscle, and diminished central and peripheral circulatory support. The performance of many functional activities, including walking and stair climbing, can be limited by both control and capacity factors. While increasing strength in elderly patients, the frequency, duration, intensity, and speed of the

procedures must be carefully monitored to work within and improve the patient's movement capacity without overtaxing the physiological capability, thereby accounting for the slower healing time after an insult.

Treatment Techniques. RC and timing for emphasis (TE) are performed to enhance motor responses and to promote overflow from stronger segments. Techniques such as AI, SRH, and AR, which are used to promote specific stages of movement control, can be performed with increasing resistance to enhance isometric, isotonic, or eccentric responses and with additional repetitions to further improve endurance. In addition, endurance can be promoted by having the patient increase the frequency of the task as part of a supervised group or home program using elastic or weight resistance. Pulleys, weights, or isokinetic devices provide a useful adjunct to the strengthening and endurance program.

Case Study

Mrs. J is a 79-year-old with increasing difficulty walking on uneven surfaces and complains of an unsteady gait. To evaluate her status, the environmental, social, and psychological factors that may be influencing her ambulation are examined during the history. Then the impairments related to the functional outcome of ambulation are determined by systems review and specific tests and measures. These impairments are then sequenced within the stages of movement control with consideration of her movement capacity. In the clinical decision-making process, the next step is to develop the intervention plan and to determine specific treatment procedures leading toward the anticipated goals and desired functional outcome.

Mrs. J's functional limitations are decreased walking speed and poor ability to climb stairs; she uses a bannister and descends step to step. The environmental, psychological, and medical factors that may positively or negatively influence her physical functioning include living in a second-floor walk-up residence, enjoying a close friendship circle with the local church group, having medical costs paid by Medicare, being an insulin-dependent diabetic, having slight hypertension, showing some evidence of osteoarthritis (OA) of the knees by radiograph, and presently being satisfied with life but concerned about a sick spouse. Measurements of the physical systems have noted reduced range in the trunk into extension and rotation; stiffness near the ends of range in the lower extremities; diminished sensation, including position sense in the feet and toes; minimal swelling around the ankles; decreased muscle strength of 4-/5 in the lower extremity extensors and 3/5 of the dorsiflexors; and decreased ability to maintain standing without vision. The patient has reduced aerobic capacity, as demonstrated by increased heart rate, respiratory rate, and blood pressure while climbing one flight of stairs (Fig. 19-12). Organizing the findings in the Evaluation Model will help the therapist dif-

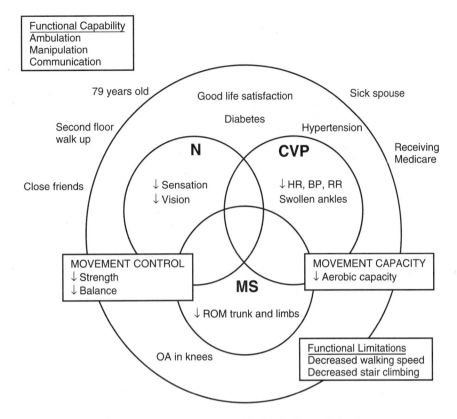

FIG. 19-12 Evaluation model with findings of Mrs. J.

ferentiate problems from environmental vs. physical origin and then determine whether the limitation is more easily rectified by modifying the environment, by teaching compensatory strategies, or by changing the person.

The impairments are classified into the intervention model and according to their control or capacity characteristics. For example, the decreased trunk and limb range would be classified under mobility-ROM; the decreased ability to maintain standing is related to the stability stage. Diminished aerobic capacity during walking comes within the duration, frequency, and intensity of this skilled activity.

The functional outcome desired by the patient is multifaceted: to maintain independent community living, including ambulation on all surfaces and stairs; to improve safety; and to increase walking speed. The therapist determines which impairments need to be changed to achieve these outcomes. The impairments that are amenable to change compared with those that may require compensatory strategies or modifications of the environment are determined. Considering these three alternatives, the degree of independence that can be achieved and the projected time required to accomplish both treatment goals and functional outcomes can then be projected.

The treatment goals sequenced within the model are stated as positive changes in the impairments. Some goals anticipate change in the individual and may include increasing ROM in the hips, knees, ankles, spine, and proximal upper extremities; improving the ability to initiate movement at a speed, frequency, and intensity necessary for static and dynamic postural responses and ambulation; improving static and dynamic stability of the postural muscles with the sequencing and duration needed for postural responses and for ambulation; and improving strength in the postural muscles during weight-bearing activities, including concentric and eccentric contractions with the needed intensity, duration, and frequency for functional activities.

If change in the person is not realistic, then adaptive and assistive strategies and environmental change may be needed and may include adding a half stair to reduce the ROM requirements of stair climbing; adding a raised toilet seat and bars if decreased lower extremity range or strength requires this modification; additional assistive devices to improve stability and speed while ambulating; increasing the stability of and adding an additional bannister to provide external support for stair climbing; and improving patient shoe support and augmenting education regarding foot care.

Plan of Care and Intervention

During intervention, many stages of movement control can be achieved simultaneously, but the procedures usually begin at the mobility stage because the other stages cannot occur without range and the ability to initiate movement. In addition, this ensures a better chance of success. With Mrs. J, intervention would begin with improving the range in her trunk and lower extremities, enhancing the holding ability of her postural extensors, and improving her ability to maintain postures. The treatment procedures can be progressed by changing any of the three units of the procedure: the activity, the posture, and movement pattern; the stage of control and particular techniques; or the exercise parameters. For example, when range in the ankle and hips has shown some improvement and static standing balance is better, then promoting eccentric control of the ankle musculature and dynamic standing balance would be logical progressions. In addition, by varying the environmental conditions, such as the chair height, the floor surface, or the treatment location, the physical demands can be altered and the ability for Mrs. J to generalize to other situations are enhanced. Her home program would include procedures that have been shown to be successful in the clinic and therefore are one stage less difficult than the procedures currently being performed by the therapist. The endurance for exercise can be improved by increasing the duration and frequency of the program. Depending on the changes occurring in her physical status, her home environment would be modified as needed.

Specific Procedures for Direct Interventions

The suggestions made for the intervention sequence incorporate progressions of the activity; the postures chosen; and the stages of movement control, beginning with the least difficult and moving to those requiring more skill. These suggestions represent a general perspective that may need to be modified for individual patients. Many of these procedures can be performed as group activities, especially with persons functioning at high levels or those with similar impairments. Group activities, in addition to improving the physical parameters, may enhance socialization and promote discussion about creative ways to overcome physical impairments. This exercise program might also be appropriate to prevent common impairments and improve or maintain functional capability.

The duration, frequency, and intensity of all of these procedures must be monitored and individually adapted. If the program developed is too vigorous, the individual may complain of tissue soreness and be discouraged from participating, or the program may stress cardiopulmonary structures, and excessive fatigue or other signs may result. Tissue changes that have occurred over a long time will take time to reverse. Many procedures are suggested so that the program can be varied and address many of the existing and anticipated problems.

The procedures are sequenced according to the difficulty of treatment activities, the postures, and movement patterns. This progression is chosen to decrease the need to move Mrs. J between postures during treatment. The stages of movement control are sequenced within each activity.

Procedures in Supine

In supine, upper trunk extension can be combined with scapula retraction and shoulder flexion, abduction, and external rotation. In the lower body, the movements that can be performed in supine include trunk flexion, extension, and rotation; hip flexion, extension, and rotation; and ankle movements.

Mobility—ROM: Goals include improving or maintaining range and decreasing tissue stiffness, particularly in the trunk, hips, knees, and ankles. Techniques to achieve these goals include heat, massage, HR, and joint mobilization.

Mobility—Initiation of Movement: Goals include improving the ability to initiate and move through the range. Although Mrs. J is ambulatory and can initiate all movements, because her ankle musculature is weak and the timing of the contraction is slowed, the initiation of ankle dorsiflexion and plantar flexion is emphasized.[53,55] HRAM, RC, and electrical stimulation are techniques that may be used to achieve these goals.

Stability-Muscle: Goals include holding an isometric contraction in the shortened range of the postural extensors. The duration of this low-intensity isometric contraction is gradually increased from 5 to 30 to 60 seconds. The level of intensity begins with gravitational resistance in spine, then external resistance may be added. In supine, the lower body extensors are resisted by placing a pillow under the knees and having Mrs. J perform quadriceps and gluteal sets by pushing into the pillow. At home, she increases the duration of the holding contraction, being careful to breathe smoothly during the exercise. The difficulty can be increased by altering the gravitational resistance and having Mrs. J roll into the prone position and hold with the postural extensors and scapula retractors. This position also is beneficial to stretch her tight hip flexors. By stretching hip flexors and strengthening trunk and hip extensors, she may be able to stand more erect and have a greater range into hip extension during gait. When positioning patients in prone, care must be taken to monitor heart rate and ease of respiration—common problems of those with hypertension. If CVP problems arise, an alternative posture in which to resist the upper trunk extensors, such as sitting, would be chosen.

Procedures in the Hooklying Posture

Mobility: Although a pelvic tilt can be performed in this posture, range into lumbar flexion is not commonly a problem. To increase range of lumbar rotation, hooklying is an appropriate posture for the spine and is not weight bearing—a consideration for those with osteopenia. The technique to increase range of the muscular tissue would be HR. Once range is gained, the patient can maintain that range by performing rhythmic rotational movements to the end of range as part of the home program. The increased lower trunk rotation is desired for improved pelvic rotation and stride length during gait.

Stability: Maintaining the posture and improving isometric ability of the lower abdominals and back extensors can be enhanced by AI with manual contacts on the knees. The patient can perform lower abdominal exercises by flattening the back, drawing in the abdomen and bringing one knee toward the chest. Most elders will not have sufficient abdominal control to maintain the lumbar spine position and bring the other leg toward the chest as well. To resist a hip abduction motion, an elastic strapping can be placed around the knees.

Procedures in the Bridging Posture

In bridging the lower trunk and hip extensors, and the hip abductors can be enhanced in their shortened ranges.

Mobility: The patient needs to have sufficient range in the hip flexors and strength in the trunk and hip extensors (3/5) so that the hips can be extended. If not, mobility is gained in non–weight-bearing postures, such as supine or prone. If the hip extensors cannot overcome the resistance of gravity, their strength is increased in supine muscle stability.

Stability: As Mrs. J maintains the position for an increasing amount of time, the endurance of the back and hip extensors is increasing. The techniques of AI and RS with resistance provided at the hips, knees, or ankles can progressively increase the difficulty of the procedure. Improving the stance phase of gait and unilateral stance for stair climbing is a goal. As part of her home program, resistance is provided by elastic material placed at the pelvis or knees to emphasize extensor or abductor control.

Controlled Mobility: Pelvic lateral shifting and rotation can be performed independently by Mrs. J as part of her home program as well as with the SRH technique. The concentric-eccentric reversal of moving into and out of bridging is designed to help her descend stairs.

Static-Dynamic: Lifting one leg from the supporting surface increases the resistance to the supporting limb and focuses on the control needed for unilateral stance and single-limb support while descending stairs.

Procedures in the Sitting Posture

The movements that can be performed in sitting include upper trunk extension, trunk extension with rotation, lumbar spine extension and flexion, hip flexion, knee flexion and extension, and ankle dorsiflexion.

Mobility: Range can be gained in the upper trunk and upper extremities and into hip flexion with the techniques of HR and joint mobilization. This range can be maintained by self-stretching movements.

Stability: Holding in the shortened range of the upper trunk extensors and scapular retractors can be performed, with resistance provided manually, by pulleys, or by elastic material.

Controlled Mobility: Weight shifting of the trunk on the hips will improve the control needed for assuming standing from sitting and the movements needed during dressing.

Skill: Lower-extremity movements can emphasize the quadriceps and dorsiflexor activity that is required for postural responses in standing and during the gait sequence. Many elders may lose their balance backward when reaching overhead or looking up. Improved dorsiflexor and quadriceps control may help to reduce this tendency. For many elders, weak quadriceps may limit stair climbing and moving between standing and sitting. Elastic band, isotonic, or iso-

kinetic resistance may be appropriate to increase quadriceps strength.

Activities in the Modified Plantigrade Position

Modified plantigrade treatment can include exercises for the lower trunk, knee extensors, and ankle. Control around these joints can be emphasized in this posture, which is also easily incorporated into the home program.

Controlled Mobility: Weight shifting and performing small-range knee extensor eccentric exercises are directed toward improving Mrs. J's ability to descend stairs. By positioning an elastic band around her knee and attaching it to an immovable object, such as the leg of a table, concentric-eccentric resistance can be added to quadriceps and hamstring contractions.

Static-Dynamic: Lifting one upper or lower extremity can be performed with gradually increasing resistance provided by an elastic band or a weight. Improved control over unilateral stance and reduced fatigue of the trunk extensors are the goals.

Procedures in Standing

In standing, trunk, hip, knee, and ankle control can be enhanced. Because these are more difficult procedures, Mrs. J may require additional support, such as the parallel bars or standing next to a stable surface.

Controlled Mobility and Static-Dynamic: During both bilateral and unilateral standing, weight shifting can be performed rocking the body in various directions and then rocking up on toes and heels. Changing the surface to a balance board will further challenge responses. If enhanced proprioceptive awareness is desired to improve her confidence in walking on uneven surfaces or in the dark, these balance tasks can be performed with the eyes closed. As this increased challenge is undertaken, the parallel bars or other supporting surfaces are used to ensure safety.

Skill: Resisted progression can emphasize the sequencing of pelvic motions during gait. At this skill stage the activity itself is practiced to enhance learning and improve endurance. A treadmill may be useful for this. To improve CVP endurance, upper and lower body ergometers (bicycles) may be appropriate.

The quadruped posture was not included in Mrs. J's treatment program because of her age, cardiac status, and arthritic knees. However, for others it may be very appropriate to increase upper extremity weight bearing and improve trunk stability.

SUMMARY

In this chapter the common ambulatory findings related to the changes in the physical systems in the elderly have been described. The clinical decision-making process related these examination findings to possible intervention strategies. The intervention related to ambulatory deficits in the elderly focused on examining the underlying impairments, evaluating the interrelationships of the impairments, and determining the most effective and efficient strategy for achieving the functional outcome. The plan followed the stages of movement control to achieve the treatment goals in a progressive and orderly sequence.

REFERENCES

1. Ades P, et al: Exercise conditioning in the elderly coronary patient. *J Am Geriatr Soc* 1987; 35:121-124.
2. Alexander B, Rivera F, Wolf M: The cost and frequency of hospitalization for fall-related injuries in older adults. *Am J Public Health* 1992; 7:1020-1023.
3. Anacker S, diFabio R: Influence of sensory inputs on standing balance in community-dwelling elders with a recent history of falling. *Phys Ther* 1992; 72:575-584.
4. Astrand P, Rodahl K: *Textbook of Work Physiology.* New York, McGraw-Hill, 1986.
5. Barbisoni P, et al: Mood improvement in elderly women after in-hosp ital physical rehabilitation. *Arch Phys Med Rehabil* 1996; 77(4):346-349.
6. Baylor A, Spirduso W: Systematic aerobic exercise and components of reaction time in older women. *J Gerontol: Psychol Sci* 1988; 43(5): P121-P126.
7. Bendall M, Bassey E, Pearson M: Factors affecting walking speed of elderly people. *Age Aging* 1989; 18:327-332.
8. Berg K, et al: Clinical and laboratory measures of postural balance in an elderly population. *Arch Phys Med Rehabil* 1992; 73:10731080.
9. Bohannon R: Comfortable and maximum walking speed of adults aged 20-79 years: Reference values and determinants. *Age Ageing* 1997; 26:15-19.
10. Borg G: Perceived exertion as an indicator of somatic stress. *Scand J Rehabil Med* 1970; 2:92.
11. Brooks V: *The Neural Basis of Motor Control.* New York, Oxford University Press, 1986.
12. Brownlee M, et al: Considerations of spatial orientation mechanisms as related to elderly fallers. *Gerontology* 1989; 35:323-331.
12a. Cavanagh PR, Molfinger LM, Owens DA: How do the elderly negotiate stairs? *Muscle Nerve (Suppl)* 1997;5:S52-55.
13. Chandler JM, Hadley EC: Exercise to improve physiologic and functional performance in old age. *Clin Geriatr Med* 1996; 12(4):761-784.
14. Chang H: *Gait Initiation in Healthy Elderly, Those with Vestibular Hypofunction and Physically Disabled Elderly.* Boston, Massachusetts General Hospital/Institute of Health Professions, 1998.
15. Chen HC, et al: Stepping over obstacles: Dividing attention impairs performance of old more than young adults. *J Gerontol: A Biol Sci Med Sci* 1996; 51(3):M116-22.
16. Chen S: *Relationship of Functional Outcomes and Physical Impairments in Patients Following TKR.* Boston, Massachusetts General Hospital/Institute of Health Professions, 1997.
17. Cunningham D, Rechnitzer PA, Pearce ME, Donner AP: Determinants of self-selected walking pace across ages 19-26. *J Gerontol* 1982; 37(5):560-564.
18. Dargent Molina P, et al: Fall-related factors and risk of hip fracture: The EPIDOS prospective study. Epidemiologie de l'osteoporose. *Lancet* 1996; 348(9021):145-149.
19. Drachman D: Memory and cognitive function in normal aging. *Dev Neuropsychol* 1986; 2:277-285.
20. Dubey A, Koval KJ, Zuckerman JD: Hip fracture prevention: A review. *Am J Orthop* 1998; 27(6):407-412.
21. Duncan P, Weiner D, Chandler J, Studenski S: Functional reach: A new clinical measure of balance? *J Gerontol: Med Sci* 1990; 45:M49-54.
22. Fiatarone M, O'Neill E, Ryan N: Exercise training and nutritional supplementation for physical fraility in very elderly people. *N Engl J Med* 1994; 330:1769-1775.
23. Fife T, Baloh R: Disequilibrium of unknown cause in older people. *Ann Neurol* 1993; 34(5):694-702.
24. Finlay O: Exercise training and walking speeds in elderly women following hip surgery 'beating the little green man'. *Physiotherapy* 1993; 79(12):845-849.
25. Frandin K, Grimby G, Mellstrom D, Svanborg A: Walking habits and health-related factors in a 70 year old population. *Gerontology* 1991; 37:281-288.
26. Friedman P, Rickmond D, Bashett J: A prospective trial of serial gait speed as a measure of rehabilitation in the elderly. *Age Aging* 1988; 17:227-235.
27. Gehlsen G, Whaley M: Falls in the elderly: Part II, balance, strength and flexibility. *Arch Phys Med Rehabil* 1990; 71:739-741.
28. Gibbs J, et al: Predictors of change in walking velocity in older adults. *J Am Geriatr Soc* 1996; 44:126-132.
29. Graafmans WC, et al: Falls in the elderly: A prospective study of risk factors and risk profiles. *Am J Epidemiol* 1996; 143(11):1129-1136.
30. Gregg EW, et al: Physical activity and osteoporotic fracture risk in older women. Study of Osteoporotic Fractures Research Group [see comments]. *Ann Intern Med* 1998; 129(2):81-88.
31. Guccione AA: Physical therapy diagnosis and the relationship between impairments and function. *Phys Ther* 1991; 71:499-509.
32. Guralnik J, Simonsick E, Ferruccil: A short physical performance battery assessing lower extremity function: Association with self-reported disability and prediction of mortality and nursing home admission. *J Gerontol* 1994; 49:85-94.
33. Hageman R, Blanke D: Comparison of gait of young women and elderly women. *Phys Ther* 1986; 66(9):1382-1387.
34. Hagerman P: Gait characteristics of healthy elderly: A literature review. *Issues Aging* 1995; 18(2):14-18.
35. Harris B, Dyreck D: A model of orthopedic dysfunction for clinical decision making in physical therapy practice. *Phys Ther* 1989; 69:548-553.
36. Hinman J, Cunningham D, Rechnitzer R, Paterson D: Age-related changes in speed of walking. *Med Sci Sports Exerc* 1988; 20(2):161-166.
37. Ho SC, et al: Risk factors for falls in the Chinese elderly population. *J Gerontol: A Biol Sci Med Sci* 1996; 51(5):M195-198.
38. House of Delegates: *House of Delegates Policies (HOD 0683-03-05).* American Physical Therapy Association, Alexandria, Va, 1989.
39. Hughes MA, et al: The relationship of postural sway to sensorimotor function, functional performance, and disability in the elderly. *Arch Phys Med Rehabil* 1996; 77(6):567-572.
40. Ihsen E, Charlton JL: The relationship between age, human factors, and stair negotiation skills in older adults. : 31-40.
41. Ikeda E, et al: Influence of age and dynamics of rising from a chair. *Phys Ther* 1991; 71:473-481.
42. Judge J, Underwood M, Gennosa T: Exercise to improve gait velocity in older persons. *Arch Phys Med Rehabil* 1993; 74:400-406.
43. Kauffman T: Posture and age. *Top Geriatr Rehabil* 1987; 2:13-28.
44. Kelly-Hayes M, et al: Functional limitations and disability among elders in the Framingham study. *Am J Public Health* 1992; 82:841-845.
45. Koski K, Luukinen H, Laippala P, Kivela SL: Physiological factors and medications as predictors of injurious falls by elderly people: A prospective population-based study. *Age Ageing* 1996; 25(1):29-38.
46. Lajoie Y, Teasdale N, Bard C, Fleury M: Upright standing and gait: Are there changes in attentional requirements related to normal aging? *Exp Aging Res* 1996; 22(2):185-198.
47. Lexell J, Taylor C, Sjostrumm M: What is the cause of the aging atrophy? *J Neurosci* 1988; 84:275-298.
48. Liston R, Brouwer B: Reliability and validity of measures obtained from stroke patients using the Balance Master. *Arch Phys Med Rehabil* 1996; 77:425-430.
49. Lord S, et al: The effect of exercise on gait patterns in older women: A randomized controlled trial. *J Gerontol: Med Sci* 1996; 51A(2): M64-M70.
50. Lord S, Clark RD, Webster I: Postural stability and associated physiological factors in a population of aged persons. *J Gerontol: Med Sci* 1991; 46:M69-M76.
51. Lord SR, Clark RD: Simple physiological and clinical tests for the accurate prediction of falling in older people. *Gerontology* 1996; 42(4): 199-203.
52. Lundgren-Lindquist B, Aniansson A, Rundgren A: Functional studies in 79 year-olds. III. Walking performance and climbing capacity. *Scand J Rehabil Med* 1983; 15(3):125-131.
53. Maki B, Holliday P, Topper A: Fear of falling and postural performance in the elderly. *J Gerontol* 1991; 46:M123-M131.

54. Manchester D, et al: Visual, vestibular and somatosensory contributions to balance control in the older adult. *J Gerontol: Med Sci* 1989; 44(4):M118-127.

55. Martin P, Rothstein D, Larish D: Effects of age and physical activity status on the speed-aerobic demand relationship of walking. *J Appl Physiol* 1992; 73(1):200-206.

56. McGavin C, et al: Dyspnea, disability, and distance walked: Comparisons of estimates of exercise performance in respiratory disease. *Fr Med J* 1978; 2:241-243.

57. McIntosh GC, Brown SH, Rice RR, Thaut MH: Rhythmic auditory-motor facilitation of gait patterns in patients with Parkinson's disease. *J Neurol Neurosurg Psychiatry* 1997; 62(1):22-26.

58. Murray M, Duthie E, Gambert S: Age-related differences in knee muscle strength in normal women. *J Gerontol* 1985; 40:275-280.

59. Murray M, Kory R, Clarkson B: Walking patterns in healthy old men. *J Gerontol* 1969; 24:169-178.

60. Myers AH, Young Y, Langlois JA: Prevention of falls in the elderly. *Bone* 1996; 18(1suppl):87s-101s.

61. Niam S, Cheung W, Sullivan PE, Kent S, Gu X: Balance and physical impairments after stroke. *Arch Phys Med Rehabil* 1999; 80(10): 1227-1233.

62. Patla A, et al: Age-related changes in balance control system: Initiation of stepping. *Clin Biomechanics* 1993; 8:179-184.

63. Peel C: Cardiopulmonary changes with aging, in Irwin S, Techlin J (eds): *Cardiopulmonary Physical Therapy,* ed 2. St Louis, Mosby, 1990.

64. Podsiadlo D, Richardson S: The Timed "Up&Go" : A test of basic functional mobility for frail elderly persons. *J Am Geriatr Soc* 1991; 39:142-148.

65. Portney L, Watkins M: *Foundations of Clinical Research: Applications to Practice.* Norwalk, Conn, Appleton & Lange, 1993.

66. Rakowski W, Mor V: The association of physical activity with mortality among older adults in the longitudinal study of aging (1984-1988). *J Gerontol* 1992; 47(4):M122-M129.

67. Rubenstein LV, et al: Improving patient quality of life with feedback to physicians about functional status. *J Gen Intern Med* 1995; 10(11):607-614.

68. Sabbahi M, Sedgwick E: Age-related changes in monosynaptic reflex activity. *J Gerontol* 1982; 37:24-32.

69. Schenkman M: Interrelationship of neurological and mechanical factors in balance control. Washington, DC, *Balance Proceedings of the APTA Forum,* 1989.

70. Skinner HB, Barrack RL, Cook SD: Age-related decline in proprioception. *Clin Orthop* 1984; April (184):208-211.

71. Smith E, DiFabio R, Gilligan C: Exercise intervention and physiologic function in the elderly. *Top Geriatr Rehab* 1990; 6:57-68.

72. Sorock G, Labiner D: Peripheral Dysfunction and falls in an elderly cohort. *Am J Epidemiol* 1992; 136:584-591.

73. Spirduso W: Reaction and movement times as a function of age and physical activity. *J Gerontol* 1975; 30:435-440.

74. Stockmeyer S: An interpretation of the approach of Rood to the treatment of neuromuscular dysfunction. *Am J Phys Med* 1967; 46:900-956.

75. Sullivan P, Markos P: *Clinical Decision Making in Therapeutic Exercise.* Norwalk, Conn, Appleton & Lange, 1995.

76. Thompson L: Effects of age and training on skeletal muscle physiology and performance. *Phys Ther* 1994; 74(1):71-81.

77. Tideiksaar R: Falls among the elderly: Community prevention program. *Am J Public Health* 1992; 6:892-893.

78. Tinetti M, Speechley M, Ginter S: Risk factors for falls among elderly persons living in the community. *New Engl J Med* 1988; 319:1707-1707.

79. Tinetti M: Performance oriented assessment of mobility problems in elderly patients. *J Am Geriat Soc* 1986; 34:119-126.

80. Topper A, Maki B, Holliday P: Are activity-based assessments of balance and gait in the elderly predictive of risk of falling and/or type of fall? *J Am Geriatr Soc* 1993; 41(5):479-487.

81. Whipple R, Wolfson L, Ameiman P: The relationship of knee and ankle weakness to falls in nursing home residents: an isokinetic study. *J Am Geriatr Soc* 1987; 35:13-20.

82. Winter D, Patla A, Frand J, Walt S: Biomechanical walking pattern changes in the fit and healthy elderly. *Phys Ther* 1990; 70(6):340-347.

83. Winter D: Foot trajectory in human gait: A precise and multifactorial motor control task. *Phys Ther* 1992; 72(1):45-56.

84. Wolfson L, Whipple R, Amermam P, Tobin J: Gait assessment in the elderly: A gait abnormality rating scale and its relation to falls. *J Gerontol: Med Sci* 1990; 45(1):M12-19.

85. Wolfson L, et al: A dynamic posturographic study of balance in healthy elderly. *Neurology* 1992; 42:2069-2075.

86. Woolacott M, Shemway-Cook A, Nashner L: Aging and posture control: Changes in sensory organization and muscular coordination. *Int J Aging Hum Dev* 1986; 23:97.

87. Woolacott M: Age-related changes in posture and movement. *J Gerontol* 1993; 48(special issue):56-60.

88. Woolacott M: Postural control mechanisms in the young and old. *Balance Proceedings of the APTA Forum,* 1989.

CHAPTER 20

LOWER EXTREMITY ORTHOTICS IN GERIATRIC REHABILITATION

LISA GIALLONARDO, PT, MS, OCS

INTRODUCTION

The use of lower extremity orthoses with elderly patients can make the difference between independent function and disability. Today's technology has made orthoses lighter and easier to don and doff. The keys to success in orthotic management are a thorough examination and evaluation that highlight the patient's impairments, functional limitations, and disability. This allows for proper matching of the orthosis to the needs of the patient.[15]

Terminology

By definition, an *orthosis* is a device that is applied around a body segment. *Orthotics* is the art and science of fabricating orthoses, and an *orthotist* is the professionally trained fabricator and fitter of these devices.

By convention, orthoses are named by the joint(s) that the device encompasses. An orthosis that fits into the shoe is called a *foot orthosis (FO)*. If this device also crosses the ankle, it is known as an *ankle foot orthosis (AFO)*. When the device spans the knee as well, it is called a *knee ankle foot orthosis (KAFO)*. However, if the orthosis only covers the knee or the ankle, it is known as a *knee orthosis (KO)* or an *ankle orthosis (AO)*, respectively.

Orthoses have characteristic components that determine function. A *stop* indicates a motion that is not allowed by the

orthosis. For example, a solid plastic AFO molded in 0 degrees of dorsiflexion (therefore not allowing plantar flexion) would be called an AFO with a *plantar flexion stop*. This can be taken one step further by indicating where in the range of motion the stop is occurring, e.g., AFO with *plantar flexion stop at 0 degrees*.

Stops can also be used to control motion rather than eliminate it altogether. A *limited motion stop* allows for a certain amount of movement while maintaining some restraint. An example of this would be an AFO with a *15 degree limited motion stop* (10 degrees dorsiflexion and 5 degrees plantar flexion).

Orthotic joints can have several characteristics. A *free joint* is one that has no limitations of motion. An *adjustable joint* is one that may be altered to allow free motion, limited motion, or no motion at all. Joints that *assist motion* have an external force that aids in *increasing* the range, velocity, or force of the desired motion. Joints that *resist motion* have an external force that *decreases* the range, velocity, or force of the desired motion. A *lock* on a joint is used to selectively stop joint motion (Fig. 20-1).

Functions

Orthoses have a variety of purposes and can be characterized based on their role. These include resting, functional, dynamic, static, and weight bearing. A *resting orthosis* provides a neutral joint position to counteract the forces of gravity or muscle imbalances. It prevents overstretching of muscle-tendon units and decreases joint irritation. Resting orthosis may be used with patients who have suffered from transient neurological problems, such as Guillain-Barré syndrome, acute head trauma, and acute stroke. These orthoses can also be used for acute orthopedic diseases and injuries, such as rheumatoid arthritis, myositis, tendinitis, and joint injuries.

A *functional orthosis* provides a substitution for muscle function through stabilization of a joint or by acting as the prime mover of a joint. It improves the functional capacity and can actually replace paralytic muscles. This is especially effective in patients with upper extremity dysfunction, such as severe arthritis, brachial plexus injuries, or quadriplegia. These orthoses are not often used in the lower extremity because of the large weight-bearing forces involved in ambulation.

Dynamic orthoses prevent or correct an ongoing deformity. Commonly seen in the treatment of patients with idiopathic scoliosis, these orthoses improve the condition or the weakness through facilitation of muscles by positioning. These orthoses also may be used in management of patients with peripheral neuropathies and transient muscle weakness.

Static orthoses work to stabilize or immobilize joints. They prevent contractures, promote healing, and sometimes relieve pain. Patients with ankle sprains, chondromalacia patella, and low back or neck pain will benefit from a static orthosis.

The *weight-bearing orthosis* affects the distribution of weight to allow proper healing and sometimes early ambulation. It is commonly used in patients with femoral and tibial fractures after open reduction internal fixation or cast removal.

Orthoses can be made out of various forms of plastic, metal, and/or leather. They can be prefabricated by size or custom molded. The more elaborate and custom the design, the greater the cost. Lower extremity orthoses require appropriate footwear to refine control and fit.

Shoes

Several characteristics are required in shoes for proper fit of an orthosis, especially in patients with lower extremity impairments. Tie shoes are most appropriate for these patients. Balmoral style shoes are stitched down in front along the metatarsal area. The Blucher shoe is not stitched down over the base of the tongue, therefore making it easier to pull the tongue forward to allow for placement of an orthosis.

A shoe is made up of three parts: the upper, the sole, and the heel. Leather uppers are preferable because leather breathes and conforms to the patient's foot. This is especially important in elders with compromised circulation. Lace stays allow for securing the shoe to the foot without pistoning. The greater the number of stays, the more secure the shoe is to the foot. Velcro is also available in closure for patients who have difficulty manipulating the laces. The sole of the shoe should be made of some form of crepe, which increases the lower extremity shock absorption during gait. Small heel height (0.5 inch for men; 0.75 inch for women) is recommended for stability and safety, as well as for distribution of forces.[28]

A shoe is constructed on a *last,* a model around which a shoe is formed. Each manufacturer has different styles of lasts, with some shoes being wider or narrower; shallow or deep; pointed, rounded, or squared toe. The shape of the shoe should conform to the person's foot. Custom made shoes with individual lasts are available for persons with deformed feet who have difficulty buying standard shoes that fit well.

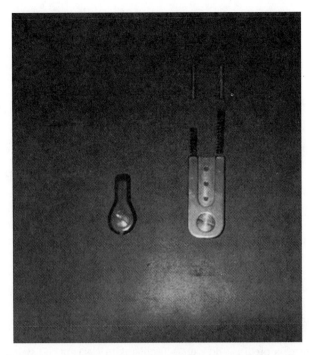

FIG. 20-1 A double-action ankle joint component has two channels for inserting pins to stabilize or springs to assist. The channels also may be kept open to allow free ankle motion.

The toe box is the reinforcement at the front of the shoe that protects the toes from injury. The shape and the depth of the box is especially important for patients with insensitive feet, where friction and pressure are dangerous to skin integrity.[9] Steel-toed shoes are made for industrial settings, but despite their safety for the toes, they are very heavy.

The heel counter is the another reinforcement available on shoes. A firm counter helps control the calcaneal rearfoot movement and is advantageous for patients with excessive calcaneal motion. Reinforcement can be built into the shoe or added as an external support.

The medial counter is the portion of the shoe between the heel and toe that reinforces the medial arch. The shank of the shoe, which is imbedded in the sole, supports it.

Shoes are made in a variety of widths, from AAAAA to EEEE, as well as lengths. There should be a ½-inch between the end of shoe and the great toe. The shape of the toe box should not squeeze the toes. Shopping for shoes should be done when the feet are more swollen; later in the day is preferable.

Gait Review

Promoting normal, efficient gait involves keeping the center of mass within a 2-inch horizontal and vertical excursion. This allows for shifts in center of mass while remaining inside the pelvis. Normal gait also involves adequate eccentric- as well as concentric-muscle force production to account for the effects of gravity. Normal gait entails having a stable base of support followed by weight shifting in a smooth, rhythmical fashion. Orthotic management should strive to improve efficiency and safety during ambulation.[21]

Disturbances can occur at any point within the gait cycle: heel strike; heel strike to foot flat; foot flat to midstance; midstance to heel off; toe off; toe off to acceleration; acceleration to midswing; and midswing to deceleration.

Inman and colleagues described six elements that reduce energy consumption during gait.[21] These determinants, discussed in the following list, are easy to examine and help identify key impairments:

1. *Pelvic rotation*—Pelvic rotation around a vertical axis is about 4 degrees in each direction and is useful for absorbing ground reaction force and minimizing excessive trunk side-to-side motion. Problems occur with too little rotation (resulting in increased hip flexion) or too much rotation (with too much energy expended).

2. *Pelvic list*—The pelvis drops slightly on the swing limb, resulting in lowering the center of mass and gives the gluteus medius a better moment arm for providing a relative abduction of the swing limb. The Trendelenburg gait (dropping of the swing side pelvis) results from weakness of the gluteus medius and causes problems in clearing the swing limb.

3. *Knee flexion in stance*—Knee flexion occurs both at heel strike and heel off, which evens out the passing from one phase to another, lowering the center of mass, and improving shock absorption. Problems occur with too much knee flexion from quadriceps weakness, resulting in a safety issue due to knee buckling. Too little knee flexion can result in difficulty absorbing shock and possible genu recurvatum with very weak hamstrings in comparison with quadriceps.

4. *Ankle dorsiflexion in stance*—The tibia moves over the foot during both foot flat to midstance and midstance to heel off, which allows for the body weight to move forward and the center of mass to be lowered for purposes of shock absorption. Too little dorsiflexion results in compensation at the subtalar and midtarsal joints in the form of excessive pronation. Weakness of the tibialis anterior, which controls the foot lowering to the ground at heel strike, will result in foot slap during this gait phase.

5. *Coordinated knee, ankle, and foot motion*—At two phases, these three joint complexes must move in concert with each other. At heel strike through midstance the knee flexes, the ankle dorsiflexes, and the foot pronates to progress the body weight forward and to lower the center of mass for shock absorption. At midstance to heel off the knee extends, the ankle plantar flexes, and the foot supinates to lengthen the limb and make the foot a rigid lever, all for efficient push off. The problems occur with too much or too little motion at one or two of the joints, requiring compensation at the other joint(s). An example of this includes too little knee flexion and ankle dorsiflexion, resulting in foot pronation to lower the center of mass, increase shock absorption, and allow the tibia to move over the foot for limb progression.

6. *Lateral trunk displacement*—The width of the base of support (stride width) and the angle of the tibia and femur (slight genu valgum) allow the feet to remain together within the base of support without excessive side to side motion. Problems occur with genu varum (bow legs), which increases the need for side-to-side motion, or excessive genu valgum (knock knees), which results in a larger stride width and excessive energy for weight shifting.

With this review of the normal gait requirements, a full examination will help identify the key impairments leading to gait deviations, some of which can be remediated with orthoses.

EXAMINATION

History and Systems Review

A good history and systems review will help the therapist decide what specific tests and measures to use in determining appropriate orthotic intervention.[17] History questions include the following:

1. General demographics
2. Social history
3. Occupation/employment
4. Living environment
5. History of current condition
6. Functional status and activity level
7. Medications
8. Other tests and measures
9. Past history of current condition
10. Past medical/surgical history
11. Family history
12. Health status
13. Social habits

The systems review will contribute to understanding the overall health status of the elderly patient. The physiological and anatomical status of the cardiopulmonary, musculoskeletal, neuromuscular, and integumentary systems and the communication, affect, cognition, language, and learning style are assessed as part of understanding the patient as a whole.

Tests and Measures

The elderly patient may present with a multitude of constraints that prevent functioning at home and in the community. These include structural lower extremity problems, muscle length and strength changes, decreased circulation and sensation, or abnormal muscle tone—all of which can contribute to functional limitation or disability.

The following tests and measures are outlined specifically in the *Guide to Physical Therapist Practice.*[17] In assessing anatomical constraints, a thorough *posture* examination should be done. This would include analysis of the resting posture of the spine and lower extremity. Examination of alignment, in weight bearing and non-weight bearing, would include the following:

1. Spinal curves (scoliosis/kyphosis)
2. Pelvic obliquity (anterior/posterior rotation)
3. Femoral torsion (anterior/posterior)
4. Coxa valga/vara

5. Genu valgum/varum
6. Tibial torsion (internal/external)
7. Tibial varum
8. Neutral calcaneal stance
9. Neutral subtalar joint position

Joint integrity and *mobility* tests and measures assess the effect of any postural deviations on the involved joints. Quality of movement, hypermobility or hypomobility, pain, swelling, and evidence of sprain of the affected and surrounding joints are evaluated.[17] Relationship to postural findings should be considered.

The constraints of muscle length and muscle strength are measured with range of motion and muscle performance techniques, respectively. *Range of motion* is evaluated using instruments such as goniometers, tape measures, and inclinometers to measure joint motion, passive muscle tension, deviations from neutral, and pain with movement. *Muscle performance* (including strength, power, and endurance) is measured with manual muscle testing or dynamometry and is helpful in assessing the patient's ability to do weight-bearing tasks.[17] Muscle performance in functional tasks is a helpful descriptive measure and may assist in highlighting orthotic needs.

The patient with a history of diabetes or peripheral vascular disease will require a complete evaluation of the constraints related to the circulatory and integumentary systems. *Integumentary integrity* involves assessment of the color, temperature, mobility, and texture of the skin as well as hair growth and signs of open wounds or blistering. The *sensory integrity* (including proprioception and kinesthesia) may also be in question and involves assessment of cortical sensations such as two-point discrimination; proprioception; and superficial sensations such as light touch, sharp/dull, and pressure. *Circulation* is assessed by pulse palpation (femoral, popliteal, posterior tibial, and pedal); capillary refill time; and evidence of edema. It is also important to include evaluation of aerobic capacity with vital signs, auscultation, and exercise testing if necessary.[17]

Abnormal tone (increased or decreased) is addressed in *motor function.* Abnormal movement patterns, muscle tone, coordination, and sensorimotor integration are all evaluated using various scales and descriptive analysis.[17] Movement patterns can provide insight on the need for orthoses and the potential for tolerance to weight bearing.

The ability to sit and stand unsupported as well as ambulate is evaluated by analyzing *gait, locomotion,* and *balance.* Good static and dynamic balance in sitting and standing is a precursor for safe and efficient transfers and gait. Characteristics of gait should be identified on even and uneven surfaces as well as on stairs. Using the determinants of gait will make the examination more efficient and help the therapist highlight functional gait difficulties. *Assistive* and *adaptive devices* should be evaluated for the their safety and effectiveness during locomotion.[17]

A complete functional assessment rounds out the examination. Analyzing *community* and *work integration* and *rein-tegration* with scales and questionnaires involves independent activities of daily living (IADL) indexes, daily activity logs, reports from family/care-givers, and a general assessment of functional capacity. Along with this, an analysis is done of *environmental, home,* and *work barriers,* including adaptations, additions, or modifications of physical space that may enhance safety, eliminate barriers, and comply with legal standards.[28] This gives the therapist an understanding of the functional deficits for which an orthoses could be useful.

EVALUATION

A correct evaluation is the key to effective treatment, including proper orthotic management. Assessing the objective findings first will lead to an accurate diagnosis and prognosis.

When reviewing the examination data the following factors should be considered: mobility, stability, controlled mobility, and skill.

Mobility is defined as having sufficient range of motion (ROM) for movement and assumption of posture.[45] The lower extremity should have functional ROM and joint mobility. If ROM is lacking, the therapist must determine whether the restriction is stemming from the joint, soft tissue, or muscle tissue. End feel is a useful guide. If joint mobility is restricted, it should be restored before gains in ROM can be achieved. Using the determinants of gait as a framework, lack of mobility is particularly problematic with pelvic rotation and ankle dorsiflexion in stance, where lack of mobility requires compensation of excessive mobility at the hip and foot, respectively.

Stability is defined as the ability of muscle to perform tonic holding and co-contraction.[45] The lower extremity muscles should have functional isometric, concentric, and eccentric strength in all positions. If muscle force production is lacking, the therapist should check whether enough range of motion exists in the joint for the muscle(s) to contract effectively. Lack of stability is an issue in knee flexion in stance, where weakness of the quadriceps can result in knee buckling. Another example would be pelvic list, in which gluteus medius weakness leads to Trendelenburg gait.

Controlled mobility is the ability of the muscles to move the proximal joints over the fixed distal end.[45] The patient should be able to bear weight and move the trunk over the foot and ankle. If the patient is unable to do these, he/she may be experiencing a continued problem in stability. The patient should also be able to accept challenges to weight bearing in both double-limb and single-limb stance. If the patient is lacking in weight-bearing ability, there may be a need for increased joint mobility to detect motion changes in the lower extremity. Coordinated knee, ankle, and foot motion allows for the tibia to move over the foot. Dysfunction in mobility and stability will either prevent this from happening or cause an inefficient gait.

Skill is the ability of the muscles to move and stabilize the proximal joint(s) with the distal end mobilized.[45] The patient should be able to walk on level and uneven surfaces as well as be able to walk step over step up and down stairs. If the patient is lacking in the ability to walk on even surfaces, mobility and stability may be lacking. If the patient is unable to walk on uneven surfaces, controlled mobility may be lacking. Problems with lateral trunk displacement make ambulating on stairs and uneven surfaces difficult and energy expensive.

Based on the relationship of all anomalous findings to each other, the therapist makes a diagnosis and a prognosis. This allows reasonable goals to be set and an intervention plan to be developed. Goals should be measurable and time related, with long-term goals related to a functional outcome. The therapist should always keep in mind the patient's goals.

ORTHOTIC MANAGEMENT

The key to effective orthotic management is understanding the impairments and functional limitations affecting the patient and whether mobility or stability is the problem.

Mobility

The purpose of orthotic intervention for impairments and functional limitations related to mobility is to support the part, provide shock absorption, and allow movement when necessary. The orthoses are generally made of flexible materials or are equipped with movable joints.

Managing patients with *impaired joint mobility, motor function, muscle performance,* and *range of motion due to capsular restriction or localized inflammation* requires both support and allowances for movement as healing progresses. The same design is also useful for patients with *impaired motor function* (generally increased muscle tone and abnormal movement patterns) and *sensory integrity* due to nonprogressive disorders of the central nervous system, such as cerebral vascular accident. The orthosis should keep the patient's joint(s) in a balanced position, allowing for a weight-

bearing pattern that is as smooth and efficient as possible. Examples of orthoses that meet this treatment goal include the following:

Soft foot orthosis: used for inflammatory conditions such as metatarsalgia, arthritis, Morton's neuroma, tendinitis, and tenosynovitis. The purpose of this orthosis is to provide rest for the joints of the foot and shock absorption for the entire lower extremity.[38] These orthoses can be very helpful with inflammatory problems in the hip and the knee as well.[8] Soft foot orthoses are made from a variety of neoprene, polyurethane, and polyethylene materials and are relatively inexpensive. They are most often found in over-the-counter styles and made in half-size increments. Because the material is soft, this type of orthosis can be cut down to fit in a patient's shoe more exactly. AliMed Corporation (Dedham, Mass.) has a large and varied assortment of soft foot orthoses that can be purchased individually or in bulk.

Rocker bottom shoe: used for capsular restriction and inflammatory disorders of the metatarsophalangeal joints, especially the great toe (e.g., hallux rigidus). This crepe device, added to the sole of the shoe just proximal to the metatarsal heads, allows for weight transference over the toes without extension of the metatarsophalangeal joints.[31] These devices can easily be added to a standard flat-soled shoe by an orthotist or an experienced cobbler (Fig. 20-2).

Metatarsal bar: designed to alleviate forefoot pressure problems, often the result of inflammatory impairments of the metatarsophalangeal joints. This bar can be made from any number of polyethylene materials and is easily and inexpensively fabricated. The bar or pad is place just proximal to the metatarsal heads and redistributes the weight-bearing forces off the metatarsal heads and onto the pad.

Flexible ankle foot orthosis (AFO): made from a flexible plastic material, this orthosis can provide proper positioning for the ankle and possibly the subtalar and the midtarsal joints as well. The flexibility allows for some motion to occur, especially a small amount of plantar flexion and dorsiflexion. This orthosis is helpful in patients with motor function impairments due to excessive tone in the lower extremity extensor group. By placing the ankle and foot in neutral, the weight bearing is more normal and the proper movement patterns are promoted. The constant pressure from the footplate may also help reduce hypertonicity.[5,18,24,39] An AFO made from metal double uprights and a joint that can be manipulated to allow or prevent movement will have the same results (Fig. 20-3).

Knee orthosis (KO) and ankle orthosis (AO): used with patients who need the support of the brace but also the mobility option of a joint or flexible material.[23] The KO and AO made of a soft elastic or neoprene material can be used with patients whose primary impairments are

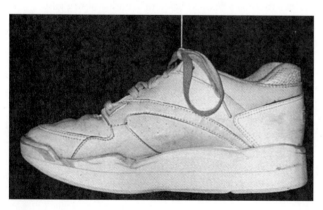

FIG. 20-2   A rocker bottom may be added to a shoe or sneaker to accommodate pressure problems in the forefoot.

inflammation, pain, or capsular restriction.[37] These orthoses are inexpensive, available in small to extra-large sizing, and provide total contact support while allowing for some movement.[29]

Knee ankle orthosis (KAFO) with a joint: used in cases in which support is needed (e.g., capsular restriction at the knee and/or ankle due to arthritis). This orthosis can be made with metal uprights and leather or uprights imbedded in plastic for more support. This orthosis is custom made and can be relatively heavy to use. Walking speed and efficiency may be negatively affected. The orthosis may be too heavy for patients with impairments in motor function and accompanying tone changes.[3] Muscle strength and endurance in the hip and knee muscles are helpful in effectively using the orthosis.

Managing patients with *impaired posture* of the forefoot and rearfoot can be effectively done using semi-rigid foot orthoses. Weight gain, increased activity, poor footwear, or swelling can all lead to further pain and dysfunction at the foot, ankle, knee, or hip.[11,42] Thermoplastic materials, such as closed cell foam or cork, can be purchased as prefabricated full-length or three-quarter length orthoses, generally available in whole sizes for men and women. These prefabricated models are considerably less expensive and can be modified by adding wedges onto the heel or metatarsal region and/or heated in a convection oven and molded to the patient's foot.[7,12] Semi-rigid orthoses may also be custom made, with a plaster mold made of the patient's foot and the orthosis molded directly over the cast. Wedging can be done very specifically and imbedded into the finished product. This type of orthosis generally has a longer wear capability and can be made to fit different types of shoes but is much more expensive to fabricate.[32]

Impaired integumentary integrity is a common and often dangerous problem in the elderly with diabetes and/or peripheral vascular disease. Proper education will help prevent breakdown and subsequent amputation. Total contact foot orthoses can also be beneficial in decreasing friction forces and increasing shock absorption. Soft or semi-rigid orthoses that have no ridges and fit compactly in the shoe diminish the negative forces and help maintain the integumentary integrity. Wedging on an orthosis can be used to offset the weight-bearing forces if toe deformities exist. For example, a metatarsal bar can be used to decrease the pressure on the metatarsal head from a claw toe deformity. Orthoses can be built up in one area of the forefoot to relieve the pressure on a toe callus or ulcer.*

Stability

The purpose of orthotic intervention for impairments and functional limitations related to stability is to act as an external stabilizer. The main problems contributing to lack of stability include *impairments in muscle performance, joint mobility, and range of motion due to ligament and connective tissue disorders and bony* and *soft tissue surgical procedures.* Patients with *impaired motor function and sensory integrity due to progressive and non-progressive CNS disorders, acute or chronic polyneuropathies,* or *peripheral nerve injuries* may also have problems with stability that require orthotic management. Examples of orthoses that meet these treatment goals include the following:

Rigid foot orthoses: used for impairments due to ligamentous and connective tissue laxity. Pes planus, or flat feet, require hard plastic orthoses such as the UCB shell pictured in Fig. 20-4. These orthoses must be custom molded over a plaster cast to ensure proper fit and supportive structure. The excessive mobility in the foot (and subsequent lack of stability) requires external assistance to act in place of the normally taut connective tissue.[10] Shoes with a firm heel counter will assist in giving support to a patient with pes planus.

Solid ankle foot orthosis (SAFO): used for patients with impairments related to lack of muscle performance at the ankle, hypermobility of the ankle joint, ligamentous and other connective tissue laxity of the ankle, or

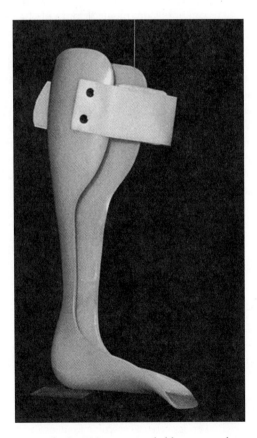

FIG. 20-3 A plastic AFO uses extended lever arms that can prevent pronation as well as assist dorsiflexion. Note the height of the wall along the medial arch, which resists the forces pushing the forefoot into pronation.

---

*References: 1,2,6,13,14,16,19,22,26,27,30,33-36,40,41,43,46,47,49

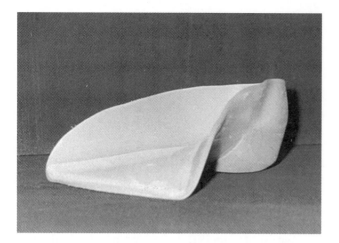

FIG. 20-4   A UCBL shell.

lack of proper motor function in the lower leg and foot. Generally constructed of a hard plastic material, the SAFO surrounds the posterior calf and ankle, acting as an external support.[20,25] These orthoses can be found in prefabricated models (sized small to extra large) or can be custom molded from a plaster cast at a much higher cost. The latter total contact orthosis is preferable for patients with impaired integumentary integrity due to diabetes or peripheral vascular disease. A similar effect can be gained by using a metal and leather orthosis with a locked ankle joint.

Knee orthosis (KO) and knee ankle foot orthosis (KAFO) with locked joint(s): used for patients with impaired muscle performance, motor function, and ligamentous and connective tissue integrity of the entire lower extremity (Fig. 20-5).[44] It is critical that the patient has good muscle control of the hip, or the orthosis will be too heavy to manipulate during gait.[4,48] Also, locking the distal joints requires compensation at the proximal joints (hip and spine) in terms of increased mobility. This orthosis can be made of plastic with metal uprights or more traditional leather and metal.

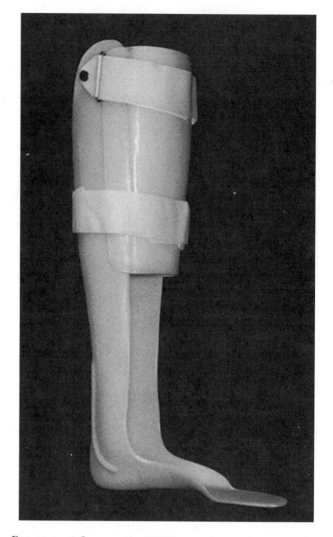

FIG. 20-5   A floor-reaction KAFO uses a three-point pressure system to prevent knee buckling.

Case Studies

Case 1: Patient with Impaired Mobility
History
General Demographics and History of Current Condition.
The patient is a 78-year-old black female who suffered a left middle cerebral artery cerebral vascular accident 1 month ago. She has right-sided hemiplegia and is currently in a rehabilitation facility for intensive physical and occupational therapy.

Social History. The patient is an active member of her local church, singing in the choir and ministering to homebound parishioners.

Occupation/Employment. The patient is a homemaker, caring for her two grandchildren 3 days a week.

Living Environment. The patient lives in a three-family home on the second floor. The staircases have two railings. No elevator is available.

Functional Status and Activity Level. The patient is able to feed, groom, and dress herself with minimum assist. She needs moderate assist to transfer bed to chair. She is currently standing with a walker but not ambulating.

Medications. The patient is currently taking furosemide (Lasix), warfarin (Coumadin), lisinopril, and colace.

Other Tests and Measures. MRI showed that the patient sustained an embolic stroke to the left middle cerebral artery.

Past History of Current Condition. The patient has a history of transient ischemic attacks for 5 years.

Past Medical/Surgical History. The patient has a 25-year history of high blood pressure that has been managed with diet, exercise, and medication.

Family History. Father died of heart disease at 50; mother died of breast cancer at 68; brother died of heart disease at 62.

Health Status. The patient admits to feeling more fatigued lately with much less energy. She does not watch her diet carefully and claims to eat a lot of red meat.

Social Habits. The patient does not drink or smoke.

Systems Review

Cardiopulmonary. Heart rate (HR), 82; blood pressure (BP), 122/74 mm Hg; respiratory rate, 12

Musculoskeletal. Left extremities have full range of motion and good strength; trunk has fair grade abdominal and back extensor muscles

Neuromuscular. Volitional movement in trunk and left extremities

Integumentary. Height, 5'4 feet; weight, 155 lbs; no swelling, discoloration noted in any extremity

Communication, Affect, Cognition, Language, and Learning. Friendly, understands and follows commands, anxious to get back home

Tests and Measures

Posture. Kyphotic cervicothoracic spine; right lower extremity held rigidly in extension

Joint Integrity and Mobility. Right knee and ankle, grade 1 mobility; right subtalar and midtarsal joints, grade 2 mobility

Range of Motion. Unable to flex knee or dorsiflex ankle voluntarily; passive motion at right knee is 0 to 100 degrees and at right ankle is 0 to 45 degrees

Muscle Performance. Good grade strength in right upper extremity; unable to test right lower extremity

Sensory Integrity (Including Proprioception and Kinesthesia). The patient has diminished proprioceptive sense with the right lower extremity

Circulation. Femoral, popliteal, posterior tibial, and pedal pulses normal in both lower extremities

Vital Signs. BP with transfer to standing, 144/78 mm Hg; HR, 86

Motor Function. Minimal voluntary motion of the right lower extremity with greatest control at the hip; movement of the right lower extremity involves extension of the hip, knee, and ankle and supination of the foot; right upper extremity has a slowed but normal movement pattern

Gait, Locomotion, and Balance. The patient comes to standing with moderate assistance; standing balance is fair with walker or parallel bars for support; poor balance without support; weight bearing on right lower extremity is on an extended foot; able to walk 5 feet with walker and maximal assistance

Assistive and Adaptive Devices. The patient is using a walker for ambulation

Evaluation

The patient is a 78-year-old female who has a right-sided hemiplegia secondary to a left cerebral vascular accident. She is beginning to get some voluntary movement of the right lower extremity but is unable to ambulate effectively because of the increased extensor tone and lack of voluntary movement in the right lower extremity. The patient will benefit from an orthosis to improve gait pattern and allow for independent ambulation.

Diagnosis

Impaired motor function and sensory integrity of the right lower extremity secondary to a left cerebral vascular accident

Prognosis

The patient will be functioning independently and ambulating with a cane in 4 to 6 weeks.

Intervention

Coordination, Communication, and Documentation. Social Services was contacted to get insurance approval for orthotic device; family was contacted to discuss options concerning discharge planning due to the stairs at home

Patient/Family Education. The patient and family were instructed in home exercises, transfers, ambulation with a cane on level surfaces and stairs, and donning/doffing the orthosis

Therapeutic Exercise. Exercise emphasized normal movement patterns of the right lower extremity in non-weight bearing and in weight bearing with orthosis; gait training performed with walker, then progressing to cane on level surfaces and stairs

Functional Training. Training involved transferring in and out a car, going to the store, maneuvering around tight spaces in a home setting

Prescription and Application of Orthosis. Patient was fitted with a *flexible AFO set in 0 degrees dorsiflexion;* her subtalar and midtarsal joints were placed in neutral in the orthosis, facilitating a more normal movement pattern when weight bearing

Outcomes

The patient was able to go home from the rehabilitation center after 4 weeks. She received 2 weeks of outpatient physical therapy to continue to improve her motor function and her gait pattern. She was given a home exercise program to prevent any secondary effects from the continued abnormal right lower extremity movement pattern. She was extremely satisfied with her rehabilitation.

Case 2: Patient with Impaired Stability
History

General Demographics and History of Current Condition. The patient is an 82-year-old white male who has been suffering with left lower leg pain and foot drop for several months. He is now unable to garden and do his daily walk because of the pain.

Social History. The patient is an avid gardener and carpenter. He walks daily with a group at the local mall. He enjoys traveling with his wife of 60 years.

Occupation/Employment. The patient is a retired stone mason.

Living Environment. The patient lives in a two-story single family home on 2 acres (he uses 1 acre for a vegetable and flower garden).

Functional Status and Activity Level. The patient is independent in all ADL. He is an early riser and does very few sedentary activities. He claims to have slowed down since the pain has increased.

Medications. The patient is currently taking insulin, furosemide (Lasix), and ibuprofen when needed for the pain.

Other Tests and Measures. Nerve conduction studies showed diminished conductivity of the left deep peroneal nerve innervating the tibialis anterior.

Past History of Current Condition. The patient has a 2-year history of pain in the left lower leg with the foot drop getting worse during the last 3 months.

Past Medical/Surgical History. The patient has a 15-year history of adult-onset diabetes mellitus for which he takes daily insulin injections. He has had periodic ulcers on both feet that healed slowly but completely. He also has a history of bilateral ankle swelling for which he takes the Lasix.

Family History. Father died of natural causes at 98; mother died in childbirth at 34; two siblings died of lung cancer in their 70s; six siblings are alive and relatively healthy.

Health Status. The patient admits to slowing down considerably because of the pain. He expressed considerable dissatisfaction with his current health status.

Social Habits. The patient smokes a cigar daily and has red wine with meals.

Systems Review

Cardiopulmonary. Heart rate, 84; blood pressure, 140/82 mm Hg; respiratory rate, 16

Musculoskeletal. Both upper extremities have full range of motion and good strength

Neuromuscular. Independent gait, transfers, and balance

Integumentary. Height, 6 feet; weight, 235 lbs

Communication, Affect, Cognition, Language, and Learning. Friendly, understands and follows commands, anxious to get back to walking and gardening

Tests and Measures

Posture. Forward head; slight genu varum bilaterally

Range of Motion. Full range of motion in both lower extremities except active left dorsiflexion limited to neutral; passive left dorsiflexion is 5 degrees

Muscle Performance. Good grade strength in both lower extremities, except left tibialis anterior tested as a fair minus grade

Sensory Integrity (Including Proprioception and Kinesthesia). Both feet were cold and hairless; decreased pin prick and two-point discrimination from the knee distally into both feet; thick calluses noted under the second and third metatarsal heads bilaterally

Circulation. Pedal and posterior tibial pulses were significantly diminished in both lower extremities; popliteal pulse only slightly diminished bilaterally; femoral pulses were normal

Gait, Locomotion, and Balance. Gait has slowed and patients states that he has been tripping when going up stairs and onto curbs during the last 3 months; foot slap on the left at heel strike to foot flat that increases as gait speed increases; slight trunk lean to the right in order to clear the left foot

Evaluation

The patient is an 82-year-old male with a long history of diabetes who now shows signs of peripheral nerve injury and diabetic neuropathy. His gait deviations are consistent with these problems. He now requires orthotic management to ambulate with a smooth and efficient gait.

Diagnosis

Impaired motor function and sensory integrity of the left lower extremity secondary to a peripheral nerve injury to the left deep peroneal nerve

Prognosis

The patient will be ambulating with less pain and be able to walk the mall and garden daily in 6 to 8 weeks.

Intervention

Coordination, Communication, and Documentation. Discussed previous foot care and education with patient's podiatrist and internist

Patient/Family Education. Instructed patient in home exercises, reviewed proper foot care, and discussed progression of activity level and use of orthosis in daily activities

Therapeutic Exercise. Exercise emphasized collateral circulation of both lower extremities (Buerger-Allen exercises) and strengthening of the left anterior tibialis; gait training performed with orthosis and emphasized bending left knee and hip to clear the left foot during swing

Functional Training. Training involved self-management of orthosis

Prescription and Application of Orthosis. Patient was fitted with a solid AFO set in 0 degrees dorsiflexion. The orthosis was custom molded and total contact to minimize friction and potential skin breakdown. The foot was set in subtalar and midtarsal neutral to maximize the normal weight-bearing pattern. A soft neoprene orthosis was added to the right shoe to decrease frictional forces and prevent skin breakdown.

Outcomes

The patient was discharged on an extensive home exercise program after 6 weeks of treatment. He did not regain any muscle function in the left anterior tibialis muscle due to his increasingly poor circulation. However, he was able to walk the mall daily and go back to gardening after an aerobic conditioning program. He lost 30 pounds with the exercise program. He was instructed in how to examine the orthosis regularly and when to call the orthotist if it was beginning to break down. He was extremely happy with his rehabilitation because of his return to his previous functional level.

Summary

Appropriate orthotic prescription requires a thorough examination, evaluation, diagnosis, and prognosis. This ensures correct style, proper fit, and a good functional outcome. Understanding whether the patient has impaired mobility or impaired stability will help determine the orthotic needs that will result in the most effective and efficient gait. In addition, consistent communication with the patient, family, and orthotist will produce the most successful outcomes.

References

1. Albert S, Rinoie C: Effect of custom orthotics on plantar pressure distribution in the pronated diabetic foot. *J Foot Ankle Surg* 1994; 33(6):598-604.
2. Armstrong DG, Lavery LA: Acute Charcot's arthropathy of the foot and ankle. *Phys Ther* 1998; 78:74-80.
3. Barnett SL, Bagley AM, Skinner HB: Ankle weight effect on gait: Orthotic implications. *Orthopedics* 1993; 16(10):1127-1131.
4. Baumann JU: [Gait changes in elderly people]. *Orthopade* 1994; 23(1):6-9.
5. Beckerman H, Becher J, Lanhorst GJ, Verbeek AL: Walking ability of stroke patients: Efficacy of tibial nerve blocking and a polypropylene ankle-foot orthosis. *Arch Phys Med Rehabil* 1996; 77(11):1144-1151.
6. Boone D, Douglas S: CAD/CAM and the Pedorthic Management of the Diabetic Foot, International Symposium CAD/CAM Systems in Pedorthics, Prosthetics & Orthotics, Clinical Perspectives and State-of-the-Art Maritim. *Abstracts.* Hotel Nuremberg, May 1997.
7. Brown GP, Donatelli R, Catlin PA, Wooden MJ: The effect of two types of foot orthoses on rearfoot mechanics. *J Orthop Sports Phys Ther* 1995; 21(5):258-267.
8. Caselli MA, et al: Evaluation of magnetic foil and PPT insoles in the treatment of heel pain. *J Am Podiatr Med Assoc* 1997; 87(1):11-16.
9. Chantelau E, Jung V: Quality control and quality assurance in therapeutic shoes for the diabetic foot, *Rehabilitation* 1994; 33(1):35-38.
10. Chao W, et al: Nonoperative management of posterior tibial tendon dysfunction. *Foot Ankle Int* 1996;17(12):736-741.
11. Conrad KJ, et al: Impacts of foot orthoses on pain and disability in rheumatoid arthritics. *J Clin Epidemiol* 1996; 49(1):1-7.
12. Cornwall MW, McPoil TG: Effect of rearfoot posts in reducing forefoot forces. A single subject design. *J Am Podiatr Med Assoc* 1992; 82(7):371-374.
13. De Keyser G, Dejaeger E, De Meyst H, Eders GC: The pressure-reducing effects of 13 different heel-protecting devices. *Adv Wound Care* 1994; 7(4):30-32, 34.
14. Evans SL, et al: The prevalence and nature of podiatric problems in diabetic patients. *J Am Geriatr Soc* 1991; 39(3):241-245.
15. Fisher LR, McLellan DL: Questionnaire assessment of patient satisfaction with lower limb orthoses from a district hospital. *Prosthet Orthot Int* 1989; 13(1):29-35.
16. George DH: Management of hyperkeratotic lesions in the elderly patient. *Clin Podiatr Med Surg* 1993; 10(1):69-77.
17. Guide to Physical Therapist Practice. *Phys Ther* 1997; 77:1163-1650.
18. Harkless LB, Bembo GP: Stroke and its manifestations in the foot. A case report. *Clin Podiatr Med Surg* 1994; 11(4):635-645.
19. Hayda R, et al: Effect of metatarsal pads and their positioning: A quantitative assessment. *Foot Ankle Int* 1994; 15(10):561-566.
20. Hill RS: Ankle equinus. Prevalence and linkage to common foot pathology. *J Am Podiatr Med Assoc* 1995; 85(6):295-300.
21. Inman VT, Raiston HJ, Todd F: *Human Walking.* Baltimore, Williams & Wilkins, 1981.
22. Janisse DJ: Prescription insoles and footwear. *Clin Podiatr Med Surg* 1995; 12(1):14-61.
23. Jansen CM, Windau JE, Bonutti PM, Brillhart MV: Treatment of a knee contracture using a knee orthosis incorporating stress-relaxation techniques. *Phys Ther* 1996; 76(2):182-186.
24. Kakurai S, Akai M: Clinical experiences with a convertible thermoplastic knee-ankle-foot orthosis for post-stroke hemiplegic patients. *Prosthe Orthot Int* 1996; 20(3):191-194.
25. King LA, VanSant AF: The effect of solid ankle-foot orthoses on movement patterns used in a supine-to-stand rising task. *Phys Ther* 1995; 75(11):952-964.
26. Landsman AS, Sage R: Off-loading neuropathic wounds associated with diabetes using an ankle-foot orthosis. *J Am Podiatr Med Assoc* 1997; 87(8):349-357.
27. Landsman AS, et al: 1995 William J. Stickel Gold Award. High strain rate tissue deformation. A theory on the mechanical etiology of diabetic foot ulcerations. *J Am Podiatr Med Assoc* 1995; 85(10):519-527.
28. Lord SR, Bashford GM: Shoe characteristics and balance in older women. *J Am Geriatr Soc* 1996; 44(4):429-433.
29. Matsuno H, Kadowaki KN, Tsuji H: Generation II knee bracing for severe medial compartment osteoarthritis of the knee. *Arch Phys Med Rehabil* 1997; 78(7):745-749.
30. Meuller MJ, Strube MJ, Allen BT: Therapeutic footwear can reduce plantar pressures in patients with diabetes and transmetatarsal amputation. *Diabetes Care Apt* 1997; 20(4):637-641.
31. Mizel MS, Michelson JD: Nonsurgical treatment of monarticular non traumatic synovitis of the second metatarsophalangeal joint. *Foot Ankle Int* 1997; 18(7):424-426.
32. Moraros J, Hodge W: Orthotic survey. Preliminary results. *J Am Podiatr Med Assoc* 1993; 83(3):139-148.
33. Morgan JM, Biehl WC III, Wagner FW Jr: Management of neuropathic arthropy with the Charcot Restraint Orthotic Walker. *Clin Orthop* 1993; 296:58-63.
34. Mueller MJ, Sinacore DR, Hoogstrate S, Daly L: Hip and ankle walking strategies: Effect on peak plant pressures and implications for neuropathic ulceration. *Arch Phys Med Rehabil* 1994; 75(11):1196-1200.
35. Mueller MJ: Use of an in-shoe pressure measurement system in the management of patients with neuropathic ulcers or metatarsalgia. *J Orthop Sports Phys Ther* 1995; 21(6):328-336.
36. Needleman RL: Successes and pitfalls in the healing of neuropathic forefoot ulcerations with the IPOS postoperative shoe. *Foot Ankle Int* 1997; 18(7):412-417.
37. Nuismer BA, Ekes AM, Holm MB: The use of low-load prolonged stretch devices in rehabilitation programs in the Pacific northwest. *Am J Occup Ther* 1997; 51(7):538-543.
38. Oddis CV: New perspectives on osteoarthritis. *Am J Med* 1996; 100:2A, 10S-15S.
39. Oshsawa S, et al: A new model of plastic ankle foot orthosis (FAFO (II)) against spastic foot and genu recurvatum. *Prosthet Orthot Int* 1992; 16(2):104-108.
40. Plummer ES, Albert SG: Focused assessment of foot care in older adults. *J Am Geriatr Soc* 1996; 44(3):310-313.
41. Richardson JK, Ashton-Miller JA: Peripheral neuropathy: An often-overlooked cause of falls in the elderly. *Postgrad Med* 1996; 99(6): 161-172.
42. Schrader JA, Siegel KL: Postsurgical hindfoot deformity of a patient with rheumatoid arthritis treated with custom-made foot orthoses and shoe modifications. *Phys Ther* 1997; 77(3):296-305.
43. Singh D, Bentley G, Trevino SG: Callosities, corns, and calluses. *BMJ* 1996; 12(7043):1403-1406.
44. Slemenda C, et al: Quadriceps weakness and osteoarthritis of the knee. *Ann Intern Med* 1997; 127(2):97-104.
45. Sullivan PE, Markos MA: *An Integrated Approach to Therapeutic Exercise: Theory and Application.* Reston, Va, Reston Publishing Company, 1982.

46. Tymec AC, Pieper B, Vollman K: A comparison of two pressure-relieving devices on the prevention of heel pressure ulcers. *Adv Wound Care* 1997; 10(1):39-44.

47. Walker SC, Helm PA, Pellium G: Total-contact casting, sandals, and insoles. Construction and applications in a total foot-care program. *Clin Podiatr Med Surg* 1995; 12(1):63-73.

48. Waring WP, et al: Influence of appropriate lower extremity orthotic management on ambulation, pain and fatigue in a postpolio population. *Arch Phys Med Rehabil* 1989; 70(5):371-375.

49. Zernike W: Preventing heel pressure sores: A comparison of heel pressure relieving devices. *J Clin Nurs* 1994; 3(6):375-380.

CHAPTER 21

LOWER LIMB PROSTHETIC REQUIREMENTS IN THE OLDER ADULT

CAROL MILLER, PT, MS, GCS

INTRODUCTION

Among the many challenges faced by older adults, the potential loss of ambulatory ability threatens independence as perhaps no other functional limitation can. One can only guess at the magnification of that threat when ambulatory abilities are compromised by lower limb amputation. Nowadays it is difficult to imagine a time when lower limb prosthetic fitting for the older patient was highly controversial before researchers were better able to elucidate the range of potential functional outcomes for an older person after amputation.[3,8,48]

Although advances in surgical intervention are not always reflected as a decrease in mortality rate after lower limb amputations,[8,53,54] surgeons are now more often able to save the knee by performing transtibial amputations. The benefit of these more distal amputations is often reflected in the research that demonstrates a decreased energy demand of prosthetic ambulation of this group when compared with persons with amputations more proximally.[36] Thus, new challenges in rehabilitation have presented themselves. Additionally, advances in prosthetic design, fabrication from light-weight material, and overall improvement in fitting a prosthesis may be able to contribute effectively to

increasing the long-term usage of a lower limb prosthesis by an older person after amputation, but that remains to be fully studied.

The overall goal of this chapter is to establish the scientific basis for clinical decision making by physical therapists regarding prosthetic management of the older adult. Furthermore, the emphasis of this chapter is on amputation as a sequelae of disease—not trauma or congenital deformity—because loss of limb from disease accounts for the greatest number of amputations among older adults. Although there are many similarities in prosthetic fabrication, fit, alignment, and training to use a prosthesis for younger patients and older adults after an amputation, critical differences in preoperative and postoperative physical therapy management of the older adult are also evident.[34]

The members of the multi-disciplinary clinical team share the responsibility for identifying key factors that affect the successful prosthetic management and rehabilitation of older persons. The physical therapist, along with the entire prosthetic team, must be able to incorporate a thorough understanding of the physiological changes that occur in the older adult into the prosthetic prescription in order to promote maximum patient satisfaction and long-term use of a prosthesis.

In addition, knowledge about psychological readiness, appreciation of socioeconomic factors, and awareness of third-party payer systems are essential to determine optimal prosthetic prescription and physical therapy intervention with a geriatric patient.

INCIDENCE OF AMPUTATION IN THE OLDER ADULT

There are approximately 270,000 persons with amputation living in the United States,[46] with an annual incidence of approximately 50,000 lower limb amputations.[32] The major causes for lower limb amputations are peripheral vascular disease, trauma, malignancy, and congenital deficiency.[36,45] The most common levels of surgical amputation secondary to ischemic vascular disease are transfemoral (25%), transtibial (50%), and transmetatarsal (25%).[51] Other types of amputation, such as the hip disarticulation, knee disarticulation, and hemipelvectomy, are much less common for the older adult with vascular disease. Transmetatarsal amputations, often a result of ischemia or gangrene of the metatarsals, may require the addition of a filler inside the shoe but do not require prosthetic intervention.

Older adults, especially those older than 55, constitute the largest proportion of individuals with lower limb amputations.[32,49] Most commonly, lower limb amputations in this group occur as a result of peripheral vascular disease (PVD), particularly PVD associated with diabetes.[49] In fact, several studies note that approximately 70% of all amputations are the result of either diabetes or PVD or a combination of both diseases.[8,21] Also, other studies suggest that the combination of diabetes and PVD accounts for 6% to 25% of all amputations, whereas only 2% to 5% of amputations occur in non-diabetic persons with PVD.[37,54] Thus, understanding the interplay between risk factors for particular diseases such as diabetes and health habits that put the individuals at risk for still other comorbidities is critical knowledge for the practitioner. For example, the older adult who has a history of diabetes and the additional risk factor of a history of smoking, which contributes to the occurrence of PVD, is at greatest risk for amputation.[28,49]

No one can doubt the serious medical condition of the individual who requires lower limb amputation. The 2-year survival rate after lower extremity amputation averages 50%, with most of the deaths attributable to cardiovascular complications.[19,44] Moreover, there is a 20% to 50% risk of losing the contralateral leg to vascular disease during the 5 years after amputation, which must be taken into careful consideration when considering prosthetic intervention.[4]

Many of these factors might appear to mitigate against providing a prosthesis to an older adult. However, it is essential to remember that the individual's goals, personal motivation, and pre-morbid status are often the strongest determinants of success with a prosthesis. Numerous studies demonstrate that many older adults with transfemoral or transtibial amputations do achieve functional prosthetic success.[3,8,48]

PROSTHETIC DESIGN

During the past several decades, numerous advances in prosthetic design have occurred. It is well-accepted that the prosthetic team strives to achieve three essential goals in prescription, fabrication, and training: comfort, function, and cosmesis. Foremost, function and cosmesis cannot readily be considered nor addressed without first achieving comfort. The increased use of modern thermoplastics, especially since the 1980s, has resulted in the fabrication of many different types of sockets and liners, knee mechanisms, and ankle/foot designs. Generally, the use of endoskeletal components to reduce the weight of a prosthesis has increased. Many companies now produce geriatric components made of titanium and other materials that allow for lighter prostheses. In addition, computerized programs such as Contoured Adducted Trochanteric-Controlled Alignment Method (CAT-CAM) and Computer Aided Design-Computer Aided Manufacturing (CAD-CAM), are available to assist the prosthetist in fabrication and follow-up fitting. Unfortunately, the optimal prosthetic design, regardless of the individual's age, has remained elusive. The daily and long-term effects of these types of prosthetic improvements on function for the older adult still require continued investigation.

The obvious impact of amputation on the gait of a person with a lower limb prosthesis is easily attributable to the substitution of prosthetic parts for the normal skeletal segments and joints.[11] Most importantly, the prosthesis must provide comfortable containment of the residual limb tissue during the stance phase of gait and provide a means of transferring the amputee's weight through the pelvis and residual limb to the floor.[42] Prosthetic factors such as fit and alignment, the type of knee unit,[18,26,42] and foot component[42,50] have been demonstrated to influence gait parameters. Yet, the relationship between prosthetic fabrication and fit, muscle activity within the prosthesis, and function for the person with amputation is still not clearly understood. The fit, alignment, and adjustment of the prosthesis to the amputee must provide maximal restoration of function with minimal gait deviation, in both the stance and swing phase of a walking cycle.[11,18,42,47]

During normal gait, lower limb stance and swing phases occur as the result of precisely timed control of joint motion and muscle action. The lower limbs easily adapt to changes in walking terrain and even naturally accommodate for obstacles, in which case, energy conservation is optimal. Lower limb amputations cause a loss of limb length; normal joint mobility; direct muscular control; and local proprioception, especially altering the precise awareness of foot contact on the floor.[39] Even with the many advances made with prosthetics, a prosthesis at best can only imitate, but certainly cannot replicate, normal gait patterns. Due to the complexity of issues that surround the older adult whose health status necessitates an amputation, these seemingly simple primary goals of providing optimal comfort, function, and cosmesis can present the medical team with a challenging clinical problem.

PHYSIOLOGICAL CHANGES

Age alone is not a sound determinant of predicting the prosthetic success of an older adult, but it is clearly considered a risk factor for increased mortality and less-than-optimal outcomes.[8,22,48] Studies have indicated for quite some time that increasing age was associated with an increased likelihood of above-knee amputation, with greater incidence of bilateral limb loss, and with lengthened time necessary for successful rehabilitation.[22] Pertinent to prosthetic selection for the older patient, studies have shown that individuals with multiple comorbidities are at highest risk for death and mortality and have the least success with rehabilitation.[3,8]

Steinberg recommends careful selection of patients appropriate for prosthetic by considering a detailed list of "clinical concerns:" cognitive dysfunction that interferes with training; advanced neurological disorders; cardiopulmonary conditions severe enough to impose limitations on effort; ulcers or infections with compromised circulation; irreducible and pronounced knee flexion contractures in below-knee candidates; and hip flexion contractures in above-knee candidates.[48]

The clinician is best able to formulate a plan for intervention and identify goals for successful prosthetic rehabilitation by completing a comprehensive examination and applying sound knowledge of the influences of the cardiovascular, musculoskeletal, neuromuscular, and integumentary systems to evaluation of these data. Physiological changes in each of these systems can affect prosthetic fit and function.

Cardiovascular

Complications related to diabetes more commonly occur when blood glucose levels are consistently elevated over time. Microvascular, or small blood vessel, complications evident in retinopathy, nephropathy, and neuropathy are discussed under neuromuscular considerations later in this chapter. Macrovascular, or large blood vessel, complications such as development of atherosclerotic narrowing of blood vessels relate to an increase in coronary artery disease and myocardial infarction, as well as cerebral vascular disease and stroke.[9,33] One significant implication of this is that the person with lower limb amputation and diabetes will have many more confounding risk factors that could increase demands on the cardiovascular system. Consequently, the medical conditions of these persons require careful monitoring by all members of the medical team to prevent undue stress to the cardiovascular system.

Energy requirements for using a prosthesis have been a major concern for decades. In earlier years, prostheses were not prescribed for the older adult due to the extensive demands on the cardiovascular system. In the past 2 decades, prosthetics has increasingly moved toward using lighter endoskeletal components, especially for the older adult. These lighter-weight prostheses, specifically fabricated for the geriatric ambulator, have been marketed by many different manufacturers; however, the effect of these lighter components on reducing stress to the cardiovascular system remains to be fully studied.

One of the best indicators of cardiovascular functional capacity is obtained through the measurement of the maximal oxygen uptake, or $\dot{V}o_2max$. Healthy older individuals in the sixth decade of life use 41% of their maximum aerobic capacity during walking.[52] Many studies have indicated that

the energy costs of using a prosthesis are substantially increased over normal bipedal locomotion, with estimates ranging from 40% to 60% with unilateral transtibial amputation, 60% to 100% with bilateral transtibial amputation, 90% to 120% with unilateral transfemoral amputation, and more than 200% with bilateral transfemoral amputation.[8,14,48,52]

Interestingly, steady state energy costs for the older persons with amputation compared with a healthy adult of similar age are not significantly different. When compared with normal gait, persons using a lower limb prosthesis will demonstrate much slower walking velocity and cadence, which continually decrease as the level of amputation increases. In effect, the person with a lower limb amputation seemingly slows down to reduce the stress on his/her cardiovascular system. Thus, when only the amount of oxygen utilization is compared between a healthy individual and one using a prosthetic limb, and time or distance is ignored, the oxygen utilization per meter can be essentially the same between the two individuals.

Monitoring the patient's heart rate (HR) during activity is absolutely essential in the clinic. English suggests that a pulse rate of approximately 130 beats per minute in a patient who has been walking at a constant rate of 5 minutes is the best indication of the patient's maximum functional physical capacity.[13] The "six minute walk-test" is often used by the physical therapist to assess the quality and integrity of a person's cardiopulmonary response to activity; however, one must take into consideration that many older adults with amputation, particularly those with transfemoral amputation, cannot walk for a total of 6 minutes until much later in the rehabilitation process, and many others are unable to ever achieve this goal. As mentioned previously, the person with amputation often slows his/her velocity and cadence significantly to reduce stress on the cardiovascular system. In light of this, the results of the six-minute walk test have to be interpreted cautiously. Monitoring vital signs during arm ergometry exercise may offer the clinician an alternative for assessing cardiopulmonary integrity in these patients.

Foremost for the clinician, knowledge of energy cost and oxygen utilization requirements is necessary to formulate an intervention with the appropriate exercise frequency, duration, and intensity. Careful attention should be paid to appropriate intensity of cardiovascular exercise before training, as well as during gait training times. Allowing the person with amputation longer periods of time to perform a task and encouragement of slower or more comfortable speeds for gait also may prove helpful.

Musculoskeletal

With each ensuing decade of life past the middle years, the likelihood is a greater that postural changes will occur, even in the absence of disease. Most often, these changes are the result of inactivity and decreased mobility. The most common types of postural changes in the lower limb joints are increased flexion at the hips and knees and loss of dorsiflexion at the ankle. In addition, physiological changes that occur with aging of the musculoskeletal system, such as a decrease in connective tissue extensibility, decline in muscle strength, and muscle imbalance, further promote these postural problems and may limit the effectiveness of the physical therapist's intervention.

Contractures occurring in the lower limb joints of the older person can negatively affect functional outcomes and even prevent prosthetic use in some cases. Contractures can influence prosthetic fit, alter postural alignment in stance, and contribute to poor gait patterns and even the inability to ambulate. Most contractures are the result of muscle imbalance, especially after the surgical division of muscles, previous impairment, or long-standing poor postural habits. Hip flexion, abduction, and external rotation contractures may occur in a patient after transfemoral amputations, with hip flexion being the most common in this patient group. Hip flexion; abduction; external rotation; and most commonly, knee flexion contractures may develop as a result of transtibial amputations.

Generally, only knee flexion contractures of no more than 10 to15 degrees for below-knee amputations and hip flexion contractures of no more than 15 to 20 degrees for above-knee amputations can be readily be accommodated for in the fabrication and fit of the prosthetic device. Persons with contractures greater than these can be fitted with prostheses; however, gait patterns may become more significantly altered with increased deformity. Furthermore, contractures greater than these often inhibit safe ambulation and diminish an individual's ability to maintain safe static and dynamic postures as well. However, to promote the ability to transfer and provide acceptable cosmesis, a prosthetist often may be able to modify a prosthesis for a person with transtibial amputation and accommodate knee flexion contractures

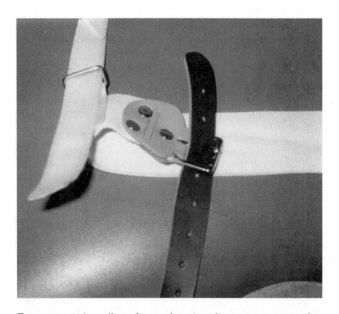

FIG. 21-1   Velcro allows for much easier adjustment as opposed to buckles, which are more cumbersome.

as great as 35 to 40 degrees. Additionally, even in the presence of these more significant contractures, some patients have been able to successfully ambulate with a modified prosthesis and an assistive device. Therefore, impaired muscle length or soft tissue extensibility should not necessarily deter the patient or clinician from pursuing a prosthetic fit. Other modifications in prosthetic design, such as a bent knee prosthesis, have been used in the presence of extreme knee flexion contractures, sometimes as large as 70 to 90 degrees. However, poor cosmesis is often a problem in these cases and may discourage long-term use of the prosthesis.

For the person with transfemoral amputation, it can be quite difficult, if not impossible, for the prosthesis to accommodate a hip flexion contracture greater than 25 degrees and allow for safe ambulation. Stability during the gait cycle can be significantly compromised in these patients, resulting in decreased safety and increased risk for falls. With significant contractures at the hip, a prosthesis is not generally provided, even to assist with transfers, but if one is requested by the patient, it may be provided for the purpose of improving cosmesis.

Prevention of these deformities from the outset is absolutely the best intervention and should be emphasized throughout the rehabilitation process. Along with patient education, early postoperative management should include stretching and strengthening the remaining lower limb joints and muscles as well as proper positioning to reduce the chances of developing contractures.

Neuromuscular

Peripheral neuropathies may result from the microvascular changes seen with PVD but can also be attributed to diabetes alone. Altered sensation in the distal parts of the extremities, especially the hands and feet, is noted in the presence of PVD and in clinical diabetic neuropathy.[9] In addition, atrophy of the intrinsic musculature of hands and feet ensues over longer periods of time. Depending on the severity, intrinsic muscle wasting in the hands can affect grasp and may prevent independent donning and doffing of the prosthesis without modification. Hand function, especially grasp, should be tested and documented as a part of the physical therapist's initial examination. Finally, retinopathy, which is often present with microvascular disease, can greatly affect vision and may impede independence in prosthetic donning and doffing without modification.

Prosthetists often are able to make different types of prosthetic modifications to accommodate decreased hand function and impaired vision. Simple modifications can be made to reduce the need for normal hand dexterity. Use of Velcro material or "D" rings on the straps, such as those used on the Silesian band or supracondylar cuff, allow for much easier adjustment than that required to use buckles (Fig. 21-1). Although used less commonly for the older adult, another modification is a prosthetic system called the "3-S system." The suspension sleeve has a pin attachment on its end and can be easily rolled onto the residual limb, requiring less fine-motor hand function. The sleeve is then simply inserted into the prosthesis until three audible clicks are heard for safe attachment of the pin in the prosthesis (Fig. 21-2).[38] This type of system may also be easier for an older adult with visual impairment. A few factors that may deter the use of this system are increased difficulty in prosthetic fit, increased fabrication costs, and a potential development of skin allergies from the liner material.

Intrinsic muscle atrophy in the unaffected lower extremity can influence lower limb alignment and the joint integrity and soft tissue structure of the remaining foot, resulting in greater risk of damage due to trauma. Consultation with appropriate team members, such as an orthotist, is recommended to provide orthoses or other types of accommodative footwear that may reduce trauma and delay, if possible, further excess strain on the muscles of the unaffected lower limb.

Any areas on the body with diminished sensation, especially due to diabetes or PVD, can potentially increase a patient's risk of developing bruises, ulcers, and other skin problems. In the long term, this patient may experience additional detrimental consequences, including further loss of limb or loss of the contralateral limb. Prosthetic fit and comfort can be particularly difficult if sensory feedback in the residual limb is affected. Teaching compensatory techniques, such as using a hand-held mirror to clearly see the entire residual limb along with careful monitoring of skin condition, will reduce the risk of skin damage to all areas affected by sensory loss.

The result of limb dysfunction secondary to cerebrovascular accident (CVA) also may affect the person's ability to control the prosthesis if worn on the involved side. Changes in muscle tone, loss of range of motion, weakness, and decreased coordination associated with CVA can also have effects on the contralateral extremities and must be carefully examined. The ability to perform coordinated tasks in a specific sequence is essential for prosthetic donning and doffing as well as functional performance. Few, if any, prosthetic modifications can accommodate for these types of problems. Unfortunately, when the impairments and functional limitations are substantial as a result of a CVA, the patient is typically not considered to be a strong candidate for safe prosthetic use.

Integumentary

In essence, the only skin surface on the human body designed to tolerate weight bearing is the plantar surface of the foot. By virtue of the design of lower limb prostheses, one must consider the impact of weight-bearing forces on the skin and soft tissue of the residual limb. Maintaining healthy skin integrity is critical because wearing a prosthesis requires an intimate fit between the socket and the person's residual limb.

Physiologically, skin changes with aging. These changes may vary by gender, race, and influence of disease; however, much greater research is needed in this area as they relate to prosthetic use by older adults. Some of the pertinent changes in skin relative to use of a prosthesis include atrophy and fragility of the dermis, decreased solubility and stiffness of collagen, decreased elasticity, reduced viscosity, less eccrine and apocrine sweat, and regression and disorganization of small vessels.[31] Rete ridges, which lie at the epidermal junction, are directly responsible for the skin's resistance to shearing forces. These ridges are thought to flatten with aging. Therefore, the skin's ability to resist shearing forces is compromised. Clinically, this is often seen as skin tears and can occur at any interface between the residual limb and the prosthesis.[25] Persons with diabetes or PVD can also present with decreased sweat gland function, decreased tolerance to shear forces, and decreased skin structural stability secondary to a compromised microcirculation.

It is also important to consider the problem of decreased sweat gland function because the socks worn within a prosthesis can be extremely warm and often hot. Alteration in perspiration within the socket can result in skin conditions such as folliculitis (inflammation of the hair follicle) that may result in pain and discomfort. If this condition persists, prosthetic use must often be temporarily discontinued, which has significant impact on the person's functional abilities. Patient education regarding personal and prosthetic hygiene and consultation with the prosthetic team are encouraged.

To understand the appropriate timing to schedule prosthetic fitting and initiate safe progression of prosthetic use, the clinician needs to be aware of normal wound healing for the older adult, including wounds that occur through surgical intervention.

Wound healing is age dependent.[46] Wound healing in the elderly follows the classical inflammatory, proliferative, and remodeling phases. However, these phases take place at a delayed rate.[10] The tensile strength of healing wounds, as defined by the force required to disrupt wounds, is decreased in persons older than 70.[7] Again, diseases such as PVD and diabetes can also delay healing time for surgical wounds. The distal end of the limb, especially along the scar line, is thus most vulnerable to damage. Dehiscence of the wound can occur if fit is improper or too much stress is placed on the

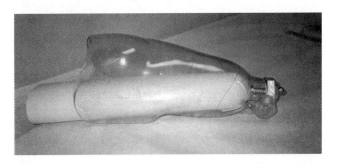

Fig. 21-2 A suspension sleeve with a pin attachment on its end can be rolled onto the residual limb, requiring less fine motor hand function.

incision site in wearing the prosthetic in the early phases of postsurgical rehabilitation. Edema reduction or control of volume of the residual limb may be difficult due to the presence of circulatory disease. Volume changes in the residual limb affect its shape and size, ultimately influencing the type and timing of initial and final prosthetic fit.

An essential part of clinical management of the patient with lower limb amputation concerns monitoring the patient's skin condition before and throughout prosthetic training. In view of the skin changes and wound healing time that occur with aging, the therapist must be certain that the wound is completely healed for training. The approximate or average time for fitting a prosthesis varies but is around 3 months after surgery.[29] Prosthetic fitting can occur as early as 3 to 4 weeks for the person with transfemoral amputation and 5 to 6 weeks for the person with transtibial amputation but remains dependent on scar healing. Early or immediate postoperative fitting is sometimes attempted but is not commonly recommended for the older adult due to the nature of amputation.

The most commonly prescribed prosthetic sockets are made of rigid materials that do not readily yield under forces during activities such as gait. Pressure and stability requirements are in opposition within a prosthesis, where a rigid support is required for stabilization during weight bearing, but a soft support is important to reduce pressure on soft tissue and enhance proprioception.[2] The material of the socket and the alignment of the prosthesis have been shown to increase the shear forces and pressure on the residual limb within a socket.[26,45] Flexible sockets, which are not commonly prescribed for the older adult because of cost, durability, and greater complexity in fitting, may allow increased comfort by reducing shear forces on the skin.[24,38] Residual limb socks or liners, which are used to create a more intimate fit, are also in direct contact with the skin. In the past, socks were made of materials such as cotton and wool. Recently, prosthetic modifications have included the use of limb socks or liners made of newer materials, such as silicone. For example, alpha liners, silipoas sleeves, among others have a gel-like feel and provide cushioning to the residual limb within the socket. This type of modification may be helpful to reduce shear on the residual limb; provide more uniform pressure; and hopefully, improve comfort, especially for the older person with fragile skin after transtibial amputation. In addition, these materials also may more readily accommodate for changes in limb volume secondary to edema.[24,38] One concern is that the materials used in certain liners or socket fabrication can cause allergic reactions in the form of a rash or dry irritated skin[25]; therefore, skin condition must be monitored carefully. As with other prosthetic modifications, research regarding the effectiveness for preventing skin breakdown and improving comfort and function in the older amputee is clearly needed.

Finally, skin integrity of the contralateral limb needs to be carefully examined. It is important to document any changes in lower limb pulses; presence of edema; and any alterations in the amount of hair, color, and degree of warmth. Padding areas of the prosthesis, such as the rivets over suspension mechanisms or over prominent areas of the socket, may be needed to reduce the risk of tearing skin on the uninvolved limb.

PROSTHETIC CLINIC TEAM

Typically, the clinic team includes a physician, a prosthetist, and a physical therapist. Each one of these members of the prosthetic clinic team contributes an important perspective. Other team members, such as the case manager and psychologist, may additionally become involved in assisting the older person to achieve optimal recovery after amputation. Unfortunately, the patient's role as a member of the team is often overlooked by the practitioners on the clinical team. Patient and family involvement are extremely important, and these members of the team should be present at each meeting whenever possible.

The physical therapist should provide the team with a thorough examination and evaluation of the patient before the prosthetic prescription. This examination should include a thorough history and systems review and objective tests and measures, with an overall emphasis on the patient's previous functional abilities and goals for the future (Box 21-1). The physical therapist should also play a role in prosthetic prescription. The initial part of the prescription process should involve all team members, including the patient. The prosthetist has particular expertise in the fabrication and alignment of a prosthesis. Furthermore, the prosthetist will bring to the attention of the team knowledge of the most recent advances in components appropriate to the older adult. Continual consultation between the prosthetist and the physical therapist ultimately creates a very effective means of caring for the patient.

Once the prosthesis is fabricated and fit to the patient, the physical therapist bears substantial responsibility for assisting the patient with adjustment to and acceptance of the device, along with continual assessment of fit and function during all of the patient's activities of daily living. Finally, the physical therapist must maintain open lines of communication with the prosthetist so that modifications can be made based on the patient's physical performance and the fit and alignment of the prosthesis.

It is unfortunate that clinical teams may not be readily available to every patient with prosthetic requirements; this may especially affect persons residing in long-term care, assisted care facilities, and at home. Quite often for persons with amputation who reside in long-term–care facilities, the therapist initially learns of problems, such as changes in the person's ability to wear and use the prosthesis safely and effectively, from the nursing staff or family members or from an annual screening process. By this time, problems such as improper fit and decreased patient satisfaction may have resulted in a decline in functional abilities. For the person living in the community, dissatisfaction with fit and function often arise when the patient obtains multiple prostheses from different prosthetists without adequate examination from rehabilitation experts or clinic teams.

Lims demonstrated a reduction of about 20 days in inpatient hospital stay, a fivefold increase in percentage of patients discharged with prosthesis, and a threefold increase in the effectiveness of long-term rehabilitation over a 5-year period among patients who received team care compared with persons treated in environments without a clinical team approach.[30] Multidisciplinary teams, functioning in a coordinated effort, offer a sound way to identify and resolve the complex problems that accompany amputations, especially among the very young and very old.[43]

PSYCHOSOCIAL IMPLICATIONS

Psychosocial issues relevant to successful prosthetic management warrant careful consideration of an individual's readiness, cognitive status, and depression. In some cases, the influence of the involvement of significant others or family may also determine whether prosthetic use is feasible. In addition, factors such as the cost of obtaining and learning to use a prosthesis may pose a significant financial burden to the patient and family and therefore must be considered.

Most importantly, the patient must have a desire to use a prosthesis. The loss of a limb is almost always considered initially devastating by the individual, and this perception exists regardless of age. A person's evaluation of his/her body image can both positively and negatively influence self-esteem, anxiety, and depression.[5] Specific education about the advantages and disadvantages of using a prosthesis for cosmesis, functional activities, and ambulation may assist the patient and others involved to understand the scope and limitations of the rehabilitation outcomes expected for that individual. Support groups, peer visitors, or volunteers who can demonstrate different prosthetic components and their level of success are sometimes psychologically beneficial to the patient who is preparing to use a prosthesis. Because psychological readiness is so extremely important to outcome, the patient may require psychological intervention before or concomitant with the physical therapist's intervention.

Although intellectual ability is normally maintained well into the mid-70s or later, other aspects of cognitive function, including the speed of memory processes and abstract thinking, decline with age. These changes, if present, have significant implications for an older individual's ability to incorporate new skills in motor behaviors to replace lost abilities.[1] In view of these changes, all members of the health care team, and especially the physical therapist, must actively become involved in consistent, ongoing education. Repetition of tasks may prove helpful for the patient and family to learn new tasks such as donning and doffing of the prosthesis. One effective tool that a physical therapist may use is an educational questionnaire that addresses all aspects of residual limb care and prosthetic management (Box 21-2). These questions can be asked frequently, to ensure safety with limb

---

BOX 21-1

PHYSICAL THERAPIST EXAMINATION FOR PROSTHETIC DETERMINATION

I. Patient History

 Past medical history:
 Prior functional abilities:
 Patients goals:

 Systems Review
  Medical diagnosis:

 Tests and Measures
  Range of motion:
  Muscle performance:
  Neuromotor development:
  Integumentary integrity:
   Sensory integrity:
   Anthropometric characteristics of residuum:
  Pain:
  Gait—locomotion and balance:
  Ambulation: Device: Assistance:
      Distance:
  Cognition:

 Footwear:

 Evaluation/Physical Therapist Diagnosis:

 Plan for Prosthetic Prescription:

II. Clinic Visits Examination

 Device:
 Patient Self-Report:
 Gait Deviations:
 Problem Areas (include the prosthetic or patient problem and source):

 Fit (document adjustments needed):

 Patient/Family Instruction (includes wearing time, skin inspection, gait, don/doff of device, exercise, other):

 Footwear (includes shoe/sneaker—modifications needed):

 Plan for Follow-Up:

---

care once the patient is independent of therapy. Home programs on videotape or with pictures can be helpful for those who have difficulty with written items. Even patients with minimal to moderate cognitive impairments have learned to use a prosthesis with consistent repetition in a structured environment.

Research has indicated that memory, attention, concentration, and organizational skills are cognitive functions necessary for effective use and maintenance of a prosthetic limb.[41] Many mental and affective assessment tools, such as the Mini-Mental Status Examination, Beck's Depression Inventory, and the Test of Mental Functions for the Elderly, are available to the physical therapist and could be

---

BOX 21-2

EDUCATIONAL QUESTIONNAIRE FOR INDEPENDENT PROSTHETIC USE

Prosthetic Socket Management

Where should your leg feel the pressure in the socket?

What does the liner do?

What is the difference between the sheath/liner and the socks?

How often should you clean the socket?

Sock Management

Name the different types of socks and how many you should wear?

What is the proper way to put on your socks?

How should you wash and dry the socks?

What do you do when your leg feels loose in the socket?

What do you do when your leg feels tight in the socket?

Why is it important to always carry extra socks with you when wearing your artificial leg?

Skin Care

What is the importance of checking your skin regularly?

How long should areas of redness last on your skin?

What do you do when you have an area of skin breakdown?

BOX 21-3

FUNCTIONAL LEVELS FOR PROSTHETICS

Level 0: Does not have the ability or potential to ambulate or transfer safely with or without assistance and a prosthesis does not enhance patient's quality of life or mobility.

Level 1: Has the ability or potential to use a prosthesis for transfers or ambulation on level surfaces at fixed cadence. Typical of the limited and unlimited household ambulator.

Level 2: Has the ability or potential to traverse low-level environmental barriers such as curbs, stairs, or uneven surfaces. Typical of the limited community ambulator.

Level 3: Has the ability or potential for ambulation with variable cadence. Typical of the community ambulator who has the ability to traverse most environmental barriers and may have vocational, therapeutic, or exercise activity that demands prosthetic utilization beyond simple locomotion.

Level 4: Has the ability or potential for prosthetic ambulation that exceeds basic ambulation skills, exhibiting high impact, stress, or energy levels. Typical of the prosthetic demands of the child, active adult, or athlete.

(Adapted from the *Region C DMERC Supplier Manual* [Summer 1997].)

---

implemented as a component of the initial examination, if deemed necessary.[15,20]

The costs associated with prosthetic fabrication, fitting, and follow-up can also be substantial. A prosthesis for a person with lower limb amputation can cost thousands of dollars; yet, many insurance policies often only cover 80% of the total amount. In an overview report on 15 persons with traumatic below-knee amputation in 1997, Lims noted that the mean number of prostheses per patient was 3.4 with a total prosthetic charge of $10,829 (range, $2,558 to $15,700) during the first 3 years of wearing a prosthesis.[30] Presently, many of the advances in socket design and liner materials are not covered by Medicare and can be costly for the patient. Many older adults live on limited incomes in their later years, especially older women whose income after retirement is generally less than that of their male counterparts. The existence of poverty, especially among older persons of racial and ethnic minority, may further prevent their ability to pay 20% of the medical bills incurred. Furthermore, those who are underinsured may need other sources of income or support from community organizations to subsidize the costs of a prosthesis. Any of these factors can create financial hardship for the older person after amputation. Thus, the decision about which type of prosthesis, or even whether to provide a prosthesis, may become quite dependent on the older adult's socioeconomic status. In many of these situations, the clinician may choose to take on an advocacy role or make a decision to refer the patient to a skilled case manager for further support.

Insurance Guidelines for Prosthetics

Insurance reimbursement guidelines for prosthetics are usually found with the rules that cover durable medical equipment. Established insurance guidelines can be useful to clinicians because they often affect the patient's, the prosthetist's, and other clinic team members' decisions before a prosthetic is prescribed. As health care changes, with the possibility of increased managed care for all older adults, the clinical team will need to consider the particulars of the individual's health insurance benefits before prescribing a prosthesis. Third-party payers typically require a physician's prescription as a part of the reimbursement process.[40] In the early 1990s, four regional medical directors for prosthetics, orthotics, and supplies collaborated with Medicare to develop criteria and coverage policies for prosthetic prescriptions. The resulting document is a detailed supplier manual for prosthetics and orthotics, whereby the four durable medical equipment regional carriers (DMERCs) follow the same policies for prosthetic prescription; however, coverage and reimbursement for similar items may vary by region.[35] The Health Care Financing Administration (HCFA), which administers the Medicare program, approved these policies as an established set of guidelines that describe the type of lower limb prosthesis that may be covered based on the person's "potential" functional level. Originally, the guidelines did not include the word "potential." This term was added in recent years and as a result allows the clinical team greater decision-making autonomy in determining the likelihood of prosthetic success. Presently, the guidelines state that the determination of "potential" functional ability is based on the reasonable expectations of the prosthetist and the ordering physician, considering factors including, but not limited to, the patient's past history (including prior prosthetic use if applicable); the patient's current condition, including the status of the residual limb and the nature of other medical problems; and the patient's desire to ambulate.[35] The "potential" functional levels from the *Region C DMERC Supplier Manual* for prosthetics is displayed in Box 21-3.[35]

COMPONENTS OF THE PROSTHESIS

Comprehensive texts and recent articles regarding specific prosthetic components and prosthetic training for diverse patient populations have been well-documented.[12,30,33,34] To ensure that the patient can properly and safely use the prosthesis, the clinician must understand how different sockets and components function. Consultation and discussion with a prosthetist is extremely helpful to develop further appreciation of the various types of components most suitable to the older adult patient. Sequences for donning and doffing and the progression of functional training with a prosthesis are quite similar for the older adult and a younger person.

Some of the more commonly prescribed prosthetic components based on functional levels as earlier described under insurance guidelines are listed in Table 21-1.[35] Most adaptations from the prostheses described in this table are made based on the decisions of the patient and clinic team to maximize a patient's independence in the use and management of the prosthesis.

A general rule regarding prosthetic prescription for the older adult is that the prosthesis should be light-weight, comfortable, safe, securely suspended, and easy to put on and take off.[27] The prosthesis should be simple, and the components used should be considered most appropriate for the "potential" functional level. The prosthesis should be fitted and aligned to maximize stability.

Insurance limitations or specific guidelines for prosthetic socket design are not as restricting as those for component parts; therefore, socket fabrication may be more dependent on the comfort of the patient and the skill of the prosthetist. Although suction is the preferred method for suspension, this is difficult for the geriatric amputee with conventional donning techniques.[1] As previously mentioned, alternative types of liners and suspension systems, such as the "3-S," may be easier for an older person. With the transfemoral prosthesis, the knee joint should be reliable, stable, and simple to use. New knee joints that combine the features of weight-activated stance as well as polycentric and pneumatic control provide greater stability in stance phase.[1] Finally, the prosthetic foot should be light-weight for all older adults. Again, all components should be considered durable, stable, simple, and cost-effective.[6]

ISSUES RELEVANT TO REHABILITATION

It is important to remember that many studies show that a high percentage of older adults discard their prosthesis within months or the first year of training.[3,8,53]

However, intensive rehabilitation efforts by an interdisciplinary team have shown positive outcomes for use of prosthesis.[17,30] Also, rehabilitation after the loss of the second

TABLE 21-1

COMMONLY PRESCRIBED PROSTHESES FOR THE OLDER PERSON

FUNCTIONAL LEVEL	TYPE OF PROSTHESIS
F0	**No** prosthesis is prescribed
F1	Suspension: Silesian for transfemoral; supracondylar for transtibial. Suction not considered.
	Socket: Quadrilateral for transfemoral; patella-tendon bearing for transtibial.
	Liner: Pelite (two per prosthesis).
	Knee: Single axis, constant friction, safety
	Ankle/Foot: SACH.
F2	Suspension: Same as for F1, suction considered
	Socket* and Knee: Same as for F1.
	Ankle/Foot: Axial rotation units, flexible-keel, and multiaxial foot.
F3	Suspension: Suction most often considered, also secondary suspension
	Socket: Same as for F1 and F2.
	Knee: Fluid and pneumatic knee.
	Ankle/Foot: Flex foot or flex-walk system, energy storing foot, multiaxial ankle/foot, dynamic response.

SACH = single axis cushion heel
*Suction socket designs, such as the narrow medial lateral, CAT-CAM or CAD-CAM, ischial containment, flexible brim, etc.
(Adapted from the *Region C DMERC Supplier Manual* [Summer 1997].)

limb is more likely to be successful if rehabilitative efforts were successfully undertaken after the loss of the first limb.[23] Finally, based on what has been reported to date thus far, the physical therapist must remember that prosthetic success is multifactorial.[3,16,53]

One of the trends in health care is that many persons are being discharged from acute care to home earlier, and their cases are being followed through home health services with or without physical therapy involvement, until wound healing is complete and the patient can be considered ready for prosthetic fitting. For the person with lower limb amputation, this may mean discharge before prosthetic limb fitting. Under optimal circumstances, the person has achieved independence in wheelchair management and mobility and independence in basic activities of daily living at a wheelchair level before this discharge.[1] In addition, the added time during wound healing allows time for the patient and the rehabilitation team to focus on the pre-prosthetic program, which can afford the best opportunity to formulate realistic treatment goals.[12] The overall costs of rehabilitation for the older adult, however, may also be increased if the patient needs an extended period to function successfully after amputation. This remains to be more fully studied.

Another issue related to rehabilitation is that a delay in prosthetic fitting can often make prosthetic training at a later date very difficult. Deviations in gait may be increased with a lower frequency of physical therapy intervention early on in the rehabilitation process and may ultimately require longer therapy. Psychological readiness can also be adversely affected with delay in fitting. Some patients become so proficient in functioning with a wheelchair that they express concerns about fear of falling and the effort needed to learn to be proficient in ambulating with a prosthesis. In the past, numerous studies have related prosthetic success to intensive in-patient rehabilitation[8,17,30,53]; however, to date, there are few, if any, studies that compare different settings to level of successful outcomes. Regardless of the setting for early intervention, once the wound is healed, successful prosthetic use will certainly be enhanced by coordinated rehabilitation team efforts.

Finally, there is no doubt that in the initial phases of prosthetic use, more frequent prosthetic revisions and patient and family training are necessary to ensure safe use and especially prevent complications of skin breakdown. Systematic methods of examining the person with amputation and his/her prosthesis not only determine whether the goals of comfort, function, and cosmesis have been met, but also serve as a basis to correct problems.[38] In the home arena, the members of the team may simply need to communicate more frequently by telephone or other means to allow constant dialogue between physician, prosthetist, and therapists. Furthermore, each member of the team and those members of the patient's immediate family affected by the limb loss need to independently examine and evaluate the patient to better determine appropriate management so that the patient achieves an optimal functional level, which attends to his/her quality-of-life needs.[40]

Case Studies

Case Study 1

Ms. M is 67 years old and had a left transfemoral amputation on Nov. 13, 1997, secondary to vascular insufficiency. She presented with multiple medical issues and significant past medical history as follows: PVD, coronary artery disease (CAD), pancreatitis, diverticulitis, chronic obstructive pulmonary disease (COPD), cervical cancer, lung cancer, hypertension, history of seizures, and status post colostomy. Patient and family goals for rehabilitation were to receive a prosthesis and learn to walk. The discharge plan was for the patient to return to her daughter's home with 24-hour supervision. Her status at admission to rehabilitation in December 1997 included the following problems:

- Range of motion: Remarkable for hip extension contractures of −25 degrees left (residual side), −15 degrees right. Left upper extremity shoulder flexion 0 to 85 degrees, abduction 0 to 80 degrees.
- Motor performance: Grossly 3+/5 left lower extremity, 4−/5 right lower extremity.
- Integument integrity: Residuum with sutures removed, healing well.

- Bed mobility/transfers (without prosthesis): Minimum assistance for bed mobility, for squat-pivot transfer bed to/from wheelchair, and to stand from chair in parallel bars.
- Cognitive status: Fluctuating confusion, follows one-step commands, emotional lability. (Upon admission, medication changes resulted in resolution of pseudo-dementia, but decreased cognition for complex tasks persisted.)

Prosthetic Clinic Assessment

The patient was evaluated in the prosthetic clinic 4 weeks after her date of amputation. Even though the patient had multiple issues, she was progressing well with functional tasks and was very motivated to walk with good family support. The patient was measured for a left quadrilateral socket, with socket flexed to accommodate her contracture, with a single axis locked knee, and single axis cushion heel (SACH) foot.

Ms. M's in-patient rehabilitation physical therapy program before she received the prosthesis involved group as well as individualized treatment sessions. Group mat activities emphasized lower extremity stretching and strengthening exercises. Patients also worked on dynamic sitting balance activities with a balloon or ball toss and performed cardiovascular training on an arm ergometer, with vital signs monitored as appropriate. Individual prosthetic training began on parallel bars with emphasis on weight acceptance on the prosthesis, dynamic weight shifting, and limb progression to prepare for ambulation with a walker. Patient and family education for prosthetic management and mobility tasks, such as transfers and wheelchair management, were addressed by all members of the team consistently and repetitively due to the patient's initial difficulty remembering complex activities.

At the time of discharge from rehabilitation, 3 weeks after receiving the prosthesis, her status was as follows: supervision for transferring to/from bed and wheelchair; supervision and occasional minimum assistance for donning/doffing the prosthesis; wearing prosthesis for 6 hours per day; supervision for gait with a standard walker and prosthesis, 80 to 100 feet; and contact guarding for negotiating 5 to 10 steps with a railing. Family members were able to safely and independently assist the patient with donning and doffing the prosthesis, transfers, gait, and stair climbing.

Follow-up prosthetic clinic assessment was continued on an out-patient basis. The assessment 1 year after in-patient rehabilitation shows that the patient continues to ambulate in her daughter's home several times per day and is able to negotiate stairs to get outside the home. She required supervision only for safety, secondary to decline in cognition. Her family also supervises her in prosthetic donning/doffing.

Ms. M had multiple medical problems, with significant physical and cognitive limitations noted. In view of these problems, she also had multiple relative contraindications for prosthetic fit. The patient and family, however, were highly motivated and willing to work with the entire rehabilitation team to achieve this level of success. A transfemoral prosthesis that is simple in design, modified to accommodate the contracture in her hip, and aligned to maximize stability allowed her to function in her daughter's home with only minimal supervision. Early rehabilitation and coordinated efforts of the prosthetic clinic team can play a significant role in promoting a person's maximum functional potential.

Case Study 2

Mr. B is 62 years old and underwent a left transtibial amputation secondary to vascular insufficiency on April 10, 1997. He was referred to the out-patient prosthetic clinic July 1997 and presented with a well healed left residuum. Past medical history included bilateral femoral-popliteal bypass grafts in 1996 and history of angina, PVD, CAD, and type II diabetes. The patient's goal was to receive a prosthesis and begin walking as soon as possible. Before his amputation, he had recently retired as a carpenter and was extremely active in fishing, sailing, and hiking.

Prosthetic Clinic Assessment

Physical therapy examination for prosthetic determination noted the following problems:

- Range of motion: Remarkable for knee flexion contracture of −10 degrees residual side; +10 degrees left Thomas test.
- Motor performance: Grossly 5/5 throughout.
- Integument integrity: Residuum scar well healed, bulbous shape with mild edema noted distal end of residuum.
- Bed mobility/transfers (without prosthesis): Independent.
- Gait: Ambulates independently more than 2000 feet with axillary crutches in home and community; independently ascends/descends 24 steps with crutches and railing.
- Cognitive status: Intact.

Mr. B was examined in the prosthetic clinic 3 months after his date of amputation. Since he had recently retired, he was having difficulty with his insurance company and could not begin prosthetic fitting until his coverage plan was corrected. He was extremely frustrated with his company and was extremely anxious to walk. Even though the patient was progressing well with functional tasks and the surgical site was well healed, he had not been performing any methods for edema control, stretching exercises, or desensitization techniques for the residuum. Emphasis was placed on education for the use of a shrinker, hamstring stretching for his left leg, and massage techniques to assist with desensitization. A follow-up clinic visit was established for 2 weeks with a goal of making a cast for a left patella-tendon bearing prosthesis with a supracondylar suspension strap and a carbon copy II foot.

Mr. B was fitted with his prosthesis 3 weeks after the initial visit and was referred for out-patient physical therapy intervention. On the follow-up clinic visit, he reported doing hamstring stretching, but he was not performing the stretches at the recommended consistency and thus the contracture had only decreased by 5 degrees. The prosthesis was aligned to accommodate this knee position; the socket fit was acceptable with no areas of redness noted in pressure-sensitive areas on the residuum. He was educated in management of use of limb socks and proper skin inspection and was instructed to wear the prosthesis 1 hour twice a day while sitting, then increase wearing time 1 hour each day if no skin problems were observed. He was instructed not to ambulate with the prosthesis until he began physical therapy.

He reported to his first physical therapy session 2 days later and stated that he had worn his prosthesis 6 hours after the prosthetic clinic session and was trying to walk on it because he was really anxious to "get moving." The physical therapist noted on examination several blistered areas along the incision/scar line and grafted site and contacted other members of the clinic team. This area of skin breakdown necessitated that Mr. B stop wearing the prosthesis for 10 days. He was offered support regarding his progress thus far and was encouraged by the team to carefully attend to the recommended program.

The patient was seen again by the clinic team 10 days after the wounds had healed. The team decided to provide him with a gel sock to decrease friction over the distal end of the residuum and skin graft site and therefore increase his prosthetic wearing tolerance. He then began gait training with physical therapy. At this time, he carefully complied with his wearing schedule and continued to progress without further complications.

The evaluation 3 months after the initial clinic visit showed that the patient achieved independent community ambulation on all surfaces without an assistive device. Mr. B's case continues to be followed by the prosthetic clinic every 3 to 6 months, as needed, for monitor of fit, alignment, and wear. He returned to fishing, sailing, and hiking.

This patient had issues related to limited insurance coverage after amputation, resulting in a delay in prosthetic fit. In addition, his anxiety about "being behind" and wanting to "get moving" compromised his skin integrity and further delayed the process. A simple modification of using a gel liner, instead of a standard limb sock, reduced friction on the residuum and allowed him to progress more rapidly with wearing time and ambulating with the prosthesis. The coordinated efforts of the out-patient physical therapist and the prosthetic clinic team, who included support and encouragement to comply with the prescribed program, allowed him to maximize his functional potential as quickly as possible.

SUMMARY

Many factors influence the successful use of a prosthesis for the older person who has experienced a lower limb amputation. Careful examination of the person's psychosocial, socioeconomic, and physiological status assists the clinician and entire prosthetic clinical team in formulating a prognosis and designing appropriate interventions that lead to successful prosthetic functional outcomes. Improvements in surgical techniques for amputation and advancements in prosthetic design occur each year. Yet the effects that these scientific advances have on the quality of life and functional mobility of the older adult who uses a lower limb prosthesis remain to be studied fully. Physical therapists may encounter older adults who require prosthetic prescription and application more often in the home setting than ever before, given the present trends in health care service delivery. Advocacy and consultation with other members of the prosthetic team are essential to assist older adults to achieve their maximum functional potential using a prosthesis.

REFERENCES

1. Andrews KL: Rehabilitation in limb deficiency. 3. The geriatric amputee. *Arch Phys Med Rehabil* 1996; 77:s-14-17.
2. Appoldt F, Bennett L, Contini R: Stump socket pressures in lower extremity prostheses. *J Biomech* 1968; 1:247-257.
3. Beekman CE, Axtell LA: Prosthetic use in elderly patients with dysvascular above-knee and through-knee amputations. *Phys Ther* 1987; 67:1510-1516.
4. Bodily K, Burgess E: Contralateral limb and patient survival after leg amputations. *Am J Surg* 1983; 146:280-287.
5. Breakey JW: Body image: The lower-limb amputee. *J Prosthet Orthot* 1997; 9(2):58-65.
6. Brown PS: The geriatric amputee. *Phys Med Rehabil: State of the Art Rev* 1990; 4(1):67-76.
7. Carter DM, Balin AK: Dermatological aspects of aging. *Med Clin North Am* 1983; 67(2):531-543.
8. Cutson TM, Bongiorni DR: Rehabilitation of the older lower limb amputee: A brief review. *J Am Geriatr Soc* 1996; 44:1388-1393.
9. Drasch AL (ed): Diabetes care—American Diabetes Association: Clinical practice recommendations 1996. *J Appl Rsch Educ* 1996; 19(suppl):s67-s72.
10. Eaglstein WH: Wound healing and aging. *Clin Geriatr Med* 1989; 5:183-188.
11. Eberhart HD, Inman VT, Bresler B: The principle elements in human locomotion, in Klopsteg PE, Levison PD (eds): *Human Limbs and Their Substitutes.* New York, McGraw-Hill, 1954.
12. Edelstein JE: Preprosthetic management of amputation, in Kraft GH, Friedman LW (eds): *Physical Medicine and Rehabilitation Clinics of North America: Prosthetics.* Philadelphia, WB Saunders, 1991.
13. English E: The energy costs of walking for the lower extremity amputee, in Kostuik JP (ed): *Amputation Surgery and Rehabilitation.* New York, Churchill Livingstone, 1981.
14. Fisher SV, Gullickson G: Energy of ambulation in health and disability: A literature review. *Arch Phys Med Rehabil* 1978; 59:124-133.
15. Folstein MF, Folstein SE, McHugh PR: "Mini Mental State"—a practical method for grading the cognitive state of patients for the clinician. *J Psychiatr Res* 1975; 12:189-198.
16. Grise ML, Gauthier-Gagnon C, Martineau GG: Prosthetic profile of people with lower extremity amputation: Conception and design of a follow-up questionnaire. *Arch Phys Med Rehabil* 1993; 74:862-870.
17. Harris KA, et al: Rehabilitation of elderly patients with major amputations. *J Cardiovasc Surg* (Torino) 1991; 32:463-467.
18. Inman VT, Ralston HJ, Todd F: *Human Walking.* Baltimore, William & Wilkins, 1981.
19. Kald A, Carlsson R, Nilsson E: Major amputation in a defined population: Incidence, mortality and results of treatment. *Br J Surg* 1989; 76:308-310.
20. Kane RA, Kane RL: *Assessing the Elderly: A Practical Guide to Measurement.* Lexington, MA, Lexington Books, 1981.
21. Kay HW, Newman JD: Relative incidence of new amputations: Statistical comparison of 6000 new amputees. *Orthot Prosthet* 1975; 29:3-16.
22. Kerstein MD, et al: What influence does age have on rehabilitation of amputees? *Geriatrics* 1975; 12:67-71.
23. Kihn RB, Warren R, Bebe GW: The geriatric amputee. *Ann Surg* 1972; 176:305-314.
24. Krebs DE, Tashman S: Kinematic and kinetic comparison of the conventional and ISNY above-knee socket. *Clin Prosthet and Orthot* 1985; 9:3:28-36.
25. Lake C, Supan TJ: The incidence of dermatological problems in the silicone suspension sleeve user. *Prosthet Orthot Int* 1997; 9(3):97-104.
26. Leavitt LA, et al: Gait analysis and tissue-socket interface pressures in above-knee amputees. *South Med J* 1972; 65:1197-1207.
27. Leonard JA Jr: The elderly amputee, in Felsenthal G, Garrison SJ, Steinberg FU(eds): *Rehabilitation of the Aging and Elderly Patient.* Baltimore, William & Wilkins, 1994.
28. Levy LA: Smoking and peripheral vascular disease. *Clin Podiatr Med Surg* 1992; 9:165-171.
29. Lilja M, Oberg T: Proper time for definitive transtibial prosthetic fitting. *J Prosthet Orthot* 1997; 9(2):90-95.
30. Lims PA: Advances in prosthetics: A clinical perspective. *Physical Medicine and Rehabilitation: State of the Art Reviews* 1997; 11(1):13-38.
31. Loescher LJ: The dynamics of skin aging. *Progressions* 1995; 7(2):3-13.
32. Malone JM: Complications of lower extremity amputation, in Moore WS, Malone JM (eds): *Lower Extremity Amputations.* Philadelphia, WB Saunders, 1989.
33. Margolis S, Saudek CD: *Diabetes Mellitus: John Hopkins White Papers.* New York, Medletter Associates, 1997.
34. May BJ: *Amputations and Prosthetics: A Case Study Approach.* Philadelphia, FA Davis, 1996.
35. Medicare: Prosthetics and Orthotics Coverage and Payment Rules, in *Region C DMERC Supplier Manual: Durable Medical Equipment Prosthetics, Orthotics and Supplies.* Palmetto Government Benefits Administrators, 18:18.25-18.28, Summer 1997.
36. Moore TJ, et al: Prosthetic usage following major lower extremity amputation. *Clin Orthop* 1989; 1(236):219-223.
37. Moss SE, Klein R, Klein BE: The prevalence and incidence of lower extremity amputation in a diabetic population. *Arch Intern Med* 1992; 152:610-616.
38. Norman B, Fishman S (eds): *Lower Limb Prosthetics: 1998.* New York, Prosthetics-Orthotics Publications, 1998.
39. Perry J: *Gait Analysis: Normal and Pathological Function.* Thorofare, NJ, SLACK Incorporated, 1992.
40. Pike AC, Nattress LW: The changing role of the amputee in the rehabilitation process, in Kraft GH, Friedman LW (eds): *Physical Medicine and Rehabilitation Clinics of North America: Prosthetics.* Philadelphia, WB Saunders, 1991.
41. Pinzur MS, Graham G, Osterman H: Psychologic testing in amputation rehabilitation. *Clin Orthop* 1988; 29:236-240.
42. Radcliff CW: Functional considerations in the fitting of above-knee prosthesis. *J Prosthet Orthot* 1955; 2:35-60.
43. Redford JB: Rehabilitation team, in Banerjee SN (ed): *Rehabilitation Management of Amputees.* Baltimore, William & Wilkins, 1982.
44. Rudolphi D: Limb loss in the elderly peripheral vascular disease patient. *J Vasc Nurs* 1992; 10:8-13.
45. Sanders JE, Colin DH, Burgess EM: Interface shear stresses during ambulation with a below-knee prosthetic limb. *J Rehabil Res Dev* 1992; 29(4):1-8.
46. Scremin AME, et al: Effect of age on progression through temporary prostheses after below-knee amputation. *Am J Phys Med Rehabil* 1993; 72:350-354.
47. Skinner HB, Effeney DJ: Gait analysis in amputees—a special review. *Am J Phys Med* 1985;64(2):82-89.
48. Steinberg FU et al: Prosthetic rehabilitation of geriatric amputee patients: A follow-up study. *Arch Phys Med Rehabil* 1985; 66:742.

49. Stern PH: The epidemiology of amputations. *Phys Med Rehabil Clin North Am* 1991; 2:253-263.

50. Torburn L, Powers CM, Guiterrez R, Perry J: Energy expenditure during ambulation in dysvascular below-knee amputees: A comparison of five prosthetic feet. *J Rehabil Rsch Dev* 1995; 32(2):111-119.

51. U.S. Department of Health and Human Services: *Vital and Health Statistics: Detailed Diagnosis and Procedures for Patients Discharged from Short-Stay Hospitals. United States.* Series 13(118):130, 1992.

52. Waters R, et al: Energy cost of walking of amputees: Influence of level of amputation. *J Bone Joint Surg* 1976; 58A:42-45.

53. Weiss GN, et al: Outcomes of lower extremity amputations. *J Am Geriatr Soc* 1990; 38:877-883.

54. Yeager RA, et al: Surgical management of severe acute lower extremity ischemia. *J Vasc Surg* 1992; 15:385-392.

CHAPTER 22

Urinary Incontinence and Impairment of the Pelvic Floor in the Older Adult

Julie Pauls, PT, PhD, ICCE

INTRODUCTION

The stigma of urinary incontinence (UI), combined with professional lack of awareness regarding options for intervention, result in gross undertreatment of this disabling condition with serious consequences for the older individual. Unfortunately, symptoms tend to become progressively worse with age, especially in women reaching the postmenopausal years. Thomas identified that only 1 in 10 women will seek professional services for incontinence.[31] Furthermore, a survey by Lewis indicated that 75% of 827 women subjects with incontinence aged 40 to older than 70 had remained silent for 3 or more years before consulting help.[24] Ultimately, the severe restrictions on trips from home and concerns over the detection of odors prompted these women to seek medical assistance. Fortunately, several forms of treatment are effective in improving or curing UI, including common physical therapy interventions such as therapeutic exercise, weight training, biofeedback, and electrical

stimulation. Depending on individual circumstances, physical therapist management of the patient with incontinence is an important adjunct, or even an alternative, to pharmaceutical or surgical interventions.

DEFINITION OF URINARY INCONTINENCE

A straightforward definition of *incontinence* is the passing of urine in an undesirable place as this problem frustrates involved men or women who, unless severely depressed, have the inevitable desire to maintain continence.[36] A normal urination pattern in adults includes (1) maintenance of dry underclothes at all times; (2) urination volume of approximately 300 to 400 ml at each void; (3) urination frequency of approximately 4 to 6 times during the day and no more than once at night; and (4) urination without any discomfort, excessive effort, or false starts and stops.[10]

According to Laycock, several components are needed to maintain continence.[23] The continent individual must recognize the need to urinate, locate the proper place to urinate, reach that place to urinate in an efficient time period and retain the urine until the place is securely reached, and be able to urinate once arriving at the proper place. In older adults, particularly those who are disabled or hospitalized, incontinence may result more from the inability to reach the desired place than from any true urological impairment. Many facilities have beds or chairs that are hard get out of and toilets that are difficult to reach, which exacerbate this problem.

PREVALENCE

Undesirable leakage of urine ranks as one of the earliest medical complaints recorded in the Papyrus Ebers, dated 1550 BC;

the curative concoction was based on berries.[37] Current statistics demonstrate the continuation of this symptom through the ages, with incontinence currently afflicting an estimated 13 million men and women in the United States. Women experience incontinence twice as often as men, with 15% to 30% of women in all age groups affected.[9] Among middle-aged women, research indicates that 58% reported some urine loss, but only 25% sought treatment.[7] Among non-institutionalized women older than 60, it was found that 37.7% suffered from incontinence.[13] Low-end estimates of the prevalence of incontinence among nursing home residents start at 50% and at a cost of $3.3 billion each year (of the $7 billion spent on total direct costs incontinence). Lack of control over urination is one of the five main reasons for admission to a nursing home, along with immobility, cognitive impairment, falls, and the consequences of stroke.

ANATOMY AND PHYSIOLOGY

Pelvic Floor Anatomy

The pelvic floor is a group of tissues that covers the opening created at the base of the bony pelvis in much the same way that the diaphragm attaches between the ribs. Complex and often misunderstood, the role of pelvic floor in supporting pelvic organs was long underappreciated. This was partly due to study based on dissections of cadavers lying in a supine position.[27] The supine position of the cadaver, along with the embalming process, gave a false bowl-like appearance to the pelvic floor that is more accurately described as shelf-like. DeLancey's research divides this region into three main layers, going from inner layer to outer layer, known as the *endopelvic fascia,* the *levator ani muscles,* and the *external anal sphincter,* and a fourth layer relating to sexual function via the external genital muscles.[11]

The pelvic muscles play a key role in supporting the bladder. These muscles must not only be able to contract voluntarily (and rapidly at times) but also maintain a continuous resting tone. Primary pelvic organ support lies on the levator ani. When the levator ani contracts, it not only lifts the bladder neck but also helps resist force from any increase in intraabdominal or intraurethral pressure. Fascial attachments, such as pelvic and endopelvic fascia, assist in maintaining proper bladder support. From a muscular standpoint, continence maintenance is most affected by medial fibers of the levator ani.[22] These pelvic muscles include a combination of slow- and fast-twitch fibers; the former handle the postural response, whereas the latter act reflexively in response to a sneeze, cough, or other sudden stimulus. Thus, both fast- and slow-twitch muscles need to be considered during examination.

The levator ani can be subdivided into four regions whose anatomical names suggest their location: pubococcygeus, also known as the pubovisceral muscle; iliococcygeus; pubovaginalis; and both the puborectalis and puboanalis.[11,17] The specific anatomical relationship of the pubococcygeus to the pelvic organs is depicted in Fig. 22-1. Other muscles of the pelvic diaphragm include the obturator internis and the piriformis.

Physiology of Micturition

Micturition, or the process of urination, is controlled by phases of storage and emptying. During the storage phase the bladder, a muscular vesicle situated behind the symphysis

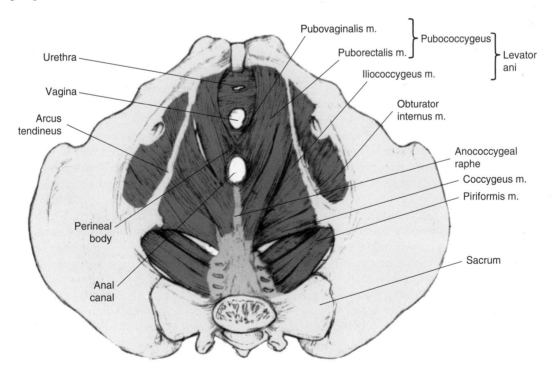

FIG. 22-1   The pelvic muscles. (From Mathers LH: *Clinical Anatomy Principles.* St. Louis, Mosby, 1996.)

pubis, slowly fills with fluid from the kidneys via the tube-shaped ureters. Promotion of storage is assisted by sympathetic relaxation of the bladder muscle (the detrusor) and by contraction or closure of both the pelvic muscles and the urethral sphincter.

Like a faucet valve, the urethral sphincter surrounds the urethral outlet and must exert enough pressure to withstand the effects of the bladder filling with urine. Thus the urethral sphincter has a reciprocal relationship with the bladder; it is contracting while the detrusor muscle of the bladder is relaxing. This mechanism maintains continence until the bladder is full, approximately 375 ml, and/or until ready for the emptying stage.

During the emptying phase the bladder detrusor parasympathetically contracts, pushing the urine out while the urethral sphincter and pelvic floor muscles relax to allow passage. After the bladder is empty, the pelvic floor returns to a contracted state and the urethral outlet is closed shut. As long as this outlet pressure is stronger (using the support of the pelvic muscles) than the pressure from the bladder, there is no unwanted urine leakage.

Causes of Urinary Incontinence

Subtypes

There are six subtypes of UI: urge, stress, mixed, overflow, function, and reflex. The pathophysiology of each subtype varies along with particular signs and symptoms (Table 22-1). Transient, or reversible, incontinence may be triggered by infection, such as a urinary tract infection, delirium, medications, or stool impaction.[26,33] Serious conditions that may present as incontinence include brain and spinal cord lesions, carcinoma of the bladder or prostate, bladder stones, and hydronephrosis.[5]

Incontinence and Aging

The older old (older than 75 years) are more likely as a group to suffer from incontinence, but this condition is not automatically linked with aging, and contrary to common belief, has nothing to do with dementia. Aging in general has an impact on UI partially because of obstruction of the bladder outlet (urethra) in older adults, which is probably due to diminished or absent urethral compliance or lack of detrusor contractility.[25] Szonyi and colleagues, for example, reported that a typical cause of urinary incontinence in elders is detrusor instability.[30] Older people may be more susceptible due to side effects of pharmaceuticals, lack of necessary social and or medical support, or an interaction of various pathologies that can lead to functional disability.[16]

As the urinary system ages, the kidneys have diminished urine concentration, which leads to increased volume of urine passing through the bladder. In conjunction with other effects of aging such as hypotrophic changes in collagen, elastic tissue, and smooth muscle of the bladder, this change in urine volume results in more frequent micturition. Decreased muscle tone in bladder, internal and external

sphincters, bladder outlet, and pelvic muscles also contributes to an elderly women's tendency toward UI, accentuated by diminished reaction time. Other age-related changes in women are reduced urethral closure pressure that is possibly due to lower estrogen levels, which leads to decreased submucosal blood supply and decreased muscle thickness around the urethra.

Bladder capacity remains the same over a lifetime unless affected by an acute illness, such as stroke, or a chronic illness, such as Parkinson's disease. Neurological disorders can trigger bladder instability primarily because they interfere with normal parasympathetic control of urination. The inability to completely empty the bladder leads to increase in residual urine volume that may promote urinary tract infections, which themselves can stimulate incontinence.[18]

In summary, age-related urinary changes include decreased maximal urethral closure; greater incidence of uninhibited contraction; increase in postvoiding residual; and altered patterns of excretion of fluid, with excretion of majority of urine at night (one to two episodes of nocturia are typical of the of the older adult).[5] It is clearly inaccurate to describe age-related changes as causes of UI, but they can further the likelihood that older adults will experience this problem. Fortunately, the problem is often transient and can be rectified promptly with the appropriate intervention.

Gender-Specific Causes of Urinary Incontinence in Women

Houston reports the most common type of incontinence for females is stress urinary incontinence (SUI) due to weak pelvic muscles or a urethral sphincter defect.[18]

In addition to the causes of stress incontinence listed in Table 22-1, other factors specific to women that result in UI are: childbirth; gynecological surgeries, such as hysterectomy; menopause; weakened pelvic support; anatomical hypermobility and tissue laxity, resulting in less urethral pressure due to a shorter urethral lumen; and organ prolapse, such as cystocele, rectocele, or prolapse of the uterus.[5,18,34] About 80% of women with one child have had some trauma during the birth process that resulted in at least partial denervation (although subsequently re-innervated).[1] Lack of pudendal innervation weakens pelvic muscle support so that the urethra cannot withstand any stress, such as straining. With time, muscle tone can get gradually weaker and weaker. Submucosal folds inside the urethra provide a very efficacious sealing effect that is most efficient when the folds are estrogenized.[14] There are two times when estrogen levels are lower: menopause and just before onset of menstruation. At these times lowered levels of estrogen diminish these previously effective folds with a resulting increase in the incidence of incontinence. Although diminished control of urination is often linked to a lack of estrogen, this has not been proven in any rigorous controlled study. Often, a good history will reveal that the incontinence started well before menopause. Interestingly, Benness and colleagues report that estrogen deficits after menopause were not an important factor in eti-

Table 22-1
Subtypes of UI

Subtype	Definition	Pathophysiology	Signs and Symptoms
Urge	Involuntary loss of urine associated with a strong sensation of urinary urgency	Involuntary detrusor (bladder) contraction, or detrusor instability (DI)	Loss of urine with an abrupt and strong desire to void; usually loss of urine on way to bathroom
		Detrusor hyperactivity with impaired bladder contractility (DHIC)	Elevated post-void residual (PVR) volume
		Involuntary sphincter relaxation	Involuntary loss of urine without symptoms
Stress	Urethral sphincter failure usually associated with increased intraabdominal pressure	Urethral hypermobility due to anatomical changes or defects, such as fascial detachments (hypermobility)	Small amount of urine loss during coughing, sneezing, laughing, or physical activity
		Intrinsic urethral sphincter deficiency (ISD), or failure of the sphincter at rest	Continuous leak at rest or with minimal exertion, including postural changes
Mixed	Combination of urge and stress UI	Same as for urge and stress UI	Combination of urge and stress UI signs and symptoms
			Typically one symptom more bothersome to individual than others; common in women, especially older women
Overflow	Bladder overdistention	Acontractile detrusor, hypotonic or underactive detrusor secondary to drugs, fecal impaction, diabetes, lower spinal cord injury, or disruption of the motor innervation of the detrusor muscle	Variety of signs and symptoms, including frequent or constant dribbling, urge or stress UI signs and symptoms, or urinary urgency and frequent urination
		Secondary obstruction due to prostatic hyperplasia, prostatic or urethral stricture in men	
		Obstruction due to severe genital prolapse, or surgical overcorrection of urethral detachment in women	
Functional	Consequence of chronic impairments of physical or cognitive function	Not pathophysiological in origin; secondary to functional limitations or impairments	Similar to UI
Unconscious or reflex	Neurological dysfunction	Decreased bladder compliance with risk of vesicourethral reflux and hydronephrosis	Postmicturitional or continual incontinence, severe urgency with bladder hypersensitivity (sensory urgency)
		Secondary to radiation cystitis, inflammatory bladder conditions, radical pelvic surgery, or myelomeningocele	
		No demonstrable DI in many non-neurogenic cases	

Adapted from Fantl JA, et al: Managing Acute and Chronic Urinary Incontinence. *Clinical Practice Guideline. Quick Reference Guide for Children, No. 2, 1996 update.* Rockville, Md, U.S. Department of Health and Human Services, Public Health Service, Agency for Health Care Policy and Research, AHCPR Pub. No. 96-0686, 1996.

ology of incontinence.[2] On the contrary, Benness found SUI more common in women receiving hormone replacement therapy (HRT) than women without HRT, implicating progesterone as a trigger that has a relaxing effect on urinary sphincter and increases frequency, urgency, and nocturia.

EXAMINATION, EVALUATION, AND DIAGNOSIS
Examination
Usually incontinence in older adults is multifactorial, necessitating thorough history, systems review, and tests and measures. A patient can self-identify the pattern of urinary symptoms in a log/diary form (Boxes 22-1 and 22-2). Bowel patterns can also be useful, especially to identify any chronic constipation that can lead to muscle denervation due to excessive stretching of the pudendal nerve with resultant demyelination.

Proper examination of the pelvic floor muscles lays the foundation for a plan of intervention.[23] Oftentimes, internal measures of pelvic muscle strength can be determined with special assessment tools, such as a pneumatic or electronic device, many with a digital readout. The position of the American Physical Therapy Association's Section on Women's Health on internal assessment states:

Internal examination of the pelvic floor muscles is consistent with physical therapy practice. It complies with national physical therapy policies requiring the performance of tests and measurements of neuromuscular function as an aid to the evaluation or treatment of specific medical conditions.[20]

There are several methods for measuring impaired pelvic muscle strength (Table 22-2). Although all are similar, one of the most commonly used is the modified Oxford scale, which uses a number to represent a certain grade of muscle power. The scale measures contractions from a low of 0 for no contraction (nil) to a high of 5 for a strong contraction. Intermediate scores of 1, 2, 3, and 4 correspond to muscle ratings of flicker, weak, moderate, and good. This scoring system can be adapted to measure muscle endurance by determining the duration and repetition of contractions and fast-twitch muscle activity by counting the number of quick contractions. Visual inspection of proper contracting and lifting activity of the pelvic floor also can be used to assess impairment.

Self-assessment can be performed by the stop test. A stop test simply tests the ability to stop the flow of urine. This test is best performed during the second void of the day to avoid any sense of urgency that may accompany the first void of the morning. It is recommended as an occasional-use test only. Performing this measure of urine control on a regular basis is contraindicated because it may trigger bladder instability or infection.

Urodynamic testing and other examination procedures to assess the extent of leakage in response to increased abdominal pressure, such as the pad test, may be performed by the therapist or other health care professionals. During a pad test the subject is asked to wear a pre-weighed pad and to drink 500 ml of fluid in a set period of time, such as 15 minutes. Next, the subject performs a variety of set functions for 30 minutes, including sit to stand, walking, jumping, reaching for an object on the floor, and running water over the hands. The pad is then re-weighed to collect data on urine loss during activity.

The extent of the examination process depends on the subject's age and contributing factors, such as presence of urinary tract infection, neurological deficit, diabetes, or respiratory disease. Prior treatment and surgeries; medications;

Box 22-1
INCONTINENCE PROFILE

The following questions are useful in the initial identification and examination of urinary incontinence:
- Can you tell me about the problems you are having with your bladder?
- Can you tell me about the trouble you are having holding your urine (water)?
- How often do you lose urine when you don't want to?
- When do you lose urine when you don't want to? What activities or situations are linked with leakage? Is it associated with laughing, coughing, or getting to the bathroom?
- How often do you wear a pad for protection?
- Do you use other protective devices to collect your urine?
- How long have you been having a problem with urine leakage?

Box 22-2
SAMPLE BLADDER RECORD

NAME: _____
DATE: _____

INSTRUCTIONS: Place a check in the appropriate column next to the time you urinated in the toilet or when an incontinence episode occurred. Note the reason for the incontinence, describe your liquid intake (e.g., coffee, water), and estimate the amount (e.g., 1 cup).

Time interval	Urinated in toilet	Had a small incontinence episode	Had a large incontinence episode	Reason for incontinence episode	Type/amount of liquid intake
6-8 AM					
8-10 AM					
10 AM-noon					
Noon-2 PM					
2-4 PM					
4-6 PM					
6-8 PM					
8-10 PM					
10 PM-midnight					
Overnight					

No. of pads used today: _____
No. of episodes: _____
Comments: _____

From Fantl JA, et al: Managing Acute and Chronic Urinary Incontinence. *Clinical Practice Guideline. Quick Reference Guide for Clinicians, No. 2, 1996 update.* Rockville, Md, U.S. Department of Health and Human Services, Public Health Service, Agency for Health Care Policy and Research, AHCPR Pub. No. 96-0686, March 1996.

such as diuretics or antidepressants; level of fitness; and support systems should also be considered.

Intervention

A common behavioral strategy of the individual with UI is to increase frequency of urination (micturition), but this urge to urinate can be consciously suppressed and the time interval between voids lengthened with training. Non-invasive approaches for functional training of the individual with UI include bladder training, habit (or timed) voiding, and prompted voiding (Table 22-3). Bladder retraining is often performed by a nurse or continence specialist.

Beginning with exercise, techniques are listed from least invasive to more invasive. Therapists are advised to consult appropriate manufacturer's guidelines before treatment. Establishing tissue integrity in the older patient is critical before physical agents are applied.

Therapeutic Exercise for Pelvic Muscle Rehabilitation

In a review of the literature on the effectiveness of pelvic muscle exercise (PME), Wells reported rates of incontinence improvement ranging from 31% to 96%.[35] Burns and colleagues used a sound research design on 123 community-dwelling older women.[8] PME (consisting of four sets of 20–10 quick and 10 sustained contractions–with increases of 10 per set during a 4-week period to reach a minimum daily repetition of 200) coupled with biofeedback were found to be effective in decreasing incontinence. The benefits of PME were maintained, and functional improvement continued for at least 6 months after the intervention.

Nygaard and colleagues found that 56% of persons who completed a course of PME had an improvement rate of more than 50%; this improvement continued when the subjects were assessed 6 months after the initial course of treatment.[28] These researchers strongly recommend initiating treatment with PME regardless of a patient's age, other health problems, surgical history, or location from treatment facility.

There is no hard and fast rule on the frequency, duration, and intensity of PME.[18] Using the same principles of muscle training for other areas of the body, muscle re-education of the pelvic floor should include overloading the muscle, training specific to each of the muscle groups capturing both the phasic and tonic capabilities of the muscle, and preventing decline by recognizing the need to continue an exercise maintenance program throughout the life span.

When instructing a patient on how to contract the pelvic muscles, the therapist should first have him/her assume a

---

Table 22-2
Comparison of Four Methods to Record Pelvic Muscle Strength

Numerical	Modified Oxford Grading Scale	Traditional	Descriptive
0	Nil	No initiation of movement	No contraction
1	Flicker	Rapid fatigue after initiation of movement	Just perceptible contraction
2	Weak	Not full range, not against gravity	Slight bulge in posterior wall as pelvic floor moves forward
3	Moderate	Full range in gravity-eliminated position	Feel some lift
4	Good	Full range against gravity	Feel firm lift
5	Strong	Full range against resistance	Strong squeezing in, with a strong lift

Adapted from Pauls J: *Therapeutic Approaches to Women's Health: A Program of Exercise and Education.* Gaithersburg, Md, Aspen Pub, 1995.

Table 22-3
Management Options: Functional Training Programs

Type of Intervention	Definition	Target Population
Scheduled toileting/habit training	Timed schedule voiding Habit training scheduled to catch patient's voiding habits Care-giver dependent	Cognitively impaired Functionally limited Incomplete bladder emptying Care-giver available
Prompted voiding	Scheduled voiding that requires prompting from care-giver Care-giver dependent	Functionally able to use toilet or toileting device Able to feel urge sensation Able to request toileting assistance Care-giver available
Bladder training	Systematic ability to delay voiding through the use of urge inhibition Active rehabilitation and education	Cognitively intact Able to discern urge sensation Able to understand or learn how to inhibit urge Able to toilet independently or with assistance

Adapted from Fantl JA, et al.: Managing Acute and Chronic Urinary Incontinence. *Clinical Practice Guideline. Quick Reference Guide for Clinicians, No. 2, 1996 update.* Rockville, Md, U.S. Department of Health and Human Services, Public Health Service, Agency for Health Care Policy and Research, AHCPR Pub. No. 96-0686, March 1996.

comfortable supine position with the legs well-supported and apart. The patient should be instructed to tighten or draw up the muscles around the openings of the vagina, urethra, and rectum as if he/she were trying to prevent the flow of urine. The therapist then encourages the patient to notice the muscle tension and hold the contraction as long as possible (striving for a goal of a 10-second contraction). The patient should then allow the muscle to relax or rest for twice as long as it contracted, i.e., if contraction is held for 3 seconds, the patient should rest for at least 6 seconds.

The therapist should then have the patient repeat the cycle of contraction and relaxation and increase his/her awareness of the muscle action. At this point the patient should be able to feel the pelvic muscles working. (Palpation or feedback with a mirror done privately can enhance understanding of the pelvic muscle action, especially if the patient is unable to feel any contraction.)

The baseline muscle performance should be measured by recording how long a contraction can be held and how many times it is repeated. After noting this baseline assessment of performance, the patient should be encouraged to increase the repetitions, duration, and frequency of the exercises. Addition of quick contractions and contractions performed in a variety of postures, such as sitting and standing, will enhance the functional training aspect of a treatment regimen. This exercise prescription is individualized to patient performance, but a plethora of predetermined regimens are offered in the literature.

Various recommendations range from a high of 300 to 400 repetitions per day[19] to as few as three to four maximal contractions performed three times a week.[4] Other protocols have been developed around other training schedules. One protocol uses three to four sets of 8 to 12 repetitions of high-resistance, slow-controlled contractions to be performed 3 times a week.[12] Another exercise prescription recommends 10-second contractions of the pelvic muscles followed by 10 seconds of relaxation 2 to 3 times a day for 20 minutes at each bout of exercise.[29] Other clinical approaches use intensive pelvic floor muscle contractions by initiating sustained contractions (6 to 8 seconds each) with another three or four quick contractions followed by a sustained contraction. Each sustained contraction is then followed by another set of quick contractions. Other exercise regimens can be performed in a group exercise setting using several positions with the legs abducted, in which 8 to 12 contractions are performed by the patient in each position followed by relaxation. This exercise prescription is recommended for use as a home program of 8 to 12 repetitions in a set performed 3 times per day.

Tries notes that patients with impaired mobility, neurogenic bladder, and/or severe stress incontinence often lose urine when moving from sitting to standing, such as during a toilet transfer.[32] To counteract this tendency, she recommends reinforcing pelvic floor contraction during such a change in position. This bracing action helps generalize the skill of recruiting the pelvic floor muscle in the supine position to actual function.

Usually, women do not notice improvement in incontinence for the first 6 to 8 weeks of an exercise program.[28] This may be too discouraging for some. Physical therapists should take care to note that 30% of women are unable to contract their pelvic floor muscles voluntarily.[22] Bump and colleagues warn that performing the exercise improperly can have an undesired effect by increasing intra-abdominal pressure.[6] Many women actually bear down by holding their breath and performing a Valsalva's maneuver or substitute for the appropriate muscle contractions by contracting muscles in the thighs or buttocks. Consequently, mere verbal or written instruction may be inadequate preparation to undertake a home program, which is sometimes known by some patients and health professionals as a *Kegel exercise program.* PMEs are often called Kegels, named for the obstetrician who performed the seminal research that postulated that pubococcygeus muscle activity provides critical support for the bladder.

Weight Training

Resistive exercise for the pelvic muscles can be performed using weighted vaginal cones. Cones are usually packaged in sets of five that gradually increase in weight, ranging from 20 to 70 grams. A woman inserts the heaviest cone that can be retained for at least 1 minute and then progresses to heavier cones and increased duration and difficulty of retention during activity as her strength improves. One treatment regimen recommends that the patient insert a cone twice a day and walk around for 15 minutes. If the cone slips, the patient should reinsert the cone. When the cone can be retained, the cone with the next highest weight can be used, or the patient can try to use the same cone with more challenging activities, such as jumping.[29] Some research suggests a 70% success rate in 30 women who were cured or whose conditions were significantly improved using cones. Kondo, however, reported a much lower success rate of 13% for 45 women.[21] Excess lubrication, such as that which occurs at ovulation, may affect cone retention. Other precautions indicate that cones should not be used during a patient's menstrual cycle. Furthermore, women with prior permanent neurological damage to the pelvic floor are poor candidates for resistive exercise that uses cones.

Biofeedback

Visual and auditory feedback can be provided using a perineometer (Fig. 22-2) or electronic biofeedback (BF) modalities (Figs. 22-3 and 22-4). The perineometer transmits pressure changes relating to pelvic muscle contractile forces. Electronic devices during examination can pick up a very sensitive range of signal from the musculature using external or internal electrodes. The success rate of visual and/or auditory feedback in muscle re-education resulting in diminished episodes of urine leakage has been estimated as ranging from 54% to 90%.[8]

Benson has proposed that four conditions contribute the successful use of this modality: an easily measurable and detectable response; an ability to detect change in that response; a cue to control need; and motivation of the patient to be actively involved in the treatment.[3]

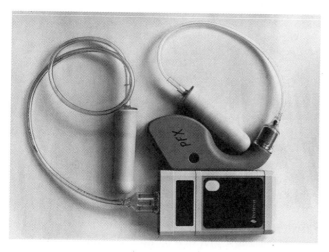

Fig. 22-2 One example of a perineometer, the Peritron precession perineometer, along with the PFX Pelvic Floor eXerciser. (Photo courtesy North American Distributors, Inc.)

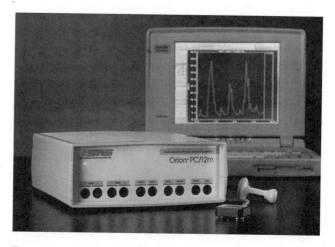

Fig. 22-3 The Orion PC office system from SRS Medical Systems, Inc., Redmond, Washington, shows a typical biofeedback display during pelvic floor contractions. Note multiple biofeedback modalities are possible with this unit, including monitoring temperature and respiration as well as multiple simultaneous muscle groups with electromyography. The "gold standard" PerryVaginal sensor is also shown. (Photo courtesy SRS Medical Systems, Inc.)

Tries concluded that not enough research has been undertaken to differentiate the effects of BF from exercise and other therapeutic interventions.[32] BF does not always require a therapist to have sophisticated electronic equipment. One of the simplest forms of visual BF can be instituted by handing the woman a mirror so that she can observe the desired lifting effect when the pelvic muscles contract appropriately.

Electrical Stimulation

Electrical stimulation uses faradic or interferential current delivered via internal and/or external electrodes to recruit muscles fibers, beginning with large-diameter fibers and eventually engaging the small-diameter fibers. Electrical stimulation can be used to achieve the following anticipated goals: enhance storage of urine by altering bladder sensation via afferent fiber stimulation, stimulate detrusor muscle activity to contract the bladder via efferent stimulation, improve circulation to the muscles and capillary network, and promote muscle hypertrophy.[3,33]

Treatment protocols vary, and intensity is determined according to patient tolerance. A stimulation frequency of 35 Hz provides muscle feedback and can elicit a cortical response. A frequency that is too high may unduly fatigue a muscle. Pulse width is generally set at 200 to 400 microseconds. An adequate rest period, usual at least equal to or longer than the stimulation phase, is mandatory.

Studies on the clinical effectiveness of electrical stimulation in treating incontinence have produced widely varying results. Pelvic floor stimulation was investigated by Sand to shore up the lack of research on this modality as standard treatment. Significant improvement was noted on several dimensions: leakage episode, urodynamic testing, and vaginal muscle strength. Furthermore, SUI improved at least 50%, and voiding diaries substantiated similar improvement. Electrical stimulation is contraindicated during menstruation or pregnancy and in patients with malignancy, metal implants, or a pacemaker.

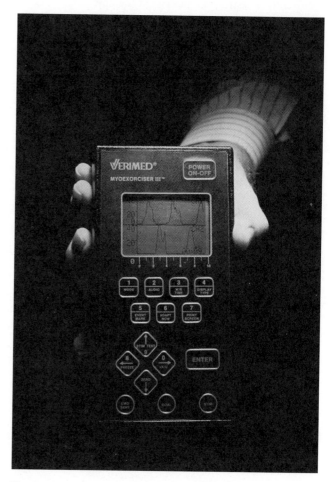

Fig. 22-4 The portable Myoexorciser III from Verimed International provides both auditory and graphical SEMG biofeedback for pelvic floor muscle re-education. (Photo courtesy Verimed International, Inc.)

Case Study

This case study describes the initial evaluation of a woman with the diagnosis of urinary stress incontinence.*

Examination
History
General Demographics: Ms. S is 67 years old. She is a retired teacher and YMCA volunteer and an occasional child-care provider for relatives.

History of Current Condition: She complains chiefly of urine leakage with coughing, laughing, or sneezing; the leakage has occurred for the last 5 years. Ms. S has previously used pads to deal with problem. She was referred by her urologist, Dr. PF, with a medical diagnosis of urinary stress incontinence.

Medications: Her current medication use includes Premarin.

Other Tests and Measures: Genuine urinary stress incontinence has been confirmed by urodynamic testing.

Past Medical/Surgical History
Endocrine: Ms. S had surgically induced menopause and is currently on estrogen replacement therapy.

Cardiopulmonary: She has a history of allergies.

Gastrointestinal: She notes frequent constipation.

Urogenital: A grade 1 uterine prolapse has been noted.

Pregnancy and Delivery: Gravida, 2—para, 2 at age 22 and age 25 with vaginal deliveries.

Gynecological Surgery: She underwent a hysterectomy at age 37. There is no other surgical history.

Health Status: Incontinence survey revealed the following:

Attitude: She scored 4 on a scale of 1 to 4, indicating a major problem.

Number of wet episodes: Ms. S reports eight wet episodes per day (wets underwear and outer clothes, but urine does not progress past clothes)

Number of pads per day: 7
Number of drinks per day: 3

Tests and Measures
Anthropometric Characteristics: Her height is 5'4 feet; and she weighs 144 lbs

Muscle performance:

Stop test: Grade 1

Pelvic muscle grading: Muscle grade of 2, with hold time of 3 seconds.

Number of repetitions of sustained contractions: 3
Number of repetitions of fast contractions: 4
Perineometer reading: 0 (Introitus too lax to contract around diameter of perineometer.)

Pain: None

Posture: Normal; kyphosis absent

Self-Care and Home Management
Urolog frequency/volume chart
Frequency: Day 10, night 2
Maximum volume voided: 200 ml
Minimum volume voided: 50 ml

Sensory Integrity: Perineal sensation intact.

Evaluation and Diagnosis
Ms. S has substantial functional limitations due to stress UI. Her major problem underlying functional limitation is impaired pelvic muscle performance.

Prognosis
During the course of 4 to 6 months, she will demonstrate a reduction in the episodes of urine leakage and increase in pelvic muscle strength.

Expected Range of Number of Visits Per Episode of Care: 12 to 18 visits during this episode of care.

Factors That May Modify the Episode of Care: Obstetrical history, motivation, increased pelvic muscle stress due to sneezing related to allergies, and chronicity of constipation may all influence the duration of the intervention; strong family support is noted.

Intervention
Ms. S. will be started on a home program designed by her physical therapist that consists of patient-related instruction in therapeutic exercise and electrotherapeutic modalities.

Patient-Related Instruction
Anticipated Goals of Patient-Related Instruction
- Ability to perform physical task without increased urine leakage
- Improved awareness of incontinence resources
- Behaviors that foster healthy bladder habits
- Reduction in disability associated with chronic incontinence
- Increased patient knowledge of personal and environmental factors associated with incontinence
- Improved physical function and health status
- Enhanced progress through patient participation
- Decreased risk of recurrence of the condition
- Reduced risk of secondary impairments
- Improved self-management of symptoms
- Decreased use and costs of health care services

Specific Interventions for Patient-Related Instruction
- Show video on bladder health from Family Life Media
- Instruct patient in pelvic muscle exercise using computer-assisted program
- Provide printout with customized written and pictorial instruction
- Have patient begin program by performing 5 repetitions of contractions with a 3-second hold, 5 times a day
- Use pelvic model to explain location of pelvic muscles and relationship to bladder function

*Adapted from Pattern C: Impaired Muscle Performance. Guide to Physical Therapist Practice. *Phys Ther* 1997; 77(11):1252-1257.

Electrotherapeutic Modalities

Due to a muscle grade of less than 3, Ms. S will be started on daily electrical muscle stimulation at 15 Hz for 15 minutes and then progress as indicated on bi-weekly phone reports.

Anticipated Goals of Electrotherapeutic Modalities

- Improved ability to perform physical tasks related to self-care
- Reduced complications
- Improved motor function and sense of well-being
- Increased muscle performance (strength, power, and endurance)
- Decreased risk of secondary impairments
- Reduced stress
- Increased tolerance to positions and activities

Re-Examination

Ms. S will be re-examined in the clinic after 6 and 12 weeks of home treatment, unless otherwise indicated through bi-weekly phone assessments. The patient is expected to demonstrate increased muscle performance as a clinical indicator of remediation of the impairment.

Outcomes

The following are expected outcomes of care:

- Patient has measurable decrease in quantity of accidental voidings
- Patient wears fewer pads
- Patient voids fewer times each day

Criteria for Discharge

The patient has satisfactory reduction in urine leakage, achieves normal pelvic muscle strength function, and has surpassed goals.

Summary

Incontinence has a severely negative impact on the lives of many older Americans. Sufferers fall prey to rashes, ulceration, infection, urosepsis, and falls leading to fracture. This problem can also lead to depression and sometimes stifling isolation from negative psychosocial effects. Fortunately, significant relief and, often, cure can be found through physical therapy treatment.

In summary, the treatment option of PMEs is strongly recommended for women with stress urinary incontinence (SUI).[15] PMEs are recommended in men and women in conjunction with bladder training for urge incontinence. PMEs may also benefit men who develop UI after prostatectomy. Pelvic muscle rehabilitation and bladder inhibition using biofeedback therapy are strongly recommended for patients with stress UI, urge UI, and mixed UI. Vaginal weight training for SUI in premenopausal women is supported by scientific evidence. Pelvic floor electrical stimulation has been shown to decrease incontinence in women with SUI and may be useful for urge and mixed incontinence. Table 22-4 offers a summary of treatment options.

Table 22-4

Management Options: Pelvic Muscle Rehabilitation

Type of Intervention	Definition	Target Population
Pelvic muscle exercises	Planned, active exercises of pelvic muscles to increase periurethral muscle strength Active rehabilitation and educational interventions	Able to identify and contract pelvic muscles Adherence to instructions
Vaginal weight training	Active retention of increasing vaginal weights to increase pelvic muscle strength Active rehabilitation and educational interventions	Cognitively intact Adherence to instructions Able to stand Sufficient pelvic floor strength to contract muscle and retain lightest weight Relative contraindication: pelvic organ prolapse
Biofeedback	Use of electronic monitoring instruments to display information about neuromuscular or bladder activity, particularly with pelvic muscle exercises Active rehabilitation and education interventions Can be used in association with other programs	Able to understand analog or digital signals using auditory or visual displays Motivated to learn voluntary control through biofeedback technique Health care provider who can appropriately assess the UI problem and provide behavioral interventions
Electrical stimulation	Application of electrical current to sacral and pudendal afferent fibers via intra-anal or intravaginal electrodes to inhibit bladder instability and improve contractility and efficiency of striated sphincter and levator ani Able to discern stimulation Active rehabilitation and educational interventions Can be used as adjunct therapy in identification of pelvic muscles	Relative contraindication: vaginal soreness, constipation, hematoma with needle stimulation

Adapted from Fantl JA, et al: Managing Acute and Chronic Urinary Incontinence. *Clinical Practice Guideline. Quick Reference Guide for Clinicians, No. 2, 1996 update.* Rockville, Md, U.S. Department of Health and Human Services, Public Health Service, Agency for Health Care Policy and Research, AHCPR Pub. No. 96-0686, 1996.

REFERENCES

1. Allen R, Hosker GL, Smith ARB, Warrell DW: Pelvic floor damage and childbirth: A neurophysiological study. *Br J Obstet Gynaecol* 97:770-779, 1990.
2. Benness C, et al: Do progestogens exacerbate urinary incontinence in women on HRT? *Neurourol Urodyn* 1991; 10(4):316-331.
3. Benson JT: *Female Pelvic Floor Disorders.* New York, Norton Medical Books, 1992.
4. Bo K: Isolated muscle exercises, in Schussler B, Laycock J, Norton P, Stanton S (eds): *Pelvic Floor Re-Education: Principles and Practice.* London, Springer-Verlag, 1994.
5. Bregg KJ, Nitti VW, Raz S: Female incontinence, in Steg A (ed): *Urinary Incontinence.* New York, Churchill Livingstone, 1992.
6. Bump RC, Hurt WG, Fantl JA, Wyman JF: Assessment of Kegel pelvic muscle exercise performance after brief verbal instruction. *Am J Obstet Gynecol* 1991; 165:322-329.
7. Burgio K, Matthews KA, Engel BT: Prevalence, incidence and correlates of urinary incontinence in healthy, middle-aged women. *J Urol* 1991; 146:1255.
8. Burns P, et al: A comparison of effectiveness of biofeedback and pelvic muscle exercise treatment of stress incontinence in older community-dwelling women. *J Gerontol: Med Sci* 1993; 48:M167-M174.
9. Cardozo LD, Cutner A: Is disturbed bladder function after pregnancy normal? *Matern Child Health* 1993; June:180-183.
10. Chiarelli PA: *Women's Waterworks: Curing Incontinence.* Australia, Gore & Osmet, 1992.
11. DeLancey J: Functional anatomy of the pelvic floor and urinary continence mechanism, in Schussler B, Laycock J, Norton P, Stanton S (eds): *Pelvic Floor Re-Education: Principles and Practice,* London, Springer-Verlag, 1994.
12. DiNubile: Strength training. *Clin Sports Med* 1991; 10(1)33-62.
13. Diokno AC, Brock BM, Brown MB, Hersog AR: Prevalence of urinary incontinence and other urological symptoms in the noninstitutionalized elderly. *J Urol* 1986; 136:1022.
14. Dolman M: Mostly female, in Getliffe K, Dolman M (eds): *Promoting Continence: A Clinical and Research Resource.* London, Bailliere Tindall, 1997.
15. Fantl JA, et al: Managing Acute and Chronic Urinary Incontinence. *Clinical Practice Guideline. Quick Reference Guide for Clinicians, No. 2, 1996 update.* Rockville, Md, U.S. Department of Health and Human Services, Public Health Service, Agency for Health Care Policy and Research, AHCPR Pub. No. 96-0686, 1996.
16. Green MF: Old people and disorders of incontinence, in Mandelstam D (ed): *Incontinence and Its Management,* ed 2. Dover, NH, Croom Helm, 1986.
17. Herman H, Wallace K: Female urogenital and musculoskeletal anatomy, in Wilder E, ed: *The Gynecological Manual.* Alexandria, Va, American Physical Therapy Association, 1996.
18. Houston K: Incontinence and older women. In Care of the Older Woman. *Clin Geriatr Med* 1993; 1:157-171.
19. Kegel AH: Physiologic therapy for urinary incontinence. *JAMA* 1951; 146:915-917.
20. Kennedy E: Minutes of Executive Committee Meeting OB/GYN Section. *J OB/GYN PT* 1993; 17:2, 19-20.
21. Kondo A: Prospective analysis of the vaginal cone treatment for stress incontinence, in Smith ARB (ed): *Urogynaecology: The Investigation and Management of Urinary Incontinence in Women.* London, RCOG Press, 1995.
22. Laycock J: Conservative management of stress and urge incontinence, in Smith ARB (ed): *Urogynaecology: The Investigation and Management of Urinary Incontinence in Women.* London, RCOG Press, 1995.
23. Laycock JO: *International Incontinence Conference Seminar, Section on Obstetrics and Gynecology of the APTA.* Boston, August 28-29, 1992.
24. Lewis D: Incontinence survey report. London, England, 1993, cited in White H: Incontinence in perspective; in Getliffe K, Dolman M (eds): *Promoting Continence: A Clinical and Research Resource,* London, Bailliere Tindall, 1997.
25. McGuire EJ, DeLancey JO: Postmenopausal women, in Buchsbaum HJ, Schmidt JD (eds): *Gynecologic and Obstetric Urology,* ed 3. Philadelphia, WB Saunders, 1993.
26. National Institute on Aging: Urinary incontinence—A vocabulary. *Clin Bull* 1, 1992.
27. Norton P: Summary and paramount anatomy and physiology of the pelvic floor, in Schussler B, Laycock J, Norton P, Stanton S (eds): *Pelvic Floor Re-Education: Principles and Practice.* London, Springer-Verlag, 1994.
28. Nygaard I, et al: Efficacy of pelvic floor muscle exercises in women with stress, urge, and mixed urinary incontinence. Part 1. *Am J Obstet Gynecol* 1996; 174(1):120-125.
29. Pauls J: *Therapeutic Approaches to Women's Health.* Gaithersburg, Md, Aspen, 1995.
30. Szonyi G, Collas D, Ding Y, Malone-Lee J: Oxybutynin with bladder retraining for detrusor instability in elderly people: A randomized controlled trial. *Age Ageing* 1995; 24(4):287-291.
31. Thomas T, et al: The prevalence of fecal and double incontinence. *Comm Med* 1984; 6:216-220.
32. Tries J, Eisman E: The use of biofeedback in the treatment of urinary incontinence. *Phys Ther Practice* 1993; 2(2):49-56.
33. U.S. Department of Health and Human Services, Agency for Health Care Policy and Research: Urinary Incontinence in Adults, *Clinical Practice Guidelines.* Pub No. 96-0686. Rockville, Md, Department of Health and Human Services, 1992.
34. Wallace K: Female pelvic floor functions, dysfunctions, and behavioral approaches to treatment. *Clin Sports Med* 1994; 13:459-481.
35. Wells TJ: Pelvic (floor) muscle exercises. *J Am Geriatr Soc* 1990; 38:333-337.
36. Willington FL (ed): *Incontinence in the Elderly.* New York, Academic Press, 1976.
37. White H: Incontinence in perspective, in Getliffe K, Dolman M (eds): *Promoting Continence: A Clinical and Research Resource.* London, Bailliere Tindall, 1997.

CHAPTER 23

CONSERVATIVE PAIN MANAGEMENT FOR THE OLDER PATIENT

JOHN O. BARR, PT, PHD

INTRODUCTION

Interest in the management of pain experienced by older individuals has grown dramatically,* as most recently demonstrated through the publication of clinical practice guidelines for management of chronic pain in older persons by the American Geriatrics Society (AGS).[5] Although pain has been recognized to be the most common symptom for which health care is sought by the general population in the United States,[19,157] this observation may be even more applicable to the elderly. The validity of this premise, however, is based on a number of factors, including predisposing physical and mental conditions and on the elderly individual's willingness to report pain and to seek health care. This chapter is concerned with conservative management of pain experienced by the older patient. Noninvasive, nonsurgical, and nonpharmacological approaches to patient care are emphasized.

INCIDENCE OF PAIN

It has been established that over 85% of older adults have at least one chronic disease that may result in a range of discomforts, including pain.[26] Arthritis, which has a high rate of occurrence across older age-groups, is likely the most common cause of pain.[34,139] Other physical conditions that commonly result in chronic pain for the elderly include cancer, osteoporosis with compression fracture, degenerative disk disease, diabetic neuropathy, post-herpetic and trigeminal neuralgias, and residual neurological deficits.[66,89,135,164] Acute postoperative pain is becoming a major concern as an increasing number of elderly individuals are undergoing surgery.[164] Pain associated with athletic injuries will become more common as a growing number of older persons pursue active recreational interests.[16]

Instances of atypical presentation of clinical pain have contributed to a controversy about the general occurrence of pain in the elderly. Acute myocardial infarction often occurs without significant pain in elderly persons. Appendicitis, gangrene of the bowel, peptic ulcer disease, and pneumonia may produce only mild discomfort. However, these conditions can contribute to observable behavioral changes, e.g., confusion, and nonspecific symptoms, e.g., fatigue. Although headaches are less common in the elderly, their presence may be associated with serious medical problems such as temporal arteritis or stroke.[26] Signs of inflammation, including redness, pain, elevated temperature, and swelling, may be much less marked in older individuals.[42] Information from major medical centers in the United States has suggested that only 7% to 10% of pain clinic patients are older than 65,[63] although this proportion was recently reported to approximate 20% at one Canadian center clinic.[56] It is important to recognize that data obtained through pain clinics may be skewed by age limits, by large numbers of younger patients, or by individuals with complex social and psychological problems.[56,169]

---

*References 20,24,45,47,48,56,69,89,162,174

The actual occurrence of pain in the elderly has been demonstrated using a number of approaches. Perhaps most relevant are surveys and interviews of elderly persons at different levels of functional independence. Nearly 70% of the 205 healthy elderly surveyed by Roy and Thomas reported some type of pain problem.[139] However, no significant differences were seen in social and physical/recreational activities when compared with respondents without pain. Lavsky-Shulan and associates interviewed 3097 elderly living in rural settings and found 22% to have had low back pain in the prior year, with 15% to 42% experiencing some type of functional limitation.[92] Most recently, a Louis Harris and Associates telephone survey of 500 individuals who regularly took pain medications determined that 64% of respondents older than 60 experienced chronic pain that prevented performance of routine tasks and hobbies.[34]

In contrast, a survey by Roy and Thomas of 132 elderly nursing home residents and day-program participants revealed 83% to have pain-related problems and 74% to claim that pain interfered with daily activities.[138] Although 50% of these individuals noted moderate to high levels of pain, analgesics were the only type of treatment reported. Surprisingly, 16% of respondents were not treated for their pain. Weekly interviews were used by Brody and Kleban to document physical and mental health symptoms for 120 elderly people having at least one chronic condition and a range of cognitive capabilities, i.e., normal mental function, functional mental disturbance, and senile dementia.[22] Pain was reported at least once by 73% of all participants, although it was noted by significantly more subjects diagnosed with functional mental disturbance than by those with normal mental function (83% vs. 63%). Most frequently reported, pain accounted for 38% of symptoms overall, and it was the greatest cause of activity disturbances. Parmalee, however, determined that compared with cognitively intact elders significantly fewer cognitively impaired elderly nursing home and congregate apartment residents reported one or more chronic pain complaints and had significantly fewer localized pain complaints and lower pain intensity ratings.[128] These findings were tentatively attributed to a reporting bias whereby cognitive impairment was associated with a decreased propensity to report pain. The potential effect of dementia on the pain experience has recently been reviewed by Farrell and associates.[43]

From these few studies, it can be appreciated that pain is experienced with significant frequency by elderly persons. A trend also begins to emerge that implies that older individuals who have less functional independence are more incapacitated by pain-related problems. These relationships require clarification through further epidemiological research. Caution should be used in interpreting studies on the prevalence of pain in relation to age. For example, it has been suggested that the lower incidence of pain with age for community-dwelling adults may be based on the increased institutionalization of older individuals having chronic pain.[56] Ferrell and Ferrell have noted that, overall, population-based studies suggest that the prevalence of pain increases with age, although *reports* of pain tend to decrease slightly among the oldest.[48] Additionally, Harkins has provided evidence that acute nociceptive sensations from deep body structures are reduced with age but that the frequency of chronic pain from the same structures increases with age, e.g., an acute myocardial infarction is less painful, but angina of effort increases.[63]

EVALUATION OF CLINICAL PAIN

Concern for the proper evaluation of pain experienced by older individuals has become more apparent in the professional literature.[5,56,63,66,69,70] Indeed, AGS practice guidelines recommend that at initial presentation to any health care service, an older person should be assessed for evidence of chronic pain.[5] It is critical that pain be accurately evaluated. Evaluation represents a synthesis of information derived from the patient's history, subjective interview, objective physical examination, and special tests, e.g., blood chemistry, roentgenograms, computerized tomographs, and electrodiagnostic studies. Other references should be consulted for information concerning comprehensive patient evaluation, including physical, psychological/psychiatric, and special testing procedures related to pain.[157] The evaluation should clarify the underlying basis for the pain and guide proper therapeutic interventions. Appropriate referrals should be made for specialized services, e.g., psychiatric, addiction management, and multidisciplinary pain management.[5] The evaluation also provides baseline information needed to determine the effectiveness of treatment. Ongoing re-evaluation of pain is necessary to disclose a change in the patient's physical status and to document response to treatment. The frequency of follow-up re-evaluation is related to the severity of the clinical problem and to the potential for adverse effects from treatment.[5]

Pain has been defined as an unpleasant sensory and emotional experience associated with actual or potential tissue damage or described in terms of such damage.[111] More simply, pain has been defined as a hurt that we feel.[149] Unfortunately, the assessment of pain is confounded by its private and subjective character.[29] The way in which an individual reports pain is related to a number of factors including age, gender, personality, ethnic/cultural heritage, behavioral needs, and past pain experiences.[106,149] Elderly persons often believe that pain is an inevitable consequence of aging that must be endured without complaint. The presence of pain may be denied out of fear of medical procedures and expenses, loss of autonomy, and possible institutionalization. Conversely, pain complaints may be used to conceal or rationalize other functional impairments. Boredom and loneliness may contribute to increased perception and complaints of pain.[69]

The patient's history should include information about concurrent medical problems and present medications, including prescription, over-the-counter, and natural/home remedies. Utilization of pain medications may be evaluated, with the type, amount, route, and frequency being documented. A standard "morphine equivalent" dose can be calculated, thus providing a basis for comparison among a range of pain medications.[126] Elderly persons have been found to consume nearly 25% of all prescription medications used in the United States.[88] Analgesic drugs are the most common treatment for pain in older adults.[5] One study found that analgesics were the third most frequent prescription drug and the most frequent nonprescription drug used by a community sample of nearly 3500 persons aged 65 and older.[65] Interestingly, another study demonstrated that older postsurgical patients had less analgesic medication both prescribed and administered.[41] Although these latter findings may have been related to concern by physicians and nurses for the physical status of older surgery patients with more concurrent illnesses, adequacy of pain management must be questioned. Dramatic pain relief may be attained by pharmacological means in the elderly, e.g., the use of high doses of steroids for the treatment of temporal arteritis. However, the hazards of medication use by the elderly are well-known. These include multiple drug use, drug interactions, adverse drug reactions, medication errors, and the narrowing of the margin of safety between therapeutic and toxic doses.[88,89,117,163] Proper pharmacological management of acute postoperative[129] and chronic[5] pain has recently been described. One goal of conservative treatment for the elderly is the appropriate reduction of medication usage.

Information concerning past remedies or treatments that have been both successful and unsuccessful in managing pain should also be included in the history. Through such inquiry, it may be possible to learn about patient biases for or against certain interventions and also to gain further insight as to why a prior treatment was a success or a failure. Previous inadequate patient education may have contributed to a lack of enthusiasm for, and compliance with, a prior pain management program.

During the subjective interview, the patient should be given the opportunity to voluntarily verbalize complaints of pain and related symptoms, e.g., aching, burning, discomfort, joint warmth, paresthesia, and stiffness. The examiner should follow up with specific questions concerning the onset, occurrence, intensity (current vs. greatest vs. least), quality, distribution, and duration of pain. Pain at multiple sites, such as arthritic joints, may require that specific assessment tools be referenced to the worst or to multiple joints. Pain at rest should be distinguished from pain with movement.[17] A body diagram may be coded by the patient to document the quality and distribution of pain.[106] Factors that the patient believes to aggravate and relieve the pain should be identified, e.g., movements, postures, and rest.

The initial examination should include a comprehensive physical examination that places particular emphasis on the neuromuscular and musculoskeletal systems.[5] The objective examination typically focuses on physical signs or characteristics thought to be associated with a given pain problem.

Sternbach has observed that patients with acute pain often present with increases in pulse rate, systolic blood pressure, and respiratory rate. Dilation of the pupils, perspiration, nausea, and pallor of the skin also may be present.[149] Others have cautioned that such physiological correlates of pain are general responses to stress that are not unique to pain and that these responses habituate with time.[110] Behavioral indicators of pain such as facial expression, crying, and mood changes may be especially useful for documenting pain in patients with severely limited verbal abilities. Numerous physical criteria have been evaluated in relation to clinical pain problems, including duration of joint-loading time,[104] edema,[127] gait,[39] grip strength,[120] joint range of motion,[127] joint tenderness,[17] muscle strength and endurance,[144] posture,[175] pressure threshold and tolerance,[52] pulmonary functions,[137] skin temperature,[130] tissue compliance,[52] and tissue healing.[51]

Patients in pain typically have reduced activity levels, so it is important to assess physical function, including activities of daily living (ADL) and physical performance.[5] Portable automated timer systems have been used to measure functional aspects of patient movement such as "uptime"[140] and activity patterns,[54] but these systems have not been validated with older individuals experiencing pain.[59] It is important to note that lack of sensitivity to, or limited correlation with, pain has been noted for some physical criteria,[17] including some criteria that are more functional in character.[25,75] Some measures of functional activity, e.g., the Barthel Index and the Katz Index of ADL, do not include the range of activities in which community-dwelling elderly individuals are typically engaged. Gibson and colleagues have suggested that the Human Activity Profile and the Sickness Impact Profile are more useful for this sub-population since both also assess social activities.[59] Weiner and associates determined that observational analysis of relevant simulated ADL performance was sensitive and valid in assessing pain behavior in older persons with chronic low back pain.[165]

In the attempt to more objectively document patients' subjective pain experiences, a number of pain assessment tools have been developed.[108,110] A select sample of these tools that have particular relevance to the elderly will now be discussed.

Perhaps the simplest unidimensional tool for the measurement of pain intensity is the Verbal Rating Scale[125] (also called the Verbal Descriptor Scale[68]). With this approach, patients are required to label their pain with a single word descriptor, e.g., no, mild, moderate, severe, or unbearable pain. Such adjectival scales may be preferred by patients who find them easy to understand, which may be associated with low scoring failure rates.[87] The major limitation of this approach is its lack of sensitivity in detecting changes based on a limited number of word categories.[75]

Using the Pain Estimate[152] (also called the Numeric Rating Scale[110]), patients rate the severity of their pain on a scale of 0 to 10, or 0 to 100. On this scale, 0 indicates no pain, and end points of 10 or 100 represent the worst possible pain that the patient could ever imagine.[152] It is critically important that the patient understand the definitions related to these end points. If, for example, the patient thought that a rating of 100 corresponded to "the worst pain I've ever had," then pain that was even more severe the next day could not be properly rated. Primary advantages of this approach are that it is easy to understand and that patient ratings can be done verbally. The 0 to 10 format has less sensitivity than its 0 to 100 counterpart.

The Visual Analogue Pain Rating Scale consists of a 10-cm line with typical verbal anchors of "no pain" at the left and "pain as bad as it could be" at the right when the scale is oriented horizontally (Fig. 23-1, *A*).[141] Patients place a vertical mark at one location on the line that corresponds to the severity of their pain. This scale also may be used in a vertical orientation (Fig. 23-1, *B*). A new unmarked scale is presented to the patient each time pain is to be rated, although there has been controversy about showing the patient prior ratings.[17] It has been suggested that the scale should more appropriately be constructed to rate pain relief by using anchors of "complete pain relief" and "no pain relief" (Fig. 23-1, *C*).[73,74] Such an approach relies on memory of the earlier pain and may introduce a bias toward expected pain relief.[110] Visual analogue scales have also been constructed to evaluate limitations in physical function that may be related to pain.[75] Unfortunately, visual analogue scales

rely on vision and motor control, which may be compromised in the elderly patient. Although some studies have suggested that elderly individuals may have difficulty with abstract thought processes needed to understand and use visual analogue scales,[27,77,87] other studies with elderly patients have found these scales to be useful and reliable.[18,68] Vertical presentation of the scale in the format of a "pain thermometer" may be more effective with some elderly patients.[69]

The Graphic Rating Scale (Fig. 23-1, *D*) consists of a visual analogue pain rating scale with additional word descriptors, e.g., mild, moderate, and severe. Placement of these words without spacing along the line between anchors helps to improve the distribution of patient responses when using this type of scale.[141]

The McGill Pain Questionnaire is probably the best known of the multidimensional tools for measuring pain.[56,107] The questionnaire includes a body diagram for information concerning the location of pain. Sensory, affective, and evaluative qualities of the pain experience are assessed via a pain rating index based on word descriptors. Pain intensity is measured with a five-category present pain intensity scale. A short-form version of the questionnaire has been developed, reducing the amount of time needed to administer this tool to 2 to 5 minutes.[109] The short form may be less fatiguing for elderly patients who have problems with maintaining concentration. Difficulty may still be encountered with complex word descriptors.[69] This difficulty may be more related to educational level, verbal intelligence, and cognitive impairment than to age.[56]

For the general population, the visual analogue scale and the McGill Pain Questionnaire are probably the most commonly used self-rating pain measurement tools.[110] A number of studies have compared methods of rating pain,[38,77,125,164] including some that have specifically examined elderly individuals with pain.[18,66,68,87] Helme and colleagues have suggested that appropriately screened patients older than 70 may actually be more reliable than younger individuals in reporting pain, mood, and activity using psychometric tools.[66] Herr and Mobily determined that older adults in the community with leg pain preferred and found the verbal descriptor scale easier to use in comparison with the visual analogue scale (in horizontal or vertical presentations), the numeric rating scale, and a pain thermometer tool.[68] With the exception of the McGill Pain Questionnaire, the pain rating scales described in the preceding text have been criticized for focusing primarily on the intensity of pain while excluding other qualitative characteristics. Gagliese and Melzack have advocated that comprehensive evaluation of pain should include both unidimensional measures, e.g., VAS, and multidimensional measures, e.g., McGill Pain Questionnaire, because each samples an important part of the overall pain experience.[56] There has been controversy concerning appropriate mathematical and statistical analyses to be used with these scales.[29,110,164,166] Most recently, Herr and colleagues have provided preliminary support for the use of the Faces Pain Scale with cognitively intact elderly individuals.[70]

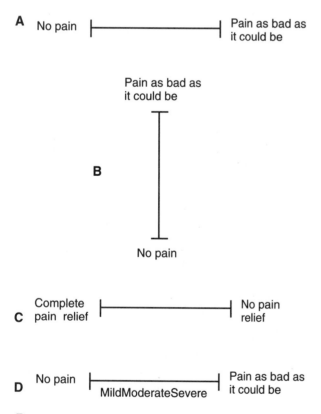

FIG. 23-1   Simple pain rating scales. **A,** Visual Analogue Pain Rating Scale (horizontal). **B,** Visual Analogue Pain Rating Scale (vertical). **C,** Visual Analogue Pain Relief Rating Scale. **D,** Graphic Rating Scale.

This scale consists of seven cartoon facial depictions arranged in order from least to most distressed.

Herr and Mobily have reviewed the complexities of clinical pain assessment with elderly persons and offered numerous practical suggestions.[69] A person's health status, severity of pain, and ability to cooperate will dictate the number and detail of evaluation sessions needed to adequately assess pain. It is critically important to establish good rapport and to avoid being rushed during examination sessions. Suspected impairments in vision, hearing, speech, and mental processes should be evaluated. Nursing home residents may have less formal education than elderly in the community. Pain measurement tools should be selected or modified to account for these factors, which might limit the validity and reliability of testing procedures. The clinician must be assured that the patient understands and can successfully use a pain measurement tool, with supervision if necessary, especially if the tool is to be used in the home setting.[17] A pain log or diary should be used by patients and care-givers to regularly document pain intensity, medications, response to treatment, and associated activities.[5] Family members, friends, and other health care workers can provide useful information about changes in behavior or functioning.[69] Observational assessment of pain, with inferences drawn from facial expression, body language, and other nonverbal behaviors, can be used to identify pain affecting severely demented older persons.[128] No one pain measurement tool will meet the needs of all elderly individuals. The patient's physical and cognitive abilities[55,69] and tool preferences[68] must be kept in mind during the selection of pain measurement tools. Certain diagnoses associated with aging, e.g., dementias, including Alzheimer's disease, will require the development, validation, and reliability testing of new measurement tools.

In rendering an evaluation of pain, the health care professional usually labels or further classifies pain experienced by the patient. Pain of less than 3 months' duration have been termed *acute,* whereas pain persisting for 3 or more months is referred to as *chronic.*[111] Acute pain occurs as a result of mechanical trauma, ischemia, or active inflammation. It is often associated with increased autonomic nervous system activity and anxiety. Chronic pain is not merely a time extension of acute pain. Indeed, chronic pain may lack a demonstrable physical basis. It is often associated with nonfunctional pain behaviors, e.g., attention-getting pain displays such as grimaces, guarded motion, or knee buckling, and depression in the general population.[147,151,163] The interdependence of chronic pain and depression has generally been noted to be even greater in the elderly.[163] Because of the higher occurrence of pain, chronic stress and depression has been thought to be more likely in the elderly.[63] However, Middaugh and associates did not find depression to be more prevalent in older as compared with younger patients with chronic pain.[113] Most recently, Wright and colleagues determined that in persons with rheumatoid arthritis, younger individuals were more likely to report depressive symptoms and to have higher levels of daily stress and higher levels of pain.[173]

Additional varieties of pain differ based on a number of characteristics including time frame, severity, quality, distribution, and likely basis. Acute recurrent pain is experienced when there is recurrent nociceptive stimulation associated with chronic pathology, as in rheumatoid arthritis and osteoarthritis. Acute ongoing pain occurs with continued nociceptive stimulation from uncontrolled malignancy.[163] Subacute pain is often noted at 72 or more hours after trauma or inflammation. It may persist for 2 to 3 weeks.[98] It has been suggested that elderly patients have the tendency for pain to be referred from a site of origin to other regions of the body.[26] As discussion of other types of pain, e.g., radiating, myofascial, thalamic, and phantom, is beyond the scope of this chapter, the reader should consult other sources.[105,106,111,158,162]

THEORETICAL BASIS FOR PAIN

It has been widely proposed that pain is not simply a direct consequence of the normal aging process.[59,63,90,168] This position has been supported by ambiguous results from psychophysical studies that have induced pain by various means, e.g., heat, electrical shocks, and mechanical pressure, while assessing behavioral responses, e.g., pain threshold, reaction, or tolerance, in human volunteers of different ages. On the balance, earlier studies of pain did not indicate age-specific changes in pain sensation.[64] More recent studies, however, have begun to lend support to age-related changes contributing to pain in the elderly.[35,63]

Mechanisms for modulating pain portrayed in Fig. 23-2 are thought to be operational within the dorsal horn of the spinal cord.[57,91,161,163,176] Nociceptors attached to small-diameter afferents are activated by intense mechanical or thermal stimuli and by various chemical sensitizing or depolarizing agents liberated with trauma or inflammation, e.g., bradykinin, prostaglandin, histamine, substance P, lactic acid, and potassium ions. Some of these agents may become concentrated in the vicinity of nociceptors due to circulatory impairment or to muscle spasm. Nociceptive excitation of small-diameter afferents (myelinated A delta and unmyelinated C fibers) results in the release of neurotransmitters that stimulate second-order neurons, ultimately resulting in the perception of pain at higher brain centers. Sensory input from large-diameter afferents (myelinated A beta fibers) associated with mechanoreceptors has an inhibitory effect on input from the smaller afferents conveying nociceptive input. Inhibitory descending control from higher centers and the brainstem also can act to minimize the effects of nociceptive input. This descending inhibition is mediated by neurotransmitters such as norepinephrine (NE; noradrenaline) and serotonin (5-HT).

Anatomical studies have demonstrated that nociceptors, i.e., free nerve endings, in the skin undergo little structural change with age.[28] Age-related decreases in responsiveness of nociceptors and small unmyelinated fibers to noxious chemical stimulation have been described.[59] Based on slowed re-

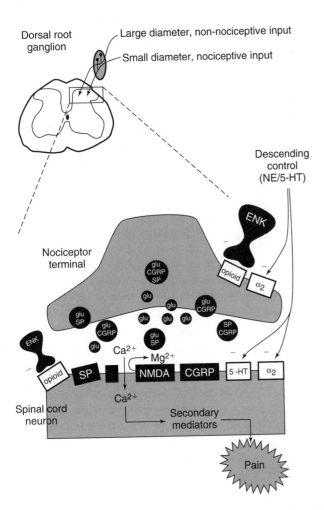

FIG. 23-2 Diagram of a primary afferent nociceptor (e.g., C fiber) terminal in the spinal cord dorsal horn (see *boxed area,* upper left), illustrating the storage and release of neurotransmitters from the nociceptor terminal in the spinal cord and presynaptic and postsynaptic receptors. Nociceptor neurotransmitters substance P (SP), calcitonin gene-related peptide (CGRP), and glutamate (glu) are stored in vesicles and released when the nociceptor is depolarized by a peripheral noxious stimulus. Note that these peptide and non-peptide neurotransmitters are typically co-contained in and co-released from presynaptic vesicles. The postsynaptic receptors at which SP, CGRP, and glutamate act are identified as *filled and labeled boxes.* The glutamate receptor is named the N-methyl-D-aspartate (NMDA) receptor and is an ion channel that permits entry of calcium into the postsynaptic spinal cord neuron. Calcium activates a variety of secondary mediators that can ultimately result in the perception of pain, a supraspinal event. The activity of nociceptors and of spinal cord neurons can be inhibited by a variety of means, including actions of descending noradrenergic (NE) and serotonergic (5-HT) systems acting presynaptically and/or postsynaptically at α_2 adrenoceptor and 5-HT receptors, respectively. Also illustrated are opioid receptors at which endogenous opioids such as enkephalin (ENK) released from small interneurons or exogenously administered opioids such as morphine can act to inhibit the nociceptive signal. (Courtesy GF Gebhart, Department of Pharmacology, College of Medicine, University of Iowa.)

sponse times to noxious thermal stimulation, an age-related decrease in conduction of small myelinated fibers consistent with selective peripheral neuropathy has been suggested.[63] Aging is indeed associated with increased incidence of certain chronic neuropathic pain problems, e.g., post-herpetic neuralgia and trigeminal neuralgia. Based on changes seen in animal preparations, Devor speculated that these conditions could be based on age-related loss of dorsal root ganglion cells, increased ectopic impulse discharge, and increased cross-excitation of adjacent dorsal root neurons.[35] Additional research is needed concerning possible changes in A delta and C afferent fibers associated with nociceptors.

Studies have shown age-related decreases in sensation of touch and vibration[160] that would otherwise oppose nociception. Age-associated decreases in the number of mechanoreceptors such as Merkel's disks, Meissner's corpuscles, and pacinian corpuscles have been demonstrated. Structural changes have also been noted in these receptors and in their related large-diameter afferents.[28,160] However, the confounding role of inactivity has not been ruled out as a basis for these changes.[28]

Oxidative deactivation of amines involved in descending inhibitory control is done by the enzyme monoamine oxidase (MAO). Interestingly, human hindbrain, plasma, and platelet MAO activity is increased after about age 60.[136] The resultant age-related increase in the deactivation of key neurotransmitters might increase pain perception and affective disorders such as depression or mania.[64,136] Endogenous opiate-like transmitters play a role in initiating one type of descending inhibition (via endorphins) and in local inhibition at the spinal cord level (via enkephalins). Decreases in concentrations of endorphins and enkephalins and a reduction of endogenous opiate receptors have been noted in old age.[42,163] Keefe and associates have recently noted that older adults who have impaired cognitive functions may lose the benefits of descending pain modulation systems.[81]

Thus, there are a number of anatomical and physiological changes associated with aging that on the balance may actually predispose elderly individuals to both a greater incidence of clinical pain and to less effective pain relief with various conservative treatment interventions.

STRATEGIES FOR PAIN CONTROL

Pain management may be either the short- or long-term goal of a comprehensive treatment plan. Whenever possible, conditions underlying a clinical pain problem should be the focus of treatment. Those who care for elderly patients with pain have come to appreciate the importance of a comprehensive multidisciplinary approach to evaluation and treatment.* A multidisciplinary approach is specifically indicated in cases in which the underlying cause of pain is not remediated or only partially treatable.[5] Such an approach may integrate the involvement of numerous health care professions including medicine, nursing, occupational therapy, orthotics and prosthetics, physical therapy, psychology, recreational therapy, social work, and others. Gibson and colleagues have summarized and critiqued studies involving the multidisciplinary management of chronic nonmalignant pain in older adults.[58] A frequently cited study by Middaugh and associates determined that patients 55 and older benefited as much, if not more than, younger patients participating in a multidisciplinary chronic pain rehabilitation program.[113] A multidisciplinary approach is also valuable in identifying and initiating management of comorbidity that occurs with older individuals who experience chronic pain, e.g., patients with cardiovascular, gastrointestinal, and psychiatric problems.[67]

It has been noted that the selection of pain management strategies by health care professionals varies with the age of the patient.[24] Burke and Jerret surveyed student nurses for their perceptions of the best interventions for acute pain.[24] Breathing and relaxation, imagery, and distraction techniques were selected less frequently for elderly persons as compared with younger adults. However, touch or massage, physical comfort approaches, verbal reassurance, and medication were more commonly selected for the elderly than for younger adults. Although these results were not analyzed statistically, different patterns of strategy selection were associated with patient age. Barta Kvitek and colleagues determined that physical therapists who were given hypothetical patients were significantly less aggressive in goal setting for older patients.[14]

A wide array of conservative treatment approaches for pain control have been developed over the years. By way of an overview, Box 23-1 (p. 358) summarizes select conservative interventions used in pain management for the general population. Traditionally, these interventions have been used singly or in various combinations in the attempt to more completely treat factors underlying a clinical pain problem. The value of combined use of conservative interventions for the management of chronic pain in the elderly is gaining recognition.[3,5] Primary theoretical mechanisms of action are suggested relative to the mechanisms for modulating pain depicted in Fig. 23-2. The reader is encouraged to consult other sources for detailed descriptions of specific treatment procedures.[4,5,85,105,112,122,147,155,162]

General Safety Precautions and Contraindications

Even conservative treatment of elderly patients requires following a number of general safety precautions and being alert for contraindications to treatment. In general, the patient should have adequate sensation of temperature and pain in the area being treated in order to provide feedback to the clinician. A body region must also be sentient if peripheral sensory input is critical to a particular mechanism for pain relief. For example, sensation of light touch should be present where electrodes are applied for conventional low-intensity transcutaneous electrical nerve stimulation (TENS). Potential for increased bleeding, hemorrhage, disruption of fragile tissues, fracture, spread of infection, cardiovascular or neurological compromise, and enhanced growth or metastasis of cancer represent general contraindications for treatment. Special considerations are necessary to

ensure safety of the elderly patient when using specific conservative treatment interventions, as is discussed in the following paragraphs.

Establishing Treatment Effectiveness

Recent clinical guidelines have suggested that many nonpharmacological interventions provide only short-term pain relief, with few studies showing greater benefit than placebo controls in randomized trials for long-term management of chronic pain.[5] As discussed previously, age-associated changes may render the elderly person less responsive to treatment. It is important to appreciate that a patient's response to treatment will be based on a number of factors, including the natural history of the underlying clinical problem, a placebo effect, and a specific treatment effect. Fig. 23-3 illustrates these factors and emphasizes that in order for a treatment to be deemed "effective" its impact must be greater than that attributable to natural history and the placebo effect.[49] The periodic worsening and improvement

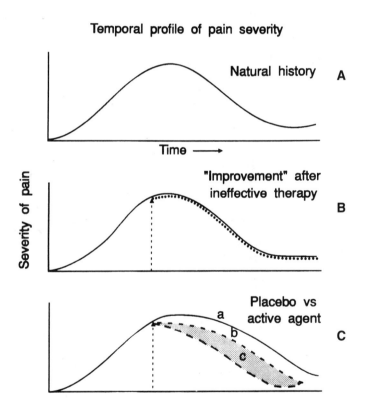

FIG. 23-3 Determination of treatment effectiveness. **A,** The natural history for the severity of pain associated with a clinical problem. **B,** "Improvement" after an effective therapy is begun at the time indicated by the *arrow.* If it is not appreciated that a remission is expected to occur, the remission will be attributed to the therapy. **C,** The natural history of pain severity *(a)* is compared with results from placebo therapy *(b)* and somatically active therapy *(c).* The analgesia attributable to active therapy (i.e., treatment effectiveness) is represented by the difference between *b* and *c.* The placebo component of the therapy is the difference between *a* and *b.* (Adapted from Fields HL, Levine JD: Placebo analgesia—A role for endorphins?, in *Trends in Neuroscience,* 1984; 7:271-273.)

BOX 23-1

PRIMARY THEORETICAL MECHANISMS OF ACTION FOR CONSERVATIVE TREATMENT INTERVENTIONS USED TO MANAGE PAIN

I. Decrease activity of nociceptors or their afferent nerve fibers.
  A. Limit mechanical stresses through:
    1. Prevention of acute edema formation with ice, compression, elevation, or electrical stimulation
    2. Assistive gait device (e.g., cane, walker, and orthotics)
    3. Rest from stressful function
    4. Limitation of the effects of gravity via hydrotherapy
    5. Immobilization (e.g., orthotics, traction)
    6. Resorption of chronic edema via mild heat, massage, elevation and compression, or electrical stimulation
    7. Elongation of restrictive connective tissue using vigorous heat (as with diathermy or ultrasound) and prolonged stretch
    8. Restoration of normal joint arthrokinematics through joint mobilization, stretching or strengthening exercise, or biofeedback
    9. Application of ergonomic principles
  B. Limit effects of chemical depolarizing and sensitizing agents through:
    1. Enhanced local circulation produced with mild to moderate heat, massage, exercise, or electrical stimulation
    2. Decreased local metabolic activity with cryotherapy (e.g., cold pack or ice massage)
    3. Decreased muscle spasm via select physical agents, massage, exercise, or biofeedback
  C. Create local anesthetic or anti-inflammatory effects through:
    1. Iontophoresis (e.g., with Lidocaine or Dexamethasone)
    2. Phonophoresis (e.g., with hydrocortisone)
    3. Cryotherapy (e.g., cold pack or ice massage)
    4. TENS
    5. Low-intensity laser
II. Increase activity of mechanoreceptors or their afferent nerve fibers.
  A. Stimulate mechanoreceptors through:
    1. Passive and active joint range-of-motion exercise
    2. Joint mobilization
    3. Comfortable massage strokes (i.e., mild to moderate intensity)
    4. Voluntary (e.g., walking, swimming, bicycling) and electrically stimulated exercise
  B. Directly stimulate large-diameter afferents from mechanoreceptors through:
    1. Comfortable low- to moderate-intensity TENS (e.g., "conventional," "pulse-burst," or "modulated" TENS modes)
    2. Comfortable submaximal intensity NMES
III. Increase descending control via cortical or reticular formation inhibition.
  A. Reduce patient anxiety through:
    1. Progressive relaxation exercises
    2. Inducing relaxation with biofeedback (e.g., EMG or thermal modes)
    3. Patient education concerning basis for pain and the plan for its successful treatment
  B. Maximize a placebo effect.
  C. Increase physiological and psychological stress through use of uncomfortable "counterirritants" such as:
    1. Intense massage (e.g., strong friction, acupressure, connective tissue massage)
    2. Acupuncture or electroacupuncture
    3. Uncomfortable but maximally tolerated NMES
    4. Uncomfortable but maximally tolerated TENS (e.g., "strong low rate," "brief intense," "pulse-burst," or "hyperstimulation" modes)
    5. Uncomfortable brief ice massage

TENS = transcutaneous electrical nerve stimulation; NMES = neuromuscular electrical stimulation; EMG = electromyography.

---

of symptoms that reflect the natural history of some disease processes, such as rheumatoid arthritis, often present a confusing picture to the clinician attempting to assess the impact of a therapeutic intervention. Did the patient's status improve because of effective treatment or in spite of ineffective treatment?

It has been determined that 30% to 70% of patients will obtain satisfactory pain relief from a placebo treatment.[15,37,49] Classically, placebo effects have been assessed in experimental research by randomly assigning patients to either active drug or sham drug, i.e., sugar pill placebo, groups under double-blind conditions. This methodology requires that neither the patient nor the clinician knows which treatment

has been given. In some investigations it is impossible to disguise treatments so that the patient or clinician is unaware of which treatment is active or placebo. For this reason, non-crossover designs, in which a subject receives only one experimental treatment intervention, have been favored.[91] In any event, the person performing patient assessments should not be aware of the treatment given.[62]

A placebo can be effective for anyone under the right conditions. It has been suggested, however, that older persons respond more frequently to placebos.[26] The placebo effect is not simply based on a reduction in a person's anxiety. Larger placebo effects have been associated with patients having high anxiety, severe pain, or expectation of a good treatment outcome. The attitude of the health professional, communicated by personal enthusiasm or skepticism about a treatment, can also influence the magnitude of a placebo response.[15,49] It is important to recognize that investigators may inadvertently provide a suggestion of treatment effectiveness for a control or placebo treatment that is psychologically stronger than that given with an active treatment intervention. Such an influence might have occurred in the study by Deyo and colleagues that reported TENS to be ineffective for chronic pain in the general population.[36] The use of neutral or permissive instructions to all research subjects regardless of group assignment should help to minimize this problem.[8] In clinical practice, however, the health professional may choose to take advantage of the placebo effect as a means of maximizing pain relief. Controversy exists as to the effective duration of a given placebo effect.[37] Sternbach has suggested that placebos do not work for longer than 1 to 2 weeks.[150] The physiological basis for the placebo effect involves both endorphin and nonendorphin mechanisms.[90]

Unless involved in research to establish the true effectiveness of a treatment intervention, practitioners will not give placebo treatments to their patients. Under clinical conditions, however, it is certainly desirable to establish the efficacy of a treatment in decreasing pain, improving limited function, and saving health care dollars. Valid and reliable testing procedures, including those discussed for the assessment of clinical pain, must be used at regular intervals during the course of patient treatment and follow-up examinations in order to establish the efficacy of an intervention.

Review of Select Treatment Interventions

Review articles concerned with pain management for elderly individuals have most commonly recommended the conservative treatment interventions of assistive devices and orthotics; exercise; thermal agents, i.e., heat or cold; and TENS.* More recently, the true importance of psychoeducational interventions has been recognized.[3,41,81] In the following review of select treatment interventions for pain management, it is valuable for the reader to consult Box 23-1 regarding theoretical mechanisms of action. Well-controlled studies done with individuals aged 55 years and older are highlighted. It is important to recognize, however, that many studies have used small experimental group samples. This has greatly contributed to the inability to statistically discern a difference between experimental treatment groups.[133,167]

Assistive Devices and Orthotics

Assistive devices and orthotics are used to control pain by limiting mechanical stresses to nociceptors in affected structures. Ambulatory aids such as canes and walkers are probably the most common assistive devices used by the elderly with pain. Foot, knee, and leg pain were the most frequent

complaints reported by 457 individuals older than 50 surveyed by Finsen.[50] A two-point cane gait (cane in hand opposite to involved hip) can reduce pain-inducing hip contact force by 36%.[21] Care must be taken, however, not to improperly overload the joints of the upper extremity when using these devices. Pressure on hip and knee joints during push-off may also be controlled through the use of raised seats on toilets and chairs. Appropriate shoe orthoses, including inserts and heel lifts, can be used to minimize pain of the foot, knee, hip, and back.[72,101,124]

Varying degrees of immobilization can be attained for neck and back pain with spinal orthoses. The limited temporary immobilization from a soft cervical collar may be appropriate for a patient with mild cervical spondylosis, whereas a patient with rheumatoid arthritis and atlantoaxial subluxation would benefit from a more rigid Philadelphia collar[119] or a sternal-occipitomandibular immobilizer (SOMI).[112] A thoracic lumbosacral orthosis (TLSO) may be used to manage compression fractures associated with spinal osteoporosis.[142] In older women, kyphosis is related to spinal osteoporosis, and it commonly causes chronic upper and middle back pain.[40] Spinal flexion can be controlled with a Jewett hyperextension orthosis or a cruciform anterior spinal hyperextension (CASH) orthosis.[124] Finsen has suggested that serious morbidity from back pain associated with osteoporotic fractures does not begin to occur until 80 years of age.[50] Pain from spinal stenosis can be addressed with orthoses that limit extension, such as the Williams flexion orthosis.[124]

Exercise

Exercise involves the performance of physical exertion for improvement of health. Various forms of exercise may be used to modulate pain either directly or indirectly, as depicted in Box 23-1. A direct effect on pain may be achieved in some cases by increasing comfortable mechanoreceptor input to the central nervous system via active or passive exercise. Indirect effects of exercise on pain may be related to increased blood flow, which disperses chemical depolarizing/sensitizing agents; decreased edema; inhibition or fatigue of muscle spasm; enhanced range of motion, flexibility, strength, or endurance, which may improve biomechanical factors; and relaxation and reduction in anxiety. The importance of combining exercise with other therapeutic interventions, e.g., thermal agents and patient education, to attain significant clinical outcomes, including pain relief, is well-recognized.[3,61,85,93]

Although it has been known for some time that elderly persons are capable of significant strength gains from voluntary resistive exercise,[118] published literature dealing with the effectiveness of exercise in controlling pain experienced by elderly persons is surprisingly sparse. Unfortunately, even fairly recent studies have been poorly controlled, have not been appropriately blinded, and have used small numbers of subjects that have limited the power of statistical analyses.[53,133] The following studies are examples of some of the

---

*References 5,45,47,59,89,119,124,131-133,163,172

better research that supports the use of exercise in pain management for older adults.

Minor and associates assessed the relative efficacy of three exercise protocols for patients with chronic rheumatoid arthritis or osteoarthritis.[116] The mean age of the 120 subjects who entered the study was 59 years. After baseline testing, subjects were stratified by diagnosis and randomly assigned to one of three groups: aerobic walking, aerobic aquatics, and nonaerobic active range of motion (ROM) and relaxation exercise control. Additionally, subjects in all groups participated in exercises for flexibility and isometric strengthening. All exercise groups were supervised and met for 1 hour, 3 times per week, for 12 weeks. At the conclusion of the 12-week period, all subjects were consistently encouraged to continue exercise, including participation in community programs (aquatics, walking, and fitness). It was not noted whether the assessors were blinded to subjects' group assignments. At the end of the 12-week period, the aerobics groups showed significant improvements over the nonaerobic group relative to aerobic capacity, 50-feet walking time, physical activity, anxiety, and depression. No significant between-group (aerobics vs. nonaerobic) difference was seen for pain. However, both the walking and nonaerobic groups demonstrated significant within-group improvements in pain. Three months later only aerobic capacity significantly differed between the groups. The nonaerobic group no longer had a significant improvement in pain. At the 9-month follow-up, no significant between-group differences were seen. Numerous significant within-group differences existed, including decreases in pain for the aquatic and nonaerobic groups. Significant changes in the intensity of medication regimens could not be disclosed at 12 weeks or 9 months. This study demonstrates that supervised exercise can successfully motivate elderly individuals to improve fitness and control pain without significantly exacerbating arthritic symptoms.

Kovar and colleagues completed a study of supervised fitness walking with 92 patients (mean age of 69 years) having osteoarthritis of the knee.[86] After initial assessment, outpatients participated in an 8-week program based on randomized assignment to one of two groups: a fitness-walking and patient education group or a control group receiving standard medical care. Walking/education sessions were conducted by a physical therapist 3 times per week for 90 minutes. Supervised indoor fitness walking using supportive athletic or walking shoes on a tile floor was done for up to 30 minutes. Patient education consisted of guest speakers and group discussions; instruction in proper walking techniques; light stretching and strengthening exercises; and supportive encouragement. In addition, self-efficacy and behavioral psychology concepts were used to ensure adherence with the walking regimen. Patients in the control group were only contacted each week by telephone to discuss their activities of daily living. All patients were assessed before and after the intervention period using a 6-minute test of walking and select subscales of the Arthritis Impact Measurement Scale (AIMS). The assessor was not blinded to

subject group assignment. Results of the study indicated that patients in the walking/education group had significant improvements in comparison with control subjects regarding increased walking distance, i.e., an average improvement of 70 meters vs. a 17 meter decrease; a 39% increase in physical activity; and a 27% decrease in pain. Although medication was used less frequently in the walking/education group, there was no significant difference from the control group. This study indicates that an intervention program consisting of supervised fitness walking and patient education can have significant impact on the management of osteoarthritis.

Singh and colleagues evaluated the responsiveness of 32 depressed community-dwelling older persons (mean age of 71 years) to a randomized controlled trial of progressive resistance exercise training.[143] After baseline assessment, subjects were assigned by randomization to either the training group or the control group for 10 weeks. All outcome measures, except that for strength, were conducted by a blinded assessor. Progressive resistance training, done 3 days per week, consisted of chest presses/pull-downs, leg presses, and knee extension/flexion. Resistive load was set at 80% of the one-repetition maximum load (initially and at the fourth week) and was increased at each session as tolerated. Training sessions consisted of three sets of eight repetitions for each exercise (lasting approximately 45 minutes total; followed by 5 minutes of stretching). The control group met 2 days per week for a 1-hour program of interactive health education, i.e., lectures, videos, and discussion, on topics including nutrition, heart disease, first aid, falls, home safety, incontinence, medical ethics, and eye/ear disease. In comparison with subjects in the control group, subjects in the training group had significant improvements in strength, i.e., 33% increase vs. 2% decrease; all measures of depression; bodily pain; vitality; and social functioning. There were no significant changes in measures of self-efficacy or activities of daily living. This study demonstrates that exercise training can be a significant factor in managing patients with major or minor depression or dysthymia, including pain.

Appropriate precautions should be followed when using exercise with elderly individuals. Severe osteoporosis may even pose limitations for ROM exercises. Older hypertensive individuals who perform a Valsalva's maneuver during strenuous resistive exercise risk a dangerous elevation in blood pressure. Exercise-induced muscle damage and soreness occur especially after vigorous eccentric exercise in both young and old subjects. Although rates of tissue repair are similar for healthy active subjects, older subjects show significantly greater muscle shortening.[32] This may predispose the older individual to a greater risk of further injury from exercise.

Thermal Agents

Traditionally, a wide range of thermal agents have been used to treat painful conditions affecting the elderly. Thermal effects leading to the modulation of pain may be directly and/or reflexly mediated. It would thus seem important to know the effective depth of penetration into the body of the common thermal agents. Table 23-1 summarizes this information, as has been described by others.[60,84,85,93,98,112,170] A number of sources can be consulted for specific descriptions of thermal agent treatment procedures.[60,84,85,93,112]

During the past 40 years a large number of studies have been concerned with establishing the efficacy and effectiveness of thermal agents in controlling pain and related clinical problems. Unfortunately, only a small number of published reports have specifically included elderly individuals as subjects. Representative studies that have included individuals aged 55 and older are summarized in Table 23-2. Overall, treatment efficacy was demonstrated for the thermal agents used. However, significant treatment effectiveness—albeit short term—was only shown in the study by Clarke.[31] As can be seen from Table 23-2, opposing thermal agents, i.e., cold vs. heat, have been shown to have equivalent efficacy with some clinical pain problems.[61,167] This may be related to separate but equally potent mechanisms of pain relief, which when combined with exercise act to further control pain and enhance function. Proposed theoretical mechanisms of action may not be supported, however. For example, Klemp and colleagues determined that ultrasound treatment of chronic fibromyotic upper trapezius muscles resulted in a significant **decrease** in muscle blood flow during treatment.[83]

Kauffman has reviewed physiological factors that need to be considered when therapeutic heat and cold are used with the elderly.[79] The following factors contribute to increased risk of thermal injury for the elderly: decreased reactivity of the hypothalamic thermoregulatory system; decreased autonomic and vasomotor responses; impairments of the circulatory system; loss of sweat glands; atrophy of skin, with reduction in circulation; lessened sensation of thirst; and decreased perception of thermal gradients. Common medications can further impair thermoregulatory control. Vasodilation in the skin may be hampered by diuretics, which limit volume expansion. Sweating in the skin may be inhibited by anticholinergic drugs. Various dermatological conditions and spinal cord lesions may impair sweating as a mechanism of heat loss. Skin vasodilation associated with heating of a large body surface area may place hazardous demands on cardiac output.[79] Conversely, cold may produce a temporary increase in systolic and diastolic blood pressure, which poses a risk for hypertensive patients. It has been recommended that blood pressure be monitored and that treatment with cold be discontinued if blood pressure becomes elevated.[112] Increased mechanical stiffness of joints, aversion to cold, and cold intolerance may limit applications of cold with some older patients.[93,112] Long-term use of steroids can produce fragile capillaries, which are easily damaged by thermal or mechanical agents.[112]

Precautions exist for the use of electromagnetic energy generated by a number of therapeutic heating modalities, e.g., microwave and shortwave diathermy.[33,78,112] Of major concern for the elderly is the potential for interference with the functioning of cardiac pacemakers and other electromedical de-

TABLE 23-1

DEPTH OF EFFECTIVE PENETRATION INTO THE BODY BY COMMON THERAPEUTIC THERMAL AGENTS

THERMAL AGENT	DEPTH INTO SOFT TISSUES
Cold pack	2 mm–4 cm
Hot pack	2–5 mm
Hydrotherapy (warm)	2–5 mm
Paraffin	2–5 mm
Fluidotherapy	2–5 mm
Infrared	
Nonluminous	2–5 mm
Luminous	5 mm–1 cm
Shortwave diathermy (27.12 MHz; subcutaneous fat < 2 cm thick)	1–3 cm
Microwave diathermy (2450 MHz; nondirect contact applicator; subcutaneous fat < 0.5 cm thick)	1–5 cm
Ultrasound	
3 MHz	1–2 cm
1 MHz	1–5 cm

vices, e.g., urinary bladder stimulators, electrocardiographs, and electromyographs. Jones reported on numerous cases of adverse physiological dysfunction associated with electromagnetic field interference in patients who have cardiac pacemakers. Significant interference occurred at distances of up to 15 feet.[78] Improvements in pacemaker design have eliminated this hazard for some pacemaker units.[112,146] Based on electrocardiographic changes in experimental animals, it has been recommended that treatment be avoided over the heart with ultrasound, which is not an electromagnetic form of energy. Cardiac pacemakers should not be directly exposed to ultrasound, which may interfere with electrical circuitry.[112] Metal components of objects external to patients, e.g., jewelry, clothing zippers or snaps, and furniture, or implanted within patients, e.g., joint prostheses and surgical rods, plates, and screws, act to focus electromagnetic energy in a manner that can produce burning of contiguous tissue. A similar focusing effect is produced by moisture on the skin or in dressings and clothing. The patient's eyes, fluid-filled joints, inflamed tissues, and excessive adipose tissue should be avoided for similar reasons. Such problems are encountered most often with microwave and shortwave diathermy. Although therapeutic ultrasound does not produce dangerous heating of metal like the diathermies, it should not be applied over the eye. Further research on the effects of ultrasound on nonmetallic prosthetic joint components has been advocated.[112]

The following are specific precautions that should be taken to prevent thermal injury of the older patient when using thermal agents:[79,93,112]

1. Heating can act to increase the inflammatory process in acute, subacute, and chronic conditions. Deep heating of joints involved with certain pathologies, e.g., the arthritides, may contribute to temperature-sensitive enzymatic lysis of joint cartilage.[44] Superficial moist heating for less

Table 23-2
Published Studies Assessing Thermal Agents for the Elderly with Pain

Investigators	Subjects	Design	Treatment Protocol Details	Treatment Outcome
Aldes & Jadeson[2] (1952)	N = 233 $\bar{X}$ age = 62 yrs Hypertrophic arthritis with chronic cervical or lumbosacral pain	• Not blinded, sequential clinical trials of US • Separate group same-age patients (N = 25) received sham US (unit off) in first treatment series	• All patients had poor response to prior medical and PT treatments • 3 series of 8–12 treatments, 3–10 min duration, q 48 hr, at 10-day intervals • US: 0.8 + 1 MHz, at 1.3–11.9 W, direct coupling with oil or indirect with water, moving technique; US intensity and duration increased each series • 3rd series included infrared, hot pack, and hydrotherapy • Evaluated pre and 14-day post final series, q ≤ 3.5 mo to 1 yr post ("Improvement" based on unspecified pain and ROM assessments)	Descriptive results only: 1. Sham-treated patients reported to show no improvement in first series; good response to active US in subsequent series 2. At 12 mo post, 233 active US-treated patients: 44% = "apparently permanent improvement" 27% = "partial improvement" 29% = "questionable or no improvement"
Wright[174] (1964)	N = 38 $\bar{X}$ age = 62 yrs Osteoarthritic knee	• Not blinded, noncrossover • Randomized assignment to 1 of 3 treatments: 1. Placebo tablets 2. Placebo intra-articular injections (saline) 3. SWD	• No patients had injections or SWD ≤ 6 mo prior • Treated as outpatient for 6 wk: placebo tablets B.I.D.; 4 placebo injections (1 q 2 wk); SWD 20 min 3×/wk • Evaluated pretreatment + q 2 wk (criteria: walking time, categorical evaluations of tenderness and pain; no. analgesic meds/day; "improvement" ≥ 2/4 criteria improved)	1. Placebo injections: significantly better improvement than tablets 2. Significant combined short (≤4 wk) and long-term (>10 wk) differences placebo tablets vs. SWD 3. Better long-term improvement with SWD but not significant
Clarke et al.[31] (1974)	N = 45 $\bar{X}$ age = 61 yrs Chronic osteoarthrosis of knee	• Noncrossover* • Randomized assignment to 1 of 3 treatments: 1. Ice 2. SWD 3. Sham SWD (untuned)	• Continued occasional med use • No injections or PT in prior year • Outpatient treatment × 3/wk for 3 wk • Specific treatment protocols "according to standard practice." Ice applied in bags above and below knee. • Evaluated pre- and post-treatment, and at 3 mo (4-point verbal pain and stiffness rating scales)	At conclusion of treatments: 1. Significant improvement in pain for ice vs. SWD or sham SWD 2. Significant improvement in stiffness for ice vs. SWD or sham SWD At 3 mo post treatments: 1. No significant difference between treatments 2. 82% of patients had improved pain, stiffness, knee ROM, walking time, and physician/patient assessments
Hamer & Kirk[61] (1976)	N = 31 $\bar{X}$ age = 59 yrs Chronic frozen shoulder	• Noncrossover* • Prospective assignment of patients into cryotherapy or US groups	• Patients free to continue meds (except corticosteroids) • Treated 3×/wk for 3 wk • Cryotherapy: towels dipped in crushed ice and water to shoulder for 15 min	1. Both groups improved 2. No significant differences between groups for: Number of treatments (12.4 ice vs. 14.8 US), pain grade improvement (2.0 ice vs. 2.3 US), improvement in shoulder

PNF = proprioceptive neuromuscular facilitation; PT = physical therapy; ROM = range of motion; SWD = shortwave diathermy: US = ultrasound.
*Evaluator blinded; separate therapist.

TABLE 23-2—CONT'D
PUBLISHED STUDIES ASSESSING THERMAL AGENTS FOR THE ELDERLY WITH PAIN

INVESTIGATORS	SUBJECTS	DESIGN	TREATMENT PROTOCOL DETAILS	TREATMENT OUTCOME
Hamer & Kirk[61] (1976) —cont'd			• US: ?site for US, 5–8 min continuous, at 0.5 W/cm^2 • All patients did passive and active exercise b.i.d., 10 min, for hospital and home programs • Patients discharged from outpatient therapy when pain relief attained • Evaluated pre- and post-treatment (pain assessment technique unspecified)	rotation (14.1 ice vs. 12.4 US)

Bulgen et al.[23] (1984)	N = 42
	$\overline{X}$ age = 56 yrs
	Chronic frozen shoulder
		• Noncrossover*
		• Randomized assignment to 1 of 4 groups:
		  1. Ice packs and PNF
		  2. Maitland mobilization
		  3. Injection
		  4. Non-treatment
			• All got home pendulum exercise, non-ASA analgesics and diazepam (p.r.n. at night)
			• No specific details on ice packs, PNF, or mobilization
			• Injections of 20 mg methyl prednisone acetate and 1% lignocaine hydrochloride (0.5 mL to subacromial bursa, 0.5 mL to shoulder joint)
			• Groups no. 1 and 2 treated 3×/wk for 6 wk; no. 3 injected 1×/wk for 3 wk
			• Evaluated pretreatment, 1×/wk for 6 wk, and 1×/mo for 6 mo (pain assessed by visual analogue scale; ROM)
				1. Problems noted with use of visual analogue scale to assess pain; no data given, "majority pain free at 6 mo"
				2. ROM (cumulative) improvement: greatest for injection (no. 3), with significant between-group difference at wk 4; ice with best improvement at 6 mo but nonsignificant difference between groups

Williams et al.[167] (1986)	N = 18 $\overline{X}$ age = 58 yrs Rheumatoid arthritic shoulder	• "Single-blinded,"* noncrossover • Randomized assignment to hot-pack or cold-pack groups	• Patients free to continue meds (no steroid injection in prior 3 mo) • Treated 3×/wk for 3 wk • Hot pack: initially at 138° F; 8 layers of Turkish towel between pack and skin • Cold pack: crushed ice in Turkish towel, 4 layers between ice and skin • Both heat and cold applied for 20 min, followed by supervised 20-min exercise program to cervical spine, both shoulders, and upper extremities • Evaluated pre- and post-treatment (pain assessed with McGill Pain Questionnaire, parts 1 and 4)	1. Both groups improved, but no within-group statistics performed 2. No significant differences between groups for: Pain rating index improvement: 5.7 heat vs. 6.9 cold Flexion ROM: 12.2 heat vs. 5.0 cold Abduction ROM: 26.1 heat vs. 22.8 cold
Svarcova et al.[153] (1988)	N = 180 $\overline{X}$ age = 63 yrs Osteoarthritis of hip or knee	• Not blinded, noncrossover • Patients divided into 3 treatment groups:	• US: moving 5 cm/sec, 3 fields, 5 min each • Galvanic: 0.1 ma/cm^2, 20 min; SWD: pulsed at	Between treatment comparisons only For pain relief (at treatment 10):

TABLE 23-2—CONT'D
PUBLISHED STUDIES ASSESSING THERMAL AGENTS FOR THE ELDERLY WITH PAIN

INVESTIGATORS	SUBJECTS	DESIGN	TREATMENT PROTOCOL DETAILS	TREATMENT OUTCOME
Svarcova et al.[153] (1988) —cont'd		1. US 2. Galvanic current 3. SWD • Active and placebo medications given to one-half of subjects in each group	46 MHz, 2 fields, 2 min each • Active med: 400 mg ibuprofen • US, galvanic current and SWD for 10 treatments, q 2 days, med B.I.D for 3 wk • Evaluated at treatment sessions 5 and 10 (pain by visual analogue; 4 category "therapeutic effect" rating)	1. All treatments plus active med were significantly better than treatments alone 2. No significant differences between treatment groups For "therapeutic effect": 1. No significant difference between groups 2. Overall, 89% of subjects rated treatments as "good" to "excellent"

than 20 minutes, on the other hand, has been shown to result in a lowering of joint temperature.[71] Thus, it is critical that the most appropriate treatment modality be selected for a given clinical condition.

2. Operating temperatures for heating agents should be lowered, whereas those for cooling agents should be raised. For example, if a vigorous heating effect is needed to increase connective tissue extensibility in conjunction with prolonged stretch, targeted tissue should be heated to only 40° C as opposed to 45° C.[112] Typical modality intensity settings will need to be modified, and in some cases, thermostatic controls will need to be reset, e.g., for paraffin and hot and cold pack units. Use of paraffin with a low melting point (104° F as opposed to 124° F) has been recommended.[72] Both hot and cold packs may need to be better insulated with greater thicknesses of dry toweling, which the patient should not be permitted to compress with his/her body weight.

3. A slower rate of temperature change may be more desirable. Therapeutic ultrasound, which produces the most rapid deep-temperature elevation by easily penetrating subcutaneous fat, may need to be used with a modified technique, e.g., lower intensity, faster sound head movement, and less overlap of sound head strokes.

4. Treatment times may need to be shortened. The customary 20- to 30-minute treatment time used with superficial heating agents may need to be limited to no longer than 20 minutes.[72,112] More conservative treatment times for deeper-heating agents may also be appropriate, e.g., use of ultrasound for 5 minutes for each 150 cm² of skin surface[60] rather than for an area two to three times the size of the sound head.[112]

5. Reflex-based consensual vasodilation may be used to produce less pronounced increases in skin blood flow in body regions that cannot tolerate direct heating.[93] Consensual circulatory reactions for cold have been controversial.[85]

Although these modifications may improve the safety of various treatment interventions, further research is needed to determine whether resultant therapeutic effects are lessened substantially.

A number of clinical factors should guide the health care professional in the selection and application of the appropriate thermal agent. Michlovitz has discussed key factors to consider when using thermal agents in the management of rheumatic diseases.[112] These factors, modified for a broader consideration of other pain-related diagnoses encountered with elderly patients, include the following:

1. The stage of the inflammatory/repair process is important to determine. Based on signs, symptoms, and physiological characteristics, the acute inflammatory stage may last as long as 2 weeks. Cardinal signs of local pain, redness, increased temperature, swelling, and loss of function are common. There is a predominance of neutrophils. The subacute stage of inflammation may then continue for up to 1 month and is associated with a considerable lessening of cardinal signs. The chronic stage of inflammation occurs after 1 month and is associated with the presence of lymphocytes, monocytes, and macrophages and with the proliferation of fibroblasts related to adhesion and scar formation. Within the first 24 to 72 hours after trauma or onset of inflammation, heating agents must be avoided to prevent aggravating changes in local permeability, circulation, and metabolism. Cooling the affected site results in decreased membrane permeability and vasoconstriction, which act to limit formation of edema.[112] Local tissue metabolism is also lowered, which may also act to limit secondary hypoxic injury of adjacent tissues. Concurrent compression with an elastic wrap and elevation further act to control edema formation.[85] Beyond 72 hours, mild and then more vigorous local heating may be indicated. However, the patient is always monitored for signs and symptoms of aggravated inflammation. It should be appreciated that early vigorous cooling can also worsen inflammation.[112] In addition, cold may also be used to modulate pain in subacute and chronic stages.

2. The "target tissue" for the thermal agent must be determined. In the acute stage, cooling to the site of inflammation is desired. However, mild heating superficial to inflamed tissues may successfully relieve muscle spasm

and related pain. In some chronic conditions, deep, vigorous heating combined with prolonged low-load stretch may be required to restore pain-free joint range of motion. However, it has been suggested that deep heating of subacute and chronic arthritic joints may promote cartilage destruction.[44]

3. The size of the body region, i.e., tissue volume, and number of joints involved present practical treatment considerations. The diathermies may more easily be used to heat large and relatively deep-body regions than ultrasound used on multiple fields. Unlike the diathermies, ultrasound will not dangerously heat subcutaneous fat. Hydrotherapy may be preferred to hot packs or paraffin for superficial tissue heating when multiple joints or large body regions are involved.

4. The decision to continue treatment in the clinic or via home program instruction may be guided in part by the suitability of appropriate treatment modalities. Some cooling agents, e.g., ice cubes in a plastic bag or used for massage, and heating agents, e.g., moist towels microwaved in unsealed plastic bags, timer-controlled electric moist-heating pads, and home paraffin units, may successfully be used in the home environment with proper patient education. All deep-heating agents, e.g., diathermies and ultrasound, require application by a health care professional in the clinic or home.

Transcutaneous Electrical Nerve Stimulation

The most common form of therapeutic electrical stimulation used for pain control is TENS, which involves the stimulation of cutaneous and peripheral nerves via electrodes on the surface of the skin. Six types, or "modes," of TENS have been most commonly discussed in the literature. These six modes are conventional, strong low-rate, brief-intense, pulse-burst, modulated, and hyperstimulation TENS. Each mode uses unique electrical output characteristics and a variety of electrode site options. Different perceptual-motor qualities are associated with each mode as a result of nerve and/or muscle activation. Table 23-3 introduces key features of these common TENS modes, including typical stimulator characteristics, electrode sites, and desired perceptual-motor experience. To communicate effectively, it is important that clinicians and researchers specify details of their methods rather than just relying on descriptive TENS mode labels. Other publications should be consulted for more detailed discussion of the theoretical bases for pain relief with TENS and associated clinical decision making.[9,105]

Although a number of professional publications have suggested or recommended TENS for pain control with elderly patients,* a survey by Leseberg and Schunk revealed that initiation of TENS treatment for the elderly by physical therapists was in reality quite low.[97] Despite the fact that hundreds of research papers have been published on TENS,[123] very few studies have been conducted with patients with an average age in the mid-50s and older. Table 23-4 summarizes published studies that have assessed either the efficacy or effectiveness of TENS for elderly patients with acute or chronic pain. In addition, Levy and associates used TENS to treat experimental acute arthritis induced in rat

---

*References 5,47,59,72,89,94,119,124,131,132,154,156,159,163,172

Table 23-3
Common Modes of Transcutaneous Electrical Nerve Stimulation for Pain Control

Mode Classification	Typical Stimulator Output Characteristics	Typical Electrode Sites	Desired Perceptual-Motor Experience
Conventional (Barr et al.)[12]	Frequency: 10–100 Hz Pulse duration: 50–100 µs Amplitude: low to medium*	At perimeter of painful area or over nerve to region; or at segmentally related area	Distinct paresthesia superimposed on painful areas, or in segmentally related area
Strong low-rate (Andersson et al.)[7]	Frequency: below 10 Hz Pulse duration: 100–300 µs Amplitude: high*	Over nerve related to muscle in or remote from painful area	Uncomfortable rhythmic muscle contractions at patient tolerance
Brief-intense (Leo et al.)[96]	Frequency: 60–150 Hz Pulse duration: 50–250 µs Amplitude: high*	Over nerve related to muscle in or remote from painful area	Uncomfortable tetanic muscle contraction that fatigues, at patient tolerance
Pulse-burst (Mannheimer and Carlsson)[104]	Frequency: high (60–100 Hz) modulated by low (0.5–4 Hz) Pulse duration: 50–200 µs Amplitude: low to high*	Over nerve related to muscle in or remote from painful area	Weak to strong intermittent tetanic muscle contraction and paresthesia
Modulated (Miller et al.)[115]	Frequency, pulse duration, or amplitude modulated separately or together down 60% from preset values Amplitude: Low to high*	Any of these listed sites	Weak to strong sensation, with or without muscle contraction; may minimize perceptual accommodation
Hyperstimulation (= "noninvasive" electroacupuncture) (Leo)[95]	Frequency: 1–100 Hz Pulse duration: up to 500 ms Amplitude: high*	Acupuncture points	Sharp burning sensation at tolerance; no muscle contraction

*Adequate to give desired perceptual-motor experience.

TABLE 23-4

PUBLISHED STUDIES ASSESSING TENS FOR THE ELDERLY WITH ACUTE AND CHRONIC PAIN

Investigators	Subjects	Design	TENS Mode	Electrode Sites	Protocol Details	Treatment Outcome
Acute pain						
Smith et al.[145] (1983)	N = 50 (subject subset) $\bar{X}$ age = 73 yrs Total condylar–total knee replacement surgery	• Not blinded, noncrossover • Prospective division of patients into TENS and non-TENS groups	Unspecified (likely CONV or MR) "pleasant stimulation"	2 electrodes parallel to incision	• Preoperative TENS education • Patients adjusted TENS unit controls, with b.i.d. monitoring by PT • TENS continuous until discharge • All patients had PT (exercise and gait training)	Patients in TENS group had significantly fewer injections of Demerol, lower total Demerol dosage, fewer days until straight leg raise, shorter hospital stay; no significant difference in days until ambulation
Finsen et al.[51] (1988)	N = 51 $\bar{X}$ age = 69 yrs Lower extremity amputation due to diabetes or artherosclerosis	• Not blinded, noncrossover • Randomized postoperative assignment to: 1. Active TENS 2. Sham TENS (no stimulation) 3. Sham TENS and chlorpromazine	PB (90 μs impulses at 100 Hz; burst of 7 pulses 2×/sec; amplitude to discomfort)	2 electrodes over femoral nerve, 2 over sciatic nerve	• Treated 30 min 2×/day for 2 wk • TENS unit light on • Analgesic meds on demand • Pain assessment technique unspecified	1. Self-rated analgesic effect for all active TENS and 50% of sham TENS 2. Nonsignificant difference in analgesic use or phantom pain in first 4 wk 3. Active TENS had significantly more healing at 6 and 9 wk 4. Active TENS had significantly fewer cases of phantom pain at 16 wk (10%) than sham (36%) or sham plus chlorpromazine (58%); no difference $\geq$ 1 yr later
Chronic pain						
Abelson et al.[1] (1983)	N = 32 $\bar{X}$ age = 56 yrs Rheumatoid arthritis with chronic wrist pain	• "Double-blind"* noncrossover • Random assignment to active or placebo TENS (no stimulation) treatment	BI? (frequency = 70 Hz; high intensity)	Dorsal and ventral wrist	• Anti-inflammatory meds stopped 12 hr before treatment • Neutral statement on likely effects to both groups • Treated 15 min 1×/wk for 3 wk • TENS unit light on • Visual analogue pain relief rating pre- and post-treatment	Only within-group comparisons done: 1. Active TENS gave significant improvements in resting and grip pain, power, and work 2. Placebo effect for pain averaged 17%; nonsignificant for all criteria

Study	Sample	Design	TENS parameters	Electrode placement	Procedure	Results
Lewis et al.[100] (1984)	N = 28 Median age = 61 yrs Osteoarthritis with chronic knee pain	• "Double-blind,"† crossover • Active and placebo TENS (no stimulation) treatment	CONV or BI? (frequency = 70 Hz)	4 electrodes at acupuncture points around knee	• Initial "washout" week, paracetamol only med (also available during TENS trials) • Home program: 30–60 min 3×/day for 3 wk of each treatment • TENS unit light on • Assessed weekly, including visual analogue pain relief rating	1. "> 50% pain relief" for 46% active, 43% placebo 2. Significant difference in median duration of pain relief: active (151 min) vs. placebo (110 min) 3. Significant improvement pain relief after 3 wk active, not placebo 4. Both groups had significant improvement in "pain index" based on knee ROM and weight bearing, and reduction in meds 5. Preferred treatment if continued > 3 wk: 43% active, 36% meds, 14% placebo
Langley et al.[91] (1984)	N = 33 $\overline{X}$ age = 54 yrs Rheumatoid arthritis with chronic hand pain	• "Double-blind,"* noncrossover • Random assignment to group 1 or 2 active TENS or group 3 placebo TENS (no stimulation) treatments	1. BI? Frequency = 100 Hz; pulse duration = 200 μs 2. "Acupuncture-like" (PB?) Frequency = 100 Hz, pulsed 2/sec; both no. 1 and 2 at highest tolerated intensity, displayed on oscilloscope 3. Placebo = no current but given signal on oscilloscope	1 dorsal and 1 ventral, proximal to wrist	• Initial neutral instructions to all subjects • Strong suggestion given to placebo group • No meds < 24 hr prior • Treated once for 20 min • Pre- and post-treatment assessment each 15 min, including visual analogue pain rating	1. Overall "≥ 50% pain relief": 59% in group 1; 64% in 2, 55% in 3 2. Nonsignificant group differences, as all groups had significantly decreased resting and grip pain 3. Nonsignificant group differences for overall pain relief, total joint tenderness, or number of tender joints 4. No significant changes in power or work

*Evaluator blinded; separate therapist.

†Unable to determine adequacy of "double-blind" conditions.

BI = brief-intense; CONV = conventional; MR = modulated rate; PB = pulse-burst; PT = physical therapy; ROM = range of motion; TENS = transcutaneous electrical nerve stimulation.

knees.[99] A 5-minute TENS treatment resulted in a small but significant increase in temperature (largest mean value = 0.4°C) and a significant decrease in pressure measured intra-articularly. Synovial fluid volume and total leukocyte count were also significantly less than the levels found in the opposite nontreated knee.

The author of this chapter conducted a modified double-blind crossover study with elderly individuals (N = 22, mean age = 74 ± 10 years) who had chronic musculoskeletal pain.[10] Although all subjects were informed that TENS could possibly produce pain relief, this was done with neutral instructions. Each of three TENS treatments was given to each subject for 30 minutes at 48-hour intervals for 1 week. (The three TENS treatments consisted of conventional TENS: frequency = 60 Hz, 40 μs pulse duration, amplitude to distinct paresthesia; pulse-burst TENS: seven impulses each of 40 μs duration and frequency of 110 Hz, pulsed at two per second, amplitude producing maximum tolerated muscle contraction; and sham control TENS: conventional TENS settings but stimulation on for only 10 seconds.) Stimulation via two electrodes was perceived within the painful area. Pain and simulated functional activities were assessed by a blinded investigator who used separate visual analogue scales. Significantly less immediate pain relief was seen for the sham control treatment (19.5% vs. 32.5% for true conventional and 33.9% for pulse-burst). When compared with the control treatment, both active TENS treatments produced significantly greater pain relief for up to 8 hours but had no significant effect on the simulated functional activities used in this study.

Overall, these studies indicate both efficacy[1,145] and effectiveness of TENS in controlling a range of pain problems experienced by elderly individuals under controlled short-term conditions.[10,51,100] Only when strong suggestion was provided to a placebo TENS group was active TENS seen to be ineffective for older patients,[91] as has been the case for the general population.[36] Well-controlled studies assessing pain control with long-term TENS use, i.e., for greater than 1 month, in the elderly are sorely lacking.

Demand-type (synchronous) cardiac pacemakers represent the primary contraindication for electrical stimulators, including TENS devices. Although TENS has been safely used on the body close to older-style fixed-rate (synchronous) pacemakers and on regions remote from demand-type units, a wide range of hazardous electrical stimulation characteristics and electrode placements has yet to be fully investigated.[9] At this time it is probably safest to recommend that all patients with cardiac pacemakers be electrically monitored during extended initial trials of therapeutic electrical stimulation.[9,30] If interference is noted, it may be appropriate to re-program the pacemaker to a lower level of sensitivity.[30] It also has been suggested that electrical stimulation not be performed on the anterior chest wall of patients with cardiac histories, over the carotid sinus, or close to the larynx.[105] The effects of TENS on patients with cerebral vascular accidents, transient ischemic attacks, epilepsy, and seizure disorders are not well-established.

Dry skin associated with aging and cleansing of the skin with alcohol-based products act to increase the impedance under electrodes used for electrical stimulation. This will necessitate the use of higher-intensity stimulation, which may be uncomfortable and irritating to the skin. Skin impedance can be lowered by hydration of the skin with skin cream or nonabrasive electrode gel. Use of alternate electrode sites will prevent breakdown of fragile skin from cumulative effects of allergic, chemical, electrical, and mechanical irritation. Tape and self-adhering electrodes should be peeled back slowly while underlying skin is held down to prevent skin stripping.

Although clinical procedures involved in the application of TENS have been outlined elsewhere,[9,105] factors related to successful pain control with TENS for the elderly merit specific discussion. Even though the clinician is faced with an array of stimulators, only a handful of publications have critically assessed specific brands and models of TENS units.[9] Equipment-related factors play an important role in the success or failure of treatment with TENS. These factors include reasonable cost, "user-friendly" instruction manuals and unit controls, durable unit components, independence between unit control settings and other unit output parameters, good battery life, and electrical output being limited to established safety standards. The American National Standard for Transcutaneous Electrical Nerve Stimulators should be consulted for detailed safety guidelines.[6]

A guiding concept for the treatment of all patients with TENS, regardless of age, is a modification of the "KISS" principle, i.e., **K**eep **I**t **S**imple **S**timulation. Technology incorporated into some TENS units is inappropriately designed or too complex. Unit components are easily lost or misplaced by patients. Controls may be confusing and may be difficult to see or to adjust because of their small size. For this reason an older-style single-channel TENS unit with only one control dial, i.e., on/amplitude, may be superior in some instances to the latest subminiature multiprogrammable unit. Electrode systems need to be custom fit to each patient's needs and abilities. A patient with severe hand osteoarthritis may be unable to manipulate and secure traditional carbonized silicone rubber electrodes, conductive gel, and tape; only higher-priced reusable, self-adhering electrodes may be suitable. Health care professionals need to be familiar with options available in TENS units and components, e.g., lead wires, connectors, electrode styles, adhesive materials, and battery packs, and be able to exercise reasonable freedom in selecting the optimal TENS setup for their patients.

Unfortunately, an adequate number of comparative studies have not been conducted to determine the best mode of TENS for treating specific types of pain. Wolf and colleagues have noted that some patients with peripheral nerve injuries benefit from higher-intensity stimulation.[171] Patients generally find conventional TENS and lower-amplitude versions of other modes, i.e., pulse-burst and modulated, to be most acceptable. The author of this chapter has found elderly patients with chronic pain to rate conventional low-intensity

TENS as being more comfortable than high-intensity pulse-burst TENS.[13] Although it has been recommended that initial treatment be performed with conventional TENS (frequency at 60 Hz, short-pulse duration, and amplitude that gives distinct paresthesia in the painful region),[11,12,102] alternate TENS modes may need to be used to attain successful pain control.[9,96,105]

It is critically important that the patient and significant others be given adequate instruction in self-treatment and outcome documentation, e.g., via activity logs and pain and functional rating scales. The patient **must** attain successful pain control under the supervision of the health care professional before being given a home program that has any chance of long-term success. Medicare and many insurance companies require at least a 1-month rental period before authorizing a TENS unit purchase.

Psychoeducational Interventions

Allegrante has reviewed an array of related psychoeducational interventions used to manage pain that can be of value in treating elderly patients.[3] These interventions include patient/care-giver education, cognitive-behavioral therapy, and family and social support. In relation to the theoretical mechanisms of action noted in Box 23-1, it is likely that these interventions exert their effects directly via an increase in descending inhibitory control mechanisms. Additionally, these interventions ultimately can lead to behaviors that decrease undesired activity in nociceptors or their afferents, or that increase desired input from mechanoreceptors or their afferents.

Traditionally, educational interventions have been used to enhance patient and care-giver knowledge about disease and its treatment, to modify attitudes and beliefs, and to improve a range of skills, e.g., self-management, problem-solving, coping, communication, and compliance/adherence behaviors.

Ferrell and associates have developed and tested a three-part home-based educational program for elderly patients with cancer and their care-givers.[46] Program content includes a general overview of pain and its management, specific information about pharmacological management, and discussion about and demonstration of 19 non-drug management approaches, e.g., heat, cold, massage, relaxation, distraction, and imagery techniques. Educational materials include written information and instructions and audio cassette tapes. In the third session the visiting nurse recommends a non-drug intervention, including the purchase of equipment with a total cost of no more than $50. A combination of pharmacological and non-drug interventions has been suggested to provide optimal pain relief. Key teaching principles for pain education have been outlined. These include emphasis on individualized education, with consideration of cultural influences; brief instructional sessions, with breaks as needed; sensitivity to issues of cost, e.g., the seemingly minimal cost of purchasing tape recorder batteries may be a financial burden; incorporating the patient's values and beliefs, e.g., use of prayer and inclusion of culturally sensitive methods; and involvement of care-givers in non-drug interventions, which can decrease their sense of helplessness. Throughout this well-accepted program, Ferrell has noted that pain education is essential to empower patients and care-givers to increase their involvement in pain management.

Very positive results have also been seen for patient education in conjunction with arthritis management.[3] Perhaps best known is the Arthritis Self-Management Program (ASMP), the 12-year results of which have been summarized by Lorig and Holman for more than 1000 clients.[103] The community-based program consists of 6 weekly 2-hour sessions instructed by trained lay leaders. Participants receive the *Arthritis Helpbook*. They and significant others are instructed in the following: an overview of the anatomy/physiology of different types of arthritis, medication uses and effects, designing an individualized exercise and cognitive pain management program, nutrition, patient/physician communication, and solving disease-related problems. Results from the ASMP, based on the comparison of responses from active program participants vs. wait-list control subjects in randomized trials, indicated the following: (1) program participants had significantly increased self-efficacy, significantly increased frequency of exercise and relaxation per week, significantly decreased pain, significantly decreased arthritis-related physician visits, and trends toward decreases in depression and disability; (2) self-efficacy, i.e., confidence that one has in his/her ability to perform a specific behavior or change a specific cognitive state, was enhanced by an education program that emphasized self-efficacy; and (3) without formal reinforcement, significant ASMP effects lasted as long as 4 years.

Cognitive-behavioral treatment is comprised of an array of psychosocial approaches.[3,46,81] The cognitive approaches challenge how patients perceive themselves and their pain, and help them divert their thoughts away from pain. Behavioral approaches are used to decrease pain behaviors, and to increase wellness behaviors.[81] Specific techniques are used to improve coping and problem-solving, and to reduce emotional distress associated with pain. These techniques include passive and progressive relaxation; biofeedback; rest and activity cycling; attention diversion/distraction; imagery/visualization; meditation and prayer; self-hypnosis; and cognitive restructuring.[3,46,81]

Keefe and colleagues have provided the following practical suggestions for implementing a number of these techniques with older individuals:[81]

1. During relaxation training, patients often fall asleep. This can be minimized by conducting practice when patients aren't fatigued, reducing the length of sessions, and allowing patients to keep their eyes open.
2. Brief "mini-practice" sessions of relaxation should be encouraged throughout the day, i.e., 20 to 30 seconds in duration, up to 20 times per day.
3. Activity-rest cycling is used to break the pain cycle by making activity levels contingent on time, not on pain. Over-doers should stop and rest before increased pain is

experienced; under-doers should gradually increase activity levels.

4. Imagery should involve all of the patient's senses and be preceded by relaxation.

5. In using cognitive restructuring, patients should monitor their negative thoughts. A rational coping thought should be developed to challenge each negative thought. For example, the negative thought "the pain will never end" brings feelings of depression. An appropriate coping thought might be "the pain has always lessened in the past."

Middaugh and associates assessed the efficacy of biofeedback-assisted relaxation training in comparing the responses of 20 younger (mean age of 38.5 years) and 17 older (mean age of 62.4 years) patients with chronic pain.[114] A total of 8 to 12 training sessions, with daily homework sessions, were performed. The sessions consisted of muscle relaxation—i.e., initially tense/relax muscle contractions progressed to diaphragmatic breathing and relaxation without tensing; digital skin temperature and respiratory rate were monitored—and EMG biofeedback—i.e., monitoring muscles in a specific area of pain, with relaxation practiced during actual and simulated daily activities. Testing was done before and after training. Both younger and older subjects demonstrated comparable significant improvements in skin temperature and respiratory rate responsiveness. A subgroup of patients with cervical pain showed similar improvements in EMG measures for the upper trapezius muscle. Maximum reported pain was decreased significantly for both the younger and older groups, but current pain was only decreased significantly for the older participants. This often-cited study indicates that older patients with chronic predominately musculoskeletal pain are responsive to biofeedback-assisted relaxation training.

Keefe and Williams determined that there were no significant age-related differences in the use or perceived effectiveness of pain coping strategies among patients with chronic pain.[82] Older patients who viewed themselves as effective in controlling pain and in avoiding maladaptive "catastrophizing" strategies reported significantly lower levels of pain and disability. After cognitive-behavioral training, older patients who increased their perceived effectiveness of coping (and decreased catastrophizing) were more likely to have decreased pain and disability.[81] Both daily and "time-lagged" coping effects have been determined for patients experiencing rheumatoid arthritis.[80] Patients who reported high levels of coping efficacy on one day had lower levels of pain and more positive mood the following day.

The health status and coping abilities of individuals with chronic illness can be greatly influenced by spouse, family, and social support.[3,81] Direct support can include assisting the patient to practice and in maintaining coping skills, e.g., identifying high-risk situations, identifying natural cues to assist with coping, and developing a plan for dealing with flares in pain. However, excessive or solicitous support may foster a dependent life-style that perpetuates pain behaviors.[81] Jamison and Virts determined that 1 year after completing a chronic pain management program, patients who described their families as being supportive reported significantly lower pain intensity, less reliance on medications, and less interference with activities than patients who perceived their families as nonsupportive.[76] Interestingly, Rene and associates found that supportive monthly telephone calls by lay personnel that promoted self-care were associated with improvements in joint pain and physical function over a 1-year period for patients with osteoarthritis.[134]

Case Studies

To more completely describe the application of conservative pain management principles, two case studies involving older patients are now presented.

Case 1

Mr. Jones was an 81-year-old retired electrical contractor, living alone, with severe degenerative joint disease. He was referred as an outpatient to the physical therapy department from the medical center's Geriatric Evaluation Unit (GEU). His main complaint was right hip pain on weight bearing. Mr. Jones had tripped over a curb with his right foot 1 week ago, which had resulted in immediate hip pain. His related history included blindness, moderate bilateral hearing loss, no evidence of fracture by roentgenogram taken on the day of referral, and a prescription for naproxen (375 mg, 3 times a day). The clinic physician felt that Mr. Jones should be assessed as a candidate for possible right total hip replacement by an orthopedist, but the patient vigorously opposed this idea. (Mr. Jones reported that a good friend had recently died as a result of complications associated with just such a surgery.) Evaluation in the physical therapy department revealed moderately limited active and passive ROM and 3/5 grade muscle strength of all right hip muscles (except abductors at 2/5) associated with pain. Strength at other right lower extremity joints and of other extremities and trunk was generally at 4/5. He was independently ambulatory with a slow antalgic gait using his sounding cane in the right hand. Mr. Jones noted only localized "deep" hip pain; his pain with weight bearing was rated 7/10; with active hip motion, 5/10; and at rest supine, 2/10 (by Pain Estimate Rating). It was the assessment of the physical therapist that Mr. Jones had strained the muscles of his hip (principally the abductors) and was in a subacute stage of pain. The initial treatment plan included patient education/recommendations for reduction of mechanical forces on muscles of the right hip to decrease pain and promote healing and gentle active ROM exercises to maintain and later increase hip ROM to restore safe functional gait. It was recommended that weight-bearing activity be temporarily decreased, but he refused to be fitted for a standard straight cane. He was willing to limit ambulation, especially on stairs, for a period of "a couple weeks." He was instructed in an initial home program of gentle active ROM exercises for the right hip. Since he was planning to leave the community for the next few months to visit his children out of state, he was instructed to arrange for re-evaluation upon his return.

Mr. Jones attended physical therapy after another GEU visit 5 months later. The GEU physician had increased the naproxen (375 mg) to 4 times a day. Roentgenograms remained negative. On this occasion, he reported increased right hip pain extending to the lateral mid-thigh: rated 8/10 with weight bearing, 6/10 with active ROM, and 3/10 at rest supine. He exhibited marked tenderness to palpation at the right greater trochanter only. Although not agreeable to manual muscle testing of the hip, no distal weakness was noted. Mr. Jones now accepted fitting and instruction in use of a straight cane, which he found to be safer when using in the right hand. His home ROM exercise program was modified to self-assisted ROM in pain-free range only. A future trial of TENS for pain control was suggested to Mr. Jones.

A trial of TENS for pain control was begun 1 week later. Pain rating before treatment was 8/10 during weight bearing of ambulation, even with the cane on right. TENS was begun in the "conventional" mode (frequency = 60 Hz, phase width = 40 μs, amplitude adjusted to produce a "distinct electrical sensation overlying the area of pain"). One TENS unit channel was used, with one electrode over the greater trochanter and the other at mid-lateral thigh. At the end of stimulation for 20 minutes, Mr. Jones rated pain with weight bearing and ROM at 3/10 and pain at rest 0/10. With the TENS unit turned off, significant carryover of pain reduction was seen for approximately 2 hours. A second TENS trial was done 4 days later, with initial pain again at 8/10 on weight bearing. Within 20 minutes of stimulation, this pain was reduced to 4/10, with significant post-stimulation carryover again for 2 hours. Mr. Jones was formally instructed in a home TENS program 3 days later, to be done twice a day in conjunction with the self-assisted ROM program. Reusable self-adhering electrodes could be applied and cared for by Mr. Jones after detailed instruction and supervision. He also mastered TENS unit operations (including the battery recharging procedure and use of alternate electrode sites).

After 4 weeks, Mr. Jones was admitted to the hospital with a small gastrointestinal bleed. Although taken off naproxen, he continued TENS and was regularly able to reduce his pain with weight bearing to 3/10 and had no pain at rest. Unfortunately, 1½ months later, he fractured his right hip while lifting heavy pails of water for his six dogs. He underwent a successful right total hip replacement, which included conventional postoperative physical therapy. At a return GEU visit 9 months later, Mr. Jones demonstrated a symmetrical pain-free gait without any assistive device. Strength of the right hip muscles was found to be 4-5/5, with full ROM throughout. Mr. Jones was continuing a home exercise program of resistive exercise and walking on a daily basis.

This case illustrates the practical implementation of conservative pain management interventions for a highly independent older individual. The physical therapy program involved extensive patient education and psychological support. The program included the use of an assistive device, exercise, and TENS in a manner that helped to both control pain and maintain functional independence during an 8-month period leading up to a much-feared total joint replacement surgery.

Case 2

Mrs. Smith was a 61-year-old right-hand–dominant female hospital clerk with a chief complaint of right shoulder pain. This pain prevented use of the right upper extremity for work and activities of daily living that required the finger tips to be raised higher than her ear lobe, e.g., stocking items on overhead shelves and combing her hair. She was seen initially in the physical therapy department 1 day after sudden onset of right shoulder pain that occurred while she was tearing paper from a computer printer; her recollection of the pain was rated at a level of 10/10. She was referred from the orthopedics department with a diagnosis of right subacromial bursitis and a prescription for topical 5% hydrocortisone to be used for phonophoresis. The patient was taking ibuprofen and acetaminophen as needed. Physical therapy evaluation revealed a "painful arc" of active right shoulder abduction ROM from 60 to 120 degrees in neutral rotation and from 90 to 120 degrees in full external rotation. A manual muscle test of the right deltoid and rotator cuff muscles was rated at 4/5 (with pain); left shoulder and bilateral elbow, wrist and hand muscles were all 5/5. Upon palpation of the right subacromial area, the patient noted sharp pain and rated it 9/10. Pain with active shoulder abduction was rated 7/10 and was relieved by rest and medications. Manual examination of the cervical spine did not reproduce shoulder pain. The patient reported not being allergic to cold or medications. Mrs. Smith was assessed to have acute onset right subacromial bursitis. Short-term treatment goals were to decrease inflammation and pain. Long-term goals were to restore full pain-free ROM and shoulder strength and to regain use of the shoulder for functional work activities and ADL. Physical therapy treatment consisted of rest from repeated trauma in the workplace through temporary job task reassignment; education in a home program (application of specific ergonomic principles in the home and workplace; ice massage for 7 to 10 minutes, twice a day for 1 week; and gentle pain-free ROM exercise); outpatient treatment 3 times a week consisting of phonophoresis (using 5% hydrocortisone with continuous 1-MHz ultrasound, at 0.7 to 0.8 W/cm², moving technique for 7 minutes); and exercise (ROM; progressive resistive exercise when inflammation gone).

At physical therapy re-evaluation 10 days later, Mrs. Smith reported that the right shoulder was generally feeling better. Examination disclosed a painful arc from 70 to 120 degrees in neutral and from 90 to 115 degrees in external rotation, manual muscle tests were unchanged, and medication use was still as needed. Pain with active shoulder abduction was rated 6/10. One week later, Mrs. Smith claimed that she was pleased with her progress on pain control but noted shoulder "weakness." Examination showed a painful arc of active shoulder abduction (in neutral rotation) at 90 to 110 degrees, pain was rated 4/10, and muscle strength tests were unchanged. The patient claimed less frequent medication use. She was begun on gentle progressive resistive exercise for the right shoulder using a "yellow"-coded Theraband and was monitored closely for increased inflammation. At a clinic visit 1 week later, phonophoresis was discontinued. A painful arc remained at 90 to 110 degrees, with pain rated at 4/10 and strength unchanged. Medication use was now infrequent. Mrs. Smith's exercise program progressed to a "red"-coded Theraband.

Mrs. Smith was discharged from formal out-patient physical therapy 1 week later (1 month after her initial visit), claiming to be pain free. The patient had resumed her original workload, with task modifications. No painful arc with active right shoulder abduction or to palpation was present; thus, pain was rated 0/10. Manual muscle testing showed deltoid and rotator cuff muscles at 4+/5, without pain. Medications were being used infrequently for inflammation or pain. Mrs. Smith's home progressive resistive exercise program, using a "green-" and then "blue"-coded Theraband with proprioceptive neuromuscular facilitation (PNF) patterns (D1 and D2 flexion) was reviewed, and she was determined to be independent in its application. She was assessed as having good progress with her program, which she continued at home and in the workplace. She appeared to understand that she was at risk for recurrence of this condition. A formal re-evaluation was to be done in 2 months.

This case illustrates the successful conservative management of an injured older employee. Specific outpatient physical therapy care was provided in the acute and subacute stages of her condition. A detailed home program was instituted for a 3-month period that actively involved the patient in her own recovery and set the stage for prevention of a recurrence. Clinical improvement by natural history of the healing process cannot be ruled out as a significant factor in this case. However, left untreated, it is very possible that this condition would have been exacerbated in the workplace and might have progressed to a chronic painful or frozen shoulder.

SUMMARY

A large proportion of older individuals experience significant physical pain as a result of the aging process and related illness. Fortunately, there is growing interest both in accurate assessment of clinical pain and in conservative pain management for the older patient. When properly applied, conservative treatment interventions exist that have been demonstrated to be either efficacious or effective in the control of pain associated with select problems affecting individuals aged 55 and older. However, given physiological age-related changes, concerns for patient safety and treatment effectiveness require further modifications in many treatment protocols. Additional studies of pain assessment tools, especially for older individuals who have significant cognitive impairments, are warranted. Conservative treatment interventions should continue to be examined both singly and in combination for their effectiveness in managing a wider range of pain-related problems of concern to older individuals.

REFERENCES

1. Abelson K, et al: Transcutaneous electrical nerve stimulation in rheumatoid arthritis. *N Z Med J* 1983; 96:156-158.
2. Aldes JH, Jadeson WJ: Ultrasonic therapy in the treatment of hypertrophic arthritis in elderly patients. *Ann West M & S* 1952; 6:545-550.
3. Allegrante JP: The role of adjunctive therapy in the management of chronic nonmalignant pain. *Am J Med* 1996; 101(suppl 1A):33S-39S.
4. Alon G, DeDomenico G: *High Voltage Stimulation: An Integrated Approach to Clinical Electrotherapy.* Chattanooga, Tenn, Chattanooga Corporation, 1987.
5. American Geriatrics Society, Panel on Chronic Pain in Older Persons: Clinical practice guidelines: The management of chronic pain in older persons. *JAGS* 1998; 46:635-651.
6. *American National Standard for Transcutaneous Electrical Nerve Stimulators. ANSI/AAMI NS4-1985.* Arlington, Va, Association for the Advancement of Medical Instrumentation, 1986.
7. Andersson SA, et al: Evaluation of the pain suppressive effect of different frequencies of peripheral electrical stimulation in chronic pain conditions. *Acta Orthop Scand* 1976; 47:149-157.
8. Barr JO: TENS for chronic low back pain (letter). *New Engl J Med* 1990; 323:1423-1424.
9. Barr JO: Transcutaneous electrical nerve stimulation for pain management, in Nelson RM, Currier DP (eds): *Clinical Electrotherapy,* ed 2. Norwalk, Conn, Appleton & Lange, 1991.
10. Barr JO, et al: Effectiveness of transcutaneous electrical nerve stimulation (TENS) for the elderly with chronic pain (abstract). *Phys Ther* 1989; 69:165.
11. Barr JO, Nielsen DH, Soderberg GL: Investigation of transcutaneous electrical nerve stimulation parameters for altering pain perception. *Phys Ther* 1986; 66:1515-1521.
12. Barr JO: The effect of transcutaneous electrical nerve stimulation parameters on experimentally induced acute pain (abstract). *Phys Ther* 1981; 61:582.
13. Barr JO, et al: Effectiveness and comfort level of transcutaneous electrical nerve stimulation (TENS) in elderly with chronic pain (abstract). *Phys Ther* 1987; 67:775.
14. Barta Kvitek SD, et al: Age bias: Physical therapists and older patients. *J Gerontol* 1986; 41:706-709.
15. Beecher HK: The placebo effect as a nonspecific force surrounding disease and the treatment of disease, in Janzen R (ed): *Pain: Basic Principles, Pharmacology, Therapy.* Baltimore, Williams & Wilkins, 1972.
16. Bell AT: The older athlete, in Sanders B (ed): *Sports Physical Therapy.* Norwalk, Conn, Appleton & Lange, 1990.
17. Bird HA, Dixon JS: The measurement of pain. *Baillieres Clin Rheumatol* 1987; 1:71-89.
18. Boeckstyns MS, Backer M: Reliability and validity of the evaluation of pain in patients with total knee replacement. *Pain* 1989; 38:29-33.
19. Bonica JJ: *Management of pain.* Lecture as visiting professor, Department of Anesthesiology, College of Medicine, University of Iowa, Iowa City, Dec 7, 1988.
20. Bornerman T, Ferrell BR: Ethical issues in pain management. *Clin Geriatr Med* 1996; 12:615-628.
21. Brand RA, Crowinshield RD: The effect of cane use on hip contact force. *Clin Orthop* 1980; 147:181-184.
22. Brody E, Kleban M: Day-to-day mental and physical health symptoms of older people. A report on health logs. *Gerontologist* 1983; 23:75-85.
23. Bulgen DY, et al: Frozen shoulder: Prospective clinical study with an evaluation of three treatment regimens. *Ann Rheum Dis* 1984; 43:353-360.

24. Burke SO, Jerret M: Pain management across age groups. *West J Nurs Res* 1989; 11:164-178.

25. Burton KE, Wright V: Functional assessment. *Br J Rheumatol* 1983; 22(suppl):44-47.

26. Butler R, Gastel B: Care of the aged: Perspectives on pain and discomfort, in Ng L, Bonica J (eds): *Pain, Discomfort and Humanitarian Care.* New York, Elsevier/North-Holland, 1980.

27. Carlsson A: Assessment of chronic pain. I. Aspects of the reliability and validity of the visual analogue scale. *Pain* 1983; 16:87-101.

28. Cauna N: The effects of aging on the receptor organs of the human dermis, in Montogna W (ed): *Aging.* New York, Pergamon Press, 1965.

29. Chapman CR: Measurement of pain: Problems and issues, in Bonica JJ, Albe-Fessard D (eds): *Advances in Pain Research & Therapy,* vol 1. New York, Raven Press, 1976.

30. Chen D, et al: Cardiac pacemaker inhibition by transcutaneous electrical nerve stimulation. *Arch Phys Med Rehabil* 1990; 71:27-30.

31. Clarke GR, et al: Evaluation of physiotherapy in the treatment of osteoarthrosis of the knee. *Rheumatol Rehabil* 1974; 13:190-197.

32. Clarkson PM, Dedrick ME: Exercise-induced muscle damage, repair and adaptation in old and young subjects. *J Gerontol* 1988; 43:M91-96.

33. Cook TM, Barr JO: Instrumentation, in Nelson RM, Currier DP (eds): *Clinical Electrotherapy,* ed 2. Norwalk, Conn, Appleton & Lange, 1991.

34. Cooner E, Amorosi S: *The Study of Pain and Older Americans.* Louis Harris and Associates, New York, 1997.

35. Devor M: Chronic pain in the aged: Possible relation between neurogenesis, involution and pathophysiology in adult sensory ganglia. *J Basic Clin Physiol Pharmacol* 1991; 2:1-15.

36. Deyo RA, et al: A controlled trial of transcutaneous electrical nerve stimulation (TENS) and exercise for chronic low back pain. *New Engl J Med* 1990; 322:1627-1634.

37. Doongaji DR, Vahia VN, Zharucha MPE: On placebos, placebo responses and placebo responders. A review of psychological, psychopharmacological, and psychophysiological factors. II. Psychopharmacological and psychophysiological factors. *J Postgrad Med* 1978; 24:147-157.

38. Downie WW, et al: Studies with pain rating scales. *Ann Rheum Dis* 1978; 37:378-381.

39. Ducroquet R, Ducroquet J, Ducroquet P: *Walking and Limping: A Study of Normal and Pathological Walking.* Philadelphia, JB Lippincott, 1968.

40. Ensrud KE, et al: Correlates of kyphosis in older women. The Fracture Intervention Trial Research Group. *JAGS* 1977; 45:683-687.

41. Faherty BS, Grier MR: Analgesic medication for elderly people postsurgery. *Nurs Res* 1984; 33:369-372.

42. Falck I: Observations on altered patterns of response in old age. *Methods Find Exp Clin Pharmacol* 1987; 9:149-151.

43. Farrell MJ, et al: The impact of dementia on the pain experience. *Pain* 1996; 67:7-15.

44. Feibel A, Fast A: Deep heating of joints: A reconsideration. *Arch Phys Med Rehabil* 1976; 57:513-514.

45. Ferrell BA (ed): *Clinics in Geriatric Medicine: Pain Management.* Philadelphia, WB Saunders, 1996.

46. Ferrell BR: Patient education and nondrug interventions. In Ferrell BR, Ferrell BA (eds): *Pain in the Elderly.* Seattle, IASP Press, 1996.

47. Ferrell BR, Ferrell BA: Easing the pain. *Geriatr Nurs* 1990; 11:175-178.

48. Ferrell BR, Ferrell BA (eds): *Pain in the Elderly.* Seattle, IASP Press, 1996.

49. Fields HL: *Pain.* New York, McGraw-Hill, 1987.

50. Finsen V: Osteoporosis and back pain among the elderly. *Acta Med Scand* 1988; 223:443-449.

51. Finsen V, et al: Transcutaneous electrical nerve stimulation after major amputation. *J Bone Joint Surg* 1988; 70B:109-112.

52. Fischer AA: Advances in documentation of pain and soft tissue pathology. *Med Times* 1983; 12:24-31.

53. Fisher NM, et al: Muscle rehabilitation: Its effect on muscular and functional performance of patients with knee osteoarthritis. *Arch Phys Med Rehabil* 1991; 72:367-374.

54. Follick MJ, et al: Chronic pain: Electromechanical recording device for measuring patients' activity patterns. *Arch Phys Med Rehabil* 1985; 66:75-79.

55. Forrest J: Assessment of acute and chronic pain in older adults. *J Gerontol Nurs* 1995; 21:15-20.

56. Gagliese L, Melzack R: Chronic pain in elderly people. *Pain* 1997; 70:3-14.

57. Gebhart GF: Personal communication, Department of Pharmacology, College of Medicine, University of Iowa, Aug 20, 1998.

58. Gibson SJ, Farrell MJ, Katz B, Helme RD: Multidisciplinary management of chronic nonmalignant pain in older adults. In Ferrell BR, Ferrell BA (eds): *Pain in the Elderly.* Seattle, IASP Press, 1996

59. Gibson SJ, et al: Pain in older persons. *Disabl Rehabil* 1994; 16:127-139.

60. Griffin JE, Karselis TC: *Physical Agents for Physical Therapists,* ed 2. Springfield, Ill, Charles C Thomas, 1982.

61. Hamer J, Kirk JA: Physiotherapy and the frozen shoulder: A comparative trial of ice and ultrasonic therapy. *N Z Med J* 1976; 83:191-192.

62. Hamilton M: *Lectures on the Methodology of Clinical Research,* ed 2. Edinburgh, Scotland, Churchill Livingstone, 1974.

63. Harkins SW: Geriatric pain. Pain perceptions in the old. *Clin Geriatr Med* 1996; 12:435-459.

64. Harkins SW, Kwentus J, Price DD: Pain and the elderly, in Benedetti C, Chapman RC, Moricca G (eds): *Advances in Pain Research and Therapy,* vol 7. New York, Raven Press, 1984.

65. Helling DK, et al: Medication use characteristics in the elderly: The Iowa 65+ rural health study. *J Am Geriatr Soc* 1987; 35:4-12.

66. Helme RD, et al: Can psychometric tools be used to analyze pain in a geriatric population? *Clin Exp Neurol* 1989; 26:113-117.

67. Helme RD, et al: Multidisciplinary clinics for older people: Do they have a role? *Clin Geriatr Med* 1996; 12:563-582.

68. Herr KA, Mobily PR: Comparison of selected pain assessment tools for use with the elderly. *Appl Nurs Res* 1993; 6:39-46.

69. Herr KA, Mobily PR: Complexities of pain assessment in the elderly: Clinical considerations. *J Gerontol Nurs* 1991; 17:12-19.

70. Herr KA, et al: Evaluation of the faces pain scale for use with elderly. *Clin J Pain* 1998; 14:29-38.

71. Horvath SM, Hollander JL: Intra-articular temperature as a measure of joint reaction. *J Clin Invest* 1949; 28:469-473.

72. Hunt TE: Management of chronic non-rheumatic pain in the elderly. *J Am Geriatr Soc* 1976; 24:402-406.

73. Huskisson EC: Measurement of pain. *Lancet* 1974; 2(4889):1127-1131.

74. Huskisson EC: Visual analogue scales, in Melzack R (ed): *Pain Measurement and Assessment.* New York, Raven Press, 1983.

75. Huskisson EC, Jones J, Scott PJ: Application of visual analogue scales to the measurement of functional capacity. *Rheumatol Rehabil* 1976; 15:185-187.

76. Jamison RN, Virts KL: The influence of family support on chronic pain. *Behav Res Ther* 1990; 28:283-287.

77. Jensen MP, Karoly P, Braver S: The measurement of clinical pain intensity: A comparison of six methods. *Pain* 1986; 27:117-126.

78. Jones SL: Electromagnetic field interference and cardiac pacemakers. *Phys Ther* 1976; 56:1013-1018.

79. Kauffman T: Thermoregulation and use of heat and cold, in Littrup Jackson O (ed): *Therapeutic Considerations for the Elderly.* New York, Churchill Livingstone, 1987.

80. Keefe FJ, et al: Pain coping strategies and coping efficacy in rheumatoid arthritis: A daily process analysis. *Pain* 1997; 69:35-42.

81. Keefe FJ, et al: Pain in older adults: A cognitive-behavioral perspective, in Ferrell BR, Ferrell, BA (eds): *Pain in the Elderly.* Seattle, IASP Press, 1996.

82. Keefe FJ, Williams DA: A comparison of coping strategies in chronic pain patients in different age groups. *J Gerontol* 1990; 45:P161-P165.

83. Klemp P, et al: Reduced blood flow in fibromyotic muscles during ultrasound therapy. *Scand J Rehabil Med* 1982; 15:21-23.

84. Kloth L, Morrison MA, Ferguson BH: *Therapeutic Microwave and Shortwave Diathermy. A Review of Thermal Effectiveness, Safe Use, and State of the Art.* HHS Publication FDA 85-8237. Rockville, Md, US Department of Health and Human Services, 1984.

85. Knight KL: *Cryotherapy: Theory, Technique, and Physiology.* Chattanooga, Tenn, Chattanooga Corporation, 1985.

86. Kovar PA, et al: Supervised fitness walking in patients with osteoarthritis of the knee. A randomized controlled trial. *Ann Intern Med* 1992; 116:529-534.

87. Kremer E, Atkinson JH, Ignelzi RJ: Measurement of pain: Patient preference does not confound pain measurement. *Pain* 1981; 10:241-248.

88. Krupa LR, Vener AM: Hazards of drug use among the elderly. *Gerontologist* 1979; 19:90-94.

89. Kwentus JA, et al: Current concepts of geriatric pain and its treatment. *Geriatrics* 1985; 40:48-57.

90. Langley GB, Sheppeard H: Transcutaneous electrical nerve stimulation (TNS) and its relationship to placebo therapy: A review. *N Z Med J* 1987; 100:215-217.

91. Langley GB, et al: The analgesic effects of transcutaneous electrical nerve stimulation and placebo in chronic pain patients. A double blind non-crossover comparison. *Rheumatol Int* 1984; 4:119-123.

92. Lavsky-Shulan M, et al: Prevalence and functional correlates of low back pain in the elderly: The Iowa 65+ rural health study. *J Am Geriatr Soc* 1985; 33:23-28.

93. Lehmann JF (ed): *Therapeutic Heat and Cold,* ed 3. Baltimore, Williams & Wilkins, 1982.

94. Leijon G, Boivie J: Central post-stroke pain—the effect of high and low frequency TENS. *Pain* 1989; 38:187-191.

95. Leo KC: Use of electrical stimulation at acupuncture points for the treatment of reflex sympathetic dystrophy in a child. A case report. *Phys Ther* 1983; 63:957-959.

96. Leo KC, et al: Effect of transcutaneous electrical nerve stimulation characteristics on clinical pain. *Phys Ther* 1986; 66:200-205.

97. Leseberg KA, Schunk C: TENS and geriatrics. *Clin Manage Phys Ther* 1990; 10(6):23-25.

98. Levi SJ, Maihafer GC: Traditional approaches to pain, in Echternach JL (ed): *Pain. Clinics in Physical Therapy,* vol 12. New York, Churchill Livingstone, 1987.

99. Levy A, et al: Transcutaneous electrical nerve stimulation in experimental acute arthritis. *Arch Phys Med Rehabil* 1987; 68:75-78.

100. Lewis D, Lewis B, Sturrock RD: Transcutaneous electrical nerve stimulation in osteoarthritis: A therapeutic alternative? *Ann Rheum Dis* 1984; 43:47-49.

101. Liang MH, Fortin P: The management of osteoarthritis of the hip and knees (editorial). *New Engl J Med* 1991; 325:125-127.

102. Linzer M, Long DM: Transcutaneous neural stimulation for relief of pain. *IEEE Trans Biomed Eng* 1976; 23:341-344.

103. Lorig K, Holman H: Arthritis self-management studies: A twelve-year review. *Health Educ Q* 1993; 20:17-28.

104. Mannheimer C, Carlsson CA: The analgesic effect of transcutaneous electrical nerve stimulation (TNS) in patients with rheumatoid arthritis. A comparative study of different pulse patterns. *Pain* 1979; 6:329-334.

105. Mannheimer JS, Lampe GN: *Clinical Transcutaneous Electrical Nerve Stimulation.* Philadelphia, FA Davis, 1984.

106. Melzack R: *The Puzzle of Pain.* New York, Basic Books, 1973.

107. Melzack R: The McGill pain questionnaire: Major properties and scoring methods. *Pain* 1975; 1:277-299.

108. Melzack R (ed): *Pain Measurement and Assessment.* New York, Raven Press, 1983.

109. Melzack R: The short form McGill pain questionnaire. *Pain* 1987; 30:191-197.

110. Melzack R, Katz J: Pain measurement in persons in pain, in Wall PD, Melzack R (eds): *Textbook of Pain,* ed 3. Edinburg, Scotland, Churchill Livingstone, 1994.

111. Merskey H (ed): Classification of chronic pain. Descriptions of chronic pain syndromes and definitions of pain terms. *Pain* 1986; (suppl 3):S1-S226.

112. Michlovitz SL: *Thermal Agents in Rehabilitation,* ed 2. Philadelphia, FA Davis, 1990.

113. Middaugh SJ, et al: Chronic pain: Its treatment in geriatric and younger patients. *Arch Phys Med Rehabil* 1988; 69:1021-1026.

114. Middaugh SJ, et al: Biofeedback-assisted relaxation training for the aging chronic pain patient. *Biofeedback Self Regul* 1991; 16:361-377.

115. Miller BA, et al: A comparison of modulated-rate and conventional TENS (abstract). *Phys Ther* 1984; 64:744.

116. Minor MA, et al: Efficacy of physical conditioning exercise in patients with rheumatoid arthritis and osteoarthritis. *Arthritis Rheum* 1989; 32:1396-1405.

117. Morgan J, Furst DE: Implications of drug therapy in the elderly. *Clin Rheum Dis* 1986; 12:227-244.

118. Moritani T, deVries HA: Potential for gross muscle hypertrophy in older men. *J Gerontol* 1980; 35:672-682.

119. Moskovich R: Neck pain in the elderly: Common causes and management. *Geriatrics* 1988; 43:65-70, 77, 81-82, 85-90.

120. Myers DB, Grennan DM, Palmer DG: Hand grip function in patients with rheumatoid arthritis. *Arch Phys Med Rehabil* 1980; 61:369-373.

121. Nation EM, Warfield CA: Pain in the elderly. *Hosp Pract* 1989; 24:113, 117-118.

122. Nelson RM, Currier DP (eds): *Clinical Electrotherapy,* ed 2. Norwalk, Conn, Appleton & Lange, 1987.

123. Nolan MF: *A Chronological Indexing of the Clinical and Basic Science Literature Concerning Transcutaneous Electrical Nerve Stimulation (TENS) 1967-1987.* Section on Clinical Electrophysiology. Alexandria, Va, American Physical Therapy Association, 1988.

124. Nguyen DM: The role of physical medicine and rehabilitation in pain management. *Clin Geriatr Med* 1996; 12:517-529.

125. Ohnhaus EE, Adler R: Methodological problems in the measurement of pain. A comparison between the verbal rating scale and the visual analogue scale. *Pain* 1975; 1:379-384.

126. Olin BR, et al (eds): *Drug Facts and Comparisons.* St Louis, JB Lippincott, 1989.

127. Paris DL, Bayres F, Gucker B: Effects of the neuroprobe in the treatment of second-degree ankle inversion sprains. *Phys Ther* 1983; 63:35-40.

128. Parmalee PA: Pain in cognitively impaired older persons. *Clin Geriatr Med* 1996; 12:473-487.

129. Pasero CL, McCaffery M: How aging affects pain management. *Amer J Nurs* 1998; 98:12-13.

130. Pochaczevsky R: Assessment of back pain by contact thermography of extremity dermatomes. *Orthop Rev* 1983; 12:45-58.

131. Portenoy RK: Optimal pain control in elderly cancer patients. *Geriatrics* 1987; 42:33-41.

132. Portenoy RK, Farkash A: Practical management of non-malignant pain in the elderly. *Geriatrics* 1988; 43:29-40, 44-47.

133. Puett DW, Griffin MR: Published trials of nonmedicinal and noninvasive therapies for hip and knee osteoarthritis. *Ann Intern Med* 1994; 121:133-140.

134. Rene J, et al: Reduction of joint pain in patients with knee osteoarthritis who have received monthly telephone calls from lay personnel and whose medical treatment regimens have remained stable. *Arthritis Rheum* 1992; 35:511-515.

135. Roberto KA: Chronic pain in the lives of older women. *J Am Med Womens Assoc* 1997; 52:127-131.

136. Robinson D, et al: Relation of sex and aging to monoamine oxidase activity of human brain plasma and platelets. *Arch Gen Psychiatry* 1971; 24:536-539.

137. Rooney SM, et al: A comparison of pulmonary function tests for postthoracotomy pain using cryoanalgesia and transcutaneous nerve stimulation. *Ann Thorac Surg* 1986; 41:204-207.

138. Roy R, Thomas MR: A survey of chronic pain in an elderly population. *Can Fam Physician* 1986; 32:513-516.

139. Roy R, Thomas MR: Elderly persons with and without pain: A comparative study. *Clin J Pain* 1987; 3:102-106.

140. Sanders SH: Toward a practical system for the automatic measurement of "up time" in chronic pain patients. *Pain* 1980; 9:103-109.

141. Scott J, Huskisson EC: Graphic representation of pain. *Pain* 1976; 2:175-184.

142. Shurr DG, Cook TM: *Prosthetics and Orthotics.* Norwalk, Conn, Appleton & Lange, 1990.

143. Singh NA, Clements KM, Fiatrone MA: A randomized controlled trial of progressive resistance training in depressed elders. *J Gerontol: Med Sci* 1997; 52A:M27-M35.

144. Smidt GL, et al: Assessment of abdominal and back extensor function. A quantitative approach and results for chronic low-back pain patients. *Spine* 1983; 8:211-219.

145. Smith MJ, Hutchins RC, Hehenberger D: Transcutaneous neural stimulation use in postoperative knee rehabilitation. *Am J Sports Med* 1983; 11:75-82.

146. Smyth NPD, et al: The pacemaker patient and the electromagnetic environment. *JAMA* 1974; 227:1412.

147. Snyder-Mackler L, Robinson AJ: *Clinical Electrophysiology: Electrotherapy and Electrophysiological Testing.* Baltimore, Williams & Wilkins, 1989.

148. Sorkin BA, et al: Chronic pain in old and young patients: Differences appear less important than similarities. *J Gerontol* 1990; 45:P64-P68.

149. Sternbach R: *Pain: A Psychophysiological Analysis.* New York, Academic Press, 1968.

150. Sternbach R: Evaluation of pain relief. *Surg Neurol* 1975; 4:199-201.

151. Sternbach RA: Psychophysiology of pain. *Int J Psychiatry Med* 1975; 6:63-73.

152. Sternbach RA, et al: Measuring the severity of clinical pain, in Bonica JJ (ed): *Advances in Neurology,* vol 4. New York, Raven Press, 1974.

153. Svarcova J, Trnasky K, Zvarova J: The influence of ultrasound, galvanic currents and shortwave diathermy on pain intensity in patients with osteoarthritis. *Scand J Rheumatol Suppl* 1988; 67:83-85.

154. Swezey R: Low back pain in the elderly: Practical management concerns. *Geriatrics* 1988; 43:39-44.

155. Tappan RM: *Healing Massage Techniques: Holistic, Classic, and Emerging Methods,* ed 2. Norwalk, Conn, Appleton & Lange, 1988.

156. Thorsteinsson G: Chronic pain: Use of TENS in the elderly. *Geriatrics* 1987; 42:75-77, 81- 82.

157. Tierney LM, McPhee SJ, Papadakis MA (eds): *Current Medical Diagnosis and Treatment,* ed 36. Stamford, Conn, Appleton & Lange, 1997.

158. Travel JG, Simons DG: *Myofascial Pain and Dysfunction. The Trigger Point Manual.* Baltimore, Williams & Wilkins, 1983.

159. Tyler E, Caldwell C, Ghia JN: Transcutaneous electrical nerve stimulation: An alternative approach to the management of postoperative pain. *Anesth Analg* 1982; 61:449-456.

160. Verrillo RT: Age related changes in the sensitivity to vibration. *J Gerontol* 1980; 35:185-193.

161. Wall PD: The gate control theory of pain mechanisms. A re-examination and re-statement. *Brain* 1978; 101:1-18.

162. Wall PD, Melzack R: *Textbook of Pain,* ed 3. New York, Churchill Livingstone, 1994.

163. Wall RT: Use of analgesics in the elderly. *Clin Geriatr Med* 1990; 6:345-364.

164. Walsh TD, Leber B: Measurement of chronic pain: Visual analog scales and McGill Melzack pain questionnaire compared, in Bonica JJ, Lindblom U, Iggo A (eds): *Advances in Pain Research and Therapy,* vol 5. New York, Raven Press, 1983.

165. Weiner D, et al: Pain measurement in elders with chronic low back pain: Traditional and alternative approaches. *Pain* 1996; 67:461-467.

166. Wewers ME, Lowe NK: A critical review of visual analogue scales in the measurement of clinical phenomena. *Res Nurs Health* 1990; 13:227-236.

167. Williams J, Harvey J, Tannebaum H: Use of superficial heat vs ice for the rheumatoid arthritic shoulder: A pilot study. *Physiother Can* 1986; 38:8-13.

168. Witte M: Pain control. *J Gerontol Nurs* 1989; 15:32-37.

169. Witters D, Lapp A, Hinckley SM: A descriptive study of transcutaneous electrical nerve stimulation devices and their electrical output characteristics. *J Clin Electrophysiol* 1991; 3:9-16.

170. Wolf SL, Basmajian JV: Intramuscular temperature changes deep to localized cutaneous cold stimulation. *Phys Ther* 1973; 53:1284-1288.

171. Wolf SL, Gersh MR, Rao VR: Examination of electrode placements and stimulating parameters in treating chronic pain with conventional transcutaneous electrical nerve stimulation (TENS). *Pain* 1981; 11:37-47.

172. Workman BS, Ciccone V, Christophidis N: Pain management for the elderly. *Aust Fam Physician* 1989; 18:1515-1521, 1524-1525, 1527.

173. Wright GE, et al: Age, depressive symptoms, and rheumatoid arthritis. *Arthritis Rheum* 1998; 41:298-305.

174. Wright V: Treatment of osteoarthritis of the knees. *Ann Rheum Dis* 1964; 23:389-391.

175. Zacharkow D: *Posture: Sitting, Standing, Chair Design and Exercise.* Springfield, Ill, Charles C Thomas, 1988.

176. Zimmerman M: Peripheral and central nervous mechanisms of nociception, pain and pain therapy, in Bonica JJ, Liebeskind JC, Albe-Fessard DG (eds): *Advances in Pain Research and Therapy,* vol 3. New York, Raven Press, 1979.

CHAPTER 24

CHRONIC DERMAL WOUNDS IN OLDER ADULTS

Rita A. Wong, PT, EdD

INTRODUCTION

Advanced Age and Chronic Dermal Wounds

Chronic dermal wounds occur most commonly in the older population. This higher prevalence in the elderly corresponds to a higher proportion of older adults who have health problems commonly associated with increased risk of ulcer development and delayed wound healing: (1) peripheral circulatory diseases (either arterial or venous), (2) diabetes mellitus, and (3) hypertension. Frail elders, with multiple medical problems and decreased activity level, often have numerous risk factors for developing dermal wounds and for delayed wound healing. Box 24-1 lists factors commonly associated with delayed wound healing.

Normal Age-Related Changes in Wound Healing

Current research indicates that healthy older adults experience a somewhat slower rate of wound healing than younger persons[12,13,60,144] but that the quality of the wound scar may actually be better in the healthy older person.[11-13,144] Normal age-related changes in skin, immune system, and microcirculation are believed to influence the rate of wound healing, although the exact mechanisms are unclear.[11,14,60,144] Overwhelmingly, the individual with a chronic dermal wound is not simply "old." This individual has an illness or injury related to one or more of the risk factors identified in Box 24-1. It is the presence of the disease state, not old age, that leads to markedly delayed wound healing (chronic wounds). The inability of a dermal wound to heal represents a pathological state that warrants vigorous intervention and should not be considered a "normal" consequence of the aging process.

Normal Tissue-Healing Process

When a tissue is injured, the body's natural response is to activate the inflammatory process. This process guides each sequential step of tissue repair and protects the wound against invading microorganisms.[123] The *acute inflammatory phase* is an essential first step in tissue repair, usually lasting about 2 days, and is carefully orchestrated to provide the correct physiological stimulus for the level of injury. If an inadequate inflammatory response occurs, the healing process will be delayed; if an excessive response occurs, enhanced scarring can occur. Typically, the tissue moves into the *prolifera-*

tive phase within about 3 days of onset of injury. In this stage, wound contraction and epithelialization occur. In the final stage of wound repair, the *remodeling stage,* the wound is no longer open. The connective tissue, which is usually laid down in a fairly random manner in the proliferative stage, becomes better aligned with the stresses put upon it, resulting in a strong, pliable scar. This process can take up to 1 year to complete. As discussed previously, in the absence of pathology, the healing time for older adults is slightly longer than for younger adults, and the quality of the scar should be generally similar (if not better) than scars of younger adults.[12,13] Comorbid disease states may affect both the rate of wound healing and the quality of the scar tissue.

Wound Classification

In general, chronic dermal wounds are classified according to the predominant underlying cause of their occurrence: arterial insufficiency, venous insufficiency, pressure (decubitus), and neuropathy (insensitivity). For a given patient, an ulcer may fit into more than one classification category. Ulcers are also categorized according to their severity. Two different classification systems are commonly used. The more general classification, often associated with pressure and venous insufficiency ulcers, assigns the ulcer to one of four stages dependent on the depth of the ulcer (Table 24-1).[116] An alternative system, described by Wagner and often associated with neuropathic and arterial insufficiency ulcers, considers depth of the ulcer as well as the health of the surrounding tissues (Table 24-2).[147]

This chapter discusses the epidemiology, etiology, and clinical signs and symptoms for each of the four general causes of chronic ulcers: arterial insufficiency, venous insufficiency, pressure induced, and neuropathy. Tests used to identify high-risk patients are described as well as general treatment approaches and interventions.

TABLE 24-1
NATIONAL PRESSURE ULCER ADVISORY PANEL'S CLASSIFICATION SYSTEM FOR PRESSURE ULCERS

STAGE	DESCRIPTION
Stage 1	Non-blanchable erythema of intact skin. In individuals with darker skin, discoloration of skin, warmth, edema, induration, or hardness also may be indicators.
Stage 2	Partial-thickness skin loss involving epidermis, dermis, or both.
Stage 3	Full-thickness skin loss involving damage to or necrosis of subcutaneous tissue that may extend down to, but not through, underlying fascia.
Stage 4	Full-thickness skin loss with extensive destruction; tissue necrosis; or damage to muscle, bone, or supporting structures.

From Panel for the Prediction and Prevention of Pressure Ulcers: Pressure Ulcers in Adults: Prediction and Prevention. *Clinical Practice Guideline No. 3, AHCPR Publication No. 92-0047.* Rockville, MD, Agency for Health Care Policy and Research, US Public Health Service, US Department of Health and Human Services, 1992.

Regardless of the underlying cause of the ulcer, the general treatment approach includes removal of risk factors that impede the normal healing process (see Box 24-1), augmentation of normal wound healing, and prevention of injury recurrence.[52,145] The final section of the chapter identifies common physical therapy interventions for the treatment of dermal wounds, reviews the rationale for their use, and discusses any special considerations when applying these interventions to older adults. The ultimate goal of intervention is complete closure of the wound with a strong, resilient scar.

Wound Examination

Examination of the patient with a chronic dermal wound includes identifying and quantifying factors that contribute to wound development and/or delayed wound healing as well as obtaining objective information about the wound itself. Examination activities can be organized into three broad categories: (1) medical and social history; (2) review of related physiological systems, e.g., cardiopulmonary and vascular, musculoskeletal, neuromuscular; and (3) objective tests and measures of the integument, including wound characteristics, and quantification of factors contributing to

---

BOX 24-1
FACTORS THAT MAY DELAY WOUND HEALING

1. Inadequate blood supply to the wound
2. Wound infection
3. Inadequate nutrition
4. Adherent scab or eschar
5. Wound edema
6. Venous hypertension
7. Anemia
8. Cigarette smoking
9. Systemic hypertension
10. Decreased capillary membrane diffusion
11. Increased blood glucose levels
12. Medications—steroids, certain immunosuppressive drugs, high doses of antimicrobial agents (e.g., >0.001% povidone-iodine; >0.5% sodium hypochlorite)

From Feedar J, Kloth L: Conservative management of chronic wounds, in Kloth L, McCulloch J, Feedar J (eds): *Wound Healing: Alternatives in Management.* Philadelphia, FA Davis, 1990.

TABLE 24-2
WAGNER CLASSIFICATION SYSTEM OF ULCER STAGES

STAGE	DESCRIPTION
0	Intact skin
1	Superficial ulcer involving skin only
2	Deep ulcer involving muscle and, perhaps, bone and joint structures
3	Localized infection—may be abscess or osteomyelitis
4	Gangrene, limited to forefoot area
5	Gangrene of the majority of the foot

wound development and delayed wound healing, such as circulatory insufficiencies or sensory deficits.[9,102,140]

The *Guide to Physical Therapist Practice* identifies the general tests and measures applicable to the physical therapy management of patients with integumentary system dysfunction.[9]

Treatment approach will be influenced by the wound characteristics. Therefore, the general appearance of the wound should be noted. Is the wound open or closed? If it is open, what color is the tissue? Is granulation tissue evident? Does the wound look clean and free of necrotic tissue and pus? Is there any drainage from the wound? If yes, is the drainage clear and thin, purulent and thick, or bloody? How much drainage is there? A wound culture should be taken from the deepest part of the wound, not simply from the surface tissue.

If the wound is covered, what is covering it? Is it covered by thick, crusty material; tightly adherent eschar; thick, purulent material; or healthy granulation tissue? Adherent eschar, purulent materials, and necrotic tissue need to be removed for wound healing to progress. Wound infection needs to be eliminated, and excessive fluid loss needs to be brought under control.

What is the size and depth of the wound? The external dimensions of the wound can be reliably traced by placing a material such as transparent acetate sheets, plastic wrap, or sterile x-ray film against the wound and tracing its outline.[101,102,140] Graph paper can then be used to calculate the approximate size of the wound. The depth of the wound can be determined by placing a sterile, cotton-tipped probe into the wound and recording the depth of penetration of the probe. A detailed discussion of wound examination procedures can be found in recent wound management texts by Sussman and Gogia.[102,140]

The Health Care Team

Physical therapists working with patients with chronic dermal wounds are usually working as part of an interdisciplinary team. Each team member brings unique skills and knowledge. The team may include, but is not limited to, a family practitioner or other physician, vascular surgeon, nurse, dietitian, physical therapist, occupational therapist, orthotist, and podiatrist. One team member is often identified as the "case manager." This individual coordinates services among the multitude of health care team members involved in the patient's care. The physical therapist may serve in this role in some health care settings.

The family practitioner (or internist) will evaluate and treat the patient for general medical conditions that may impede the overall healing process. A vascular surgeon will determine the location and severity of vascular insufficiencies and the appropriateness of various surgical approaches for re-establishing more normal vascular hemodynamics (either arterial or venous) as well as the need for skin grafting to close the wound. Nursing will develop and implement a care plan to monitor the wound environment; minimize risk factors for delayed wound healing; and make dressing changes

as needed to maintain a clean, healthy tissue environment supportive to healing. A dietitian should plan the specific dietary needs of the patient to ensure adequate nutritional support during the healing process. Other health professionals can be consulted as needed, depending on the patient's specific needs. For example, an orthotist may fabricate appropriate footwear for the patient with an ulcer on the foot.

The role of physical therapy can be very narrow and focused (providing one specific direct intervention in concert with a broad team involvement) or quite broad (serving as case manager, coordinating services, and providing multiple interventions). Through the use of physical agents, gait modifications, selective therapeutic exercise activities, functional training, and patient education, physical therapists provide important augmentation of the healing process. The physical therapist's role in the interdisciplinary team must always be considered in the overall treatment planning.

Additionally, both patient and care-givers must become an integral part of the health care team because the healing of a chronic dermal wound is a long-term process. Both care-givers and the patient need to understand the purpose of each intervention, accurately and consistently follow through with all patient and family-directed interventions, and recognize inappropriate treatment responses.

Good communication between all members of the team is essential. Each team member should understand the unique perspective of other members of the team and work to build a consistent, effective overall treatment approach. Since the purpose of this chapter is to address the specific role of physical therapy in wound management, the specific activities of other team members have only been mentioned briefly. This does not imply less value for the role of other team members but simply reflects the main focus of the chapter.

CHRONIC DERMAL WOUNDS FROM ARTERIAL INSUFFICIENCY

Epidemiology

Arteriosclerosis obliterans (ASO) represents about 90% to 95% of all cases of chronic occlusive arterial disease.[50,105] ASO is also known as *atherosclerotic vascular disease* and *obliterative arteriosclerosis*. Most dermal ulcers associated with arterial insufficiency are secondary to ASO.[50] Ulcers related to ASO indicate a severe compromise of local circulation and thus tissue nutrition. Typically, the distal foot, particularly the tips of the toes, is the first area to undergo ischemic damage.

ASO affects men more commonly than women, and prevalence increases with age. Paris and colleagues in a study of nursing home residents found that 35% of the subjects who were between 76 and 80 years old had significant arterial disease.[117] This number gradually increased with increasing age. Approximately 65% of patients older than 90 had significant arterial disease. Petermans evaluated 261 older adults admitted to one acute care hospital in Belgium for medical problems not associated with vascular disease.[118]

In this sample, with a mean age of 81, 58% were found to have ASO.

Etiology

The formation of atherosclerotic plaques begins in childhood with the laying down of fatty streaks within the intimal wall of the medium and large arteries. Over time, fibrous plaques develop. The progression to atherosclerotic vessel occlusion with onset of symptoms generally occurs very slowly over many decades.[50,75] The body accommodates to this chronic, slowly progressive decrease in perfusion by producing collateral circulation in the area served by the occluded vessel and by decreasing peripheral vessel resistance so that blood can pass through the artery more easily. These adaptations delay the onset of ischemic symptoms until substantial narrowing of the lumen of the vessel occurs.[84,105]

In the person with severe arterial insufficiency, minor trauma can result in a non-healing ulcer. Tissue injury from a poorly fitting shoe, an ingrown toenail, or stubbing one's toe are examples of situations that can lead to a serious dermal wounds in the person with ASO. In this individual, the increased oxygen demand that accompanies the normal inflammatory response to tissue injury may go unmet due to the inability to increase blood flow into the area. Unmet oxygen demands lead to further tissue ischemia and, eventually, cell death.

Risk factors for the development of ASO include cigarette smoking, diabetes mellitus, high intake of saturated fats, being male, and sedentary life-style.[50,76,87,117] Although the exact mechanism through which cigarette smoking exacerbates ASO is unknown, it is clear that individuals who smoke at least 20 cigarettes per day have much greater risk of developing symptomatic ASO than do non-smokers.[37,87,91,105] The elimination of cigarette smoking is very important in controlling the progression of ASO. One recent large prospective study suggests that non-smokers who consume moderate amounts of alcohol (seven glasses per week) are at lower risk of peripheral arterial disease than individuals who have less than one drink per week.[37] Smokers, however, do not receive a circulatory benefit from moderate alcohol consumption. The negative circulatory effects of cigarette smoking cannot be counteracted with moderate alcohol consumption.

Individuals with hypertension have a greater risk of complications from ASO than do non-hypertensive persons.[50,75] In patients with diabetes mellitus a high association between peripheral vascular insufficiency and distal lower extremity neuropathy exists.[61,65] Lower extremity neuropathy is a major contributing factor to the development of foot ulcers of patients with diabetes. The vascular insufficiency that occurs concurrently with neuropathy in many patients with diabetes appears to be a key factor in delayed healing (or non-healing) of neuropathic ulcers.[61,65] Neuropathic ulcers are discussed later in this chapter.

Clinical Signs and Symptoms of ASO in the Elderly

Older adults, particularly those older than 70, may have atypical presentation of ASO. It is common in the elderly to have substantial pathology, even leading to gangrene of the part, without any complaints of intermittent claudication—one of the first and most commonly observed signs of ASO in the younger population.[76] Intermittent claudication pain stems from inadequate blood flow through the exercising muscle. This pain is usually felt in the calf but can occur in the thigh, hip, or buttocks.[127] The pain is first noted during ambulation and, characteristically, quickly disappears once the person sits down and stops contracting the involved muscles.

Older patients may complain that their legs feel heavy or cold, rather than painful, with ambulation. Characteristic changes in the skin below the level of circulatory compromise are commonly observed. Ulcers may develop on the toes (Fig. 24-1).

Objective Tests for Arterial Insufficiency

Noninvasive hemodynamic assessment of blood flow can be done through flow-detecting Doppler ultrasound, volume-detecting plethysmography, or tissue oxygen tension tests ($TcpO_2$). Doppler ultrasound is a simple, reliable, noninvasive test of arterial circulation. The frequency of the ultrasound unit is such that the pattern of sound waves reflected from the moving blood provides a very sensitive indicator of blood flow in the area being sonated. The test is performed by first occluding blood flow to the lower leg with a blood pressure cuff. The ultrasound is applied as the cuff deflates, and the systolic pressure is recorded.[105,140] Meaningful values are obtained by comparing the blood pressure response of the arm with that of the ankle, creating the ankle/arm, or the ankle/brachial, index (ABI). In young adults the ratio of ankle to arm pressure is 1:1, giving a pressure "index" of "1." In normal older adults the ankle pressure may be slightly higher than the arm pressure, thus increasing the index to slightly greater than 1. However, an ABI greater than 1.1 may indicate calcific changes in arterial walls that impede compression of the vessel and thus greatly decrease the accuracy of the test.

Although researchers and clinical experts differ somewhat in their interpretation of critical values of the ABI, the following are general guidelines. An ABI of less than 0.9 is suggestive of vascular disease.[117,140] It is commonly believed that a value less than 0.7 or 0.75 confirms arterial disease and is associated with intermittent claudication.[44,57,117] A value less than 0.4 to 0.5 indicates severe impairment, is usually associated with rest pain, and serves as an indicator for avoiding exercise to the involved limb.[57,105,140] An ABI of greater than 0.45 is believed necessary for a foot ulcer to heal.[22] An ABI of less than 0.25 is associated with ischemic ulceration and impending gangrene.[57]

Transcutaneous tissue oxygen tension tests measure the partial pressure of oxygen across the skin when the skin is heated to a pre-determined level (typically 43° to 44° C). When the skin is warm, the transcutaneous oxygen value has been found to closely approximate the blood value.[102,132] The test has limited reliability in the presence of infection or edema.[132]

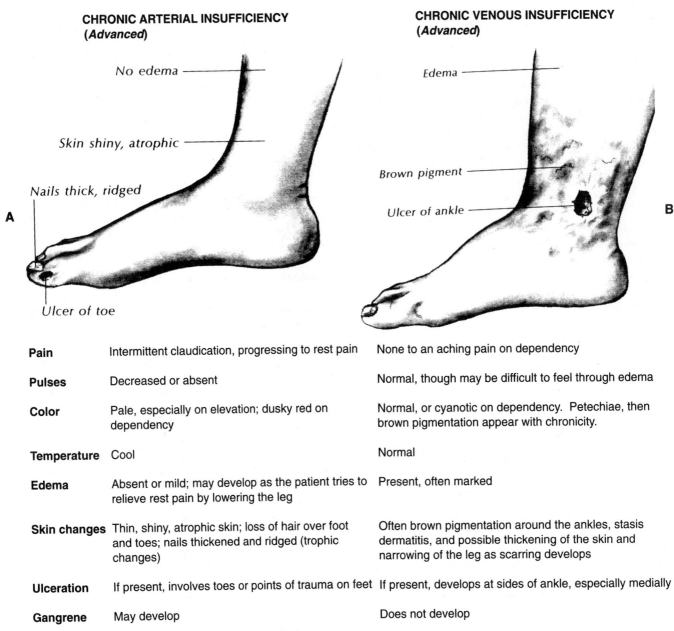

CHRONIC ARTERIAL INSUFFICIENCY
(*Advanced*)

No edema

Skin shiny, atrophic

Nails thick, ridged

A

Ulcer of toe

CHRONIC VENOUS INSUFFICIENCY
(*Advanced*)

Edema

Brown pigment

Ulcer of ankle

B

Pain	Intermittent claudication, progressing to rest pain	None to an aching pain on dependency
Pulses	Decreased or absent	Normal, though may be difficult to feel through edema
Color	Pale, especially on elevation; dusky red on dependency	Normal, or cyanotic on dependency. Petechiae, then brown pigmentation appear with chronicity.
Temperature	Cool	Normal
Edema	Absent or mild; may develop as the patient tries to relieve rest pain by lowering the leg	Present, often marked
Skin changes	Thin, shiny, atrophic skin; loss of hair over foot and toes; nails thickened and ridged (trophic changes)	Often brown pigmentation around the ankles, stasis dermatitis, and possible thickening of the skin and narrowing of the leg as scarring develops
Ulceration	If present, involves toes or points of trauma on feet	If present, develops at sides of ankle, especially medially
Gangrene	May develop	Does not develop

FIG. 24-1   Characteristics of chronic insufficiency of (**A**) arteries and (**B**) veins. (From Bates B: *Guide to Physical Examination and History Taking*, ed 4. Philadelphia, JB Lippincott, 1997. Used by permission.)

Arteriography is the most invasive of the evaluative procedures and is usually reserved for patients for whom vascular reconstructive surgery is contemplated. Arteriography requires the injection of radiopaque dye into an artery with subsequent radiographic visualization of restrictions to the flow of dye through the arteries. This is considered to be a very reliable method of evaluating the specific location and severity of the vascular occlusions.

General Treatment Approaches

When the dermal wound is triggered by arterial insufficiency, improving arterial circulation as well as eliminating risk factors for delayed wound healing (see Box 24-1) take

priority. Arterial bypass surgery, endarterectomy, and percutaneous transluminal angioplasty with or without placement of endovascular stent are frequently utilized.[141] Arterially insufficient chronic dermal wounds do not usually occur until the occlusion is severe, potentially threatening limb viability. If the ABI is less than 0.45 or substantial gangrene is present, the probability of wound healing with conservative intervention is low. Therefore, surgical intervention for the reestablishment of blood flow through the occluded segment usually takes precedence at this time. Surgical intervention is the treatment of choice if the patient has no substantial contraindications to surgery and the location of the occlusion is amenable to this intervention.[50,141] These procedures com-

Table 24-3

Summary of Physical Therapy Modalities for Wound Healing

Therapeutic Modality	Treatment Goals	Physiological Effects of Modality	Expected Treatment Outcome			
			Arterial	Venous	Pressure	Neuropathic
Low-intensity electrical stimulation	Augment wound healing ↓Wound infection	Stimulate endogenous bioelectrical activity Bactericidal	+	+ +	+ +	?
Compression devices Dressings Elastic bandages Elastic stockings Pumps	↓Wound and limb edema ↑Wound nutrition	↑Lymphatic and venous return ↓Tissue colloid osmotic pressure Normalize fluid dynamics ↑Fibrinolytic activity at wound margins	NI	+ +	+*	+†
Whirlpool	Clean wound and prepare for debridement Ease wound dressing removal	Water agitation helps remove debris, topical medications residue Softens necrotic, adherent tissue and bandages	+‡	+‡§	+	+
Nonthermal ultrasound	Augment wound healing	Accelerates or reactivates normal wound-healing process	?	+	+	?
Hyperbaric oxygen	↑Wound nutrition	↑O_2 saturation at the wound	+	+	+	?
Total contact casting/walking splint	↓High plantar pressures to allow safe PWB gait Enhance wound healing	Redistributes plantar pressures to unload high-pressure areas Immobilizes irritated tissues to foster healing Minimizes deconditioning by allowing ambulation	NI	NI	NI	+ +
Consensual heating of low back	↑Blood flow to feet	Induces reflex vasodilation of distal blood vessels by temperature of low back	+	NI	NI	NI
Patient/care-giver education	Maximize wound healing Prevent wound recurrence	Patient and/or care-givers able to take an active role in achieving wound healing and preventing wound recurrence	+ +	+ +	+ +	+ +

*Compression dressing if wound edema is present.
†Use compression devices if limb edema is present.
‡Use neutral water temperature.
§Avoid dependent limb position.
+ = some, but limited, evidence of positive outcomes; + + = substantial evidence of positive outcomes; ? = insufficient evidence to determine outcome; NI = modality is not indicated for this wound type; PWB = partial weight bearing.

monly provide at least temporary circulatory patency (1 to 3 years). If surgery is contraindicated or has proven unsuccessful, a sympathectomy is often used to inhibit vasorestrictive tone in the lower extremities.

Physical Therapy Intervention

A number of physical therapy interventions may be used in the attainment of treatment goals (Table 24-3). Low-intensity electrical stimulation for tissue repair (ESTR) applied directly over the wound may augment normal healing and decrease wound infection. Whirlpool at neutral skin temperature will assist in wound cleaning and debridement. Hot packs placed over the low back may reflexly enhance blood flow to the feet. There is some, but limited, evidence that hyperbaric oxygen therapy (HBO) will enhance healing of ul-

cers caused by arterial insufficiency. Also, patient and care-giver education in wound care and prevention of reinjury are essential components of any intervention.

CHRONIC DERMAL WOUNDS FROM VENOUS INSUFFICIENCY

Epidemiology

Fitzpatrick notes that "chronic venous insufficiency (CVI) of the legs is one of the most common medical problems in the elderly."[70] Coon and colleagues in a 1973 study found that CVI affected 7 million people in the United States and that more than 500,000 of these individuals suffered from chronic ulcerations of their lower extremities.[46] Venous ulcers make up between 70% and 90% of all ulcers of the foot and lower leg.[77] Predisposing factors for the development of CVI are a history of thrombophlebitis, family history of venous insufficiency, and trauma.[4,7]

Unlike ulcers of arterial origin, venous ulcers rarely lead to limb amputation. However, venous ulcers tend to be very chronic problems, with a high incidence of recurrence.[4,111] The ulcers are easy targets for infection. The decreased movement of blood through venous varicosities and incompetent valves increases the risk of acute thrombophlebitis with its potentially life-threatening consequences.

In a comprehensive study of the population of Goteborg, Sweden, 1377 patients sought medical care for leg or foot ulcers in 1980.[77] At least 70% of these ulcers were believed to be of venous origin. The median age of the patients with ulcers was 73, and the majority was women. Men developed ulcers on average 5 to 10 years earlier than women. The incidence of ulcers increased rapidly with increasing age—1% of the 70-year-old population compared with 5% of the 90-year-old population. The Goteborg study also indicated that patients with ulcers had double the mortality rate of matched individuals without ulcers, primarily due to a higher-than-average rate of ischemic heart disease in those patients.

Etiology

In the lower extremities, the venous system is made up of deep, superficial, and communicating (also called perforating) veins. In general, blood from the superficial veins returns to the heart by flowing through the communicating veins into the deep veins and is prevented from flowing backward by the bicuspid venous valves, which allow blood only to move toward the heart. Typically, competent venous valves can withstand 200 mm Hg pressure without allowing retrograde blood flow.[143]

Unlike arteries, veins have very little smooth muscle. Therefore, active venous constriction is minimal. Veins also have a lower resistance than arteries to passive dilation from elevated local blood pressure. Movement of venous blood is dependent on blood flow pressure gradients and external compression of the deep veins by contraction of the calf muscles, particularly when the legs are in the dependent position. Competent venous valves are essential in controlling the unidirectional flow of blood toward the heart.

When the calf muscles contract, the deep veins are constricted and push the blood in them toward the heart. Relaxation of the calf muscles allows reopening of the deep veins, which provides a low-resistance pathway for blood to be drawn from superficial into deep veins.[4,34] During active calf muscle contraction, the blood pressure in the superficial veins drops from its normal value of 90 mm Hg with quiet standing to 20 to 30 mm Hg.[34] Damage to a venous valve may make this blood flow pattern ineffective, thus allowing blood to move in both directions.[106] This abnormal blood flow pattern results in unremitting hypertension in the affected superficial veins.

This unremitting hypertension leads to a "stretching" of the interendothelial pores of the venules (Fig. 24-2). With an increase in the size of these pores, larger molecules are allowed to diffuse out of the vein, changing the colloidal osmotic pressure gradients with resultant interstitial edema.[4,34] The chronic presence of interstitial edema sets the stage for the development of a non-healing wound.

The traditional belief that venous ulcers result from inadequate oxygenation due to blood stagnation,[25] although still taught, was proven incorrect many years ago.[33,34] Indeed, blood flow in the area of a chronic venous wound is generally good. Rather, the ability to diffuse nutrients and waste products into and out of the wound area appears impaired.[4,8,34]

The exact cause of decreased diffusion across the venous ulcer is unclear. There are several theories, all with some support but no definitive answer. One theory implicates the diffusion of large-molecule fibrinogen into the interstitial space.[7,33,34] Sustained venous hypertension fosters a gradual build up of fibrin, which forms a pericapillary fibrin cuff.[4] This fibrin cuff impedes diffusion across capillary membranes. Another theory is commonly called the "white blood cell trapping theory." With sustained venous hypertension and decreased diffusion across capillary membranes, white blood cells become trapped. These blood cells are 2000 times stiffer than red blood cells, forming a neutrophil barrier in the microcirculation.[8] Additionally, when "trapped," the white blood cells release potent proteolytic enzymes that are intended to stimulate a healing inflammatory response. However, excessive amounts of the enzyme are released, according to the theory, which results in capillary tissue damage and subsequent wound development and delayed wound healing.[4,8,143] Much work still needs to be done to better delineate the underlying cause of non-healing venous ulcers.

Clinical Examination for Venous Insufficiency

The International Consensus Committee on Chronic Venous Disease has recently agreed to a clinical classification of chronic venous disease that uses four different classifications of the ulcer: clinical description, etiology, anatomical, and pathophysiology.[18] The signs and symptoms of CVI are outlined in Fig. 24-1. The most common site of ulcer development is just above the medial malleolus. Typically, the ulcer is shallow, irregularly shaped, and persistent and often becomes worse with prolonged walking or sitting with the legs dependent.

Tests for Venous Insufficiency

Strain gauge plethysmography, air plethysmography, and photoplethysmography are noninvasive procedures traditionally used to provide objective assessment of venous valve competence.[18,92,121] However, these tests have limitations in their ability to provide specific information about the exact location or extent of the venous problem. With increasing frequency, duplex Doppler ultrasound, particularly with color-flow Doppler scanning, is being used for non-invasive assessment of the peripheral venous system. This test can detect both the anatomical distribution of a blockage or narrowing as well as the severity of venous reflux in specific veins.[8,18,64,92] The test is still not 100% accurate but does increase specificity and accuracy over plethysmography techniques.

Continuous Doppler ultrasound provides a simple and quick screening for both arterial and venous insufficiencies and is often part of a routine vascular assessment. Typically, a significant finding with continuous Doppler is an indicator for further, more-sophisticated assessments. Since studies have demonstrated that approximately 20% of patients with peripheral venous disease also have peripheral arterial disease, screening for arterial insufficiency should be a standard part of the assessment of the patient with venous dysfunction.[92]

If surgical intervention is contemplated, then the more invasive venography is performed. The injection of radiopaque dye into the vein is followed by radiographic visualization of the vein. This technique outlines the exact locations of occlusions and valve incompetencies.

General Treatment Approaches

Decreasing superficial venous hypertension is the key to preventing and healing venous ulcers. Queral and Dagher caution that "CVI of the lower extremities, leading to ulceration, is largely an incurable disease. However, treatment is possible and amelioration of the ulcer and the insufficiency is achievable."[121]

Conservative management of a CVI ulcer focuses on strategies to decrease limb edema. Complete bedrest with the legs elevated will accomplish this goal, but this strategy is neither practical nor safe for most elderly patients.[74] The use of various external compression devices when the legs are dependent is effective for many individuals. Surgical interventions to correct venous incompetency are occasionally used. Superficial vein ligation and stripping are the most common surgical procedures used for incompetent venous valves.[8,121] Successful treatment is temporary, however, unless the patient complies with strategies to minimize lower extremity edema and hypertensive stress on a long-term basis.[56]

Physical Therapy Intervention

An array of treatment approaches summarized in Table 24-3 and discussed in detail later in this chapter are available to the physical therapist to meet the goals outlined in the preceding text. Edema may be controlled through the long-term use of compression devices such as custom-fit or ready-made elastic stockings, standard or specialized elastic bandages, Unna's paste boots, and compression orthoses. In the presence of moderate or severe edema, the use of an intermittent, or sequential, compression pump may be warranted in addition to external compression garments or boots.[2] Use of these pumps is contraindicated in the presence of marked arterial insufficiency, local infection, acute thrombophlebitis, or lymph node infection.

Athermal (nonthermal) ultrasound has been used to enhance the normal healing process. In selected cases, whirlpool

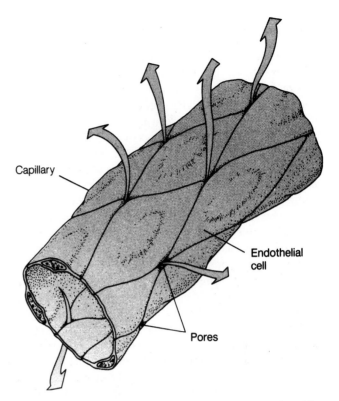

FIG. 24-2 Interendothelial pores of capillaries. As theorized by Browse, these pores can be stretched by prolonged, increased capillary pressure, thus allowing plasma proteins to escape into interstitial fluid. (From Sherwood L: *Fundamentals of Physiology: A Human Perspective.* St Paul, Minn, West Publishing, 1991. Used by permission.)

may be beneficial to soften eschar before debridement or to clean the wound. Whirlpool should be used judiciously, however, to avoid increasing lower extremity edema and should not be continued once the wound is clean and debrided. Hyperbaric oxygen also has been used successfully to treat CVI ulcers.

Complete bedrest with limb elevation fosters wound healing, but this is neither practical nor safe for most elderly persons. The use of compression devices combined with frequent bouts of limb elevation is considered the hallmark of wound healing in CVI.

PRESSURE (DECUBITUS) ULCERS

Epidemiology

There is little doubt that pressure sores are a major problem confronting health practitioners in nearly every geriatric setting in the United States. Eighty-two percent of patients with decubitus ulcers are older than 70 years.[146] Prevalence estimates of pressure ulcers in the nursing home population have ranged from as low as 2.6% to as high as 24%.[29] In a study that included 19,889 nursing home residents in 51 nursing homes, Brandeis and colleagues found that 17.4% of the residents had pressure ulcers upon admission; 11.3% of the ulcers were classified as stage 2 or worse.[29] This figure contrasts with an 8.9% prevalence of pressure sores among residents, which included 6.8% of residents with ulcers classified as stage 2 or worse. The presence of a pressure sore upon admission is an important clinical finding with grave implications. Berlowitz and Wilking found that patients who were admitted to a nursing home with a pressure sore were nearly twice as likely to die within 6 weeks of admission as patients who did not have a similar lesion upon admission.[20] In another study of almost 5000 nursing home residents, Spector and colleagues concluded that the following factors significantly related to having a pressure ulcer: older age; being a male, nonwhite, or unable to bathe; needing help to transfer; wearing a catheter; experiencing fecal incontinence; being confined to bed; having been recently hospitalized; and having no rehabilitation potential.[137]

Decubitus ulcers are not confined to nursing homes. Indeed, in the majority of persons (57% to 60%) who develop pressure ulcers, the ulcer first developed in the acute care hospital. Estimates of the prevalence of pressure ulcers in acute care settings varies from 2.5% to 29.5%.[5,142] Some evidence suggests that a number of factors influence the development of pressure sores in hospitalized elderly: fractures, fecal incontinence, hypoalbuminemia, and cognition.[5] Pressure ulcers can involve intensive therapeutic efforts by a multiplicity of professionals. The costs of total patient care for treatment of these lesions have ranged from $4,000 to $40,000, depending on the stage of the wound.[29]

Etiology

Prolonged pressure and shear forces, particularly over bony prominences, can impair blood flow, leading to tissue ischemia and ulcer formation.[19,51] The duration of the pressure load, degree of accompanying shear forces, and general health status of the patient have substantial impact on the amount of pressure needed to provoke ulcer formation.[19]

Normal capillary pressure ranges from 20 to 35 mm Hg.[19] Individuals with normal circulation can tolerate prolonged pressures much higher than 35 mm Hg without tissue damage. Part of the reason for this is that the pressure through the capillaries can increase up to diastolic levels in response to an outside pressure stress.[83] The skin, in particular, with its inherent ability to shunt blood, has a high tolerance for anoxia. However, in the presence of shearing forces, which cause a distortion of small blood vessels, less external pressure is needed to occlude blood flow.[67] A very common source of shear force is lying in bed with the head of the bed elevated, particularly at an angle greater than 45 degrees (Fig. 24-3). In this position, the skin overlying the ischium and sacrum stays in one position, and the underlying tissue moves in response to the forces of gravity and the weight of the body.

Deeper structures are more susceptible than the skin to ischemic damage in response to high shear forces.[19,131] This often results in an ulcer that, although small in appearance, has a deep sinus tract. It is estimated that the typical pressures exerted by lying on a bony prominence will cause tissue damage within 2 to 6 hours.[126] Damage may occur sooner in the high-risk, frail individual.[17] Common risk factors for the development of pressure ulcers are identified in Box 24-2. Advanced age, per se, does not increase one's risk of developing a pressure ulcer, but many chronic conditions common to old age commonly place older people in a high-risk category.[19,107] Additionally, normal skin changes of advanced age, such as decreased extensibility of the skin and decreased skin blood flow, may compromise the tissue's ability to adapt to a compressing force.[49]

Schubert has implicated low systolic blood pressure, particularly prevalent in ill individuals older than 70 years, as an additional risk factor for the development of pressure ulcers.[130,131] In ill elders, lower systolic pressure was significantly correlated to low peak skin blood cell flux and a slower circulatory recovery after occlusion. This suggests

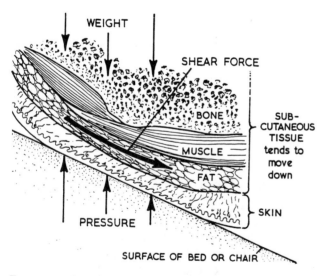

FIG. 24-3 Shear forces occurring when lying in bed with head of bed angled up. The skin overlying the trunk remains stationary as the body shifts downward, resulting in torsion of underlying tissue, including blood vessels. (From Fernandez S: *Physiotherapy* 1987; 73:451. Used by permission.)

Box 24-2
RISK FACTORS FOR THE DEVELOPMENT OF PRESSURE ULCERS

1. Immobility
2. Decreased sensation
3. Muscle atrophy
4. Decreased circulation
5. Positioning allowing high shear forces
6. Poor nutritional status
7. Incontinence
8. Site of a previous ulcer
9. Edema at the site of increased pressure
10. Anemia

that low blood pressure may be an important risk factor for the development of a decubitus ulcer in the frail elderly patient.

Clinical Signs and Symptoms of Decubitus Ulcer Formation

Pressure ulcers do not occur spontaneously. At least one and often multiple risk factors for pressure ulcers are present (see Table 24-5). The patient who develops a decubitus ulcer is usually ill and probably has limited mobility, often including limited bed mobility. Sensory loss or decreased cognition may impair the patient's awareness of excessive pressure. Skin redness over areas exposed to pressure, particularly bony prominences, may indicate damaging pressure levels. A transitory hyperemic response occurs any time pressure is removed from the skin. Normally, this redness should disappear within 1 hour.[17] Redness that lasts longer suggests a stage 1 decubitus ulcer (see Table 24-1). Because of the tendency for damage in deep structures before superficial structures, the presence of prolonged hyperemia, even in the absence of observable tissue damage, should be taken very seriously. The potential damage beneath the skin may be very difficult to identify. Areas at greatest risk of pressure ulceration are illustrated in Fig. 24-4.

The Norton Scale, first proposed in 1962, and the Braden scale, described in 1988, are commonly used tools to assess the extent to which an individual is "at risk" of developing a pressure ulcer.[28,113] The Norton scale provides a numeric score between 1 and 4 for each of five factors: physical condition (very bad to good), mental condition (stupor to alert), activity (bed to ambulant), mobility (immobile to full), and incontinent (doubly to not). A lower score indicates a greater risk of pressure ulcer. A score of 16 indicates "onset of risk," and score of 12 or less indicates "high risk."[113] The Braden scale also provides a numeric summary of "risk of pressure ulcer." This scale has six factors, each with a fairly detailed written description of characteristics of each score within each factor. The factors included in the Braden scale are sensory perception, moisture, activity, mobility, nutrition, friction or shear.[28] The test forms, with further descriptions, have been collected by Sussman and Bates-Jensen.[140]

Objective Evaluation of Decubitus Ulcer Risk

Few clinical tools are readily available to measure the effects of external pressure on blood flow through the involved tissue. Laser Doppler fluxmetry, which measures microcirculatory changes, may be of some value. This device measures the number of skin blood cells in a given portion of skin. *Skin blood cell flux (SBF)* is defined as "the product of the number of skin blood cells and their velocities within the measuring volume."[130] When this technique is applied, blood flow is temporarily occluded, and when pressure is released, the rate of blood-flow change is measured. This technique can identify individuals with sluggish postpressure responses and low occlusive pressures, which may help to identify high-risk patients. The limita-

tions of this technique are that it only measures very superficial skin blood flow and it is not readily available in clinical settings.

If arterial or venous insufficiency is suspected, the vascular tests identified in previous sections of this chapter should be performed. No evaluation technique is clinically avail-able to reliably measure the shear forces that are strongly implicated in tissue breakdown, particularly at the sacrum and ischium.

General Treatment Approaches

The key to preventing decubitus ulcers and reversing the delayed wound healing associated with them is pressure relief. The patient or the care-givers need to ensure frequent positioning changes and consistent use of the appropriate pressure-relieving cushions and mattresses prescribed for the patient. A summary of the various pressure-relieving devices, with discussion of the benefits and drawbacks of each, is discussed in detail by Rappl.[122]

As with other types of ulcers, the factors that may delay wound healing need to be addressed if a healthy wound environment is to be achieved (see Box 24-1). If the patient's medical condition will support involvement in a muscle-strengthening program, consequent increases in muscle mass may assist in decreasing the threat of decubitus formation as well as in increasing mobility.

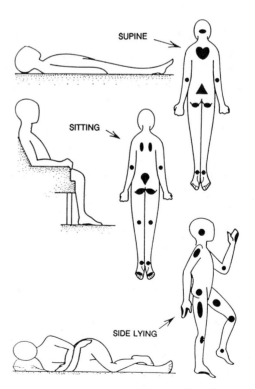

FIG. 24-4 Areas at greatest risk for pressure ulcer formation. (From Fernandez S: *Physiotherapy* 1987; 73:450. Used by permission.)

Physical Therapy Intervention

Patient and care-giver education is an important primary intervention. Thorough instruction in proper positioning procedures to avoid excess time in one position and effective use of individualized pressure-relieving devices are essential. Since immobility is a major contributing factor to pressure ulcers, all patients who are capable should receive therapeutic exercise and functional training to maximize their ability to move, thus decreasing the time periods of sustained tissue pressure. Even small improvements, such as improving the patient's ability to roll from side to side, can be very beneficial. Low-intensity electrical current or non-thermal ultrasound may be used to enhance wound healing. Whirlpool may be used for wound cleaning and debriding.

NEUROPATHIC PLANTAR ULCERS

Neuropathic plantar ulcers are a special category of pressure ulcer. These ulcers do not develop in response to prolonged periods of maintained pressure, as with decubitus ulcers. Rather, these ulcers develop in response to repetitive pressure stresses on weight-bearing surfaces of the foot in persons with peripheral neuropathy.

Epidemiology

The vast majority of plantar ulcers occur in persons with diabetes mellitus (DM).[38,133] The National Center for Health Statistics identifies diabetes mellitus as one of the five most common chronic diseases of persons older than 65 years.[78] The incidence of DM gradually increases with increasing age until about age 65, when it levels off to 9.3% of the population.[78] The prevalence of DM in the elderly black and Hispanic populations is, however, as high as 20% to 24%.

The increased prevalence of DM in the older population combined with the long time period between onset of disease and onset of neuropathic changes increases the probability that plantar ulcers will be most evident in old age. Foot pathologies associated with DM are frequently responsible for long periods of inactivity, illness, hospitalization, and limb amputation.[78,98,133] An estimated 25% of persons with a 10-year history of DM and 50% of persons with a 20-year history of DM have distal neuropathic changes.[133] Distal neuropathy and impaired peripheral circulation often coexist in individuals with long-standing diabetes.[53,61]

Etiology

Repetitive mechanical stress on weight-bearing structures of the insensitive foot is the primary precipitating factor in the development of plantar ulcers.[22,134] A lack of protective sensation in the foot impedes the individual from sensing excessive plantar pressures during ambulation.

Normal foot biomechanics allow considerable force to be safely placed across the foot because weight-bearing forces are distributed over a large surface area. In a normal upright posture the body's weight rests primarily on the heel and the five metatarsal bones, with the midfoot and great toe assuming a lesser amount of weight and the four smaller toes assuming very little weight.[40]

If biomechanical abnormalities exist, the weight-bearing surfaces may become malaligned, leading to abnormally large loads being carried over small surface areas. Individuals with intact sensation feel discomfort from these abnormal weight-bearing forces and alter their gait or their footwear to relieve this repetitive mechanical stress. However, the person who lacks protective sensation will, unknowingly, continue to submit the foot to these excessive stresses, thus placing the foot at risk for injury. Even minor biomechanical abnormalities can, over time, lead to substantial trauma in the person with neuropathy. The metatarsal heads and the great toe are common sites of increased plantar pressures and ulceration.[22,120,134]

Foot deformities and biomechanical abnormalities are common in diabetic patients and may arise from many sources. Motor neuropathy may accompany sensory neuropathy, leading to weakness in the intrinsic and extrinsic muscles of the foot.[47] Resultant muscle imbalances foster the development of deformities such as claw and hammer toes, both of which increase pressures under the metatarsal heads.[26,27,82,139] Foot deformities associated with age-related biomechanical dysfunction may also be present in this population and may include hallux valgus, hammer toes, plantar-flexed first ray, and pes planus.[62] These deformities are commonly associated with increased pressure over the metatarsal heads and the great toe.

Decreased range of motion (ROM) in the ankle is commonly observed in the elderly person with DM. Decreased joint flexibility will alter dynamic joint movement, possibly leading to abnormal weight-bearing pressures during gait.[109,110] Hallux limitus has been associated with high pressures under the great toe and ulcers of the great toe.[21] Decreased dorsiflexion and subtalar joint movement have been implicated in increased forefoot pressures and history of plantar ulcers in patients with peripheral neuropathy.[109]

The risk of ulceration is further enhanced by changes in the forefoot fat pad. Foot deformities, such as claw and hammer toes, often result in distal slippage of the fat pad. Gooding and colleagues found that patients with DM have significantly thinner forefoot fat pads than age-matched subjects without diabetes.[73] These changes result in decreased cushioning over the metatarsal areas most likely to be exposed to high plantar pressures.

Autonomic neuropathy is also implicated in increased risk of ulceration. The patient with an autonomic neuropathy lacks natural skin hydration, resulting in skin that is very dry and easily fissured. The autonomically denervated limb will be unable to "deactivate" the arteriovenous shunting mechanism. This neuropathic change is believed to be the mechanism responsible for the fivefold increase in foot blood flow reported by Archer and colleagues in their study of persons with nonpainful autonomic denervation of the foot.[10] Despite this high blood flow, the adequacy of local tissue nutrition is unclear because the blood is being shunted through the arteriovenous system and away from the nutritive capillaries.[10,133] A secondary complication of this high blood flow is osteopenia, resulting in increased risk of neuropathic fracture at the foot. This is a very serious complication of autonomic neuropathy that greatly compromises the individual's ability to ambulate.

Persons with DM have a risk of large-vessel occlusion similar to that of age-matched persons without diabetes. However, atherosclerosis in medium-sized vessels, particularly the tibial and peroneal, occurs much more frequently in persons with DM than in nondiabetics.[82,84,133] In contrast to traditional teachings, little evidence exists that blood flow compromise in the foot is related to microcirculatory disease.[98,133] Circulatory compromise in the foot appears to stem primarily from compromised blood flow through the peroneal and tibial arteries, not from microcirculatory changes.[98]

Clinical Signs and Symptoms of Neuropathic Ulcer

Signs of high plantar pressure may include localized areas of increased warmth, redness, discoloration, hematoma, callous formation, or swelling, particularly if these changes occur on a weight-bearing surface. A traumatized area may have a "boggy" feeling to it. An overt ulcer may be superficial or deep and may or may not involve tissue necrosis. The ulcer may be open or covered with a scab, eschar, or thick callus. A large callus overlying the ulcer may mask underlying tissue damage. Removal of the callus is necessary to adequately evaluate the underlying tissue.[133] Wagner's six-stage classification system is often used to categorize the severity of plantar ulcers (see Box 24-2). The patient should also be evaluated for signs of autonomic dysfunction, including increased warmth and redness of the entire foot; very dry, cracked skin; and loss of sweating in the foot.

Tests for Neuropathy and High Plantar Pressure

The presence of protective sensation can be reliably measured using Semmes-Weinstein monofilaments.[53,93] These thin nylon monofilaments are calibrated according to the force required to cause them to buckle when they are briefly pressed against the skin at a right angle to the skin (Fig. 24-5). The thinner the filament, the lower the monofilament number and the lower the force needed to induce buckling. The thinner filaments are, therefore, considered more sensitive. Protective sensation in the foot is considered absent if an individual cannot feel the 5.07 monofilament.[22] Monofilament testing should be performed at several sites on the foot, with emphasis on areas exposed to high weight-bearing pressure (Fig. 24-6).[22,93]

Motor nerve conduction velocity testing, described in most basic electrotherapy texts, can provide important information regarding the state of innervation of the muscles of the foot and, therefore, the practicality of potential muscle-strengthening programs and risk of foot deformity. Muscle testing, ROM testing, and biomechanical evaluation of the foot should all be included in the evaluation of the insensitive diabetic foot. If an ulcer is not present, then a careful gait analysis, both static and dynamic, should be performed. This evaluation should focus on identifying any gait abnormalities, subtle or obvious, that may predispose the patient to areas of high plantar pressures. If the patient with an insensitive foot currently has a plantar ulcer, the gait evaluation must be deferred until the ulcer is healed or until an acceptable pressure-relieving device is in place.

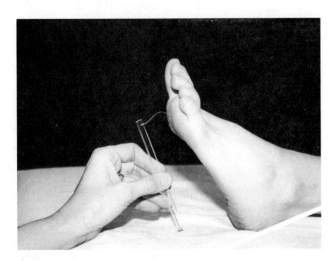

FIG. 24-5 Correct pressure to use for testing protective sensation using Semmes-Weinstein monofilaments. Note the "C" curve of the filament and the positioning of the filament perpendicular to the skin surface.

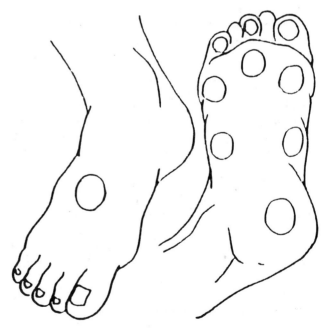

FIG. 24-6 Sites to test for protective sensation when using Semmes-Weinstein monofilaments. (From Birke J, Sims D: The insensitive foot, in Hunt G [ed]: *Physical Therapy of the Foot and Ankle.* New York, Churchill Livingstone, 1998. Used by permission.)

Qualitative assessment of high plantar pressure can be obtained with an inexpensive ink mat. An ink impression is obtained when the patient stands on a three-layered mat. The top layer is dry and does not absorb any ink. The middle layer contains an even layer of ink. The lower layer is a clean paper surface onto which the ink impression is made. The greater the pressure, the darker the ink impression.

Presently, quantitative measurements of plantar pressures are performed primarily with research-focused, expensive equipment not readily available in most clinics. Microprocessor-controlled imaging systems are used to provide a computer-driven visual image of the forces a person places across an illumination plate, or force transducer, as the person stands or walks across the device.[26,40] With improvements in computer technology it is realistic to anticipate the development of a relatively inexpensive and "user-friendly" computer-assisted pressure measurement device that can be used for patient assessment of plantar pressure sites in general clinical practice.

If there is any indication of concurrent arterial or venous insufficiency, then vascular testing, as described in previous sections of this chapter, should also be obtained.

General Treatment Approaches

As with other ulcers, wound care is the first step in the care of a plantar ulcer. The wound must be clear of infection, necrotic tissue, and excessive callous formation for healing to progress.[138] Plantar pressures must also be substantially decreased. This can be achieved by placing the patient on complete bedrest, by allowing ambulation but with a strict non–weight-bearing (NWB) status, or by using an external limb-support device, e.g., cast or walking splint.[22,24,74,95,114] External support will substantially decrease the pressure over the ulcer site and decrease movement at the foot and ankle while allowing the patient to partial weight bear on the foot.

Each approach has benefits and drawbacks. If the patient complies with strict bedrest, the ulcer will usually heal and ulcer changes can be monitored easily.[43] However, the negative physiological effects of bedrest are well-documented, and elderly patients in particular are vulnerable to these negative effects.

Allowing ambulation but requiring a strict NWB status will also foster wound healing, allow the wound to be easily monitored, and eliminate the need for bedrest. However, even short periods of unprotected weight bearing may delay healing. If the patient lacks the physical strength, balance, or determination to remain strictly non-weight bearing, this treatment approach may fail.

Total contact casting (TCC) is an effective wound-healing approach for many patients with neuropathic ulcers.[95] The primary drawback is the inability to inspect the ulcer visually at frequent intervals. A walking splint or a cutout shoe, which allow frequent inspection of the skin, may be more beneficial for patients with substantial circulatory compro-

mise. The drawback of these latter devices is the higher risk of shearing and friction forces with weight bearing due to the less precise fit of these devices.

Physical Therapy Intervention

Physical therapists are often involved in the evaluation for and fabrication of external pressure-relieving devices such as TCC, walking splints, and cutout shoes. The fabrication of these devices, particularly the TCC, requires a great deal of training and practice.[24] The entry-level physical therapy practitioner should understand the principles behind TCC, recognize appropriate patients for this approach, and effectively communicate this information to other members of the health care team. Fabricating TCC is an advanced clinical competency.

As with other types of ulcers, a team approach is needed to adequately treat these patients. Preventing infection, ensuring adequate nutrition for ulcer repair and control of diabetes, removing calluses and adherent eschar, maximizing distal circulation, ensuring compliance with recommended weight-bearing status, providing patient education opportunities, prescribing and fabricating protective footwear and orthotics, and providing gait training will be a joint effort of many health professionals.

PHYSICAL THERAPY INTERVENTIONS TO AUGMENT WOUND HEALING

A wide variety of modalities are used by physical therapists to treat patients with chronic dermal wounds. Each modality is focused on one of two overall goals: (1) to directly amplify the body's natural healing process or (2) to eliminate factors that block the activity of the body's natural healing processes, e.g., wound infection and inadequate wound nutrition.

Electrical Stimulation of the Wound Site

For many years, low-intensity ESTR has been advocated for the augmentation of wound healing, regardless of the underlying cause of the ulcer. Several studies, each using slightly different pulse generators, have demonstrated the substantial benefit that accompanies this intervention.[3,16,39,66,71,89,152] Despite the demonstrated effectiveness of ESTR, adoption of this technique by clinicians has been slow. Physical therapists are appropriate health care professionals to introduce this technology to the health care community and establish the scientific credibility of the technique.

In Wolcott and co-workers' classic study, 20 elderly patients with ulcers from either arterial or venous insufficiency received ESTR.[149] For these 20 patients, the median decrease in ulcer size was 100% for the patients with venous insufficiency and 96% for those with arterial insufficiency. In both cases, these previously non-healing ulcers healed at a rate of 14% per week once the electrical stimulation was begun. Researchers who used similar protocols at a later date reported even more rapid healing rates.[39,71,89] Carley and Wainapel tested Wolcott's protocol using a matched-control design in which control subjects received sham electrical stimulation.[39] They found that the 35.6% per week healing rate of patients in the electrically stimulated group was twice that of patients in the sham treatment group.

Kloth and Feedar, using a well-controlled design, demonstrated that high-voltage pulsed stimulation (HVPS) at very low output levels can be used successfully to heal stage 4 decubitus ulcers.[89] In their study of 16 elderly patients, the wounds in the electrical stimulation group healed completely within 7.3 weeks, at an average weekly healing rate of 45%. During this same period, the wounds of subjects in the control group increased in size 29%. In all these studies, both experimental and control subjects received the same ulcer care. Kloth states that pressure was relieved from ulcer sites, a high-protein dietary supplement was used, wound tissue was debrided as needed, and the wounds were kept clean and free of infection.[89] All wounds were debrided before electrical stimulation was initiated, and elimination of any wound infection was the initial treatment priority. Baker and colleagues found the rate of healing of chronic ulcers in patients with diabetes increased twofold when an asymmetrical biphasic electrical current was added to standard wound care.[16] Treatment occurred 5 to 7 days per week for 30 to 90 minutes per day at an amplitude less than the muscle contraction level. The underlying causes of the dermal wounds were not identified in the study.

Although it is clear that electrical stimulation can be very effective in wound healing, the ideal electrical stimulation parameters remain elusive.[72] A variety of parameters have proven effective. One set of parameters, those used by Kloth and Feedar in their recent examination of wound healing with HVPS, is outlined in Table 24-4.[89] Most investigators have used unidirectional current, either pulsed or uninterrupted, both of which provide a means of controlling the polarity of each electrode. The polarity of the electrical current is implicated in both augmentation of wound healing and inhibition of infection. Placing the positive electrode over the wound is generally believed more effective in augmenting healing than placing the negative electrode over the wound. In contrast, the negative electrode over the wound may be more effective in inhibiting infection.[31,32,136]

The underlying rationale for enhanced tissue repair in response to ESTR is unknown, although many theories have been proposed. Increased adenosine triphosphate (ATP) production as well as enhanced cellular migration at the wound site, increased collagen synthesis, increased wound blood flow, and bactericidal effect have been reported in skin wounds treated with electrical stimulation.[6,16,41,88,112] Experimentally induced wounds treated with electrical stimulation have been found to have a greater tensile strength in addition to faster healing rates.[112]

Regardless of the underlying triggering mechanism, the effectiveness of the low-intensity current used with ESTR in

TABLE 24-4
PROTOCOL FOR ESTR UTILIZING HIGH-VOLTAGE PULSED CURRENT

PARAMETER	PROTOCOL
Pulse rate	105 pulses per second
Intrapulse interval	50 μs
Amplitude	Sensory only; no muscle contraction
	If serous drainage after 1 hour of stimulation, increase amplitude
	If bloody drainage after 1 hour of stimulation, decrease amplitude
Duty cycle	Continuous
Treatment time	45 minutes, 5 times per week
Polarity	"+" over the wound for healing
	"−" over the wound if infected
	"Switch polarity" if healing plateau is reached

Adapted from Kloth L, Feedar J: *Phys Ther* 1988; 68:503–508.

reinitiating stalled wound healing is consistent with the Arndt-Schultz law of biological response:

> Weak stimuli excite physiological activity, moderately strong stimuli favor it, strong stimuli retard physiological activity, and very strong stimuli arrest physiological activity.[48]

Compression Techniques

Control of edema is a major factor in attaining healing of chronic lower extremity ulcers complicated by insufficient venous function.[8,97] In the presence of venous insufficiency, compression devices assist in decreasing interstitial fluid volumes. The pressure shift encourages the movement of fluids and proteins from the interstitial spaces into veins and lymphatics. There is less venous reflux, and the calf muscle pump can work more effectively.[104] This maintained external compression at the wound site also has been associated with increased fibrinolytic activity at the wound, thus improving wound nutrition.[35]

Many devices have been used to provide controlled compressive forces to the lower extremity. Among these are a variety of elastic bandages, ready-made and custom-fit gradient-pressure elastic stockings, Unna's boots, and intermittent pneumatic compression devices.[2,8,42,97,128,129] Two recent studies have found no relationship between patient age and success of compression therapy for healing chronic venous ulcers.[97,128]

The degree of compression needed and the patient's tolerance and activity level dictate the specific device. Typically, the goal of compression devices is to provide sufficient compression to overcome the existing excessive outward capillary pressure gradients, thus stimulating fluid resorption.[129] Devices using graded pressures, greater distally than proximally, enhance this movement of fluids. For patients with chronic venous insufficiency it is important that they continue to wear a compression device even after the wound is healed. Typically, the underlying venous circulatory problem that lead to a chronic ulcer still exists, and the maintenance of external pressure when the legs are dependent is an essential component of preventing recurrences.[128]

The compression found in elastic compression stockings varies from about 8 to 50 mm Hg at the ankle. A pressure of 30 to 40 mm Hg at the ankle with a 15- to 20-mm Hg decrease proximally is common. A pressure of 40 to 50 mm Hg may occlude blood flow in some. Very light compression may be ineffective. If the edema and ulceration are limited to the distal extremity, knee-high compression wrap may suffice. If the edema extends above the knee, full-length compression will be required.

Standard elastic wraps are inexpensive and fairly easy to don but commonly do not provide appropriate levels of compression. Standard elastic bandages can be applied too loosely or tightly. These bandages frequently shift position with limb movement, resulting in inconsistent pressure application. Ready-made compression stockings are convenient and usually come in three to four "standard" sizes, thus with limited range of patients for whom they are appropriate.

Standard compression stockings are much less expensive than custom-fit stockings. Custom-fit gradient-pressure stockings are often needed to obtain appropriate amount and placement of compression. Although these stockings provide a very precise fit, a common drawback of the snug fit is the inability of the individual to don the stockings independently. This is particularly common in older persons who may require higher levels of external compression to counteract the venous hypertension.[135] Custom-fit stockings are available in variety of pressures and with zippers for easier donning.[128] The development of very absorbent hydrophilic dressing materials that can be used under the stocking has decreased, but not eliminated, the risk of skin maceration.[63,124]

In general, elastic compressive devices should be put on before getting out of bed in the morning and taken off once the patient is in bed at the end of the day. This ensures that external compression is applied at all times when the legs are in a dependent position.

Compression pumps are often needed in addition to gradient elastic stockings to enhance fluid resorption.[104] Two different inflation modes are commonly available, single- and multiple-chamber compression. The single-chamber unit inflates the entire chamber (distal and proximal portions) simultaneously. A newer variation, the multiple-chamber unit, inflates sequentially, beginning distally and moving proximally. Evidence suggests that the sequential mode of inflation results in more effective edema reduction in a shorter time period than the single-chamber method.[2,104] Typical parameters for compression pumps used to treat chronic venous insufficiency are listed in Table 24-5.

Total Contact Casting and Other Protected Weight-Bearing Devices

Unna's boot, TCC, and a variety of walking splints and shoes are available to allow selected patients with foot ulceration to remain ambulatory while fostering wound healing. Unna's boots are used primarily with patients with venous insufficiency ulcers who have intact sensation in the foot. The Unna's boot maximizes the muscle-pumping capability of the calf by providing an unyielding surface against which compressive forces on the interstitial tissues can develop. Thus, each muscle contraction promotes effective pumping of fluid into veins and lymphatics.

Unna's boot, first described more than 100 years ago, consists of a "nonstretchable, pliable, adhesive mold" that is applied to the ulcered lower extremity somewhat like a cast.[96] These boots are left on for days or weeks, and patients are allowed to partial weight bear on them. Contraindications to the use of Unna's boot include large amounts of wound drainage, wound infection, and arterial insufficiency. Unna's boot eliminates the need for daily donning and doffing of tightly fitting stockings and has been associated with more rapid ulcer healing than custom-fit gradient-pressure stockings.[81,96] The major disadvantage is the inability to perform a daily visual check of the wound for signs of skin irritation or wound deterioration.

TCC is used primarily for the treatment of patients with Wagner's stages 1 and 2 neuropathic plantar ulcers (see Table 24-2). The goal of these devices is to redistribute the weight-bearing forces across the foot and immobilize inflamed tissues to allow healing to occur. The patient's lack of sensation makes proper fit of these devices crucial.

The TCC contours the foot much more precisely than the Unna's boot. Plaster is very carefully molded around the foot and lower leg to conform very closely to the contours of the limb, thus providing very even pressure distribution with minimal shearing or rubbing forces. A rocker-bottom heel is applied to the cast to minimize metatarsal pressure. This type of casting was introduced to this country by Brand in the 1960s for the treatment of plantar ulcers in patients with neuropathy related to Hanson's disease (leprosy). This intervention has since been expanded to include patients with di-

Table 24-5
Compression Pump Parameters Commonly Used for Venous Insufficiency Wounds of the Lower Extremity

Parameter	Intermittent Pump	Sequential Pump
Compression	30–60 mm Hg (most often 30–40 mm Hg)	30–60 mm Hg (most often 30–40 mm Hg)
Duty cycle	90 sec "on"; 30 sec "off"	190 sec "on" with 60-sec sequential inflation of three areas: distal to proximal; 50 sec "off"
Treatment time	1–3 hr, 2 to 3 times daily	20 min–2 hr, 2 to 3 times daily

abetic neuropathy. The effectiveness of TCC in healing diabetic neuropathic plantar ulcers has been demonstrated by several researchers.[79,94,119,134] In these studies, 73% to 100% of the ulcers treated with TCC healed completely within 5 to 6 weeks of initial casting. On average, these healed ulcers had been present from 9 to 14 months before initiation of TCC and had shown no evidence of healing. The lack of control groups weakens these studies slightly. However, the complete healing of ulcers of 9 to 14 months' duration within 5 to 6 weeks of the application of the TCC suggests that the intervention, not the passage of time, was the major influence in these successful outcomes. Mueller and colleagues, in a controlled clinical study, supported the hypothesis that TCC is more effective than alternative conservative techniques in the treatment of plantar ulcers.[110] Helm and colleagues reported a low ulcer recurrence rate (19.3%) over a 2-year period in patients treated with TCC and careful post-ulcer reinjury prevention training.[80] Nearly 50% of the ulcers that did recur were attributed to patients' nonadherence to the post-ulcer prevention plan.

The TCC is changed at least every 2 weeks. It is changed more frequently if loosening, large amounts of drainage, or damage to the cast is noted. For TCC to be effective, the cast must fit very precisely, and the patient needs frequent follow-up and thorough training in care of the foot and cast. Birke and co-workers sum up the goals of TCC as follows: "The casts redistribute walking pressures, prevent direct trauma to the wound, reduce edema, and provide immobilization to joints and soft tissue."[24] A more detailed description of the fabrication techniques for TCC are found in several publications.[22,24,43]

Total contact casting is contraindicated for individuals who have cellulitis, hypotrophic skin changes, infection, or severe arterial insufficiency (A/A index less than 0.45). Individuals classified by Wagner as having stage 3, 4, or 5 ulcers need medical or surgical intervention before TCC should be considered.[24] Efforts should be made to decrease lower leg edema before the application of a TCC.

For the patient for whom TCC is contraindicated, a custom-molded walking splint may be appropriate.[23,24,55] This splint follows the general principles of the TCC except that it can be removed easily to check on the condition of the skin. This advantage is tempered by the fact that the fit is not as snug as the TCC, allowing more shearing forces on the ulcer, which may impede healing.

Birke and co-workers also describe the use of a walking sandal for patients with ulcers on the weight-bearing surfaces of their toes.[24] These sandals remove pressure and shear forces from the toes but are less successful in redistributing weight throughout the foot and in decreasing joint movement at the foot and ankle. For selected patients, however, these may be very valuable tools.

Any technique that allows continuation of walking while the ulcer is healing is of great benefit to the elderly patient. The detrimental effects of bedrest can be devastating, particularly to an individual on the verge of frailty. The techniques of Brand, Birke, and Sims should be given strong consideration in the overall treatment of neuropathic plantar wounds.

Whirlpool

Whirlpool is commonly used to clean and debride wounds because its agitation and moisture are believed to loosen, debride, and soften adherent eschar. Wet to dry dressings, often used to facilitate the separation of eschar and thickened exudate, may be very painful to detach and may remove good granulation tissue along with eschar. Soaking the wound in the whirlpool before removal of dressings may greatly decrease this discomfort. Antimicrobial agents can be added to the water to help fight wound infection. Warm water is often used to increase blood flow, induce relaxation, and decrease pain. However, although widely used, almost no information exists on which to judge objectively the effectiveness of whirlpool for enhancing wound healing. Some precautions to the use of whirlpool with chronic wounds, however, are well-delineated.

In patients with severe arterial insufficiency, the whirlpool temperature should not be raised above a neutral water temperature, 92° F to 96° F (33.5° C to 35.5° C). One must remember that any modality that increases tissue temperature also increases tissue metabolism, which increases the tissue's need for oxygen. Typically, the body meets this increased oxygen demand by vasodilation, thus increasing blood flow through the tissue. Persons with severe arterial insufficiency have inadequate blood flow at neutral tissue temperatures and are unlikely to be able to meet this increased demand for blood as tissue temperature rises. Thus, this increased metabolic demand may result in further tissue necrosis rather than healing. In addition, the arterially insufficient limb will allow greater local heat build up than normally perfused tissue because of the lack of insufficient blood flow to conduct heat away from the local tissue.

Whirlpool also needs to be used cautiously for persons with venous insufficiency. Placing a leg with chronic venous hypertension into the dependent position, then inducing vasodilation by circulating warm water around it, does not make any sense physiologically. This activity will simply promote further engorgement of the veins. For this same reason, Birke and Sims discourage use of whirlpool for neuropathic ulcers.[22] In very limited situations, use of a large whirlpool or Hubbard tank may be appropriate. However, patient positioning in the tank should eliminate the dependent position, and a neutral water temperature should be used. Readers are referred to entry-level texts on physical agents for detailed descriptions of whirlpool application techniques.[90,108]

Wound irrigation and wound lavage using either a low-pressure syringe system or a high-pressure lavage system (with or without return suction) is becoming increasingly popular to debride and clean wounds.[99,103] These systems, which use jets of water (usually saline solution) rather than a full whirlpool bath, allow greater selectivity of treatment location. Areas needing debridement or sinus tracts needing cleaning can be focused on while healthy granulation tissue is avoided. Typically, these devices take less time to set up and clean than a whirlpool and have a lower risk of cross-contamination because most use disposable materials. The more sophisticated units have a "return suction" feature that collects the saline solution after it is ejected. These types of devices have been used in surgery for years and in some specialized burn units. Their popularity in basic wound care is fairly recent, however. Clinically, many wound care specialists are now using these devices frequently and anecdotally reporting good results. However, there is virtually no published evidence of their general effectiveness or of the relative effectiveness over traditional whirlpool. Much work is needed in this area.

Nonthermal Ultrasound

Several researchers have found nonthermal ultrasound more effective than sham ultrasound in enhancing wound healing, particularly ulcers of venous origin.[36,59,125] In general, however, ultrasound appears to be less effective than several alternative treatment approaches. Three separate studies each reported 33% to 35% decreases in wound size during a 4-week trial of 3-MHz, pulsed, nonthermal ultrasound at an intensity of 0.2 to 1 W/cm² delivered to the periphery of the wound for 5 to 10 minutes, 1 to 3 times weekly. However, within the same time frame, other studies of the effects of TCC, ESTR, Unna's boot, and compression garments plus compression pumps all report much greater wound healing. The 3-MHz, rather than the standard 1-MHz, ultrasound is purported by Dyson to be the most effective frequency for dermal wounds because more energy is absorbed in superficial tissues.[58,59] Indeed, one study that concluded that ultrasound was ineffective for wound healing used a 1-MHz frequency.[100] Parameters commonly identified as effective for wound healing are listed in Table 24-6.

Ultrasound seems to enhance the patient's ability to move through the inflammatory stage of repair. It does not interfere with the inflammatory stage, which Dyson reminds us is the body's natural mechanism for stimulating and guiding the tissue repair process, but rather it enhances the body's ability to use the inflammatory stage to stimulate repair.[58,59] In patients with normal wound hemodynamics, the use of nonthermal ultrasound has been associated with a stronger, more resilient wound scar.[59] The exact mechanism by which this occurs, however, remains elusive.

Despite the fact that the impact of ultrasound on wound healing may be less pronounced than with some other modalities, there are advantages to this modality. The treatment time is very short (about 10 minutes), and treatment frequency may be as low as 1 to 3 times per week. This technique does not require enclosing the leg in a cast or boot for long periods. It also does not require advanced skills to apply the modality competently, and most patients find the modality very comfortable. Systematic study needs to be undertaken to evaluate the possibility of combining nonthermal ultrasound with other modalities to further enhance wound healing, e.g., using custom-gradient elastic stockings and intermittent compression devices daily plus ultrasound 3 times per week in the patient with chronic venous insufficiency ulcers.

Much remains unknown about the effectiveness of ultrasound for wound healing. The few studies to date have all examined venous insufficiency ulcers. No reason was given in any of these studies for the exclusion of ulcers from other pathologies. Except for the recognition that very low intensities of current are preferable, very little information is given to justify the arbitrary parameters used for treatment. Much further work is needed to determine whether these are the "best" parameters.

Hyperbaric Oxygen

Hyperbaric oxygen (HBO) has been used successfully to treat venous insufficiency ulcers and decubitus ulcers but has a low success rate with arterially insufficient ulcers.[54,68,69,115] With this technique, the ulcerated limb is placed into a pressurized chamber, and pure oxygen is circulated within the chamber at a rate of 4 to 8 L/min. The pressure within the chamber is either held steady at 1.03 atm of pressure (22 mm Hg) or varies cyclically from 1 atm of pressure up to 3 atm (810 mm Hg). Pressures greater than 22 mm Hg may occlude capillaries; therefore, any pressures greater than this level must be cyclic. The majority of studies of HBO have used the constant 22 mm Hg pressure. Large increases in the partial pressure of oxygen (Po_2) have been noted during HBO treatment.

It is unclear as to whether the increased Po_2 values, external compression, in-patient nursing care, or an interaction of these factors were the key(s) to success. The effectiveness of Unna's boots, compression pumps, and other compression devices has been well-documented. It may be that the 1.03 atm of pressure that was applied for several hours daily was the salient feature of successful ulcer healing, not the increased atmospheric oxygen. Also, in the majority of studies reviewed, patients were admitted as hospital in-patients for 2 to 8 weeks to receive HBO. The in-patient setting alone, with its ready access to high-quality, frequent wound care

Table 24-6
Ultrasound Parameters Commonly Used for Chronic Dermal Wounds

Parameter	Guidelines
Frequency	3 MHz for stage 2 ulcers 1 MHz for stage 3 or 4 ulcers
Intensity	0.2–1.0 W/cm²
Duty cycle	20% pulsed
Treatment time	1–2 min per area 1½ times the size of the soundhead; 3 times weekly
Treatment location	Around the edges of the wound or directly over the wound with water-based occlusive dressing as conducting medium

and the increased potential for longer periods of bedrest and decreased limb dependency, probably contributed to wound healing. The relative benefits of increased oxygen tensions, which is the unique aspect of HBO, cannot be ascertained from these studies. Will compression devices; bedrest; and good, frequent wound care be just as effective as HBO? Will a home program be just as effective? Much more research needs to be done to identify the comparative role of this modality in the treatment of ulcers.

Treating the Low Back for Vasodilation of the Feet

In the 1960s, the use of superficial heat to the low back was suggested as an effective adjunct to the treatment of peripheral vascular disease because of observations made by Abramson and Wessman that heating of the low back resulted in a reflex vasodilation of the skin vessels of the feet.[1,148] No further evaluation of the effectiveness of this method of consensual heating for patients with PVD has been found in the literature. Further evaluation of this simple and safe technique is warranted.

Another indirect approach to increasing blood flow to the feet is through epidural electrical stimulation at the T10 spinal cord level using standard transcutaneous electrical nerve stimulation (TENS) parameters. This modality requires a surgical procedure to implant electrodes into the epidural space. Once implanted, the stimulation is given for many hours daily and has been found to be very effective in decreasing pain and avoiding limb amputations in patients with severe arterial insufficiency. Owing to the implanted nature of the electrodes, physical therapists are not currently involved in this form of indirect stimulation.[15,30,45,85,86]

SUMMARY

Healthy elders have little risk of developing non-healing ulcers. Ill and frail elders, however, are at a much higher risk, as all four leading causes of dermal wounds—arterial insufficiency, venous insufficiency, pressure, and neuropathy—are closely associated with illnesses that are most prevalent in the older population.

Effective treatment of chronic dermal ulcers requires careful evaluation and an individualized treatment approach based on team collaboration and involvement. The underlying cause of initial ulceration needs to be determined as well as the factors that are currently impeding the healing process. The health care team needs to develop a coordinated treatment approach that focuses first on removing the factors that are contributing to the non-healing status, e.g., infection, eschar, and poor nutrition, and then use interventions that will foster healing. The intervention is modified, as needed, to ensure continual movement toward healing. Once healing is achieved, it is essential that the patient and care-givers be fully educated in strategies to prevent wound recurrence.

In situations in which the physiological effects of the modality have been carefully matched with the physiological needs of the wound, many physical therapy modalities have been found to be effective in fostering wound healing. Electrical stimulation for tissue repair; compression pumps; and external support devices, such as total contact casts, are examples of modalities with strong clinical and research support for their effectiveness. Nonthermal ultrasound and hyperbaric oxygen have shown some evidence of effectiveness, particularly for patients with venous insufficiency ulcers. However, the extent of their benefit seems less pronounced than some alternative modalities available to us.

Whirlpool, although widely used for chronic wounds, has almost no research data to support or refute its usefulness. Clinically, it is often the preferred modality for cleaning wounds and preparing them for debridement. The ability of whirlpool to stimulate healing or disperse medication into the wound is questionable. Wound irrigation and lavage techniques are replacing whirlpools in many clinics. There is no evidence to judge the relative benefit of this much more localized treatment, but the perceived benefits in terms of cost savings, ease of care of equipment, and decreased risk of cross-infection have made these products popular.

Physical therapists have a great deal to contribute to the care of patients with chronic ulcers. It is essential, however, that the intervention chosen fits the specific physiological needs of the patient and blends well with the overarching treatment approach of the involved health care team.

REFERENCES

1. Abramson D: Indirect vasodilation in thermotherapy. *Arch Phys Med Rehabil* 1965; 46: 412-420.
2. Airaksinen O, Kolari P: Intermittent pneumatic compression therapy. *Crit Rev Phys Rehabil Med* 1992; 3:219-237.
3. Akers TK, Gabrielson AL: The effect of high voltage galvanic stimulation on the rate of healing of decubitus ulcers. *Biomed Sci Instrum* 1984; 20:99-100.
4. Alguire PC, Mathes BM: Chronic venous insufficiency and venous ulceration. *J Gen Intern Med* 1997; 12:374-383.
5. Allman RM, et al: Pressure sores among hospitalized patients. *Ann Intern Med* 1986; 105: 337-342.
6. Alvarez OM, Mertz PM, Smerbeck RV, Eaglstein WH: The healing of superficial skin wounds is stimulated by external electrical current. *J Invest Dermatol* 1983; 81:144-148.
7. Angel MF, et al: The causes of skin ulcerations associated with venous insufficiency: A unifying hypothesis. *Plast Reconstr Surg* 1987; 79: 289-297.
8. Angle N, Bergan JJ: Chronic venous ulcer [see comments]. *Br Med J* 1997; 314:1019-1023.
9. APTA: Guide to Physical Therapist Practice. *Phys Ther* 1997; 77: 1163-1650.
10. Archer AG, Roberts VC, Watkins PJ: Blood flow patterns in painful diabetic neuropathy. *Diabetologia* 1984; 27:563-567.
11. Ashcroft GS, Horan MA, Ferguson WJ: The effects of ageing on cutaneous wound healing in mammals. *J Anat* 1995; 187:1-26.
12. Ashcroft GS, et al: Age-related changes in the temporal and spatial distributions of fibrillin and elastin mRNAs and proteins in acute cutaneous wounds of healthy humans. *J Pathol* 1997; 183:80-89.
13. Ashcroft GS, Horan MA, Ferguson WJ: Aging is associated with reduced deposition of specific extracellular matrix components, an up-regulation of angiogenesis, and an altered inflammatory response in a murine incisional wound healing model. *J Invest Dermatol* 1997; 108:430-437.
14. Ashcroft GS, Horan MA, Ferguson M: Aging alters the inflammatory and endothelial cell adhesion molecule profiles during human cutaneous wound healing. *J Lab Invest* 1998; 78:47-58.

15. Augustinsson LE, et al: Epidural electrical stimulation in severe limb ischemia: Pain relief, increased blood flow, and a possible limb-saving effect. *Ann Surg* 1985; 202:104-110.

16. Baker LL, Chambers R, DeMuth SK, Villar F: Effects of electrical stimulation on wound healing in patients with diabetic ulcers. *Diabetes Care* 1997; 20: 405-412.

17. Bates-Jensen B: Pressure Ulcers: Pathophysiology and prevention, in Sussman C, Bates-Jensen B (eds): *Wound Care-A Collaborative Practice Manual for Physical Therapists and Nurses.* Gaithersburg, Md, Aspen Publications, 1998.

18. Beebe H, et al: Classification and grading of chronic venous disease in the lower extremity: A consensus statement. *Eur J Vasc Endovasc Surg* 1996; 12:487-492.

19. Bennett L, Lee B: *Chronic Ulcers of the Skin.* New York, McGraw-Hill, 1985.

20. Berlowitz DR, Wilking SV: The short-term outcome of pressure sores. *J Am Geriatr Soc* 1990; 38:748-752.

21. Birke J, et al: Relationship between hallux limitus and ulceration of the great toe. *J Orthop Sports Phys Ther* 1988; 10:172-176.

22. Birke J, Sims D: The insensitive foot, in Hunt G, McPoil T (eds): *Physical Therapy of the Foot and Ankle.* New York, Churchill Livingstone, 1995.

23. Birke JA, Sims DSJ, Buford WL: Walking casts: Effect on plantar foot pressures. *J Rehabil Res Dev* 1985; 22:18-22.

24. Birke JA, et al: Methods of treating plantar ulcers. *Phys Ther* 1991; 71:116-122.

25. Blalock A: Oxygen content of blood in patients with varicose veins. *Arch Surg* 1929; 19:898-905.

26. Boulton AJ, et al: Dynamic foot pressure and other studies as diagnostic and management aids in diabetic neuropathy. *Diabetes Care* 1983; 6:26-33.

27. Boulton AJ, et al: Abnormalities of foot pressure in early diabetic neuropathy. *Diabet Med* 1987; 4:225-228.

28. Braden B, Bergstrom N: Clinical utility of the Braden Scale for predicting pressure sore risk. *Decubitus* 1989; 2:44-51.

29. Brandeis GH, Morris JN, Nash DJ, Lipsitz LA: The epidemiology and natural history of pressure ulcers in elderly nursing home residents [see comments]. *JAMA* 1990; 264:2905-2909.

30. Broseta J, et al: Spinal cord stimulation in peripheral arterial disease. A cooperative study. *J Neurosurg* 1986; 64:71-80.

31. Brown M, Gogia P: Effect of high voltage stimulation on cutaneous wound healing in rabbits. *Phys Ther* 1987; 67:662-667.

32. Brown M, McDonnell M, Menton D: Electrical stimulation effects of cutaneous wound healing in rabbits: A follow-up study. *Phys Ther* 1988; 68:955-960.

33. Browse NL, Burnand KG: The cause of venous ulceration. *Lancet* 1982; 2:243-245.

34. Browse NL: The etiology of venous ulceration. *World J Surg* 1986; 10:938-943.

35. Burnand K: Venous lipodermatosclerosis: Treatment by fibrinolytic enhancement and elastic compression. *Br Med J* 1980; 280:7-11.

36. Callam M, et al: A controlled study of weekly ultrasound therapy in chronic leg ulceration. *Lancet* 1987; 8552:204-206.

37. Camargo C Jr, et al: Prospective study of moderate alcohol consumption and risk of peripheral arterial disease in US male physicians. *Circulation* 1997; 95:577-580.

38. Caputo G, et al: Assessment and management of foot disease in patients with diabetes. *N Engl J Med* 1994; 331:854-860.

39. Carley PJ, Wainapel SF: Electrotherapy for acceleration of wound healing: Low intensity direct current. *Arch Phys Med Rehabil* 1985; 66:443-446.

40. Cavanagh PR, Rodgers M, Liboshi A: Pressure distribution under symptom-free feet during barefoot standing. *Foot Ankle* 1987; 7:262-276.

41. Cheng H, et al: The effects of electric currents on ATP generation, protein synthesis and membrane transport in rat skin. *Clin Orthop* 1982; 171:264-272.

42. Christopoulos DG, et al: Air-plethysmography and the effect of elastic compression on venous hemodynamics of the leg. *J Vasc Surg* 1987; 5:148-159.

43. Coleman WC, Brand PW, Birke JA: The total contact cast. A therapy for plantar ulceration on insensitive feet. *J Am Podiatry Assoc* 1984; 74:548-552.

44. Coni NK: Posture and the arterial pressure in the ischaemic foot. *Age Ageing* 1983; 12:151-154.

45. Cook AW, et al: Vascular disease of extremities. Electric stimulation of spinal cord and posterior roots. *NY State J Med* 1976; 76:366-368.

46. Coon WW, Willis PW, Keller JB: Venous thrombo-embolism and other venous diseases in the Tecumseh community health study. *Circulation* 1973; 48:839-846.

47. Ctercteko GC, Dhanendran M, Hutton WC, Le Quesne LP: Vertical forces acting on the feet of diabetic patients with neuropathic ulceration. *Br J Surg* 1981; 68:608-614.

48. Cummings J: Role of light in wound healing, in Kloth, LC, McCulloch, JM, Feedar, JA, (eds): *Wound Healing: Alternatives in Management.* Philadelphia, FA Davis, 1990.

49. Czerniecki JM, et al: The effects of age and peripheral vascular disease on the circulatory and mechanical response of skin to loading. *Am J Phys Med Rehabil* 1990; 69:302-306.

50. Dagher FJ, Queral LA: Ischemic ulcers of the lower extremities, in Dagher FJ (ed): *Cutaneous Wounds.* New York, Futura Publishing, 1985.

51. Daniel RK, Priest DL, Wheatley DC: Etiological factors in pressure sores: An experimental model. *Arch Phys Med Rehabil* 1981; 62:492-498.

52. Dayton PD, Palladino SJ: Electrical stimulation of cutaneous ulcerations. A literature review. *J Am Podiatr Med Assoc* 1989; 79:318-321.

53. de Sonnaville JJJ, Colly LP, Wijkel D, Heine RJ: The prevalence and determinants of foot ulceration in type II diabetic patients in a primary health care setting. *Diabetes Res Clin Pract* 1997; 35:149-156.

54. Diamond E, Forst MB, Hyman SA, Rand SA: The effect of hyperbaric oxygen on lower extremity ulcerations. *J Am Podiatry Assoc* 1982; 72:180-185.

55. Diamond JE, Sinacore DR, Mueller MJ: Molded double-rocker plaster shoe for healing a diabetic plantar ulcer. A case report. *Phys Ther* 1987; 67:1550-1552.

56. Dickey JWJ: Stasis ulcers: The role of compliance in healing. *South Med J* 1991; 84:557-561.

57. Donaldson MC, Olin JW: Peripheral arterial disease: 5 steps to a better outcome. *Patient Care* 1999; 30:22-36.

58. Dyson M: Non-thermal cellular effects of ultrasound. *Br J Cancer Suppl* 1982; 45:165-171.

59. Dyson M: Stimulation of tissue repair by therapeutic ultrasound. *Infect Surg* 1982; 1:37-44.

60. Eaglstein WH: Wound healing and aging. *Clin Geriatr Med* 1989; 5:183-188.

61. Edelman D, Hough DM, Glazebrook KN, Oddone EZ: Prognostic value of the clinical examination of the diabetic foot ulcer. *J Gen Intern Med* 1997; 12:537-543.

62. Edelstein JE: Foot care for the aging. *Phys Ther* 1988; 68:1882-1886.

63. Elder DM, Greer KE: Venous disease: How to heal and prevent chronic leg ulcers. *Geriatrics* 1995; 50:30-36.

64. Erickson CA, et al: Healing of venous ulcers in an ambulatory care program: The roles of chronic venous insufficiency and patient compliance. *J Vasc Surg* 1995; 22:629-636.

65. Faglia E, et al: Angiographic evaluation of peripheral arterial occlusive disease and its role as a prognostic determinant for major amputation in diabetic subjects with foot ulcers. *Diabetes Care* 1999; 21(4): 625-630.

66. Feedar JA, Kloth LC: Chronic dermal ulcer healing enhanced with monophasic pulsed electrical stimulation. *Phys Ther* 1991; 70:639-649.

67. Fernandez S: Physiotherapy prevention and treatment of pressure sores. *Physiotherapy* 1987; 73:450-454.

68. Fischer BH: Topical hyperbaric oxygen treatment of pressure sores and skin ulcers. *Lancet* 1969; 2:405-409.

69. Fischer BH: Treatment of ulcers on the legs with hyperbaric oxygen. *J Dermatol Surg* 1975; 1:55-58.

70. Fitzpatrick JE: Stasis ulcers: Update on a common geriatric problem. *Geriatrics* 1989; 44:19-26, 31.

71. Gault WR, Gatens PFJ: Use of low intensity direct current in management of ischemic skin ulcers. *Phys Ther* 1976; 56:265-269.

72. Gogia PP: Physical therapy modalities for wound management. *Ostomy Wound Manage* 1996; 42:46-52, 54.

73. Gooding GA, et al: Sonography of the sole of the foot. Evidence for loss of foot pad thickness in diabetes and its relationship to ulceration of the foot. *Invest Radiol* 1986; 21:45-48.

74. Gupta PD, Saunders WA: Chronic leg ulcers in the elderly: Treated with absolute bedrest. *Practitioner* 1982; 226:1611-1612.

75. Haak S, Richardson S, Davey S: Alterations of cardiovascular function, in Heuther S, McCance K (eds): *Understanding Pathophysiology.* St Louis, Mosby, 1996.

76. Halperin JL: Peripheral vascular disease: Medical evaluation and treatment. *Geriatrics* 1987; 42:47-61.

77. Hansson C: Studies on leg and foot ulcers. *Acta Derm Venereol Suppl* (Stockh.) 1988; 136:1-45.

78. Harris M: Epidemiology of DM among the elderly in the United States. *Clin Geriatr Med* 1990; 6:703-719.

79. Helm PA, Walker SC, Pullium G: Total contact casting in diabetic patients with neuropathic foot ulcerations. *Arch Phys Med Rehabil* 1984; 65:691-693.

80. Helm PA, Walker SC, Pullium GF: Recurrence of neuropathic ulceration following healing in a total contact cast. *Arch Phys Med Rehabil* 1991; 72:967-970.

81. Hendricks WM, Swallow RT: Management of stasis leg ulcers with Unna's boots versus elastic support stockings. *J Am Acad Dermatol* 1985; 12:90-98.

82. Holewski JJ, et al: Prevalence of foot pathology and lower extremity complications in a diabetic outpatient clinic. *J Rehabil Res Dev* 1989; 26:35-44.

83. Holstein P, Nielsen PE, Barras JP: Blood flow cessation at external pressure in the skin of normal human limbs. Photoelectric recordings compared to isotope washout and to local intraarterial blood pressure. *Microvasc Res* 1979; 17:71-79.

84. Husn EA: Skin ulcers secondary to arterial and venous disease, in Lee BK (ed): *Chronic Ulcers of the Skin.* New York, McGraw-Hill, 1985.

85. Jacobs MJ, et al: Epidural spinal cord microvascular blood flow in severe limb ischemia. *Ann Surg* 1988; 207:179-183.

86. Jacobs MJ, et al: Foot salvage and improvement of microvascular blood flow as a result of epidural spinal cord electrical stimulation. *J Vasc Surg* 1990; 12:354-360.

87. Juergans J, Barker N, Hines E: Arteriosclerosis obliterans: Review of 520 cases with special reference to pathogenic and prognostic factors. *Circulation* 1960; 21:188-195.

88. Kincaid CB, Lavoie KH: Inhibition of bacterial growth in vitro following stimulation with high voltage, monophasic, pulsed current. *Phys Ther* 1989; 69:651-655.

89. Kloth LC, McCulloch JM, Feedar JA: Acceleration of wound healing with high voltage, monophasic, pulsed current. *Phys Ther* 1988; 68:503-508.

90. Kloth LC, Feedar JA: *Wound Healing: Alternatives in Management.* Philadelphia, FA Davis, 1990.

91. Knighton DR, Fylling CP, Fiegel VD, Cerra F: Amputation prevention in an independently reviewed at-risk diabetic population using a comprehensive wound care protocol. *Am J Surg* 1990; 160:466-471.

92. Korstanje MJ: Venous stasis ulcers-diagnostic and surgical considerations. *Dermatol Surg* 1995; 21:635-640.

93. Kumar S, et al: Semmes Weinstein monofilaments: A simple effective and inexpensive screening device for identifying diabetic patients at risk of foot ulceration. *Diabetes Research and Clinical Practice* 1991; 13:63-67.

94. Laing P, Cogley D, Kenerman L: Neuropathic foot ulceration treated by total contact casting. *J Bone Joint Surg* 1991; 74B:133-136.

95. Lavery LA, Vela SA, Lavery DC, Quebedeaux TL: Total contact casts: Pressure reduction at ulcer sites and the effect on the contralateral foot. *Arch Phys Med Rehabil* 1997; 78:1268-1271.

96. Lippmann HI, Briere J: Physical basis of external supports in chronic venous insufficiency. *Arch Phys Med Rehabil* 1971; 52:555-559.

97. Lippmann HI, et al: Edema control in the management of disabling chronic venous insufficiency [see comments]. *Arch Phys Med Rehabil* 1994; 75:436-441.

98. Lipsky BA, Pecoraro RE, Ahroni JH: Foot ulceration and infections in elderly diabetics. *Clin Geriatr Med* 1990; 6:747-769.

99. Loehne H: Pulsatile lavage with concurrent suction, in Sussman C, Bates-Jensen B (eds): *Wound Care: A Collaborative Practice Manual for Physical Therapists and Nurses.* Gaithersburg, Md, Aspen, 1998.

100. Lundeberg T, et al: Pulsed ultrasound does not improve healing of venous ulcers. *Scand J Rehabil Med* 1990; 22:195-197.

101. Majeske C: Reliability of wound surface area measurements. *Phys Ther* 1992; 72:138-141.

102. Marquez RR: Wound evaluation. In Gogia PP (ed): *Clinical Wound Management.* Thorofare, NJ, SLACK Incorporated, 1995.

103. Marquez RR: Wound debridement and hydrotherapy, in Gogia P (ed): *Clinical Wound Management.* Thorofare, NJ, SLACK Incorporated, 1995.

104. Mayberry JC, Moneta GL, Taylor LMJ, Porter JM: Fifteen-year results of ambulatory compression therapy for chronic venous ulcers. *Surgery* 1991; 109:575-581.

105. McCulloch JM: Peripheral vascular disease, in O'Sullivan S, Schmitz TJ (eds): *Physical Rehabilitation Assessment and Treatment.* Philadelphia, FA Davis, 1994.

106. McEnroe CS, O'Donnell TFJ, Mackey WC: Correlation of clinical findings with venous hemodynamics in 386 patients with chronic venous insufficiency. *Am J Surg* 1988; 156:148-152.

107. Meijer JH, et al: Method for the measurement of susceptibility to decubitus ulcer formation. *Med Biol Eng Comput* 1989; 27:502-506.

108. Michlovitz S: *Thermal Agents in Rehabilitation.* Philadelphia, FA Davis, 1996.

109. Mueller MJ, Diamond JE, Delitto A, Sinacore DR: Insensitivity, limited joint mobility, and plantar ulcers in patients with diabetes mellitus. *Phys Ther* 1989; 69:453-459.

110. Mueller MJ, et al: Total contact casting in treatment of diabetic plantar ulcers: A controlled clinical trial. *Diabetes Care* 1989; 12:384-388.

111. Nelzén O, Bergqvist D, Lindhagen A: Venous and non-venous leg ulcers: Clinical history and appearance in a population study. *Br J Surg* 1994; 81:182-187.

112. Nessler J, Mass D: Direct-current electrical stimulation of tendon healing in vitro. *Clin Orthop* 1987; 217:303.

113. Norton D: Calculating the risk: Reflections on the Norton Scale. *Decubitus* 1989; 2:24-31.

114. Novick A, et al: Effect of a walking splint and total contact cast on plantar forces. *J Prosthet Orthot* 1991; 3:168-178.

115. Olejniczak S, Zielinski A: Low hyperbaric therapy in the management of leg ulcers. *Mich Med* 1975; 74:707.

116. Panel for the Prediction and Prevention of Pressure Ulcers: Pressure Ulcers in Adults: Prediction and Prevention. *Clinical Practice Guideline No. 3*, AHCPR Publication No. 92-0047. Rockville, Md, Agency for Health Care Policy and Research, US Public Health Service, US Department of Health and Human Services, 1992.

117. Paris BE, et al: The prevalence and one-year outcome of limb arterial obstructive disease in a nursing home population. *J Am Geriatr Soc* 1988; 36:607-612.

118. Petermans J: Prevalence of disease of the large arteries in an elderly Belgian population: Relationship with some metabolic factors. *Acta Cardiol* 1984; 39:365-372.

119. Pollard J, LeQuesne L: Method of healing diabetic forefoot ulcers. *Br Med J* 1983; 286:437-438.

120. Pollard J, LeQuesne L, Tappin J: Forces under the foot. *J Biomed Eng* 1983; 5:37-40.

121. Queral LA, Dagher FJ: Venous ulceration in the lower extremity, in Dagher FJ (ed): *Cutaneous Wounds.* New York, Future Publishers, 1985.

122. Rappl L: Management of pressure by therapeutic positioning, in Sussman C, Bates-Jensen B (eds): *Wound Care: A Collaborative Practice Manual for Physical Therapists and Nurses.* Gaithersburg, Md, Aspen, 1998.

123. Reed B, Zarro V: Wound healing and the use of thermal agents, in Michlovitz S (ed): *Thermal Agents in Rehabilitation.* Philadelphia, FA Davis, 1996.

124. Rijswijk R, et al: Multicenter clinical evaluation of a hydrocolloid dressing for leg ulcers. *Cutis* 1985; 35:173-176.

125. Roche C, West J: A controlled trial investigating the effect of ultrasound on venous ulcers referred from general practitioners. *Physiotherapy* 1984; 70:475.

126. Romanus M: Microcirculatory reactions to local pressure induced ischemia. A vital microscopic study in hamster cheek pouch and a pilot study in man. *Acta Chir Scand Suppl* 1977; 479:1-30.

127. Rutherford RB, et al: Recommended standards for reports dealing with lower extremity ischemia: Revised version. *J Vasc Surg* 1997; 26: 517-538.

128. Samson RH, Showalter DP: Stockings and the prevention of recurrent venous ulcers. *Dermatol Surg* 1996; 22:373-376.

129. Sayegh A: Intermittent pneumatic compression: past, present and future. *Clin Rehabil* 1987; 1:59-64.

130. Schubert V, Fagrell B: Evaluation of the dynamic cutaneous postischaemic hyperaemia and thermal response in elderly subjects and in an area at risk for pressure sores. *Clin Physiol* 1991; 11:169-182.

131. Schubert V: Hypotension as a risk factor for the development of pressure sores in elderly subjects. *Age Ageing* 1991; 20:255-261.

132. Siegal A: Noninvasive vascular testing, in Sussman C, Bates-Jensen B (eds): *Wound Care: A Collaborative Practice Manual for Physical Therapists and Nurses.* Frederick, Md, Aspen, 1998.

133. Sims DSJ, Cavanagh PR, Ulbrecht JS: Risk factors in the diabetic foot. Recognition and management. *Phys Ther* 1988; 68:1887-1902.

134. Sinacore DR, et al: Diabetic plantar ulcers treated by total contact casting. A clinical report. *Phys Ther* 1987; 67:1543-1549.

135. Smith PC, Sarin S, Hasty J, Scurr JH: Sequential gradient pneumatic compression enhances venous ulcer healing: A randomized trial. *Surgery* 1990; 108:871-875.

136. Snyder-Mackler L: Electrical stimulation for tissue repair, in Robinson A, Snyder-Mackler L (eds): *Clinical Electrophysiology: Electrotherapy and Electrodiagnostic Testing.* Baltimore, Williams & Wilkins, 1995.

137. Spector WD, Kapp MC, Tucker RJ, Sternberg J: Factors associated with presence of decubitus ulcers at admission to nursing homes. *Gerontologist* 1988; 28:830-834.

138. Steed DL, et al: Effect of extensive debridement and treatment on the healing of diabetic foot ulcers. *J Am Coll Surg* 1996; 183:61-64.

139. Stokes IA, Faris IB, Hutton WC: The neuropathic ulcer and loads on the foot in diabetic patients. *Acta Orthop Scand* 1975; 46:839-847.

140. Sussman C, Bates-Jensen B: *Wound Care: A Collaborative Practice Manual for Physical Therapists.* Gaithersburg, Md, Aspen, 1999.

141. Tetteroo E, van der Graaf Y, Bosch JL, van Engelen AD: Randomized comparison of primary stent placement versus primary angioplasty followed by selective stent placement in patients with ilia-artery occlusive disease. (Dutch Iliac Stent Trial Study Group). *Lancet* 1998; 351:1153-1160.

142. Thomas DR: Pressure ulcers, in Cassel CK, et al (eds): *Geriatric Medicine.* New York, Springer-Verlag, 1997.

143. Thulesius O: The venous wall and valvular function in chronic venous insufficiency. *Intl Angiol* 1996; 15:114-118.

144. Van De Kerkhof PC, Van Bergen B, Spruijt K, Kuiper JP: Age-related changes in wound healing. *Clin Expr Dermatol* 1994; 19:369-374.

145. van Rijswijk L: General principles of wound management, in Gogia PP (ed): *Clinical Wound Management.* Thorofare, NJ, SLACK Incorporated, 1995.

146. Versluysen M: Pressure sores in elderly patients. The epidemiology related to hip operations. *J Bone Joint Surg* [Br.] 1985; 67:10-13.

147. Wagner F: The dysvascular foot: A system for diagnosis and treatment. *Foot Ankle* 1981; 2:64-122.

148. Wessman HC, Kottke FJ: The effect of indirect heating on peripheral blood flow, pulse rate, blood pressure, and temperature. *Arch Phys Med Rehabil* 1967; 48:567-576.

149. Wolcott L, et al: Accelerated healing of skin ulcers by electrotherapy: Preliminary clinical results. *South Med J* 1999; 62:795-801.

PATIENT EDUCATION AS AN INTERVENTION WITH THE OLDER ADULT

DALE L. AVERS, PT, MSED AND DAVIS L. GARDNER, MA

OUTLINE

tion strategies grounded in sound theory and research may make the difference between the patient's success or failure in achieving rehabilitation goals. In this chapter, patient education and the physical therapist's role as a patient educator are emphasized in terms of a practical yet philosophically based experience that can influence older patients' self-direction in prescribed treatment regimens. A review of learning theories is presented, followed by a philosophical approach to learning and patient education. Characteristics of older adult learners and some common barriers to their learning also are summarized. The role of the care-giver and teaching strategies to enhance this role are discussed, and selected assessment methods are presented. The chapter concludes with three typical patient education scenarios that illustrate some of the concepts presented relative to patient education as a treatment modality.

CHAPTER OBJECTIVES

As a result of studying this chapter, the reader should be able to do the following:

1. Identify the characteristics of older adult learners that influence the planning and implementation of patient education sessions
2. Identify typical obstacles to effective patient education interaction with older adults
3. Apply instructional strategies to improve interaction with older adult learners in patient education settings
4. Develop and apply a patient education philosophy

LEARNING THEORIES

Learning by its very nature defies easy definition and simple theorizing. The concepts of behavioral change and experience are central to learning theories. *Learning* is defined as the

INTRODUCTION

Imparting information to a patient is one of the most common interventions a physical therapist uses. However, patient education is often the least addressed topic in physical therapy schools and the least understood concept as far as effective methodology. Rehabilitation professionals often do not perceive themselves as educators despite of the fact that the therapist spends much of any treatment session instructing patients in new techniques or home programs or facilitating relearning of motor skills. Using appropriate educa-

capacity to behave in a given fashion, which results from practice or other forms of experience that causes an enduring change in behavior.[32] Learning as a process, rather than an end product, focuses on what happens as learning takes place. Explanations of this process are called *learning theories*. It is necessary to understand the components of how learning occurs to effectively address specific learning situations. The organization schema of Merriam and Caffarella[26] has been adopted in this chapter to explore the development and application of learning theories through four learning orientations: behaviorist, cognitive, humanist, and social.

Behaviorist Orientation

Behaviorism is a familiar theory credited to John B. Watson (1878-1958) but also loosely encompasses other researchers such as Thorndike, Tolman, Guthrie, Hull, and Skinner.[30]

Behaviorism focuses on observable behavior shaped by environmental forces. Learning occurs when there is a change in the form or frequency of observable performance.[14] The key elements in learning are the stimulus, the response, and the association between the two. The environment plays the most important role in the behaviorist theoretical approach. Behavioral theorists believe that the teacher's role is to design an environment that elicits desired behavior and to extinguish behavior that is not desirable. An example in physical therapy patient education would be the therapist verbally reinforcing a correct transfer technique as it is being performed while ignoring the behavior when the transfer technique is done incorrectly. Another example might be when the therapist instructs a patient in stair climbing and consistently reinforces the "correct technique," such as the right foot advancing first. The patient eventually performs according to the therapist's instructions but may not know why.

Important concepts of learning that are derived from a behaviorist orientation are Thorndike's Law of Exercise and Law of Readiness. The Law of Exercise asserts that the repetition of a meaningful connection between a situation and a response results in substantial learning when simultaneous reinforcement is present. Sheer repetition on its own does not strengthen learning. The Law of Readiness states that if the learner is ready for the connection, learning is enhanced; if not, learning is inhibited. The systematic design of instruction, behavioral objectives, notions of the instructor's accountability, programmed instruction, computer-assisted instruction, and competency-based education are strongly grounded in behavioral learning theory.

The behaviorist orientation is thought to be ideal for learning that requires rote responses and recalling of facts. Behaviorism is not appropriate for higher order thinking skills, such as problem solving.[14]

Cognitive Orientation

In the late 1950s, learning theory began to shift away from behaviorism, in which the emphasis was on promoting the student's performance by manipulation of the stimulus, to a cognitive orientation, in which the emphasis was on promoting mental processing. Cognitive processes such as thinking, problem solving, language, and concept formation were stressed in the cognitive approach. Learning is equated with discrete changes between states of knowledge rather than in the probability of response. Cognitive theories focus on the conceptualization of students' learning processes and address the issues of how information is received, organized, stored, and retrieved by the mind.[14] The cognitive approach focuses on the mental activities of the learner that lead up to a response and acknowledges the processes of mental planning, goal-setting, and organizational strategies. A cognitive theorist who is relevant to older adult learning is Jerome Bruner.

Bruner developed a theory about the act of learning involving the following four simultaneous processes: (1) ability to use specific skills in acquiring knowledge; (2) developing an attitude toward learning that involves a "sense of discovery" of relationships and a "need to know" feeling; (3) transformation, or the process of manipulating knowledge to make it fit new tasks; and (4) evaluation, or checking whether the way information is manipulated is adequate to the task.[7] These learning principles became the foundation for an instructional theory that emphasizes the need for the instructor to (1) implant a desire to learn (to motivate); (2) organize the body of knowledge to be taught (to enhance memory, storage, and retrieval); (3) sequence the presentation of materials to be learned (to enhance storage and retrieval); and (4) specify the nature and spacing of rewards and punishments (to provide feedback). Each learner has a unique sequence preference based on past learning, stage of development, the nature of the material, and individual differences.

One concern of a cognitive researcher would be how aging affects an adult's ability to process and retrieve information and how aging affects an adult's internal mental structures. An example of applied cognitive theory in geriatric physical therapy would be demonstrated in how the therapist organizes a treatment session with the goal of instructing the patient how to weight shift prior to ambulation. In such an example, the therapist would build on the simple to more complex tasks of supine weight shifting and to sitting weight shifting before proceeding to standing weight shifting. Progression would then advance from bipedal weight shifting to unilateral weight shifting to advancing a foot forward. Concern for the proper pacing of instruction would be addressed throughout the treatment session.

Humanist Orientation

Humanist theories consider learning from the perspective of the human potential for growth. From a learning theory perspective, humanism emphasizes that a person's perceptions are centered in experience, as well as the freedom and responsibility to become what one is capable of becoming. These tenets underlie much of adult learning theory that stresses the self-directedness of adults and the value of experience in the learning process. Two psychologists who have contributed much to the understanding of learning from this perspective are Abraham Maslow and Carl Rogers.

Maslow interpreted the goal of learning to be self-actualization or the full use of talents, capacities, and potentialities. Carl Rogers described his philosophy of learning and teaching in his book *Freedom to Learn for the 80's.*[29] He defined the elements of learning as a "quality of personal involvement"—with both feeling and cognitive aspects being part of the learning event. Learning is self-initiated so that even when the impetus or stimulus comes from an external source, the senses of discovery, of reaching out, and of grasping and comprehending come from within. Learning is so pervasive that behavior, attitudes, and perhaps even the personality of the learner are affected. Learning is evaluated by the learner. The learner knows whether the instruction is meeting a need and is leading toward a goal.[29] Rogers states that significant learning combines the logical and the intuitive, the intellect and the feelings, the concept and the experience, the idea and the meaning.

Perceptual Theory

The perceptual theory suggests that views or perceptions of people, objects, and events in the individual's environment will have much to do with behavior. Adults have lived in the world for a given number of years and have gained many perceptions of their environment and of all its objects and events. Five concepts that affect an individual's perception of environment are beliefs, values, needs, attitudes, and self-experience.

Beliefs are what adults perceive to be true, whether these take the form of faith, knowledge, assumption, or superstition. Beliefs are reality to individuals, and individuals behave as if the beliefs are true. *Values* identify people's feelings about what is important to them and could be related to ideas, a way of life, material things, or people. *Needs* are what individuals require to maintain or enhance themselves. According to this concept, needs can be divided into two kinds: (1) physiological needs, such as food, water, air, shelter, and (2) social needs, such as the need for approval and acceptance, status, prestige, or power. *Attitudes* reflect an emotionalized belief about the degree of worth of someone or something. *Self-experience (self-concept)* is how people see themselves, how they feel about being that person, how they think others see them, how they see other people, and how they feel about this.

People are most threatened when they are forced to change the ways in which they seek to maintain or enhance their concept of self. Threat then causes defensive behavior and a narrowing and constricting of the perceptual field. When threatened, people are resistant and seek to maintain themselves instead of seeking growth or enhancement of self-concept. Rogers advocated that external threats should be kept to a minimum when learning is perceived as threatening to the self. A corollary is that self-evaluation and self-criticism are more acceptable to adults than evaluation by

others. Humanist orientation emphasizes the individual's choice, responsibility, and internal motivation (locus of control). For example, the patient's desire to become independent after a severe stroke becomes the internal motivation for going through intense rehabilitation and discomfort. This motivation coupled with self-evaluation may lead the patient to develop new ways of doing things independent of the therapist.

Social Learning Theory

Social learning theory is a system of thought based on imitation or modeling. Bandura postulated that one can learn from observation without having to imitate what was observed.[5] He further explored self-directed behaviors. In order for people to regulate their own behavior, well-defined objectives or goals are selected; contractual agreements are negotiated to further increase goal commitment; objective records of behavioral changes are used as additional sources of reinforcement for their self-controlling behavior; and the stimulus condition under which the behavior customarily occurs is altered. For example, for the older adult who has difficulty adhering to his/her diabetic diet, removing the source of temptation or storing the forbidden food in a different place would alter stimulus conditions. The progressive narrowing of stimulus control, for example, may initiate change over a period of time instead of creating a total change at one time. A commitment to monitor food intake would also be important from the social learning viewpoint.

The term *locus of control* is used to explain which behavior in the individual's repertoire will occur in a given situation. Typically, people with an internal locus of control will adhere more consistently and longer than those with an external locus of control, which requires external motivation such as praise and material rewards. Social learning theories provide an additional factor in how adults learn by acknowledging the importance of context and the learner's interaction with the environment to explain behavior.

Adult Learning Orientation

Andragogy is a term popularized by Knowles to explain a philosophical orientation for adult education.[21] His four main assumptions of changes in self-concept, role of experience, readiness to learn, and orientation to learning lay the foundation for the instruction of older adults.

Changes in self-concept occur as individuals grow and mature. Their self-concept moves from one of total dependency (as is the reality of an infant) to one of increasing self-directedness. Any experience that adults perceive as putting them in a position of being treated as a child will interfere with their learning, commonly resulting in expressions of resentment and resistance.

Role of experience defines the role of lifetime experiences. As individuals mature, they accumulate an expanding reservoir of experience, producing an older adult who has a *rich* and varied background to facilitate new learning and knowledge. Any situation in which adults' experiences are perceived to be devalued or ignored may be perceived as rejecting their experience and even their person.

The concept of *readiness to learn* explains the shift from an external stimulus to an internal stimulus. As individuals mature, their readiness to learn is decreasingly the product of biological development and academic pressure and is increasingly the product of the developmental tasks required for the performance of evolving social roles. Learning experiences must be timed to coincide with the learners' developmental tasks. For example, a geriatric patient may need to attempt ambulation before comprehending the importance of general strengthening or balance activities.

Orientation to learning reflects the adult's purpose for learning. Adults tend to have a problem-centered orientation to learning. Real-life problems are the purpose for seeking educational opportunities. The immediate application of information learned is a primary need of the adult learner.[21]

In conclusion, the following principles developed by Darkenwald and Merriam summarize the principles applicable to patient education as a treatment modality:[11]

- Adults' readiness to learn depends on their previous learning.
- Intrinsic motivation produces more pervasive and permanent learning.
- Positive reinforcement is effective.
- Material to be learned should be presented in an organized fashion.
- Learning is enhanced by repetition.
- Tasks and materials that are meaningful are more fully and more easily learned.
- Active participation in learning improves retention.
- Environmental factors affect learning.
- Adults learn throughout their lifetime.
- Adults exhibit learning styles that illustrate various learning theories such as the following:
  a. Having personal strategies for coding information.
  b. Perceiving in different ways—cognitive procedures.
  c. Perceiving learning activities to be problem-centered and relevant to life.
  d. Desiring some immediate appreciation.
  e. Having a concept of themselves as learners.
  f. Being self-directed.

The learning theories and principles presented in this section are diverse but can also compliment each other. The effective health care provider will use a variety of patient education interventions based on the outcomes desired.

PSYCHOLOGICAL FACTORS OF THE LEARNING SITUATION

To develop a philosophical approach to patient education, physical therapists must understand their own motivations and biases toward their role as the helper, their attitudes toward their patients, and their attitude toward the informa-tion they are sharing. Understanding the older adult's perceptions of self and of learning is also important. This section discusses factors that contribute to the therapist's and patient's attitudes toward teaching and learning.

Therapist's Perception of the Patient Educator

One motivation for entering the health care field is to help people. This avowed motive is sincere in most cases. People become helpers because they really enjoy helping others and want to impact their lives positively. Although the motive to help others focuses on the needs of the patient, the needs of the "helper" must be acknowledged as a philosophy of patient education is developed. The helper's need to be needed and the helper's needs as a person both exist, i.e., "I want to be needed and wanted but not to be completely responsible for a person." Another common but deeper, less obvious thought that can shape the physical therapist's attitudes is the "there but for the grace of God go I" reaction when the patient becomes a disturbing mirror image of the helper's real or potential suffering. Asserting authority is often the helper's defense against this phenomenon.

Two less apparent reasons for entering a health field are the desire to learn about oneself and the desire to exert control. The desire to exert control, to be in charge, and to have some noticeable impact on the world is particularly relevant when attempting to "teach" a patient. This attitude of control can make the physical therapist the "high priest" of the learning situation, perhaps inhibiting the learning situation.

To understand the effect of this attitude of "control" or dominance, a common model prevalent in the U.S. health care system, Parsons' sick role model, is discussed. This model often shapes therapists' initial attitudes toward their professional responsibilities. The sick role model was described by Parsons in 1951 as made up of four aspects that permeate the attitudes and behaviors of both the patient and the health care professional. The first is that the sick person is relieved of normal social responsibilities, e.g., he/she does not have to get dressed or may need help to go to the bathroom or to be fed. The second is that the sick person must be taken care of and thus assumes a dependent role. The third is that the sick person should regard getting well as an obligation, i.e., to be motivated. And the fourth is that the sick person should seek out expert help and cooperate with the process of getting well.[27]

This model implies that the health care professional is in a position of authority and the patient is in a role of dependency, obligated to get well according to the methods and desires of the health care professional. The patient hands the problem over to the professional and becomes passive, whereas the professional takes charge of all aspects of that patient and whatever problems are present. When the acuity of the situation lessens, Parsons[27] and Silver-stone[33] describe the sick role as evolving into a patient role characterized by conformity, dependency, and receptivity to care that excludes patient aggressiveness and attempts at self-reliance.

Another model similar to the sick role model and very prevalent in today's health care environment is the cure model of health care. Paternalism is the framework for this view of the patient, placing the health care provider in the role of decision maker about the type and amount of information the patient receives. Paternalism is most often associated with the traditional medical model, which uses authority, power, and superior knowledge to act on the patient's behalf. Paternalism tends to reinforce the passiveness of the patient and communicates expectations of compliance and unquestioning obedience. The role of the health care provider is a "father" figure, i.e., authoritarian and all knowing. The limitation is that the health care provider may be perceived as overbearing. The patient's needs, concerns, and choices may not be considered and therefore the health care provider may act incompletely or inappropriately.[25]

An alternative to the cure model of health care is the care model. The care model values patient autonomy and mutual collaboration between the patient and the health care provider. The role of the health care provider is one of consultant and enabler, peer and adviser, facilitating the patient's needs and desires. In this model, the type and amount of information are determined by the patient with a commitment from the health care provider to be honest and forthcoming. Individualized care, compassion, warm personal regard, and open communication are additional values. Limitations of the care model involve the need for patients to make decisions for themselves. A patient may not be able to make his/her own decisions in times of grief or extreme stress or with certain medical conditions. This approach also takes longer, making it less efficient. Finally, the health care provider may not use his/her extensive knowledge as overtly as in the cure model, perhaps putting the patient at a slight disadvantage.[25]

Older Adults' Perception of Self

Human beings are complex and whose behavior, attitudes, and conditioning are affected by multiple internal and external forces. Any number of these forces can affect how older adult patients respond to medical situations and their attitudes toward the learning situation. This section briefly presents several of the forces that affect the geriatric patient.

Self-Concept and Self-Esteem

The view one has of one's self is called *self-concept,* and the value placed on that self-concept is *self-esteem.* Life experiences, attitudes toward self and others, beliefs, and value systems all factor into the self-concept/self-esteem equation of the older adult. Multiple losses are common as a person grows older and can reinforce any existing negative self-perception or may negatively affect a life-long positive self-perception. Losses can include the death of a spouse, adult children, grandchildren, friends, and peers or loss of

health or of one's home. Retirement from the work force may be viewed as the loss of a productive role when no valued activities exist to replace the former occupation or profession. In addition to any or all of these, the geriatric patient participating in rehabilitation has experienced some degree of trauma and may have serious self-doubts concerning the ability to function again in the home, community, or work environment.

Sensitivity to Failure

Many therapists treating older adults will be a significant number of years younger than their patients. An older adult's sensitivity to failure may be affected by the age difference and by the perceived ease with which the younger therapist performs complicated tasks and physical movement. The therapist also must realize the patient may be comparing current performance with previous normal performance, which can enhance the perception of failure. A negative self-concept and the older adult's view of his/her own personal crisis, e.g., disability, illness, or personal loss, also may accentuate the sensitivity to failure.

Resistance to Change

Resistance can be a normal coping strategy to change and fear and should not be viewed as a rigidity of attitude or behavior and thus result in a person being unamenable to change. Rogers stated resistance may be observed when the individual feels threatened. The geriatric patient also may express total hopelessness for improved function and exhibit a resignation to accepting the present limitations. This attitude may be manifested in resistance to suggestions, change, or help. Skepticism and even some degree of fear may underlie resistance.

In summary, the geriatric patient in treatment sessions is an individual with a complex psychosocial profile that will influence the degree of willingness to learn. The therapist also has complex attitudes and beliefs regarding the role of the health care professional that affect the tone, manner, and flexibility of the therapist in the teaching/learning situation. The initial step in becoming an effective patient educator is to recognize underlying attitudes affecting the learning situation.

MOTIVATION AND LEARNING

When the underlying attitudes and values of both the older patient and the therapist are recognized and accepted, the therapist can develop strategies for facilitating and affecting the desired learning from a psychological perspective. This section discusses the role of motivation and choice as well as specific techniques to deal with the psychological attitudes of both the older adult and therapist that are discussed in the preceding section.

Eliciting patient compliance is often a perceived goal of patient education. The lack of compliance or motivation is also a common reason to refer an older adult to psychological services. The physical therapist often requests that a psychological referral include: "Increase their motivation so that they'll comply with my instructions" or concludes: "This patient isn't motivated because my instructions on practicing transfer techniques aren't being followed." Compliance and motivation are sometimes used interchangeably, although they are very different concepts. In order to develop appropriate goals for patient education, an understanding of the terms and implications of compliance and motivation is important.

The term *compliance* implies that the older adult follows medical orders and does what the health care professional has instructed. Compliance is authoritarian in tone and implies that the patient must do as the therapist instructs in order for the patient education session to be successful. Compliance is a natural goal when operating under the sick role model because it implies the patient's subservience, dependence, and unquestioning obedience to authority.[12] The sick and patient role models foster the idea that the patient is dependent on the health professional to get better. These models put enormous responsibility on the therapist to make the patient better and may be one cause of therapist burnout.

Adherence, on the other hand, is a term that implies independent choice and action on the part of the patient; therefore a willingness to participate is implied. Adherence can be defined as a consistent behavior that is accomplished through an internalization of learning, enhanced by independent coping and problem-solving skills.[2]

Motivation, as used by Kemp,[20] is a complex attitude composed of wants, beliefs, and rewards versus cost of the behavior. Motivation is not on a continuum of poor, average, or high. Rather, motivation is a characteristic of all adults that is manifested in behavior. Therapists incorrectly assess a patient's motivation as poor because the patient is not being "compliant" when, in fact, the patient might be "highly" motivated for another activity of greater value to the patient. The therapist who facilitates patient learning must discern the distinct differences in compliance and adherence and also must develop an understanding of these psychological implications and attitudes.

Goals of Patient Education

D'Onofrio contends that the goals of education are to equip the learner with problem-solving skills whereby the learner can gain greater control over the directions of his/her own life.[12] Rogers goes further and suggests that the goal of education is to facilitate learning.[29] He states that instruction must develop the learner to decrease dependence on the instructor. Consistent with this philosophy, education is viewed as the process of facilitating the learner's problem-solving skills with the goal that the learner will gain control over any specific problem. Learning places the responsibility on the learner, the patient. To teach does not imply learning. Teaching is one-sided and asks nothing of the patient except that

the patient be present. An example of this concept is seen in motor learning. Motor learning uses the strategy of the patient's internal feedback to provide stimulus for learning, rather than the therapist's stimulus of telling the patient his/her movement is "right or wrong." For instance, while assisting a patient with the task of stair climbing, instead of directing the patient in a certain "technique" of stair climbing, the therapist may instead suggest that the patient begin to climb the stairs and that facilitate the patient's internal feedback mechanism by asking questions such as "how did that feel" when the patient starts to lose his/her balance or "did you notice the difference" when the patient tries a technique that was more complex.[9,10]

Payton asserts that only the patient can make the decision that a goal is worth working for attainment.[28] Lindgren states that older patients should be viewed as individuals who are capable of making their own decisions—not as dependent recipients of medical care.[22] These two statements clearly convey the important message that older adults can and do exercise choice in whether they will participate in treatment sessions.

Rogers believes that it is impossible to "teach" anyone anything unless the learner wants to learn.[29] Think of the patient who sits through a detailed exercise program. A strong feeling is transmitted that the patient really is not listening to the therapist and is, in fact, in a hurry to leave. No matter how great a "facilitator of learning" the therapist is, if the patient does not want to learn, he/she will not.

Basically, one learns what one wants to learn. When one wants to learn, one is described as being "motivated," an internal phenomenon. Bille relates Maslow's needs hierarchy to patient motivation in an interesting and relevant manner.[6] Maslow theorized that one's basic physiological needs (air, food, water, movement, sex, avoidance of pain) and safety and security needs (assurance that the world is regular and predictable; that death, destruction, or physical/social/emotional/economic harm is not imminent) must be met before affiliation and esteem needs can be met.

Bille applies this concept to the patient who has experienced physical trauma and whose current needs basically are physiological and safety-oriented. The patient may find it difficult to focus on adjusting to the trauma and the necessary rehabilitation and may not be able to envision managing the changes that may result from that trauma. Motivation will be enhanced, therefore, when instruction is centered on procedures that are, in the patient's perspective, physiological and safety-oriented, such as strength, mobility, ambulation, or activities of daily living (ADL). When these needs are met, self-esteem increases as progress is made.

Bille relates the need for esteem to the motivation to learn and states that as self-esteem increases, motivation to learn will increase. The therapist can foster the patient's self-esteem, and therefore motivation, when open, two-way communication exists. The patient needs to feel free and unthreatened to tell the therapist what has affected or lowered his/her self-esteem. The basic characteristics a teacher needs to exhibit to facilitate this open communication as described by Rogers are realness or genuineness; prizing the learner; acceptance; trust; and empathic understanding.[29] When the health care professional exhibits realness or genuineness, the facade is lifted, and the therapist comes into a direct personal encounter with the learner and meets the learner on a person-to-person basis, as peers or equals. There is no hiding behind an authoritarian role; there is no sterile facade. The physical therapist can express emotions and attitudes and becomes, to the patient, a real person with convictions and feelings.

Rogers describes prizing the learner as valuing the learner's feelings, opinions, and the person as a whole. Prizing is caring for the learner, accepting the learner as a separate person, appreciating the learner's differences, and exhibiting a belief that the learner is fundamentally trustworthy. The physical therapist who exhibits this attitude can fully accept the fear and hesitation of the older adult as the patient approaches his/her own personal crisis. This attitude allows the therapist to accept the "poor motivation" of the older adult and to make attempts to understand the factors contributing to the motivational problem. Empathic understanding is the therapist's ability to appreciate the patient's reactions from the patient's perspective and to have a sensitive awareness of the way the processes of education and learning seems to the patient. The likelihood of significant learning is increased when these characteristics are exhibited by the therapist.[29]

To increase the patient's self-directedness, the therapist should provide opportunities for the patient to make decisions about treatment and to identify what is to be learned. Payton presents excellent examples of this process in his chapter the "Patient as Planner."[28] To increase the patient's motivation, the therapist should lead the patient to explore the range of concerns and then to identify the primary concern. Goal setting by the patient becomes a motivator because a greater degree of choice is exercised.

Payton also outlines four levels of patient participation in goal identification that range from the patient's free choice, with open-ended questions, to no choice, with the therapist prescribing and telling the patient what to do. The free-choice level is possible when the therapist does not suggest answers. This allows the patient autonomy, an important aspect of self-esteem and motivation. Payton uses the following as an example of the free-choice process:[28]

Therapist:	What bothers you?
Patient:	I have a tingling on my left side.
Therapist:	Is there anything else bothering you?
Patient:	I have trouble using my left ankle.
Therapist:	Is there anything else?
Patient:	I can't move my toes.
Therapist:	What bothers you the most?
Patient:	It's hard for me to walk.

By allowing the patient to explore several concerns, identification of the walking difficulty provided the basis for a goal statement that was generated by the patient. Therefore, the patient's motivational level was enhanced for treatment sessions because the therapist addressed the primary concern of the patient.

At the next level, the therapist asked questions and offered several options or suggestions, with permission to offer those options first being elicited from the patient. The resulting multiple-choice question still allowed the patient to exercise choice and control among the options. This level is in contrast with the lowest level, in which the question to the patient is followed by the therapist's immediate answer or recommendation. Thus, the patient's participation is excluded, self-esteem is questioned, and motivation is diminished.

Older adults may exhibit some resistance to becoming partners in treatment decisions and sessions. Anderson suggests that this reluctance may be based on their perceptions of health care professionals as "high priests" whose wisdom is all encompassing and whose decisions are not to be discussed or questioned.[1] This perception was described earlier in the discussion of the sick role model. Obviously in acute cases, this perception of the medical model may be the most appropriate one. However, in many situations the patient's progress will depend more on the helping process than on the sick role model of health care delivery.

In the sick role model, the patient has a more passive role in treatment sessions, whereas the therapist is the activist. In contrast, in the helping process, the patient is more active in identifying the problem, setting goals, exploring alternative solutions, and assessing the results. When the patient is active in the helping process, the patient's ability to appropriately cope with any problems that arise is strengthened. Coping may involve consulting with the therapist for opinions on the proposed solutions, but the intent is for the patient to become more of a partner than a passive recipient in the health care regimen.[1]

In summary, the helping process appears to be more congruent with the geriatric patient's need for self-esteem, autonomy, the exercise of choice, and the partnership that Payton advocates. To be an effective patient educator requires an approach of empowering the patient rather than assuming an authoritarian role. An effective patient educator facilitates the learner's learning, appreciates the learner's differences, and helps the learner establish goals and responsibility for learning. A patient whose ideas, interests, concerns, and feelings have been heard and responded to by others is much more likely to enter into active, cooperative planning for necessary treatment. A patient who is actively involved in treatment planning is more likely to adhere to those cooperative plans and guarantee the success of treatment. The importance of self-esteem and choice relates closely to the geriatric patient's motivational level. Lasting gains are possible when the geriatric patient perceives the therapist as a supportive partner in treatment sessions. The therapist's degree of success when working with a geriatric patient is related to the perception of that patient as a person against a background of cognitive and psychosocial characteristics.

Strategies to Affect Learning

The therapist's actions and behaviors are keys in working with an older patient whose negative self-concept presents a significant obstacle to treatment progress. To attempt to counter these doubts and to modify the patient's perception of self to a positive rather than a negative view, the therapist should emphasize the successful experiences the patient has had as an adult in overcoming other difficult experiences. Other techniques include guiding the patient to identify the reason(s) for any past failures and assisting the patient to recognize that the reason(s) for failure may not be a factor in treatment. If, however, the reason(s) for past failure may be present in the therapeutic environment, the therapist should help the patient identify the factors that can be controlled at this time.[35] For example, consider the patient with previously treated low back pain who starts physical therapy. The patient's behavior indicates a reluctance to try the exercises. As the therapist explores this reluctance, the patient indicates, "No one really explained the previous exercises." The therapist indicates that doing an exercise incorrectly can cause increased pain. Extra care and a thorough explanation of the exercises are indicated to address the patient's history of perceived failure.

Creating a successful instructional environment and providing opportunities for successes, no matter how small they may be, are valuable tools. Any contributions the patient may make should be recognized, and establishing a partnership relationship in the treatment goals and sessions is helpful.[35] However, psychological counseling is best done by counseling professionals.

During the treatment session, the therapist should provide tasks that the patient can do successfully. Focusing on relevant information in an organized, clear manner, and providing adequate time for skill practice can enhance successful performance. The therapist should sensitively give adequate, honest feedback and encouragement for correct responses and performance to diminish the chances for and perception of failure. The patient's positive contributions and correct performance of any tasks[35] should be stressed; be aware that depressed patients may demonstrate an increased sensitivity to failure and heightened self-criticism.

Accepting the patient's existing attitudes and recognizing that new attitudes, behaviors, and values cannot be forced on the geriatric patient may help temper any resistance to change of treatment. Creating constructive dialogue and reasoning instead of participating in arguments that tend to further entrench negative attitudes may help prevent these natural reactions of resistance and resignation. Discovering the source of patient motivation is paramount. Exploring the elements of Kemp's model for motivation described earlier may help the therapist address the patient's concerns or fears.[20]

The older adult's performance and learning can be affected by past experiences of mastering earlier developmental tasks. Havighurst succinctly identified six developmental tasks of old age: (1) adjusting to decreasing strength and health, (2) adjusting to retirement and reduced income, (3) adjusting to the death of a spouse, (4) establishing an explicit affiliation with members of one's own age-group, (5) meeting social and civic obligations, and (6) establishing satisfactory physical living arrangements.[18] Mastery of these six tasks for the older adult is dependent, to some degree, on how successfully the earlier developmental tasks through the childhood, adolescent, and young and middle adult years were mastered. Any deficits in mastery of earlier tasks or of these tasks for the older adult can affect the geriatric patient's motivation, learning, and performance.

Educational and Cultural Background

The number of years between earlier instructional activities and present instructional activities, previous level of education, and past experiences with learning are components of the geriatric patient's psychosocial profile. Instruction related to job and profession or participation in adult education and community education courses may be factors that will influence the patient's positive predisposition toward learning new tasks. However, if the patient primarily remembers negative experiences in earlier educational situations, these unpleasant memories may make it more difficult for the geriatric patient to be a cooperative and a willing participant in treatment sessions. The therapist should make every effort to ensure that the patient experiences success in the initial treatment sessions and to assist in the differentiation of any earlier negative experiences from present therapeutic procedures.

Low literacy skills may be a barrier to successful learning and should be recognized by the physical therapist. Many older adults have deficient learning skills and can be proficient at hiding them because of embarrassment. Using a variety of teaching methods, simple vocabulary, and repetition of key points can enhance the learning opportunities of the older adult with low literacy skills.

Many ethnic populations reside across the United States—with African-Americans, Native Americans, Asian-Americans and Pacific Islanders, and Hispanics being the standard four major groups. The therapist must remember that in addition to the patients having lived many years, their ethnic environment will influence their predisposition toward, perception of, cooperation with, and follow-up of treatment. Traditional tribal and home treatment methods are influential in all four ethnic populations. Illness is not a word in some Pacific/Asian languages, and in others, illness is synonymous with acute conditions and death, and hospitals may be viewed with fear.[4]

Another consideration with ethnic geriatric patients is level of English proficiency and education. Language barriers are common for therapists working with the Pacific/Asian ethnic group, which is composed of 18 subgroups of

Pacific Islanders and Asian-Americans. Using translators if the therapist—or another member of an interdisciplinary team—does not have bilingual-bicultural skills is very helpful. Although family members and friends may appear to be the most logical choice for this important task, the recommended choice is an interpreter who has a background in medical terminology as well as in language and cultural expertise. Cultural differences must be translated in culturally appropriate terms. The same recommendation is made when selecting Hispanic translators. Many large institutions have employees who are willing to serve as translators. When working with an African-American elder, the therapist must remember the earlier segregation of health care facilities and must respect the black elder as a survivor of a health care system that was not accessible and perhaps was even hostile.[4]

Patient education materials for geriatric patients of ethnic groups must be designed with cultural diversity as one of several important considerations. The translator should examine the text carefully for any words or phrases that might be incorrectly interpreted. Illustrations should reflect ethnic customs when possible. Any number of reliable methods to test for appropriate reading level can be used. Field testing patient education materials using a sample of the intended audience before final production is recommended to determine the effectiveness of the material.

The extended family as care-givers to the elderly is common among other cultures. A lack of familiarity with health care resources and the bureaucratic processes for access often results in underutilization by minorities. Among Hispanics, the use of formal health care services can be viewed as the family's failure to take care of its own. The health care an individual family member is allowed to receive may be subject to the approval or disapproval by the elder dominant family member.[4]

The norm for health care delivery in the United States evolved from the middle-class northern European models of care. The health care system in the United States will have increasing numbers of ethnic patients. Building a level of trust through demonstration of sensitivity to their history and cultural view of illness and health care in order to negotiate successful treatment regimens with ethnic elders is effective.[4] The therapist should regard this interaction as an opportunity for learning and increasing cultural sensitivity and awareness.

THE OLDER ADULT AS A LEARNER

This section relates patient education as a treatment modality to the knowledge of the process by which older patients "learn." The statement "you can't teach old dogs new tricks" can be a negative influence on a new therapist who is beginning a career and who has not yet had enough experiences with older adults to recognize the fallacy of such a generalization. Older adults can and do learn. To work with older adults successfully, a new therapist must develop a dual role as a caring and competent therapist and as a skillful facilita-

tive instructor. This discussion examines the cognitive and physical aspects that influence the ability and the predisposition of older adults to be effective and efficient learners in treatment sessions.

Cognitive Aspects

Cognition refers to intellectual processes, whereas learning generally is considered the acquisition of knowledge or skills achieved by study, instruction, practice, and experience. An individual's performance becomes the basis for inferring the level of learning that has been achieved. Two aspects must be considered in discussing cognitive learning—the end product and the process. Many research studies focus only on the end product. Therefore, when a person's performance improves in an intellectual or physical task, the inference is that learning has occurred. Failure in performance, however, does not infer that learning has not occurred or has been lost. Many factors affect an older adult's performance, including motivation and physical and emotional states. The physical therapist must be sensitive to the fact that multiple variables affect the learning situation and avoid concluding that the older adult cannot learn.

Several areas relate to the cognitive abilities of older patients. Intelligence as measured by standard testing procedures has been shown to decline with increasing age. However, when adjusted for time, i.e., when increased time (pacing) is allowed, no significant decline is observed.

Research generally concludes that memory does decline with age. However, this conclusion can be challenged because of methodological considerations and multiple variables as well as the lack of a functional corollary with skills and tasks in everyday life. Studies that show declining memory changes in older adults may have used artificial tasks that were not relevant to the subject's everyday tasks. Babins states, therefore, that careful examination is needed of studies that show a decline in older adults' memory functions.[3] In other words, evidence exists to suggest that memory involving skills and tasks used frequently does not decline to the degree that infrequently used information decreases. The adage "if you don't use it, you lose it" can be appropriately applied to cognition. Other research studies focus on the process, and results show that when new information can be related to older adults' existing knowledge, their new learning is facilitated. Some factors involved in the cognition or intellectual processes can be accommodated by the physical therapist. These factors are assessment of learning level, learning readiness, and learning styles.

Learning Level

Assessment of each patient's learning level is important for instructional planning, implementation, and patient education procedures and materials. Although the educational level of the older adult has been steadily increasing, one study reported about one half of adults older than 65 years did not complete high school. Within this group, women were more likely to have continued in school to junior high or high school, whereas men were more likely to have attended only some elementary grades.[15] Mayeaux and colleagues report that almost one half of American adults have deficient literacy skills, a problem further compounded by limited knowledge of medical terminology.[23] The authors report that this deficiency can translate into poor comprehension of oral and written communication. The patient history provides an excellent opportunity to gain information about the learning level of the patient. An estimate of learning level can be obtained by talking, in a conversational manner, about current or former employment positions. Duties and responsibilities at home, in the community, or in volunteer work and information on hobbies can give further assessment data on the cognitive functional level of the patient. Other indicators are the vocabulary used by the patient and the level of understanding demonstrated in response to questions and to the general conversation initiated to establish rapport with the patient. The physical therapist should use an assessment of the patient's learning and functional literacy level in patient education.

Learning Readiness

Learning readiness means that until basic skills are mastered, the mastery of more complex behavior is not possible. A number of factors can affect the patient's readiness to learn, some of which are closely related to the patient's motivational intensity discussed earlier.

Gage and Berliner reported studies conducted by Levinson and Reese with four age-groups—preschool, fifth graders, college freshmen, and the aged.[13] These studies found that extensive practice was necessary for older adults to develop learning readiness. Learning was less effective if practice was discontinued before the learner gained sufficient competence and confidence in the task. For older adults to process information into their first or primary memory store, application, practice, and rehearsal are essential.

To assess the patient's learning readiness for psychomotor activities, the therapist must determine the existing level of physical strength and skills and build from those points. To assess the patient's understanding of the reasons and need for therapy, the therapist would determine the patient's level of understanding of the particular physical condition and prescribed treatment. The therapist should sequence instruc-tion from simple skills and concepts to the more complex ones, with sufficient supervised practice to ensure the correctness of performance and to develop the patient's learning readiness to progress to more difficult and complex tasks.

Learning Styles and Information Processing

Learning style refers to how information is processed and is unique to each individual. An individual's learning style determines the consistent way the individual receives, retains, and retrieves information. Learning style also includes how an individual feels about and behaves in instructional experiences. An individual's learning style often is identified at one extreme or the other of any given learning style continuum—a classification that is probably too rigid to be realistic.

An individual's typical mode of perceiving, thinking, problem solving, remembering, selecting, and organizing information and educational experiences defines how that individual processes information. McLagan describes three primary dimensions of information processing as continua: content, initiative, and tactics—each of which has its own continuum.[24] She also emphasizes that a profile that responds to specific functions is more descriptive and realistic than labeling an individual at a fixed point on any of the three continua. These three continua are described next.

Content, the first dimension, ranges from a detail learner to a main idea learner. The detail learner will be attentive to the step-by-step explanation of a procedure but is less attentive to the overall goals of the therapy. The main idea learner will be eager to hear about the overall goals but may be less attentive to specific instructions and details.[24] For example, a detail learner will be more interested in the number of repetitions and appropriate time of day to perform the exercise, whereas a main idea learner will want to know the purposes and possible outcomes of the exercises.

Initiative, the second dimension, ranges from an active/aggressive/energetic learner to one who is passive in instructional sessions. The active/aggressive/energetic learner exerts a high degree of initiative and questions many aspects of the treatments, causes, and effects. However, conclusions may be reached erroneously. At the other extreme, the passive learner is one who exhibits little initiative and who must be encouraged to participate actively in treatment sessions.[24] A passive learner is a greater challenge to the instructor and does not necessarily indicate an unwillingness to learn.

The third dimension, tactics, refers to how information is processed in terms of organization and structure. The analytic learner processes best when structure is present and when step-by-step explanations and demonstrations are presented sequentially. The intuitive/creative learner, on the other hand, responds best to instruction that is less structured and more open-ended. Problem solving and shared decision making in treatment sessions are more productive with the intuitive/creative information processor.[24]

In summary, Cassata condensed a number of findings related to cognitive aspects of the older adult learner:[8]

- Patients forget much of what the doctor tells them.
- Instructions and advice are more likely to be forgotten than other information.
- The more patients are told, the greater the proportion they will forget.
- Patients will remember (a) what they are told first and (b) what they consider most important.
- Intelligent patients do not remember more than less intelligent patients.
- Older patients remember just as much as younger ones.
- Moderately anxious patients recall more of what they are told than highly anxious patients or patients who are not anxious.

- The more medical knowledge patients have, the more they will recall.
- If patients write down what the doctor says, they will remember it just as well as if they only hear it.

Physiological Aspects

A number of changes occur with aging that can be accommodated by the therapist to facilitate the geriatric patient's learning. These changes may involve neurological functions, vision and hearing impairment, and diminished motor dexterity. Worcester relates these physiological changes to patient education.[36]

Neurological Changes

Neurological changes that may affect learning are slower nerve transmission, which affects pacing; decreased short-term memory; and a larger store of existing information that must be integrated into the treatment setting. Slower nerve transmission can slow the reception of information and reaction times of the patient and therefore creates the need for more time in the treatment session. Implications for instruction include sensitivity to the pacing of instruction and speech and frequent assessment of the patient's level of understanding.[36]

Decreased short-term memory can cause difficulty in retaining new material and necessitates repetition and adequate practice time. Short-term memory can be enhanced through multisensory approaches, i.e., visuals, models, demonstrations, and patient education materials. The volume of information accumulated over a lifetime can interfere with learning when the new information is not congruent with prior information and experiences. Cognitive overload—too much information—also is a potential factor. Strategies for effective instruction can be used to assess the patient's knowledge base about the particular physical condition, make connections between prior knowledge and new knowledge, clarify any misconceptions, and present less material in each treatment session.[36]

Visual Changes

Decreases in acuity, accommodation to dim lighting, and lens transparency are significant visual changes that may affect the patient's ability to learn effectively. The decreased sharpness of vision, or acuity, implies that details in print materials and illustrations are more difficult for the geriatric patient to see clearly. Therefore, illustrations in patient education materials need bold lines, a minimum of detail, and a plain print style. The use of larger, simple type styles and uppercase/lowercase letters for the text material is recommended strongly. In the same manner, decreased accommodation creates difficulty in the lens adjusting to different light intensities and to color differentiation. Bright overhead lights in the clinic may create accommodation difficulties for the geriatric patient, just as dim lights may make visual perception more difficult. The patient should not be placed in a position that faces any source of glare. For patient educa-

tion materials, black ink on nonglare yellow paper for optimum acuity and accommodation should be used. Decreased lens transparency may be due to external as well as to internal causes. The therapist should make certain the patient's glasses are clean and should provide magnifying aids, if needed, when referring to patient education materials.[36]

Hearing Changes

High frequencies, such as the *c, ch, f, s, sh, t*, and *z* sounds, are more difficult for older adults to distinguish clearly. By asking the patient to repeat what was heard, the therapist can detect problems and correct errors. The therapist's pace of speech and clear enunciation are more important than volume because slow or loud speech does not necessarily increase reception. Background noises need to be controlled because the geriatric patient may have difficulty screening sounds. Patient education materials that have illustrations and audio/videotapes with individual headsets can assist the hearing-impaired patient.[36]

Motor Changes

A number of changes in the musculoskeletal condition of the geriatric patient may affect his/her ability to respond to treatment. Adequate time must be provided to accommodate slower movement and responses, and adaptive equipment, as appropriate, should be available. The therapist should plan to have the patient begin with simple tasks that can be accomplished, then build to more complex tasks.[36]

Implications for Patient Education Materials

This discussion of the cognitive aspects and physical changes has particular implications for patient education materials. The vocabulary level, sentence length, complexity, and organization of content should be examined carefully for comprehension. Reading level for print materials should approximate fourth- to sixth-grade level for maximum patient comprehension. Visual changes experienced by older adults dictate using clear, simple print styles. Black ink on nonglare paper and distinctly contrasting colors are recommended. Patient education materials should be tested with a representative sample of the audience for whom they are designed for clarity, comprehension, and readability before production—an instructional and cost-effective strategy.

In summary, the therapist ideally facilitates the older adult patient's move toward self-direction, adherence, independent problem solving, and error detection. Therefore, consideration should be given to the positive impact that occurs when learning style and information processing are investigated, assessed, and used. Awareness of the physical changes that occur in the older adult patient can enhance the learning experience when appropriate techniques are applied. Time spent in careful assessment of the many cognitive aspects of learning and the physical changes can create a more productive instructional time for each patient. Geriatric patients in treatment sessions will exhibit characteristics of older adult learners. The therapist who is aware of the cognitive and physiological aspects discussed in this section is better prepared to work more effectively and efficiently with geriatric patients and to facilitate their progress in treatment sessions.

THE CARE-GIVER

Illness and disability present a serious crisis not only for the patient but also for the family. Responses to illness will affect the current family interactions and establish new interactions with the health care team. A responsibility of the health care provider is to assist the patient and the family in responding to this crisis.

Assessment of the family should occur at the beginning of the rehabilitative process. Assessment will provide information on the individual dynamics of the family, identifying dysfunctions that may need special interventions. Observing interactions between key family members and the patient may reveal dependence issues, fear of the disability, or fatalism. Assessment also will reveal cultural or emotional issues that may be barriers to learning. The therapist must realize that the family will be experiencing grieving in similar ways to the patient.[19] The family may exhibit a resistance to instruction at this time. Often they feel powerless and worry excessively about the patient. These feelings and behaviors may be in part because of a lack of knowledge about the patient's future, current disability, illness, or anticipated needs, resulting in fear and feelings of inadequacy.

Smith and Messikomer reported a study about family care-givers of 39 geriatric patients discharged from a rehabilitation center in Pennsylvania.[34] Of those who provided ADL support, one half reported the tasks as burdensome. Giving baths and dealing with incontinence were particularly troublesome, with burden attributed to the amount of time required for the former and to the unpleasantness of the latter. The most prevalent problem expressed by care-givers was fear about the impaired person's condition, followed by the uncertainty about the illness and its treatment and the conflict between the needs of the care-giver and the needs of the disabled individual.

The family's fears and apprehensions regarding care-giving must be addressed as soon as they are recognized. Fear is a great source of stress for families. Fears identified by Hamberger and Tanner include the following:[16]

- Accidentally injuring the patient
- Not knowing what to do in an emergency situation
- Receiving criticism from the patient and/or nursing staff
- Losing leisure or career time to become the care-giver
- Accepting more responsibility than they can handle
- Causing adverse effects on the family as a unit

Teaching basic care-giving techniques using the principles of andragogy can alleviate these fears. Studies have indicated providing thorough information about the disease or disability can significantly decrease stress in care-giving. Providing the family with clear, necessary information in written or media format, such as a videotape, provides the family with the needed information that can be absorbed in the care-giver's own time and environment. Allowing time for the care-giver to absorb the information presented will enhance learning. The family gains confidence as they participate in care-giving (repetition) and eventually learn to carry out the treatments independently.

Modeling by the therapy staff can be a valuable teaching tool to instruct the family care-giver in necessary care. Always approaching a stroke patient from the affected side to encourage the patient to look to that side is an example. Practicing hands-on training provides the care-giver with active participation and the potential for problem solving, using the professional's input. Often the care-giver will verbalize that the professional therapists "perform the tasks easily" and "are more successful" with the patient. The therapist needs to acknowledge to the care-giver that success is due to familiarity with, and repeated use of, the appropriate techniques. The care-giver often may find a better way to perform the same task and share it with the therapist.

Hamberger and Tanner identify six educational objectives for the family:[16]

- Knowledge of illness
- Knowledge of patient's functional potential
- Knowledge of patient's functional limitations
- Knowledge of needed treatments (theory, practical application, and complications)
- Knowledge of prescribed medications
- Knowledge of available resources

The therapist's awareness of these six objectives can ensure that the family has adequate information relevant to the care-giving responsibilities.

Conflicts within the care-giver can create internal stresses that conflict with the ideal environment needed to optimize the rehabilitation goals. Two stresses identified by Hasselkus relevant to patient education are (1) a sense of personal causation ("If only I had gotten to him quicker") and (2) a fear of inadequacy or "goofing up," which can make accompanying the patient to therapy sessions a frightening and threatening experience.[17] During the period before discharge, an attitude of "they know best" prevails, with family members passively accepting the therapist's instructions and recommendations despite fears and doubts about their own capabilities.

During the period immediately after discharge to home care, the sense of failure on behalf of the family may shift from concern about long-term solutions to a focus on day-to-day problem solving. Some care-givers describe this period in terms of "busy-ness" with multiple services being provided in the home, whereas other care-givers describe these services as intrusive: "I was always waiting for someone" or "my days were never my own." While observation by the therapist of the care-giver is an appropriate part of a treatment session, care-givers may perceive such observation as threatening and respond with agitation and irritation.

The theme of managing can become predominant as care-givers struggle to establish routines, to learn new tasks, and to bring a semblance of comfort to the new situation. During this period, learning behaviors can reflect tension between the previous pattern of "they know best" and an emerging pattern of critique and modification. Initial efforts to do what they were "supposed to do" are gradually, or sometimes quickly, modified to be compatible with what the care-givers perceive to be their own capabilities and their sense of coping. For many care-givers, their growing sense of special knowledge may provoke the need to "teach the professional how." An eagerness to share what is successful can prevail. This tension between the care-giver's views and the therapist's views may derive from the professional's view of care-giving. The perspective based in professional training and theoretical background and the care-giver's view of the situation as a personal experience may be in conflict. Treatment may not succeed unless discrepancies are recognized and resolved. To minimize this clash of perspectives, the therapist should focus on the family as the integrating agency and the primary source of help. According to Hasselkus, the therapist's role then becomes a facilitator, a supporter, and an assistant to the family as the family develops self-help strategies.[17] A specific strategy presented by Payton and colleagues is a learn-use-teach model whereby the care-givers learn a skill, practice the skill, and then teach the skill to others.[28]

In summary, families as care-givers have unique worries, concerns, fears, coping mechanisms, and experiences as a result of their care-giving responsibilities. The physical therapist would be remiss to ignore these concerns or the wealth of knowledge and experience that result from daily "hands-on" care. All experienced therapists probably have learned some of their most "functional" hints from a care-giver or a patient. In understanding the characteristics of an older adult learner, the significance and importance of allowing the care-giver to be self-directed are clear.

Assessment of Learning

Patient education is only as effective as the results of the education and learning experiences. Because instruction has occurred, it cannot be assumed that learning has been accomplished. Without evaluation, the instructor has no information on the success of the instructional activity. Successful evaluation not only indicates achievement but also reflects and provides information on the degree of instructional effectiveness.

For purposes of this section on assessment, *learning effectiveness* is defined as a change in behavior directed toward achieving the goals agreed upon in the initial patient session. The effectiveness of the educational experience can be evaluated in many ways that vary from traditional tests. Variations of the question-and-answer format include learning contracts, self-report, interview, diaries,

checklists, and return demonstration. Several are described in this section.

Learning Contract
One very significant finding from adult learning research states that adults who are internally motivated, as contrasted with being taught something, are highly self-directing. Learning that is engaged in for purely personal development can be independently planned and carried out completely by an individual on his/her own terms and with only a loose structure. Learning that has the purpose of improving one's competence to perform a given task or activity must take into account the needs and expectations of the learner, the therapist, the institution, and any medical or environmental concerns that may affect the activity. Learning contracts provide a means for negotiating a reconciliation between these external needs and expectations and the learner's internal needs and interests.

Knowles recommends that several steps be followed to develop a learning contract:[21]
- Identify the learning need
- Specify the learning objectives
- Specify learning resources and strategies
- Specify evidence of accomplishment
- Carry out the contract
- Evaluate the learning

The imposed environment and structure that inhibit the older adult's deep psychological need to be self-directing may result in resistance, apathy, and withdrawal. Learning contracts provide a vehicle to make the planning of learning experiences a mutual undertaking between the physical therapist and the patient. By participation in goal setting, resource identification, strategy choice, and evaluation of the accomplishments, the patient develops a sense of ownership of, and commitment to, the plan. Furthermore, the basis for assessment of learning is evident.

Self-Report
Self-report often is discounted as a reliable method of evaluation because of its subjective nature. However, self-report assessments of noncompliance have been found to be reliable, and patients often respond favorably to intervention techniques. Advantages of the self-report method of assessment are the speed and ease of administration and, if used correctly, its facilitation of the patient-therapist relationship. The supportive, empathetic approach discussed earlier is recommended to obtain valid information and to develop a rapport with the patient so that inappropriate behaviors can be investigated and modified, if indicated.

The issue of empowering the older adult and allowing him/her to be self-directing may entail giving the patient permission to be noncompliant. Acknowledging that adherence to a particular activity is difficult for the patient provides a supportive environment so that the patient feels comfortable in admitting any problems that may be occurring.

Schunk states that self-report may lack some of the validity and objectivity of other methods in assessing adherence, but it can provide instant valuable information in the clinical setting.[31]

Checklist

A checklist can be used to assist in the evaluation of performance based on specific criteria. A checklist is an observational tool that allows for observing and recording the presence or absence of behaviors, characteristics, or events in specific learning situations. Activities on the checklist should be stated clearly and should reflect the most important components of the task. The more clearly the actions are described, the more accurate the learning assessment will be. The checklist can be used by family members in teaching each other specific tasks and care-giving responsibilities and also can be used as a reminder of important components within a treatment plan.

Return Demonstration

Return demonstration or checkout after instruction is usually some variation of "What did you hear me say?" or "Show me what you are going to do." The therapist checks for accuracy and completeness of what the patient understood from the instruction. A checkout is important not only immediately after instruction but also at a later date. By observing the patient perform the activity without cuing from the therapist, an accurate assessment of learning can be determined. Asking the patient to show how the home exercises are being done provides valuable information on the accuracy of the patient's understanding—without which adherence to the program is impossible. Care must be made to avoid a threatening or ridiculing atmosphere in order to allow the adult learner the choice to be self-directing or to be noncompliant.

Self-Assessment Questions for the Therapist

The following questions, identified by Freedman and adapted by Gardner and colleagues, may be helpful in a self-assessment of instruction and interaction:[15]

1. *Have I correctly assessed what my patient knows?* What has been taught before, and how much does my patient remember? What technical terminology needs to be reviewed or clarified?
2. *Am I certain that I know what needs to be taught and what my patient should be able to do as a result of my instruction?* Do the objectives reflect our negotiated goals? Are they in the appropriate sequence?
3. *Have I planned an introduction to the instruction?* Have I planned how to communicate clearly what will be taught and what my expectations are in this session?
4. *Did I present the information clearly and give pertinent examples?* Did I confuse my patient in my instruction? Was my instruction in logical sequence, with pauses for my patient to assimilate the information and to ask questions? Were my directions clear? Were there clear-cut guidelines for my patient to follow?
5. *Did I present information and examples that were relevant to my patient?* Did I keep the instruction focused on the main points without cluttering my patient's information-processing mode with extraneous material? Were my examples clear and to the point?
6. *Did I prevent or avoid an information overload for my patient?* Did I present information appropriate for the time I had with my patient? Did I limit my instructional aids or handouts to those that emphasized the major points?
7. *Were my handouts and other instructional aids appropriate?* Were my handouts organized, clear, simple, and legible? Was the reading level appropriate for my patient? Did they accommodate any vision impairment?
8. *Did my patient have enough practice time?* Did I remember that older learners do not respond well under pressure or on timed tasks? Did I help my patient develop a sense of confidence in the task? Were my verbal and nonverbal feedback reinforcing?
9. *Did I help my patient by providing cues to proper performance?* Did I coach my patient during the practice period? Did I point out any specifics that my patient could monitor to determine correct or incorrect performance?
10. *Was I sensitive to my patient?* Was I aware of my patient's reaction to the information I presented? Did I try to see things from the patient's perspective?

The effectiveness of instruction is greatly enhanced by clear, concise, and direct verbal expression. The therapist's nonverbal communication through body language, voice tone, and eye contact should inspire confidence in the therapist without limiting interaction or intimidating the patient. The therapist's verbal and nonverbal behaviors can contribute significantly to creating a positive learning environment that is conducive to positive and productive interaction between the patient and the therapist.

Case Studies

The following three scenarios illustrate selected principles that have been presented in this chapter. As the reader reviews "The Incident" and "The Dialogue" sections, significant points that relate to the chapter's content should be noted. The reader should also check to see whether these points are included in the "Discussion" and "Summary" sections. The reader should identify more points than are included in those sections.

Scenario 1: The Inattentive Learner

The Incident

Mr. Smith, a 75-year-old white male, was admitted to a rehabilitation facility 3 weeks ago for stroke. Although he has been willing to work toward his goals in all previous sessions, today he is inattentive to the therapist, as observed by his lack of eye contact, fidgeting, head movement, and other body language indicators. The therapist has to repeat instructions and questions, and basically no progress is being made.

The Dialogue

Therapist:	Mr. Smith, you seem to be preoccupied today. What's on your mind?
Patient:	Well, as a matter of fact, I've got a problem I need to take care of at the bank, and I don't know how or when I can take care of it.
Therapist:	I can understand why you are preoccupied. Anytime my bank calls me, I get worried, too! What could we do to help you with this problem?
Patient:	Well, I really need to personally talk with my banker as soon as possible. But I just don't see how I can do it. (Pause.) Do you really mean that you can help?
Therapist:	The best we can do is to at least try. What do you need?
Patient:	I need a ride because I have to take care of this in person. But I don't know if I can get in and out of the car!
Therapist:	If I can arrange a car and driver for this afternoon, would you be willing this morning to work on how to get in and out of a car?
Patient:	Do you really think I can learn how to do that this morning?
Therapist:	Yes, I think you can with some hard work. You already have worked hard on improving your balance, and besides, you've been getting in and out of cars all your life. Let's go do it.

Discussion

The therapist recognized that the patient was distracted and preoccupied and that there was an obvious obstacle to a productive treatment session. The therapist provided an opportunity for the patient to communicate the factors that were creating interference with this treatment session by asking an open-ended question that gave the patient the opportunity to state his need. The therapist further demonstrated authenticity and empathy to the patient's concern in agreeing that a call from his banker also would concern this therapist.

With encouragement and another open-ended question, the therapist facilitated the patient's problem-solving skills. The patient was allowed to maintain autonomy and self-empowerment and was allowed to determine how specific needs could be met. The therapist also demonstrated valuing (prizing) of the patient by addressing the patient's need and by referencing the patient's accomplishments in therapy as well as past experiences.

Summary

The therapist recognized that the patient's problem was primary to the patient and that the therapy was low on his priority list. Therefore, the patient was not ready to learn. By having the patient identify the reason for inattentiveness and then using those needs and concerns, the therapist was able to negotiate the activity for this treatment session. Therefore, the patient's goals were accommodated and progress toward the discharge goals was made.

Scenario 2: Learned Helplessness

The Incident

Mrs. Bailey, a 69-year-old black female, has an above-knee amputation and has been referred to physical therapy for prosthetic training. She is accompanied by her husband who appears impatient and unwilling to let his wife attempt any task. She appears passive and willing for, if not expectant of, his assistance. During the evaluation, her passiveness and helplessness also appear to be her pattern of behavior in the home setting.

The Dialogue

Therapist:	Mrs. Bailey, what would you like to be able to do at home that you aren't doing now?
Patient:	Well, I'd like to be able to do things in my kitchen.
Therapist:	What kind of things do you want to do?
Patient:	I want to be able to cook dinner and do the dishes.
Therapist:	Is your husband doing those things now?
Husband:	Yeah. I cook and do the dishes because my wife can't stand up.
Therapist:	What would you like for your wife to be able to do?
Husband:	I'd like for her to be able to stay by herself so I can get out in the fields and do my work. But that would mean I'd have to leave her alone, and I just can't do that.
Therapist:	Mrs. Bailey, do you think that you could be able to stay by yourself?
Patient:	Well, my husband does everything for me now. I don't know if I can or not.
Therapist:	Mr. Bailey, it is important to realize that your wife can learn to do a number of things for herself if she is given the opportunity. However, it means that you have to allow her enough time to perform a task in her way without interfering or taking over.
Husband:	That's really hard to do. It is easier and quicker for me to do it for her. Besides, she was so sick that she really needed my help.
Therapist:	I understand that. You obviously have done a terrific job, and lots of husbands would not have done as well as you have. However, she's progressing so well that she is ready to learn to walk on her artificial leg. For both of you to regain the independence you both want, she needs the opportunity, the time, and the encouragement to begin practicing those things that together we decide are the next steps in her treatment program.

Discussion

The therapist recognized that some social barriers prevented Mrs. Bailey's willingness to participate fully in a treatment program designed to promote her independence. Chief among these barriers was her husband's overt willingness to assist in her every movement. The therapist was sensitive that this level of care-giving was required initially and positively acknowledged the husband's care-giving.

The therapist recognized that in order to achieve the level of independence that both the Baileys desired, less assistance would be required from the husband and more initiative from Mrs. Bailey. The therapist achieved this in a supportive manner by focusing on both of their goals while describing the process in achieving those goals. In this way, goal negotiation is a mutual agreement rather than a unilateral decision by the therapist.

Summary

The therapist recognized the husband's care-giving in a positive manner and then literally gave the husband permission to decrease the level of care-giving as part of the treatment program, thus avoiding the exclusion the husband might feel as his wife worked toward greater independence. The therapist also made the wife aware that her physical condition now will safely accommodate increased activity and encouraged the patient's initiative by focusing on the patient's goal of being able to work in her kitchen.

Scenario 3: The Dominant Hurried Therapist
The Incident

Mrs. Miranda, an 80-year-old Hispanic female, checks in for her scheduled appointment at an out-patient clinic. She tells the receptionist in a thick accent that her granddaughter insisted she come and see about the pains in her right shoulder but that her granddaughter couldn't come with her. After a considerable period in the waiting room, she was shown to a treatment cubicle by the receptionist and was told to wait for the therapist. The therapist eventually rushed in to the cubicle and, without introduction, told the patient that he was here to "fix her shoulder."

The Dialogue

Therapist:	So, honey, the receptionist tells me your left shoulder hurts. I think we can fix you up in a jiffy if you'll just do what I tell you to do.
Patient:	(Hesitantly with accent.) Well, really, it's my—
Therapist:	(Interprets.) Wudja say? Here, let's look at your shoulder. (Therapist proceeds to examine left shoulder.) I'm going to get a hot pack to put on your shoulder. Wait here.
Patient:	Si, si.
Therapist:	Wudja say?
Patient:	Si.
Therapist:	Oh, well, whatever. (Therapist returns with the hot pack and places it on left shoulder.) While the heat's on your shoulder, here's a sheet of exercises I wantcha to do. Eyeball these, and I'll be back in a flash.
Patient:	(Looks at the sheet, but her lack of proficiency in English impedes her understanding. Folds sheet and puts it in her lap.)
Therapist:	(Returns and removes heat.) Well, I know your little ole shoulder feels lots better now. Like I told ya, sweetie, you just do these exercises like it says, and I'll see ya next week.

Discussion

Mrs. Miranda represents an ethnic population whose knowledge of health care in the United States is sketchy at best. Her granddaughter, on the other hand, as a third-generation Hispanic, has become enculturated and recognized that her grandmother's traditional home remedies could be supplemented by professional care. Mrs. Miranda has some suspicion about people caring for her in an unfamiliar environment, but to please her granddaughter, she agreed to go to the clinic. In addition, Mrs. Miranda is aware of her limited English proficiency and her thick accent and is reluctant to speak when away from her community environment.

Often an older person has a greater comfort level with a nonauthoritarian person than with one who represents power and expertise. Mrs. Miranda told the receptionist and her granddaughter about her right shoulder pain; however, she did not persist in her attempt to correct the therapist when he placed the heat pack on the wrong shoulder. Further, she did not tell the therapist that she could not read the exercises on the paper that he gave her. No effort was made to determine her understanding or to demonstrate and practice the exercises.

This lack of communication occurred not only because of Mrs. Miranda's natural reluctance but also because of the therapist's dominant behaviors. The lack of an introduction, the ageist remarks, and no elicitation of the patient's needs or reasons for being at the clinic are examples of these behaviors. The therapist's body language also communicated to the patient that time was not available for attention to her situation. The numerous slang words used in the therapist's hurried speech only confounded Mrs. Miranda's difficulty with English. No directions were given concerning how she would make an appointment for next week.

Summary

This scenario attempts to present a negative role model for patient interaction that could result in, at the very least, ineffective treatment perhaps even to the wrong shoulder, and at the very most, the patient could actually be harmed if she didn't understand safety instructions. When communicating with an older person of an ethnic population, care must be given to adequately assess the level of English proficiency. The possibility that cultural perceptions of health care delivery can impede treatment necessitates the therapist's increased sensitivity. A willingness to assess the patient's understanding, the rate of speech, diction, attention to the patient's nonverbal reactions, and courtesy demonstrate this sensitivity.

SUMMARY

A therapist with competencies in the various treatment modalities can be successful with a geriatric patient only to the degree that the patient chooses to participate fully in the treatment regimen for the necessary time period. Given a therapist with the appropriate knowledge and skills in treatment techniques and modalities, the degree of success with a majority of geriatric patients will depend (1) on the patient's physical condition, level of motivation, care-givers, and support systems and (2) on the therapist's skill as a patient educator.

A therapist who is a successful geriatric patient educator has developed the following:

- A philosophy of patient education based on (a) some knowledge of learning theories from which a dominant orientation has evolved and (b) clarification of the therapist's approach as one of patient empowerment instead of authoritarian
- An awareness of the characteristics of and sensitivity to the geriatric patient as an older adult learner
- The ability to develop negotiated goals with patients
- The ability to facilitate patients' learning
- A willingness to regularly and honestly assess the quality and results of the instruction provided

Patient education as a treatment modality has a solid base in educational psychology and instructional theories as well as in everyday experience and practice. Geriatric patients need and deserve therapists who recognize the importance of this treatment modality and who will work to develop and enhance their competency as patient educators.

REFERENCES

1. Anderson T: An alternative frame of reference for rehabilitation: The helping process versus the medical model, in Marinelli RP, Orto AEO (eds): *The Psychological and Social Impact of Physical Disability.* New York, Springer, 1977.
2. Avers D, Wharton MA: Improving exercise adherence: Instructional strategies. *Top Geriatr Rehabil* 1991; 6(3):62-73.
3. Babins L: Cognitive processes in the elderly: General factors to consider. *Gerontol Geriatr Educ* 1987-1988; 8:9-22.
4. Baker FM, et al: Rehabilitation in ethnic minority elders, in Brody SJ, Pawlson LG (eds): *Aging and Rehabilitation: The State of the Practice.* New York, Springer, 1990.
5. Bandura A: *Principle of Behavior Modification.* New York, Holt, Rinehart and Winston, 1969.
6. Bille DA: *Practical Approaches to Patient Teaching.* Boston, Little, Brown, 1981.
7. Bruner J: *Toward a Theory of Instruction.* Cambridge, Mass, Harvard University Press, 1966.
8. Cassata DA: Health communication theory and research: An overview of the communication specialist interface, in Nimmo D (ed): *Communication Yearbook II.* New York, ICA, 1978.
9. Cech D, Martin S: *Functional Movement Development Across the Life Span.* Philadelphia, WB Saunders, 1995.
10. Crutchfield CA, Barnes MR: *Motor Control and Motor Learning in Rehabilitation.* Atlanta, Stokesville Publishing, 1993.
11. Darkenwald G, Merriam S: *Adult Education: Foundations of Practice.* New York, Harper & Row, 1982.
12. D'Onofrio CN: Patient compliance and patient education: Some fundamental issues, in Squires W (ed): *Patient Education, Inquiry Into the State of the Art.* New York, Springer-Verlag, 1980.
13. Gage NL, Berliner DC: *Educational Psychology.* Chicago, Rand-McNally College Publishing, 1975.
14. Ertmer PA, Newby TJ: Behaviorism, constructivism: Comparing critical features from an instructional design perspective. *Performance Improvement Q* 1993; 6(4):50-71.
15. Gardner DL, Greenwell SC, Costich JF: Effective teaching of the older adult. *Top Geriatr Rehabil* 1991; 6(3):1-14.
16. Hamberger SG, Tanner RD: Nursing intervention with families of geriatric patients. *Top Geriatr Rehabil* 1988; 4(1):32-39.
17. Hasselkus BR: Rehabilitation: The family caregiver's view. *Top Geriatr Rehabil* 1988; 4(1):60-70.
18. Havighurst RJ: History of developmental psychology: Socialization and personality development through the lifespan, in Baltes PB, Schaie KW (eds): *Life Span Developmental Psychology.* New York, Academic Press, 1973.
19. Hibbard MR, et al: Cognitive therapy and the treatment of poststroke depression. *Top Geriatr Rehabil* 1990; 5(3):43-55.
20. Kemp BJ: Motivation, rehabilitation, and aging: A conceptual model. *Top Geriatr Rehabil* 1988; 3(3):41-51.
21. Knowles M: *The Adult Learner: A Neglected Species.* Houston, Gulf Publishing, 1978.
22. Lindgren CL: Understanding and promoting compliance in older patients. *The Older Patient* 1989; 3:28-30.
23. Mayeaux EJ, et al: Improving patient education for patients with low literacy skills. *Am Fam Phys* 1996; 53(1):205-211.
24. McLagan PA: *Helping Others Learn: Designing Programs for Adults.* Reading, Mass, Addison-Wesley, 1978.
25. Mellert RB: Cure or care? The future of medical ethics. *The Futurist* 1997; 31(4):35-38.
26. Merriam SB, Caffarella RS: *Learning in Adulthood.* San Francisco, Jossey-Bass, 1991.
27. Parsons T: *The Social System.* New York, Free Press, 1951.
28. Payton OD, Nelson CE, Ozer MN: *Patient Participation in Program Planning: A Manual for Therapists.* Philadelphia, FA Davis, 1990.
29. Rogers C: *Freedom to Learn for the 80's.* Columbus, Charles E Merrill, 1983.
30. Sahakian WS: *Introduction to the Psychology of Learning,* ed 2. Itasca, Ill, Peacock Publishing, 1984.
31. Schunk C: Prediction and assessment of compliant behavior. *Top Geriatr Rehabil* 1988; 3(3):15-20.
32. Schunk, DH: *Learning Theories: An Educational Perspective.* New York, Macmillan, 1991.
33. Silverstone B: Social aspects of rehabilitation, in Williams TF (ed): *Rehabilitation in the Aging.* New York, Raven Press, 1984.
34. Smith V, Messikomer C: A role for the family in geriatric rehabilitation. *Top Geriatr Rehabil* 1988; 4(1):8-15.
35. Staropoli CJ, Waltz CF: *Developing and Evaluating Educational Programs for Health Care Providers.* Philadelphia, FA Davis, 1978.
36. Worcester MI: Tailoring teaching to the elderly in home care. *Home Health Q* 1990; 11:69-120.

PART IV

THE SOCIAL CONTEXT OF GERIATRIC CARE

CHAPTER 26

REIMBURSEMENT ISSUES IN GERIATRIC PHYSICAL THERAPY

JEAN OULUND PETEET, PT, MPH

INTRODUCTION

In 1994, the federal government took a significant step toward reforming the American health care system. On a national level, legislators, consumers, and providers debated about our health care system. Many issues surfaced in this debate—the most important being whether health care is a right for all citizens. It was generally agreed that everyone has a right to health care, but no consensus was reached on how to finance and structure a system for delivering care. Consumers, legislators, and providers still differ about the mix of private and public fiscal responsibility for health care, in particular, long-term care.

A second important step was made in 1997, when the federal Balanced Budget Act (Public Law 105-33) was passed.[2] This was considered to be the most important bill affecting health care since Medicare was enacted in 1965. For the first time since 1969, the federal deficit was eliminated. This was be-

ing achieved by spending cuts that included $115 billion in Medicare and $13.6 billion in Medicaid over 5 years.

As various aspects of the BBA began to be implemented in 1998, health care providers and patients began to experience the effects of these spending cuts. After extensive lobbying by all affected groups, the Balanced Budget Refinement Act of 1999 was passed, which restored $12 billion in cuts to providers and made adjustments to better implement the original bill.[3,5] The American Physical Therapy Association (APTA) and physical therapists formed a grassroots effort to impose a moratorium on a previously instituted $1500 cap on outpatient physical therapy. That process was a dramatic example of the importance of the physical therapist's role, both individually and collectively, as legislative advocate.

Health care is changing rapidly. The reader is directed to the Medicare, Health Care Financing Administration (HCFA), and the APTA web sites to read up-to-date information on legislation, regulatory interpretation, and opportunities for professional legislative advocacy.

INSURANCE PROGRAMS

The federal government provides about 80 programs to assist the elderly either directly or indirectly with long-term–care problems. There is no one program, however, designed to address all long-term–care problems in a comprehensive and coordinated manner. There is uniformity among states only in the Medicare program. Benefits in other insurance programs, such as health maintenance organizations (HMOs), vary from state to state. A major concern for elderly patients is the confusion and changes in services and reimbursement as these patients transition from and to different settings for their care.

Primarily four funded programs provide elder care: Medicare, Medicaid, Title III of the Older Americans Act, and Social Security Block Grants. An overview of the programs that offer physical therapy services to the elderly are discussed here.

Medicare

In 1965 the federal government became directly involved in health care in its enactment of Title 18 of the Social Security Act, known as the Medicare program, which provided for funding for acute medical care for persons 65 years or older and certain persons with disability. Medicare was not intended to be a program for long-term–care needs. Persons advocating national health insurance thought that a comprehensive system for the United States would soon be developed. However, to date, such a system is not in place, and both practitioners and administrators are faced with working with the Medicare program as the major source of funding for elder care.

The federal government, through HCFA, administers Medicare. HCFA contracts with private insurance organizations called *intermediaries* and *carriers* to process claims and make Medicare payments. Medicare is a two-part program consisting of (1) Hospital Insurance (Part A), which helps to pay for inpatient hospital care, some care in a skilled nursing facility (SNF), home health care, and hospice care and (2) Medical Insurance (Part B). Medicare B helps to pay for physicians' services, outpatient hospital services, durable medical equipment, and some services not covered under Part A.[9]

The Balanced Budget Act (BBA) of 1997 added Part C, the Medicare+Choice Program. This program allows beneficiaries a wider choice of benefit programs that can include HMOs, plans offered by provider-sponsored organizations, or use of a medical savings account (MSA) or private fee-for-service plans. *MSAs* are accounts with fixed amounts of money determined by the insurance companies for the insured to control for payments of certain types of health care. These have been used by some insurers in the private sector, but not until now with Medicare recipients.

Box 26-1 lists criteria for some of the items most often needed by physical therapists for their patients. Equipment is covered under Part B of Medicare. A physician's prescription is necessary for all items, but this alone will not guarantee coverage by Medicare. Medical necessity must be documented, and it is often the physical therapist who is most able to address why equipment will improve the patient's functional outcome.

Generally, Part A Hospital Insurance coverage includes deductibles and co-insurance, but most persons older than 65 years do not pay premiums if they receive benefits under Social Security or the Railroad Retirement system. In addition, persons younger than 65 can receive Part A benefits without paying premiums if they have been receiving Social Security or Railroad Retirement Board disability payments for more than 24 months.

Part B Medical Insurance includes premiums, deductibles, and co-insurance amounts that the individual pays himself/herself or through coverage by another insurance plan. Table 26-1 shows a comparison of benefits under Medicare parts A and B.

The federal government pays groups of practicing physicians and other health care professionals to review the care given to Medicare patients. These groups are called Peer Review Organizations (PROs), and they have the authority to deny payments if care is deemed not medically necessary or has not been delivered in the most appropriate setting. PROs are also responsible for investigating beneficiary complaints about poor-quality care.

Although review of care should serve to improve quality and reduce costs, it can also have a negative financial impact on health care providers. Medicare reviewers may determine retrospectively that based on the provider's documentation, a claim for physical therapy services is not medically necessary and deny payment to the therapist. If the therapist or facility has a large Medicare population

---

BOX 26-1
DURABLE MEDICAL EQUIPMENT (DME)

To be covered by Medicare, all the following conditions must be met. The equipment must be:
1. Prescribed by a physician
2. Rentable from a supplier (the method preferred by Medicare), returnable, and therefore, reusable by other patients
3. Used for a primarily medical purpose
4. Useful only to individuals who are sick or injured
5. Appropriate for use in the patient's home

Examples of equipment that may be covered:
  Walker, cane
  Wheelchair
  Prosthetic device for limb
  Prosthetic device for internal body organ
    Corrective lenses after cataract surgery
    Colostomy or ileostomy bags
    Breast prostheses
  Leg, back, neck brace
  Orthopedic shoes only if an integral part of a leg brace
  Surgical dressings, splints, casts
  Oxygen equipment
Examples of equipment never covered:
  Orthopedic shoes without a brace
  Dental devices

TABLE 26-1
BENEFITS UNDER MEDICARE

TYPE OF INSURANCE	HELPS TO PAY FOR
Part A Hospital Insurance	
No premiums if benefits under Social Security	Inpatient hospital care
	Skilled nursing facility care
Must pay deductibles and coinsurance	Home health care
	Hospice care
Part B Medical Insurance	
Must pay premiums to receive it	Doctors' services
Must pay deductibles and coinsurance	Outpatient services
	Durable medical equipment

and payment denials occur frequently, the therapist or facility may be unable to meet costs. Later in this chapter, suggestions for addressing this issue with patients and with Medicare are discussed.

Costs have escalated in the Medicare program, making it imperative for the government to closely scrutinize the care being provided. An important change in reimbursement in the Medicare program occurred in 1983 when a Prospective Payment System (PPS) was enacted. Initially implemented in the acute care setting, with the enactment of the Balanced Budget Act, the PPS was extended to be adapted to skilled nursing and rehabilitation facilities, outpatients, and home health agencies. Under this system, specific predetermined rates are set for each discharged patient. Diagnosis-related groups (DRGs) are the basis for this reimbursement system. In the DRG system, inpatients who are medically related in terms of diagnosis and treatment and who are statistically similar in their length of hospital stay are grouped in the same category. Diagnoses are categorized into a total of 467 groupings, and a dollar amount is assigned for reimbursement for each of the groups. Hospitals are paid a fixed amount for each patient based on the principal diagnosis for each Medicare hospital stay. In some cases, the Medicare payment is more than the hospital's costs; in other cases, the payment is less than the hospital's costs. Hospitals can keep the excess payment, but patients are not required to make up the difference if the hospital is paid less than the cost of providing service for a specific hospitalization. The hospital can receive additional payment for "outlier" days, which extend the length of stay due to medical complications. Although in theory the enactment of the PPS has not reduced benefits for Medicare recipients, there is the potential for hospitals to decrease the amount of service and quality of care to patients as they attempt to keep the length of stay of the elderly as short as possible to achieve maximum reimbursement from Medicare.

Medicare defines *benefits* under benefit periods. The first benefit period begins the first time a patient enters the hospital. It ends when the patient has been out of a hospital or other facility that primarily provides skilled nursing or rehabilitation services for 60 days in a row. Ninety days of care are allowed in each benefit period. There is no limit to the number of benefit periods a patient can have for hospital and skilled nursing care.

As of 2000, Part A pays for all but the first $768 of covered services for days 1 to 60 of a hospitalization. For days 61 to 90, Part A pays for all except $192 per day. If a patient goes beyond the 90 days of care in a benefit period, up to 60 lifetime reserve days can be applied toward care. The patient must pay a co-insurance of $384 per day for each lifetime reserve day used.

Deductibles and co-insurance are a part of the Medicare plan. The patient pays the first $100 annually for covered medical expenses under Part B. The co-insurance for most outpatient services was 20% of "approved" or "reasonable" charges. Medicare has specific guidelines on approved care and ceilings on the amount considered "reasonable" as a charge.

Reimbursement in all settings that provide treatment to Medicare patients is in a period of transition as rules and regulations are implemented based on the Balanced Budget Act. It seems inevitable that ethical dilemmas will be encountered more frequently as less service is reimbursable for patient care through the Medicare program, as providers see that services are needed, will not be covered by Medicare, and cannot be afforded by the patient (see also Chapter 27).

Prepaid Health Plans

Prepaid health plans such as HMOs contract with Medicare to provide service to Medicare beneficiaries. Medicare pays these organizations directly for services. Elders may also choose to enroll in a prepaid health plan, if there is one available in their area, rather than receive benefits under Medicare's traditional fee-for-service system. These prepaid health plans charge the beneficiary fixed monthly premiums and minimal co-insurance payments. The benefits to the elderly are (1) minimal paperwork since they generally do not have to file any claims and (2) additional services offered by many organizations at minimal or no cost, such as preventive care, dental care, hearing aids, and eyeglasses. In addition, since 1991, most HMOs that enrolled Medicare beneficiaries were required by the Medicare program to provide, at no additional charge, extended hospital and skilled nursing facility stays, expanded home health benefits, respite care, and coverage for certain drugs.[9,10]

A potential disadvantage for beneficiaries who choose an HMO is that they may have a limited choice in doctors, therapists, and hospitals. The HMO usually specifies which providers can be used in order to receive benefits. Since income received by the HMO is on a prepaid basis, there is increased incentive for the organization to minimize costs. A "gatekeeper," often a nurse or physician, may be used to control unnecessary use of services. HMOs ration physical therapy services by requiring physician authorization for a fixed number of visits. An elderly patient with a chronic problem requiring long-term physical therapy may find limited coverage authorized for a specific problem. This is more likely to occur in this setting than under the Medicare fee-for-service program.

Provisions in the Balanced Budget Refinement Act have helped to lessen the financial burden on HMO providers who are Medicare providers, recognizing that there needs to be adequate reimbursement to providers who agree to participate with the Medicare program.

Medicaid

The federal government became involved with health care for low-income individuals through the 1965 congressional enactment of Title 19 of the Social Security Act. Financial assistance for low-income elderly is available through a joint federal and state program called *Medicaid* in most states. In contrast with the Medicare program, Medicaid does support long-term services, principally nursing home care, but only for specified low-income persons or only after persons have exhausted their own resources. Medicaid also covers adult day care, which allows supervision of elders who are not safe alone all day, prepares meals, and provides socialization. The PACE program described in the following text is an example of how the services of adult day centers are being expanded to be more comprehensive.

To qualify for Medicaid, annual income level generally must be at or below 133% of the national poverty level and the individual cannot have access to many financial resources such as bonds, stocks, or bank accounts. This would mean in 2000 that a family of three would qualify for Medicaid if their income were less than $16,032.[8,11] The state governments assist individuals by paying for health insurance premiums. Each state sets its own guidelines as to who qualifies for assistance. Physical therapists must know the specific requirements of each state in which they practice.

Supplemental Insurance, or Medigap, Policies

Elders under Medicare are responsible to pay a co-payment of 20% for many of the services provided under parts A and B. This can be a significant amount of money for an elder with frequent hospitalizations and ongoing medical problems. This has prompted the need for supplemental, or "Medigap," policies: policies underwritten by private insurance companies to cover such costs. This supplemental insurance may be purchased to cover the 20% co-payment. The future of Medigap policies is in question given the high cost of the premium, making the policy available only to elders with substantial financial resources.

Private Long-Term–Care Insurance

Elders primarily have two choices to pay for long-term care. One is to pay out-of-pocket until their resources are depleted and apply for Medicaid, under which nursing homes are a covered service, or to purchase private insurance. Neither choice provides a comprehensive solution for elders. Long-term care raises issues about relationships, roles, and responsibilities as much as it does about health, illness, or regulations.

Medicare does not cover any long-term–care needs identified as "maintenance" care in any setting. *Maintenance care* is defined by Medicare as any care that does not significantly increase the patient's function but only maintains the condition of the patient.

Cost estimates of a 1-year stay in a nursing home averaged $46,000 per year in 1995, a staggering cost for elders and families.[4] Costs to keep an elder at home are not necessarily less than costs in a nursing home. To stay at home, patients may need nursing care, homemaker, aide, medical social services, rehabilitation therapies, medical supplies, education, and training and counseling for themselves and care-givers. Full-time home health care can easily cost $250 per day or upwards of $45,000 if a patient needs full-time care for 6 months.

Although the number of individuals buying long-term–care insurance is increasing, barriers still exist. There is still confusion about what is covered by the federal government, concerns about how to choose the product, cost, and insufficient knowledge about the risk of needing long-term care. The Kennedy-Kassenbaum Bill, passed in 1994, gives a tax advantage for purchase of long-term–care insurance and may provide incentive for purchasers.

The cost of individually purchased long-term–care insurance rises dramatically with age, approaching the cost of long-term care itself. This raises the issue of the need for public funding for such coverage.[7]

Long-term–care policies need to be reviewed carefully before purchase. There can be exclusions specifically for the care needed. For example, coverage might require the home-care provider to be state licensed or Medicare certified. Although this might first appear beneficial to the patient and no immediate barrier to services, many states do not license all home health care providers. If a state does not license home care, benefits would be unavailable to the patient. In evaluating any long-term–care policy, one should consider such things as whether there is a required hospital stay to receive benefits, guaranteed renewability, inflation coverage, coverage for home health care, and specific coverage of Alzheimer's and other organic-based mental illness.

A good policy should pay for benefits when the insured cannot perform basic activities of daily living (ADL). Who should buy these policies? These types of policies most likely help persons in the middle-income range. Elderly persons who have exceptional financial resources and could afford to pay out of pocket for a nursing home for several years usually do not need a such policy. Elderly persons who have very little money usually cannot afford the policy premium. Individuals should be cautioned in purchasing policies because these policies are relatively new, and it is not clear, given the escalating costs of health care, whether insurance companies will be able to fulfill the obligations of the policy.

DOCUMENTATION REQUIREMENTS FOR REIMBURSEMENT

There are three important requirements for reimbursement to physical therapists under the Medicare program. First, services must be prescribed by a physician. Second, services must be "reasonable and necessary" to the individual's illness or injury and under accepted standards of medical practice; they must be of a level of complexity and sophistication such that only a licensed physical therapist can provide the services; and the expectation must exist that the condition will improve significantly in a reasonable time period. Third, physician re-certification is required every 30 days. Certification can be accomplished by written communication between the therapist and physician.

These documentation requirements might seem easily met, even though the requirement for physician referral and continued authorization negates any direct access to physical therapy where allowed by state laws. In practice, documenting so that reimbursement is received for service not only requires a knowledge of Medicare guidelines but also additional help from therapists experienced in documentation and articles, such as those published in APTA publications, that address practical issues and offer "how-to" suggestions.

Examples of documentation that would support reimbursement for physical therapy for Medicare patients include the following:

1. Range of motion (ROM) measurements show loss of motion compared with the unaffected side.
2. Strength shows significant loss—in zero, trace, poor, fair range.
3. Type of exercise includes resistive exercises with weights or manually, muscle re-education, proprioceptive neuromuscular facilitation, and stretching.
4. Patient is treated for more than just pain, i.e., loss of ROM and/or strength.
5. Examination is complete with measurement of ROM, strength, and functional assessment, and patient shows steady progress with objective evidence of improvement in baseline tests and measures (strength, ROM, functional assessment).
6. Patient shows functional gains as a result of treatment.

The following example of an initial examination summary meets the requirements for Medicare reimbursement:

This 70-year-old female patient suffered a fall 2 weeks ago, sustaining a left ankle eversion strain. She has rheumatoid arthritis, diagnosed 10 years ago, and has hypertension for which she is on daily medication. Patient presents in physical therapy with impaired ROM and strength on manual muscle test (see details in initial examination) in the left ankle, impaired joint position sense in the left ankle, and a compensated gait pattern secondary to ligamentous instability of the lower extremity. Unsupported standing balance is Fair. Patient requires contact guarding in ambulation using a walker. Patient was previously ambulating up to two blocks without an assistive device. She was independent in all ADL. She is at risk for falls due to her impaired balance. The goal of physical therapy is to return patient to previous level of functioning. It is anticipated that she will need physical therapy intervention two to three times per week for 4 to 6 weeks consisting of therapeutic exercise, muscle re-education instruction in safety, balance and gait training, community mobility training, and a home exercise program.

Jan. 10, 1999
J. Jones, P.T. License #1111

It is important to specify the impairments and functional limitations of the patient. Other medical diagnoses or complicating factors may be included to help explain why progress might be slow. The reader is referred to the APTA *Guide to Physical Therapist Practice* for understanding the elements of patient management and intervention strategies for particular patient diagnostic groups.

Examples of physical therapy services that would not be covered under Medicare include:

1. Maintenance therapy that includes a program in which expected improvement is insignificant in relation to the extent and duration of the service
2. General strengthening exercises that maintain strength and endurance
3. Hot packs and paraffin
4. Passive ROM

At issue for physical therapists are those patients who require the skills of a physical therapist to "maintain" their condition because of the complexity of their medical/psychological status. For example, patients with medical conditions such as multiple sclerosis or Parkinson's may have a need for periodic re-examination to change a maintenance plan rendered by an unskilled provider (family member, nursing aide, physical therapy aide). Careful documentation is necessary to demonstrate that such care should be covered under Medicare.

It is important that physical therapists understand insurance regulations to assist the patient and family in determining whether Medicare or other insurance programs might cover the needed therapy. The therapist cannot assume because a physician (or podiatrist or dentist) has requested physical therapy service that an insurer will cover it.

REIMBURSEMENT METHODS IN DIFFERENT SETTINGS

Acute Care

Reimbursement for physical therapy services in acute care settings is included in the fixed payment assigned to the particular DRG under the PPS. Thus, whether a hospital provides physical therapy once a day or twice a day for 7 days a week, the reimbursement stays the same. It is therefore in the hospital's financial interest to determine the intensity of service that can reduce hospital length of stay and to provide no more than that minimum.

Physical therapists in acute care settings must demonstrate their value in reducing hospital length of stay. New models of care are being created as providers attempt to provide the quality and amount of care to the patient within the constraints of reimbursement allowed for care.

One such model is termed *subacute care* and is provided in a transitional care unit or in some instances in an SNF. Some consider this model to be a variation on care that has been provided for years, but it has been given a new name. Subacute care is comprehensive inpatient care designed for a patient who has had an acute illness. Care is generally more intensive than that provided in an SNF but less intensive than that provided in an inpatient rehabilitation facility. Physical therapists provide care in this setting as part of a multidisciplinary team.

Although the PPS is not affected by the BBA in the acute care sector, a transfer rule is part of the law. Patients considered for transfer are those with select diagnoses—stroke; amputation; major joint replacements; hip, femur, and pelvic fractures; skin grafts—and those receiving ventilator care, those with organic disturbances, and those discharged earlier than average from an acute care hospital to any post-acute inpatient program. The acute care hospital does not receive all of the DRG payment. This has created an incentive for acute care hospitals to develop subacute units in order to keep patients and thus maximize reimbursement.

Inpatient Rehabilitation

The elimination of a cost-based system between 1999 and 2001 has resulted in a transition to a PPS in all settings. Because of this, these settings, each to varying degrees, will no longer be able to increase the intensity of physical therapy and other rehabilitation services or add programs and receive additional reimbursement.

This change significantly affects staffing patterns in these settings. Like acute care settings, inpatient rehabilitation hospitals will now need to stay within cost limits as they receive pre-established fixed fees for patient care. It is probable that facilities will question whether less costly personnel, such as physical therapist assistants, or even aides, can be substituted for physical therapists. The impact of the BBA was positive to the extent that it eliminated overuse of health care resources. The potential for a negative impact exists if poor patient outcomes result due to insufficient or inadequate care.

Skilled Nursing Facility

An SNF has staff and equipment to provide skilled nursing care or rehabilitation services and other health services. Most nursing homes are not SNFs, and many SNFs are not Medicare certified. If certified as a Medicare provider, the SNF provides care under Part A coverage. As part of the BBA, SNFs are transitioning to a PPS. Skilled nursing facilities have the financial incentive to provide care at the least cost. It is increasingly important for physical therapists to actively examine the necessary mix of rehabilitation staff (aides, physical therapist assistants, physical therapists) and to demonstrate the relationship between functional outcomes and skilled service in order to financially justify service.

Outpatient Rehabilitation

Medicare requires certification for any facility or independent practitioner who provides care to Medicare patients. Certification requirements include such areas as quality assurance, safety, nondiscrimination, and documentation standards. Medicare can withdraw certification from a facility or individual if standards are not met.

The $1500 cap per calendar year previously imposed on Medicare recipients receiving PT, OT, and SP in outpatient care in all but acute care outpatient hospitals was suspended until 2002. During this time of suspension, the HHS secretary will be examining a mechanism to ensure appropriate use of services and payment based on criteria that includes such elements as diagnosis and functional status. This suspension, as part of the BBA Refinement Act, was a remarkable demonstration of the effectiveness of lobbying efforts by individual providers, individual patients, and our professional association who were seeking legislative change. The $1500 cap in the BBA, even though raised from $900, was inadequate for Medicare patients with complex rehabilitation problems. Physical therapists should be encouraged that it is possible to achieve positive social change in a complex reimbursement system.

Home Health

Home health care not only provides skilled care services such as nursing, physical therapy, home health assistance, and speech therapy but also includes sophisticated services such as nutritional feeding via feeding tubes; intravenous, antibiotic, and pain therapy; and chemotherapy. This has increased the level of complexity of the patient conditions with which physical therapists work.

While the BBA legislated a PPS for home health and a 15% reduction in payment to home health agencies, the Refinement Act delayed its implementation. Additionally, the BBA required that home health agencies complete the Outcome and Assessment Information Set (OASIS) questionnaire to patients beginning in fiscal year 2000. The PPS is similar to the system already used in acute care settings. The home health agency receives a fixed amount of money for an admission and is expected to provide all necessary care, rather than bill for individual services it provides. Some of the challenges in home care are to develop a case-mix that will accurately determine patient characteristics that are predictive of home health resource utilization, enabling a basis for adequate reimbursement in the PPS, and to demonstrate patient outcomes related to provision of physical therapy.

The Medicare definition of *homebound* is important in determining benefits to homebound elders. Generally, the homebound requirement is met if at least one of the following characteristics are present:

1. If a patient has a condition due to an illness or injury that restricts his/her ability to leave home except with the aid of supportive devices, such as crutches and canes, or the assistance of another person
2. If leaving home is medically contraindicated
3. If a patient has a psychiatric problem that would make it unsafe for him/her to leave home unattended, even if he/she has no physical limitations

Patients may still be considered homebound if absences are infrequent, for short time periods, or are for the purpose of obtaining medical treatment.

Currently, Medicare will pay for covered home health service by a physical therapist employed by a participating home health agency or an independent Medicare-certified physical therapist. Medicare currently has a requirement that an independently practicing therapist must maintain an office with equipment that is surveyed by a Medicare representative before certification is issued. This is a disincentive to physical therapists who wish to have only home health patients as their population, as it adds an increased financial investment to meet the Medicare rule of an office. Private insurers that cover physical therapy in the home may only require that a therapist be licensed in that state.

As each health care setting attempts to be more cost-effective and cost-efficient, it is likely that patient length of stay will decrease. The need for home health services may increase dramatically as patients are discharged sooner.

Hospice Care

Hospice care offers an important choice to patients. A hospice is a public or private organization that provides supportive services and pain relief to terminally ill patients in a home setting. Medicare Part A helps to pay for these services when the following conditions are met: (1) a doctor certifies that a patient is terminally ill, (2) a patient chooses to receive care from a hospice instead of standard Medicare benefits for the terminal illness, and (3) care is provided by a Medicare-participating hospice program. Physical, occupational, and speech therapy are covered under Medicare, as are all other services, when treatment is for pain relief and symptom management.[9,10]

Nursing Home/Chronic Care

Nursing homes do not receive reimbursement under the Medicare program if they provide only maintenance care. Some nursing homes, however, are licensed as SNFs and receive Medicare reimbursement for care provided at the skilled level.

The joint state-federal Medicaid program covers care in nursing homes that do not qualify for Medicare because they provide a lesser level of skilled service. In these settings, the physical therapist's role is usually to evaluate patients for their ability to make functional gains and to develop programs for nursing or physical therapy aides or assistants to perform. The therapist may be an employee and receive a salary or, as in a growing number of instances, provide service under a contractual agreement with the facility.

A major legislative change that addressed nursing home needs was the Nursing Home Reform Amendments of OBRA, '87, effective October 1990.[1] This legislation focused on a new philosophy whereby nursing homes were required to focus on each individual's highest potential for physical, mental, and psychosocial well-being by assessing these abilities and developing plans of care for individuals. Most of an elder's needs for long-term care are primarily for physical and personal care. Many elders reside in a nursing home because no coverage for this costly care is provided.

Retirement Communities

Retirement communities can be divided into two categories. They either (1) provide health services directly or indirectly or (2) provide no health services at all. Those that offer health services are becoming known as *continuing care retirement communities*. These communities may provide long-term nursing care or limited emergency care. They may finance these services through a rental fee, on a fee-for-service basis, or through an entrance fee. Similarly, the housing units may be rental, cooperative, condominium, or entrance-fee type.

Some retirement communities, realizing the benefit to attract the elderly, offer preventive exercise programs. Reimbursement for this service, which might be provided by a variety of individuals including dance instructors, health club instructors, or physical therapists, can be by contractual arrangement with the retirement community. Physical therapists need to increase their involvement particularly in these communities because this is an ideal setting for prevention and wellness education and exercise.

REIMBURSEMENT ISSUES

The enactment of the BBA has raised significant policy issues regarding the adequacy of reimbursement for health care services. The complexity of insurance programs, lack of long-term–care elder coverage insurance funded through the health care system, and the need for an integrated system of care delivery are three of many issues requiring debate.

Complexity of Insurance Programs

Legislative changes will affect care to elders in all settings, and the Medicare and Medicaid programs may become even more complex both for providers and patients as rules and regulations change. Dramatic changes have been legislated with providers given little time to prepare for these changes.

There may be more instances in which disagreements over health care coverage are taken to court. While adding documentation requirements may seem burdensome, it is in effect the only means of demonstrating the necessity of the care that is given, that significant functional outcomes are achieved, and the only means of eliminating arbitrary decisions regarding coverage of services. Resorting to legal venues to resolve disputes with insurers certainly cannot be the preferred method for creating change. The physical therapy profession has made significant progress in developing a framework of its examination and intervention skills through the APTA's *Guide to Physical Therapist Practice.* It is essential that therapists incorporate this framework and terminology into practice to improve the ability as a professional body to be consistent in documentation and understood by other providers and insurers.

Lack of Long-Term–Care Coverage

The United States needs continued philosophical debate about long-term care to establish agreement about America's values and expectations. Funding issues will include what mix of public and private coverage is acceptable. If coverage is primarily public, there will be the difficult task of deciding the absolute level of expenditure, trying to estimate the amount of expenditures needed by elders in the future, and how individual states will participate in the administration of long-term–care benefits. It is crucial that there be advocacy for women and their unique health needs in this debate. The majority of long-term–care beneficiaries are frail, elderly, single women, and most of the care providers (registered nurses, licensed practical nurses, certified nursing assistants, housekeepers, dietary staff, and physical therapists) are women as well.

NEED FOR INTEGRATED CARE

Patient length of stay in all settings is decreasing as elders are quickly transferred to the least costly settings for each phase of their care. For elders and their families, this can be perceived as discontinuity of care with sometimes abrupt and frequent transfers. This lack of integrated care is a problem that must be addressed.

ADVOCACY ROLE OF PHYSICAL THERAPISTS

Programs for populations such as the frail elderly, well elderly, older athletes, and adults with developmental disabilities are discussed in other chapters in this text. In the current health care system, health insurers do not often cover programs that address prevention and wellness. Most insurance policies create a financial incentive for patients to wait to seek help until sickness occurs. For example, carriers will pay $30,000 for coronary artery bypass surgery but will not pay $2,000 for a cardiac rehabilitation prevention program. Many programs should be expanded if physical therapists are to prevent many injuries and subsequent illness from occurring.

Arguments are made supporting both the need to have such programs covered under health insurance policies and the need to have some costs borne by the patient. Therapists cannot, however, wait until insurance companies cover a program to develop it. Active involvement is necessary through state and national organizations to convince insurers and patients of the value of physical therapist's services. Many programs to the elderly can be provided at low cost, and supportive personnel can be used to assist in the program. All practitioners are being increasingly challenged to become more efficient in their delivery of care and to ensure insurers that they are providing care at the least possible cost. Therapists will need to be increasingly creative as to how to develop, market, and financially support programs that are vital to the elderly and require a physical therapist's knowledge and skills.

NEW MODELS

The economist Victor Fuchs has estimated that if the trends we have experienced in the past years continue, health care consumption by older persons in 2020 will approximate $25,000 per person (in 1995 dollars) compared with $9200 in 1995.[6] New models for delivery of care are needed.

There may be more creative ways to provide service to functionally and cognitively impaired elderly persons. We already know that the current structure has not been serving the American people well. Increasing the number of residentially based services and the flexibility of such services may offer the elderly more privacy, freedom of choice, and dignity.

New models for living situations are being developed for the elderly. One model is that of a "full-service" life care retirement community where elderly persons can use the equity from a home purchased years ago, which is now too large, to purchase a smaller living unit in a complex that offers meals, nursing care, activities, medical supervision, and transportation. This can be ideal for a single person or even a couple in which one partner is frail and may have nursing needs. It allows the elderly the independence of owning their own living quarters but having services readily available. Unfortunately, this approach does not serve economically disadvantaged elders who don't own a home and have few resources to stay independent.

There also are new initiatives to integrate the primary, acute, and long-term–care services funded by Medicaid and Medicare. These integrated systems should be more cost-effective than the current system of care. One such integrated program is called the Program of All-Inclusive Care for the Elderly (PACE). The federal government has funded 10 of these sites across the country. The elders served by PACE must be at the point to which they otherwise would be admitted to a nursing home. Instead of placement in a nursing home, this program allows the elder to stay at home but attend a day-care center where he/she receives comprehensive medical care, physical therapy if needed, meals, personal care, and socialization. The Medicare and Medicaid reimbursements are pooled, minimizing cost shifting between these programs.

States also are pursuing reform in their long-term–care financing and delivery systems through funding under private foundations. These initiatives are encouraging and may result in models of care that can be expanded to be effective across the country.

Physical therapists will increasingly need to be involved in the development of regulations, quality assurance, and reimbursement criteria for physical therapy as it is provided in all settings. The Balanced Budget Act established reimbursement for the provision of care through high-capacity computing and advanced networks, termed *telehealth service,* in rural health manpower shortage areas. This presents an opportunity for physical therapists to creatively address health care needs. As written, the BBA does not identify physical therapists as providers to be reimbursed for telehealth. Therapists will need to advocate participating in this service.

Physical therapists will also need to further educate patients and insurers about what the profession can offer with more evidence that it is cost-effective. Physical therapists will need to develop a better understanding of all needs of the elderly and a positive definition of "maintaining function" as they work with patients who have diseases that may span decades. It may be that the physical therapist's role as a patient educator increases and that is where a substantial portion of the "skill" of the profession will lie in the future.

SUMMARY

This chapter has provided a framework for understanding the planning and financing of long-term–care services and explored some of the issues surrounding the need for changes in reimbursement systems. Legislators, insurers, and health care providers have the task of interpreting current reimbursement regulations, advocating change for legislation that is not serving elders, and developing a comprehensive system for financing services for the elders.

Escalating health care costs have been an impetus for physical therapists to critically review care. Physical therapists are facing a critical opportunity to further define the profession through the legislative process, more effectively use physical therapist assistants, and expand settings in which therapists provide care in order to participate as an efficient and effective providers in health care delivery.

REFERENCES

1. American Physical Therapy Association: *Summary: Omnibus Budget Reconciliation Act of 1990.* Washington, DC, APTA Governmental Affairs Committee, 1990.
2. Balanced Budget Act of 1997. Medicare and Medicaid Provisions. PL105-33. Available at: http://www.hcfa.gov/regs/regs/htm. Accessed March 20, 2000.
3. Balanced Budget Refinement Act. HR3075.RFS. Available at: http://thomas.loc.gov/cgi-bin/query/z?c106:H.R.3075. Accessed March 20, 2000.
4. Binstock RH, Spector WD: Five priority areas for research on long-term care. *Health Serv Res* 1997; 32:715-730.
5. Garland N: Highlights of the Medicare Balanced Budget Refinements Act of 1999. *PT Magazine* 2000; 8:2.
6. Iglehart J: The American health care system–Medicare. *N Engl J Med* 1999; 340(4):327-332.
7. Kuttner R: The American health care system. Employer sponsored health care coverage. *N Engl J Med* 1999; 340(3):248-252.
8. U.S. Department of Health and Human Services, Health Care Financing Administration: *Medicaid.* Available at: http://www.hcfa.gov/medicaid/meligib.htm. Accessed March 22, 2000.
9. U.S. Department of Health and Human Services Health Care Financing Administration. Medicare and you 2000. 1999; Pub No HCFA-10050.
10. U.S. Department of Health and Human Services Health Care Financing Administration. *Medicare questions and answers.* 1999; Pub No HCFA-10117.
11. U.S. Department of Health and Human Services. *The 2000 HHS poverty guidelines.* Available at: http://aspe.hhs.gov/poverty. Accessed March 22, 2000.

ADDITIONAL READINGS

American Physical Therapy Association: Guide to physical therapist practice. *Phys Ther* 1997; 77(11):1163-1150.
Annas GJ: When should preventive treatment be paid for by health insurance? *N Engl J Med* 1994; 331(15):1027-1030.
Barry K: Status report: The continuing process of developing Medicare's outpatient PT screens. *Phys Ther Today* 1988; II (spring):18-22.
Bodenheimer T: Longterm care for frail elderly people—the On Lok Model. *N Engl J Med* 1999; 340(1):70-76.
Cain TD, Webster JR: Health care delivery for the elderly—reform or revolution? *Compr Ther* 1994; 20(9):481-484.
Carney K, Burns N, Brobst B: Hospice costs and Medicare reimbursement: An application of breakeven analysis. *Nurs Econ* 1989; 7:41-48.
Cohen MA, Jumar Nanda AK: The changing face of long-term care insurance in 1994: Profiles and innovations in a dynamic market. *Inquiry* 1997:34:50-61 (Blue Cross and Blue Shield Association and Finger Lakes Blue Cross and Blue Shield 0046-9580/97 3401-0050).
Dombi WA: Legal issues in home care. *Caring* 1994; 13(5):12-16, 18-20.
Ellwood P: Shattuck lecture: Outcomes management, a technology of patient experience. *N Engl J Med* 1988; 318:1549-1556.
Entoven A: Consumer-choice health plan. *N Engl J Med* 1978; 298:650-658.
Eubanks P: LTC advocate proposes part C for Medicare. *Hospitals* 1990; 64(3):62.
Freedman S: Coverage of the uninsured and underinsured. *N Engl J Med* 1988; 318:843-847.
Gillick M: Long-term care options for the frail elderly. *J Am Geriatr Soc* 1989; 37:1198-1203.
Ginzberg E: The reform of Medicare—if I were king. *J Med Pract Manag* 1987; 3:151-153.
Ginzberg E: The destabilization of health care. *N Engl J Med* 1986; 315:757-760.
Harrington C: Public policy and the nursing home industry. *Int J Health Serv* 1984; 14:481-490.
Hillman A, et al: Managing the medical-industrial complex. *N Engl J Med* 1986; 315:511-513.
Hsiao W, et al: Results and policy implications of the resource-based relative-value study. *N Engl J Med* 1988; 319:881-888.
Hudson T: NAIC (National Association of Insurance Commissioners) chief pushes LTC reform. *Hospitals* 1990; 64(4):72-73.
Iglehart J: The American health care system—expenditures. *N Engl J Med* 1999; 340(1):70-76.
Infante MC: Options for long-term care financing reform: A view from the inside out. *J Long Term Care Adm* 1993; 21(3):60-65.
Jennings MC: Financing long-term care. *Top Health Care Financ* 1991; 17:49.
Kane R, Kane R: A nursing home in your future. *N Engl J Med* 1991; 324:627-629.
Kemper P, Murtaugh CM: Lifetime use of nursing home care. *N Engl J Med* 1991; 324:595-600.
Magary J: The fundamental elements of Medicare documentation. *Phys Ther Today* 1988; II(spring):23-27.
Marlowe JF: Long-term care insurance: A private sector challenge. *Empl Benefits J* 1996; 21(4):8-12.
Mefford J: Funding alternatives for home care agencies. *Caring* 1994; 13(4):4, 7, 58-60.

National Citizen's Coalition for Nursing Home Reform: Summary of nursing home amendments in the 1990 budget act (newsletter). Nov 2, 1990, pp 1-5.

O'Shaughnessy C: Financing and delivery of long-term care services for the elderly. Adapted from O'Shaughnessy C, et al: *Financing and delivery of long-term care services for the elderly.* Library of Congress Pub No 85-1033 EPW, Oct 17, 1985.

Purtilo RB: Saying "no" to patients for cost-related reasons. *Phys Ther* 1988; 68:1243-1247.

Ricker-Smith KL: A challenge for public policy: The chronically elderly and nursing homes. *Med Care* 1982; 20:1071-1079.

Shen J, et al: PACE: A capitated model towards long-term care. *Henry Ford Hosp Med J* 1992; 40:1, 2, 41-44.

Weisset WG, et al: Models of adult day care: Findings from a national survey. *Gerontologist* 1989; 29:640-649.

CHAPTER 27

ETHICAL AND LEGAL ISSUES IN GERIATRIC PHYSICAL THERAPY

RON SCOTT, PT, JD, MS, OCS AND ANDREW A. GUCCIONE, PT, PhD, FAPTA

INTRODUCTION

Not all the difficult decisions in physical therapy are related to choices about therapy. Sometimes the therapeutic choice appears quite simple, yet there are other questions regarding the patient whose answers do not lie within the typical boundaries of physical therapy. These questions include the following:

- When should the professional's opinion outweigh the concerns of the patient?
- How do I decide how much time to give one patient and take away time from another?
- What rights do patients have to control their care even when they are mentally incapacitated?
- What do I do if I suspect someone has physically abused a patient?

Professional ethics and health care law provide the principal rules by which practitioners decide how they ought to act toward patients, other professionals, and one another as interdependent human beings. Specifically, ethics raises questions about the rightness or wrongness of actions on the basis of the self-chosen principles that an individual uses to guide conduct. The law deals with a smaller set of behaviors, including actions performed in a professional role, and judges their legal rightness or wrongness according to the rules agreed upon by specific legislative and judicial bodies. Often, law and ethics overlap, as their concerns are similar even if their scopes and processes are different. In the present day, law and ethics have largely been blended into common standards of professional conduct (Fig. 27-1). Almost without exception, professional conduct that constitutes a breach of ethics also constitutes a violation of law, and vice versa. Many decisions by health care professionals regarding health care delivery require thorough knowledge and careful analysis of professional ethical and legal duties, as well as compliance with professional ethical and legal standards. As with legal requirements pertaining to physical therapist practice, ignorance of professional ethical responsibilities is no excuse for noncompliance.

The advent of managed health care delivery in the 1980s and its exponential growth during the 1990s have resulted in both problems and promise for health care professionals. Managed care is an amorphous concept that has been defined in different ways by various authorities. Everyone agrees, however, that managed care is a system of health care service delivery that focuses significant attention on cost-containment, as well as the quality of patient care delivered by the system. Managed care in the 1990s has become the private sector analogue to the failed federal public-sector health care reform initiatives of the early part of the decade.

Managed care has created profound challenges for professionals in all health care disciplines and significant ethical concerns. Of principal concern is the fact that, for the first time, the health care delivery system under managed care has made cost-containment a co-equal (but hopefully not a higher) consideration with optimal quality.

It is always possible for the health practitioner to evaluate whether professional actions meet ethical and legal standards, even those activities that are routine behaviors. This

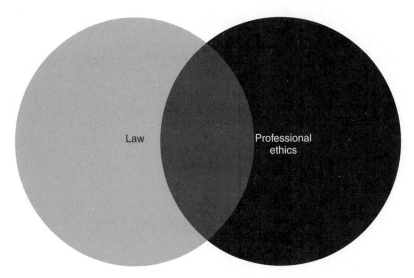

FIG. 27-1   The interface between law and professional ethics. (Adapted from Scott RW: *Professional Ethics: A Guide for Rehabilitation Professionals.* St Louis, Mosby, 1998.)

chapter has two purposes. The first is to outline the ethical dimensions of professional practice and discuss the ethical issues that a physical therapist may confront as a practitioner to the elderly. The second is to identify the laws that have been passed and legal opinions that have been rendered to address these ethical issues from a legal perspective. These laws provide boundaries to the social context of geriatric care and place important constraints on professional actions.

PRINCIPLES OF ETHICS

There are situations in clinical practice that are so overwhelming in their consequences that no one doubts their ethical importance. Often, these cases are literally "life-and-death" issues, such as who can decide what medical care is appropriate for a terminally ill elder with senile dementia. While it is easy to assume that only unusual circumstances generate ethical problems, any professional action that a physical therapist might take toward another individual can be examined in light of its ethical impact. The day-to-day practice of physical therapy contains many instances in which physical therapists must consider what their ethical duties are and how they may act toward their patients. Because of the issues confronting elders, the need to make ethical decisions as part of one's clinical practice is particularly evident in geriatric physical therapy. Models of ethical decision making that govern patient care are based on the foundational ethical principles of autonomy, nonmaleficence, beneficence, and justice and reflect the professional duties of competency, confidentiality, fidelity, and truth. Conducting oneself in conformity with these principles and duties can seem even more challenging under the current health care delivery paradigm of managed care, which may present significant conflicts of interest.

There are two ways in which we may understand autonomy as it relates to ethics.[1,3] The first notion of autonomy comes from Immanuel Kant, whose view was that all individuals must always be treated as ends in themselves and never as means to an end. Kant believed that individuals are rational agents who freely impose upon themselves universal moral standards to which they will hold themselves accountable.[21] In comparison, John Stuart Mill developed the concept of autonomy from the perspective of freedom.[26] Mill thought that people should be limited in their actions only to the degree necessary to prevent harm to others and to allow everyone else a similar amount of freedom.

The second major category of ethical obligations draws attention to the probable consequences of an action and how these outcomes influence our decisions about what is the right thing to do. The primary consideration for physical therapists, as it is for all health professionals, is that the physical therapist do no harm (the principle of nonmaleficence). This cardinal rule of ethical health care is one that all health professionals cannot ethically and legally ignore. In its broadest form, nonmaleficence means: "Do no harm yourself, and protect individuals under your care from harming themselves or others." Nonmaleficence means that health care professionals will not intentionally cause harm to patients under their care.

In addition to preventing harm, physical therapists are obliged to do as much good as they can (the principle of beneficence). Many individuals are initially attracted to physical therapy for the opportunity to do good by alleviating suffering and assisting patients to develop their fullest human potential. The promotion of well-being among individual elders extends the ethical dimensions of physical therapy to the societal level because the optimal health of all elders contributes to the common good of society.[18]

Next, there are general ethical obligations of fidelity that pertain to the professional-patient relationship. Commitment to truth telling and confidentiality, which is essential to good communication, provides a solid ethical foundation between a physical therapist and a patient. This relationship of trust assumes that the professional is committed to providing competent and compassionate care to all individuals and demonstrates commitment to patient autonomy. Although physical therapists can sort out the difference between being a professional care-giver and being a friend to someone in need, elders who are lonely and often very vulnerable when they are sick may not make this distinction quite so easily. Therapists need to recognize that when an elder is sick, there may be a need for this person to feel safe among "friends." Even though professional care-givers are "friendly" and honestly concerned about the patient's welfare, they are, in reality, not friends. For example, friends share their most troublesome problems with each other and derive support from each other. Professional care-givers, on the other hand, would never burden a patient with their own personal problems or seek to have a patient provide emotional support for them.

It is not unusual for a therapist to develop a relationship with a patient in which many personal facts about the patient are shared openly with the therapist. This may include information about the elder's past or current medical history, personal relationships, and financial affairs. Family members and friends may seek to obtain information about the patient from the therapist, just as they would from any other member of the family or friend. Physical therapists are obligated to protect this information as a professional committed to confidentiality, divulging only essential information with only those who need to know such information and sharing personal information only with the prior explicit approval of the elder. Also, if patients believe that historical information conveyed by them to health care providers will be kept confidential, they are more likely to freely and openly communicate information to their health care providers. That, in turn, facilitates the formulation of accurate diagnoses, which inures to the benefit of patients, providers, the health care organizations and third-party payers, and society. Finally, maintenance of patient confidentiality (absent the exceptions discussed in the following text) is required by state practice acts and implementing regulations, other health-related statutes, and by professional codes of ethics. Failure to comply with these directives is a basis for imposition of disciplinary sanctions against providers bound by law and ethics to follow them.

The most obvious type of permissible disclosure of otherwise confidential information involves disclosure pursuant to a valid waiver signed by a person whose privacy is affected by the disclosure of information. Patients typically expressly, i.e., explicitly and unambiguously, authorize release of health-related information to third-party payers, health care professional consultants, next-of-kin, and others. Patients may impliedly, i.e., by implication, authorize release of confidential information to other entities, e.g., to governmental and accreditation reviewers and researchers, among others.

Because, on average, 75 people have access to each patient's confidential health record,[37] patient authorizations for release should clearly state the expected types of professionals and others privileged to invade the patient's privacy and learn confidential information about the patient. Unfortunately, most health-related general releases are woefully inadequate in this regard.

Mandatory disclosures of personal information occur without regard for permission of the subject of the information disclosed. Most such disclosures are authorized by state or federal law. Such disclosures include among others: release of information concerning infectious and sexually transmitted diseases to governmental entities; release of information to law enforcement officials upon request or in compliance with reporting statutes; and release of information to third parties pursuant to the federal Freedom of Information Act[42] or state freedom of information or open records statutes.

A special case of mandatory release involves the situation in which a patient has communicated a threat of inflicting serious bodily harm or death upon a specified victim. In the case of *Tarasoff vs. Regents of the University of California*,[39] a psychotherapist employed by the University of California was treating a mentally ill patient, who threatened bodily harm against his former girlfriend during his therapy sessions. Although the psychotherapist reported the threats to his supervisor, neither the psychotherapist nor his supervisor reported the patient's threats to the potential victim or law enforcement authorities. When the patient murdered his former girlfriend, her parents brought this legal action against the Regents of the University of California, alleging professional negligence on the part of their agent, the psychotherapist. In ruling in favor of the victim's parents, the California Supreme Court ruled that a psychotherapist owes a legal duty to identifiable third parties threatened by mental patients under their care to warn them of the threats. The court reasoned that, on balance, the duty of confidentiality owed by psychotherapists to patients under their care was outweighed by the court-imposed duty to identifiable third parties to take reasonable steps to warn them of foreseeable serious bodily harm or death at the hands of such patients. This legal duty has been extended to physicians and other health care professionals in many states.

"Routine" disclosures involve releases of personal information not deemed (by legislatures or regulatory agencies) to be confidential to enumerated third parties, made either without a subject's consent or in the absence of an express directive by the subject not to release such information. Examples of routine releases of information include "directory information," such as the presence of a person in a medical facility and that person's condition, place of residence, gender, and age.

A third facet of professional confidentiality concerns "discretionary" disclosure of information. The issue of discretionary disclosure of confidential information largely applies to attorneys, who traditionally have been disallowed by professional ethical and state bar rules from disclosing any patient confidence, even a patient's plan to commit a future crime involving serious bodily harm or death to an identified third party. The concept of discretionary disclosure of confidential information might also apply to a rehabilitation professional who is not protected by a Tarasoff law and who discovers, in the course of care delivery, a patient's intent to commit serious bodily harm or death against an identifiable third party. Before breaching patient confidentiality in such cases, health care professionals are urged to consult with facility or personal legal counsel for advice.

Very closely related to the ethical duty of confidentiality owed by health care professionals to patients are the duties of fidelity and truthfulness in dealing with patients and their significant others. Every health care professional who accepts a person into care is a fiduciary, i.e., a person in a special position of trust in relation to the patient. Not only is the health care professional obligated under professional ethical standards to act in patients' best interests, i.e., with beneficence, but also as a fiduciary who places patients' interests above all others, including the financial and other interests of the provider himself/herself.

It may seem a truism that health care professionals owe patients the duty always to be truthful. Yet there are situations in which health care providers, professional disciplines and organizations, the legal system, and society accept deception of patients as legitimate. One such example involves therapeutic privilege, an exception to the requirement for patient informed consent, in which a primary care physician imposes a gag order on health professional team members, disallowing them to disclose diagnostic or prognostic information to a particular patient who the physician believes is incapable of handling the disclosure psychologically. Other examples of deception in health care clinical practice involve situations more focused on provider self-interest. Examples of such deception include the nondisclosure to patients of actual provider conflicts-of-interest and provider compliance with managed care "gag clauses" in employment or participation contracts that impede full disclosure of treatment-related information to patients.

Finally, there is the principle of justice. The formal concern of justice is to ensure that individuals without relevant differences between them are treated equally. Rawls has argued for a concept of justice as fairness, whereby essential goods and services must be distributed equally unless an unequal distribution works in favor of the disadvantaged.[29] Physical therapists frequently concern themselves with issues of justice when they decide how to allocate resources to patients, including the time they spend with some individuals, which lessens the time they can spend with others. Considering only an individual's need for intervention, a therapist may opt to spend more time with a more therapeutically challenging patient who has the less overall potential, rather than the patient who actually needs less therapy to realize a greater rehabilitation potential. Given that there are always a limited number of hours in a therapist's work week as well as different requirements set by each insurer to authorize care, it is impractical to believe that each patient will receive an optimal amount of physical therapy based solely on the need for intervention. Physical therapists, especially those who work with elders, must increasingly consider the outcome of treatment in relationship to the investment of resources when choosing to provide more physical therapy resources to one patient than to another.

RIGHTS

When a therapist needs to determine what ought to be done to act ethically in a particular situation, there is often a need to consider a patient's rights and their relevance to a decision about what to do. A *right* is a claim by one individual or group that can be made upon another person or group. Some rights are protected by law.

Rights and duties are correlative. If a person has a particular right or claim that can be made on someone else, then the person or group on whom that claim has been made has an obligation or duty to the person invoking that right. Rights take two forms: liberty rights and entitlement rights. The American notion of life, liberty, and the pursuit of happiness are well-known examples of liberty rights. Each person is free to engage in the exercise of these rights as long as an individual's actions do not infringe on the rights of others. The duty attached to a claim based on liberty rights requires that another party refrain from acting or interfering with the exercise of those rights.

Entitlement rights entail a different set of concerns. A claim made on another as an entitlement right requires that another party not only refrain from acting but also take positive actions to assist or enable another person to exercise that right. Social rights are often presented as entitlement rights. The debate over the right to health care has often hinged on the question of whether the government has a positive obligation to provide health care for all persons. Some ethicists and politicians argue that the government has no such obligation to assist others in exercising their right to health care. Conceived as a liberty right, the right to health care obligates the government not to pass laws or allow regulations that prohibit individuals from receiving health care. Statutes against discrimination in the provision of health care on the basis of age, gender, race, creed, national or ethnic origin, or disability are an example of how a liberty right to health care corresponds to the government's duty to honor this claim made upon it. Presented as an entitlement right, the right to health care requires the government to do more than eliminate discrimination in order for a person to exercise the right to health care. One of the major barriers to receiving health care services, including physical therapy, is the ability to pay for these services. Therefore, some would argue that if an elder is unable to pay for health services, then the government must facilitate a person's entitlement right to health care by underwriting these services. To some extent, the government has already honored the right to health care as an entitlement by creating Medicare and Medicaid. These programs, however, do not allow all elders to receive all the services that might be recognized as "basic" to the health care of the elderly and essential for the humane treatment of our nation's elderly. The argument in the next few years over the right to health care as an entitlement will seek to establish a national consensus on what kinds and amounts of services constitute acceptable treatment of elders. Physical therapists who participate in this discussion and share their clinical expertise and experience can influence public policy in a way that will benefit everyone, including elders, through a just distribution of resources.

In health care, the right to privacy may be conceived as both a liberty and an entitlement right. One has the right to have the details of one's medical care kept private, and therefore others must refrain from infringing on that privacy. Patients may also make a special claim on health care providers to maintain confidentiality. Conceived as an entitlement right, the right to privacy requires that professionals take appropriate actions to safeguard this entitlement in their record-keeping procedures and enable patients to exercise their right to privacy.

AUTONOMY AND PATERNALISM

Physical therapists have professional expertise that can promote good consequences for many individuals. Beneficence means that a health care professional's conduct relative to a particular patient will be carried out in accordance with that patient's best interests, as ascertained from the perspective of the health care professional. The desire to do good and the knowledge of how to do it are strong motivations for physical therapists and a substantial consideration in their decisions about what they owe their patients. Therefore, physical therapists often refer to the principles of nonmaleficence and beneficence as justification for the actions that they may take to prevent negative consequences for their patients and promote their well-being. The desire to do good, however, often subtly encourages physical therapists to act paternalistically toward their patients. Paternalism has been defined as "interference with a person's liberty of action justified by reasons referring exclusively to the welfare, good, happiness, needs, interests or values of the person being coerced."[13] In short, paternalism denies the autonomy of the individual.

As described elsewhere in this text, physical therapists frequently experience situations in which patients ignore their home exercise programs or disregard safety instructions about how to use an assistive device. Sometimes, the physical therapist may believe that the patient should be "forced" into following the therapist's recommendations based on the reasoning that these suggestions were provided in the patient's best interests. Autonomy recognizes the inherent human right of self-determination in every individual who has mental capacity. Placing a professional's judgment of "what's best" for the individual ahead of the expressed desires of the individual suggests that honoring a person's own choice (the principle of autonomy) should not count as much as the consequences that will follow (the principles of nonmaleficence and beneficence).

Autonomy cannot always be reconciled with the principles of nonmaleficence and beneficence in matters of health.[18] The consequences of some decisions that a patient might make may very well result in harm. For example, a patient's decision not to follow a physical therapy home program for range of motion might result in additional pain for the patient or further diminish function. Although this is distressing to the therapist, there is always the opportunity for the patient to reconsider. Sometimes, however, the exercise of autonomy may result in irreparable harm to the patient, or even death. For example, an elderly patient may refuse to take a cardiac medication that prevents a life-threatening arrhythmia. A complete discussion of the complex ethical and legal issues surrounding this sort of situation is far beyond the scope of this chapter. It is, however, important to realize that a patient's mental status, mood, and outlook on life are essential data in such decisions. Every individual has a unique history and self-concept that has been developed over the years (Fig. 27-2). Although the ongoing process of aging may begin to strip away physical or mental capacities, a person cannot lose one's history that unites all the progression through the life span or the values and attitudes that have created history. Therapists who have an ongoing, and often long-term, association with their geriatric patients may contribute much to understanding whether an elder is purposely choosing negative consequences, is merely uneducated about the potentially harmful effects of not adhering to the health professional's recommendations, is depressed to the point of contemplating suicide, or is exhibiting signs of cognitive decline.

A physical therapist must then also consider whether interfering in an elder's autonomy is a temporary decision that will allow the individual increased autonomy in the future or if the paternalistic act diminishes the person's autonomy on an ongoing basis for an unlimited time period.[8,9] For example, consider the ethical questions presented to the physical therapist in the case of Esther R. Esther R is an 84-year-old never-married female who has recently suffered a stroke and was transferred to a rehabilitation hospital within 1 week of the event. Although she generally cooperates with her therapist, she shows little interest in her program and often states emphatically that she would rather "just go home to die." Should the therapist stop treatment and facilitate Ms. R's discharge home out of respect for her autonomy as an individual, or should the therapist continue to encourage her to participate as long as the patient offers no physical resistance to treatment in order for her to realize her full potential for rehabilitation?

The therapist may choose to act in a weakly paternalistic way and continue to coax and cajole Ms. R to receive treatment. On the grounds of preventing harm in the interim, the therapist might argue that the patient will be in a better

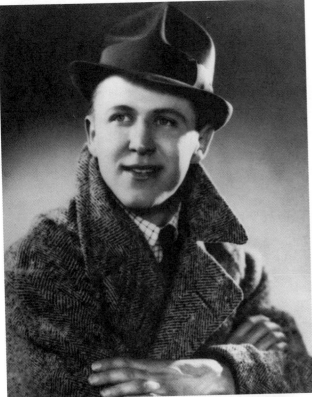

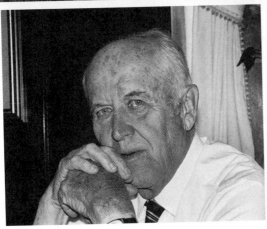

FIG. 27-2   Despite the physical changes of aging that alter identity, the history of the individual forms a continuous personal identity.

the discharge plan can be implemented, if necessary. Hospitals function to at least some degree, as the sociologist Erving Goffman put it, as "total institutions," controlling how the time of the individual will be spent, with whom, and under what conditions the "inmate" is free to leave.[14] Total control over all aspects of an elder's life may be even more predominant in the nursing home setting.[20] Once the patient has been taken into the system, time, energy, and money are invested in the process to make the person "better." It can be very difficult to reflect on what is happening to the patient, whether the patient has freely chosen to continue treatment or perhaps to terminate treatment, when the patient still has rehabilitation potential. However, when members of the rehabilitation team forget to let the patient's own goals direct the team's efforts, the individual becomes a prisoner to the "good consequences" intended by others.

The conflict between the ethical principles of autonomy and the principles of nonmaleficence and beneficence in the case of Esther R underscores the nature of an ethical dilemma. An ethical dilemma exists whenever an individual is confronted with two or more mutually exclusive obligations in a single situation. Therapists confronted by an ethical dilemma find themselves proverbially "caught between a rock and a hard place." In fact, when a therapist weighs the alternatives, it is quite possible to find that no one alternative satisfies all ethical obligations at the same time. For example, one cannot always adhere to the principle of autonomy while simultaneously preventing all bad consequences from befalling a patient. In choosing what to do, one course of action will uphold one principle at the expense of another equally important and valued principle. Therefore, moral obligations, as specified by the general ethical principles outlined in the preceding text, have come to be recognized as prima facie obligations, each needing to be recognized as relevant to the situation at hand on the first look.[32] None of these principles in itself, however, represents a final and absolute obligation. Otherwise, no decision in which a therapist weighted the importance of one ethical principle greater than another would be ethically defensible.

SOURCES OF ETHICAL CONFLICTS

Some situations with an ethical dimension require us to determine exactly where the ethical concern lies. Sometimes a therapist may need to reconcile personal and professional beliefs. For example, although working with elders is a rewarding experience, this experience is not found with every elder. Try as one might, no physical therapist will be able to relate in a humanly meaningful way to every patient. However, every patient, regardless of the quality of the interaction for the therapist, deserves the best care that the therapist can render. The therapist in such a case must resolve the conflict between personal feelings and professional responsibilities.

Conflict can also occur between professionals or professional groups.[6] Other therapists, nurses, and physicians all

position to make autonomous choices in the future when her depression is resolved and she has had sufficient time to adjust to the sudden changes in her life brought on by the stroke. On the other hand, at some later point in her rehabilitation, the therapist may also need to recognize that a patient's verbal request to be discharged from the hospital does represent the patient's own choice, regardless of the negative consequences that may ensue. In that instance, the therapist is obligated to communicate this fact to the rehabilitation team so that the appropriate discussions can take place and have expectations of the physical therapist on the team. Some of these expectations facilitate a high level of performance among all the team members; other expectations are based on misinformation, misunderstanding, and mistrust. Such situations force us to consider what we owe our colleagues and what kinds of implicit promises have been made to each other by virtue of working together as a team.

Some ethical conflicts originate at the societal level. There is a wide difference of opinion within our society about how we ought to act toward elders, particularly in allocating health care resources. These differences are inevitable in a society that tolerates a range of political philosophies and also is composed of many cultures with different ideas about aging and the elderly. Some therapists, frustrated in their genuine desire to help their patients, may be tempted to do whatever is necessary on a case-by-case basis to achieve "justice" for each individual in their care. Justice reflects the desire to achieve fundamental fairness in health care delivery at individual, group, societal, and global levels. Just as laws do not resolve intrapersonal or interpersonal conflicts, problems in the society at large must be addressed at the appropriate level and through the appropriate channels. Physical therapists who refrain from sharing their expertise delay recognition of unjust distributions of resources, where they exist, and perpetuate the conditions that hamper physical therapists in their efforts to allow all individuals to reach their full potential for rehabilitation.

The managed care model of health care delivery presents a myriad of potential ethical dilemmas for health care professionals, who may face issues of ever-more sharply divided loyalties involving their employers and patients. Health care professionals self-identify as being altruistic and, specifically, focused on the welfare of their patients. They are governed in their professional conduct with patients and their families and significant others by fundamental ethical principles.[3] A growing backlash of legislative initiatives at the state and federal levels, designed to curb managed care practices that restrict patient access to and funding of health care, challenge the perpetuation of managed care in its extreme forms.[24] Some health policy makers are particularly critical of the fundamental tenets of managed care, arguing that its clear purpose is managing, i.e., minimizing, monetary outlays for health care, rather than managing the health of patients.

PROFESSIONAL ETHICAL STANDARDS

Some ethical analyses tend to focus only on the relationship between patient and professional and tend to divorce ethical problems from the larger social context in which they are found. As Beauchamp and Childress have commented:

> Moral principles. . .are not disembodied rules, cut off from their cultural setting. . . . "Morality," as we understand the term, emerges from shared experiences and social arrangements (tacit or otherwise).[3]

Assistance to health care professionals facing ethical dilemmas is often provided in health care organizations by institutional ethics committees, bringing the individual's problem under the scrutiny of the local professional community. These multidisciplinary committees may have several roles, including policy making, education, and provision of consultation services. Furthermore, the professional community of physical therapists, the broad cultural setting of our ethical problems, has codified its shared experience and values in the Guide for Professional Conduct of the American Physical Therapy Association (APTA) based upon APTA's *Code of Ethics*.[15] Professional codes of ethics have four primary purposes.[30] First, a professional code of ethics is directive, i.e., it provides guidance for mandatory behavior by members of a profession. Professional ethics codes may also provide nondirective guidance for permissive or recommended conduct of members of a profession. Second, a code must be protective of the rights of patients and subjects, their significant others, and the public at-large. Third, a professional code of ethics must be specific, i.e., address areas of ethical problems, issues, and dilemmas particular to the discipline(s) governed by the code. Finally, a professional ethics code must be enforceable and enforced.

By endorsing a code of ethics, the physical therapy profession publicly states that certain ethical ideals should be implicit in every professional action committed by a physical therapist. A patient reading the APTA Code of Ethics can determine what ethical standards can be expected from physical therapy practitioners. For example, a patient who goes to any physical therapist can expect to be treated in a manner that supports personal dignity and maintains confidentiality. These Code of Ethics do not provide specific answers to particular ethical problems, but they do emphasize for the individual therapist or assistant those factors that the professional group believes are important to take into consideration when making an ethical decision. These ethical standards of the profession may also be used by others to formulate a legal decision as well. Failure to understand what is contained in these documents may adversely affect a physical therapist. The APTA's Code of Ethics ethically binds APTA members to its principles. Failure to meet these standards could result in sanctions such as being expelled from the Association. The APTA's Code of Ethics can also affect nonmembers as well. Many state practice acts reference the Code of Ethics as the standard of ethical practice for all physical therapists licensed in that state, not just APTA members. Ignoring the Code of Ethics in these states may result in disciplinary action by a state board of licensure, which may even revoke a therapist's license. A licensing board when conducting an official review of a therapist's actions may also look to the Patient's Bill of Rights to define what standard of care has been legally accepted.

On rare occasions, conduct by health care professionals may constitute a violation of professional ethical standards, but not violate the law. Consider the following example: An employment contract between a health care professional and a Medigap managed care organization contains a provision that prohibits the health care professional from discussing treatment options with geriatric patients that are not offered by the managed care organization. Such a contractual provision is commonly referred to as a "gag clause."[7] While compliance by the health care professional with the gag clause might be upheld by a court as a legally acceptable course of action, such conduct might still constitute an actionable breach of professional ethics. Under traditional ethical standards governing patient informed consent to treatment, a competent patient must be informed by a clinical health care professional of all reasonable alternatives to recommended interventions, irrespective of whether a managed care entity elects to offer them as a matter of its business judgment. The health care professional in this case might, therefore, face adverse administrative or association action for a breach of professional ethics, in spite of the hypothetical legality of the contract.

LEGAL PROTECTION OF THE AUTONOMOUS INDIVIDUAL

Informed Consent

The essence of a clinical encounter between a physical therapist and a patient involves physically touching a patient for assessment and treatment. Although the physical therapist's "hands-on" actions are undeniably in the patient's best interests, a therapist may not touch a patient without that individual's permission to be touched. Touching without consent is known as battery, and a therapist may be sued when this occurs.[36] Most professional malpractice, however, does not involve touching without consent. Rather, allegations of malpractice tend to be made when the patient has consented to being touched without having received enough information to give or refuse consent to the touching. When a therapist does not provide the patient with sufficient information to make a decision to receive or refuse treatment, the therapist may be held negligent for not allowing the patient to exercise the right to informed consent. Informed consent is a legal and professional ethical prerequisite to physical therapy examination and intervention. From a professional ethical perspective, the making of relevant disclosures and the obtaining of patient informed consent is premised, not on beneficence or paternalism, but on respect for patient autonomy over treatment-related decision making. Under the biomedical ethical principle of autonomy, it is the patient (or surrogate decision maker) who decides whether to accept or to reject a recommended health intervention.

The history of patient informed consent has been rocky and precarious. Health care professionals never willingly chose to involve patients or surrogates in treatment-related decision making or to give them veto power over professional recommendations until an activist judiciary in the 20th century imposed such requirements upon health care providers.[36]

The term *informed consent* has been used in a legal context for the last 40 years, since a California court ruled that a physician had a positive obligation to disclose any information regarding the risks and dangers of tests or treatments

that was essential for an individual to make an informed decision.[33] The legal right to self-determination, however, was articulated earlier in the century when Judge Cardozo ruled that surgery performed on a mentally competent adult without the patient's consent was an assault for which the surgeon was liable.[34]

Disclosure of relevant intervention-related information by health care providers to patients empowers patients to make knowing, intelligent, voluntary, and unequivocal decisions to accept or decline recommended interventions, based on what individual patients believe to be in their best interests. In a sense, respect for patient autonomy, as applied to the law and ethics of informed consent, is the antithesis of the traditional paradigm of paternalism.

The legal concept of informed consent institutionalizes several of the ethical concepts described in the aforementioned text and places particular legal obligations on the physical therapist. Respecting personal autonomy usually obliges a practitioner to assist an individual in the exercise of free choice by providing appropriate information and allowing the patient to develop sufficient understanding to make an informed decision.[3] From the moral point of view, informed consent is one way in which physical therapists respond to the principle of autonomy.[11] Although most actions that a physical therapist might take toward an elder are not as risky as those of a surgeon, every individual has a right to information that might lead the patient to reject the treatment, and the therapist has the correlative duty to furnish it. As Purtilo has noted, informed consent is a type of contract that is knowingly entered into by the physical therapist and the patient.[28] Under the law, contracts may only be made between equals and by those individuals who are legally free to enter into such binding agreements. Therefore, the physical therapist must share information with the patient to counteract the imbalance of knowledge between the two parties and legally ensure the patient's capacity for self-determination. Purtilo also identifies failure to inform an individual as a possible form of harm, which would be a violation of the principle of nonmaleficence. Furthermore, informed consent defines the patient's reasonable expectations to which the physical therapist must respond, a component of the principle of fidelity. Despite the legal recognition of these concepts, most patients do not understand the purpose of informed consent. In a now classic study, Cassileth and colleagues found that nearly 80% of 200 cancer patients believed that informed consent was a method of protecting physicians and not patients.[10]

As the term implies, informed consent involves two separate elements: information and consent. Legally, the information provided to the patient must satisfy four conditions. The information provided to the patient should outline the nature and the purpose of the treatment, alternatives to that particular treatment that the patient might choose instead, the risks and consequences of the proposed treatment, and the likelihood of success or failure of the treatment. One recommendation is that physical therapists provide patients with information checklists covering the most common physical therapy procedures or use them to guide discussion with a patient as a practical method of meeting the ethical and legal requirements of informed consent.[36] While the precise litany of disclosure elements for legally sufficient patient informed consent may vary from state to state, the following list of disclosure elements is representative of what is typically required of physical therapists: information about a patient's condition and diagnosis; information about the recommended intervention(s); discussion of risks of serious harm or complication associated with the recommended intervention(s), if any; discussion about reasonable alternatives or options to the recommended intervention(s), if any; and discussion of the goals of intervention.[35] This disclosure must be imparted at the patient's (or surrogate's) level of comprehension and be made in a language that the patient (or surrogate) understands.

In addition to the conditions set on the information provided to the patient, the consent must be obtained from someone who is competent to consent, who clearly understands the information provided, and who agrees without coercion. In the case of the elderly individual, each of these three conditions may pose barriers to informed consent. Special communication problems may affect geriatric physical therapy patients, including a decline in visual acuity that alters a patient's ability to read information on an informed consent form and age-related hearing loss that alters a patient's ability to receive disclosure information. Elders also suffer from the stereotype of declining mental competence. Present-day elders also often do not have the educational backgrounds of most members of society. Therefore, it is erroneously assumed that an older person is incapable of understanding complex information. Taking the time to explain to the patient is not merely educating the patient for therapeutic reasons, but ethically, it allows the individual to exercise autonomy and legally to enter freely into a relationship with the therapist after an informed decision. Some elders are, in fact, mentally incapable of making decisions for themselves; however, this does not mean that their rights to informed consent can be completely abrogated. Kapp stresses that there are degrees of mental incapacitation.[22] Even though an elder may be unable to make all decisions, there may be some decisions that are simple enough to be within the elder's grasp, particularly if environmental factors such as time of day or medications are controlled to present the information to the patient during a period of lucidity.[22] While it is clear that geriatric patients who lack mental capacity to make informed decisions must be represented by surrogate decision makers, the health care, legal, and political professional communities have not effectively addressed the problem of confused geriatric patients or long-term-care (LTC) residents for whom surrogate decision makers have neither been sought nor appointed.

Extreme forms of managed care have created a myriad of legal and ethical dilemmas relevant to informed consent, including the advent of "gag clauses" in provider-employer contracts that purport to disallow providers from engaging in free and full communications with patients; incentive compensation schemes for providers that severely curtail intervention choices for subscribers; and productivity standards that limit providers' time to impart information carefully and patiently to patients under their care.

Three APTA documents also serve as sources of legal obligation to establish a standard of care regarding informed consent for physical therapists in clinical practice: the Standards of Practice for Physical Therapy,[38] which delineates in detail the universal disclosure elements for legally sufficient patient informed consent; the Guidelines for Physical Therapy Documentation,[16] which address acceptable methods for documenting patient informed consent and restate the practice standard requiring patient informed consent as a prerequisite to intervention; and the Guide for Professional Conduct,[15] which enunciates the professional ethical duty that "physical therapists shall obtain patient informed consent before treatment."

LEGAL DIMENSIONS OF PATIENT SELF-DETERMINATION

In addition to the precedent-setting judge-made case law establishing the legal duty to obtain patient informed consent, the Consumer Bill of Rights and Responsibilities of 1998 (CBRR)[41] and the Patient Self-Determination Act of 1990 (PSDA)[45] take the moral and ethical underpinnings of the informed consent duty and transform them into a binding legal obligation. The CBRR and the PSDA are grounded in respect for patient self-determination as are the modern legal and ethical dimensions of patient informed consent generally. The CBRR states in pertinent part that:

> Consumers have the right to receive accurate, easily understood information and some require assistance in making informed health care decisions about their health plans, professionals, and facilities. Consumers have the right and responsibility to fully participate in all decisions related to their health care. Consumers who are unable to fully participate in treatment decisions have the right to be represented by parents, guardians, family members, or other conservators.[41]

The PSDA is a federal statute that codifies into law the right of patients and residents of LTC facilities to exercise control over health care decision making, both routine and extraordinary. The PSDA provides in pertinent part that:

> [A health care] provider [must] maintain written policies and procedures with respect to all adult individuals receiving medical care...to provide them written information to each such individual concerning an individual's rights under state law (whether statutory or recognized by the courts of the state) to make decisions concerning...medical care, including the right to accept or refuse medical or surgical treatment.[46]

The PSDA obligates the range of health care organizations that receive federal funds to fulfill its provisions. The fundamental purposes of the PSDA are to (1) educate patients and residents of LTC facilities about their rights (consistent with state law) to execute and enforce advance directives; (2) facilitate the making of advance directives by patients, LTC residents, and others; (3) cause health care organizations and providers to honor patients' and LTC residents' wishes concerning life-sustaining medical interventions; and (4) help to address the enormous economic costs of end-of-life health care interventions. Advance directives are legal documents that memorialize an individual's personal desires concerning life-sustaining measures that may be undertaken in the event of that person's subsequent incapacitation. Advance directives are completed while the affected person has legal capacity to make decisions for himself/herself. There are two principal types of advance directives: the living will and the durable power of attorney for health care decisions.

The main premise undergirding the PSDA is respect for a person's inherent right of self-determination or autonomy over health care treatment decision making. This same premise forms the basis for requiring primary health care providers (including physical therapists treating geriatric patients) to make legally sufficient disclosure of relevant treatment-related information so as to allow the patient (or a surrogate decision maker) to give informed consent to a recommended intervention.

Although the PSDA does not create any new substantive individual rights, it does obligate health care providers and facilities to do the following: provide written information to patients and LTC residents concerning their rights under applicable state law to make and have enforced enumerated advance directives; provide copies of institutional policies concerning patient-informed decision making and advance directives to patients and LTC residents; and document in patient or resident records whether patients have executed any advance directives concerning their care.

Larsen and Eaton carried out an exhaustive investigative analysis of the PSDA and reported that this statute has been relatively unsuccessful in safeguarding individual rights concerning the making of health-related advance directives.[23] The reasons for the lack of success of the PSDA include a lack of awareness on the part of patients and others of the existence of the PSDA; reluctance on the part of patients and LTC residents to execute advance directives; and recalcitrance on the part of health care professionals to honor valid advance directives involving patients under their care.

Physical therapists treating geriatric patients should become more involved in educating patients, significant others, and professional colleagues of their rights and duties pursuant to the PSDA by direct communications with patients, LTC residents, surrogate decision makers, and others and through participation in relevant teams and committees.

Living Wills

One event that most individuals wish to retain complete control over is paradoxically enough the circumstances of one's death. The ability of technology to maintain the human body has created ethically troublesome questions of immense importance to most adults. Society has recognized that most of us wish to be able to tell our care-givers how we want to be treated when we might otherwise be unable to communicate our choices. The Omnibus Budget Reconciliation Act of 1990 requires all health care facilities receiving Medicare or Medicaid funds to facilitate a patient's right to formulate advance directives about treatment in the event that the individual is no longer able to control the direction of treatment after loss of mental capacities. A living will is one type of advance directive that is recognized in most states. It is a legal instrument, signed by its drafter, that states the person's wishes concerning permissible and impermissible life-sustaining measures to be undertaken in the event of the person's subsequent incapacitation. By executing a living will while still mentally competent, an individual indicates personal preferences for treatment; how treatment should be used to sustain life; and the conditions, if any, under which that person would find continuation of life unacceptable. Thus, elders have the opportunity to express how they wish to be treated, even if refusal of treatment may eventually lead to death if that is one's preference. A living will may be called by other names, depending on state law, most notably a "directive to physicians" or a "natural death act instrument." Living wills are recognized as valid in a majority of states. Most jurisdictions require that a person be both legally incapacitated and terminally ill, i.e., have a condition expected to directly result in the person's death, in order for a living will to become legally operative. Some states also permit a living will to become effective when a person is in a persistent vegetative state.

Durable Power of Attorney

Many health decisions do not concern prolonging life. These choices and decisions, some as simple as whether to participate in physical therapy or act as a research subject, also require the consent of the elder. Durable power of attorney is another method for ensuring that the patient retains a degree of autonomy, even though the patient's mental status prevents communication. The durable power of attorney for health care decisions is the second principal type of advance directive. Its meaning is best ascertained by defining its component parts. "Durable" indicates that decision-making power endures after the drafter loses mental capacity to make legally enforceable decisions. "Power of attorney" is a term of art for surrogate, or substitute, decision making by a designated third party. Durable power of attorney implies control over a broad array of decisions. "Health care decisions" limits the scope of the decision making power of the designated third party to health-related decisions affecting the maker of the legal instrument. Some states, therefore, specifically identify a durable power of attorney for health care decisions. This agent is not always the same person who has durable power of attorney over other matters, e.g., handling finances.

A person normally may designate anyone to be a substitute decision maker under a durable power of attorney for health care decisions, including a spouse, relative, friend, or other trusted person. Ideally, the surrogate is one who knows the individual very well, such as a spouse, child, or close friend, and can articulate what the incapacitated individual would say if able to do so. In comparison with living wills, durable power of attorney has the advantage of allowing the mentally compromised individual to direct all forms of medical treatment, not merely those related to death and dying. Unfortunately, even the closest spouse or friend may not have discussed every decision that might need to be made or know what the incapacitated person's views would have been on a particular issue. Doukas and McCullough recommend that elderly patients record their preferences through a values history, which establishes the general values that should underlie the decisions made on that individual's behalf by a proxy agent.[12]

What occurs in the case in which a person fails to execute a living will or durable power of attorney and a life-and-death medical decision must be made? The states each treat this situation differently. One prominent example of how this dilemma is addressed involves the Texas Consent to Medical Treatment Act, under which the following list of persons, in descending order of priority, are empowered to consent to medical interventions for incapacitated hospitalized patients or residents of a LTC facility: a spouse; an adult child as a sole decision maker (with the consent of all siblings); a majority of reasonably available adult children; a parent; another surrogate decision maker clearly identified by the patient; the nearest living relative; and a clergy-person.

ELDER ABUSE

One of the most distressing facts about the elderly is that they can be the victims of violence by criminals and abuse perpetrated by their care-givers, including their family. Elder abuse may take many forms, but it generally involves some infliction of physical pain or mental anguish, confinement, deprivation, or financial exploitation. The characteristics of an elder abuser are unclear. Sometimes the abusing spouse or child is continuing a tradition of family violence. The abuse may also stem from a care-giver's own substance abuse problem, which predisposes to violence in stressful situations. Abusers may also have distinctly negative attitudes toward the elderly and unrealistic expectations of how much an elder can cooperate with the care-giver. These negative attitudes are not limited to family members. Sometimes paid care-givers with little training in geriatrics or appreciation for the elderly abuse patients. Physical therapists may assist in the prevention of elder abuse by carefully guiding and educating all care-givers in the proper treatment of the elder and establishing realistic expectations of an elder's dependency.

When a physical therapist suspects elder abuse, he/she should report it to the appropriate authorities for investigation of the complaint and the initiation of adult protective services for the elder. These services differ geographically. Each state has its own statutes that define who is responsible for reporting abuse and to which agency. Therefore, it is the responsibility of therapists to know the procedures specific to the states in which they practice.

The therapist may have learned of the abuse as part of confidential information or may have been instructed by the patient not to reveal the situation. Although regulatory statutes that mandate reporting can be used to justify breaking the patient's confidentiality, such breaches of trust cannot be taken lightly.

Health care professionals and their assistants and extenders have the professional ethical and (in most states) the legal duty to identify and report suspected patient abuse to law enforcement authorities.[47] Patient abuse categories reflect patient age or relational status to the abuser, as follows: child, domestic (spousal), and elder abuse.

Research reports indicate that health care professionals do not report suspected abuse involving their patients as often as they are required to, even when failure to do so constitutes a criminal offense.[2] Reasons proffered for failing to report include lack of training on the signs and symptoms of abuse, overwork, and fear of defamation liability exposure. Professional associations, including the American Physical Therapy Association, offer guidelines and risk management seminars focused on recognizing and reporting patient abuse.[17]

Patient abuse may be physical (including sexual) and psychological (including neglect). In the absence of other explanations, common signs that may be indicators of patient abuse include the following: untreated or unexplained injury; skin irritation, scratches, burns, lacerations, or bruising; patient reticence; failure to make eye contact; annoyance over personal questions during the taking of a patient history; inappropriate withdrawal from touch; malnutrition or dehydration; poor hygiene; soiled clothes; and clothing inappropriate for the season or setting. As a matter of professional ethical and legal duty and prudent liability risk management, every health care clinical manager should ensure that all clinical health care providers receive recurrent instruction on patient abuse by competent professionals. The act of reporting suspected patient abuse should not give rise to liability (although it might give rise to litigation), because health care providers are afforded qualified or limited immunity from defamation liability for making good faith reports of suspected patient abuse to adult protective services or other authorities. State legislatures should also provide for anonymity and express release from confidentiality provisions in mandatory abuse reporting statutes.

Reporting abuse does not always lead to the consequences that the therapist might intend. One way in which an elder may be protected against further abuse is to be removed from the environment in which it occurs. Some elders will, however, refuse to leave their homes, even to escape violence. Elders may be reluctant to talk to investigators, fearing reprisals from the perpetrator of the abuse. Revelation of abusive conditions at home may unfortunately prompt additional abuse from the care-giver who maltreated the elder in the first place.

PATIENT RESTRAINTS

The use of physical and chemical restraints has also come under intense ethical and legal scrutiny in recent years as a potential form of elder abuse. The Health Care Financing Administration (HCFA) surveys LTC facilities for Medicare and Medicaid certification, based on compliance with more than 100 requirements delineated in the Nursing Home Reform Act, part of the Omnibus Budget Reconciliation Act of 1987 (OBRA).[43] OBRA greatly expanded the rights of LTC residents, including a prohibition on the use of physical and chemical restraints with nursing home residents except under certain conditions.[19] Physical restraints may never be used for discipline or the convenience of the nursing home staff, and a resident may refuse to be placed in a restraint. Restraints include not only traditional arm and leg cuffs and lap belts but also bedding materials such as sheets, when they are used to limit a patient's free movement, and side-rails, if used to prevent a patient from exiting the bed.[5] Restraints such as safety vests may be used to protect the patient or others from harm but should be as least restrictive as possible. A patient should be able to remove any physical restraint used as a safety reminder, such as a lap board on a wheelchair, without assistance from the staff. Proper record keeping is essential when restraints are used because the professional applying the restraint may be held legally accountable if one is used without appropriate documentation and authorization.

Whenever physical restraints are to be used, providers must justify their use through clear documentation in a patient's treatment records, including a physician's order for restraints; patient or surrogate informed consent for their use; clinical justification; and a statement that less restrictive alternatives to physical restraint have been tried and found to be inadequate. The physician's order to restrain the patient must specify the purpose of the restraint, the type of restraint to be used, and the length of time it is required. If the patient is awake, a restraint must be released every 2 hours. While patient safety is a paramount consideration for every patient care provider, many professionals regard the attempt to reduce the use of physical and chemical restraints as a creative challenge that allows an elderly person an optimal amount of freedom of movement as well as protection from harm. Since OBRA's implementation, the former widespread use of physical restraints in long-term–care facilities has decreased significantly; moreover no controlled study has concluded that physical restraints prevent falls or fall-related patient injury.[5]

LEGAL PROTECTION OF THE OLDER WORKER

Employment Protection

Not all ethical situations confronting patients and therapists occur during illness or at the end of life. As the American population "grays," more and more older workers are participating in the labor force; some by choice, others by economic necessity. Data indicate that 30% of the total population older than 55 years are employed.[31] In 1996, 57.9% of Americans aged 55 to 64 years were employed.[4] Older work-

ers face a dichotomy in their treatment by employers and co-workers. On one hand, their perceived experience, dedication, and loyalty are viewed as positive attributes, whereas their perceived diminished physical abilities and lack of technological savvy create a negative impression, which may subject these workers to employment discrimination.

Physical therapists not only examine and intervene with these patients, but they may also act as advocates, or at least as initial resources for older patients, who are facing possible employment discrimination. With a basic understanding of key employment law protections for older workers, physical therapists can inform their patients of the right to seek legal counsel for potential problems threatening their work lives, as warranted.

The Age Discrimination in Employment Act

The Age Discrimination in Employment Act of 1967 (ADEA) prohibits employment-related discrimination by private- and public-sector employers of workers aged 40 or older.[40] This broad prohibition against discrimination of older workers encompasses the entire employment continuum from recruitment and selection to training, promotion, and conditions of employment.

The ADEA was augmented in 1990 by the Older Workers Benefit Protection Act, which clarified congressional intent that benefits protection was included in age-related federal anti-discrimination statutory law.[44] The amendment also permits employers to ask dismissed older workers to waive their rights to sue for age discrimination under the ADEA in exchange for compensation.

The Equal Employment Opportunity Commission (EEOC) is the federal agency that administers and enforces the ADEA (as well as other key federal civil rights laws). State statutes and judicial case law may afford additional protection to older workers. In 1991, the EEOC and state agencies responsible for protecting older workers' rights processed 27,748 age-discrimination claims.[27]

In the current political climate, older workers are finding it more difficult to prevail in age-discrimination claims and lawsuits brought against employers. For example, federal appellate courts have ruled that older workers claiming violations of the ADEA must prove intentional discrimination by their employers, and not merely a disproportionate disparate adverse impact of employer actions on older workers.[25]

MAKING ETHICAL DECISIONS

Despite the intricacies of the issues that have been presented in the aforementioned text, physical therapists do actually have to make difficult ethical decisions as part of their professional practice, just as they make difficult therapeutic choices. No matter how difficult this task may be, the need to decide can be inescapable. Fortunately, the overall process used to make choices about physical therapy procedures is the same as the process that is used to make other kinds of decisions in the clinical setting. In general, there are four steps to determine what is the ethically right thing to do: identifying the problem, formulating possible responses, weighing the alternatives, and choosing a course of action. The first step in the decision-making process requires us to determine what the facts of the case are, what are the relevant assumptions, and what are the unknowns associated with the problem. Specifically, it is essential to define just what the ethical problem is and what prima facie ethical principles are relevant to the situation. Often there are also additional facts about the context of the situation that are helpful to make a decision. Does the situation raise legal questions as well as ethical ones? It is quite possible that legal requirements prohibit or mandate certain actions by the therapist in response to the situation, as in the case of elder abuse previously discussed. Identifying these in advance might decrease some of the uncertainty that accompanies many ethical judgments.

Because ethical problems can evoke strong emotions very quickly, it is often thought that there is only one right thing to do. Physical therapists are fortunate in that most of the ethical decisions that they must make are not split-second life-or-death decisions. Although in some cases there is only one right thing to do, it sometimes happens that there are several equally acceptable and equally defensible things to do. The second step in ethical decision making is to list all the possible responses that may be made to a situation without prejudging the suitability of any one of them. Often the range of possible responses is much broader than originally thought, and careful consideration of all possible responses may yield an alternative plan that reflects more of the principles and values of the decision maker than the alternative that was conceived first. Once again, the law's constraints on professional behavior must also be considered.

Having set down the broadest array of responses, the decision maker must then proceed to weigh each of these options in light of the principles of ethics, the ideals of the professions, and the values of the individual therapist. In the case of a true dilemma, any option will compromise one principle while upholding the other. Furthermore, there may be sociocultural, economic, and political ramifications that may need to be taken into consideration.

Finally, one must settle on an alternative and implement a course of action. Resource constraints will rule some choices out of consideration. This is particularly true in matters of allocating scarce resources. For example, one way to provide physical therapy to every patient solely on the basis of need would be to hire as many therapists, physical therapist assistants, and aides as necessary in every physical therapy clinic. While this solution is ethically justifiable and obviates the need to ration resources, it is impossible to implement. In choosing to act, the therapist must be ready to take responsibility for acting. Although some ethical decisions are made with the same degree of uncertainty as other professional choices, following these four steps to make a decision can ensure that each therapist has made a reasonable and justifiable decision.

Case Study

A Day in the Life

Jennifer Radisson is the physical therapist assigned to the 18-bed geriatric rehabilitation unit at Village Falls Medical Center. She also works at a nursing home two blocks away from the hospital, which has contracted for services with Jennifer's physical therapy department of five therapists. Most of the patients on the geriatric unit are on active physical therapy programs. The therapists in this facility rarely have a slow day. Jennifer usually sees eight or nine patients at the nursing home for active therapy as well. Given her caseload, she is grateful for physical therapist assistants Bill Montoya, who works at the hospital, and Sabrina Jefferson, who works part time at the nursing home. The nursing home has hired a physical therapy aide, Vivian Lesko, for a few hours each day to assist Jennifer, which also has helped her meet the needs of so many patients.

As Jennifer sits at the nurses' station at the hospital early one morning, sipping coffee and reviewing patient records, Dr. Virgilio stops by to inquire about the progress of Mrs. Godfrey, whose husband had been chief of medicine 30 years ago and was a major fund-raiser for the hospital's building campaign in the late 1960s. Although Jennifer is pleased with Mrs. Godfrey's progress, it has been slow. Dr. Virgilio reminds Jennifer how important the Godfreys have been to the medical center and suggests emphatically that Mrs. Godfrey's progress might be more substantial if Jennifer would increase the amount of time spent with her each day. Jennifer responds that she will do the best she can and makes a mental note to review Bill's caseload for openings.

Brian McSweeny, the head nurse on the unit, overhears the conversation and sits down next to Jennifer after Dr. Virgilio leaves. "Pushing for another donation, I bet," he whispers, "but don't give all your time away. There's a new patient in Room 1212, who was admitted last night. Seems like the poor guy lives alone with his son, who is known to the social worker down in detox. This new patient, whose last name is Gunther, is severely dehydrated, incontinent, and hasn't been out of bed for a week. The son says that he was fine until then."

"Thanks," Jennifer replies. "I'll put him right near the top of my priorities today."

Jennifer reviews her patient caseload. There is Mrs. Godfrey, the new patient Mr. Gunther, and two patients whose evaluations are still in progress. Jennifer is still not very clear about what their needs might be. In addition, Mrs. Reedy needs her discharge evaluation and referral because she will be leaving the hospital for further rehabilitation for her hip fracture closer to her daughter's home. Mr. Stevenson and Ms. Sanborn are patients whose treatment goals and programs are well established. Jennifer co-treats

Ms. Sanborn with Bill, the physical therapist assistant. She has used this opportunity to develop Bill's skills in treating patients with neurological disorders. Bill has been carrying a full caseload of patients with diverse needs for the past 2 weeks.

As Jennifer is walking down the hall to meet the new patient, Mr. Gunther, she spies Mrs. Godfrey looking forlornly out the window.

"How are you doing today, Mrs. Godfrey?" she asks. "Is anything the matter?"

"Well, dear, I know my family is pushing everyone around here to wait on me hand and foot and to get me to therapy even more often than you do," Mrs. Godfrey replies. "But frankly, I don't even want to do what I'm doing now. Please don't take offense. You are a talented young woman, but I just really want to go home. I can afford to pay someone to help me."

Unsure of how to respond, Jennifer says, "Maybe we can talk about it later."

Jennifer introduces herself to Mr. Gunther, who is a thin, malnourished-looking man. As he responds to Jennifer's questions about his home life, Jennifer notices some small inconsistencies that suggest the need for a closer examination of his mental status. Given the number of other patients she has to see today, she decides to defer this issue until tomorrow.

As she is examining the skin on his lower extremities, she notices multiple cuts and several large areas of ecchymosis.

"Did something happen to you recently?" she asks.

"Yeah, that lousy son of mine got stinking drunk and pushed me to the floor when he was supposed to be helping me," Mr. Gunther replies, almost with a laugh.

Jennifer is immediately unsure whether to believe him based on his questionable mental status. She concludes her examination and heads for the nurses' station to begin her note writing. When her beeper goes off, Jennifer responds immediately. The department secretary is transferring a call from Sabrina, the part-time physical therapist assistant at the nursing home.

Sabrina rapidly tells her that she was in a car accident on the way to work. "I'm shaken, but I'll be better by tomorrow. The car is the problem—it's a wreck. Look, I won't be in for the rest of the week. Maybe Vivian can do something with the patients. She really does know a lot about what I do with them," she says.

"Well, I agree," Jennifer says, "but I have to think about giving her so much responsibility, even if they really need the care."

As Jennifer heads toward the elevators and down to the department to discuss the situation with the department's chief physical therapist, she begins to review her predicament. She has a full caseload and now needs to cover for Sabrina or let an aide provide the care. She's not sure what to do about Mrs. Godfrey and Dr. Virgilio, nor what she should do with the information about Mr. Gunther's bruises. Bill cannot possibly increase his caseload without taking on a few patients whose problems exceed his expertise. As the elevator doors close in front of her, she wonders aloud, "What am I going to do now?"

If you were Jennifer, what would you do?

SUMMARY

Physical therapists in geriatric practice interact with patients, families, and co-workers in complex situations that can require careful ethical and legal analyses. A physical therapist is guided in the decision-making process by a concern to adhere to the ethical obligations of all health care practitioners and the rights of the patient. Specifically, with respect to the elderly patient, the therapist must seek solutions to ethical problems that conserve the individual's autonomy and promote well-being. Legally, autonomy is recognized through the requirements of informed consent. A strong commitment to ethical behavior and a sound knowledge of the laws governing professional actions are essential components of a geriatric physical therapist's clinical practice.

REFERENCES

1. Appelbaum PA, Lidz CW, Meisel A: *Informed Consent: Legal Theory and Clinical Practice.* New York, Oxford University Press, 1987.
2. Arispe R: It's the law: Health professionals required to report abuse and neglect. *San Antonio Medical Gazette,* October 10-16:4, 1996.
3. Beauchamp TL, Childress JF: *Principles of Biomedical Ethics,* ed 4. New York, Oxford Press, 1994.
4. Bleakley FR: More unemployed are returning to labor pool. *Wall Street Journal,* Jan 22, 1997; A2.
5. Braun JA: Legal aspects of physical restraint use in nursing homes. *Health Lawyer* 1998; 10(3):10-16.
6. Bruckner J: Physical therapists as double agents: Ethical dilemmas of divided loyalties. *Phys Ther* 1987; 67:383-387.
7. Bursztajn HJ, Saunders LS, Brodsky A: Medical negligence and informed consent in the managed care era. *Health Lawyer* 1997; 9(5):14.
8. Caplan AL: Informed consent and provider-patient relationships in rehabilitation medicine. *Arch Phys Med Rehabil* 1988; 69:312-317.
9. Caplan AL, Callahan D, Haas J: Ethical and policy issues in rehabilitation medicine. *Hastings Cent Rep* 1987; (special suppl):17(4):1-20.
10. Cassileth BR, et al: Informed consent—why its goals are imperfectly realized. *N Engl J Med* 1980; 302:896-900.
11. Coy JA: Autonomy-based informed consent: Ethical implications for patient non-compliance. *Phys Ther* 1989; 69:826-833.
12. Doukas DJ, McCullough LB: Assessing the values history of the elderly patient regarding critical and chronic care, in Gallo J, Reichel W, Anderson L (eds): *Handbook of Geriatric Assessment.* Rockville, Md, Aspen Publishers, 1988.
13. Dworkin G: Paternalism. *Monist* 1972; 56:64-84.
14. Goffman E: *Asylums.* Garden City, NY, Anchor Books, 1961.
15. *Guide for Professional Conduct.* Alexandria, Va, American Physical Therapy Association, Judicial Committee,1996
16. *Guidelines for Physical Therapy Documentation. 1996.* Alexandria, Va, American Physical Therapy Association, 1996.
17. *Guidelines for Recognizing and Providing Care for Victims of Domestic Abuse.* Alexandria, Va, American Physical Therapy Association, 1997.
18. Hayley DC, Cassel CK: Overview of ethical issues, in Cassel CK, et al (eds): *Geriatric Medicine,* ed 3. New York, Springer-Verlag, 1997.
19. Janelli LM, et al: What nursing staff members really know about physical restraints. *Rehabil Nurs* 1991; 16:345-348.
20. Kane RA: Ethics and long-term care, in Sachs GA, Cassles CK (eds): *Clin Geriatr Med* 1994; 10:489-499.
21. Kant I: *Foundations of the Metaphysics of Morals.* Indianapolis, Bobbs-Merrill, 1956.

22. Kapp MB: Medical treatment and the physician's legal duties, in Cassel CK, et al (eds): *Geriatric Medicine,* ed 3. New York, Springer-Verlag, 1997.

23. Larsen EJ, Eaton TA: The limits of advance directives: A history and assessment of the patient self-determination act. *Wake Forest Law Review* 1997; 32(2):249-293.

24. McGinley L: Clinton to prohibit HMO gag clauses under Medicaid. *Wall Street Journal,* Feb 20, 1997:A22.

25. McMorris FA: Age-bias suits may become harder to prove. *Wall Street Journal,* Feb 20, 1997:B1.

26. Mill JS: *On Liberty.* Indianapolis, Bobbs-Merrill, 1956.

27. Perry PM: Don't get sued for age discrimination. *Law Practice Management* 1995; (May/June):36-39.

28. Purtilo RB: Applying the principles of informed consent to patient care: Legal and ethical considerations for physical therapy. *Phys Ther* 1984; 64:934-937.

29. Rawls J: *A Theory of Justice.* Cambridge, Mass, Harvard University Press, 1971.

30. Richardson ML, White KK: *Ethics Applied.* New York, McGraw-Hill, 1993.

31. Rix SE: Older workers—not a rosy picture for either gender. *Aging Today* 1997; Jan/Feb:10.

32. Ross WHD: *The Right and the Good.* Oxford, Clarendon Press, 1930.

33. *Salgo vs Leland Stanford, Jr, University Board of Trustees.* 154 Cal App 2d 560, 317 P 2nd 170 (1957).

34. *Schloendorff vs Society of New York Hospital.* 211 NY 127, 129, 105 NE 92, 93 (1914).

35. Scott RW: *Professional Ethics: A Guide for Rehabilitation Professionals.* St Louis, Mosby, 1998.

36. Scott RW: *Promoting Legal Awareness in Physical and Occupational Therapy.* St. Louis, Mosby, 1997.

37. Siegler M: Confidentiality in medicine—a decrepit concept. *New Engl J Med* 1982; 307:1518.

38. *Standards of Practice for Physical Therapy.* Alexandria, Va, American Physical Therapy Association, 1996.

39. *Tarasoff v. Regents of the University of California,* 17 Call.3d 425 (1976).

40. *The Age Discrimination in Employment Act of 1967,* 29 United States Code Sections 621-634.

41. *The Consumer Bill of Rights and Responsibilities of 1998: Report to the President of the United States.* Advisory Commission on Consumer Protection and Quality in Health Care.

42. *The Freedom of Information Act,* 5 United States Code Section 552.

43. *The Nursing Home Reform Act, Omnibus Budget Reconciliation Act of 1987,* 42 United States Code Sections 1395i-3, 1396r.

44. *The Older Workers Benefit Protection Act of 1990,* 29 United States Code Section 623.

45. *The Patient Self-Determination Act of 1990,* 42 United States Code Sections 1395cc, 1396a.

46. *The Patient Self-Determination Act of 1990,* 42 United States Code Section 395cc(f)(1)(A)(i).

47. Velick MD: Mandatory reporting statutes: A necessary yet underutilized response to elder abuse. *Elder Law Journal* 1995; 9(2):165-190.

PART V

PROGRAMS FOR PARTICULAR POPULATIONS

CHAPTER 28

THE FRAIL AND INSTITUTIONALIZED ELDER

KATHLEEN KLINE MANGIONE, PT, PhD, GCS

INTRODUCTION

The term "frailty" describes a subset of older persons who have multiple deficits. Despite its widespread use in the literature, there is no accepted definition of frailty. Nevertheless, clinicians report anecdotally that "they recognize a frail elder when they see one." Although imprecise, this statement may not be far from the truth. Strawbridge and colleagues have described frailty as a loss of capabilities that make the individual more vulnerable to environmental challenges.[44] Furthermore, they suggest that frail elders demonstrate deficiencies in at least two of the following domains: physical, nutritive, cognitive, and sensory. This framework supports the notion that frailty can manifest itself in many forms.

Institutionalization is a term that unfortunately conjures up images of an older person being abandoned forever at the door of some dark building. However, admission to long-term–care institutions is not permanent in many cases. If permanent residence is required, a wide variety of services are available to residents to ensure quality of life for the remainder of life. This chapter describes the profile of frail elders who reside in long-term facilities, describes the physical therapy examination and interventions commonly used with these elders, and provides a case example.

PROFILE OF RESIDENTS IN LONG-TERM CARE

Permanent residence in long-term care has typically been associated with demographic factors, economic factors, and functional status. Unmarried, aged white women who live alone, are poor, and are impaired in activities of daily living (ADL) and cognitive statuses are most likely to reside permanently in long–term-care facilities.[10] The Health Care Financing Administration (HCFA) reported demographic characteristics of residents in long-term care.[30] More than 4500 residents from 177 nursing homes in six states were categorized by diagnostic groups and stratified on the need for complex care. The most common diagnostic categories were (1) major stroke; (2) depression; (3) coronary vascular disease (CVD), diabetes, dementia; (4) midstage dementia; (5) late-stage dementia; (6) Alzheimer's disease; (7) comatose and pulmonary; (8) multiple chronic disease, osteoporosis, and fracture; (9) debilitated CVD; (10) post-acute CVD convalescence; and (11) stable. They reported that the majority (73.9%) of residents in nursing homes were female, and the mean age varied by diagnoses. The youngest residents were those who had experienced major stroke (mean age, 77.5 years), whereas the oldest residents were those with multiple chronic disease, osteoporosis, and fracture (mean age, 90.4 years). Most residents were in the 85 to 94 age-group category.[30]

Approximately 46% of the residents were admitted from an acute care hospital, whereas another 31% were admitted from private dwellings. The majority of subjects (80.3%) were not married. Medicaid was the major payer source (57.3%), followed by self-pay (29%). The mean length of stay (LOS) for the entire sample was 636 days but varied greatly by diagnoses. A LOS of 1 to 180 days was typical for 76% of patients with multiple chronic diseases, osteoporosis, and fracture and for 69% of residents with post-acute CVD convalescence. These stays are in marked contrast to patients with late-stage dementia, who had a mean LOS of approximately 5 years, and those with depression, who had an LOS of 3 years.[30] From these data, one can see that many of the residents who reside in long-term care have the potential to benefit from physical therapy.

PHYSICAL THERAPY EXAMINATION AND INTERVENTION

The challenges of working with frail elders in long-term care are teasing out the many intervening factors that affect function and determining which factors are remediable by intervention.[41] Fig. 28-1 depicts the commonly measured impairments and the physical, psychological, and cultural factors that affect function. Clinicians working with frail elders must recognize that measuring impairments and functional limitations will give only a partial description of the older person. The modifying factors should also be considered in the evaluation process.

Examination

The examination entails taking a history, performing a systems review, and using specific tests and measures, such as tests for strength, flexibility, endurance, and balance/ coordination.[2]

History

The history is obtained from the medical record and from the resident and/or the resident's family or friends. A thorough history is essential to prognostication and to the cre-

ation of a realistic plan of care. The patient's prior functional or activity level may be the most useful information in setting long-term goals for the resident. Even in long-term care, returning the resident to the prior level of function may still be the ultimate goal. The goal or time frame to achieve the goal may be modified by the other information provided in the chart, such as the history of the current illness, nutritional status, and laboratory values. For example, if a resident was independent in ADL and ambulation before hospitalization for a fractured hip, an appropriate expectation would be a return to independent level of functioning. Therapists make this decision based on knowledge about bone healing. However, if a patient with metastatic prostate cancer who was dependent in ADLs and was becoming increasingly confused was hospitalized for a fractured hip, the therapist would not set a goal for independence in ADL and ambulation. Likewise, if the patient who was previously independent at home experienced a stroke, the goal would need to be modified from independence in function, based on the therapist's knowledge of recovery from stroke. These pieces of information are critical to gather a clinical impression of the person and establish realistic, obtainable goals.

History of falls should be noted in the history. The mean incidence of falls in nursing homes is 1.5 falls/bed per year. This rate is approximately 3 times the rate of that of community-dwelling older adults. The fracture rate is about 4%, whereas the serious injury rate is approximately 11%.[38] The most common causes of falls among institutionalized elders are gait impairments, balance impairments, or lower extremity weakness; dizziness or vertigo; environment-related factors; confusion; and others (including arthritis, acute illness, drugs, pain, epilepsy, and falling from bed). In long-term–care institutions, the risk for falls include (in decreasing order): weakness, balance deficit, gait deficit, impaired mobility or use of walking aid, functional impairment, visual

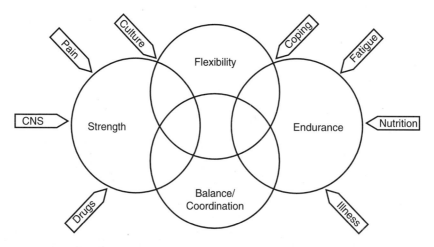

FIG. 28-1 The complex intereactions of physiological capabilities and other modifiers that define functional behavior. (Modified from Scwartz RS: Sarcopenia and physical performance in old age: Introduction. *Muscle Nerve* S5:S10-S12, 1997.)

impairment, use of anti-depressants, postural hypotension, and use of sedative hypnotics.[38] Luukinen and colleagues investigated the independent risk factors for recurrent fallers among an ambulatory sample of nursing home residents. They predicted 83% of the recurrent fallers by the variables of slow walking speed, a change in living conditions during the previous 2 years, reduced quadriceps strength, and existence of an ophthalmic disease.[28] By knowing the demographics of those who fall and the risk factors for falling, clinicians may be able to be proactive in their institutions by implementing fall prevention programs.

Systems Review

A systems review can provide additional information about various body systems. For example, a resident's cognitive status should be assessed if there is reported confusion or history of depression, since these conditions can affect treatment. For example, the Mini-Mental Status Examination may be administered as part of the systems review of these individuals.[17] This 30-point, untimed test will screen for gross impairments in orientation; registration; attention; and calculation, recall, and language. Scores less than 24 out of a total of 30 points indicate some form of cognitive impairment, and consultation with the health care team is indicated.[17]

The special senses of vision and hearing should also be included in the systems review. Since most residents are in their 80s, it is highly likely that they have experienced age-related changes in vision and hearing. Residents often wear corrective lenses. However, approximately 25% of residents in long-term–care settings who wear corrective lenses still have moderate vision impairment, i.e., vision less than 20/70.[22] Hearing losses are the most prevalent of all sensory losses.[1] In a sample of 198 nursing home residents, researchers asked residents whether they had difficulty hearing in a group, while watching television, or while talking on the telephone. This three-question method was significantly more effective than the use of a single hearing loss question in predicting which residents had hearing loss as measured by audiometric assessment.[48] Details about the visual and auditory status of frail elders will help the clinician plan the treatment sessions.

Control of bowel and bladder functioning also can be noted. Approximately 49% of residents in long-term care are incontinent of urine.[7] Incontinence is reported to be highly associated with impairment in ADL, the presence of dementia, restraint use, the use of bedrails, and the use of anti-anxiety/hypnotic medications.[7] Incontinence, for many residents, may likely be due to impairments in ADL. Once functional status improves, one should expect incontinence also to improve.

Before the appropriate tests and measures can be selected, the clinician synthesizes the information obtained from the history and systems review. Oftentimes, frail elders have acute disease superimposed on several chronic conditions and comorbidities. A disease, e.g. pneumonia, may be re-

solved; however, the bedrest accompanying the disease most likely will have caused impairments and functional limitations. Bedrest is known to impair many systems. For example, bedrest is associated with decreased muscle strength,[5] increased incidence of orthostatic intolerance,[25] and decreased bone density.[33] Superimposing bedrest on an individual with multiple comorbidities, e.g. arthritis and CHF, drastically increases the potential for functional loss. This information is synthesized to formulate a clinical picture of the patient before collecting more detailed information.

Tests and Measures

Tests and measures performed on frail elders residing in nursing homes are not geriatric-specific, with the possible exception of some of the performance-based measures. Commonly used tests address aerobic capacity and endurance, range of motion (ROM), muscle performance, motor performance, and self-care activities.[2] Aerobic capacity and endurance tests include vital signs at rest and after activity, autonomic responses to positional change, and functional tests of endurance. Ooi and colleagues reported that greater than 50% of more than 900 nursing home residents studied had at least one episode of orthostatic hypotension.[34] Their operational definition for orthostasis was a 20 mm Hg or greater decline in systolic blood pressure (BP) 1 or 3 minutes after changing from a supine to a standing position. These researchers measured BP in supine and standing after 1 and 3 minutes before and after breakfast and lunch. Frequency of orthostatic hypotension was greatest before breakfast. Those patients with persistent orthostasis tended to complain of dizziness or light-headedness, be independent in ambulation, have hypertension (systolic greater than 160 mm Hg or diastolic greater than 95 mm Hg) or mood disorders, be taking psychotropic medications, and have multiple comorbid conditions.[34]

Range of motion is often limited in nursing home residents. Molinger and Steffen measured knee flexion contractures in nursing home residents for 10 months.[31] They reported that 75% of their sample of 112 residents had unilateral knee flexion contractures of greater than 5 degrees. The presence of knee flexion contractures were associated with resistance to passive motion, cognitive impairment, impaired ambulation, and complaints of knee pain. Their results suggested that residents whose knee flexion contractures approached 20 degrees may also develop subsequent ambulation impairment, therefore intervention may be indicated in these patients.[31]

Deficits in muscle performance are commonly multifocal. Muscle weakness can result from age-related changes in strength (especially the lower extremity),[45] a history of hip fracture or arthritis,[11,42] or from bedrest during recovery from an acute disease process.[5] Whatever the rationale, most residents will need a strengthening program.

Motor function (motor control and motor learning) as well as impairments in gait, locomotion, and balance and gait deficits can be assessed by a variety of balance and physical performance tests described in the following text. The Romberg test is a static timed test in which the person stands with the feet together. It was not originally designed for frail elders. However, the Romberg is included as part of the balance screening assessment used for all residents in nursing homes. This screening assessment is called the Minimum Data Set 2.0 (MDS 2.0) (see Chapter 7). The MDS uses a threshold of 10 seconds for advancing to higher-level tests such as the semi-tandem or tandem Romberg. The tandem test requires that the patient's feet are in a heel-to-toe position, and the semi-tandem test requires that the person's feet are between the Romberg and tandem positions. These tasks also use 10 seconds as the upper limit of performance for both the tandem and semi-tandem tests. Iverson and colleagues compared tandem Romberg times among three groups of community-dwelling elders and found that those who were sedentary or moderately active were able to maintain the tandem position for approximately half the time of very active elders; 19 seconds versus 38 seconds in the active group.[23] Another static balance test that is used alone or as part of a physical performance test is the one-legged standing (OLST) test. Bohannon originally reported that in a small sample of healthy, community-dwelling persons in their seventh decade, the mean OLST was 14 ± 9 seconds.[6] When OLST is used in physical performance measures such as the Tinetti or Berg scales, described in the following text, a more conservative approach is taken, and 5 seconds is the upper limit of testing.

Physical performance measures include a variety of tools that vary in length and complexity. The "Timed Up and Go" test is a simple procedure devised for frail elders in a geriatric day hospital.[35] The test starts with the patient sitting in an arm chair. The timing begins as the patient stands up, walks 3 meters, turns around, walks back to the chair, and sits down. Preliminary data from 60 subjects (mean age, 79.5 years) suggested that if it took the subject more than 30 seconds to complete the task, he/she would likely need much more assistance in transfers, climbing stairs, and going out alone. On the other hand, if the person took less than 20 seconds to complete the test, the person would likely be independent in the aforementioned activities.[35] Using an entirely different approach to measuring risk for falls and thus dependence in ADLs, the functional reach test measures the amount of forward reach and estimates the margins of stability.[13] Predictive validity studies conducted with more than 200 elderly male veterans indicated that persons with a mean reach of 6 inches or less had the greatest risk of recurrent falls.[12]

Other performance-based tests include the Tinetti Test, or Performance Oriented Assessment of Mobility (POMA),[47] and the Berg Balance Test.[4] The tests are similar in that they require the person to go through a variety of maneuvers that involve both balance and function. The POMA includes a balance segment and a gait assessment segment. The balance portion of the POMA evaluates a person's performance from a chair (sitting balance, arising from a chair, sitting down, and immediate standing balance in the first 5 seconds) and from a standing position (Romberg position, eyes open and closed, sternal nudge, and turning 360 degrees). Scoring is ranked as 0 = unable, 1 = able but requires assistance or more than one attempt, and 2 = able to completely independent. The maximum score that one can achieve on the balance portion is 16. Reliability has been established for novice and experienced physical therapists.[8] Scores of less than 10 appeared to differentiate between recurrent fallers and non-fallers in a retirement community.[46] The gait assessment includes initiation of gait, step length, step height, step continuity, step symmetry, walking stance, amount of trunk sway, and path deviation. These items are graded as normal or abnormal.[47]

The Berg Balance Test includes the activities of going from sitting to standing, standing unsupported, sitting unsupported, standing to sitting, transfers, standing with eyes closed, standing with feet together, reaching forward with outstretched arm, retrieving object from the floor, turning 360 degrees, placing alternate foot on stool, standing with one foot in front, and standing on one foot. Scoring is rank ordered from 0 to 4, with 0 being "unable to perform" and 4 being "able to complete task independently and in a timely fashion." The maximum score is 56. Reliability and validity were established and found to range from good to excellent in a sample of community-dwelling and institutionalized elders. Scores on the Berg test differentiated between groups of subjects and corresponded to qualitative ratings given by physical therapists. Persons who scored between 0 to 20 tended to be wheelchair bound and were rated as having poor balance by other physical therapists. Those who scored between 21 and 40 tended to walk with assistance, corresponding with a designation of fair balance by physical therapists in the study. Those who scored between 41 and 56 were usually independent in gait and were rated as having good balance. Likewise, subjects who used walkers had a mean score of 31, those who used canes had a mean score of 39, and those who did not use assistive devices had a mean score of 47.[3,4]

Reuben and Siu developed the Physical Performance Test (PPT) as a measure of fine upper extremity (UE) function, gross UE function, balance, mobility, coordination, and endurance.[37] Scoring is based on time and is ranked from 0 (unable) to 4 (most capable). The test can be used as a 9-item (max = 36) or 7-item form (max = 28). Subjects are asked to complete the following tasks:

1. Write the sentence "Whales live in the blue ocean."
2. Simulate eating by moving five coffee beans from a bowl to a coffee can using a teaspoon.
3. Lift a heavy book from a table, and place it on a shelf above shoulder height.
4. Put on and remove a jacket, sweater, or laboratory coat.
5. Pick up a penny from the floor.
6. Turn 360 degrees.
7. Walk 50 feet by walking 25 feet out and 25 feet back.

8. *Climb a flight of steps (9 to 12 steps)**
9. *Walk up and down a flight of stairs as many times as possible (max = 4).**

Gait speed is an easy and objective performance measure that has been shown to correlate with functional ability[27] and incidence of falls[49] in elders. Many of the exercise intervention studies have used gait speed as a functional outcome variable. Although the methods for measuring gait speed, distances walked during the tests, and instructions to the subjects vary from study to study, the range of gait speeds reported for institutionalized elders vary from 0.40 to 0.50 m/sec.[15,20,39] Interventions that report improvements in gait speed report changes in the range of 0.03 to 0.06 m/sec. The meaningfulness of these changes are not well-understood.

The data obtained from the tests and measures are used to make a clinical judgment (evaluation) and to establish a diagnosis and prognosis.[2] The examination findings often suggest that frail elders have cardiovascular, musculoskeletal, and neuromuscular impairments. The diagnosis (label encompassing a cluster of signs and symptoms) is multi-system impairment. Factors that may modify the frequency or duration of visits include age, chronicity of condition, comorbidities, psychosocial and socioeconomic stressors, and accessibility of resources.[2] However, for many frail residents, returning to the prior level of function is a reasonable goal.

Intervention: Coordination, Communication, and Documentation

Intervention has three components: coordination, communication, and documentation; patient-related instruction; and direct interventions.[2] Coordination, communication, and documentation include documentation and patient care conferences. Patient care conferences are conducted with all team members to discuss the patient's plan of care. The conferences are held for all new admissions or whenever a significant change in functional status or medical condition occurs. The team also is involved in decisions about restraint use. In the past, restraints have been used to keep elderly residents from falling and injuring themselves. However, the Omnibus Reconciliation Act of 1987 specifies that residents have the right to be free from restraints and therefore restraints can be used only when all other alternatives to prevent injuries have failed.[1] Since the time the act was enacted, restraint reduction programs have proliferated in nursing homes and national rates for restraint use have dropped from 35% to 15.5%.[50]

The rules that are used to reduce restraints have varied from institution to institution. Physical therapists promoting mobility often find that they are the strongest advocates for keeping elders restraint-free. Results from balance assessments and the fact that only 5% of falls result in fractures are information the therapist uses to keep elders mobile. However, more objective tools exist. Schnelle and colleagues described a tool that measured the behavioral factors related to falls and injuries among institutionalized elders.[40] The tool, called "Safety Assessment for the Frail Elderly" (SAFE), is a performance assessment of transitional tasks and of walking. The items assess safety awareness or physical functioning. The transitional activities include 10 tasks comprising an elder's ability to stand safely from a sitting position and then to return to sitting. The 13 tasks involved in the walking assessment include standing, walking, turning, and picking up objects from the floor. The items are scored from 0 to 4 and are represented as a percentage of the total possible scores. The 23 tasks can be expressed as four subscales and an overall SAFE score. In a sample of 112 residents who were able to stand and walk without assistance, the subjects who were restrained had a judgment subscale score of 60.9%, whereas subjects who were not restrained had a score of 87.3%. Likewise, the overall SAFE score for restrained residents was 71.2% and for unrestrained residents was 90.0%. Reliability has been established for SAFE.[40] This tool is an example of how coordination, communication, and documentation can be used to keep the resident as mobile as possible.

Intervention: Patient-Related Instruction

Patient-related instruction is common in long-term care of frail elders, especially in the form of verbal and pictorial instruction to assist nursing staff in correct positioning of residents or correct guarding techniques. Box 28-1 contains a

---

> **Box 28-1**
> ## RESTORATIVE NURSING IN-SERVICE CURRICULUM
>
> A. Introduction
>   1. Principles of geriatric rehabilitation and restorative care
>   2. Goals of restorative program
>   3. Role of the restorative aide
> B. Positioning and bed mobility
>   1. Dangers of prolonged bedrest and immobility
>   2. Abnormal posturing in bed and chair
>   3. Positioning techniques and aids for proper positioning
>   4. Body mechanics for positioning and bed mobility
> C. Transfers
>   1. Body mechanics
>   2. Types of transfers (including use of Hoyer lift and emergency transfer techniques)
>   3. Exercises to increase mobility in bed or chair
> D. Exercise and ROM
>   1. Definition of types of exercise
>   2. Principles of exercise and ROM
>   3. Incorporating exercise into ADL
> E. Ambulation and assistive devices
>   1. Preparation for ambulation
>   2. Guarding techniques for ambulation
>   3. Weight-bearing status and other precautions
> F. Working as a rehabilitation team
>   1. Roles of occupational therapy and speech-language pathology
>   2. ADL techniques

ADL = activities of daily living; ROM = range of motion.

---

*The italicized areas are omitted for 7-item scoring. Reported reliability and validity are good.[37]

suggested curriculum that may be provided to nursing staff who are involved in providing care to residents who are no longer receiving skilled physical therapy interventions. (See also the discussion on secondary prevention later in the chapter.)

Intervention: Direct Interventions

Direct interventions most typically occur in the following categories: therapeutic exercise, functional training in ADL and IADL, and prescription and training with assistive devices.[2] Therapeutic exercise interventions may include aerobic endurance activities, posture awareness training, strengthening exercises, and stretching exercise. The literature is beginning to describe effective interventions for working with frail, institutionalized elders. Some interventions report the effectiveness of training to address a specific impairment, such as strengthening of the quadriceps. Fisher studied the effects of isometrically strengthening the quadriceps at 90 degrees of knee flexion and three different hip flexion angles in a sample of 14 institutionalized men and women.[16] The exercise consisted of five isometric contractions, held for 5 seconds at three different hip angles. The frequency and duration were 3 times per week for 6 weeks, respectively. This minimal exercise produced changes in isometric quadriceps strength for this sample.[16] Connelly and Vandervoort studied the effects of strength training the quadriceps on strength, "timed up and go" speed, gait speed (slow, habitual, and fast), and grip strength. The subjects were 10 frail women with a mean age of 82 years who took an average of six medications. The training consisted of knee extension exercises at 30% to 50% of their one-repetition maximum (1-RM). The subjects performed three sets of 10 repetitions 3 times per week for 8 weeks. The intensity was upgraded weekly to maintain the 30% to 50% of their 1-RM. After the training, the subjects showed increases in isometric quadriceps strength, increases in 1-RM, increases in slow and fast gait speeds, and improved "timed up and go" speeds.[9] These data suggest that lower extremity strengthening can impact the function of frail, institutionalized elders.

The largest controlled trial of a strengthening regimen for frail elders was conducted by Fiatarone and colleagues.[15] In this study, 100 nursing home residents (mean age, 87 years) were randomly assigned to one of four groups: high intensity strengthening, nutritional supplementation, strengthening and nutritional supplements, or a placebo exercise/nutrition control group. Strengthening was targeted to the hip and knee extensors, and the intensity was 80% of the subjects' 1-RM. The residents performed three sets of eight repetitions 3 times per week for 10 weeks. The outcome measures included strength (1-RM), gait speed, stair-climbing power, nutritional intake, body composition, and physical activity. The strengthening intervention significantly improved muscle strength and increased quadriceps cross-sectional area, habitual gait speed, stair-climbing power, and overall

level of physical activity. The nutritional supplement did not provide additional benefit to the changes seen with exercise alone.[15] The design and number of subjects in this study provide the most convincing evidence that high-intensity strengthening exercises in frail, institutionalized elders is safe and effective in improving both impairments and functional limitations.

Aerobic training has not been as thoroughly investigated in nursing home residents. However, Foster and colleagues compared the effects of moderate- and low-intensity exercise in women residing in retirement homes.[18] The mean age of this relatively healthy sample was 78.4 years. The women were randomly assigned to walk 3 times a week at a heart rate that corresponded to 60% or 40% of their heart rate reserve. After 10 weeks of training, both groups showed improvements in maximal oxygen consumption, but there was no difference between groups. Similarly, MacRae and colleagues performed a randomized controlled trial investigating the effects of a walking program on walk endurance capacity, physical activity level, mobility, and quality of life in nursing home residents.[29] The 22-week intervention required that the residents in the intervention group walk at their habitual pace for a maximum of 30 minutes per day. The results showed that the daily walking routine improved residents' walking endurance but did not improve the other outcome measures.[29] The results of these studies suggest that low-intensity exercise (of sufficient duration) may be enough of a stimulus to produce cardiovascular and functional changes.

Impairments in range of motion can lead to contractures in frail residents in long-term care. Light and colleagues investigated an intervention for decreasing knee flexion contractures in institutionalized elders by comparing high load brief stretch (HLBS) to low load prolonged stretch (LLPS).[26] The protocol suggested by Light and co-workers consisted of a 1-hour duration of stretch, twice a day for 4 weeks. The intensity of the stretch was such that the slack was taken up in the muscle. The stretch was maintained by a traction unit that hung off of a plinth. High load brief stretch consisted of proprioceptive neuromuscular facilitation (PNF) technique to hold the muscle at its end range for 1 minute, followed by a 15-second rest, and then the process was repeated 3 times. LLPS techniques was found to be more effective than HLBS in reducing knee flexion contractures.[26]

Physical therapists do not generally treat single impairments in frail elders due to the presence of multiple comorbidities. Research has begun to describe the effects of individualized physical therapy on function. Harada and colleagues studied the effects of range of motion, strengthening, balance, gait, and transfer training on 27 residents of a residential care facility.[20] The outcomes were three physical performance measures: habitual gait speed, Berg Balance Test scores, and POMA scores. The residents received individualized therapy 2 to 3 times per week for 4 to 5 weeks. Each session lasted 20 to 40 minutes. After the individually determined intervention, the subjects demonstrated significant increases in Berg and POMA scores but no significant increase in gait speed.[20] The authors suggested that a longer intervention period may have been needed to observe changes in habitual gait speed.

Mulrow and colleagues conducted a randomized controlled trial with 197 residents from a skilled nursing facility. The residents were randomized to an intervention or control group. The intervention group performed individualized exercise 3 times a week for 30 to 45 minutes for 16 weeks. The exercises consisted of passive range of motion (PROM), active range of motion (AROM), progressive resistive exercises (PREs), endurance exercises, balance training, bed mobility, transfer, and wheelchair and gait training. The control group received friendly visits for the same frequency and duration. The outcomes measures included fall rate, Physical Disability Index (PDI) scores, ADL scores, and health status as measured by the Sickness Impact Profile.[32] The PDI is a performance-based measure for use in frail nursing home residents.[19] The 65 items in the scale measure performance in range of motion, strength, balance, and mobility. The items are converted to scaled scores (0 to 100, with 100 being the best performance).[19] During 16 weeks of exercise, the subjects spent the majority of sessions (69%) doing strength and endurance activities, 33% of the time doing functional training, and 40% of the time doing ROM exercises. The only differences between the intervention and control groups at the end of the 16 weeks was a 15.5% improvement in the mobility subscale of the PDI.[32] Considering the evidence from the strength training research, the clinician should question whether the intensity of the strength training was sufficient and why a relatively small percentage of sessions included functional training.

Balance is usually implicitly studied with falls research because of the strong association between balance impairment and fall risk. Ray and colleagues evaluated a falls prevention intervention in nursing home residents who were at a high risk of falling.[36] The 267 control subjects resided in different nursing homes than the 232 residents who received the intervention. An interdisciplinary falls consultation team conducted the intervention and attempted to decrease unsafe practices in the following four domains: environmental and personal safety, wheelchairs, psychotropic drugs, and transferring and ambulation. Residents' rooms were assessed for environmental hazards, wheelchairs were assessed and modified as needed, psychotropic drug use was evaluated in ambulatory residents, safety in transfers and gait was evaluated, and in-services were given to all nursing home staff regarding causes and consequences of falls and for recognizing environmental hazards. The outcome measures were the number of recurrent fallers and the number of injurious falls. An average of 15 recommendations were made per patient. The intervention group showed 19% fewer recurrent fallers and 31% fewer injurious falls. The program was more effective among the residents who had three or more falls the prior year and when compliance with the recommendations was achieved. These results suggest that high rates of falls can be lowered through interdisciplinary approaches in long–term-care settings.[36]

Secondary Prevention

Secondary prevention refers to decreasing the risks of functional decline and impairment progression. In most long-term–care settings, the risk of decline is addressed by the use of restorative nursing programs. Restorative nursing programs are generally carried out by certified nursing aids and/or physical therapy or occupational therapy aides and can include programs such as supervised ambulation or ROM exercise programs. These programs can flourish if both nursing and rehabilitation staff are committed to their success. Programatic features that should be present include (1) a method of screening to assess functional abilities or to classify patients according to program requirements or guidelines, (2) a means of reassessment to determine whether residents continue to need the services, (3) a documentation/communication system to convey information about patients to all staff involved in the program on an ongoing basis and to ensure accountability, and (4) a method of objectively evaluating the effectiveness of the program and determining whether program goals have been met.[21]

Physical therapists often refer patients to these restorative nursing programs upon discharge from skilled physical therapy as a type of "step-down" program for the residents. Alternatively, residents will be referred to restorative programs if they require physical assistance with walking but will not achieve independence. Other suggestions for restorative programs include turning and positioning programs, wheelchair mobility and endurance programs, ADL programs, active range of motion programs, and restorative dining programs. Recreational therapists, occupational therapists, and nursing aides may all be involved with these programs. Programs that encourage walking as part of the resident's daily routine, e.g., walking to the dining room, have been reported to increase overall ambulatory endurance,[24,29] decrease fall rates,[24] decrease incidences of incontinence,[29] and inhibit functional decline.[43]

Case Study

The physical therapist received a referral from the staff physician to evaluate and treat a resident in the skilled nursing facility who has just completed medical treatment for pneumonia.

History

Demographics: The patient is a 75-year-old English-speaking male.

Social history: The patient is a retired clergyman. He has telephone contact with several colleagues and has one regular social friend who visits almost daily.

Living environment: The resident has lived in the skilled nursing facility for the last year and plans on remaining there for the rest of his life.

History of current condition: He was treated with IV antibiotics and bedrest for 10 days. The referral was received 2 weeks after the initial diagnosis of pneumonia was made. The patient is incontinent of urine. The patient understands what has occurred and is anxious to return to his prior activity level.

Functional status and activity level: Before this illness, he was ambulating daily with a rolling walker for approximately 500 feet. He was usually accompanied by his friend during these walks. The patient was independent in all other ADL, except putting on his shoes.

Medications: amitriptyline (Elavil), multivitamins, colase, carbidopa-levodopa (Sinemet)

Other test and measures: Lungs clear on radiographs taken 4 days before referral.

Past medical/surgical histories: Parkinson's disease, osteomyelitis; of the left lower extremity (LLE) for the past 50 years; depression; left hip fracture with ORIF 3 years ago; right CVA with mild left hemiparesis 2 years ago; wears ankle foot orthosis on LLE; history of multiple falls.

Health status: Before the episode of pneumonia, the patient reported his health status as good. He now reports that his physical functioning is poor to fair. The medical record indicates that the patient's psychological function is fair since he has episodes of confusion and hallucinations.

Screening

Cognition: The resident scored 28/30 on the Mini-Mental Status Examination, suggesting that cognitive function should not interfere with treatment.

Skin: This patient has been in bed, inactive, and has a history of osteomyelitis. Upon further questioning, the patient reported that he was shot in World War II and has had a wound in his LLE ever since; he denied experiencing pain in the area. Further consultation with nursing staff and visual inspection indicated that there was a quarter-size open area on his left shin that had not changed in size or drainage since he was first admitted to the facility. The patient had no other areas of skin redness.

Special senses: The patient wears corrective lenses to read. The patient reported that he has difficulty hearing when using the telephone; this information would suggest that the patient uses non-verbal cues to increase his understanding of the spoken word.

Continence: The patient's incontinence occurred since the pneumonia. Because the patient reported that he was aware of the need to void and pneumonia was the only new disease, the incontinence is most likely due to his impairment in ADL. Once his functional status improves, his incontinence also should improve.

Tests and Measures
Aerobic capacity and endurance
- Vital signs at rest and after activity
  Resting heart rate (HR): 76; BP 130/70 mm Hg; respirtory rate (RR), 18
  After activity (25 feet ambulation with rolling walker)
- HR: 98, BP: 125/72 mm Hg, RR: 28
- Autonomic responses to positional changes
  Supine HR: 72, BP: 125/70 mm Hg
  After standing 1 minute: HR: 76, BP: 102/74 mm Hg
- Performance-based test of endurance: unable to perform 6-minute walk test

Sensory integrity: Proprioception is impaired in left great toe, intact proximally; superficial pain and light touch are intact in both LEs

Reflex integrity: +Babinski

Passive range of motion: Upper extremities (UE): within functional limits (WFL); hip and knee flexion: WFL; hip extension: −15 degrees from neutral bilaterally; knee extension: −20 degrees on left and −15 degrees on the right

Muscle performance
- Muscle tone: No resting tremor, mild rigidity left greater than right; UE greater than LE
- Muscle strength: (0-5 grading)
- Hip extension: Unable to formally test; functionally appears 3+ bilaterally
- Hip flexion: Left, 3+/5; right, 4−/5
- Knee extension: Left, 3+ to −35 degrees extension; right, 4− to −20 degrees extension
- Knee flexion: Left, 4/5; right, 4/5
- Dorsiflexion: Left, partial anti-gravity motion in synergy; right, 4−/5
- Triceps: Left, 4/5; right, 5/5
- Grip strength: Left, 5/5; right, 5/5

Motor Function
- Balance testing: Functional reach, 3.2 inches; Romberg eyes open, 10 seconds; semi-tandem Romberg, 2; tandem Romberg, unable
- Physical performance tests
  Timed Up and Go, 68 sec (with rolling walker)
  Berg Balance test, 25/56
- Gait Assessment: Patient uses rolling walker and requires contact guard; stopped after 25 feet secondary to complaints of shortness of breath and fatigue. Patient remains in hip and knee flexion throughout all phases of gait. He exhibits shortened step length bilaterally. His gait speed is 0.65 m/sec.
  Wheelchair parts management and safety: Patient is independent in propelling short distances (50 to 100 feet) indoors using both arms and legs. Patient is limited by overall fatigue, can lock and unlock wheelchair brakes independently, and exhibits safe behavior with wheelchair brakes.

Self-Care (including ADL and IADL)
- Transfer ability: Sit to stand from wheelchair with minimal to moderate assistance; patient tends to fall posteriorly.
- Bed mobility: Patient rolls side to side with rail independently supine to short sit independently.

Orthotic, Protective, and Supportive Devices

Alignment and fit of AFO: Post-leaf spring orthosis fits patient appropriately and does not cause reddened skin after ambulation.

Intervention

This resident was treated 5 days per week for 1 month. Before his sessions began, he would lie supine on a plinth for 1 hour. An aide placed hot packs under his thighs and weights on the anterior aspect of his thigh to provide a low load long duration stretch to his bilateral knee and hip flexors. The patient then performed high-intensity strength training for his quadriceps and hip extensors (2 times per week) and an upper and lower body active range of motion aerobic program for 20 minutes at an RPE of 14 (3 times per week). Transfer training and gait training with a rolling walker occurred daily. Nursing staff was instructed to put knee immobilizers on the resident's knees during his hours in bed. After 2 weeks of physical therapy, the resident was started on an ambulation program on the nursing unit so that he ambulated every afternoon. After 1 month, the resident had returned to his prior functional level of independent ambulation with a rolling walker for 500 feet.

SUMMARY

The complexity of frail, institutionalized elders necessitates the use of an organizational framework to analyze patient problems. Existing literature and the *Guide to Physical Therapist Practice*[2] can help the clinician change what is depicted in Fig. 28-2. This figure depicts a theoretical decline in vigor with aging.[41] What is not represented in this graph is the impact of physical therapy on the slope of projected decline. Preliminary research has demonstrated that frail, institutionalized elders can improve both impairment level measures as well functional status through rigorous, well-designed exercise programs. Our challenge is to continue to define and deliver effective physical therapy with frail, institutionalized elders.

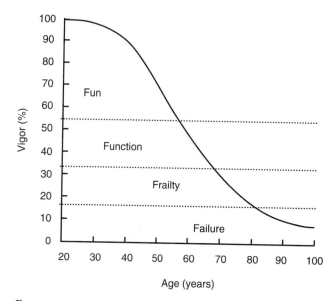

FIG. 28-2 The loss of functional ability with aging. As subjects age and lose "vigor," they move progressively from a life-style that includes having fun, to a functional life-style, to a state of frailty and finally to failure. (Modified from Scwartz RS: Sarcopenia and physical performance in the old age: Introduction. *Muscle Nerve* S5:S10-S12, 1997.)

REFERENCES

1. Abrams WB, Beers MH, Berkow R (eds): *The Merck Manual of Geriatrics.* Whitehouse Station, NJ, Merck Research Laboratories, 1995.
2. American Physical Therapy Association: Guide to physical therapist practice. *Phys Ther* 1997; 77:1155-1674.
3. Berg K, et al: Clinical and laboratory measures of postural balance in an elderly population. *Arch Phys Med Rehabil* 1992; 73:1073-1080.
4. Berg K, Wood-Dauphinee S, Williams JI, Gayton D: Measuring balance in the elderly: Preliminary development of an instrument. *Physiotherapy Canada* 1989; 41:304-311.
5. Bloomfield SA: Changes in musculoskeletal structure and function with prolonged bed rest. *Med Sci Sports Exerc* 1997; 29:197-206.
6. Bohannon RW, et al: Decrease in timed balance test scores with aging. *Phys Ther* 1984; 64:1067-1070.
7. Brandeis GH, et al: The prevalence of potentially remediable urinary incontinence in frail older people: A study using the Minimum Data Set. *J Am Geriatr Soc* 1997; 45:179-184.
8. Cipriany-Dacko LM, Innerst D, Johannsen J, Rude V: Interrater reliability of the Tinetti balance scores in novice and experienced physical therapy clinicians. *Arch Phys Med Rehabil* 1997; 78:1160-1164.
9. Connelly DM, Vandervoort AA: Improvement in knee extensor strength of institutionalized elderly women after exercise with ankle weights. *Physiotherapy Canada* 1995; 47:15-23.
10. Coughlin TA, McBride TD, Liu K: Determinants of transitory and permanent nursing home admissions. *Med Care* 1990; 28:616-631.
11. Craik RL: Disability following hip fracture. *Phys Ther* 1998; 74:387-398.
12. Duncan PW, Studenski S, Chandler J, Prescott B: Functional reach: Predictive validity in a sample of elderly male veterans. *J Gerontol* 1992; 47:M93-M98.
13. Duncan PW, Weiner DK, Chandler J, Studenski S: Functional reach: A new clinical measure of balance. *J Gerontol* 1990; 45:M192-M197.
14. Fiatarone MA, et al: High-intensity strength training in nonagenarians: Effects on skeletal muscle. *JAMA* 1990; 263:3029-3034.
15. Fiatarone MA, et al: Exercise training and nutritional supplementation for physical frailty in very elderly people. *New Engl J Med* 1994; 330:1769-1775.
16. Fisher NM, Pendergast DR, Calkins E: Muscle rehabilitation in impaired elderly nursing home residents. *Arch Phys Med Rehabil* 1991; 72:181-185.
17. Folstein MF, Folstein SE, McHugh PR: "Mini-Mental State": A practical method for grading the cognitive state of patients for the clinician. *J Psychiatr Res* 1975; 12:189-198
18. Foster VL, et al: Endurance training for elderly women: Moderate vs low intensity. *J Gerontol* 1989; 44:M184-M188.
19. Gerety MB, et al: Development and validation of a physical performance instrument for the functionally impaired elderly: The physical disability index (PDI). *J Gerontol* 1993; 48:M33-M38.
20. Harada N, et al: Physical therapy to improve functioning of older people in residential care facilities. *Phys Ther* 1995; 75:830-839.
21. Herr RA, Mangione KK: Monitoring ambulatory status in a skilled nursing facility population. *Top Geriatr Rehabil* 1995; 11(2):55-60.
22. Horowitz A: Vision impairment and functional disability among nursing home residents. *Gerontologist* 1994; 34:316-323.
23. Iverson BD, Gossman MR, Shaddeau SA, Turner ME: Balance performance, force production, and activity levels in noninstitutionalized men 60 to 90 years of age. *Phys Ther* 1990; 70:348-355.

24. Koroknay VJ, Werner P, Cohen-Mansfield J, Braun JV: Maintaining ambulation in the frail nursing home resident: A nursing administered walking program. *J Gerontol Nurs* 1995; 21(11):18-24.

25. Levine BD, Zuckerman JH, Pawelczyk JA: Cardiac atrophy after bedrest deconditioning: A nonneural mechanism for orthostatic intolerance. *Circulation* 1997; 96:517-525.

26. Light KE, Nuzik S, Personius W, Barstrom A: Low-load prolonged stretch vs. high-load brief stretch in treating knee contractures. *Phys Ther* 1984; 64:330-333.

27. Lundgren-Lindquist B, Aniansson A, Rundgren A: Functional studies in 79-year-olds: Walking performance and climbing capacity. *Scand J Rehabil Med* 1983; 15:125-131.

28. Luukinen HM, Koski KM, Laippala PP, Kivela SM: Risk factors for recurrent falls in the elderly in long-term institutional care. *Public Health* 1995; 109:57-65.

29. MacRae PG, et al: A walking program for nursing home residents: Effects on walk endurance, physical activity, mobility, and quality of life. *J Am Geriatr Soc* 1996; 44:175-180.

30. Manton KG, Cornelius ES, Woodbury MA: Nursing home residents: A multivariate analysis of their medical, behavioral, psychosocial, and service use characteristics. *J Gerontol* 1995; 50:M242-M251.

31. Mollinger LA, Steffen TM: Knee flexion contractures in institutionalized elderly: Prevalence, severity, stability, and related variables. *Phys Ther* 1993; 73:437-446.

32. Mulrow CD, et al: A randomized trial of physical rehabilitation for very frail nursing home residents. *JAMA* 1994; 271:519-524.

33. Nishimura Y, et al: Bone turnover and calcium metabolism during 20 days bed rest in young healthy males and females. *Acta Physiol Scand* 1994; 616:27-35.

34. Ooi WL, et al: Patterns of orthostatic blood pressure change and their clinical correlates in a frail, elderly population. *JAMA* 1997; 277:1299-1304.

35. Podsiadlo D, Richardson S: The timed "up & go": A test of basic functional mobility for frail elderly persons. *J Am Geriatr Soc* 1991; 39:142-148.

36. Ray WA, et al: A randomized trial of a consultation service to reduce falls in nursing homes. *JAMA* 1997; 278:557-562.

37. Reuben DB, Siu AL: An objective measure of physical function of elderly outpatients: The physical performance test. *J Am Geriatr Soc* 1990; 38:1105-1112.

38. Rubenstein LZ: Preventing falls in the nursing home. *JAMA* 1997; 278:595-596.

39. Sauvage LR, et al: A clinical trial of strengthening and aerobic exercise to improve gait and balance in elderly male nursing home residents. *Am J Phys Med Rehabil* 1992; 71:333-342.

40. Schnelle JF, et al: Safety assessment for the frail elderly: A comparison of restrained and unrestrained nursing home residents. *J Am Geriatr Soc* 1994; 42:586-592.

41. Scwartz RS: Sarcopenia and physical performance in old age: Introduction. *Muscle Nerve* 1997; S5:S10-S12.

42. Slemenda C, et al: Quadriceps weakness and osteoarthritis of the knee. *Ann Intern Med* 1997; 127:97-104.

43. Spier BE, Meis M: Maintenance ambulation: Its significance and the role of nursing. *Geriatr Nurs* 1994; 15:277-281.

44. Strawbridge WJ, et al: Antecedents of frailty over three decades in an older cohort. *J Gerontol* 1998; 53B:S9-S16.

45. Thompson LV: Effects of age and training on skeletal muscle physiology and performance. *Phys Ther* 1994; 74:71-81.

46. Tinetti ME, Williams TF, Mayewski R: Fall risk index for elderly patients based on number of chronic disabilities. *Am J Med* 1986; 80:429-434.

47. Tinetti ME: Performance-oriented assessment of mobility problems in elderly patients. *J Am Geriatr Soc* 1986; 34:119-126.

48. Voeks SK, Gallagher CM, Langer EH, Drinka PJ: Self-reported hearing difficulty and audiometric thresholds in nursing home residents. *J Fam Pract* 1993; 36:54-58.

49. Wolfson L, Judge J, Whipple R, King M: Strength is a major factor in balance, gait, and the occurrence of falls. *J Gerontol* 1995; 50A:64-67.

50. Wynn KE: Of dignity and mobility. *PT Magazine* 1998; 6(7):52-57.

CHAPTER 29

THE WELL ELDERLY

Marybeth Brown, PT, PhD

INTRODUCTION

Because the older adult population is growing at such a rapid rate, it is more important than ever for physical therapists to become involved in promoting wellness for these men and women. In the past decade it has become apparent that physically active older adults are the ones who advance into old age successfully, without physical infirmity.[10,12, 27-29,49] Indeed, exercise has been described as the most potent modifier of physical frailty of any modality available, which provides our profession with unlimited opportunity.[1,35,54] There is no other discipline with the potential to influence the destiny of so many older adults as can physical therapy.

It is also becoming apparent that older men and women are capable of adapting to an exercise stimulus at any age. There is a growing body of literature that clearly demonstrates that the elderly can make substantial gains in strength,[19,37,43,44,52,55] flexibility,[5,8] balance,[11,34,58] endurance,[11,16,32] and physical functional capacity,[15, 18,53,54] which often results in enhanced psychological well-being and self-efficacy.[18] These gains have been made in men and women

without infirmity and in those who have less-than-optimal health.

Several other factors should influence the course of action of physical therapists. Older adults also are living longer, and because women tend to outlive men, most of those who need assistance with exercise planning are women. On average, women live with physical infirmity 4 years longer than do men, a dismal scenario for the end of life.[36,46,47,51,56] Thus, much of the targeting done by physical therapists should be directed toward women and before they functionally decline.

Adults who experience physical limitation are generally older. Reportedly, more than one half of adults older than 85 years are unable to complete activities of daily living without help.[46,56] The physical difficulty most frequently reported is walking,[22,42,60] which suggests that one of the primary goals of exercise should be improvement in walking capacity.

What is the implication of these findings for the well elderly? A substantial proportion of the physical difficulty experienced by the older adult population can be prevented by adherence to a program of simple physical activity, prescribed and promoted by a physical therapist. If exercise, in any capacity, were incorporated into the daily routine, a shift to a more capable older adult population would occur.[10,12,27-29,49]

It is ironic that exercise must be added to the daily routine. Until World War II, the completion of chores was sufficiently challenging physically to preclude the need for exercise. Since that time, more and more modern conveniences have eliminated the need for muscle contraction and movement. It is this increased sedentary life-style that has contributed to the loss of function in our society.

This chapter was written with the intent of providing some of the tools for determining what is needed in a program of exercise for the well elderly. This chapter also provides some suggestions for exercise prescription for elders. Because those in the young old category (65 to 75 years) tend to have different needs and deficits than men and women older than 75 years, some attention is given to evaluative procedures and exercise modes that are somewhat age and capability appropriate.

What constitutes "well elderly?" Definitions vary, including those that exclude pathology (very few elders) to those that exclude current hospitalization (nearly all elders).[6,7] For purposes of this chapter, *well elderly* is defined as someone living in the community who is accomplishing all or most ADL independently and does not need rehabilitation. Typically, well elderly have chronic diseases—mostly arthritis, diabetes, and coronary artery disease—but the disease does not preclude participation in physical activity.

THE NEED FOR EXERCISE IN THE WELL-ELDERLY POPULATION

As indicated in other chapters of this text, normal age-related changes occur in all tissues. Of particular relevance to physical therapy is the decline in muscle mass and strength that has been associated with difficulty in performing selected activities and with placing elders at a higher risk for falling.[2,30,38,41,45,57] Even though strength and muscle mass begin to decline in the third decade,[3] the loss in mass and strength seems to accelerate after the age of 65 years.[3,21] This accelerated decline suggests that intervention in the young old years is even more important to prevent the superimposition of the negative effects of inactivity on top of normal aging and to maintain muscle mass and strength as long as possible. The author's experience in working with men and women between the ages of 60 and 100 years suggests that intervening in the young old years yields bigger gains in the long run, before losses are irretrievable, than trying to gain something from nearly nothing.

The rate of decline in strength and muscle mass varies from muscle group to muscle group. In general, a faster and larger decline occurs in the muscles of the lower extremity, particularly those needed most for posture, such as the gluteals, quadriceps, and plantar flexors.[3] If disease is present, the degree of strength decline is even greater, particularly when pain is present, as in some cases of osteoarthritis. It should be noted that strength decline with aging has been reported to be ~1% per year in healthy subjects.[3,26] Thus, those with disease, painful conditions, and physical inactivity probably have an even greater rate of decline.

Does muscle strength decline in physically active individuals? The answer unequivocally is yes, but the decline is far less than that seen in sedentary persons. For example, power lifters in their 60s and 70s who came into a clinic for testing generated approximately one half the torque as lifters in their 20s.[9] Torque values for the older lifters, however, were nearly 30% higher than those of inactive elders of the same age. It appears that continuous resistance exercise training markedly attenuates strength losses with aging but does not eliminate loss altogether.[9] Klitgaard and co-workers found strength and muscle fiber area values for older lifters to be comparable to those of young sedentary men.[31] What these data suggest is that a significant portion of the strength loss

that occurs with age is due to disuse. A number of studies of humans and animals supports the contention that an unacceptably large proportion of the change in strength and function with age is due to inactivity.[17,47,53]

THE UTILITY OF EXERCISE FOR THE OLDER ADULT

During the past decade a number of studies documenting the positive effects of exercise for the older adult have been published. These reports overwhelmingly confirm the "trainability" of the older adult for endurance, strength, balance, and flexibility. For example, Frontera and associates trained men aged 60 to 72 years on a universal gym for 12 weeks. The training load was 80% of an individual's one-repetition maximum (1-RM), and three sets of eight repetitions were performed 3 times per week. An enormous (109%) increase in the 1-RM was obtained.[20] Probably the most exciting study to date demonstrates that frail men and women can gain strength. Fiatarone and colleagues weight trained 10 long-term–care residents ranging in age from 86 to 96 years.[19] An 8-week program of three sets of eight repetitions of knee flexion and extension at 80% 1-RM was performed 3 times a week. Initial quadriceps strength averaged 9 kg at the beginning of the study. The average strength gain at 8 weeks was 174%. Total muscle mass as determined by computerized tomography increased an average of 9% in the quadriceps. Furthermore, changes in functional mobility, e.g., time taken to rise from a chair, correlated with the improvements in muscle strength. The 174% increase in strength compared with the 9% increase in muscle mass strongly suggests that disuse accounted for the majority of the decline in strength. More recently, Chandler and colleagues demonstrated that improvements in lower extremity strength were directly related to enhanced functional ability in a group of men and women who were frail.[13] Their strength training program of Theraband exercises in the home setting 3 times per week for 10 weeks resulted in a significant increase in chair rise time, preferred walking speed, and falls efficacy.[13] Cress and colleagues strength trained older men and women for up to 1 year and demonstrated that strength gains occurred continuously throughout that time period.[16] The greatest gain occurred within the first 3 months, but the lack of plateau in strength after 1 year was unexpected. There are several other studies that demonstrate that strength gains of a more modest nature are possible with lower-intensity programs,[2,34,38] which is important because strength increases are often needed in patients; however, because of the pathology commonly present, traditional methods of strengthening are not appropriate. In summary, the studies cited indicate that the potential to gain strength is present at all ages.

It is important to note that most of the subjects involved in the studies by Fiatarone[19] and Cress[16] had medical problems: arthritis, coronary artery disease, osteoporosis, and hypertension. Yet strength training was feasible in this population and was associated with significant gains in strength and an increase in functional ability. All subjects safely completed the protocols, even those with cardiovascular disease.

Flexibility also is amenable to change in the older adult. Range of motion (ROM) increases have been observed in the neck, shoulder, hip, and other joints as the result of an 8-week program of dance therapy,[38] a 10-week program of Feldenkreis exercises,[53] and with more traditional exercises emphasizing the end range of motion.[8,34,39] Whether the increases in passive range of motion translated to improvements in active range was not demonstrated in any of these studies.

In-house experience with a somewhat frail older adult population ($\bar{x} = 83 \pm 4$ years) indicates that (1) ROM increases do not translate into major changes in functional capacity and (2) improvements vary tremendously (range 0 to 22 degrees) given all the joint pathology present in this population. Twenty-five men and women who performed daily stretching exercises at home for 3 months had significant improvements in ROM, as expected, but performance on a physical performance test did not change. The time taken to put on and take off a laboratory coat was improved, but overall scores on the test did not increase.[8]

Cardiovascular endurance changes in response to exercise have been studied the least in older adult populations. Cardiovascular adaptation to exercise has been observed in older adults between the ages of 60 and 79 years,[1,32] but very little is known about the potential for adaptation for those older than 79 years. High-intensity aerobic training interventions have not been described at all in the frail elderly. In a young old group of men and women (61 to 67 years), Seals found that the 11 subjects increased their VO_2max an average of 30% in response to a 1-year endurance exercise program.[48] More importantly, these investigators also observed that a program of walking at 40% of heart rate reserve increased VO_2max by 12%. Forty percent of heart rate reserve is well within the capability of most men and women older than 60 years, even those with mild hypertension, pulmonary disease, congestive heart failure, arthritis, and other limitations. Hagberg and colleagues demonstrated that 70- to 79-year-old men and women who trained 3 times per week at 75% to 85% of VO_2max increased VO_2max an average of 22%.[25] Subjects in this study, however, were above average in fitness and ability.

More recently, it has been reported that older adults are able to improve balance, even subjects who are at risk for falls. Important studies by Wolf,[58] Shumway-Cook and colleagues,[50] and others[33,55] clearly indicate that older men and women are able to improve standing and walking balance significantly. Wolf and associates, for example, noted that men and women at risk for falling decreased their risk and were less afraid of falling after a 15-week program of Tai Chi exercise.[58] Wolfson examined subjects who underwent 3 months of intensive balance training followed by 6 months of low-intensity Tai Chi. Subjects improved on all measures of balance and also maintained their exercise-related gains in balance at the 6-month follow-up.[59] Shumway-Cook and

colleagues used an individualized multi-dimensional exercise approach—e.g., balance, mobility, strengthening, and flexibility, if indicated—to improve balance, mobility, and falls risk. This approach was very successful. Significant improvements in the Tinetti Mobility assessment, functional balance test, and falls risk were among the results achieved.[50] Thus, exercise appears to be efficacious for the improvement of balance, and some studies seem to indicate that exercise can have a beneficial effect on falls risk.

In studies conducted by the author and colleagues of frail older adults aged 80 years and older, significant improvements on the Berg test for balance, the Romberg test, in the ability to negotiate an obstacle course, and to stand on one limb were noted in response to a low-intensity exercise program that included balance training. Functional reach did not change during the 3 months of physical therapy-type exercise but did improve significantly after 3 months of strength training, which also resulted in an increase in calf strength (unpublished observations).

In summary, the recent literature overwhelmingly supports the efficacy of exercise for improving strength, flexibility, balance, and other factors associated with reduced physical function, even for the oldest old. In addition, studies are beginning to indicate that improvements in strength (but not other risk factors for frailty as yet) have a direct impact on function. Increases in strength have been related to increases in chair rise time, self-selected gait speed, stair climbing, and stopping. Clearly, exercise has the potential to keep older adults from losing their independence and to maximize their remaining abilities.

HOW TO GET STARTED
Initial Observations
Appropriate exercise prescription for the well elderly is based, like all of physical therapy care, on information obtained from examination and evaluation. Whether the desired outcome for exercise is improved strength, enhanced flexibility, or ability to run a marathon, examination is imperative.

An evaluation for an exercise program begins immediately with patient introduction. The first 30 seconds of contact often provide the necessary information to get started at the proper level of examination. For example, if the patient has difficulty getting out of the waiting room chair, ambulates at a slow rate of speed to the examination area, and is breathing heavily with the little bit of effort required for this task, it is immediately recognized that strength, gait, and cardiovascular endurance must be examined at the start. Once lower extremity gait, strength, and cardiovascular endurance have been examined, other areas that need to be examined will be obvious, e.g., range of motion, balance, and function (ADL and IADL). These observations also will make it apparent to the therapist whether the patient's desired exercise outcome is feasible. For example, if the aforementioned person desired to resume square dancing, the therapist would have sufficient information to disabuse the patient from attending dance classes immediately. Rather, a remedial program of strengthening activities with an emphasis on standing and walking for endurance might better serve this individual as a first step. Perhaps the next step could be a course in ballroom dancing.

The therapist's immediate observations can provide the majority of information needed to determine what additional specific examination tests and measures are appropriate. Sharp observations skills are imperative as well as close attention to detail in observing functional activities such as climbing steps, rising from a chair, walking, and turning—all of which are indicators of strength and range deficits and limitations in balance. Any hesitancy in doing what is requested should be noted. It is important to note whether the patient is lean, tall, stout, or disproportioned in some way and whether posture is of concern. Other things to notice when meeting with a patient for the first time is whether he/she uses an assistive device, has apparent swelling, avoids use of a body part, wears clothes and shoes that were selected for ease of application, wears glasses and/or hearing aid, has appropriate skin color and hair on the extremities, or has obvious joint deformity. Again, this information serves as the basis for the remainder of the examination.

If older adults are simply coming into the clinic for exercise, the 30-second evaluation can often provide adequate information to get started at an appropriate level of activity. For example, if most of the adults coming to the clinic use an assistive device, are slow to get started, and appear a little deficient in balance, perhaps exercises should be done, at least initially, sitting or holding onto the wall or chair. If a patient is robust, has a substantial amount of muscle mass to work with, and is in good health, then a fairly rigorous program of exercise can be initiated, once baseline measures of heart rate and blood pressure are established.

History

During the course of examination, some form of history taking is indicated. Some suggestions for inclusion that are over and above the usual information related to age, date, gender, and weight include the following:

1. *Exercise history.* Is the patient accustomed to physical activity or is this the first time he/she ever participated in exercise? Caution is indicated when progressing someone with no exercise background. Sense of body, particularly body in space, may be remarkably limited.
2. *Medical problems.* It is rare that an older adult does not have multiple medical diagnoses. Even though medical compromise is usually a given, there are conditions for which care must be taken, such as heart disease, arthritis, diabetes, osteoporosis, and hypertension.
3. *Medications.* Is the patient taking a medication that will alter exercise responses, e.g., beta blockers?
4. *Painful conditions.* Does the patient have chronic conditions such as back or hip pain that require referral to a physician or accommodation in an exercise program?
5. *Recent injuries or surgeries.*

Cardiovascular System Review

Another imperative for working with older adults is some test of the cardiovascular system. The facility in which the author works does not have the means to do sophisticated stress testing, therefore patients must receive approval from their physician before the physical therapist's examination. Most of the referring physicians are helpful in providing a safe or target heart rate range. During the other parts of the physical therapist's examination, blood pressure and heart rate are monitored to get some idea of how much challenge the cardiovascular system can tolerate.

The author's clinic is not readily accessible, requiring patients to walk a considerable distance from the parking lot, and then they must ascend a flight of stairs just to get to the waiting room. If a 70-year-old patient is sweating profusely by the time he/she arrives and has a heart rate of 130 beats per minute (bpm) and a blood pressure of 180/90, data suggest that a walking program to increase cardiovascular endurance is probably more than adequate initially.

Even when a target heart rate or heart rate range is provided, it is hard to know where to start without some notion of what type of activity will generate such a heart rate response. Follow-up tests and measures typically include walking at normal speed, fast walking, or walking on a treadmill; heart rate and blood pressure are monitored throughout. If a patient wants a home exercise program for a specific piece of equipment, heart rate and blood pressure monitoring are done on that piece of equipment. A large number of persons who go to the author's clinic have exercise bikes, rowing machines, and so forth that are gathering dust in the basement. These items typically were gifts because "the patient needed to get some exercise." Now the patient needs proper guidelines on how to use his equipment appropriately.

One of the most useful tests of cardiovascular capability is the 6-minute walk.[24] This test requires the therapist to record a baseline heart rate while a patient is sitting quietly and then to have the older adult walk (or propel a wheelchair), using whatever assistive device is required, as far as he/she is capable for 6 minutes. If rests are needed, they are included in the 6-minute data collection period. A markedly deconditioned patient, for example, might walk while pushing a wheelchair for 15 feet, sit down and rest, push the chair another 15 feet, sit down and rest, and so forth. The total distance achieved during the 6-minute walk might be 75 feet (in contrast to the 1800 feet accomplished by a young adult without running). Immediately after the 6 minutes, heart rate is measured and used as another indicator of the stress of the test. Improvements in cardiovascular endurance may be noted in both the distance traveled and the heart rate response. If someone walks farther at the same heart rate, obvious improvement has taken place.

To summarize, elsewhere in this text are specific exercise tests for examination of the cardiovascular system. Some type of follow-up may be indicated to determine how the heart will function during an actual exercise intervention. In other words, patients will probably need information related to how fast they should walk, whether to incorporate an incline on the treadmill, how much resistance to use on a bicycle, and how long to exercise. Supplemental information, over and above that gained from stress testing, typically is required.

EXAMINATION TESTS AND MEASURES
Flexibility

Most healthy young old adults have ranges of motion within acceptable limits; the older old are more likely to show deficits in range that limit functional performance. Thus, exercises for ROM enhancement are more important for those in the eighth and ninth decades. Regardless of age, ROM needs to be assessed functionally—during walking, getting up and down from a chair (preferably one that is lower than usual, e.g., 16 inches), getting up and down from the floor (if appropriate), reaching for an object overhead, and reaching for something on the floor. If specific ranges are needed for billing purposes, a goniometric measurement can be made of the joints that were identified as deficient with functional assessment. For example, even though the majority of older adults fall each year, many do not have enough knee ROM to get up off the floor should they come in contact with the ground.

Personal observations of numerous older adults throughout the years have revealed problem areas that are often gender specific. Women are more likely than men to have significant ROM deficits in ankle dorsiflexion, knee flexion, and shoulder elevation. Men are more likely than women to have deficits in the hip and trunk. Both men and women are likely to have major deficits in neck range (severe enough to make driving an unsafe activity), hip extension, and trunk rotation.

If a young older adult is a candidate for walking, fast walking, or jogging, two tests of flexibility are strongly recommended. They are the Thomas test for hip flexor tightness and a check for dorsiflexion range. More than 60% of older walking/jogging exercise participants observed by the author experienced hip or back pain if hip flexor tightness was greater than 10 degrees. Once the tightness was reduced, the pain subsided, which suggests a strong relationship between the two. The other possible limitation, dorsiflexion, is more often seen in women because of a long history of wearing high-heeled shoes. Unless dorsiflexion range is at least zero degrees (neutral), walking for exercise cannot be done comfortably. A good walking shoe can accommodate for the 10 degrees of dorsiflexion usually required during gait, but again, neutral ankle dorsiflexion is a minimum.

In the old older adult, ROM deficits may be tied to postural instability. Significant hip flexor tightness, for example, may result in an anterior pelvic tilt and forward trunk lean, placing the center of mass farther forward than normal. Inadequate dorsiflexion may place the center of mass behind the malleoli, thus placing the responsibility for the maintenance of balance on the dorsiflexors, which are usually too weak to handle the demand. ROM deficits that undermine a patient's ability to maintain good balance under static and dynamic conditions must be remediated.

Strength

An imperative component of any physical examination is strength. An assessment of strength can be made in a multitude of ways, all of which have advantages and disadvantages: manual muscle testing (MMT), isokinetic testing, speed of movement, gait, functional testing, hand-held dynamometry, force transducer tests, and 1-RM.

Manual Muscle Testing

MMT has the major disadvantage of only identifying strength deficits when patients have lost 40% to 50% of pre-existing strength. MMT is difficult in an older adult population, since some strength loss with aging is normal, but current methods are too crude to distinguish between age-associated strength losses and those sustained secondary to disuse and disease. MMT by break testing is rather static; whether patients can use their strength during an activity requiring a large arc of motion cannot be discerned with this mode of testing.

Positive aspects of muscle testing include being able to obtain specific information about select muscle groups and getting some insight into functional loss. No other form of testing provides this data about individual muscles (although for healthy older adults, this information is not particularly useful). Selected muscle tests, e.g., rising up onto the toes to test calf strength, will immediately indicate whether a patient is likely to have difficulty with heel rise during gait.

There are three muscle test items recommended for inclusion in the initial examination. The first, rising up on the toes 10 to 20 times (one leg at a time), is performed to determine strength for the gastrocnemius-soleus group. If a grade of F+ or better cannot be achieved, the utility of a walking program is limited, i.e., strengthening must be done to bring patients into the F+ or better category. The second item examined is gluteus medius capability. Patients are asked to hold onto a chair or wall with one finger and then slowly lift a foot from the ground. If the pelvis drops, indicating gluteus medius weakness, remedial exercises are begun. Again, a walking program is not appropriate if the pelvis drops every time a step is taken. The final muscle test performed is for hip extension strength. The traditional prone posture is assumed, and patients are asked to raise the entire lower extremity against gravity through full ROM. Those with weakness of the hip extensors tend to walk with the trunk forward, which often results in back pain.

These muscle test items are offered as suggestions only. Strength can be determined in other ways that are equally as effective but cannot provide a "grade," which may be important for documentation purposes. For example, lack of heel rise during gait implicates the calf as being weak, but whether it falls in the trace, poor, or fair category cannot be determined by gait observation alone.

Isokinetic Testing

Isokinetic testing has the disadvantages of being nonfunctional and difficult for some older adults to learn. In addition, results are hard to interpret because there are few age-appropriate norms available. For information related to expected torque ranges for older adults, however, the studies of Bemben and colleagues are recommended.[3] There are two advantages to isokinetic testing: (1) being able to determine movement capability at different speeds and (2) being able to identify point of fatigue. Older adults often test reasonably well during a static form of muscle testing but perform poorly when speeds of 180 or 360 degrees/second are requested. Normally, the speed of 300 degrees per second is used by most persons routinely in daily activities, and if a patient is incapable of moving that fast, a significant deficit has been identified. The knee moves at 360 degrees per second during normal velocity walking; the arm may move at 1200 degrees per second or more to throw a ball. Older men and women who cannot move quickly are at risk for falling. Thus, if isokinetic testing reveals inability to perform at faster speeds, exercise to correct this deficit should be instituted. For example, one patient, age 79 and with a history of falling, was found to have no protective reactions (arms or legs) when asked to perform a balance maneuver. Isokinetic testing revealed a total inability to move the arm of the isokinetic equipment faster than 180 degrees per second with either the upper or lower extremities. Exercises (dance per the patient's preference) to emphasize control, balance, and speed were instituted.

Isokinetic dynamometry can be used to identify persons who fatigue quickly. Protocols vary, but typically, patients are asked to perform maximum contractions repetitively to look at the slope of decline after a certain number of contractions or to maintain a certain proportion of output, e.g., 50% of a maximum isometric voluntary contraction for about 30 seconds. Fatigue protocols are not appropriate for many older patients, particularly those who are frail. Elders with hypertension, joint deformity or pain, and cardiac compromise should probably not be tested using the protocols described.

Fatigue

Many older men and women complain of muscle fatigue, yet muscle endurance is rarely tested in this population, primarily because tests and measures to routinely assess this element of performance are not in place. Ignoring muscle fatigue is not an acceptable approach, and thus each clinic should embrace a simple protocol that can be easily reproduced quickly and reliably. Suggestions for a fatigue protocol include having the patient lift a small weight with the upper extremity to a target distance overhead, then recording the number of times the patient can achieve the target or having the patient hold a position or weight until he/she is "fatigued" and then recording the amount of time that the patient maintained the position or weight. Examples include a wall sit, a partial chair stand, holding a weighted ankle or wrist against gravity, and standing.

Speed of Movement

Another aspect of strength that needs to be evaluated is the speed with which the activity is accomplished. Some older adults have adequate passive ROM, but the speed with which they move within that range is unacceptable. Unless the arms can be raised in time to prevent a fall or the knees can be moved quickly through normal 70-degree arc of motion during gait, strength is not adequate. Recognition of patients' willingness to use their strength in a dynamic, functional way is important.

Functional Testing

Functional testing is important to perform, especially in the older old category. Functional testing for the lower extremities may include having the patient get up and down from a seated position, sometimes from chairs of different heights. Some investigators advocate repeated bouts (five times) of rising and sitting. Another functional test is having the patient walk up and down curbs of different heights. Testing may include curb heights of 4, 6, and 8 inches. Walking devices are used if needed, and the level of ability is recorded appropriately as well as any loss of balance during the testing. Stair climbing is a third functional test that may be requested. Steps should be of normal height and include a handrail. Ability to negotiate steps, with or without rails or assistive devices, is noted. If appropriate, getting up and down from the floor may be included in the testing. Other options include having the patient pick up an object from the floor, stoop down into a cupboard, and walk up and down a ramp. Upper extremity tests may include having the patient put on a sweatshirt (overhead, no buttons), reach up into a cupboard, and pick up a weighted object and move it a short distance.

A physical performance test that puts together nine functional items was described by Reuben.[40] The advantages of this approach is that it can be used in a variety of settings, e.g., home, assisted living, and community, and enables the examiner to determine performance times that can be converted to a score. Thus, improvements in performance, e.g., putting on a sweater or picking up a penny from the floor, can be graded—something a third party payer can understand. The physical performance test described by Reuben and Siu is easy to perform, requires little equipment, and takes 10 to 15 minutes to complete.[40] Another test, the continuous-scale physical performance test, developed by Cress and associates, requires approximately 45 minutes to complete but provides a fairly comprehensive overview of community capability. This test requires the patient to lift groceries, get in and out of a car, and make a bed, among other items.[14]

The obvious advantage of functional testing is that it identifies areas of ADL that need remediation. A major disadvantage is that functional testing is nonspecific; strength deficits may be obscured by ROM or other problems and none of the probable strength deficits identified on functional testing can be quantified. The experienced therapist can usually recognize what is balance, strength, or range limited, but a great deal of learning and expertise are required to reach that level of clinical competence.

Hand-Held Dynamometry

Hand-held dynamometry rapidly provides information regarding the capability of any major muscle group. Another advantage is that side-to-side differences can be discerned, and the process of data collection is time efficient. Disadvantages of dynamometry include the fact that some instruments are more reliable than others, the strength of the tester is vitally important (if the patient is stronger than the therapist, the data are useless), and values reflect static strength only. Still, dynamometry can provide an index of patient capability. For example, if quadriceps strength is less than 50% of body weight, some compensation or deviation is to be expected.

Force Transducer Tests

The advantages and disadvantages of using force transducer are similar to those of using hand-held dynamometer. Differences between the two are ease of application (positioning requirements for using a force transducer are cumbersome), number of muscle groups that can be tested (fewer with force transducer), and the nature of testing. The strength of the tester is not a factor when a force transducer is used.

One-Repetition Maximum

A 1-RM test is an accepted, but time-consuming, test to administer. Not all muscle groups can be evaluated this way, and many persons need to be tested several times before a true 1-RM is determined. If older adults are very deconditioned, the testing sometimes results in a lot of muscle soreness. Nonetheless, the 1-RM test provides data that may serve as a useful guide for improvement and can be correlated with changes in functional performance as well.

A number of options for strength testing have been presented, all of which have positive and negative aspects about them. What works best for a clinic will be based on mode of practice (is the patient base composed of average senior citizens or are there master athletes), the space available, machinery available, amount of time that the physical therapist can devote to the evaluation, amount of data necessary, patient expectation, and need for documentation.

Gait

Gait assessment is useful for all kinds of evaluative purposes, e.g., strength, ROM, endurance, and balance. Some strength deficits can be identified on the basis of deviations in the gait cycle. Lack of heel rise during terminal stance has already been identified as one indicator of inadequate calf strength. Other aspects of gait to note include pelvic drop, forward trunk lean, diminished or absent knee flexion during loading, and reduced knee flexion. Pelvic drop in the frontal plane indicates that muscles stabilizing the pelvis (gluteus medius, gluteus minimus, tensor fascia latae) are not strong

enough to meet the demand. Forward trunk lean commonly indicates inadequate hip extensors. Diminished or absent knee flexion right after heel strike suggests that the quadriceps are not strong enough to absorb the shock of loading, which requires an F+ or better grade. Finally, reduced knee flexion during swing may indicate weakness of the gastrocnemius or hamstrings.

A proper examination of gait also should include an assessment of velocity (strength deficits result in reduced gait speed), stride length, stride width, and variability in stride characteristics. Diminished stride and so forth may indicate reduced strength but also may be indicative of balance problems, sensory loss, or cardiovascular compromise.

Gait assessment is quickly performed (10 seconds of the 30-second initial observation) and reveals an enormous amount of information. Suspected strength deficits are identified, and follow-up testing on functional items such as rising from a chair or MMT can be performed to confirm inadequate strength. Gait deficits do not provide much information regarding deficits in strength.

Balance

Balance testing can be static or dynamic, and both have advantages and disadvantages. Examples of static testing include the stand-on-one-leg test, the sharpened Romberg, the postural stress test, and the reach test. Dynamic tests include walking, walking through an obstacle course, and platform testing.

Static Balance

Standing on one leg with the eyes open (and closed if indicated) is an easy test to administer and provides a number value in less than 1 minute. Care must be taken not to allow the patient to accommodate by placing the swing leg on the stance leg, shifting position of the stance leg, or hopping. Several trials are required to make the patient feel comfortable with the testing and to ensure reliable data. The ability to stand on one leg for long periods (30 to 40 seconds) is not particularly meaningful. However, whether a patient can stand on one leg for less than 10 seconds is indicative of significant deficit. In the author's clinic, most of the adults tested are unable to stand on one leg for more than 1 to 3 seconds. These values do not mean much in an absolute sense, but they at least indicate whether the task can be accomplished at all. Attempting to stand on one leg with the eyes closed will give some insight as to whether the individual being tested should be counseled about walking around in the dark (e.g., walking to the bathroom along a darkened corridor).

The sharpened Romberg is a popular test of static balance with progressively difficult postures to maintain. The first segment of the six-part test is to stand with the feet together and with the eyes open for 10 seconds. Grading is simple: able or not able to complete the requested task. The second segment requires the patient to stand with the feet together for 10 seconds but with the eyes closed. The third component of the test requires standing in the semi-tandem

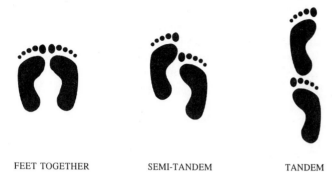

FEET TOGETHER   SEMI-TANDEM   TANDEM

FIG. 29-1   Foot placements for sharpened Romberg test.

position (Fig. 29-1) for 10 seconds with the eyes open. The fourth component is standing in the semi-tandem position for 10 seconds with the eyes closed. The fifth and last segments require the patient to stand in the full tandem position (one foot immediately in front of the other, heel to toe [see Fig 29-1]), first with the eyes open and then with the eyes closed. This test is easy to administer, reasonably reliable, and does not require much time to complete. One small problem with the test is that no instructions are provided as to how a patient should be graded if the individual falls while getting into the test position but then passes that particular segment of the test.

The reach test has been found to be reliable and valid and is simple to perform. Subjects stand comfortably and reach forward (not down) as far as they can along a yardstick that is placed on the wall next to them. Distance reached is recorded. Reaching distances of less than 10 inches are of concern.

One test of balance that can be included in both the static and dynamic portions of examination is the Berg test.[4] This 14-item test challenges balance in a progressively more difficult approach. The easiest item, for example, is to sit without losing balance. The test progresses through transfers without loss of balance to actually standing on one leg. Each task is graded on a 4-point scale, and thus a judgment of the safety and skill of the patient is provided. The total test is worth 56 points, and there are cut-offs for performance that indicate whether a patient is at risk for falling.

Dynamic Balance

Examples of dynamic tests include movable platforms, the "get-up-and-go" test, walking an imaginary balance beam, and completing an obstacle course. None of these tests has norms, but the platform developed by the Nashner group has been evaluated extensively. The platform, however, is extremely expensive and beyond the means of most clinics. Results apparently provide information that is no more useful in predicting falling behavior than the simple, no-cost one-legged stance test and functional reach test. The get-up-and-go test requires the patient to rise from a chair and go toward a destination as quickly as possible. Usually, turns are incorporated into the protocol. Trials are timed, and difficulties with performing the test are noted.

Similarities exist between the obstacle course, get-up-and-go test, and the imaginary balance beam. All are timed trials and challenge the patient to operate within a discrete base of support. For example, the imaginary balance beam typically is a dark line painted on the floor. Trials are usually videotaped, and the number of times a patient misses the "beam" is noted, as is the amount of time needed to complete the trial. Obstacle courses vary in difficulty but usually incorporate a number of functional tasks. The one used by the author has three levels of difficulty. The first task requires the patient to rise from a chair, walk 12 feet, step up a 4-inch step, turn around, step down the step, return to the chair, and sit. Practice trials are permitted for safety sake, although in real life no one gets two chances to prevent a fall. The second task requires standing from a seated position, walking forward, stepping over an obstacle (a 2- × 2-foot piece of wood), ascending a 6-inch step (no rail), turning, and repeating the process in reverse.

As with the other tests presented so far, what is selected to incorporate in the clinic will depend on time, money, the nature of the clientele, and how much information is needed. These tools will at least provide a start.

Activities of Daily Living

Any evaluation of the older adult must include some sort of ADL assessment. A number of options have been presented in Chapter 7 and are not elaborated here.

The assessment to be chosen will again depend on the patient and the patient's capabilities. For example, a 93-year-old woman who is barely getting by may be having difficulty with everything on the test sheet, but a healthy 67-year-old may simply have trouble taking heavy garbage cans to the curb. If the ADL assessment does not capture whatever difficulty the patient is experiencing, make a notation in the record. Identifying the needs of the patient is crucial.

Posture

In many instances, a detailed posture examination is not indicated. Paying attention to deviations from the norm is necessary, but this component of the examination can be taken care of during the initial 30-second sweep or at any other point in the initial assessment. Items to note are hip asymmetry; genu valgus or varus; pronated or supinated feet; excessive lordosis, kyphosis, or scoliosis; and extremes of pelvic tilt. Postural faults that are likely to result in a painful condition must be accommodated. Someone with severe flat and painful feet, for example, is not likely to respond to a walking program. Postural faults that are probable contributors to balance instability also need to be addressed.

EXERCISE PRESCRIPTION

The information gathered during the examination needs to be integrated by evaluation into a total picture from which an exercise plan will evolve. Successful exercise planning takes into account all the subtle and not-so-subtle changes that have occurred with aging, the patient's goals, chronic diseases (if present), physical capabilities, and painful conditions and is based on a common-sense approach. The following case histories are presented to illustrate these ideas. Four patients are presented, one for each of the seventh, eighth, ninth, and tenth decades of life. These men and women were chosen to illustrate the differences in approach to the oldest old and to demonstrate that age is not always indicative of capability.

Case Studies

Mr. P

Mr. P is 67 years old, 5 feet, 10 inches, and weighs 267 pounds. He is very sedentary. Physical examination revealed a forward head posture, 30 degrees of hip flexor tightness (Thomas test), bilateral iliotibial band tightness with knee pain, probable knee arthritis bilaterally, and grade 3 flat feet. His gait was slow (48 m/min) with a foot flat approach at heel strike, no toe-off, and a bilateral pelvic drop during stance. Muscle testing revealed good strength throughout, with exception of plantar flexors (F+) and abdominals (P). Because the patient weighed so much, he had difficulty getting out of chairs and up stairs. This man was very awkward, giving the impression of someone with little sense of body awareness. Although Mr. P had had a nonremarkable stress test before coming in for evaluation, he was asked to walk on a treadmill so that heart rate (HR) and blood pressure (BP) responses could be determined. The patient walked on the treadmill for 5 minutes (until fatigue) at a speed of 3.0 mph with no incline. HR increased to 134 bpm, which was estimated to be about 90% of his Vo_2max. Systolic BP rose to more than 200 mm Hg during the 3.0-mph test.

Mr. P came into the clinic for an exercise program at the behest of his wife, who had been urging him for months to "do something." His expectation was that a walking program would be prescribed, and he was not enthusiastic at the prospect. This patient was rather unenthusiastic about the prospect of exercise, particularly walking, but he was aware of his need for activity. The week before the evaluation he had experienced extreme difficulty getting out of the seat of a theater, and this provided some motivation to seek care.

The patient and therapist agreed on the following: for the first 2 to 3 months he would park in the lot farthest from the facility (2/10 mile) and walk in at a slightly-faster-than-usual pace. Mr. P would participate 3 times per week in a flexibility and strengthening program aimed particularly at the trunk and lower extremities. Orthotics and good shoes would be obtained to accommodate for his flat feet and to decrease strain on the knees. The walking and exercise plan was designed to provide some cardiovascular stimulation and improved strength and ROM, respectively. At the end of 3 months, lower extremity strength and flexibility were adequate for the next phase of training. Walking for more than a short distance really was not indicated for Mr. P, given his painful knees, excess weight, marginal strength, and lack of desire to do this type of exercise. Instead, a home cycle program was chosen because the patient had a bike, and he was interested in pursuing this form of activity.

A very modest program was begun and consisted of biking at 100 W for 15 minutes. Over time the patient progressed steadily, and program modifications were instituted once a month. He is currently cycling for 1 hour using 150-W protocol for 10 minutes as a warm up, a 300-W intensity for training, and a 15-minute cool-down at 100-W. The exercise cycle is in front of the television, and the patient barely notices that 1 hour has passed. Mr. P performs his exercise regularly; he is very proud of himself and his ability to get from place to place without difficulty.

Mrs. M

Mrs. M is 75 years old, 5 feet, 4 inches, and weighs 96 pounds. She is sedentary but is engaged all day long managing her own linen business. Her 105-year-old mother is in a nursing home because of osteoporosis and frailty. Mrs. M smokes 1 pack of cigarettes a day and has mild hypertension. She is cleared for exercise by her physician but is allowed a maximum heart rate of 110 bpm as long as her diastolic blood pressure does not rise beyond 90 mm Hg. Physical evaluation reveals a mild kyphosis but no other postural faults. Strength and range are good, and there are no gait or balance deficits. She was able to perform all ADL without difficulty. Mrs. M has a treadmill at home that she would like to use.

Treadmill walking was performed during the testing session to determine HR and BP responses. Treadmill speed was 2.0 mph initially and was increased by 0.5 mph every 2 minutes until an HR of 110 bpm was reached. Blood pressure was within acceptable limits. A walking program of 2.5 mph at a 2% incline for 20 minutes a day was begun. Within 6 weeks the patient could walk at 3.0 mph at a 2% incline with the same HR and BP response. Ultimately, the amount of treadmill time was increased so that the patient was walking 40 minutes a day. It should be noted that proper footwear was procured before the walking program began.

Four months into the program, Mrs. M broke her toe (unrelated to exercise), which did not heal for months because of her low bone density and possibly her smoking. Once healing occurred, she resumed her walking program but needed to start over from the beginning. In addition, 10 flights of stairs per day were added to provide loading through the long bones in an attempt to promote bone growth. Exercise seems to have checked the mild hypertension, and the patient is now allowed a higher exercise intensity (125 bpm). Mrs. M exercises daily, but whether the program has affected bone density is unknown.

Mrs. B

Mrs. B is 83 years old and regards herself as a "typical" octogenarian. She lives with her husband in an apartment, is busy with her social activities, accomplishes all ADL independently, and drives her car approximately 2000 miles per year. A 30-second observation revealed a kyphotic woman who walked slowly with a wide-base, with no arm support, clutching her purse, and looking down at the floor. Further examination revealed a woman with reaction times slower than those required for safely driving a car in the community, compromised balance, poor cardiovascular and muscular endurance, barely adequate strength, and upper extremity limitations in range. Although "independent" in the community, it became apparent that if Mrs. B had a luncheon engagement, it took her the entire morning to bathe and dress for the occasion. Although she shopped for groceries, she had the check-out clerks take the groceries to the car and the apartment doorman to bring the groceries into her apartment. Frequently, she had groceries delivered by a local store that caters to older patients. She ambulated only in familiar areas as she knew where all the walls, hand-holds, and chairs were, and she could ambulate safely within the learned environment. She did not go out at night or during periods of higher traffic. Physical activity consisted of playing cards with friends and neighbors.

Physical therapist examination revealed a score of 40/56 on the Berg test for balance, a 7½-inch functional reach, strength scores suggesting F+ throughout, inability to move the isokinetic machine arm faster than 180°/s, 120 degrees of shoulder flexion, 45 degrees of shoulder external rotation, a 48 M/min gait speed, 220 feet covered with the 6-minute walk (estimated $\dot{V}O_2$peak is approximately 13 ml O_2/kg/min), reaction times of 550 ms (normal for young adult is approximately 160 ms), non-existent balance reactions, inability to turn and maintain balance, and impaired lower extremity sensation. The patient and physical therapist determined that her initial exercise program should be performed on an outpatient basis so that supervision could be provided, particularly during balance activities. Her exercises consisted of activities on a mat that required numerous position changes, included prone lying; exercises to encourage proximal muscle involvement, e.g., straight leg raise; standing and sitting balancing; activities to promote increased speed of reaction, e.g., playing catch with a sponge ball; and walking. Once Mrs. B developed better body handling skills and muscle "tone," she progressed to a modest program of weight training.

Mr. C

This remarkable 90-year-old moved to St. Louis from Montana, where he had maintained a horse ranch for the last 50 years. Reasons for the move from a rural to urban setting included death of his spouse and a fall from his horse. Επvaluation revealed a robust-appearing man with no apparent deviations from the norm upon observation of chair rise, gait, hand-shaking, and placing his coat on a rack. History was extraordinary in that he did not smoke or drink, had always engaged in rigorous activity, had no history of cardiovascular disease, did not require glasses or hearing aid, had no dependency in ADL or IADL, and could drive at night. Examination revealed a man with far better than average strength, adequate ROM with the exception of his hamstrings, and

better than average cardiovascular endurance. His problems were poor balance and suspected spinal stenosis with pain and tingling into his right lower extremity. His exercise program consisted of working at home (his request) on activities to challenge his balance, such as standing at the counter and attempting to shift balance from one side to the other, standing on one leg, rocking back and forth from heel to toe, and placing one toe in front and then shifting the leg to a position behind him, all while holding his balance as well as possible without holding on. A modified Tai Chi program was begun, and exercises to increase hamstring length were also instituted. Prone lying on the floor was strongly suggested, and exercises to eliminate hip flexor tightness were also begun. Ultimately he progressed to a modest prone press-up. Standing exercises were done barefoot instead of in cowboy boots, his usual footwear. Goals included better balance as evidence by a higher score on the Berg test, ability to negotiate an obstacle course safely in 15 seconds, a 4/6 on the Romberg test, normalization of wide-based gait and staggering, and reduced or eliminated back and leg pain.

SUMMARY

The well elderly present a rewarding therapeutic opportunity for physical therapists. They are extremely challenging because they are so diverse in their abilities. Exercise prescription for this population taxes the ingenuity of a physical therapist as no other group of patients. The potential for change is substantial, maybe more so than the change that may occur secondary to rehabilitation. Our ability to affect the well-being of the older adult population is enormous. Exercise should be available for all seniors to prevent deterioration and to keep adults maximally capable, thereby eliminating the need for dependence on others. Physical therapists have the skill and knowledge to provide healthy older adults the best care possible.

REFERENCES

1. American College of Sports Medicine: Exercise and physical activity for older adults. *Med Sci Sports Exerc* 1998; 30:992-1008.
2. Bassey EJ, et al: Leg extensor power and functional performance in very old men and women. *Clin Sci* 1992; 82:321-327.
3. Bemben MG, et al: Isometric muscle force production as a function of age in healthy 20- to 74-year old men. *Med Sci Sports Exerc* 1991; 23:1302-1310.
4. Berg K, et al: A comparison of clinical and laboratory measures of balance control in an elderly population. *Arch Phys Med Rehabil* 1992; 73:1073-1083.
5. Binder EF, et al: Effects of a group exercise program on risk factors for falls in frail older adults. *J Phys Activ Aging* 1994; 2:25-37.
6. Bortz WM: The physics of frailty. *J Am Geriatr Soc* 1993; 41:1004-1008.
7. Brown I, Renwick R, Raphael D: Frailty: Constructing a common meaning, definition, and conceptual framework. *Intern J Rehabil Res* 1995; 18:93-102.
8. Brown M, Holloszy JO: Effects of a low intensity exercise program on selected physical performance characteristics of 60- to 71-year olds. *Aging: Clin Exp Res* 1991; 3:129-139.
9. Brown M: The master athlete. *Ortho Phys Ther Clin North Am* 1997; 6:253-266.

10. Buchner DM, et al: Effects of physical activity on health status in older adults II: Intervention Studies. *Ann Rev Publ Health* 1992; 13:469-488.

11. Buchner DM, et al: A comparison of the effects of three types of endurance training on balance and other fall risk factors in older adults. *Aging: Clin Exp Res* 1997; 9:112-119.

12. Cartee GD: Aging skeletal muscle: Response to exercise. *Exerc Sci Rev* 1994; 22:91-120.

13. Chandler JM, Duncan PW, Kochersberger G, Studenski S: Is lower extremity strength gain associated with improvement in physical performance and disability in frail, community-dwelling elders? *Arch Phys Med Rehabil* 1998; 79:24-30.

14. Cress EM, et al: Continuous-scale physical functional performance in healthy older adults: A validation study. *Arch Phys Med Rehabil* 1996; 77:1243-1250.

15. Cress ME, et al: Exercise: Effects on physical functional performance in independent older adults. *J Gerontol* 1999; 5 4:M242-248.

16. Cress ME, et al: Effect of training on VO2 max, thigh strength, and muscle morphology in septuagenarian women. *Med Sci Sports Exc* 1991; 23:752-758.

17. Davis JW, et al: Strength, physical activity, and body mass index: Relationship to performance-based measures and activities of daily living among older Japanese women in Hawaii. *J Am Geriatr Soc* 1998; 46:274-279.

18. Engels HJ, Drouin J, Zhu W, Kazmierski JF: Effects of low-impact, moderate-intensity exercise training with and without wrist weights on functional capacities and mood states in older adults. *Gerontology* 1998; 44:239-244.

19. Fiatarone MA, et al: High-intensity strength training in nonagenarians. Effects of skeletal muscle. *JAMA* 1990; 263:3029-3034.

20. Frontera WR, et al: Strength conditioning in older men: Skeletal muscle hypertrophy and improved function. *J Appl Physiol* 1988; 64:1038-1044.

21. Grimby G: Muscle performance and structure in the elderly as studied cross-sectionally and longitudinally. *J Gerontol* 1995; 50:17-22.

22. Guralnik JM, et al: A short physical battery assessing lower extremity function: Association with self-reported disability and prediction of mortality and nursing home admission. *J Gerontol* 1994; 49:M85-M94.

23. Gutman GM, Herbert CP, Brown SR: Feldenkrais versus conventional exercises for the elderly. *J Gerontol* 1977; 32:562-567.

24. Guyatt GH, et al: The 6-minute walk: A new measure of exercise capacity in patients with chronic heart failure. *Canadian Med Assoc J* 1985; 132:919-923.

25. Hagberg JM, et al: Cardiovascular responses of 70- to 79- year old men and women to endurance training. *J Appl Physiol* 1989; 66:2589-2594.

26. Hakkinen K, Hakkinen A: Muscle cross-sectional area, force production and relaxation characteristics in women at different ages. *Eur J Appl Physiol* 1991; 62: 410-414.

27. Hamdorf PA, Withers RT, Penhall RK, Haslam MV: Physical training effects on the fitness and habitual activity patterns of elderly women. *Arch Phys Med Rehabil* 1992; 73:603-608.

28. Harridge S, Magnusson G, Saltin B: Life-long endurance-trained elderly men have high aerobic power, but have similar muscle strength to non-active elderly men. *Aging: Clin Exp Res* 1997; 9:80-87.

29. Holloszy JO, Spina RJ, Kohrt WM: Health benefits of exercise in the elderly. *Med Sport Sci* 1992; 37:91-108.

30. Judge JO, Schechtman K, Cress E, FICSIT Group: The relationship between physical performance measures and independence in instrumental activities of daily living. *J Am Geriatr Soc* 1996; 44:1332-1341.

31. Klitgaard H, et al: Function, morphology and protein expression of ageing skeletal muscle: A cross-sectional study of elderly men with different training backgrounds. *Acta Physiol Scand* 1990; 140:41-54.

32. Kohrt WM, et al: Effects of gender, age, and fitness level on response of VO$_{2max}$ to training in 60-71 yr olds. *J Appl Physiol* 1991; 71:2004-2011.

33. Lord SR, Ward JA, Williams P, Strudwick M: The effect of a 12-month exercise trial on balance, strength, and falls in older women: A randomized controlled trial. *J Am Geriatr Soc* 1995; 43:1198-1206.

34. Mills EM: The effect of low-intensity aerobic exercise on muscle strength, flexibility, and balance among sedentary elderly persons. *Nurs Res* 1994; 43:207-211.

35. O'Brien SJ, Vertinsky PA: Unfit survivors: Exercise as a resource for aging women. *Gerontologist* 1991; 31:347-357.

36. Ory MG, et al: Frailty and injuries in later life: The FICSIT trials. *J Am Geriatr Soc* 1993; 41:283-296.

37. Oster P, et al: Strength and coordination training for prevention of falls in the elderly. *Z Gerontol Geriatr* 1997; 30:289-292.

38. Pendergast DR, Fisher NM, Calkins E: Cardiovascular, neuromuscular, and metabolic alterations with age leading to frailty. *J Gerontol* 1993; 48:61-67.

39. Raab DM, Agre JC, McAdam M, Smith EL: Light resistance and stretching exercise in elderly women: Effect upon flexibility. *Arch Phys Med Rehabil* 1988; 69:268-272.

40. Reuben DB, Siu AL: An objective measure of physical function of elderly outpatients. The physical performance test. *J Am Geriatr Soc* 1990; 38:1105-1112.

41. Ringsberg K, Gerdehm P, Johansson J, Orbrant KJ: Is there a relationship between balance, gait performance and muscular strength in 75-year-old women? *Age Ageing* 1999; 28:289-293.

42. Rockwood K, Stolee P, McDowell I: Factors associated with institutionalization of older people in Canada: Testing a multifactorial definition of frailty. *J Am Geriatr Soc* 1996; 44:578-582.

43. Roman WJ, et al: Adaptations in the elbow flexors of elderly males after heavy-resistance training. *J Appl Physiol* 1993; 74:750-754.

44. Rooks DS, Kiel DP, Parsons C, Hayes WC: Self-paced resistance training and walking exercise in community-dwelling older adults: Effects on neuromotor performance. *J Gerontol* 1997; 52:M161-168.

45. Schenkman M, Highes MA, Samsa G, Studenski S: The relative importance of strength and balance in chair rise by functionally impaired older individuals. *J Am Geriatr Soc* 1996; 44:1441-1446.

46. Schneider EL, Guralnik JM: The aging of America: Impact on health care costs. *JAMA* 1990; 263:2335-2340.

47. Schroll M, Avlund K, Davidson M: Predictors of five-year functional ability in a longitudinal survey of men and women aged 75 to 80. The 1914-population in Glostrup, Denmark. *Aging: Clin Exp Res* 1997; 9:143-152.

48. Seals DR, et al: Endurance training in older men and women: Cardiovascular response to exercise. *J Appl Physiol* 1984; 57:1024-1029.

49. Seeman TE, et al: Predicting changes in physical performance in a high-functioning elderly cohort: MacArthur studies of successful aging. *J Gerontol* 1994; 49:M97-M108.

50. Shumway-Cook A, Gruber W, Baldwin M, Liao S: The effect of multidimensional exercises on balance, mobility, and fall risk in community-dwelling older adults. *Phys Ther* 1997; 77:46-57.

51. Simonsick EM, et al: Risk due to inactivity in physically capable older adults. *Am J Public Health* 1993; 83:1443-1450.

52. Sipila S, Suominen H: Effects of strength and endurance training on thigh and leg muscle mass and composition in elderly women. *J Appl Physiol* 1995; 78:334-340.

53. Skelton DA, Greig CA, Davies JM, Young A: Strength, power and related functional ability of healthy people aged 65-89 years. *Age Ageing* 1994; 23:371-377.

54. Strawbridge WJ, Camacho TC, Cohen RD, Kaplan GA: Gender differences in factors associated with change in physical functioning in old age: A 6-year longitudinal study. *Gerontologist* 1993; 33:603-639.

55. Topp R, et al: The effect of a 12-week dynamic resistance strength training program on gait velocity and balance of older adults. *Gerontologist* 1993; 33:501-506.

56. Torrey BB, Kinsella K, Taeuber CM: *An Aging World. International Population Reports*, ed 95. U.S. Bureau of the Census, Washington DC, 1987.

57. Whipple RH, Wolfson LI, Amerman PM: The relationship of knee and ankle weakness to falls in nursing home residents: An isokinetic study. *J Am Geriatr Soc* 1987; 35:13-20.

58. Wolf SL, Barnhart HX, Ellison GL, Coogler CE: The effect of Tai Chi Quan and computerized balance training on postural stability in older subjects. Atlanta FICSIT group. Frailty and injuries: Cooperative studies on intervention techniques. *Phys Ther* 1997; 77:371-381.

59. Wolfson L, et al: Balance and strength training in older adults: Intervention gains and Tai Chi maintenance. *J Am Geriatr Soc* 1996; 44:498-506.

60. Wolinsky FD, Callahan CM, Fitzgerald JF, Johnson RJ: The risk of nursing home placement and subsequent death among older adults. *J Gerontol* 1992; 47:S173.

CHAPTER 30

THE OLDER ATHLETE

LYNN SNYDER-MACKLER, PT, ScD, SCS, ATC AND JOHN F. KNARR, PT, MS, ATC

INTRODUCTION

Individuals are living longer and staying physically active into old age. Moreover, the fitness craze of the 1970s and 1980s included persons who came to athletics later in life. Continued or new exercise affects an aging musculoskeletal system in many ways, not all of them positive.[13,19,36] Certainly, the demand for sports rehabilitation services for the geriatric patient will increase along with the population and activity levels.

This chapter defines the geriatric athlete and describes typical musculoskeletal and cardiovascular characteristics found in these individuals. Common musculoskeletal problems are discussed, and the impact of aerobic conditioning on rehabilitation is addressed. The role of comorbidity also is considered. Designing exercise programs for the well elderly individual who is beginning an exercise program or cardiovascular conditioning is not discussed. Practical considerations such as personnel, equipment, and marketing are considered. Finally, case studies are used to illustrate the interrelationship among the variables that affect treatment of the older athlete.

DEFINING THE POPULATION

Who is the geriatric athlete? Unless the population can be defined, identification of problems and potential solutions is difficult. It is actually easier to list who the geriatric athlete is not. The average well elderly person is not discussed here. The care of former athletes also is not reviewed unless these athletes are still actively engaged in regular physical activity. Thus, there are three indistinct groups that make up this population of older athlete. Although there may be an overlap of problems, these groups have some apparent differences that influence their need for rehabilitation services. Each group is dealt with in turn.

The first group consists of former competitive athletes who have continued to exercise, e.g., the football or field hockey team player who is now conditioning on a more individual basis, using running, swimming, or cycling. (As previously mentioned, former competitive athletes who no longer exercise are not discussed in this chapter.) The group being discussed encompasses life-long athletes who trained intensively for a period in their lives and currently may or may not be training at a relative intensity that is comparable with their earlier training levels. A wide variety of sports and training intensities are included in this group; however, these athletes share some similarities that necessitate this categorization. Virtually all the athletes who played team sports as competitive performers and who are still exercising are training at some other sport. For this group, previous injury plays a large role in potential problems in old age.

The second group is composed of life-long recreational athletes. Again, these athletes are involved in quite a spectrum of activities and training intensities. Most, however, are lifetime sports people. They play tennis or squash; they run or cycle. They may even participate in several different activities, but their involvement has been primarily in one sport or group of sports. This population may have a disproportionate amount of the overuse type of injury. For these individuals, athletic activity is as much a part of their routine as dressing or eating meals. They are reluctant to stop participating in an activity, even in the face of significant pain or dysfunction.

The final group is made up of the nonathlete who began to exercise late in life (arbitrarily, after age 40). This is a smaller group but a significant one. These individuals present a unique set of problems related directly to beginning physical activity at an older age and indirectly to their reasons for beginning to exercise. In many instances, exercise has been prescribed (dictated) by a change in health status. Common examples of this type of individual may include the patient who has experienced coronary symptoms (or may be a prime candidate for them) that are the direct result of a number of controllable risk factors including improper diet (obesity) and lack of exercise. In many cases, the physician has prescribed a progressive walking program as a beginning or introduction to exercise. The fact that a person's walking program was begun as a result of a heart attack does not protect him/her from musculoskeletal injury, but it may interfere with motivation for recovery.

The three groups described may differ in the quality of their exercise. Most older athletes are involved in racquet sports, running, walking, and low-impact sports such as golf and bowling. All of these sports can be played in a highly competitive manner against an opponent, a score, or a time.[27] Competitive athletes can be found in any of the three categories of older athlete previously described. Masters athletes are those who are 40 or older. Competitive amateur Masters events have been established for years, e.g., swimming, weight lifting, road running, and track and field. Professionally, the "Senior" golf tour and Masters races for runners are the most high profile events. There was even an attempt to begin a "Senior" baseball league using professional baseball's spring training sites. The trend in population growth toward a larger number of elderly dictates that the number of events and competitors will continue to increase.

All older athletes, regardless of the category in which they fall, have experienced some generic age-related changes. Older athletes are generally less flexible[22,27,33,39] and have smaller muscle masses,[16] lower aerobic capacities,[17,32] and less well-tuned thermoregulatory mechanisms[38] than they did at a younger age. They are likely to have osteoarthritis of the weight-bearing joints. These age-related changes affect training, injury, and treatment of the older athlete and must be considered when designing their rehabilitation program.

MUSCULOSKELETAL PROBLEMS

The older athlete, as the younger athlete, incurs acute or traumatic injury and overuse injury.[27] Unlike the younger athlete, however, these injuries are superimposed on an aging musculoskeletal system, and recovery may take longer. Prevention, therefore, takes on a much more important role in this population. Proper equipment selection and use, e.g., shoes, racquet, and stretching and training techniques must be encouraged to avoid such problems.

Acute, Traumatic Injury

Acute musculoskeletal trauma is different in the older athlete than in the younger athlete. Since most older athletes no longer participate in collision sports, major contusions, fractures, and multiple ligament trauma rarely occur. However, when ligamentous sprains and muscle tears occur, these injuries can be devastating to the older athlete.

Detraining or deconditioning occurs as a result of lack of exercise and takes much less time than training for persons of all ages. The rest required after ligamentous injury or muscle tear can mean the end of athletic activity for an older athlete because of this detraining effect. Fractures, when they occur, are often pathological: osteoporosis and cancer are the most common causes. Fortunately, weight-bearing activity may serve a protective function for women in the case of bone loss and associated fractures, although the intensity and frequency of exercise necessary to achieve this effect are subject to conflicting information.[2]

Overuse Injury

Most serious athletes suffer from injuries that fall into the overuse category; older athletes are no exception. For the purposes of this chapter, *overuse injuries* will be operationally defined as those injuries resulting from training but not attributable to a single traumatic event. Older athletes may actually be more prone to this type of injury than younger athletes.[27] Several factors may contribute to this predisposition. First, older athletes are less flexible than younger athletes.[27,33,39] Second, most have at least some arthritic changes in weight-bearing joints.[15] Third, muscle mass is reduced.[16] Muscle soreness is common, especially at the beginning of an exercise program or when new types of exercise are added to an existing program. This should not be a concern to the therapist. Muscle soreness is attributed to microscopic injury to muscle and connective tissue, which is a necessary prerequisite to muscle strengthening. A certain amount of soreness is expected. Delayed onset muscle soreness (DOMS) occurs in this population as well as in younger populations and occurs 24 to 48 hours after exercise. Rest from exercise (a day off or exercise of uninvolved muscles) and, in some cases, the use of ice and aspirin or some other anti-inflammatory medication will take care of the problem and the athlete will be ready to exercise again the next day. Eccentric exercise appears to be the biggest culprit for DOMS.[1,3,35] Prolonged muscle soreness (significant pain that lasts longer than 48 hours after exercise) should be evaluated. This could indicate muscle or tendon injury that may be the result of overtraining either by frequency, duration, or intensity.

Joint pain and associated effusion also are common in this population. Joint pain as a single symptom should be attended to when it occurs without an associated change in the type or intensity of the exercise or if sharp pain occurs. Otherwise, transient joint pain should be watched and managed symptomatically. If joint effusion or other signs of inflammation occur (redness, warmth), the joint should be thoroughly evaluated because it may be indicative of a more severe underlying problem such as arthritis, infection, fracture, or tumor.

Pain with specific movements or pain that occurs after certain activities that is not "joint pain" or DOMS can occur. These types of injuries are more like the "overuse" injuries that occur in younger athletes. They usually can be attributed to a specific set of circumstances or to structural abnormalities. For example, the athlete with medial knee pain may in fact have tendinitis of the pes anserine region. Other examples may include pain in the subacromial region as a result of impingement of the suprahumeral space, or plantar fasciitis, which may indicate a need for orthotic fabrication. The injuries of older athletes are approached in a similar manner to the problems in younger athletes. In our experience, older athletes respond well to treatment, but healing takes longer and may result in more residual dysfunction.

Arthritis and the Athlete

Articular degeneration is a process that occurs over time. Characterized by joint space narrowing, articular degeneration can be accompanied by swelling, stiffness, and muscle weakness. Inevitably, pain and decreased function result from joint degeneration. The prevalence of osteoarthritis in lower extremities is high in older athletes, especially in the hip and knee.[6,7,37]

In general, treatment of osteoarthritis of the lower extremities should focus on patient education in functional activities, with emphasis on activities that minimize compression and sheer (so-called joint-sparing techniques) to avoid a progression of impairments. Exercise programs to maintain strength and range of motion are supported strongly in the literature. Exercise programs can decrease pain with functional activities, but the long-term effectiveness is somewhat unclear. Exercises should focus on those that minimize weight bearing, e.g., stationary cycling.

Degenerative arthritis of the hip is quite common in the elderly. Groin pain and hip muscle weakness are the primary problems. Patients typically have a Trendelenburg gait. Athletes with symptomatic degenerative arthritis of the hip must avoid weight-bearing athletic activities. Swimming, cycling, and other joint-sparing activities can allow the athlete to participate for a relatively long period of time. Continued progression of the degenerative joint disease, however, often results in the need for hip arthroplasty. Total hip arthroplasty is being performed in younger individuals, and the longevity of the prosthesis itself is increasing. Return to athletic activity takes about 6 months after total hip arthroplasty. This return also depends on maintenance of cardiovascular conditioning during the recovery time.

There are many new orthopedic procedures for treatment of degenerative arthritis of the knee.[29] Focal articular cartilage defects can be treated surgically in many ways. Drilling and micro-fracture techniques allow the defect to fill in with fibrocartilage. The theoretical evidence for healing (6 months to 1 year in some cases before cartilage has maximally healed) supports mitigation of weight bearing after these procedures for at least 3 months. Clinically, this is impractical. Generally, weight bearing is limited for the first 3 to 4 weeks, and joint-sparing activities are emphasized throughout the revolt patient phase.

Two new experimental techniques are being used to facilitate the healing of articular cartilage defects with normal hyaline cartilage, as opposed to fibrocartilage.[29] Autologous chondrocyte transplantation into cartilage defects and osteochondral allograft transplantation (OATS), in which cartilage is taken from a non–weight-bearing surface and transplanted into the articular cartilage defect, both demonstrate some preliminary evidence for effectiveness.[29] Patients who undergo these techniques are restricted from weight-bearing activities for at least 3 months. Return to weight-bearing athletic activity is not recommended.

Patients with focal articular cartilage defects or other types of unicompartmental arthritis can benefit from a relatively new type of functional bracing.[18,24,28] Braces that unload the medial or lateral compartments of the knee have been used throughout the past 10 years and have been studied extensively. This type of brace is designed to unload the affected compartment and to redistribute the load to the more normal or less-involved compartment. Significant pain relief in functional improvement has been demonstrated with the use of these braces.[18,24]

Progressive unicompartmental degeneration usually results in the need for high tibial osteotomy. High tibial osteotomy also can be used to allow individuals to return to a high level of activity. Severe joint degeneration is usually managed with total knee arthroplasty. Patients who have had total knee arthroplasty, unlike those with a total hip arthroplasty, are not encouraged to return to weight-bearing athletic activities. Technological advancement in this area of orthopedic surgery is exponential, and expectations for return to athletic activity is high in the near future.

The Older Shoulder

A lifetime of weightlifting, overhead activities such as baseball and tennis, or participation in collision sports such as football in early adulthood often results in a plethora of problems with the shoulder in older athletes. The most common problems are impingement, partial to full rotator cuff tears, and degenerative acromioclavicular joint problems. In all of these cases the patients usually have a gradual onset of shoulder pain that crescendos and ultimately results in a visit to a physician and then to a physical therapist in an attempt to delay or prevent surgical intervention. These cases are managed differently depending on the patient's activity, pain, and functional goals.

Non-operative management of impingement includes ensuring that the patient has full, pain-free range of motion. Subacromial impingement syndrome in this population usually is a result of some sort of subacromial spurring and may involve rotator cuff tendinitis.[4,5] Patients have symptoms of pain with shoulder motion above the horizontal. The primary problem is a lack of joint space. Physical therapy intervention should be directed at pain management. Joint mobilization can help alleviate the symptoms. In many of these cases the primary pain results from the accompanying rotator cuff tendinitis and/or rotator cuff tear.[25] The supraspinatus muscle is always involved in these cases. Dynamic retraining of the rotator cuff muscles to provide for better humeral head depression during elevation can be very effective in helping patients return to full activity. Reviewing training techniques can be critical to prevent further deterioration of the existing problems. Modifications to limit or restrict some overhead activity, especially in weight training, should be encouraged. Narrower hand spacing, the use of an underhand grip, and avoidance of any behind-the-neck lifts are the primary modifications to weightlifting for this population of patients.[12]

Non-operative management of degenerative acromioclavicular joint disease is limited by the state of the degenerative process. These injuries are usually the result of years of weightlifting as part of the athlete's training regimen, combined with overhead athletic activities. The administration of nonsteroidal anti-inflammatory drugs, modification of activity, and mobilization of the acromioclavicular joint can provide some reduction in symptoms. The use of electrotherapeutic modalities and ice also may help to control global pain. Minimizing repetitive weightlifting trauma is important in this population. Common recommendations for weightlifting modification include no lifting above nipple height and the use of a wide grip for all lifts. Quite often, corticosteroid injections and eventually surgery are inevitable in these patients to allow for their return to athletic activity.

Prevention

Injury prevention has always been an integral part of sports physical therapy. Because even a minor injury can lead to the end of an older athlete's sports participation, prevention is extraordinarily important for the older athlete. There is no substitute for an adequate warm-up before exercise. Athletes who have always avoided this aspect of training find it essential as they age. The best warm-up for a specific activity is 10 minutes or so of low-intensity engagement in that activity. If tennis is the activity, then the players should begin by hitting balls across the net, slowly at first and then with increased velocity and movement. If running is the activity, the runner should begin the first mile at an easy jog and gradually pick up speed. This rule is easily generalized to other sports.

Warm-up is often confused with stretching. Although stretching may be a component of the warm-up for some athletes, stretching can be as much of a problem as it can help. Improper or inconsistent stretching techniques, e.g., ballistic, can cause muscle strains and soreness. Stretching is often a prelude to activity. Although it may not be harmful, stretching a cold muscle is not a sensible idea. As a rule of thumb, athletes who have always stretched before exercise should not be discouraged from doing so. It is suggested, however, that other athletes engage in more global activities to warm the muscles before stretching or, even better, to in-corporate stretching into their cool-down routine. It seems logical to suggest stretching as a remedy for the flexibility changes that occur with aging.[22] However, the reason for the loss of flexibility with aging may be less a result of soft tissue tightness and more a result of joint changes. Some changes include joint surface deterioration, breakdown of the collagen fibers, and a decrease in the viscosity of synovial fluid. In these cases, stretching may not be particularly helpful.

The authors strongly endorse the philosophy of "If it ain't broke, don't fix it" in sports rehabilitation. Others have suggested that abnormal physical findings such as increased Q angle, "tight hamstrings," and excessive pronation should be treated, even in asymptomatic individuals. The authors also do not advocate preventive orthotic fittings or other types of interventions to prevent injury or interfering with an athlete's training regimen just because it might cause problems. Studies that have investigated predisposing factors for overuse injury have been remarkably unsuccessful in establishing a relationship between measurable variables, e.g., rear foot abnormalities, muscle strength, and training regimens, and predisposition to injury.[23]

CARDIOVASCULAR FUNCTION AND LIMITS TO PERFORMANCE

Longitudinal studies of cardiovascular fitness show a decline with increasing age. Physically active individuals, however, demonstrate less of a decline than sedentary individuals (Fig. 30-1).[10,30] Conventional wisdom about aerobic fitness and age is shattered almost weekly; the true limits to performance in the older athlete are largely unknown. Masters and age-group distance running, cycling, and swimming records are lowered at a staggering rate.[4] The Masters marathon record was shattered in 1990 when John Campbell (as a newly minted 40-year-old) finished among the top five runners of all age-groups in the Boston Marathon, running a 2:11:04. Although the ability to do work diminishes with increasing age, the limits are constantly being challenged.

COMORBIDITY

Systemic disease, degenerative disease, and previous injury can have a tremendous impact on athletic performance in the older adult and likely will influence the choice of activity. Systemic diseases whose incidence increases with age include cardiovascular disease and diabetes. Exercise has been shown to have a generally positive effect on these diseases.[9,14,20,21] The therapist needs to be aware of the kinds of screening necessitated by the presence of systemic disease. For example, adults with diabetes should be carefully examined for signs of foot problems related to diminished peripheral sensation secondary to degeneration of myelin and a compromised vascular system due to arteriosclerosis. Other factors associated with diabetes mellitus include coronary complications, kidney failure, blindness, cataracts, and muscle weakness. Degenerative disease, most notably os-

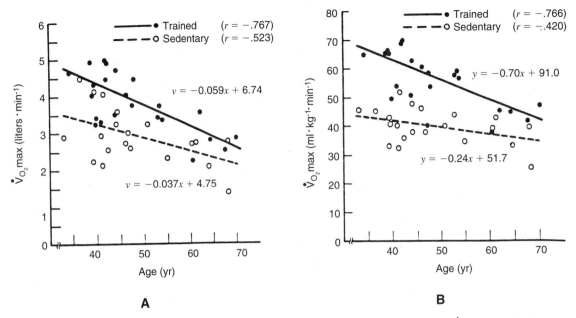

FIG. 30-1 Effects of age on $\dot{V}O_2$max in trained and sedentary men. **A,** The y axis = $\dot{V}O_2$max $1 \cdot min^{-1}$; **B,** The y axis = $\dot{V}O_2$max mL $\cdot$ kg $\cdot$ min^{-1} (From Brooks GA, Fahey TD (eds): *Exercise Physiology.* New York, Macmillan, 1985. Used by permission.)

---

teoarthritis, occurs in most older individuals.[8] However, the relationship of exercise to osteoarthritis is equivocal. Although athletes may have roentgenographic evidence of osteoarthritis, careful physical examination is essential before the osteoarthritis can be incriminated as the cause of exercise-related symptoms. Very often, the presence of osteoarthritis is sufficient for a physician or rehabilitation professional to attribute activity-related pain to arthritis, when in fact it may be merely coincidence that the patient's complaint is in the general area of a joint with osteoarthritis. Degenerative disc disease also can be a problem in the older athlete, but again, radiographic evidence is not sufficient to ascribe symptoms to its presence. Care should be taken to carefully evaluate other possible causes of pain, such as hypomobility, inflammation, and overuse.

PROGRAMMATIC CONSIDERATIONS

When the question, "What do we know about athletic injuries in the older population?" is asked, the answer is "Not much." Much of the literature is anecdotal. Few epidemiological studies have been conducted. From the literature about sedentary individuals who are beginning low- to moderate-level exercise, it can be concluded that injury rarely occurs. This, however, does not necessarily generalize to the older athlete. Therefore the next section of this chapter focuses on recommendations to rehabilitation professionals who would like to treat the older athlete regarding personnel and facilities.

Personnel

The authors, in their collective 30 years of practice of physical therapy and athletic training, have treated many older athletes for musculoskeletal problems associated with exer-

cise. Once injuries occur, regardless of their incidence in the general population or other factors, the patient needs to be treated. Many aspects of treatment of the younger athlete can be generalized to the older athlete. However, the differences inherent in an aging musculoskeletal system and other problems of aging are unique. Some of the changes affecting the skeletal system include deterioration of joint surfaces; breakdown of collagen fibers; and a decrease in the viscosity of synovial fluid, which can result in a loss of flexibility and an increase in joint stiffness. Changes affecting the muscular system include a decrease in the size, number, and type of muscle fibers. Individual motor units lose fibers, which results in a decrease in the force-generating ability of that muscle. There is an effective loss of type II fibers, which results in a higher percentage of type I fibers. Although this change in percentage may increase the muscle's ability to sustain performance during endurance activities, it may limit the muscle's ability to generate strength and power. Muscles experience a decrease in respiratory capacity and an increase in fat and connective tissues. The rehabilitation professional who expects to treat the older athlete must have experience and a good working knowledge of the mechanisms of athletic injuries. The ideal individual would have first-hand experience with caring for athletes before, during, and after athletic participation and know both the physical and psychological demands sports place on the participant. This medical care provider should be versed in a diversity of areas, including anatomy, cardiovascular and muscle physiology, nutrition, biomechanics and kinesiology, physical training, flexibility and conditioning programs, protective/preventive taping and/or bracing, and rehabilitation. Understanding age-related physiological changes and their ramifications relating to physical exercise is vital to the patient's safe and successful return to participation and, in some cases, competition. Knowledge of pathological changes and their effects on the ability to participate in athletic activities is critical in the design and implementation of a rehabilitation program for the older athlete.

Facility

Typical sports or orthopedic outpatient facilities require little change to allow for intervention with the older athlete. Traditional agents and electrotherapeutic modalities, e.g., ice, electrical stimulation, ultrasound, and moist heat, are commonly used in the treatment of the older athlete. Exercise equipment used to treat this population may require some modifications, such as the availability of lighter weights for exercise and slower velocities for instrumented treadmills. Electromechanical devices—which permit isokinetic, isotonic, and isometric exercise and passive motion exercise capabilities—and hydrotherapy also are helpful in the treatment of the older athlete.

Hydrotherapy is being used more frequently for large-joint exercise and rehabilitation of athletic injuries involving all populations of athletes. Smaller exercise tanks have allowed many facilities without room for a therapeutic pool to incorporate much of pool therapy into a smaller area of practice. Its application is especially important when treating the older athlete since it reduces the weight-bearing effects imposed on joint surfaces. The use of this modality also allows the athlete to continue to train and maintain cardiovascular fitness while decreasing the amount of stress to preexisting injuries. The facility should allow for the treatment of different aged athletes together. Interaction among athletes of various ages and sports is helpful to recovery from a motivational aspect. For this reason, a large open exercise area is preferable to small, enclosed booths or cubicles. Although some privacy is lost, the effect of the interaction with other injured athletes is invaluable.

Case Studies

Case 1

A 54-year-old left-handed college professor was referred to the clinic with right shoulder pain that was interfering with his exercise program. He had been a regular participant in an exercise program at the faculty fitness center for the past 5 years. His routine included aerobic exercise on a treadmill or stair climber that was unaffected by his pain and weightlifting. He had some articular degeneration evident on x-ray. He had been taking nonsteroidal anti-inflammatory medication for 2 weeks and noticed a marked improvement. His goal was to return to his weight-training program. He had decreased passive range of motion in glenohumeral abduction, flexion, and external rotation. His right external rotation strength was 50% of that of the left as measured isokinetically at 120 degrees/second. Otherwise, strength was equal in both extremities. All impingement test results were

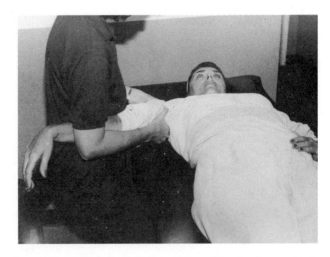

FIG. 30-2 Inferior and posterior glides of the glenohumeral joint can be used to improve range of motion.

positive on the right side.[31] He was tender to palpation of the tendon of the long head of the biceps, the supraspinatus tendon just proximal to its insertion, and the posterior joint capsule. Posterior and inferior glides of the glenohumeral joint were restricted.[31] Posterior glide was painful, and inferior glide reduced his symptoms. The therapists' hypothesis was that inflammation of the tendons and/or bursa in the suprahumeral space resulted in an impingement of these structures, causing pain during movement. The joint range of motion restriction and weakness resulted from the patient splinting and not using the arm fully. The inflammation was being managed medically, and there had been an overall improvement since the patient began to take medication. The intervention addressed the decreased range of motion and strength of the external rotators. Treatment consisted of ultrasound (1.0 W/cm^2) to the posterior capsule, followed by inferior and posterior glides of the glenohumeral joint (Fig. 30-2). Stretching using various techniques, including contract-relax, was incorporated. Transverse friction massage was applied to the bicipital and supraspinatus tendons. Progressive resistive exercises included the use of dumbbells, Theraband, and proprioceptive neuromuscular facilitation techniques for strengthening. The patient was advised to immediately return to those aspects of his athletic program that did not provoke pain in the right shoulder. He was treated twice a week for 4 weeks. The therapists observed his upper extremity weightlifting technique and made some suggestions to alter his mechanics (correcting his technique) to minimize his shoulder pain.[12] The patient was encouraged to eliminate incline and military bench press because these two exercises resulted in the most pain. His range of motion and strength returned to normal. He gradually resumed all his premorbid exercise activities, was weaned from the anti-inflammatory medication, and was discharged.

Case 2

A 73-year-old man was referred to the clinic with increasing left foot pain that was exacerbated by his running. The patient stated that he experienced excruciating pain along the bottom of his foot when he stepped out of bed in the morning that gradually got better over the first hour he was awake. However, after his daily 6-mile run, his pain was much worse. His goal was to resume his running program. He was tender to deep palpation along the plantar surfaces of both feet. Non–weight-bearing examination of his foot position showed normal rear foot and forefoot alignment bilaterally. However, in standing on the left foot as well as on videotaped walking and running sessions on a treadmill, the midtarsal joint appeared to collapse during single-limb support. Accessory motion testing of the talonavicular joints revealed hypermobility bilaterally; calcaneocuboid joints had normal mobility.[31] Ankle range of motion did not appear to be affected. Toe flexor strength was decreased slightly on the left. The therapists' hypothesis was that midtarsal joint hypermobility was causing a severe plantar fasciitis on the left and a mild case on the right foot. The patient was fitted with orthoses for use during all activities, including running. Other intervention included toe flexion exercises for strengthening and ultrasound to the plantar surfaces of both feet. He stopped running until the orthoses were fabricated. After 2 weeks, he was running 3 miles per day without discomfort. He was treated twice a week for 6 weeks, at which time he had stopped wearing the orthoses for all activities, except running. At the time of discharge, he was again running 6 miles per day.

Case 3

A 65-year-old female golfer and cross-country skier tore her anterior cruciate ligament during her first downhill skiing experience 2 weeks before her referral to the clinic. She regularly played golf (3 or 4 times per week from March through October) before her injury, and her major goal was to resume her golf schedule. She had a positive Lachman's test on the right, with no end point.[31] She also had a positive lateral pivot shift.[31] Both test results were consistent with anterior cruciate instability. All other test results were negative. She complained that her knee would give out during level walking. Peak isometric torque of the right quadriceps was 60% of that of the left. Range of motion was 0 to 135 degrees, which was comparable with her left knee. The therapists' hypothesis was that strengthening her quadriceps would help to decrease the instability during walking and that she would be able to return to golfing. She was treated with weight-bearing and non–weight-bearing progressive resistive exercise, as well as neuromuscular electrical stimulation (NMES) to her quadriceps (Fig. 30-3).[34] Although her right quadriceps strength increased to 90% of that of the left, she still had episodes of giving way during walking. She was fitted with a functional brace and began to golf. On her second day of returning to golf, she heard a "pop" at the end of her swing, felt a sharp pain in her knee, and could not straighten it out. She had torn her right medial meniscus and subsequently underwent a partial meniscectomy and a reconstruction of her anterior cruciate ligament. Rehabilitation began in the second postoperative week with passive range of motion, weight-bearing quadriceps exercises in-

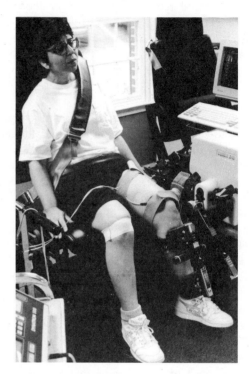

Fig. 30-3 Combination of neuromuscular electrical stimulation (NMES) and isokinetic exercise to improve the strength of the quadriceps.

cluding walking, limited-arc squats, stationary cycling, and NMES.[26] After 3 months, she was back to all daily activities and had resumed playing golf wearing a brace.

Case 4

A 58-year-old female race walker was referred to the clinic with back pain. She had a 4-month history of left-side low back pain with radiation into the left buttock and thigh. Before that time, she was a recreational race walker. She reported that "when it gets really bad," the pain extended to her knee. She had been treated at another clinic, where she received traction in the prone position and some joint mobilization treatment directed at her sacroiliac joint. At the beginning of the examination, she had only slight discomfort in the left side of her back at about the L4 level. Posterior postural evaluation revealed no obvious asymmetry; no lateral deviations or pelvic asymmetry were noted. When she was asked to forward bend, she moved easily and symmetrically into flexion with normal sacroiliac mobility and excursion. However, most of her forward bending occurred in the upper back, as her lumbar spine remained quite fixed. Her movement into extension in standing was restricted but not painful. Repeated flexion in standing caused her back pain to begin to radiate into her left buttock. Repeated extension did not worsen or lessen these symptoms. Because her symptoms were exacerbated with flexion in standing, no supine flexion tests were performed. Prone extension was restricted but again had no effect on her symptoms. Passive range of

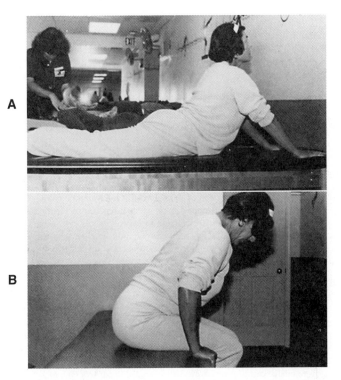

FIG. 30-4 Progession of exercise from prone back extension (A) to flexion in sitting (B).

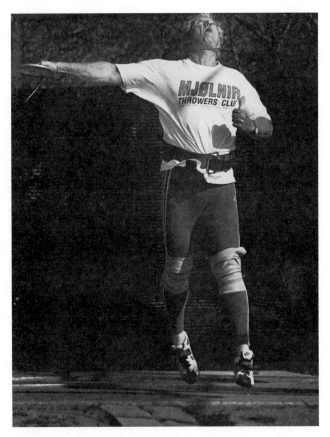

FIG. 30-5 Discus thrower described in Case 5 after recovery.

motion of the lumbar spine was examined in standing and side lying. She had very little motion into either flexion or extension as measured with inclinometers.[14] Passive intervertebral motion testing revealed significant restriction at both the L3-4 and L4-5 levels. The patient described a "stretching pain" during these tests that was unlike her typical symptoms and did not persist after the test. The results of neurological examination of the lower extremities were negative. The therapists' hypothesis was that the patient's symptoms were consistent with extension principle,[11] which appeared to be resolving. Pragmatically, the therapists believed that her problem could be treated symptomatically and that the mobility problems should be directly addressed using joint mobilization. The patient was treated with exercise including prone lying, prone back extension, and eventually back flexion with the patient sitting (Fig. 30-4). Intervertebral anterior glides and rotational mobilization techniques also were used. After 1 month, she began to walk at a slow speed on a treadmill. She gradually increased her speed to a comfortable race-walking pace on the treadmill. After 3 months her lumbar spine range of motion and intervertebral motion had improved. She was nearly pain free in all activities, and she had returned to race walking on the road/track without difficulty. As the patient's goal of pain-free activities of daily living (including race walking) was met, she was discharged.

Case 5

A 57-year-old World Class Masters discus thrower injured his right throwing shoulder while competing. He had com-

plained of a gradual onset of shoulder pain that increased over a few weeks until he was unable to continue throwing. He presented to the clinic with complaints of pain, weakness, and limited function with overhead activities. The patient reported having x-ray studies that demonstrated a hooked acromion.[4]

The initial examination revealed limited right shoulder active range of motion with a painful arc in flexion and abduction. Internal rotation was limited to 50 degrees passively. His posterior capsule was tender to palpation, and he had a decreased posterior glide. Manual muscle testing was painful and rated as a 4-/5 for both the supraspinatus and infraspinatus muscles. The results of special tests for impingement were positive.[4]

This patient began a shoulder rehabilitation program that included posterior and inferior glides and stretching of his shoulder muscles to increase range of motion. He also started an isolated rotator cuff strengthening program by restricting his scapula as he performed external rotation with the shoulder abducted between 20 to 30 degrees. He was instructed to modify his weight training to limit his overhead activities.[12] His physician prescribed a non-steroidal anti-inflammatory drugs to manage the inflammation (Fig. 30-5).

The patient was treated during six visits. His pain level decreased significantly, and he has returned to training for his Master's level competition with only minimal complaints of soreness.

SUMMARY

Older athletes who are injured present a unique set of circumstances to the rehabilitation professional. In spite of their age, they are athletes, and athletic participation is an important part of their lives. Physical therapists need to respect this importance and still understand the constraints imposed on athletic participation by injury to musculoskeletal and cardiovascular systems. This requires knowledge, patience, diplomacy, and a healthy respect for the patients' desires to return to activity.

REFERENCES

1. Abraham WM: Exercise induced muscle soreness. *Phys Sportsmed* 1979; 7:57-60.
2. Aloia JF, Cohn SH, Ostuni JA: Prevention of involitional bone loss by exercise. *Ann Intern Med* 1979; 89:356-358.
3. Armstrong RB: Mechanisms of exercise-induced delayed onset muscular soreness: A brief overview. *Med Sci Sports Exerc* 1984; 6:529-538.
4. Bigliani LU, Levine WN: Subacromial impingement syndrome. *J Bone Joint Surg Am* 1997; 79(12):1854-1868.
5. Blevins FT: Rotator cuff pathology in athletes. *Sports Med* 1997; 24(3):205-220.
6. Boyd KT, Peirce NS, Batt ME: Common hip injuries in sport. *Sports Med* 1997; 24(4):273-288.
7. Buckwalter JA, Lane NE: Athletics and osteoarthritis. *Am J Sports Med* 1997; 25(6):873-881.
8. Clark T: The Master's movement. *Runner's World* 1979; 14:80-83.
9. Costill DF, Miller JM, Fink WJ: Energy metabolism in diabetic distance runners. *Phys Sportsmed* 1980; 8:64-71.
10. Dehn MM, Bruce RA: Longitudinal variations in maximal oxygen uptake with age and activity. *J Appl Physiol* 1972; 33:805-807.
11. Delitto A, Erhard RE, Bowling RW: A treatment-based classification approach to low back syndrome: Identifying and staging patients for conservative treatment. *Phys Ther* 1995; 75(6):470-485; discussion 485-489.
12. Fees M, Decker T, Snyder-Mackler L, Axe MJ: Upper extremity weight-training modifications for the injured athlete. A clinical perspective. *Am J Sports Med* 1998; 26(5):732-742.
13. Fiatarone MA, et al: High-intensity strength training in nonagenarians, effects on skeletal muscle. *JAMA* 1990; 263:3029-3034.
14. Frontera WR, Evans WJ: Exercise performance and endurance training in the elderly. *Top Geriatr Rehabil* 1966; 2:17-31.
15. Gambert SR: Rheumatologic problems in the elderly, in Gambert SR, Benson DM, Gupta KL (eds): *Handbook of Geriatrics*. New York, Plenum Press, 1987.
16. Grimby G, Danneskiold-Samsoe B, Hvid K: Morphology and enzymatic capacity in arm and leg muscles in 78-81 year old men and women. *Acta Physiol Scand* 1982; 115:125-134.
17. Hagberg JM, et al: Cardiovascular responses of 70-79 year old men and women to exercise training. *J Appl Physiol* 1989; 66:2589-2594.
18. Hewett TE, Noyes FR, Barber-Westin SD, Heckmann TP: Decrease in knee joint pain and increase in function in patients with medial compartment arthrosis: A prospective analysis of valgus bracing. *Orthopedics* 1998; 21(2):131-138.
19. Hopp JF: Effects of age and resistance training on skeletal muscle: A review. *Phys Ther* 1993; 73:361-371.
20. Jette DU: Physiological effects of exercise in the diabetic. *Phys Ther* 1984; 64:339-341.
21. Kasch FW, et al: A longitudinal study of cardiovascular stability in active men aged 45 to 65. *Phys Sportsmed* 1988; 16:117-123.
22. Kendall HO, Kendall FP: Normal flexibility according to age groups. *J Bone Joint Surg* 1948; 30A:690-694.
23. Klein AB, et al: Comparison of spinal mobility and isometric trunk extensor forces with electromyographic spectral analysis in identifying low back pain. *Phys Ther* 1991; 71:445-454.
24. Lindenfeld TN, Hewett TE, Andriacchi TP: Joint loading with valgus bracing in patients with varus gonarthrosis. *Clin Orthop* 1997; (344):290-297.
25. Lyons PM, Orwin JF: Rotator cuff tendinopathy and subacromial impingement syndrome. *Med Sci Sports Exerc* 1998; 30(4 Suppl):S12-S17.
26. Manal TJ, Snyder-Mackler L: Practice guidelines for anterior cruciate ligament rehabilitation: A criterion-based rehabilitation progression. *Operative Tech Orthop* 1996; 6(3):190-196.
27. Matheson GO, et al: Musculoskeletal injuries associated with physical activity in older adults. *Med Sci Sports Exerc* 1989; 21:379-385.
28. Matsuno H, Kadowaki KM, Tsuji H: Generation II knee bracing for severe medial compartment osteoarthritis of the knee. *Arch Phys Med Rehabil* 1997; 78(7):745-749.
29. Minas T, Nehrer S: Current concepts in the treatment of articular cartilage defects. *Orthopedics* 1997; 20(6):525-537.
30. Nakamura E, Moritani T, Kanetaka A: Biological age versus physical fitness age. *Eur J Appl Physiol* 1983; 58:778-785.
31. Palmer ML, Epler ME: *Clinical Assessment Procedures in Physical Therapy*. Philadelphia, JB Lippincott, 1990.
32. Seals DR, et al: Endurance training in older men and women. l. Cardiovascular responses to exercise. *J Appl Physiol* 1984; 57:1024-1029.
33. Smith JR, Walker JM: Knee and elbow range of motion in healthy older individuals. *Phys Occup Ther Geriatr* 1983; 2:31-38.
34. Snyder-Mackler L, Delitto A, Bailey S, Stralka SW: Strength of the quadriceps femoris muscle and functional recovery after reconstruction of the anterior cruciate ligament. *J Bone Joint Surg* 1995; 77A(8):1166-1173.
35. Talag TS: Residual muscle soreness as influenced by concentric, eccentric and static contractions. *Res Q* 1973; 44:458-469.
36. Thompson LV: Effects of age and training on skeletal muscle physiology and performance. *Phys Ther* 1994; 74:71-81.
37. Vingard E, Sandmark H, Alfredsson L: Musculoskeletal disorders in former athletes. A cohort study in 114 track and field champions. *Acta Orthop Scand* 1995; 66(3):289-291.
38. Wagner JA, et al: Heat tolerance and acclimatization to work in the heat in relation to age. *J Appl Physiol* 1972; 33:616-662.
39. Walker JM, et al: Active mobility of the extremities in older subjects. *Phys Ther* 1984; 64:919-923.

CHAPTER 31

OLDER PERSONS WITH DEVELOPMENTAL DISABILITIES

TOBY LONG, PT, PhD AND KATHLEEN H. TOSCANO, PT, MHS, PCS

INTRODUCTION

The population of individuals older than 65 years is close to 13%.[2] Included in this group are individuals with a developmental disability who up to a few years ago would not be expected to live to the age of 65 years, much less beyond that.[16] Physical therapists are integral members of the team that serves individuals with developmental disabilities and will be expected to contribute to their care as they get older. A *developmental disability* is defined as a condition that occurs before age 22; continues indefinitely; is a substantial obstacle to the ability to function; and results in a functional limitation in three or more of the following: self-care, receptive or expressive language, learning, mobility, self-direction (or motivation), capacity for independent living, or economic self-sufficiency.[7] This definition includes individuals with mental retardation, cerebral palsy, Down syndrome, autism, and a host of other conditions that encompass a wide range of physical and mental changes that alter the functional abilities throughout the life span. The purpose of this chapter is to discuss the role of the physical therapist in providing intervention services to an elderly person with a developmental disability. Covered specifically are the legislative mandates and philosophical underpinnings of providing services to this population, the unique aspects of aging in selected disability categories, the services rendered by the physical therapist, and the facilities where services may be provided.

DEMOGRAPHICS

Programs designed to serve the general aging population define "old" as 60 years or older. In the developmental disabilities service system, a person with a developmental disability older than age 50 is considered to be "old." This discrepancy is due to the fact that most individuals with a developmental disability have a shorter life expectancy and because of the unproved assumption that individuals with developmental disabilities age more rapidly than does the general population.[24] As the general population of Americans age, so do individuals with developmental disabilities. It is anticipated that throughout the next 20 to 30 years, the number of individuals with developmental disabilities considered "old" (older than age 50) will make up approximately 1% of all persons considered "old."[24]

In the population of older adults with developmental disabilities, women tend to outlive men by about 3 to 1.[24] Surviving cohorts of women who are mentally retarded are more often mildly or moderately retarded, whereas men tend to be severely retarded. The ratio of older men to women with cerebral palsy, however, tends to be higher than that found in the general population of individuals with developmental disabilities. Also, there exists an interaction between gender, age, degree of retardation, and longevity.[16] Women with milder disabilities, such as mild mental retardation, tend to live longer.

Whereas the majority of the general geriatric population live alone or with a spouse, the majority of older adults with a developmental disability live in varied types of community residences.[27] Although the number of individuals living in state institutions has dropped significantly during the last 25 years, few older individuals with a developmental disability live at home. Estimates of persons with developmental disabilities living in their natural homes range from 2% to 31%. Of those living at home, they are often cared for by elderly parents.[16] It is likely, however, that most individuals with a developmental disability live in community-based residential facilities.

Community-based residential facilities are designed as home-like living environments that combine supervision and care with support of a family or group setting. There are four basic types of community-based residential facilities:

1. *Intermediate care facilities (ICFs):* These provide the most intensive group home setting for individuals with health problems, multiple disabilities, or very limited daily living skills. No more than eight individuals reside together in this type of setting.
2. *Community residencies (CRs):* These are group home settings for individuals with moderate abilities to care for themselves. Individuals whose primary disability is moderate mental retardation or autism often reside in these facilities. Up to 12 adults may live together in a CR.
3. *Supportive residencies:* These are for individuals with a significant level of independence. These facilities are often apartments and usually consists of two to three "roommates." Monitoring by a supervisor is done weekly or as needed.
4. *Family care homes:* These are for individuals of all degrees of disability. An individual resides with a family who has been trained and licensed to care for individuals with a developmental disability.

In addition to these community-based residencies, elderly individuals with a developmental disability may reside in skilled nursing facilities, nursing homes, or private residential facilities for persons with developmental disabilities.

THE DEVELOPMENTAL DISABILITIES SERVICE SYSTEM

The system of services for the general population of older Americans, funded primarily through federal monies, is defined as an age-based service system, i.e., the age of the individual determines eligibility for service. The services are designed focusing on the needs of the group of older citizens. In contrast, the service system for older adults with a developmental disability is considered to be needs-based and provides individualized, specialized services. Provisions for age-specialized models of service exist within this system, which is primarily state funded. The current focus of service provision is to bridge these two service delivery systems—one based on age and the other on need—and to encourage collaboration and joint planning between the systems to ensure that an individual's needs are best met in the most efficient community-based manner as possible. This contemporary

model of service provision has evolved from the "normalization " movement of the 1960s.[35] This movement was grounded in the belief that individuals would develop optimally if they were integrated into society and afforded the same experiences as those without disabilities.

The community-based model of care operationalized the normalization philosophy. By the mid-1970s states began to develop community-based residential and treatment programs. Individuals who had the opportunity to take advantage of these programs were more functional and independent than their counterparts in institutions.[6] Thus, the movement toward deinstitutionalization took hold, and by 1991 a nationwide movement took place to close all state-supported residential facilities and develop community-integrated living and vocational and leisure programming. During the last 2 decades, specific federal legislation has been passed that supports the community-based model of care and provides systems to increase the likelihood that adults and older persons with a developmental disability will become integral members of the community. The major pieces of legislation that affect service provision to older men and women with a developmental disability are outlined in Box 31-1.

BOX 31-1

LEGISLATION AFFECTING SERVICES TO OLDER ADULTS WITH DEVELOPMENTAL DISABILITIES

Older American Act Amendments (OAA) 1987

- Mandated that older persons with developmental disabilities be served under the act's provisions
- Mandated that the Administration on Aging (AOA) collaborate with the developmental disability service system to design and implement appropriate services
- OAA programs were opened to elders with developmental disabilities

Developmental Disabilities Assistance and Bill of Rights Act (1987)

- Extended the provisions of the Developmental Disabilities Services and Facilities Construction Act of 1970
- Identified service delivery models to accommodate growth in population and need for trained professionals
- Promoted community-based residential services

Americans with Disabilities Act (ADA) (1990)

- Provisions include access to and participation in senior citizen centers, day care sites, and social service centers for individuals with developmental disabilities

The Domestic Volunteer Service Act (1975)

- Authorized senior companions to assist adults with developmental disabilities

Omnibus Budget Reconciliation Act (1981)

- Before admission to a nursing home, a screening must be performed for every person with a developmental disability
- Annual review of every person with a developmental disability who resides in a nursing facility
- Persons with developmental disabilities who are found to be inappropriately placed in a nursing home must be discharged

UNIQUE ASPECTS OF AGING IN SPECIFIC DISABILITIES

As indicated previously, a developmental disability is a chronic condition that occurs before adulthood and significantly affects functional activities. The three most common developmental disabilities seen by physical therapists are mental retardation, cerebral palsy, and Down syndrome. Until recently little research documenting the changes seen in individuals with these disabilities had been conducted nor had the medical community felt the need to conduct such research since up to approximately 20 years ago, few individuals with disabilities lived beyond middle age. Longevity for individuals with Down syndrome and those with cerebral palsy is increasing. With increasing longevity, there has been a concomitant interest in the aging process for these individuals.

Down Syndrome

Age-related changes in the behavior of individuals with Down syndrome have been documented.[6,22,29] The age of onset of the decline and underlying reasons for this premature decline have yet to be determined. However, there is a growing body of literature that discusses two possibilities for this decline: Alzheimer's disease [21,26] and depression.[32]

Alzheimer's Disease

Although the exact incidence of Alzheimer's disease in individuals with Down syndrome is unknown, an estimated 40% to 45% of these individuals between 50 to 70 years of age will develop Alzheimer's disease. This incidence is three to five times greater than in the general population.[20] Furthermore, the age of onset is much earlier in those with Down syndrome (age 35 to 45 years) than seen in the general population.[25] Current research suggests a causative link between the excess material in chromosome 21 and apoliprotein production and deposition—the neuropathological finding seen in individuals with Alzheimer's who are not developmentally disabled.

Early symptoms of Alzheimer's disease in older adults with Down syndrome are similar to those in the general population: loss of memory and logical thinking, diminished abilities to perform activities of daily living, changes in gait and coordination, and loss of bowel and bladder control. Individuals with Down syndrome also develop seizure activity, a symptom not common in the general population. It is recommended that individuals with Down syndrome receive psychological testing annually starting at age 30 to determine and monitor loss of skills. Because of the known cognitive impairments of individuals with Down syndrome, declines in activities of daily living skills may be a better indicator of Alzheimer's disease than memory and cognitive loss.[22] A checklist has been developed that can be used reliably to identify early signs of Alzheimer's dementia in adults with Down syndrome.[34] Other tools, such as the Adaptive Behavior Scale,[11] the Client Development Evaluation Report,[4] and the Vineland Adaptive Behavior Scales,[30] also have been used to identify functional decline in individuals with Down syndrome.

Depression

There is indication that some individuals with Down syndrome are erroneously diagnosed as having Alzheimer's disease when, in fact, they are depressed.[32] Since depression is a treatable condition and Alzheimer's is only manageable at this time, distinguishing between the two is important for care-giving purposes. The prevalence of depression in individuals with Down syndrome is between 6% to 12%.[32] In addition to Alzheimer's, symptoms associated with other conditions such as hypothyroidism and hearing loss mask the identification of depression in individuals with Down syndrome. Although severely depressed individuals also show a loss of adaptive skills, the pattern of loss tends to be up and down rather than a continuous decline as seen in dementia. Also, individuals with depression respond positively to intervention and will regain skills that were once thought to have been lost. In addition to changes noted in adaptive skills, it is important to document changes in affective behaviors such as sadness; crying; increases in self-injurious, assaultive, or aggressive behaviors; and somatic complaints.[32]

Cerebral Palsy

Little information exists on how the aging process affects persons with cerebral palsy, and there is no reason to suspect that cerebral palsy alters the genetically driven process of aging. Life expectancy for individuals with cerebral palsy has not been studied extensively. Of the studies conducted in the 1990s, data indicate that individuals with cerebral palsy who lack mobility, are severely or profoundly mentally retarded, and cannot feed themselves have a decreased life expectancy.[10] However, the chronic physical impairments and conditions associated with cerebral palsy may affect the onset or severity of age-related changes. Box 31-2 lists the conditions that individuals with cerebral palsy identified as concerns during the National Invitational Colloquium on Aging and Cerebral Palsy held in 1993. During this colloquium, the participants also noted as concerns a decline in functioning in older adults and lack of access to appropriate health care services, including physical therapy. As indicated in the box, many complications seen in adults with cerebral palsy are re-

---

BOX 31-2

SECONDARY CONDITIONS OF CONCERN TO OLDER ADULTS WITH CEREBRAL PALSY

Musculoskeletal deformities
Pain syndrome
Cervical spine stenosis
Deconditioning
Change in skills
Falls
Osteoporosis
Fractures
Pressure sores
Emotional issues

lated to musculoskeletal changes. These impairments include contractures, scoliosis, hip subluxation or dislocation, and pathological fractures that can lead to pain (a problem not noted in young children with cerebral palsy), all contributing to a loss of independent living skills.[33] Postural pain (back or cervical) has been associated with inadequate wheelchair fitting and repair status in adults with cerebral palsy.[23]

In addition to the physical stressors listed in Box 31-2, there also are social and psychological stresses that may be evident earlier in life than what is seen in the general population due to the multiple disabilities seen in individuals with cerebral palsy. These include decreased opportunities for age-appropriate leisure and social activities, feelings of isolation, and depression.

EXAMINATION AND EVALUATION

A key role of the physical therapist working with this population is to comprehensively examine the patient because a comprehensive examination forms the basis for clinical decision making. The components of a comprehensive examination are described in the following text and listed in Box 31-3.

History

Documenting pertinent history of the patient's health and behavioral changes can help the therapist make decisions on the appropriateness of specific therapeutic strategies. In addition to the patient's developmental disability, confounding problems such as congestive heart disease, hypertension, or diabetes also may be present. These comorbidities could influence recommendations or treatment strategies. It is likely that individuals with developmental disabilities, especially cerebral palsy, will have a history of surgical intervention. As mul-

---

tiple surgical procedures may lead to scarring and deformity, it is essential to document the time frame of when the surgery occurred and how it has affected the person over time. Medications for treatment of conditions directly related to the developmental disability and those related to additional conditions should be thoroughly documented. Long-term use of anti-convulsive medications may lead to physical findings such as ataxia and tardive dyskinesia.[1] Also, behavioral changes may be related to medication use. Most individuals with a developmental disability will have had many years of various therapeutic interventions, and summarizing those interventions and their effects will prove invaluable for treatment planning. Documenting the use and effects of additional interventions, such as occupational therapy, special instruction, and therapeutic recreation that the client participates in, will assist in designing comprehensive programming that is collaborative with other disciplines and is not redundant.

Behavioral Response

Individuals with a developmental disability, especially those with severe profound mental retardation, autism, or emotional disturbance, may demonstrate behavioral characteristics that can interfere with functional use of motor skills. Documentation of the person's response to interactions and performance demands during the examination will assist with designing appropriate treatment plans. Documenting behavior also will help differentiate between behavioral characteristics that are consistent with the individual's developmental diagnosis and with those that are consistent with aging or other disabilities or medical conditions, such as depression. Documentation of antecedents to a behavioral outburst or change in behavior will assist the team in designing appropriate interaction plans and behavioral support strategies. Also, the therapist should document the method used by the individual, e.g., verbal, gestures, or sign language, to communicate needs.

Neuromusculoskeletal Status

Traditional tests of neuromusculoskeletal status, such as manual muscle tests and goniometry, may not provide the information needed to make functionally oriented habilitation plans. The physical therapist should judge through observation the client's degree of *flexibility, strength,* and *balance* within activities that are functional for the individual. It is likely that the client may have long-term limitations in range of motion and decreased strength that he/she has learned to compensate for and do not contribute to his/her functional limitations. Additionally, the therapist must be aware of the individual's interests and activity level to determine whether an impairment results in functional limitation. For example, a person with mental retardation who swims on a regular basis may consider a decrease in shoulder range of motion a significant limitation over a person who does not swim. This same approach should be taken when examining endurance and muscle strength. Assessment of strength and endurance should be performed

---

Box 31-3
COMPONENTS OF A COMPREHENSIVE PHYSICAL THERAPY EXAMINATION

History
    Medical
    Surgical
    Therapeutic
    Intervention
    Medications
    Cognition
Behavioral response
Neuromuscular status
    Flexibility
    Strength
    Muscle tone
    Posture
    Endurance
Functional skills
    Balance
    Gait
    Activities of daily living
    Use of assistive technology

within the context of functional activities that are meaningful to the individual, are age-appropriate, and are consistent with the client's desired outcomes. Table 31-1 outlines a variety of tools that are used to evaluate functional status of an individual with a disability and are discussed in depth below. One of these tools, the Functional Outcome Assessment Grid (FOAG),[5] also incorporates the assessment of neuromuscular components in the performance of specific functional activities.

Motor Function and Functional Activities

Motor function skills are those that underlie activities that the individual does or would like to do on a regular basis and are meaningful to both the client and care-givers. These skills are evident in examining mobility within the home and community and activities of daily living (ADL). The influence of gait patterns and balance on mobility also are components of motor function. Historically, elderly individuals with developmental disabilities were administered developmental motor assessments that determined the developmental age level of their skill performance.

As most clients will have documented delays in the acquisition of motor skills, it is inappropriate to test an adult with measures used to determine developmental skill level. It is, however, important to document skills that have been linked to functional activities and ADL (basic and instrumental), mobility, and recreation. In addition to the tools discussed in Chapter 7,[13,14,18,19] (Katz Index of Activities of Daily Living, Functional Independence Measure, Older American Resources and Services, the Philadelphia Geriatric Center Multilevel Assessment Instrument), elderly individuals with developmental disabilities can be assessed on the dimensions contained on the Pediatric Evaluation of Disability Inventory, The Scales of Independent Behavior, and the FOAG.

Pediatric Evaluation of Disability Inventory

The Pediatric Evaluation of Disability Inventory (PEDI) is a standardized, norm-referenced inventory that can be ad-

ministered by care-giver report, structured interview with a care-giver, or through professional observation of a client's behavior.[15] The PEDI is divided into two scales. The Functional Skill Scale has three subtests: self-care, mobility, and social function. Environmental modification and amount of care-giver assistance is systematically recorded in the Modification Scale and Caregiver Assistance Scale. Although standardized on children from 6 months old to 7 years, 6 months old, the items on the PEDI can be administered to older individuals to describe patterns of strengths and needs to assist with program planning. The Modification Scale and the Caregiver Assistance Scale also provide valuable information for program planning and documenting benefits from intervention aimed at decreasing the burden of care for an individual.

Scales of Independent Behavior

The Scales of Independent Behavior (SIB) measures functional independence and adaptive functioning in the school, home, and employment and community settings.[3] It has been specifically designed to be used with children, adults, and the elderly population. The SIB is a norm-referenced test that has been standardized on individuals aged 3 months to 90 years and older. The full scale is divided into 14 subscales, which are organized into four clusters: motor skills, social interaction and communication, personal living skills, and community living skills. Of particular interest to the geriatric population are items related not only personal care but also domestic skills, such as homemaking and community orientation. The design of the SIB also allows comparison of an individual's functional independence with cognitive status. A Screening Form and a Problem Behavior Scale are also available.

Functional Outcome Assessment Grid

The FOAG is based on the top-down model of assessing function.[5] Using the desired outcome as the starting point, the therapist determines barriers to the accomplishment of the task and strengths that will assist the client in

TABLE 31-1
ASSESSMENT TOOLS

Tool	Author	Purpose	Source
Functional Outcome Grid (FOAG)	Campbell, P*	To determine factors that limit or support the acquisition of specific skills	Allegheny University of the Health Services Broad and Vine Streets Philadelphia, PA 19102
Pediatric Evaluation of Disability Inventory (PEDI)	Haley, S, Coster, W, Ludlow, L, Haltiwarger, Andrellas, P*	To determine functional capabilities and performance, monitor progress, and evaluate therapeutic or rehabilitative program outcome	PEDI Research Group Department of Rehabilitative Medicine New England Medical Center Hospital 751750 Washington St. Boston, MA 02111-1901
Scales of Independent Behavior (SIB)	Bruininks, R, Woodcock, R, Watherman, R, Hill, B*	To measure functional independence and adaptive functioning across settings	Riverside Publishing Co. 8420 Bryn Mawr Ave. Chicago, IL 60603

*See References 3,5,15 at the end of the chapter.

accomplishing the task. Using this model, the purpose of the FOAG is to assist the team in developing and implementing functional outcomes. The FOAG is individualized, based on team consensus of desired outcomes for the client. Although there are six functional outcome areas that can be assessed, each area can be assessed independently. The six areas—caring for self, communication, learning and problem solving, mobility, play, and leisure— are associated with four disability categories: physical, sensory, special health care needs, and other. The patient is observed attempting the desired outcome, and the therapist rates components skills, such as muscle tone, strength, and flexibility, on a five-point scale from no problem to significant problem that affects or prevents skill performance. Program plans are then designed that bypass obstacles, promote strengths, and/or improve deficits.

Gait, Balance, and Locomotion

In addition to using specific assessment tools, documenting the *gait* pattern of the client is important. Individuals with developmental disabilities, especially those with cerebral palsy, have well-documented gait deviations and neuromuscular impairments. Gait assessment should document those impairments but more importantly determine the functional limitation imposed by the gait deviations. It is preferred that a gait assessment be performed in various natural settings and over a variety of terrains to determine the impact of the gait characteristics on the ability of a person to maneuver functionally. As noted in the elderly population without developmental disabilities, the client may show a decrease in speed of ambulation and an increase in energy expenditure as he/she ages.[31] Increased energy expenditure may be more pronounced in individuals with postural deviations.[12]

Balance also should be assessed. Again, traditional balance tools used with younger individuals with developmental disabilities, such as the ability to walk a balance beam or stand on one foot, may not be the most appropriate methods to determine balance in the context of function. Maintenance of balance within functional activities, such as individuals maneuvering in their own environments during routine activities, may be more helpful for program planning. The Functional Reach Measure[8] or the Progressive Mobility Skills Assessment Task,[11] as discussed in Chapter 18, may be appropriate for some individuals. Although these measures have not been validated on individuals with developmental disabilities, their use may provide additional clinical information to assist with decision making.

Assistive Technology

Many individuals with developmental disabilities use *assistive technology*. Assistive technology consists of simple adaptive equipment devices, such as adaptive spoons, to very complex computer-driven communication systems. The use of assistive technology may increase for adults with developmental disabilities as they become older. As seen in elders without developmental disabilities, the use of mobility devices will increase. This is especially true for the use of wheelchairs for individuals with cerebral palsy. A thorough assessment of the fit and appropriateness of a wheelchair or ambulatory device should be part of a comprehensive examination. The assessment of the use of assistive technology should be performed within the environment that it is to be used. Assessing the devices also will require assessment of the environment to determine whether it is conducive for the size, shape, and weight of the device. Before a person is placed in a community residential facility, the physical therapist may be asked, as part of the team, to assess the environment to ensure appropriateness for an individual's needs.

The evaluation of an older adult with a developmental disability must be comprehensive and meaningful to the person's activity level and living situation and must be individualized to meet specific needs. The therapist must consider the client's impairments, functional limitations, skill acquisition, environment, and desired functional outcomes in planning the evaluation strategies and procedures. Functionally based examinations are clinically useful.

PROGRAM PLANNING AND IMPLEMENTION

Habilitation vs. Rehabilitation

Older adults with developmental disabilities generally necessitate habilitation programs. *Habilitation,* as distinguished from rehabilitation, refers to services that assist an individual in gaining skills and abilities.[28] Rehabilitation attempts to restore skills that have been lost due to injury or medical condition.[21] Habilitation is required by law, under Medicaid regulations, and financed by Title 19 of the Social Security Act. Habilitation services for the older adult are generally provided by an interdisciplinary team. The *Individualized Habilitation Plan (IHP)* is the document that records the outcomes and goals and programmatic strategies decided by the team to be necessary for the client to attain or maintain an optimal level of independence.

The interdisciplinary team is the team approach that is most commonly used with older persons with developmental disabilities.[17] The team consists of various professionals—e.g., occupational therapists, medical doctors, speech-language pathologists, nurses, psychologists, nutritionists, special education teachers, and social workers—who independently evaluate the individual and then meet together and share their findings with each other and the individual. Based on this information and the desired outcomes of the patient and/or care-givers, the team formulates a comprehensive plan that will best meet the needs of that individual.

The role of the physical therapist on the team is determined by the needs of the client and the priority outcomes established on the IHP. The therapist may be a direct provider of service, a consultant to other team members, or a monitor of programs carried out by direct care providers. Although individuals have long-term disabilities, the role of *direct provider* of physical therapy may be intermittent. The level of intensity will be related to the prioritized outcomes of the IHP or the need for services after an acute illness or injury. More often, the therapist may be an indirect provider of service. As a *monitor* of services, the therapist establishes functional goals that are consistent with the outcomes prioritized on the IHP and trains other individuals (usually direct care providers) in a specific program aimed at achieving goals. The therapist creates a data collection system for the person implementing the program and monitors the client's progress at an appropriate frequency. Figs. 31-1 and 31-2 are examples of simple data collection systems designed for individuals living in an intermediate-care facility. The data collection system must be very simple to increase the likelihood that it will be completed by the staff. Also, the staff carrying out the program implementation must be trained and supervised. Monitoring of the program data collection and intermittent retraining must be performed on a regular basis with adaptations to the program as necessary.

The role of *consultant* requires the therapist to respond to specific requests of the client, care-givers, or program staff. Unlike monitoring services, the therapist providing consultation is not directly responsible for the outcomes of the individual client.[9] The therapist is responsible for providing to the consultee information that is helpful to assist the client in meeting the outcomes. Dunn and Campbell describe three types of consultation.[9] *Case consultation* focuses on the needs of an individual client. The therapist, for example,

may provide a care-giver suggestions on how to involve a client with cerebral palsy in leisure activities. *Colleague consultation* targets the needs of other service providers. Discussing with direct care-givers proper body mechanics to prevent back injury when transferring a patient would be an example of colleague consultation. The purpose of *system consultation* is to effect system change, with the focus being on the service delivery system rather than a specific client. In-service training, program development, or evaluation are examples of system consultation.

Regardless of the role the physical therapist takes in implementing the therapeutic program, an appropriate documentation system must be established. Documentation is important and should meet the needs of those involved in the program, third party payers, and the service system (developmental disabilities or aging). If the therapist is acting as a direct service provider, progress and the response to treatment should be documented at each visit. The plan for future treatment also should be included. If service is being provided on an indirect basis, a system for documentation must be created for those implementing the program (see Figs. 31-1 and 31-2). As indicated previously, this documentation should provide an objective measurement of the individual's progress, and the system must be clear and concise so that it is not burdensome to the care-givers. Therapists also must follow the regulations of the Medicaid and Medicare systems (see Chapter 26). Unfortunately, this may require duplication of documentation in

Goal: Tom will ambulate with his walker from the living room to his bedroom in 5 minutes.

Date	2/1	2/2	2/3	2/4	2/5	2/6	2/7	2/8	2/9	2/10
Record time in minutes	10	10	9	10	9	8	9	8	8	8
Initial										

Questions/concerns - please call E. Becker, PT, MS 202-555-7121

FIG. 31-1 Data collection system for Tom Charles, a 77-year-old man with mild-moderate mental retardation and decreased endurance due to acute emphysema.

Goal: Chris will transfer from a chair into his walker independently.

Date	2/1	2/2	2/3	2/4	2/5	2/6	2/7	2/8	2/9	2/10
Assistance needed to steady the chair Y/N	Y	Y	Y	Y	Y	N				
Assistance needed at the arms to pull up Y/N	Y	N	Y	N	N	N				
Initial										

Questions/concerns - please call C. McIntyre, DPT, 508-555-4425

FIG. 31-2 Data collection system for Chris Allen, a 59-year-old with moderate spastic diplegia.

various formats to meet the requirements of the various regulatory systems.

Resources

Since the challenge of providing services to this population is an emerging area of service delivery, it may be helpful to consult current journals in geriatrics and developmental disabilities. Periodicals such as *Mental Retardation, American Journal of Mental Retardation,* and *Journal of the Association for Persons with Severe Handicaps* may be helpful. Also, the Administration on Developmental Disabilities has funded selected University Affiliated Programs to develop training and service programs specifically for older persons with developmental disabilities. These programs offer multimedia information and are available to train service providers in providing appropriate care to elders with developmental disabilities (Box 31-4).

Box 31-4

UNIVERSITY AFFILIATED PROGRAMS WITH SPECIFIC PROGRAMS FOR OLDER PERSONS WITH DEVELOPMENTAL DISABILITIES

- *University Affiliated Program for Developmental Disabilities*, University of Arkansas, James L. Dennis Development Center, 1612 Maryland, Little Rock, AR 72202, (501) 569-3184.
- *Mailman Center for Child Development*, University of Miami, School of Medicine, P.O. Box 016820, D-820, Miami, FL 33101, (305) 547-6635.
- *Institute for Study of Developmental Disabilities*, Indiana University, 2853 E. 10th St., Bloomington, IN 47408-2601, (812) 855-6508.
- *Eunice Shriver Center*, 200 Trapelo Road, Waltham, MA 02115, (617) 734-7509.
- *Institute for Human Development*, Univeristy of Missouri-Kansas City, 22200 Holmes St., Third Floor, Kansas City, MO 64108, (816) 235-1770.
- *Strong Center for Developmental Disabilities*, University of Rochester Medical Center, 601 Elmwood Ave., Rochester, NY 14642, (716) 275-2986.
- *North Dakota Center for Developmental Disabilities*, Minot State University, 500 University Ave. W, Minot, ND 58071, (701) 857-3580.

Case Studies

Case 1

Zachary is a 67-year-old man with mild-moderate mental retardation and cerebral palsy of the spastic diplegic type. He is able to communicate verbally. He lives in an intermediate-care facility and attends a day treatment program. As a child, he walked with crutches and long leg braces. He had hamstring lengthenings and heelcord lengthenings at age 10 years and again when he was 14 years old. As he got older,

he continued to walk with crutches but without the braces. By the time Zachary reached 60 years old, his gait had slowed considerably and he was encouraged to use a wheelchair by the staff at his day treatment program. A manual wheelchair was purchased for Zachary when he was 62 years old. By 67, Zachary had gained 17 pounds and his wheelchair needed to be replaced. The range of motion in Zachary's legs had become more limited, making even stand-pivot transfers difficult.

Planning and implementing a program appropriate for Zachary involved a comprehensive examination as previously described. Through an interview with Zachary and his care-givers, it was found that Zachary was somewhat depressed regarding his inability to walk. He also was found to have an interest in improving his ability to manage transfers to and from the toilet independently. The care-givers stated that Zachary enjoyed swimming and was independent in the shallow water at the pool.

The information gained from the informal interview was enhanced by the structured interview of the PEDI. This data coupled with the information gained from the neuromuscular assessment allowed the therapist to create appropriate goals and a realistic plan that involved the desires of Zachary and his care-givers.

Independence in stand-pivot transfers was one goal. To achieve that goal, the therapist instructed Zachary's care-givers on performing transfers with the client and encouraging greater assistance from Zachary. The plan involved having Zachary practice this transfer each time he needed to use the bathroom. To create a program that was more likely to help Zachary reach his goals, the staff at the day treatment program also received training and agreed to follow the plan as designed. The therapist monitored progress weekly for 1 month and then monthly for another 2 months to ensure progression toward the goal. Additionally, building on Zachary's interest in swimming, the team designed a swimming program that would (1) promote cardiovascular fitness and weight loss and (2) improve lower extremity strength. Both of these goals would assist him in reaching his stand-pivot goal as well. Activities included swimming laps and practicing standing and walking in the water. The recreational therapist monitored the program monthly with an agreement to contact the physical therapist with any questions or concerns.

In collaboration with the social worker and physician, a new, appropriate wheelchair was prescribed and obtained for Zachary. Zachary and his care-givers were consulted to ensure that the chair was functional for him and would be easily transportable. The therapist assessed the wheelchair on a quarterly basis for safety, fit, and function. The therapist taught the staff appropriate wheelchair care and maintenance.

Zachary and his care-givers were pleased with the program because it took into consideration everyone's needs and Zachary's desired outcome. Zachary was pleased because he was able to practice "walking" in the water, which he enjoyed. He was motivated to practice the stand-pivot transfer because he wanted to regain the ability to transfer independently. This intervention program proved to be quite successful. At the end of 3 months, Zachary had lost weight; was able to complete a standing-pivot transfer with only stand-by assistance; and his new wheelchair was modern and streamlined, allowing him to maneuver in his home more efficiently. The success of this program was due to the collaboration among all team members including Zachary and the fact that it was based on Zachary's desired outcomes.

Case 2

Lisa is 71 years old and has a diagnosis of mild mental retardation. She lives in a community residential facility and attends an integrated adult day care program at a local nursing home. Lisa ambulates independently on all surfaces including stairs. She is independent in activities of daily living. She is able to take a bus to a destination, after she has been shown three to four times. Lisa has always enjoyed riding a stationary bike, but her knees and hips have begun to bother her. She has been diagnosed as having osteoarthritis, and her physician suggested that she find an alternate activity to replace the stationary bike riding.

Upon interviewing Lisa and the supervisors of her CRF, it was discovered that Lisa once enjoyed swimming, but since she had moved to this particular facility 7 years ago, there had been no opportunity for this activity. The physical therapist realized that Lisa was not in need of his direct services, but he felt that she could benefit from a non–weight-bearing exercise program. The physical therapist collaborated with the group home supervisor, recreational therapist, and social worker to involve Lisa in a regular swimming program. The social worker found a companion to accompany Lisa on the bus to a local indoor pool. The recreational therapist arranged with the staff at the pool to have Lisa participate in a water aerobics class. The adult day care staff were made aware that Lisa would be coming in late on Wednesdays and Fridays—the days she would participate in the aerobics program. The physical therapist was available to consult with the home care providers, recreational therapist, and pool staff, if necessary.

Lisa and the staff were pleased with the progress. Lisa experienced a problem often seen in the aging population, but her developmental disability made it difficult for her to access appropriate care and activities. The therapist in consultation with other members of the interdisciplinary team found an activity that Lisa enjoyed and created an effective program for her. Through a collaborative effort, a program was implemented that met the patient's needs.

SUMMARY

Information regarding aging individuals with developmental disabilities has recently begun to receive attention in the literature. Older persons with developmental disabilities have begun to be recognized by service providers and policy makers as a large heterogeneous group who require specialized services integrated into the service system of the general population of elders.

This chapter reviewed the legal mandates and social policy impetus guiding service to this group. The role of the physical therapist in examining individuals and assisting team members with designing appropriate, holistic habilitation plans was presented. Although little information is available on specific aspects of the aging process in developmental disabilities, aspects of aging in persons with Down syndrome and cerebral palsy were discussed.

Physical therapists are in a unique position to assume leadership roles in the care of elders with developmental disabilities and develop integrated programs of habilitation. Additionally, a critical role for physical therapists will be to design and foster leisure skill programming for these persons that will promote and maintain functional skills. Physical therapists also are in a position to effect system change, specifically recognizing the importance of leisure skill programming and creating reimbursement strategies that will take leisure skill programming into consideration.

REFERENCES

1. Bodfish JW, et al: Akathisia in adults with mental retardation: Development of the Akathisia Ratings of Movement Scale (ARMS). *Am J Ment Retard* 1997; 101:413-423.
2. Brock DB, Guralnik JM, Brody JA: Demography and epidemiology of aging in the United States, in Schneider EL, Rowe JW (eds): *Handbook of the Biology of Aging*, ed 3. San Diego, Academic Press, 1990.
3. Bruininks R, et al: *Scales of Independent Behavior*. Circle Pines, Minn, American Guidance Service, 1985.
4. California State Department of Developmental Services: *Client Developmental Evaluation Report*. Sacramento, Author, 1978.
5. Campbell PH: Supporting the medical and physical needs of students with deaf-blindness in inclusive settings, in Haring NG, Romer LT (eds): *Including Students with Deaf-Blindness in Typical Educational Settings*. Baltimore, Paul H Brookes, 1995.
6. Collacot RA: The effect of age and residential placement on adaptive behaviour of adults with Down's syndrome. *Brit J Psych* 1992; 161: 675-679.
7. *Developmental Disabilities Bill of Rights and Assistance Act*, 1987.
8. Duncan PW, et al: Functional reach: A new measure of balance. *J Gerontol* 1990; 45:M192-197.
9. Dunn W, Campbell PH: Designing pediatric service provision, in Dunn W (ed): *Pediatric Occupational Therapy: Facilitating Effective Service Provision*. Thorofare, NJ, Slack, 1991.
10. Eyman RK, Grossman HT, Chaney RH, Call TL: The life expectancy of profoundly handicapped people with mental retardation. *New Engl J Med* 1990; 323:584-589.
11. Fogelman CJ: *AAMD Adaptive Behavior Scale Manual*. Washington, DC, American Association of Mental Deficiency, 1975.
12. Gage JR: *Gait Analysis in Cerebral Palsy*. London, MacKeith Press, 1991.
13. George LK, Fillenbaum GG: OARS methodology: A decade of experience in geriatric assessment. *J Am Geriatr Soc* 1985; 33:607-615.
14. Granger CV, Keith RA, Hamilton BB: *Functional Independence Measure*. Buffalo, State University of New York, 1993.
15. Haley S, et al: *Pediatric Evaluation of Disability Inventory*. Boston, PEDI Research Group, New England Medical Center Hospital, 1992.
16. Hayes A, Bain LJ, Batshaw ML: Adulthood: What the future holds, in Batshaw ML (ed): *Children with Disabilities*, ed 4. Baltimore, Paul H Brookes, 1997.

17. Hernan JA: Teamwork for programs for older persons, in Garner HG, Orelove FP (eds): *Teamwork in Human Services: Models and Applications Across the Life Span.* Boston, Butterworth- Heinemann, 1994.

18. Katz S, et al: Progress in the development of the Index of ADL. *The Gerontologist* 1970; 10:10-30.

19. Lawton MP, et al: A research and service orientated multilevel assessment instrument. *J Gerontol* 1982; 37:91-99.

20. Lott I: Alzheimer's disease, www.ndss.org, 1998.

21. Machemer RH: Alzheimer's disease and Down syndrome—The connection, in Machemer RH, Overeynder JC (eds): *Understanding Aging and Developmental Disabilities: An In-service Curriculum.* Rochester, University of Rochester, 1993.

22. Miniszek NA: Development of Alzheimer's disease in Down's syndrome individuals. *Am J Men Def* 1983; 8:377-385.

23. Murphy KD, Mulnar EE, Lankaskey K: Medical and functional status of adults with cerebral palsy. *Dev Med Child Neurol* 1995; 37:1075-1084.

24. Nenno RJ, Overeynder JC: Aging and developmental disabilities service systems, in Machemer RH, Overeynder JC (eds): *Understanding Aging and Developmental Disabilities: An In-service Curriculum.* Rochester, University of Rochester, 1993.

25. Prasher VP, Chowdhury BR, Rowe BR, Bain SC: ApoE genotype and Alzheimer's disease in adults with Down syndrome: Meta-analysis. *Am J Ment Retard* 1997; 102:103-110.

26. Prasher VP, Chung MC: Causes of age related decline in adaptive behavior of adults with Down syndrome: Differential diagnoses of dementia. *Am J Men Def* 1996; 101:175-183.

27. Roth SP, Morse JS (eds): Preface, in Roth SP, Morse JS (eds): *A Life Span Approach to Nursing Care for Individuals with Developmental Disabilities.* Baltimore, Paul H Brookes, 1994.

28. Russell FE, Free TA: The nurse's role in habilitation, in Roth SP, Morse JS (eds): *A Life Span Approach to Nursing Care for Individuals with Developmental Disabilities.* Baltimore, Paul H Brookes, 1994.29.   Silverstein AB, et al: Effects of age on the adaptive behavior of institutionalized adults with Down syndrome. *Am J Men Def* 1988; 92: 455-460.

30. Sparrow SS, Bulla DA, Cicchetti DV: *Vineland Adaptive Behavior Scales.* Circle Pines, Minn, American Guidance Service, 1984.

31. Studenski S, et al: *Progressive Mobility Skills.* Presented at the American Geriatric Society Annual Meeting, May 12, 1989, p 41.

32. Sung H, et al: Depression and dementia in aging adults with down syndrome: A case study approach. *Ment Retard* 1997; 35:27-38.

33. Thometz JF, Simon SR: Progression of scoliosis after skeletal maturity in institutionalized adults with cerebral palsy. *J Bone Joint Surg, FOA* 1988; 70A:1290-1296.

34. Visser FE, et al: Prospective study of the prevalence of Alzheimer-type dementia in institutionalized individuals with Down syndrome. *Am J Ment Retard* 1997; 101:400-412.

35. Wolfensberger W: *The Principles of Normalization in Human Services.* Toronto, National Institute on Mental Retardation, 1972.

GLOSSARY

adherence Consistent behavior that is accomplished through an internalization of learning, enhanced by independent coping and problem-solving skills.

aerobic exercise training Therapeutic exercise and activities of sufficient intensity, duration, and frequency to improve the efficiency of oxygen consumption during work.

Alzheimer's disease Diagnostic label for a cluster of symptoms, including confusion and diminished mental capacity, after other diagnoses have been ruled out. Confirmation of the diagnosis can only be made with a brain biopsy, most usually on autopsy.

andragogy Philosophical orientation for adult education.

arteriovenous oxygen difference (a-$\bar{v}O_2$ difference) The difference between the oxygen content of blood in the arterial system and the amount in the mixed venous blood. At rest the normal a-$\bar{v}O_2$ difference averages 4 to 5 mL of oxygen per 100 mL of blood. With vigorous exercise, this value may increase to 15 mL of oxygen per 100 mL of blood.

arthrokinematics The relative rotary and translatory movements that occur between joint surfaces.

arthrokinesiology The study of the structure and function of skeletal joints.

assignment Process through which a provider agrees to accept the amount the insurer pays as payment in full. The only amounts the patient may be billed for are co-payments and deductibles.

assisted living settings A type of living situation in which persons live in community housing with attendant care provided for those parts of the day or those activities in which assistance is required. One attendant may provide for a number of patients.

automatic postural responses Refers to a set of muscle responses characterized by latencies of approximately 100 to 150 ms, which are longer than monosynaptic reflexes but shorter than voluntary muscle responses. They occur in response to balance disturbance (expected or unexpected) and are important in postural control. Evidence exists that these responses become delayed with age.

balance billing Procedure for billing the patient for the balance of amounts not covered by insurance. This can be done only with certain insurers for which the provider does not accept assignment.

cardiac output ($\dot{Q}$) The product of heart rate and stroke volume.

chronotropic response Influencing the rate of the heartbeat.

close-packed position The point in a joint's range of motion where maximal stability exists due to the stretch placed on periarticular structures.

cocontraction Simultaneous contraction of agonist and antagonist muscles.

compliance Subservient behavior that implies following orders or directions without self-direction or choice.

creep A measure of the deformation in a material as a result of a constant load applied over a specific time interval.

deinstitutionalization A movement that started in mental health that shifted the location of treatment from hospital to community. This philosophy has extended to current practice in general health care as seen in the move from hospital to home care.

delirium Acute and reversible changes in mental status. Causes include fever, shock, and drug overdose.

dementia Impairment of intellectual functioning, occasionally due to a treatable condition.

depression Affective disorder divided into various separate diagnoses by the fourth revised edition of the *Diagnostic and Statistical Manual of Mental Disorders (DSM-IV)*. Two diagnoses of particular interest to physical therapists are major depressive episode and adjustment disorder with depressed mood.

developmental disability A physical or mental handicap or combination of the two that becomes evident before age 22, is likely to continue indefinitely, and results in significant function limitation in major areas of life.

diagnosis-related groups (DRGs) System of categorizing acute care inpatients who are medically related in terms of diagnosis and treatment for the purpose of assigning dollar amounts for reimbursement to hospitals for care of these individuals under the Prospective Payment System.

disability Refers in the model of the process of disablement developed by Nagi to inability to fulfill specific role obligations in a particular sociocultural and physical environment. Defined by the International Classification of Impairments, Disabilities and Handicaps as limitations in functional activities.

disease Pathological condition of the body that presents as a group of characteristic signs and symptoms that indicates the condition is abnormal.

drug half-life The time required for half the drug remaining in the body to be eliminated.

durable medical equipment (DME) Equipment covered by the Medicare program for patient use. Equipment must meet specific criteria and may be rented or purchased.

durable power of attorney Designation by a mentally competent individual of the person who should make decisions for that individual in the event of mental incapacitation. Durable power of attorney may be restricted to certain kinds of decisions, and different individuals may be designated to make different types of decisions.

ejection fraction The fraction of the end-diastolic volume that is ejected with each heartbeat.

elastic stiffness The amount of tissue force produced when a tissue is deformed and held at a given length.

elder *See* older person.

end-diastolic volume The amount of filling of the ventricles during diastole.

end-systolic volume The amount of blood remaining in each ventricle after each heartbeat.

evaluation Process of making a professional clinical judgment about the data collected on examination.

examination Process of obtaining data on a patient's condition through taking a history, conducting a systems review, and performing specific tests and measures.

extrapyramidal signs Motor symptoms that mimic Parkinson's disease, dyskinesia, and other lesions in the extrapyramidal tract.

feedback control Refers to the postural control mechanism of automatic responses that occurs when there is a displacement of one's center of gravity that is not under voluntary control, e.g., a slip or a trip. Automatic postural responses that occur in response to this balance disturbance are critical in the recovery of balance and are not under voluntary control.

feedforward control Refers to the postural control mechanism of automatic responses that occurs during an intentional displacement of the center of gravity, as during voluntary movement, e.g., lifting arms overhead. Automatic postural responses occur before activation of the prime movers, are not under voluntary control, and are critical to the successful execution of the movement. Persons with impaired balance may have difficulty with the feedforward mechanism of postural control.

FEV1 The percentage of the vital capacity that can be expired in 1 minute.

functional limitation Inability to perform a task or activity in the typical or anticipated fashion as the result of impairment.

functional reach A simple clinical measure of functional balance that quantifies one's forward reach. This measure assesses one's ability or willingness to move his/her center of gravity to the margins of his/her base support. Reach is known to diminish slightly with age, but markedly restricted reach (less than 6 inches) can be a marker of frailty and signal that a person is at increased risk for falls.

functional reserve Refers to the excess or redundant function that is present in virtually all physiological systems. This is diminished in the older adult, lowering the threshold for clinically observable loss of function.

gyral atrophy Decreases in the gray or white matter of the brain or both.

health status Summary of a person's physical, psychological, and social function. May be determined by data from multiple sources, including clinical examination, self-report, or care-giver responses.

impairment Any loss or abnormality of anatomical, physiological, or psychological structure or function. Secondary impairments may be the result of primary impairments. Composite impairments may be the result of interactions between and among primary and secondary impairments.

indemnity insurance Type of insurance based on payments only when an illness or accident has occurred.

individualized habilitation plan (IHP) A written multidisciplinary plan of care for a developmentally disabled adult that identifies needs, strategies for meeting those needs, and the individuals involved in providing the program. This may be a part of a referral to physical therapy.

informed consent A process by which a mentally competent individual is given sufficient information to develop adequate comprehension about the risks, benefits, and alternatives to treatment in order to choose a treatment option voluntarily.

intermediate care facility (ICF) One that provides intermediate care, which is the care most often required in a nursing home. This may include help with activities of daily living. This type of care does not require the constant involvement of licensed professional staff.

kinematics The study of the motion within a joint or between bones, without regard to forces or torques that have caused the motion.

kinetics Describes the joint forces and torques that cause motion at a joint.

learning A change in behavior resulting from an acquisition of knowledge directed toward achieving predetermined goals.

lipofuscin A dark, pigmented lipid found in the cytoplasm of aging neurons.

locus of control An individual's orientation toward internal motivation, autonomy, and control of decisions.

mainstreaming A philosophy of incorporating individuals with special needs into programs in which peers their age participate rather than developing special programs. Has usually been used in relation to educational programs for children but is now being extended to work and leisure.

maximal voluntary ventilation (MVV) The greatest volume of air that can be exhaled in 15 seconds.

microneurography A technique for the recording of action potentials from individual peripheral nerve fibers.

minute ventilation ($\dot{V}E$) The volume of air inspired and exhaled in 1 minute. The highest minute ventilation achieved during exercise is also called the *maximum breathing capacity.*

motor time (MT) In a reaction time (RT) test, the time from onset of electromyographical activity to the initiation of the movement.

motor unit (MU) Single alpha motoneuron and all the muscle fibers it innervates.

muscle fiber types Classification of muscle fibers based on anatomical, physiological, and functional characteristics.

mutability The muscle fiber's ability to change in response to a new demand.

neuritic plaque A discrete structure found outside the neuron that is composed of degenerating small axons, some dendrites, astrocytes, and amyloid. Neuritic plaque is found in normal aging brains. Also known as *senile plaque.*

neurofibrillary tangle (NFT) A darkly stained, thick, and twisted band of material found in the cytoplasm of aging neurons.

older person Term used to refer to individuals in the later years of the life span. Arbitrarily set between 65 and 70 years old in American society for the purpose of age-related entitlements.

orthostatic hypotension A sudden decline in blood pressure that occurs on standing. Also known as *postural hypotension.*

oxygen consumption ($\dot{V}O_2$) The difference between the oxygen inspired and the oxygen exhaled is the amount of oxygen used. Maximum oxygen consumption ($\dot{V}O_2$ max): the highest amount of oxygen used during exercise. The oxygen consumption will not increase even if the exercise intensity increases. This value is often used to measure maximal exercise capacity.

pacing Accommodating for time in a test or treatment session; the rate at which instruction is given or practice is provided.

pain An unpleasant sensory and emotional experience associated with actual or potential tissue damage, or described in terms of such damage.

pharmacodynamics The study of how drugs affect the body.

pharmacokinetics The study of how the body handles drugs, including the way drugs are absorbed, distributed, and eliminated.

plasticity *Neuroscience:* Adaptive structural or physiological change in the central nervous system in response to a neuron's disturbed environment. *Biomechanics:* Defined as continued elongation of a tissue without an increase in resistance from within the tissue.

plethysmography Use of a plethysmograph to measure the volume of a body part.

polypharmacy The excessive and unnecessary use of medications.

postural hypotension *See* orthostatic hypotension.

premotor time (PMT) In a reaction time (RT) test, the time between the stimulus to the onset of electromyographical activity.

prepaid health plan An insurance plan provided by health maintenance organizations (HMOs) and competitive medical plans. Preventive and wellness services are available in addition to care for illnesses.

presbyastasis Age-related disequilibrium in the absence of known pathology.

presbycusis Age-related decline in auditory function in the absence of known pathology.

Prospective Payment System (PPS) A process under which acute care and inpatient rehabilitation hospitals, skilled nursing facilities, and home health agencies are paid fixed amounts by Medicare based on the patient's principal diagnosis or medical condition.

pseudodementia Term used to describe the misdiagnosis of depression as dementia in the elderly.

pseudoelastin A protein found in aging elastin tissue. The essential constituent of yellow elastic connective tissue.

reaction time (RT) The time required to initiate a movement after stimulus presentation.

resistance exercise training Exercise that applies sufficient force to muscle groups to improve muscle strength.

resource-based relative value system (RBRVS) A system of reimbursement being developed by Medicare for outpatient service based on assessing the intensity and complexity of a service and assigning a numerical value and dollar amount related to that value.

restorative aide A nursing assistant who works in a rehabilitation capacity and assists nursing home residents in carryover of learned functional mobility, e.g., ambulation and transfers, and activities of daily living on the patient floors.

senile plaque *See* neuritic plaque.

skilled nursing facility (SNF) Provides care that must by rendered by or under the supervision of professional personnel, such as a registered nurse. The care must be required daily and must be a continuation of the care begun in the hospital.

somatosensory evoked potential (SEP) Peripheral nerve stimulation produces potentials that can be recorded from the scalp, over the spine, or in the periphery. The potentials are called SEPs.

strain Refers to the percent change in original length of a deformed tissue.

stress The force developed in a deformed tissue divided by the tissue's cross-sectional area.

stroke volume (SV) The amount of blood ejected from the left ventricle on one beat. *Maximum stroke volume* is the highest volume of blood expelled from the heart during a single beat. This value is usually reached when exercise is only about 40% to 50% of maximum exercise capacity.

synaptogenesis The formation of new synapses.

tensile force Resistive force generated within a tissue in response to elongation or stretch.

tetany A syndrome manifested by sharp flexion of joints, especially the wrist and ankle joints; muscle twitching; cramps; and convulsions, sometimes with attacks of difficult breathing.

transcutaneous electrical nerve stimulation (TENS) Generically, refers to all forms of therapeutic electrical stimulation to intact nerve/muscle done via skin surface electrodes. Most commonly refers to electrical stimulation used specifically for pain management.

viscosity Describes the extent to which a tissue's resistance to deformation is dependent on the rate of the deforming force.

visual acuity Measure of visual discrimination of fine details of high contrast.

visual evoked response (VER) Presentation of a particular visual stimulus evokes consistent electrocortical activity that can be recorded from electrodes placed on the scalp. The potentials that are recorded are known as VERs.

vital capacity The total volume of air that can be voluntarily moved in one breath from full inspiration to maximum expiration.

$\dot{V}O_2$max The point at which oxygen consumption plateaus and shows no further increase with an additional work load. It is generally assumed that this represents a person's ability to synthesize adenosine triphosphate aerobically.

INDEX

NOTE: Page numbers in italics indicate an illustration; page numbers followed by *t* indicate a table

Buckley

The
Right
Word

Buckley:
The Right Word

ABOUT THE USES AND ABUSES
OF LANGUAGE, AND ABOUT
VOCABULARY; ABOUT USAGE,
STYLE & SPEAKING; FICTION,
DICTION, DICTIONARIES; WITH
REVIEWS AND INTERVIEWS;
A LEXICON; ON LATIN &
LETTERS, ELOQUENCE &
JOURNALISM; AND MORE,
ALL DRAWN FROM THE
WORKS OF

William F. Buckley, Jr.,

HIS CORRESPONDENTS, HIS
CRITICS, FRIENDS, AND OTHERS

SELECTED, ASSEMBLED, AND EDITED BY
Samuel S. Vaughan
WITH AN INTRODUCTION & SUNDRY
COMMENTARIES

 RANDOM HOUSE   NEW YORK

Library of Congress Cataloging-in-Publication data is available.
ISBN 0-679-45214-1

Random House website address: http://www.randomhouse.com/

Printed in the United States of America on acid-free paper
98765432
First Edition
Book design by Debbie Glasserman

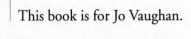 This book is for Jo Vaughan.

(This dedication is the joint idea of author, WFB, Jr., and editor, SSV, who arrived at the same thought independently.)

Editor's Acknowledgments

My gratitude is great for the limitless help, and loyal but not uncritical commentary of Mr. Buckley's peerless assistant Frances Bronson, who still finds music in his writing; to Liz Altham, who made the first gathering of WFB's words on words, and for other important contributions; to Chaucy Bennetts, copy editor extraordinaire, who has come out of retirement more times than Sinatra to work on WFB's manuscripts; to Joseph Isola; and to the hard-pressed production, art, and design talents at Random House, who took a manuscript that looked as if it had been through a Cuisinart and baked a good-looking book.

And of course to the maestro himself, for proving me right once more.

Contents

What's It Like to Edit William F. Buckley, Jr.?

This is a book Bill Buckley didn't realize he had written. Or at least was unwilling to believe he had. For years, as editor of his books, I had urged him to do a book on language—that is, a book that could be drawn from his letters, columns, essays, fiction, and lectures.

He would reply, "I haven't written enough to make up a book."

Finally he agreed to let me explore the possibilities. I had saved many copies of pieces he had written. He engaged Liz Altham, a lively, enthusiastic researcher, to gather material. Though retired as an active editor to become an active mother, she turned to the task with a will and imagination, and in due course delivered a box twelve inches high, fat with Xeroxes, here and there annotated. This book, reduced by some inches, is the result.

He needs no introduction but, as with after-dinner introducers, will get one anyhow. The voice you will hear most often in the pages following is that of Mr. Buckley, who nonetheless insists that this is "my" book.

To be clear about that point: Though the great majority of the words are his, or those of his correspondents, critics, friends, enemies, and fellow word mavens, it is my book in that I initiated the idea and I chose what to include or not. I organized and made notes on the contents. As he wrote while we were discussing the possibilities: "The liberating perspective, in my judgment, is the relationship between the project and its executioner . . . [Suddenly I saw myself in a black hood, ax in hand. Ed.] We are talking about a book you conceived, gathered, even lassoed, and it is vital to know whose eye is at work here . . . The task then becomes entirely your own, also the responsibility." Thus, following his wishes, it is fair to say that this is not a book about words that Bill himself might have gathered; his would be far different—and shorter. It is my book of his words about words and related matters.

In it you will find largely the apolitical, although hardly neutered, Buckley. The point is to show not his politics but his language in action. Much of it has appeared in print, but a considerable portion has never been in book form.

What is it like to edit William F. Buckley, Jr.? Some might think it daunting, even terrifying. After all, he is a famous debater, an enthusiastic opponent, quick to beat plowshares back into swords; he is remarkably fluid, fluent, formidable; respected and/or feared; well educated, well traveled, worldly. Before I came to the vocation as Buckley's editor, he was already the author of hundreds of thousands of published words, including at least a dozen books. The first, *God and Man at Yale,* made him a national figure before the ink was dry on his diploma.

Accordingly, I set about editing his first novel cautiously. Editing him, I would soon find out, is more terrific (or, as he would say, "Turrr-ific!") than terrifying. For one thing, he is a pro. You never get an uninteresting manuscript. There are stimulating ideas in the air, constant surprises, a narrative rush, and a voice entirely his own. Some of his books are more serious than salable, such as *Gratitude,* his short 1990 book about patriotism and national service, or *In Search of Anti-Semitism* (1992). But in general, the success rate with the public is high and has been sustained for decades.

Bill is among the most appreciative of authors. He welcomes editing and copyediting, in part because they require first of all an attentive reading. He has informal advisers—family members and trusted friends and colleagues. They serve as a sort of Greek chorus of coeditors, contributing usefully to early drafts. Buckley writes quickly (see "What's So Bad About Writing Fast?," page 185. He is open but hardly docile about just any suggestion, let alone one that proposes he rewrite the entire manuscript. This is because he abominates ennui much more than he shrinks from work. The First Great Commandment for Buckley is: Thou Shalt Not Bore, and he obeys it faithfully. He cuts his own stuff with the joy of a surgeon. Happily his drafts do not require organic rearrangement, and he accepts a multiplicity of ideas for revision. The fact that he is an editor himself is lifesaving. He is demanding of his editors only as he is demanding of himself. Writing speedily, he feels the need to be read quickly, and wants reactions promptly (almost universal among authors). His routine for years has been to produce, while on "holiday" for six weeks in winter, a draft of a book, ready to deliver to me. He does not undertake revisions until three months later when, in early summer, his demanding schedule permits. Meanwhile the manuscript has cooled.

He is ever so grateful (that phrase is his; I fall into the locutions of authors I like) for useful editorial suggestions, responsive to reactions on word, sentence, paragraph, punctuation, chapter changes, to thoughts about characters, plot, length. He is at all times considerate, a man of manners, rather than mannered.

Editing Buckley is akin to reaping the pleasures of his friendship: he is fun to be with, and to correspond with; full of enthusiasm, humor, insight, opinion. You become a part of his informal extended family, which brings the great good fortune of getting to know those who really are family, starting with the remarkable Pat Buckley, his wife, who speaks *entirely* in italics, followed by a splendidly smoky laugh; their son, the phenomenal Christopher Buckley, himself a prodigious author and editor; and on and on through sisters, brothers, friends and colleagues.

Why does Buckley write so much?* First, because duty calls: the deadlines of his syndicate, his magazine, and the newspapers and magazines that commission his work; deadlines for his TV and lecture dates; and, overarchingly, a sense of duty to his ideas and ideals. Second, to earn a living (though lecture fees go to support *National Review*). But then also to keep from being . . . yes, bored. And therefore to amuse, entertain, educate, instruct, illuminate and seek to influence events; and, at times, to infuriate or simply provoke.

Bill Buckley said somewhere, sometime, that he cannot "think" without a pen or a keyboard at hand. He writes in a sort of parallelism to the much quoted *Cogito, ergo sum*—I think, therefore I am. He claims to be not at all introspective, yet clearly he is always thinking. Which would then give us a case of *Scribo, ergo sum*—I write, therefore I am. His writing is one with his identity and sense of self.

---

* These are my speculations. WFB speculates, much more authoritatively, in the chapter on columnists, page 189.

Though not intended as such, this became in part a book on the subject of Buckley himself. For all his celebrity, not enough is really known about him. The man seen for so long on television, leaning away from his discussants, pen by jowl, at the ready, sighting down his nose at the target, eyes occasionally glittering, smile intermittently flashing—none of this reveals much about the "whole" man. His astonishing generosity to all sorts of individuals, more than a few of whom do not share his politics, religion, or "lifestyle"; his capacity to be instructed as much as to instruct; his deep-dyed loyalties—such qualities are not readily apparent in the pixels of the omnipresent living-room box that supposedly brings us the news.

And he discovers writers. Working for him early were—in addition to those noted by Charlie Rose in the book's interview chapter—Joan Didion, George Will, Arlene Croce . . .

To show William F. Buckley, Jr., fully engaged at work is to display language itself in full deployment. (I had called him an Equal Opportunity employer of words but Bill winced, understandably, preferring the sentence that follows.) The man is a comprehensive employer of words, spoken by himself, through his characters in fiction, in his paradigmatic political and philosophical fancies. The reader will find many and varied examples of thought and writing by him and by others: curious, amused and amusing, witty and barbed, sometimes pugnacious, smug, slashing. He is infinitely resourceful in his own defense, yet in style usually responsive and gracious, even to those who would score points off his own hide. There are examples in what follows of language too snappish for my taste. But most often he writes to attract interest, to inform, to heal, and, sometimes, to serve as a lingering last kiss or salute. (See "On Saying Good-bye.")

Buckley can, in my own judgment, be wrong, or overload a sentence, but it is the brio that one notices, rather than any bravado. He antagonizes but does not wrong; more often he is wronged. There are in these pages samples of Early Buckley, Middle Period Buckley, and Late Buckley. (No Blue Period: Buckley represses depression, as well as most profanity.)

To show his words in action and his consideration of others' concern for words is to document that to be intricately, intimately involved with language is more than merely a transient affair; it is a lifelong marriage. He gives himself up to his belief in the power of words, by which we live or die. Auden wrote, "Poetry makes nothing happen." What is under the surface here is the assumption that you might just change minds, even change the world, with words—words thoughtfully, lovingly assembled.

Buckley is one writer whose words have stimulated curiosity, scorn, legal action, reaction, reform, and affection. They have helped to educate and elect Presidents. His language continues to generate exasperation and admiration for the man behind them.

"My" book? This book may show what it is like to be a person, perhaps like the reader, who loves words, lives by and stands by them.

—Sam Vaughan

Samuel S. Vaughan was president, publisher, and editor in chief of Doubleday & Co. for many years, and later senior vice president at Random House, Inc., for which company he is currently editor at large. He has edited most of William F. Buckley's books since Saving the Queen *(1976).*

Buckley

The
Right
Word

Chapter 1

Usage I:
"Notes & Asides"

Some of WFB's time and a considerable portion of his correspondence is taken up with word usage—his own and that of others. Correspondents curious, combative, or admiring may disagree on who/whom and such, but most write out of a conviction that words, as the expression has it, can make a difference; that words can affect the way we perceive, think and act.

This continuing concern for just the right word is not common in our age.

Most of Buckley's correspondence is disposed of in the *National Review* column "Notes & Asides," which, although not wholly devoted to questions of language, is one of the longest-running features in journalism to give usage such attention.

Buckley relies for answers not only on his own knowledge but on friends and correspondents. They act as resources and also as antagonists. These masters have included the august critic Hugh Kenner, the newspaperman James J. Kilpatrick, and the late author and editor William F. Rickenbacker, as well as experts on his own staff, the longtime *NR* managing editor (his sister) Priscilla Buckley, Linda Bridges, his editors and writers, and others.

Samples from "Notes & Asides" (the format of which has changed over the years) introduce us to his resourceful concern for the language and continue throughout the book, showing the stimulation he provides his readers—and vice versa.

———

Dear Mr. Buckley:

What, pray tell, is a quantum jump?

This phrase has annoyed me for years, and I was most displeased to see it appear in my favorite journal. I am well aware that the expression is commonly used to indicate an upward change in the order of magnitude of whatever phenomenon interests the user, but this is not the meaning of quantum. A portion jump? A jump of a portion? A jump of the element unit of energy? An elemental unit of energy jump? The physicists would be aghast.

> *Quantum sufficit.*
> TERRENCE J. MCGHEE
> LAWRENCE, KAN.

Dear Mr. McGhee:

Webster recognizes the use of "quantum" meaning "large quantity." The OED does not. We suggest reader McGhee exorcise his rhetorical demons with Robbie Burns's song:

> *I waive the quantum o' the sin,*
> *The hazard of concealing;*
> *But och, it hardens a' within,*
> *And petrifies the feeling!*

Cordially,

—WFB   AUGUST 8, 1967

Dear Mr. Buckley:

Please, please elucidate. If you are too busy writing on world problems, perhaps some fellow reader of *National Review* will solve my problem, not shared by a single one of my friends.

What bothers me is the phrase "by and large," used constantly by both the literate and the illiterate. What do people think they are saying, with a preposition and an adjective connected by a conjunction? Take "by." By what? Now take "large." What is it that is large?

For over a year I have waited for a break in terrible world events to bend your ear about this. Now, although a born optimist, I've been forced to conclude that I'd better wait no longer.

Sincerely,

HELEN W. SANBORN

EL CERRITO, CALIF.

Dear Mrs. Sanborn: Well now, you might have reason to be dismayed at its use, but not surprised. See, e.g., *A Dictionary of American Usage,* Bergen Evans, Random House: "**by and large.** In the sense of 'generally speaking, in every aspect': *by and large (By and large, the worries of summer residents concerning snakes are far out of proportion to the dangers that exist)* is standard in American usage, though not very often used in England. Apparently it is becoming more common there, for Sir Ernest Gowers states that this 'current usage . . . exasperates the sailor' who knows the true meaning of the phrase—'alternately close to the wind and with the wind abeam or aft.' An even stronger reason for avoiding the phrase than the fear of exasperating sailors is that it is often meaningless, used simply as conversational filler." You will be happy to learn that *NR* never uses the phrase in the last, condemned, sense. Cordially,

—WFB   NOVEMBER 15, 1985

Dear Billic:

Silly Question #1: Is there a difference between Democratic and democratic?

Silly Question #2: Is there a difference between Democrat and democrat?

Then why?

An ic before the big D I could tolerate.

Sincerely,

ANDREI KOVEN

SUPREME EXAULTED PRESIDENT

PTUI FAD

(PEOPLE TOGETHER TO UNSTICK IC

FROM AFTER DEMOCRAT)

BETHEL, CONN.

Dear Mr. Koven: As far as we're concerned, it's the Democratic Party, the alternative sounding phony-baloney.

—WFB   SEPTEMBER 17, 1976

Dear Mr. Buckley:

Almost as "removed from matters of the day" as Nelson Algren, I was going through last May's *Times* this weekend and was stopped cold by the enclosed piece of your writing. The context is of course much too momentous for such a trivial point to cause Reader Arrest, but you are getting a reputation as a Word Man and hence have a certain potential for influence, for good or ill, upon the few and precious literate young. Besides, I happen to have heard you commit the same mistake recently on the air. The word in question may just possibly be on the way to being a favorite with you.

Authorities you surely respect as I do insist upon a distinction between *restive* and *restless*—the first meaning "stubbornly standing still . . . resisting control, intractable, refractory," conservative to the point of rebellion, as it were. Quotations in the OED include examples where the refractoriness is coupled with violent action: "His lordship's horse became restive and attempted to throw its rider." But resistance in the face of real or imminent compulsion is surely an implication that respect for the language would have us preserve in the use of this word. I enclose a couple of other clippings: you and Anthony Burgess seem to me to be abusers; Michener seems O.K.

Sincerely,
CLEM C. WILLIAMS, JR. (YALE '42)

(Enclosed: "Can the present-day cinema audience watch without restiveness a film in which a couple fall deeply in love without taking off their clothes?"—A. Burgess, *N.Y. Times,* July 1, 1973. "Many felt him to be unqualified to lead the nation, and when, that summer, meat prices rose, the nation grew restive."—J. Michener, *N.Y. Times,* July 1, 1973.)

Dear Mr. Williams: "Restive" also means "balky." So that it can be used halfway between restless and mutinous.

—WFB (YALE '50)   FEBRUARY 15, 1974

Dear Mr. Buckley:

Tch-tch . . . you'll never learn.

I don't really mind your dipping into your pathetic little treasury of Shakespeare quotes . . . the effect is nice and you don't overdo it. But, please . . . get them right.

On page 622 of *NR* [June 8], you reply to a letter from reader S. Manning with the most threadbare of your quotes stock thus: "Dear Mrs. Manning: That would be gilding the lily. Yrs. Cordially, etc.," and that rumbling sound you've been hearing ever since is ol' Bill Shakespeare spin-ning like a top. Ol' Bill *never* said anything about gilding the lily, and were you playing hooky during the term they taught *King John*?

Act IV, Scene 2, Earl of Salisbury in reply to Earl of Pembroke:

> *"Therefore, to be possessed with double*
> * pomp,*
> *To guard a title that was rich before,*
> *To gild refined gold, to paint the lily,*
> *To throw a perfume on the violet,*
> *To smooth the ice, or add another hue*
> *Unto the rainbow, or with taper light*
> *To seek the beauteous eye of heaven to garnish,*
> *Is wasteful and ridiculous excess."*

Did you get any other letters on this? Or am I the only Shakespearean hawkeye among your readers?

Cordially,

SAUL GLEMBY

NEW YORK, N.Y.

Dear Mr. Glemby: (1) To call to the attention of anyone over fourteen that Shakespeare didn't say gilding the lily is like calling to the attention of anyone over ten that Voltaire didn't say the one about how he would fight to the death for your right to say it. Come to think of it, I doubt very much that Voltaire would fight to the death for the right of anyone to re-mind anyone that Shakespeare didn't himself use the phrase gild the lily. (2) The phrase gild the lily, and a number of other phrases, can be used even though Shakespeare did not originate them. (3) When we use a cliché around these parts, boy we mean to use a cliché, understand, Glemby? (4) Of the four editors of *National Review,* one used to teach Shakespeare, one still does, and, when I retire, I intend to.

Cordially,

—WFB   JULY 20, 1973

Dear Mr. Buckley:

Your three columns on the *Titanic* were extremely moving and splen-didly written. I have one acidulous comment to make and here goes: Why, oh why, do you assume that when a ship dies *she* loses *her* gender? Time and again, you refer to the corpse of a majestic, devastated lady as "it"! I'd consider you, therefore, guilty of an unmitigated solecism, all the more horrendous in coming from you, a seasoned salt.

Sincerely,

CONSUELO IVES, M.D.

NEW YORK, N.Y.

Dear Dr. Ives: It was unconscious. But not uninteresting, Freudian-slipwise. Maybe a fallen lady isn't any longer a lady??? Cordially,

—WFB   DECEMBER 18, 1987

Dear Mr. Buckley:

In the editorial "Cruelest Month" [May 8, 1987], *NR* has it "*shoures soote.*" Has Chaucer been revised since the 1929 edition of *The Student's Chaucer* (The Clarendon Press, Oxford), which has it "*shoures sote,*" or has someone been guilty of carelessness?

Cordially,

ROBERT E. KOHLER

KOHLER, WIS.

Dear Mr. Kohler: It is an old rivalry (Oxford *v.* Cambridge). The Chaucer we use around here (at *National Review* we always speak in Middle English until noon) we get from the New Cambridge Edition, ed. F. N. Robinson (Houghton Mifflin), a fine book in which all *shoures* are *soote.* Cordially,

—WFB   SEPTEMBER 11, 1987

Dear Mr. Buckley:

No! No! No! No!

I will not be "convinced" to do anything by your ad for *Firing Line* video cassettes [March 27]. The word is *persuade.*

Respectfully yours,

HUGH M. FITZPATRICK

CHEVY CHASE, MD.

Dear Mr. Fitzpatrick: Quite right. Moreover, your conviction is persuasive. Cordially,

—WFB

Dear Mr. Buckley:

John Roche's contrast between a trustful Ronald Reagan and a mistrustful Lyndon Johnson ["Taming the NSC," March 27] points up the virtues of an underrated human quality that is often confused with *dis*trust. Despite the fact that so much of our Constitution was founded upon healthy mistrust, there is a part of us all that yearns to trust, freely and completely, in accordance with Henry L. Stimson's maxim that "the only way to make a man trustworthy is to trust him." But for an executive, the problem arises when trust is so all-encompassing that it leaves no room for in-house review and oversight. In the best of trusting relationships, critical review is viewed not as an intrusion but as a welcome antidote to human fallibility. Indeed, it is the keen awareness of one's own fallibility that seems to spawn the quality of mistrust in the first place. Quite simply, to be mistrustful is to be intellectually honest. Bill, as someone who counts so many bright people among his acquaintances, would you say mistrust, of themselves and others, is a common denominator?

Sincerely,

WILLIAM E. COOPER, PH.D.
PROFESSOR OF PSYCHOLOGY
UNIVERSITY OF IOWA
IOWA CITY, IOWA

Dear Professor Cooper: The difficulty is semantic. I would not use the word "mistrust" to do the work you assign it. So far as I know, the word that reaches out for your inflection does not exist. You would need to make a verb out of "blind trust." The English language, as Clifton Fadiman once wrote, is wonderfully versatile, but there are some things you simply can't do with it. Cordially,

—WFB   MAY 8, 1987

Dear Mr. Buckley:

I take exception to your sentence in "Full Circle" [June 2] that ends the episode of the incorrect baggage tally, i.e., too many bags aboard the plane. "Whose they were, we never knew; and, being a genial lot [of bags or people?], there has been no public speculation over the question." I think your participle dangles.

WARREN SNYDER
CHICAGO, ILL.

Dear Mr. Snyder: You are quite right. Introducing the word "we" before "being" would have fixed it up grammatically, though there is, you will concede, a little euphonic damage left over. Cordially,

—WFB   AUGUST 18, 1989

Dear Mr. Buckley:

Admittedly, you are articulate and fluent to the point that any attempt at criticism has to descend to mere nit-picking.

Accordingly, in my opinion, you could be more precise in your positioning of limiting adverbs, e.g., "The government can *only* do something for the people, in proportion as it can do something to the people" ["State-loving in the GOP," Dec. 18, 1987] might have been better were you to have said: The government can do something for the people, *only* in proportion etc. . . . *D'accord?*

JOHN A. HEINLEIN, M.D.

GREAT NECK, N.Y.

Dear Dr. Heinlein: You're right, but remember I was quoting Jefferson, though granted it was Jefferson who spoke of making a "more perfect" union. On the general point, see Richard Weaver's *The Ethics of Rhetoric* for the flexibility of adverb placement. Only John is sick. John only is sick. John is, only, sick. John is sick, only. All can be used accurately to communicate that only John is sick, but there are kind and less kind ways of treating the ear. Cordially,

—WFB   MARCH 18, 1988

Dear Mr. Buckley:

Don't start a sentence with "and." In the last paragraph of your column I see this, and apparently the *Star-Ledger* proofreader did not. (She sleeps a lot.)

I am beginning to wonder just how good (or bad) your high school was, and how good (or bad) a student you were.

Very truly yours,

DAVID DEARBORN, JR.

ELIZABETH, N.J.

Dear Mr. Dearborn: Verses 2–26 and 28–31, Chapter I, Genesis, all begin with "And." The King James scholars went to pretty good high schools. Cordially,

—WFB   JUNE 10, 1991

Dear Mr. Buckley:

Please be assured that there is not now, nor has there ever been, a rule against beginning a sentence with *and,* although there have been a good many admonitions to that effect by soi-disant arbiters of usage. Most of this nonsense originated among the late Victorians and their turn-of-the-century successors (but not including the brothers Fowler).

This silliness survives in some high schools, apparently, but not, I should think, in the better ones. Surely, one of the characteristics of a good high school is that it teaches its students to pay attention to what they read. Anyone who believes that there is a "rule" against beginning a sentence with *and*—or with any other coordinating conjunction—simply isn't paying attention.

To convince yourself that I'm telling the truth, all you need do is grab the first half-dozen books at hand and begin turning pages at random. You'll quickly find examples in good plenty of sentences beginning with *and*.

Sincerely yours,
DOUGLAS CRENSHAW
ANTIOCH, TENN.

P.S. To save you some trouble, I herewith append some examples culled from the books nearest my own hand. In the event that these fellows aren't sufficiently authoritative for Mr. Sidorsky to acknowledge your "high scholarly right to begin a sentence with an 'and' " ["Notes & Asides," July 29], I also append examples from a longer list I keep for another purpose (including sentences from the prose of Wordsworth, Coleridge, Shelley, Lamb, Hazlitt, De Quincey, Carlyle, Mill, Dickens, George Eliot, Arnold, Newman, Ruskin, T. H. Huxley, Pater, Wilde, Shaw, Conrad, Yeats, Joyce, Lawrence, T. S. Eliot, Beckett, Forster, Woolf, Lessing, Hulme, Richards, and Empson). After all, high scholars shouldn't be denied rights everybody else has.

1. And then the fog rose from the ground and from the very leaves and through the fog I saw the body.

—William Goyen, "In the Icebound Hothouse"

2. And the strategy worked.

—Paul Johnson, *Intellectuals*

3. And would you write "The worst tennis player around here is I" or "The worst tennis player around here is me"? The first is good grammar, the second is good judgment—although the *me* might not do in all contexts.

—Strunk & White, *Elements of Style*

4. And, for a good fisherman, the object was not to bring home a mess of fish.

—Franklin Burroughs, *Billy Watson's Croker Sack*

5. And although it is arguable that a faction might insinuate itself into the control of a legislature, this will be the less likely in proportion to the greater size of the area represented.

—Max Beloff, introduction, *The Federalist*

6. And a further reason for caution, in this respect, might be drawn from the reflection, that we are not always sure that those who advocate the truth are actuated by purer principles than their antagonists.

—The Federalist (#I Hamilton)

7. And what inspired guesses there have been!

—Malcolm Muggeridge, *Confessions of a Twentieth-Century Pilgrim*

8. And wearily, but not *simply* wearily, he returned that look.

—John Barth, *The Last Voyage of Somebody the Sailor*

Dear Mr. Crenshaw: Crenshaw! Stop! I can't stand any more, and you have sent along sixty-two! Massive retaliation was repealed at the Summit last week. Cordially,

—WFB   AUGUST 26, 1991

Dear Mr. Buckley:

As a nine- or ten-year-old reading Dear Abby, Charlie Brown, and the Royals' scores, I found your columns incomprehensible. In high school I discovered you were simply boring.

Early in my college days at Kansas State University in the journalism department and political-science classrooms I learned to admire your style but could not understand how you could be so wrong on so many issues. As a cub reporter for the *Topeka Capital-Journal* I frequently found myself agreeing with your positions but resented your patronizing tone and use of big words and foreign phrases. You abuse the reader, I thought.

Now, as a twenty-eight-year-old homeowner; underpaid, overworked director of communications for the Kansas Republican Party—concerned about over-taxation, over-spending, and under-presence in the world—and newly wed, I find we share opinions on most critical issues and that I enjoy your writing savoir-faire.

Boy, Bill, have you changed!

Yours,

ROGER AESCHLIMAN

TOPEKA, KAN.

P.S. Please, please, let's do something about the non-word "factoid." An item of information is either a fact, or it is fiction. It can not be "like a fact," even if it is trivial. It is either a trivial fact or trivial fiction, but not a "factoid." HELP!

Dear Mr. Aeschliman: We don't use "factoid" here at *NR,* but I promise to *slay* the first person I hear using it, now that I'm confident you will find my action mature. Cordially,

—WFB   AUGUST 18, 1989

The preceding letter from Mr. Aeschliman, which is reminiscent of the discovery of how one's parents get wiser as one gets older, did not end the healthy discussion of "factoids" (which sounds like a disease—and is). A subsequent correspondent suggested that the word, and perhaps the practice, originated with Norman Mailer, while another disputed Aeschliman's charge that factoid is a nonword (as it more than suggests a nontruth) because it is in The Random House Dictionary of the English Language, and proposed a "factoid" contest. Such exchanges can go on and on. And that's a fact.

Dear Mr. Buckley:

What is a fell swoop, and why is there always one fell swoop? Do fell swoops ever come more than one at a time? For example, can democracy be established in South Africa in two or three fell swoops (see "First Step to Democracy," *NR,* Nov. 25)?

Sincerely,

RICHARD PICKRELL

BERKELEY, CALIF.

Dear Mr. Pickrell: Interesting question. I haven't asked Bill Safire, but my intuitive feeling is that a swoop can't be fell unless it is consummated, even as one can't, oh, vault a pole in two or three stages. Besides, don't you get the feeling that there is an onomatopoeic imperative at work here—that the word "swoop" suggests a beginning, and requires an end? Let's think about it. Cordially,

—WFB   FEBRUARY 24, 1989

Dear Mr. Buckley:

Tell me it isn't so. Tell me the typesetter goofed. Tell me a ghostwriter improvised. Tell me anything except that you really wrote about "hot air rising *upward.*" I don't believe it. I can't believe it. I *won't* believe it.

Hopefully,

ELLEN D. PARKER

NORFOLK, VA.

Dear Mrs. Parker: Even reactionaries don't believe that hot air descends downward!

—WFB   APRIL 18, 1980

Dear Mr. Buckley:

Shame on you! See page 1113 of *NR,* Oct. 13, for the following words attributed to you in a letter to JKG [John Kenneth Galbraith] the Harvard Prof:

"It raises implicitly two points, the one, *Ought anyone* to sue for libel; the second, Is the Vidal suit, assuming the answer is yes, *to be one of them?*" [Emphasis supplied.]

I ask: One of *what?* The only plausible antecedent to "them" is "anyone," and a person (even if unspecified) can hardly *be* a libel suit, although he may perhaps initiate one. Have I caught you with your antecedents down? Or, perhaps, this Mr. Anyone will shortly sue *you* for libel (in that you asserted he *was,* or ought to be, a *libel suit* against Gore Vidal—fighting words beyond a doubt).

Have you anything to say for yourself?

> Chidingly,
> BILL WINGO
> BIRMINGHAM, ALA.

No, nothing. Chidedly,

> —WFB JANUARY 19, 1973

Dear Mr. Buckley:

There is an irritating mannerism of speech, an affectation of style, used all too frequently these days—so pernicious that it has even found its way into the "On the Right" pages of *National Review.* I have always admired your elegant and expressive use of English, and now that I find even you to be slipping into this style I feel the time has come to launch a protest.

In "The Irreverent Dr. Graham" [*NR,* June 11] you say: ". . . one might excuse a Chamberlain's making flattering references to Adolf Hitler, or a Nixon's praising Mao Tse-tung." *A* Chamberlain? *A* Nixon? How many Chamberlains and Nixons have there been? And of these, how many made flattering references, etc.? (And why not "a Hitler," or "a Mao Tse-tung"?)

I really am surprised to see this from the pen of a William F. Buckley, although if it could be shown that the device was ever used by a Chesterfield or a Chesterton, a Samuel Johnson or a Samuel Clemens, a Wolfe, a Woolf, a Wylie, or a Wilde, a Beerbohm, a Benchley, a Mencken, a Maugham, a Lardner, a Lippmann, an A. P. Herbert, or an F. P. Adams, I would consider retracting my criticism.

Meantime, do you know if this maddening mannerism has a name? Indefinitization, perhaps?

> Sincerely,
> JILL CLISBY
> SANTA MONICA, CALIF.

Dear Mrs. Clisby: "A Chamberlain" is here used, obviously, to convey: "someone situated as Chamberlain was situated." It's not called indefinitization. It is called antonomasia. Cordially,

—WFB   AUGUST 20, 1982

Buckley contributes a Foreword to Kilpatrick's book *The Writer's Art*, published by Andrews, McMeel & Parker, Inc., 1984, and even there gets involved in a spot of disagreement. But he does not shrink from an uninhibited admiration for some of his contemporaries, and "Kilpo" is one of them.

WELCOME: THE WRITER'S CRAFT

. . . Those of us disinclined to biological curiosity experience no temptation to look at pictures of livers, upper intestines, or tonsils, let alone the real thing. And we all know about those many who having experienced grammar at school, and been made to parse sentences, and to distinguish between dependent and independent clauses, subjunctive and indicative moods, have no more curiosity about the morphology of English than most of us have about the innards of a diesel engine. But now listen.

Spring is coming to Scrabble, Virginia. There is the profusion of flowers. Among them "the trillium, loveliest of them all, which kneels as modestly as a spring bride, all in white, beside the altar of an old oak stump. If you're not familiar with the trillium, imagine the flower that would come from a flute if a flute could make a flower. That is the trillium, a work of God from a theme by Mozart."

I shouldn't really need, in order to make my point that prejudices about anatomical structures are not always warranted, to do much more than to say that the man who brought off those lovely sentences—casual commentary on a natural cycle in an earlier book—has up and written an engrossing and majestic treatise on the English language. He calls it *The Writer's Art.* It is not only the best book of its kind I have ever experienced (the incomparable Fowler wrote a different kind of a book), it is the most compelling reading about writing I have ever seen. If such a book were written about human biology, I would be tempted to become a doctor. But never mind if you have a vocation: James Jackson Kilpatrick's book will be read for the sheer pleasure of the experience; read by people who intend to make no special effort to improve their writing, let alone harbor any ambition to write belletristically. But I warn that Mr. Kilpatrick's book is so seductive that the temptation to improve is not easily resisted.

It requires a chastity belt on the spirit to read and not experience temptation in the voluptuous delights of language.

It requires only a reading of a few paragraphs of the book to know that you are embarked on an important trip, under the direction of a guide who (most important) has labored intensively to understand what it is that works in English, what it is that does not work in English; moreover, a writer whose aptitude (indispensable) for words, and for the composition of sentences, is so marked that the distinctions he makes convince us in .part because they hit with revelatory force, in part because we have come to trust him deeply. Kilpatrick engages at first attention; then respect; finally devotion. This last is done, I think, because he insinuates his own veneration for the proper sentence and, sensing now what it is that we may have been missing, we are grateful to the man (person?—see Chapter 4) who helped open our eyes.

Notice that JJK has named his book *The Writer's Art*. It is art he speaks of in two senses. The first is that fine writing—he speaks of Rebecca West, for instance; Lawrence Durrell, Hemingway, and Twain—is not something we can master in the sense that, say, we can master a word processor. But it is also true, where art is the object of our scrutiny, that differing judgments can be made. It required many centuries before the aesthetic consensus crystallized that Notre Dame de Chartres was possibly the most beautiful thirteenth-century cathedral in Europe and that Westminster Abbey was possibly the ugliest thirteenth-century cathedral in Europe. Some questions about English are unresolved ("It's I" or "It's me"?). And then, too, there is the matter of usage. Although the overwhelming majority of technicians may agree that a particular usage is offensive and should be quarantined, manacled, deported—maybe even executed, if only the Supreme Court will go along—that use will at some point overwhelm us, like old age. JJK is sensitive to the autonomous inertia of words and for that reason accepts the likes of "access" as a transitive verb. But his ear is so good, his good sense so gratifyingly reliable, that we find ourselves volunteers in the good usage army, disposed to spend blood, sweat, and tears.

Over the years I have been much interested, and frequently amused, by the author's Hundred Years' War against Unusual Words. Interested because he makes his case so well; amused because he is not particularly constrained by it. He tells several amusing stories in this volume, one of them about stumbling into the word *limicolous,* which is to say, "living in mud."

He found himself using the word, and woke the next day with a most dreadful hangover. "No advice is more elementary, and no advice is more difficult to accept: When we feel an impulse to use a marvelously exotic word, let us lie down until the impulse goes away. . . . My brother pundit, Bill Buckley, falls into sin even more easily than I. He has had affairs with *decoctable, anfractuosity,* and *endogamous.* He has taken to bed with *chiliastic, phlogistonic, sciolism, incondite,* and *osmotically.* He has fallen for *hubristic, otiose, repristinate, adumbrated,* and *synecdoche.*" Two sentences later, the author uses in a dense little cluster, *arcane, syntactically,* and *bibulousness.* And this notwithstanding that there are those who believe that *arcane* is an arcane word, that *syntactically* can be made to sound like the malapropism of someone far gone in bibulousness.

I have a private theory about unusual words so simple it is embarrassing, in such august auspices, to disclose. It is as simple as that, say, we tend to conclude that people who use words with which we happen not to be familiar are using unfamiliar words. If John knows 8,000 words and Susan knows 8,000 words, inevitably John will know 250 words that Susan does not, and Susan will know 250 words that John does not, and John will think Susan exhibitionistic, and Susan will think John affected. I like to cite the waiter of a restaurant in Garden City who approached me twenty-five years ago to complain that he had subscribed to *National Review* and was absolutely certain that its circulation would greatly increase if only it stopped tolerating such unfamiliar words. Exactly two years later I was at the same restaurant, same table, same waiter, who greeted me joyfully, congratulating me on having taken his advice.

There are reasons for using words even when they are unfamiliar, a term which has to mean unfamiliar to those unfamiliar with them, a description whose geographical coordinates I would hate to have to specify. It can be a matter of rhythm, it can be a matter of the exact fit—and it can be something by way of obeisance to the people whose honed verbal appetites created the need for such a word, which therefore came into being. Call it supply-side linguistics; but whatever you call it, pray be thankful that someone invented the word *velleity* and that a few refuse to permit it to die, even as others would die to preserve the lousewort. Kilpo tells us that "as writers, we ought to take advantage of all the glorious riches of the English tongue, and to use them as best we can, but always taking into account one thing: the audience we are writing for." I would not dispute the relevance of this injunction directed at those terrible people who write those inscrutable instruction manuals (the computer-folk now call this "documentation"), but I think that writers also have an obligation to keep the frontiers of language open, else the weeds grow, the tall trees out there atrophy, and our patrimony is eroded.

———

I would not have thought it possible for someone other than a professional bibliographer to gather so many pointed examples of the kind of thing that is awfully wrong, that is less than quite right, that is okay, that is quite beautiful. In one section, JJK gives us Version One of a paragraph he wrote, lets us see its weaknesses even as he slowly descries them; lets us trace his corrections, on into drafts four and five. This is truly exciting stuff, like seeing a documentary on Picasso painting a canvas. And listen to the titles of the subchapters in Chapter 4, which are: "The Things We Ought Not to Do." They are: 1. "We ought not to use clichés." 2. "We ought never to fall into gobbledygook." 3. "We ought not to mangle our sentences." 4. "As a general rule, we ought not to use euphemisms." 5. "We ought not to pile up our nouns as adjectives." 6. "We ought not to coin words wantonly." 7. "We must not break the rules of grammar." 8. "We ought not to write dialect or slang unless we are certain of both our ear and our audience." 9. "We ought not to be redundant." 10. "We ought not to use words that have double meanings." 11. "We ought not to write portmanteau sentences." 12. "We ought not unintentionally to give offense by sexist words or phrases, but we ought not to be intimidated either." 13. "We ought not to make mistakes in spelling."

Right there we have the plainspokenness that characterizes Kilpatrick together with evidence of the ear that exactly catches what it is he wants to say, and, I guess I should add, a whiff of the imperial manner. If you feel strongly about words, it is downright offensive when someone says "hopefully," unless he is referring to a whaler's wife, looking hopefully out over the horizon from her widow's walk. Kilpatrick, while understanding and flexible to the point of acknowledging the dynamic imperative, is a firm custodian. I would trust the family treasure with him, you bet. There will be no attrition of the language at the gravesite of the collected works of James Jackson Kilpatrick.

He confesses that this is in some ways a personal book. I would guess that most proficient word-users would agree with somewhere between 90 and 95 percent of what he pronounces upon. But some things aggrieve him more than others, and that is both to be expected and, in a sense, welcomed, because once again it reminds us of the factor of art. He provides a huge chapter devoted to at least a hundred personal crotchets, of which the initial dozen are "A" AND "AN"; A.M. IN THE MORNING; ABSOLUTE WORDS; ABSTRACT/ABSTRACTION; ACCESS (v); AD HOC; AD NAUSEAM; ADAGES, OLD; ADAPT/ADOPT; ADVERSE/AVERSE; AFFECT/EFFECT; and AFFI-

DAVIT. Under ABSOLUTE WORDS we read, "My own modest list of words that cannot be qualified by 'very' or 'rather' or 'a little bit' includes *unique, imperative, universal, final, fatal, complete, virgin, dead, equal, eternal, total, unanimous, essential,* and *indispensable.*"

I dunno. Wouldn't the idiomatic ring of "altogether unique" strike you as okay? Or how about, "It was, so to speak, rather a final gesture when Dominguin dedicated the bull to his loyal public and proceeded to get killed." But . . . we are taking advice from a man whose ear is a Stradivarius, and there is reason to give him the benefit of the doubt, always allowing for the supremacy of one's own conscience. And again, everyone has his own crotchets. While I was reading Kilpo's manuscript aboard an airliner, the captain's voice rang in, "We will land at La Guardia in approximately fifty-nine minutes." *Approximately?* What's approximately for, if not imperatively conjoined to one hour, or forty-five minutes; or, at most, fifty-five minutes?

But this kind of thing can go on and on. For instance, we can agree that the "h" is not pronounced, requiring therefore "an" as the indefinite article. But then doesn't a difference come in precisely in the emphasis the individual elocutionist gives to the "h" sound? *I* would say, "a historical novel" because it happens that when I pronounce the adjective, the aitch is definitely present and accounted for. Again, mightn't a historian, even one so sure of tone that he would never think heedlessly of an "old cliché," find himself so situated as desiring to distinguish between a new and an old cliché? ("The arsenal of democracy, that very old cliché, has given way to a new cliché, namely the military-industrial complex.")

If you wish to pursue the game, the list of demurrals grows (I said I agreed with 95 percent, and 5 percent is, really, a whole lot). Consider the author's dislike for such locutions as "with deference to the learned opinion of my able and distinguished friend." But, don't you see, there is a rhetorical point to be served in occasional tushery. You are reminding the reader—and your distinctly unlearned and undistinguished colleague—that you are aware of the boundaries of diplomatic exchange, and willing to observe them, even as Winston Churchill would have addressed a communication to his German counterpart, "Dear Mr. Hitler."

While I am at it, Mr. Kilpatrick uses the exclamation *aargh!* to communicate disgust: wrongly, I think, influenced as I was when thirty years ago, reading the letters of Swinburne, I came upon him using it to express orgasmic delight in one of his vapulatory fantasies. (Mr. Kilpatrick is reaching for ugh!) Again, do we proper word-users need to stay away from the "long day" on the martinet's grounds that a day cannot have more than a fixed number of hours, and didn't Galileo or somebody go to jail to prove Kilpo's point?

On the matter of *expertise* I get deadly serious. It happens that I learned the word from a scholar bilingual in French, and that I was present when he and a renowned philosopher discussed ruefully the deterioration in the use of the word, whose corruption has been depriving us of a marvelously useful resource. Invited formally to define the word, they came up with: "*Expertise* is the body of operative knowledge" (that attaches to the subject under discussion). So that, for instance, you can say, "There is expertise in politics up to a point, after which it becomes an art." There is no way of saying this if you attach to *expertise* the vulgar meaning Mr. Kilpatrick correctly advises us would justify throwing the word away altogether. Throw out the bad word, struggle to reclaim the good one.

And then, as lagniappe, I am amused by the author's insistence that *remains to be seen* is tolerable only when you are talking about a corpse awaiting inspection in a funeral parlor. I see (and use) the phrase intending to inject doubt. Man-from-Missouri-wise-kind-of-thing. "It remains to be seen whether Harry Truman's bid for the farm vote is going to pay off." Remember that by authorizing one usage you are not committed to preferring it. "I am not so sure that Harry Truman's bid for the farm vote is going to work" would satisfy whatever doubt I desire to invest in the observation.

But what a barrel of fun. The author wrote to me that this would be his "last book." Then we find, under Number 10 above ("Avoid Words That Have Double Meanings"), "Another word that occasionally gives trouble is *last*. Its first meaning, unmistakably understood, is *final, terminal, ultimate*. But *last* also can mean 'most recent.' If we fall into a sentence involving *the last few months* or *his last book,* we may cause a flicker. By contrast, *past* admits of no confusion in a context of time: the *past few* months. Instead of *his last book,* I would suggest *his latest book.*"

Just so. It may be that James Jackson Kilpatrick will never write another book at once so charming, instructive, resourceful, and useful. But something will gestate in his mind, you watch. You know what? Something like the coming of spring we began with. This is a spring that

> . . . tiptoes in. It pauses, overcome by shyness, like a grandchild at the door, peeping in, ducking out of sight, giggling in the hallway. "Heather!" I want to cry, "I know you're out there. Come in!" And April slips into our arms. The maples do not come forth in green; they are flowering red, soft as slippers, in tassels like a jester's scepter. The flowering almond is pink, absurdly pink, little-girl pink, as pink as peppermint and cream. The apples display their milliner's scraps of ivory silk, rose-tinged. All the sleeping things wake

up—primrose, baby iris, candytuft, blue phlox, the Scotch heather that had seemed dead beyond resurrection. The earth warms—you can smell it, feel it, crumble April in your hands.

Kilpatrick was writing about the coming of spring, but as much could be written about the materialization of another book in the mind of a man who cannot stop making poetry, whether he is writing about the spring, the Supreme Court, or the English language.

Chapter 2

On Vocabulary

Speaking of the right word, let's get right to it. The word for today is on the blackboard: *vocabulary*. WFB's Introduction to the Kilpatrick book in the preceding chapter is the first of several comprehensive essays on the subject. These are needed because more people know William F. Buckley, Jr., for his vocabulary than know the details of his politics. Some are amused by it, some bemused, some attempt to equal or exceed his abilities (few succeed) while others are annoyed and a number are outright hostile. Some are simply bothered by his use of a word that the "ordinary" reader might not know and others are apt to confuse or conflate their opposition to his political views with opposition to his vocabulary.

Over the decades, Buckley has had to defend his use of what he considers the right word. There are those who have come to his defense. Some of these defenses—or, given the American theory of sports that a good offense is the best possible defense, some of his most offensive pieces—are grouped here. They are largely but not always in chronological order, as will be obvious.

Quite apart from the merits of the say-it-plainly, say-it-simply school versus the use-the-word-you-need faction, there are some splendid words involved in the never-ending debate. Many correspondents simply ask questions; others suspect Buckley of having misused or perhaps having invented a word. Whichever, there are words contained in this running debate to admire, puzzle over, or cause that delightful shock of definition.

Here is an early example, a newspaper column from the early sixties.

THE HYSTERIA ABOUT WORDS

Have you noticed that the use of an unusual word sometimes irritates the reader to such a point that he will accuse the user of affectation, than which there is no more heinous crime in the American republic? The distinguished political and social philosopher and columnist Mr. Russell Kirk used the word "energumen" to describe in his Introduction to my book *Rumbles Left and Right* who it is I agitate against, and one reviewer fairly exploded with annoyance. Now the word in question means "someone possessed by an evil spirit," and fanatically addicted to a particular idea. Can you think of a better word to describe certain kinds of people who seek to reorder public affairs according to their hypnotic visions? Should one refuse to use a venerable word for which there is no obvious synonym, simply because it is a word that does not regularly appear in the diet of the average reader?

I raise the problem because I am often accused of an inordinate reliance on unusual words, and desire—as would you in my shoes, I think—to defend myself against the insinuation that I write as I do simply to prove that I have returned recently from the bowels of a dictionary with a fish in my mouth, establishing my etymological dauntlessness. Surely one must distinguish between those who plunder old tomes to find words which, in someone's phrase, should never be let out . . . and such others as Russell Kirk, who use words because (a) the words signify just exactly what the user means, and because (b) the user deems it right and proper to preserve in currency words which in the course of history were coined as the result of a felt need.

There is a sort of phony democratic bias against the use of unusual words. Recently I heard a young movie actress being interviewed on a radio station. She was asked by her interrogator what it meant to be an actress, and replied that an actor's life is "multifaceted."

"What are you trying to pull on me?" demands the radio announcer.

She ran panicked from the argument—what else, in the democratic age, when it is deemed an effrontery on the democratic ideal to use a word that is not used twice a week by Little Orphan Annie? "I'm sorry I used such a fancy word—I guess I don't really know what it means—I should have said, there are lots of aspects to being an actress." Democracy won the day, and the show droned on.

A while ago I was on Jack Paar's television program, and he asked me a number of questions having to do with this and that, which I tried vainly to answer, as best I knew how. I wrote about that experience . . . and described the ensuing tantrum of Mr. Paar and his associates, who steamed on and on about my ideological vices, expressing special outrage at my unintelligibility.

It is a curious thing, this universal assumption by a number of prominently situated opinion- or rather mood-makers, that the American people are either unaware of the unusual word or undisposed to hear it and find out what it means, thus broadening not merely their vocabulary—that isn't the important thing—but their conceptual and descriptive powers. Those who say that the average American is incapable of appreciating the meaning of the word "energumen" are, in my humble judgment, nuts. The average American is, in Franklin P. Adams's phrase, a bit above average, and his intelligence is not tied umbilically to Jack Paar's anti-intellectualist muse.

It is curious, too, that a man who is offended by the use of the word "multifaceted" or "energumen" is perfectly capable of expressing a sentence of death-defying mechanical complexity. I am unfortunately innocent in the world of science and I wish I knew what in the world the TV hawker is talking about when he reels off something having to do with a "double action injector system in the valve mechanism" but it does not occur to me to suggest that he is putting on airs; it occurs to me to rue my patently inadequate knowledge of the mechanical a b c's.

The point about unusual words is that they are as necessary to philosophy, economics, aesthetics, and political science as they are necessary in the world of higher mechanics, in which so many people displaying the natural American genius are so much at home. It is possible, I suppose, to describe the refinements of an Astrojet fan injection through-ventilated engine in words understandable to me, but the exercise is not often resorted to because the manufacturers assume a level of mechanical literacy, even as they assume that those who do not have it ought not to set the standards for those who do have it. So it is in other fields, which is why, in my judgment, when Mr. Russell Kirk uses the word "energumen," he should be allowed to use it, and the thing for book reviewers to do when they come upon it, if they are unfamiliar with it, is not to pout, but to open a dictionary and see if the word is one whose meaning they wish to learn. They must guard against going about like anti-literate energumens.

—WFB   JUNE 15, 1963

. . . What the blazes is the meaning of the "bloviations" indulged in by Attorney William Kunstler?

The Random House Dictionary gives *blouse, blouson, blousy, blow.* The New Imperial Reference Dictionary gives *blot, blotch, blouse, blow.* And a 1928 edition of the Concise Oxford Dictionary gives *blotch, blottesque* (well done, Oxford!), *blouse* and *blow.* But I'm blowed if I could find *bloviation* anywhere.

I believe you made the word up and it is nothing more than a lot of blatant blather.

Bless you.

R.N. USHER-WILSON

BRONXVILLE, N.Y.

Yes, we did make it up—and don't think it was easy!

—ED. (WFB)   OCTOBER 22, 1968

R. N. Usher-Wilson's letter raises my eyebrow, but the response of "Ed." my hackles. The good dominie (for Usher-Wilson, in modesty, forbore to flaunt his cloth) has simply consorted with the lower class of dictionary. Had he consulted a good workmanlike Funk & Wagnalls (e.g., New Standard Dictionary of the English Language, 1913 edition as revised in 1938), he would have found, much to his delight, the following exquisite gem of unbloviated lexicography: "*blo'via'tion . . . n. Loud, defiant, boastful talk; blowing.* Literary Digest *Oct. 23, '09, p. 666.*" The word was particularly popular as an elegant variation in the United States during the second half of the nineteenth century. I believe Mark Twain indulged a certain fondness for it.

Now I pass to the more heinous lapse, the editor's claim to having invented this fulsome lip-shaping word. Many things, among them not a few both noble and sightly, the "Ed." and his merry crew may rightly lay claim to having introduced into civil discourse—but bloviation never. Bloviation belongs exclusively to publishers.

WILLIAM F. RICKENBACKER

BRIARCLIFF MANOR, N.Y.

. . . Judging from the tone of your editorials, which I enjoy very much, I'm sure that you are indeed capable of making up the word, especially if you discover at a critical moment that none of the other several hundred thousand English ones don't seem to fit the occasion. I admire your zeal.

I wonder, however, whether in this instance you may have overlooked the fact that one of our Presidents, the late and hardly lamented Warren G. Harding, is reputed to have used the word "bloviate" to describe some of his own utterances.

Mr. Harding's chief qualification for public office was considered by many to have been a something more than modest talent in chuffing wind into the small end of a bass horn, a "tin grunt," or a "helicon," to some of the older devotees. This process was accomplished by pressing down one or more of the valve buttons installed partway along such cumbrous but useful plumbing. By dint of years of devoted practice of this art Mr. Harding found that he could attract much attention by this use of his personal wind, especially if he pressed the right valves down.

After assuming high office, in the parlance of other days, Mr. Harding achieved some notoriety as a "blow-hard," i.e., a strenuous exuder of flatulence accompanied by speech. Turning such a questionable compliment to happier use, he used to say that he would "bloviate" a little bit for various assemblages. Thus came into some modest usage the term which you have turned into a sort of noun when originally it was a verb.

Although I can't cite chapter, book, verse, page, or line, I believe you will find corroboration of this essay's central theme if you will refer to Mr. Harding's usually unflattering biographies.

I hope this doesn't break your rice bowl, or spoil your day.

Yours for more neologisms and some new adaptations of the old words to tell things as they are.

ROBERT J. DEMER

HARRISBURG, PA.

———

As the drumfire—dumbfire?—increased, suggesting strongly that Buckley dumb down his language, he fired back, via another author of impressive vocabulary and returning again to his friend Kilpatrick's book, in a column this time, making a few new points.

———

THE STUDENTS, WHAT IS THEIR PROBLEM?

I spotted the scholarly and irrepressible Anthony Burgess, the English novelist essayist fantasist (author of *A Clockwork Orange,* among other things) giving advice publicly to his students (he is visiting America, teaching at the City College of New York). And what he said to the students, among other things, was: "I would ask you only to expand your vocabularies, develop a minimal grace of style, think harder, and learn who Helen of Troy and Nausicaa were. And for God's sake, stop talking about relevance. All we have is the past."

Mr. Burgess was musing about the college student he comes in contact with, at a university that practices an open admissions policy. Mr. Burgess was tactful about the whole thing, but he gave away his meaning, which is that the adulteration of education results in phony education. And when that happens, what you develop is new universities. When egalitarian ideology overtakes these, then "super universities will be built"; and after that, "super super universities . . . This can go on forever. Ultimately, the gods of learning are not mocked. The term 'university' may be rich in noble connotations, but it means only what we want it to mean."

Professor Burgess gave an example of a student essay on *Macbeth* "to which soon I must give a pass mark: 'Lady Mackbet says she had a kid not in so many words but she says she remembers what it was like when a kid sucked her nipple so I reckon she was a mother some time and the kid must have died but we dont hear no more about it which is really careless of Shakesper because the real reason why Macbeth and his wife are kind of restless and ambitious is because they did not have a baby that lived and perhaps this is all they really want and S. says notin about it.' "

Mr. Burgess provokes us by juxtaposing against that passage one from another student, presumably in the same class, whose grade—one assumes—is going to be indistinguishable from that of the young man who penetrated to the heart of Mr. and Mrs. Macbeth's difficulty. The other student wrote: "The weakly placed negatives in Dr. Faustus's penultimate line—'Ugly hell, gape not, come not, Lucifer'—may conceivably be taken as expressive of a desire, not implausible in a Renaissance scholar, to dare even the ultimate horrors for the sake of adding to his store of knowledge."

Now hang on to the point for a minute please, and reflect on one of the recommendations of Mr. Burgess. He believes that "the division between a scientific discipline and a humanistic one is already manifesting itself in undergraduate life-styles. The banner-waving students who hold protest meetings are merely indulged. They will, regrettably perhaps, never rule America; America will be controlled by the hard-eyed technicians who have no time for protest."

We should shrug off those intimations that fuel the superstition that we are being managed by a military-industrial complex. (It would appear plain that this is not the case.) But one hears plaintively the call of Mr. Burgess to his students to "expand" their vocabulary. I note among the Christmas advertisements lying around, one for a new radio receiver: "There's 150 watts IHF power, a loudness compensating switch, power output/heat sinks, IF/FM/multiplex decoder, FM muting, FM Stereo."

Now, the advertising agency that wrote those words is not putting on the dawg. The ad was, as they say, "communicating." Communicating, one supposes, not only to the "hard-eyed technicians" who are getting educated in the colleges, but to students in general. It is not afraid to use words and terms which are demanding—I, for instance, deficient in the appropriate education, do not have the least idea what the manufacturer is talking about: "power output/heat sinks" indeed! Lady Macbeth was never so inscrutable.

The moral is that the resistance to a rich vocabulary is inconsistently exercised. When the talk is of scientific or mechanical things, the public is altogether acquiescent to strange and minutely differentiated terms. Is this what Mr. Burgess is saying?—that the difficulty in making distinctions in human and social affairs leads people to Tarzan-talk in the classroom? The same people who can talk to the hi-fi people with maximum scientific sophistication? Worth musing, between the holidays.

—WFB   DECEMBER 28, 1972

THE WRITER'S CRAFT: PART TWO

Someone recently sent along an editorial from a newspaper in Wisconsin denouncing me and all my works, or I suppose more accurately denouncing all my works, on the grounds that they are strewn with unusual words. And I am glad the whole subject came up because I have been looking for a peg to celebrate the publication of a book that is useful, exciting, and beautiful, namely James Jackson Kilpatrick's *The Writer's Art.*

The protocols of full disclosure require that I instantly communicate that I wrote the Introduction to that book, but also quickly to add that I was not paid for it and have no financial stake in the book's success. But we all have a huge cultural stake in the book's success if we care about the dearest part of our patrimony, which is our language.

But first, on the matter of the unusual word. "My brother pundit, Bill Buckley, falls into sin even more easily than I. . . ."

I quarreled with him in my Introduction. . . . I said that I have a private theory, a theory so simple, so rudimentary, that it almost embarrasses me to trot it out. But think it over. It is that we tend to believe that a word is unfamiliar because it is unfamiliar to us . . .

Concede, of course, that there are words neither you nor I know. Should those words be quarantined? I wrote in my Introduction: "There are reasons for using words even when they are unfamiliar. It can be a matter of rhythm, it can be a matter of the exact fit—and it can be something by way of obeisance to the people whose honed verbal appetites created the need for such a word, which therefore came into being. Call it supply-side linguistics." . . . How is that for a defiant gesture?

But the whole business amuses. Kilpatrick knows the names of more flowers and trees and shrubs than I know names appropriate to describe Soviet policy. Are we supposed to admire the cook whose menu is unchanged?

I have recently pursued the whole question in another connection, and found myself wondering whether it is sufficiently recognized that writing is, as Mr. Kilpatrick's book title advises us, an art. We do not expect the amateur to try to play the Grieg Concerto in A Minor for Piano and Orchestra, but should we be resentful that some can do it?

John Updike is what one ought safely to be able to call a "performing writer," at whose hands the taxing demands of language are confidently met. Whereas most people don't paint canvases or play a musical instrument, everyone writes. The mistake is to suppose that one should discourage the profusion of verbal forms.

What Kilpatrick does in his book is useful to anyone with any interest either in self-expression or in the evaluation of others' expression. He lists common errors, discourses wittily on clichés and word traps, lists common solecisms. One huge chapter is devoted to one hundred personal "crotchets," he calls them: the kind of thing he often spots in print, which violates his verbal code. No adventure story is brighter, more intriguing, more heavily charged with suspense, leading to greater delights.

The Writer's Art is in my judgment the most readable book on the English language I have ever come upon, and you should get it, read it, give it to your children to read—give it to your tailor and candlestick maker. As I say, we all have a stake in it. You will shimmer with gratitude to the author, and to our forefathers, who gave us this blessed tongue.

—WFB   MAY 15, 1984

Dear Mr. Buckley:

I am enclosing an article written by one of our local columnists for the *Maries County Gazette,* which I think you will find amusing.

Sincerely,

GAIL MALONE

VIENNA, MO.

From the Front Seat
By Henry Evans

THE OBFUSCATOR

A few years ago someone in Washington had the bright idea of asking all the government bureaus and departments there to write all their papers and memos in everyday English which everyone could understand instead of their usual "federalese" which no one but the writer could understand. When that news story came over the wire a newspaper editor decided to have a little fun with it so the heading he wrote for the story said Eschew Obfuscation, or, avoid lack of clearness.

Today I would like to nominate a new Champion of Obfuscation who is not a government bureaucrat at all but, rather, a syndicated newspaper columnist and magazine publisher and editor who ought to know better and who probably does but is being perverse. He is William F. Buckley, Jr., whose column appears in several hundred newspapers and whose magazine, *National Review,* is one of the major voices of the conservative side of the political spectrum.

To put it bluntly, Buckley is worse than a bureaucratic obfuscator; he is a lexicographical snob, to use a kind of phrase he might use himself. He is a show-off who uses words no one but himself knows the meaning of and by sending his readers to the dictionary with every other paragraph he writes he thinks he is demonstrating his superiority over us lesser mortals. For my part, I think he belongs in jail; I do not believe the freedom of speech or of the press was meant for the likes of him.

Now, we have to be a little careful here. In a book of his I read last week, *Execution Eve,* which is a collection of his columns and essays as well as some correspondence, I encountered six unfamiliar words in a matter of forty pages, pages 419 through 459. I went to the dictionary for every one of them and got madder and madder with each one of them. I started hoping I would not find them in the dictionary so I could accuse him of making them up, but I found them all. Now, he can claim he should not be blamed for using properly any word found in the dictionary, but let's be reasonable about it: I have spent all these years using the English language to earn a living and I have a reasonably good, maybe not great, but reasonably good vocabulary and when I have to go to the dictionary six times within forty pages, I can only assume I am reading the words of a lexicographical snob.

First he gives us SYNECDOCHE, a figure of speech in which the whole is used for the part or the part for the whole. Then ADUMBRATED, to darken or conceal partly, to overshadow; this was followed by VELLEITY, a mere wish with no effort to obtain it. From there he takes us to MAIEUTIC, the Socratic mode of inquiry, bringing out ideas latent in the mind. Then on to PROVENANCE, the location of a beginning such as where a painting was painted or a book written. Finally, he unloads PASQUINADE on us, a publicly posted lampoon or satire or ridicule.

At this point in the book I stopped running to the dictionary at every one of his show-off words. I just skipped them. In this same book he says that among the things he likes best is good English prose. It's too bad he did not learn to write it at Yale, which along with other Ivy League institutions specializes in making snobs out of otherwise normal people.

He did not use the words in some kind of an article discussing seldom-used words. He used them in his normal writing on a variety of subjects, for which I still think he belongs in jail. Lacking that, I still have one recourse: I am going to eschew Buckley, and that is not mere velleity; I'm actually going to do it.

Dear Miss Malone: Mr. Evans is wrong. It's not so. It's *not* the company I keep. Some of my best friends don't know the meaning of the word "provenance." But he failed to note the lexicographical snobs who created the need for the words he listed. They came into being because there was what the economists call a "felt need." (Come on, Evans, you've obviously experienced a velleity at some point in your life, but what would you say if someone asked what it was you were experiencing? See? You *can't* eschew Buckley. It's bad for you.) Cordially,

—WFB   AUGUST 4, 1989

Dear Mr. Buckley:

In the August 4 "Notes & Asides," a column by journalist Henry Evans is reprinted scolding you for using words "no one but [yourself] knows the meaning of and . . . sending [your] readers to the dictionary." He complains that he had to go to the dictionary six times within forty pages, then roundly condemns you as a "lexicographical snob." Mr. Evans seems to be the sort of columnist who keeps his dictionary—indeed, all hard-bound books—out of arm's reach and his one point of view always at his fingertips.

I can readily imagine the smile turned to despair on Mr. Evans's face were he ever to encounter (in *Dear Bertrand Russell . . . ,* 1969) Bertrand Russell's "twenty favorite words": wind, alabaster, incarnadine, heath, chrysoprase, sublunary, golden, astrolabe, chorasmean, begrime, apocalyptic, alembic, pilgrim, ineluctable, fulminate, quagmire, terraqueous, ecstasy, diapason, inspissated.

And I have found in a collection of brief book reviews (*Urgent Copy,* 1969) by the novelist Anthony Burgess, in rather less than forty pages, these wonderful literary chord progressions: collocation, demotic, antinomies, polymathy, diaspora, eponym, rarefaction, gamboge, variorum (which Bernard Shaw would have said no Englishman can pronounce), etiolations, fictile, numen, neologism, repine (E. Waugh's favorite), gulosity, carious, tragoid, tabascoid, statify, anabasis, exophthalmic, "fiery laconicism" (Keats), sempiternal, bandersnatch, palindromic, tumid, interstices, and panjandrum.

Mr. Evans's column caught me at high tide and high surf astride J.I.M. Stewart's *Eight Modern Writers* (Oxford University Press, 1963), where barely through the third author, in about two hundred pages, one hears distinctly Oxford harmonies, many requiring looking up for pronunciation: subfusc, nescience, divagation, finically, thaumaturge, hortatory, recusant, conflation, viscidity, sanative, esemplatic power, prosopopoeia, facture, concatenate, deliquesces, plangently, desuetude, homothetic, mythopoeic, chthonic . . . and proem! This from a teacher.

But there is a darker side to the Evans *v.* Buckley encounter. It is expressed nicely by the American author David Leavitt in his novel *The Lost Language of Cranes* (1986), where he writes a fine paragraph on a copy editor's addiction to crossword puzzles, "the meshing of meanings, the knitting of one set of words into another," and their creators ("the vultures of the thinking world"). Leavitt concludes . . . : "And Rose was learning that such carrion was better than alcohol. This benign activity literally tied up the brain; it blocked grief, anxiety, panic. In a burst of bitter energy, Rose thrust Thomas Mann and Timon of Athens into the fray. She fired out synonyms like bullets. But in the end, her head ached horribly . . ."

> Yours,
> THOMAS GOLDTHWAITE
> HILO, HAWAII

Dear Mr. Buckley:

I am a nineteen-year-old who knows five of the six words cited by the querulous Henry Evans as cause to nominate you "Champion of Obfuscation" [Aug. 4]. While it is true I am currently an Ivy League student (with clenched teeth I will have to look down my nose upon Mr. Evans due to the snobbery he alleges I and my fellow students have), I learned those words at my public high school in Ohio.

> ADAM R. STAUFFER
> BROWN UNIVERSITY
> PROVIDENCE, R.I.

Dear Mr. Stauffer: Perhaps Mr. Evans will forgive you if you manage to forget those words before you are his age. Cordially,

> —WFB   SEPTEMBER 15, 1989

This time, WFB takes the fight to a higher court, answering a one-two challenge: first by the respected Meg Greenfield of *The Washington Post,* and then (an edged query) by a good editor, Ed Williams, of the *Charlotte Observer,* in the pages of *The New York Times Book Review.* Even so, he starts off by setting the record straight on the matter of titles.

Newspaper and magazine editors usually arrogate to themselves the right to write titles for pieces they get from authors, a nicety not known to many unsuspecting readers. A piece the editor Harry Evans once commissioned me to write for *The Sunday Times* (London), which I called "The Londonization of New York," for that was the theme, appeared under the heading "A Tale of Two Cities."

I could have sworn another writer got there first.

Editor
The New York Times Book Review
Dear Sir:
For the record, I had nothing to do with the choice of the two headlines ("Joy of Sesquipedality" and "I Am Lapidary but Not Eristic When I Use Big Words") imposed on my essay on the use of long words and foreign phrases (*TNYTBR,* Nov. 30, 1986).

Yours faithfully,

WM. F. BUCKLEY, JR.

A Defense of the Use of Unusual Words and Foreign Words

One day in May I found on my desk my column, clipped from that morning's *Washington Post,* a red arrow—courtesy of my secretary—pointing to an editorial underneath it. It read, "ERISTIC: (i ris/tik) *adj* [Gr. *eristikos,* d. *erizein,* to strive, dispute d. *eris,* strife] of or provoking controversy, or given to sophistical argument and specious reasoning." I looked up to the corresponding asterisk in the text and there saw my sentence, "The action by Judge Robert Carter [in fining the National Conference of Catholic Bishops for contempt] has brought out a lot of smiles in judicial political circles (as a rule, you don't step up and fine the Catholic or the Protestant churches—or the Jewish synagogues) for failure to comply with eristic complaints." (The Abortion Rights Mobilization was suing to deny the bishops their tax deductibility, to which end it had persuaded the judge to subpoena the bishops' internal memos on abortion.) *Washington Post* editor Meg Greenfield was rapping me on the knuckles, a quite unusual public reproach: I couldn't remember when last she had thought to help the readers of the *Post* to understand unusual words, however much time she needs to spend explaining unusual editorial positions. Dear Meg, I thought. The instincts of the Jewish Mother just took her over this time.

And then, a week or two later, another clipping on my desk, red arrow, footnote, only this time it was the *Charlotte Observer*, explaining to its readers the meaning of "lapidary." (Their footnote: "Lapidary. Having the elegance and precision associated with inscriptions on monumental stones.") Presently there appeared a letter of explanation from Mr. Ed Williams, Associate Editor of the *Charlotte Observer*, and the challenge was now, well, lapidary. Mr. Williams wrote me:

"I oversee the *Observer*'s daily Viewpoint page, and in that capacity am in charge of preparing syndicated columns for publication in this newspaper. Sometimes I insert aids to the reader, such as the definition of 'lapidary' in your recent column, enclosed. A fellow editor asked why I didn't also define *à outrance*. I replied that I thought you use foreign words and phrases in your columns because 1) you like to show off, and 2) you take delight in irritating people. Far be it from me, I said, to deny you those pleasures. Then I realized I shouldn't presume to answer for you. So let me ask. Why do you use, in your column, foreign words and phrases, and unfamiliar English words, that are unlikely to be understood by the average reader, or at least the average editor? Surrounded by dictionaries, I await your reply."

The point here raised—When is it okay to use an unfamiliar word? When is it not okay?—is endlessly argued, yet even so, fresh insights and original formulations continue to be coined. One of these, I think, was Dwight Macdonald's distinction, made in his marvelous survey of Webster III for *The New Yorker* (March 10, 1962), in which he distinguished between unusual words (okay) and words that "belong in the zoo sections of the dictionary" (not okay). I should think most people would agree, for instance, that "arachibutyrophobia" would be an example of the latter (the word is said to define the fear of peanut butter's sticking to the roof of your mouth). James Jackson Kilpatrick . . . takes a position on the dogmatic side against the use of unfamiliar words and cites me, however kindly, as a prodigious offender (as it happened, the Lord delivered Kilpatrick into my hands, because his proscriptive passage against long and unusual words contained four long and unusual words). Kilpatrick likes to quote Westbrook Pegler, who denounced the use of what he called "out-of-town words."

The question, under the proximate prodding of Mr. Williams, is worth revisiting. And an easy way to begin is to examine the two words singled out for attention: the first one the word Mr. Williams thought that courtesy required him to translate for the benefit of his readers; the second, the French, which he let pass as arrant and provocative exhibitionism.

What happens when Mr. A. and Ms. B. flatly disagree about whether a word is "unusual"? Well, there is a problem of an obvious order, namely

that some words are unusual but widely recognized, while others are unusual and widely unrecognized. Returning to the general theme a few
weeks ago, Mr. Kilpatrick wrote in his column that he had recently published the sentence "The *Miami Herald* carried a 72-point four-column
head, DADELAND IS DOYEN OF AREA MALLS." Whereafter he received a letter from a Floridian who wanted to know "How many people know what
'doyen' means?" Observed K.: "The more pertinent question: How many
of the *Herald*'s 450,000 readers know what doyen means? Ten percent? 20
percent? 80 percent?" Kilpatrick is a man of troubled conscience. He goes
right on to say that here he himself has just finished making reference to
"72-point" type. That is workaday prose of the Dick and Jane order for
anyone who has ever engaged in editorial enterprises—but what about
those 450,000 readers? Might they not have preferred, K. tortures himself,
"inch-high type"?

Nobody is going to pay Mr. Gallup a lot of money to find out how
many people in Florida know what the word "doyen" means. And not
many people would be willing to come up with a threshold percentage:
More than X know doyen?—Okay to use. Less than X, verboten (forbidden).
That's on the order of defining the line where obscenity begins.

All of which brings me to say that I do not think of "lapidary" as a word
so unrecognizable as to interrupt the reading flow of the average college
graduate. But in saying this it is important to reiterate one of the points I
made in the public argument I had with Kilpatrick. . . . It is quite simply
this, that people with vocabularies of the same size are by no means people who know the same words. A while ago I reviewed a book by John Updike (*The Coup*), discovering over twenty words the meaning of which I
didn't know. Knocking these words around at an editors' session in my office one afternoon, I would find that, cumulatively, my five colleagues
knew them all. Sam Johnson's apothegm, "In lapidary inscriptions a man
is not upon oath," if it is not in the anthologies that circle Mr. Williams's
desk, it ought to be.

But then let's take the tougher one. Here is what I wrote in a column
on Professor Paul Weiss, the philosopher whose eighty-fifth birthday was
something of a national event. "At Yale [Professor Weiss] was the political
liberal *à outrance*, but his orderly mind made it hard for him to defend
some of liberalism's zanier forms."

This, now, is concession time. How many people are familiar with *à
outrance*? It is, no question about it, an out-of-town word, though Pegler
certainly ran into it when he was out of town covering the war in France
in 1918, where the Germans faced the French, British, and Americans,
fighting their trench warfare *à outrance*. But the French word is given in
Webster, an English dictionary. First, the inquirer gets plain "outrance," in

English ("the last extremity"), and then is invited to look at *à outrance,* a separate entry, that gives: "to the death, unsparingly." The OED also lists it in French, and cites uses of it by Tobias Smollett and Walter Scott. . . .

But why should a syndicated columnist use the word? I can hear Mr. Williams re-asking. Well, not really, just to show off—one doesn't "show off" one's workaday equipment. You see, that word, and a hundred or so others, are a part of my *working* vocabulary, even as a C augmented eleventh chord with a raised ninth can be said to be an operative resource of the performing jazz pianist.

Are we now closing in on the question, by using the exclusivist word "performing"?

Yes, in a way we are, I suppose. Because just as the discriminating ear greets gladly the C augmented eleventh, when just the right harmonic moment has come for it, so the fastidious eye encounters happily the word that says exactly what the writer wished not only said but conveyed, here defined as a performing writer sensitive to cadence, variety, marksmanship, accent, nuance, and drama.

What of the reader who misses the refinement? Well, what of the listener deaf to the special reach of the C augmented eleventh? That reader has the usual choices: he can ignore the word; attempt, from the context, to divine its meaning precisely or roughly (not hard, in the narrative above, on Professor Weiss's liberal politics); or he can look it up. Are these alternatives an imposition? Yes, if the newspaper's columnist that day is giving instructions on how to treat a rattlesnake bite. You would not instruct the reader to fight the poison *à outrance.*

But newspapers, in particular in one-paper cities, tend to acknowledge an obligation beyond merely reporting the news. The very idea of a "feature," whether designed to advise (Ann Landers), amuse (Art Buchwald), satirize (G. R. Trudeau), or opine (the syndicated columnist), presupposes that the performer should use the full range of his relevant skills, even if the percentage of readers who turn to that feature is reduced. Surely there is a corner, in spacy papers that carry five pages on sports, for Addison and Steele? It required a Pulitzer Prize to alert some editors to the very existence of Murray Kempton, the most entertaining analytical belletrist in town, and now we read him, hungrily, in the *Stamford Advocate.* Readers have diverse interests, resources, skills, appetites. The Latin Mass Committee in London petitioned for the resumption of a single mass to be said in Latin after the postconciliar ban of 1965, and was turned down—on the grounds that Latin was only "for the educated few." Evelyn Waugh said it all in a letter to the *Times:* "Surely," he wrote, "in all her charity, Mother Church can make a little room, even for the educated few?"

—WFB   NOVEMBER 30, 1986

Dear Mr. Buckley:

As a longtime reader of *NR*, I've enjoyed your ongoing flirtation with abstruse English words.

After learning the meaning of "deipnosophist" the other day, I realized that I had not seen it in *NR*. One would expect it to pop up all over the place.

How do you explain this lapse?

Puzzled,

HAL MUNN

ALHAMBRA, CALIF.

Dear Mr. Munn: The word defines someone "skilled at table talk." It is used rarely for the obvious reasons. Cordially,

—WFB

Dear Mr. Buckley:

". . . savoring the highbrow's *dysphemism* for the relatively inoffensive 'stupid.' " ("The Assault on Whittaker Chambers"—WFB, Jr., Dec. 15.)

No one minds recondite words, provided they *are* words, like calling Liberals "puberulent lotophagi"—but "dysphemism"! Come now, you wouldn't josh a guy!

T. RIEDER

TORONTO, ONT.

Actually, we would. But the word exists. See Merriam-Webster III, p. 712.

—WFB   JANUARY 12, 1965

Dear Mr. Buckley:

Pray tell us readers the difference between "certain inalienable rights," as I read in my copy of The Declaration, and "certain unalienable rights," as printed on page 554 of *National Review.*

Sincerely,

COLONEL FRED W. MILLER

SCOTTSDALE, ARIZONA

P.S.: My dictionary says that "inalienable" and "unalienable" are synonymous.

Dear Colonel: "Unalienable" is the word Jefferson used. "Inalienable" is what is nowadays used. "Alienable" is what describes the rights we fought for.

Cordially,

—WFB   JUNE 25, 1976

Aｎd still the requests come in, asking WFB to explain and also defend his use of words that seem to some eyes, as his diction seems to some ears, affected. This latest (1996) was written at the request of *Sky* magazine, Delta's in-flight publication. This invitation must have appeared to Buckley, who virtually invented frequent flying, a chance to arm himself against the guy in the next seat who begins a conversation fortified by three little bottles of vodka.

He also manages to make, even now, new explanations and elaborations, elaborating on "zoo" words, getting the same advice over and over about his magazine's style, etc.

WORDS

The editor, Mr. Duncan Christy, having bombarded the readers of this magazine for eleven months with words judged "unusual" taken from my opera (Dear Sir: What does he mean, "opera"? As in *Madame Butterfly?* CURIOUS. Dear Curious: He means "works." The word is the plural of opus—a creative work. Best, Ed. Dear Sir: Well, why didn't he *say* "taken from my 'works?' " CURIOUS AND ANNOYED. Dear C & A.: He was asked to write an essay about *words,* so you shouldn't be surprised if he starts out by using an unusual word. Let's hear him out, okay? Ed.), has now decided to end the regular sessions and invites me to write in general about words. "I hope such an essay would be an encomium to words, alloyed with some direct observations about why we should not let words like 'encomium' and 'belletristic' and 'valedictory' go." Well, sure, so let me get a few things off my chest, since the question of me and words has come up before.

1. Two people of the same approximate age and education won't have identical vocabularies. She will know the meaning of maybe one hundred words that he doesn't know. But he will know an equivalent number of words—or more—that puzzle her, when and if he runs into them.

2. The reader's attitude toward an unusual word often depends on the context in which it is used. Two stories hang on this point. Years ago a classmate took me delicately to one side and said, "Bill, *National Review* would have a much larger circulation if you would just forbid the use of so many arcane words." I told him it was his imagination that so many such words congested my magazine, and I made him a bet. Sight unseen, I said, here's ten dollars that the next issue of *Time* magazine will have

more words you judge unfamiliar than you can target in any back issue, take your pick, of *National Review.*

Well, you can guess I would not be telling you this story if I had lost the bet. I won it. Question, Why was my friend under an illusion that cost him ten bucks?

Explanation. If a sentence or paragraph of prose is analytical in nature, any unusual word springs out at you. If the identical word appears in a passage in which the writer is describing something, or telling a story, the eye leaps over a word otherwise arresting. Since *National Review* is a journal of opinion, most of its articles and features are, as one would expect, analytical and critical—which means that an unusual word, in a verbally demanding environment, comes at you more aggressively.

An example:

She was a ravishing beauty, from sunlit hair to the limpid eyes to the full lips, sparkling teeth, and curious, tectonic smile. What kind of smile? The reader doesn't know, exactly, and isn't going to ask, not unless whatever the writer goes on to say about the beautiful lady can't be understood without knowing what makes up a "tectonic" smile, whatever the hell that is.

In that plane the practiced eye can discern the tectonic disruptions of an early geological age. The word tectonic (*Relating to, causing, or resulting from structural deformation of the earth's crust*) reaches out at you, and you see in its eyes the candid stricture: Buddy, unless you know what a tectonic disruption means, you can't swing with me on this one. Go read something else; or if you want to, stick around and see if you can follow what comes next.

The context often establishes whether the unusual word can coast by without interrupting the reader's thought.

3. The law of the flexed muscle. The following episode is my all-time favorite. After a lecture, at dinner . . . , one man of about fifty was visibly excited by my presence. At the end of the meal he drew me to one side to disclose the reason. He belonged, it turned out, to a militant labor union to which he was required to pay dues. Every month the union newsletter featured proudly its most recent political activities on behalf of its membership. "They are *terribly* Democratic," he complained, "and I am a *Goldwater* Republican. So when I saw you come in I really cheered."

I thanked him, and then he leaned and whispered into my ear. "Let me tell you something, Mr. Buckley. I subscribed to *National Review* just a month ago. Now if you would do something about all those long words you will"—he stretched out his arms expansively—"double . . . no, *triple* your circulation.

"Do you agree with me, Mr. Buckley?"

"Yes, sure. We'll certainly try to do something about those words."

Flash forward, one year. Same man. Same dining room (different speech). He beams when he sees me. "You took my advice. It's made the magazine!"

I was carried away by the underlying meaning of it all and smiled back exultantly. I thanked him. "It was *very* good advice." (Like the waiter's, earlier.)

The moral here is really liberating. The unused muscle begins to work out. In January it hurts awfully, looking at all those unfamiliar words—like the first day of skiing, or tennis. In February, the incidence of such words is a little less, and you feel the relief. In March it still happens to you, but only now and again. By June?—yes. You feel no pain at all.

It isn't necessarily that your vocabulary has increased at a geometric rate. It is that the words you used to think of as alien and intimidating are less and less that, as they continue to crop up and your mind and imagination are gradually including them in your immediate-visibility range. If you are assigned the job of sportswriter (my sister was, age twenty-three, by United Press) you gradually get to feel at home with any number of words you simply could not have defined before. Exactly the same thing happens, or has happened, to the reader of the Sports Section. Or of the Financial Section. After a while you feel quite at home.

4. It's fair to distinguish between different categories of unusual words. (Again) as Dwight Macdonald wrote, . . . some words belong in the "zoo section" of a dictionary—i.e., the words do exist, but the need for them is so remote, you can—and should—keep them caged up in the zoo until absolutely necessary to take one out, which may be never.

On the other hand, it is important to remember that every word berthed in the dictionary is there because at some point one of three things happened. Either an objective thing or concept or abstraction came on the scene which hadn't been descried before and now just had to be given a name ("cyberspace"); or an artistic hand closed in on what had been a void and the new word survives the infidelity of the season, earning its way into the dictionary ("seakindly"); or an authoritative writer simply uses the word and such is his prestige that his mere enunciation of it validates its legitimacy ("tushery").

Leading to my conclusion, (5), which is that while we can be very firm in resisting people who spout zoo-words, one should be respectful and patient with those who exercise lovingly the wonderful opportunities of the language. I went downtown a dozen years ago to hear a black pianist about whom the word had trickled in that here was something really cool and ear-catching, besides which his name rolled about the tongue releasing intrigue and wry amusement, and so I heard Thelonious Monk. He struck some really, sure-enough *bizarre* chords, but you know, it would never have occurred to me to walk over and say, Thelonious, I am not familiar with that chord you just played. So cut it out please.

Chapter 3

The Interview

A good interview can be a good way to get acquainted. Never definitive, it can nonetheless open windows into a character, a style, ideas. The price is often a certain mangling of the language, especially if the transcript is presented verbatim. There are oral imprecisions as well as modulations in voice and body language that cannot be caught in transcriptions. But even with its limitations, in the world of modern "media," in congressional hearings, and in police stations, the interview is a ubiquitous and sometimes even useful way to get to know someone. William F. Buckley, Jr., has been interviewed innumerable times and has interviewed some of our most interesting and most consequential contemporary figures, although he makes the point that his long-lived (thirty years) television program, *Firing Line*, is not, strictly speaking, an interview show. It is, by charter, an "exchange of views." Alistair Cooke, in an admiring but not sycophantic introduction to a book of such exchanges, *On the Firing Line* (1989), refers to Buckley as "lover of the last word," while Buckley himself confesses to leaving the studio sometimes "with much on my mind, *en esprit d'escalier,* a wonderful French term describing what you wish you had said by way of devastating retort: typically a sunburst that hits you as you reach the bottom of the staircase."

An enjoyable and revealing interview was the exchange with Charlie Rose, the affable, courteous, intelligent, and handsome Carolinian, who came to public television via Bill Moyers. This generally positive opinion of Rose still holds despite the tendency of the charming interviewer to put words into other people's mouths, sometimes while they are speaking. (This interview has been edited.) The occasion was, as it often is, the publication of a new book, *Happy Days Were Here Again.*

Given the usual barter for banter with Buckley—we'll talk about your book, Mr. B., if we can also deal with your politics, controversial positions, and opinions on world affairs and world leaders—he was asked all sorts of questions, some even pertaining to the book. Notice how quickly the interview begins to turn on specific words and their meanings. Notice, too, the prescience of WFB in October 1993 on the likely return to popularity of communism in Russia and President Clinton in the United States, each much more apparent as this book is readied for publication in early 1996.

The interview also touches on a little-known contribution of Buckley's work as an editor and employer—his role as a discoverer of other writers, of varying political persuasions but undeniable gifts.

———

CHARLIE ROSE: Welcome to our broadcast. The columnist George Will once said about William F. Buckley, Jr., that, quote, all great biblical stories begin with Genesis. Before there was Ronald Reagan, there was Barry Goldwater. Before there was Barry Goldwater, there was the *National Review*. And before there was the *National Review*, there was Bill Buckley with a spark in his mind, and that spark in 1980 became a conflagration.

BUCKLEY: And before that there was Adam.

ROSE: [*Laughs*] . . . with a spark in his mind, too . . . Good to have you here. Lots to talk about, but let me just say why *Reflections of a Libertarian Journalist* [as a subtitle] rather than—I mean, because—are you closer to libertarian than you are conservative? With no respect for any order or any government?

BUCKLEY: The conservative movement is often thought of as composed of two parts. There are those conservatives who feel it's important not to deviate too quickly from the standing order because the implications of that can be revolutionary. And there are those others who want to hang on to what we have to the extent that it augments liberty. I'm one of the latter, rather than the former. Otherwise, you get things like conservatives in the Kremlin today threatening a return to Stalinism. So you get that misuse of the word conservative.

ROSE: That must drive conservatives crazy to know that the conservatives in the Kremlin are considered those people who want to return to Stalinism, since the battle cry for conservatives for a long time was anti-communism.

BUCKLEY: Of course, a lot of conservatives are crazy. [*Both laugh*]

ROSE: How about Republicans?

BUCKLEY: It's a nice distinction. *The New York Times* once had a real problem when they reported a news story as follows: Conservatives in the Kremlin are cracking down on books imported illegally from the West. Among the proscribed titles is *The Conscience of a Conservative* by Barry Goldwater. [*Both laugh*]

ROSE: [John Leonard] used to write for the *National Review*.

BUCKLEY: Oh, yes! I read an essay by him in 1956 in a magazine called *Ivy* in which I had an essay. I thought, "Gee, this guy can write." . . . So I called him up and said, "Mr. Leonard, would you like to work for *National Review* during the summer?" He said, "I'd like to work for it anytime since I've just been kicked out of Harvard." He was then nineteen years old, twenty years old. So he worked for us for a couple of years, and then he went to Berkeley and was radicalized.

ROSE: Garry Wills is another example of someone who came through *National Review* and then went on to seemingly reflect a very different philosophy than a Buckley libertarian philosophy or a conservative philosophy.

BUCKLEY: In the case of poor Garry, he traveled in the wrong direction. I think he wrote exclusively for us for about thirteen or fourteen years. I got a manuscript, you know . . . So I called him up and he said, well, he'd like to talk to me about it. I said, "Well, I'd love to talk to you about it." So he said, "You would have to send me the money for the ticket," so I did. He flew—it was his first flight in an airplane, first time across the Mississippi River—and he married the stewardess. And I was a proud member of the wedding party.

ROSE: And how long did he stay with you?

BUCKLEY: About ten, twelve years.

ROSE: He seems to have come to a very different place now than you are, politically. Or do you say, "I hire them for their writing ability, not for the ideology"?

BUCKLEY: Well, he happened to be a very committed conservative. He was a Catholic seminarian, and then he got a classics degree at Yale. But he was—When I knew him, he was the nearest thing I ever ran into to a sheer warmonger. He thought that the Soviet Union was a menace against which we had to consolidate and be very tough with. He was pro-McCarthy and all those good things. [*Both laugh*] Then he was radicalized at the funeral of Martin Luther King.

ROSE: By the eulogies for King, or the whole—

BUCKLEY: The whole episode. It just—

ROSE: —sense of going down the streets of Atlanta and—

BUCKLEY: It just converted him. The next thing we knew, he became sort of a flower child, grunting every time Henry Kissinger spoke. That's too bad. I don't think I have an essay on him here [in the book], do I?

ROSE: No, you don't. Do you miss not being there [at the *National Review*]? Do you miss the sense that you are no longer running the place even though you are, in the end, the ultimate, I guess, authority?

BUCKLEY: Well . . . I own it. No, I think that John O'Sullivan [the Editor] is doing a superb job.

ROSE: . . . the Clinton Administration. Give me your own assessment of this administration as it now goes forward with a number of things on its agenda: health care, reinventing government, and NAFTA—plus Bosnia on the foreign policy front.

BUCKLEY: Well, it would be difficult in a single generality to touch all four of those bases. But I think that one can say this with confidence, and that is that Mr. Clinton is a genuine statist, by which I mean he thinks of the state as the apparatus through which all reforms need to be made.

ROSE: Albeit that he wants a state that is reformed, that is more effective, that is more efficient, that is more productive—

BUCKLEY: So did Hitler. So did Stalin. [*Both laugh*] Everybody wants an efficient state. It's more fun. But the point is that he . . .

ROSE: So the state has no role for—

BUCKLEY: Well of course it has a role.

ROSE: —defense.

BUCKLEY: Adam Smith outlined its role, I think definitively, but there are people who are infatuated with the state because it becomes an instrument of their policy. And if I may say so, Charlie, this is something that tends to be distinctive to the liberal mentality because a liberal is a critic, a critic of that which is. And under the circumstances, he feels, well how can I, by simply moving my fingers, affect the shape of the clay that's spinning around there. John Kenneth Galbraith will get up in the morning and think, "How can society be bettered?" To begin with, it would be better by following his advice, but in order to exert that advice, the instrumentality of the state is indispensable. Otherwise, he has to suffer such indignities as you and I have to suffer when we do a program or write books, people can pick them up or tune in, or not. You can't decide whether to tune in on IRS. It tunes in on you.

ROSE: So Mr. Clinton is a statist and believes very much [in] using the government and believes that government should play a role in terms of bettering the citizenry, bettering the life and the quality of life and—

BUCKLEY: Yes, a critical role. Yes, he has a total appetite for using the force, the resources of government. And of course, the trouble with that is that every time one has an appetite to fix your problem through the instrumentality of the state, I am affecting his freedom because in order to do something for you, I necessarily have to use his money, or reduce his independence, or whatever. That is really the basic distinction between the libertarian and the statist.

ROSE: What do you think of him as a leader?

BUCKLEY: Well, I think more of him than the American people do. He has only a forty-one percent approval now. I think his leadership qualities are really pretty considerable. Now he's got problems. One of them is that he can't understand figures. . . . It reminds me some historian told me that Hitler was that way, that Hitler would say, "Since we came to power, the steel production used to be 54 million 490 tons. Now it's 100 million 612 tons." And in that sense, Clinton uses figures without any sense that he's on top of them, which is why there are so many contradictions and why so many people accuse him of being coy in his use of these figures. For instance, he will say, "We have effected a tax reduction in Social Security." That means he's paying, the government's paying us less. But that tax reduction—that reduction in expenditures—turns out to be an increase in tax that we have to pay. If Tricky Dick were to try that, they'd run him out of town with wet towels. So he has these problems, but those are problems which, in my judgment, he has the telegenic and theatrical resources to overcome.

ROSE: Is that the leadership quality you admire about him, the telegenic and theatrical, or is it something else that you see there that . . .

BUCKLEY: No, I'll put it this way . . . Nobody would have guessed at the equivalent period in Bush's tenure that he wouldn't be reelected. Nobody at this point believes that Clinton could be reelected. I think he might very easily be reelected because there could be a swing in national sentiment about him. It would be an act of autohypnosis by the American people, but it could happen.

ROSE: Well, let me read to you, Mr. Buckley. "President Clinton is surrounding himself with the most spectacular zoo in history. His economic advisers are the despair of the thinking world. His civil rights advisers are aberrants deserving taxonomic curiosity [*Laughs*]. He proposes to bring to the State Department someone whose views on the uses of American power perfectly reflect the utter confusion of our policies in Bosnia." That's not a ringing endorsement for reelection.

BUCKLEY: No, but I'm saying it could happen. He's very unpopular right now. I told you, he has forty-one percent, and he brings this on by this ambition to be like Noah's ark, you know: Find one of everything and stick them in the White House. So I don't withdraw that at all. Don Feder of the *Boston Herald* wrote a marvelous column in yesterday's *New York Post* in which he simply took sixteen of these characters and enumerated this sort of taxonomic curiosity. And [Clinton] does collect them. Now, whether he collects them because he has this comprehensive appetite to be surrounded by one of everything, or because he just has sort of an orientation, which is a part of his general compassion for people who have problems, it's hard to say. But it has not resulted, I think, in the creation of policies that have consolidated. Nobody will accuse anybody of having a foreign policy.

ROSE: You believe there is no foreign policy. But what was George Bush's foreign policy?

BUCKLEY: You've hit a very good point. It was not by any means something that had cohered. He kept talking about a new world order, but that new world order which one thought was to have sprung out of the seeds of the rejection of Iraq when it aggressed against Kuwait did not take hold in respect to Bosnia and Yugoslavia. There was the incursion to Somalia, which seems retrospectively to have been a bad idea.

ROSE: It sure does.

BUCKLEY: So the formulation of a new world order never happened. And I'm not sure it's at all easy to have happen.

ROSE: But do you know anybody that's articulating a new American doctrine in foreign policy . . . or who has been the architect of a new approach?

BUCKLEY: Not a new approach, no, but certainly Jeane Kirkpatrick and Henry Kissinger, for instance, and *National Review* keep insisting on, not the new, but the old.

ROSE: And the old is what? I thought the old was essentially anti-communist and support of . . .

BUCKLEY: Anti-communism was the immediate aspect of a policy that was directed towards the perpetuation of American freedom, and anti-communism necessarily superordinated over all alternatives because that was what we had to begin by doing. But the central division was the division between Woodrow Wilson and John Adams. Woodrow Wilson wanted to make the world safe for democracy, and John Adams said the American people are friends of liberty everywhere, but guardians only of their own. And JFK, of course, was very much on the Wilsonian side in his famous inaugural address, but he had to retreat from it, as did all liberals retreat from it, because Vietnam forced him to do so. So it became clear that we couldn't send the marines around everywhere, but we could at least do this: Never shrink from asserting the principles of American exceptionalism . . .

ROSE: American exceptionalism in terms of how America stands as a beacon for democracy, or how the American experience is unique in the world?

BUCKLEY: Both. Both. But the ideals of the Bill of Rights are universal; i.e., you can take the Bill of Rights and stick it anywhere in the world, and if you abide by it, you would improve the lot of the human being measured in terms of liberty.

ROSE: So . . .

BUCKLEY: So therefore, we mustn't ever, in retreating from Vietnam, come back and say, "Not only do we have no business there, who says that George Washington [was] any better than Ho Chi Minh?" But that's what they were saying in Chicago when Garry Wills was turned around; i.e., there was no difference between us and them.

ROSE: Where does that bring you on Bosnia?

BUCKLEY: Well, I think it's too late to do anything about Bosnia. I would have welcomed it if Mr. Bush had moved with lightning speed and attempted to do early what now cannot be done. However, I would have a great deal of difficulty in absolutely integrating that move in my general philosophy about the reserves, or the use of American manpower because it is not a clear, apparent—it is not a clear threat to

American vital interests. But to a certain extent, I think foreign policy is an art.

ROSE: And not a doctrine, and not sort of a rigid equation.

BUCKLEY: I think it is a transcendent vision of conservatism that recognizes that sometimes government is an art. You do something because you think *noblesse oblige,* it's the thing to do. I felt that way about Somalia.

ROSE: You thought it was the thing to do. And now, would you now acknowledge that—

BUCKLEY: I didn't want to sit around and . . .

ROSE: —it was fraught with more danger than you ever imagined at the time, and perhaps, having thought it was the thing to do, on—

BUCKLEY: It didn't work.

ROSE: —reflection, it wasn't the thing to do. Are we acknowledging mistakes here?

BUCKLEY: I didn't want to be a member of a society with a stuffed granary and have two thousand people die every day. It is the rate at which they were dying.

ROSE: But wouldn't the same argument apply for Bosnia? Early on?

BUCKLEY: Yes. I would have voted in favor of a lightning strike. But Mrs. Thatcher was marvelously consistent during that entire period. All I'm saying is that it might have worked in Somalia if a particular bullet had been lucky enough to land in a particular place, but it didn't. So now we simply have another sick war.

ROSE: If, in American politics, there is a contest—bear with me because this is hypothesis—there is a contest for the Republican nomination, knowing what you know about these two people at the height of their power, it is a contest for the Republican nomination for the presidency, and the contestants are Ronald Reagan and Margaret Thatcher. Who do you support?

BUCKLEY: I'll tell you why I don't play games like that. Because it's like saying, "If you take the best symphony of Beethoven and the best cantata of Bach—"

ROSE: You'd go Bach.

BUCKLEY: "—which do you support?" Now, I'd say, "I can't do that. They say different things to me. I can tell you why I can prefer *King Lear* to *Macbeth.* . . . But I can't tell you whether I prefer *Macbeth* to John Milton's *Paradise Lost,* because they don't compete in my judgment. And in that sense . . . Margaret Thatcher had the whole legislative authority of the Parliament. Ronald Reagan didn't. Now what would Ronald Reagan have done if he had had the authority that Margaret Thatcher—

ROSE: Let me talk about some other personalities, too. Clinton . . . can you find yourself in agreement with what he wants to do in the health care area, and the way he wants to go about doing it?

BUCKLEY: Well, yes to the former, no to the latter. He doesn't want anything that you and I don't want.

ROSE: Health care of all Americans.

BUCKLEY: Sure. We all want that.

ROSE: As a conservative, you want that, but if it means government—I mean, can you do that without a kind of statist attitude about—this is one of those problems.

BUCKLEY: You have to look at the phenomenon and say, "Okay, on the basis of experience, what is the best way to go after the problem?" Now we're spending almost twice as much for individual health—or for individual Americans—as Great Britain is spending, and they have socialized medicine. So the answer is that we have too much medicine. The answer to "Why do we have too much medicine?" Because we overtreat ourselves. Why do we overtreat ourselves? Because there are no real attractions to the practice of medical husbandry. And the reason there aren't is that all of our bills are overwhelmingly paid for after a very minor deduction. . . . But Mr. Clinton wants to put all in one great big pot and have one great big national program. I don't think that's the way to go.

ROSE: How about NAFTA?

BUCKLEY: Well, I'm very enthusiastic about NAFTA, but there's something you've got to watch for, and that is there are some people using NAFTA as a vehicle on which to graft their favorite causes. The labor unions are trying this, to a certain extent, and the environmentalists are trying it. So that it can run, conceivably, the danger of being the terrific instrument to promote free trade, which also brings you guaranteed longevity for spotted owls, and a certain—

ROSE: No sympathy for the spotted owl?

BUCKLEY: Well, I like spotted owls, but I'm not prepared to organize my life around their longevity. [*Both laugh*]

ROSE: Around the species, even if they're endangered as a species?

BUCKLEY: An estimated ninety-nine million species are extinct, and here we are. . . .

ROSE: Ross Perot. What do you think of him? How do you explain his attraction to the American public?

BUCKLEY: I think that he is a conduit for American frustration.

ROSE: He's a vessel that everybody fills their own—

BUCKLEY: Sure. Perot is the "none of the above," the incarnation of "none of the above," and people are so dissatisfied by Congress and by the Executive and to a certain extent by the courts that they want to commit acts of *lèse majesté,* and the way to do that is to back Perot. I think he's utterly irresponsible.

ROSE: In what way?

BUCKLEY: Well, anybody who says that we're going to lose five million jobs the moment we sign NAFTA is irresponsible. He cannot prove it, can't come close to proving it. The highest estimate is two hundred thousand with however many other hundred thousand new jobs we create.

ROSE: Clinton says two hundred.

BUCKLEY: He arrives to meet the press, you know, after running for President for fourteen months, and they ask him how he would reduce the deficit, and he says, "I didn't know you were going to ask me that question. I would have brought my notes." Well, I say that I wouldn't expose myself to a session with *Meet the Press* or a session with you if I didn't have my notes in my head on a matter as critical as how would I reduce the cost of government, which he had been talking about for two years.

ROSE: Turning to the other side, the Republican Party as opposition, do you think there is a known alternative agenda coming from the Party that you belong to that is convincing? And why not?

BUCKLEY: It's in part because our government is not set up that way. In England, you have a shadow government, and that shadow government always comes in with A when you come in with B, or with Z when you come in with W. We don't do that. There isn't a, quote, leader of the Republican Party with the authority to do that. So it is a situation in which you synthesize and distill when you get closer to the nomination time for a new President. Whatever you have learned from primaries, from polls, from experiences. What the shape of the Republican platform will be in ninety-six is not yet, in my judgment, discernible.

ROSE: Do you think it ought to have most of the tenets that were reflected in the Republican convention in Houston in 1992?

BUCKLEY: [*Laughing*] I know what you're leading to. I don't think the Republican Party is going to say, "Forget about family values. Go ahead and have a happy abortion."

ROSE: I just sat on a panel with Mary Matalin, who ran the Bush campaign, who thinks that the Republican convention in Houston was a disaster for their candidate. Disaster may not be her choice of words, but . . . was not helpful.

BUCKLEY: That's an extremely interesting question, and especially interesting given the fact that one week after the convention began—

ROSE: I knew you were going to say that.

BUCKLEY: —the polls rose by fourteen points.

ROSE: That's the Pat Buchanan argument, too.

BUCKLEY: Well, it's the argument, isn't it? But what then happened [during the campaign] was that the Republicans took it on the chin, and they permitted people to say this was a declaration of civil war. Well, I don't really think it was any-

	thing of the sort. I think some of the language that was used was incautiously used, but I've never . . .
ROSE:	The Buchanan speech being one prime example?
BUCKLEY:	Yes.
ROSE:	Just incautious language . . . ?
BUCKLEY:	Well, put it this way. For anything indefensible spoken in Houston, I can give you ten indefensible statements spoken in New York.
ROSE:	Like— Give me two.
BUCKLEY:	Well, the notion that the whole of the decade of the eighties was designed to make people richer who were rich. That's an indefensible statement. It is not true. But if you took the whole of everything that Clinton said in the last three years . . . and tried to write an economic history based on it, you would find he was less accurate than Karl Marx.
ROSE:	Do you find—having read Milton Friedman and promoted him—and he's a Nobel laureate now—but having listened to his articulation of the relation between government and economy and his economic views, when you look at the piling up of the deficit in the eighties, can you say that was good for the economic future of the country?
BUCKLEY:	Of course not. But—
ROSE:	I never hear you—
BUCKLEY:	Well, read my book, and you will find a hundred references to it are there. The fact of the matter is that revenues under Reagan did not decrease, but expenses—
ROSE:	And government . . .
BUCKLEY:	—expenses increased. Now they increased actually at a lesser rate than under the three preceding Presidents. But they still continued to increase. And of course, it increases geometrically. If you compensate for inflation and do the entitlements thoroughly and have an aging population, you have that much more money [committed].
ROSE:	Most economists now believe that unless you do something about entitlements, you will not deal with the deficit, and you buy that idea?

BUCKLEY: Absolutely. You can prove it mathematically. Rudman says that in the year 2004—

ROSE: Warren Rudman, the former senator.

BUCKLEY: Sorry. Only four percent of the budget at this rate will be something over which Congress has any vote.

ROSE: Everything else will be paying the interest on the debt and entitlements which are already in the law.

BUCKLEY: That's right. So something has to be done about it.

ROSE: Do you think there's a political will in the Congress, in the public today, to do it? Or what has to change to create that public will?

BUCKLEY: Well, what you run into is *force majeure*. . . . The overwhelming force is, simply, you run out of money. The only way we can ultimately get out of this debt, unless we control the rate of expenses, is through inflation. . . . There's a tricky and rather easy way to do it and that is simply capital confiscation of a percentage of what everybody owns. But if we have inflation of ten percent, we reduce our national debt by $160 billion. So that's a relatively painless way to do it, but you've mortgaged other things about your future, the kind of security that people making investments and putting up capital have to worry about.

ROSE: There's a real problem in America that we're not a saving society, that we do not save.

BUCKLEY: Yes. I disagree in the sense that the American people have been trained to believe that their pension funds, which are enormous—we're talking about three or four trillion dollars—are their savings, that plus their Social Security. So they are not encouraged to save in the sense that the Japanese are encouraged to save, who will have to look after their own needs primarily on their own. So that a lot of the squandermania that America's all about—

ROSE: There's not so much squandermania. Well, okay, we are— we consume too much and save too little, and therefore we have too little to invest in creating and making ourselves a more productive economy.

BUCKLEY: Yes, but . . . if you're a working man and you're contributing ten percent to your pension account and thirteen percent to Social Security, you might say to yourself, "Well, that's as much as I'm disposed to save." Although I'm only saving three percent [in the bank, etc.], it's three percent on top of twenty-three percent, and that's really a pretty healthy amount to save.

ROSE: I want to turn now to the book.

BUCKLEY: That's good. [*Rose laughs*]

ROSE: I knew you were waiting for that moment. You have never been to a baseball game.

BUCKLEY: That's not a major point I'm making.

ROSE: No, I know. [*Laughs*] I just want to play for a minute before we get serious.

Why not? I mean, it's part of the Ameri— You know the famous quote by Jacques Barzun: To know America, you have to know baseball.

BUCKLEY: I wasn't aware of that . . . I know Jacques Barzun . . . Well, the answer is he's obviously wrong.

ROSE: Don't you feel any . . . I mean . . . Have you ever watched a game on television?

BUCKLEY: Yes.

ROSE: Do you understand the game?

BUCKLEY: I used to play it as a boy, sure. You know, I had a debate with John Kenneth Galbraith at Harvard on Reagan. It was televised. So he called me up and he said, "You know, Buckley, you're such a dumb producer. Here you schedule this at the same time as the Super Bowl."

ROSE: And you said?

BUCKLEY: I said, "Well, you know, the truth is I had nothing to do with the scheduling. That's PBS." He said, "Nobody will see it." And so about three hours later I walked down the street and every third person, it seemed to me, said, "Gee that was interesting," or "That was terrible," or whatever. Well, the answer is there are ninety million people watching Super Bowl and ten million who don't.

ROSE: And so ten million is a pretty damn good audience! You have never had any desire to go to a game . . . I mean, does sports itself, other than skiing and sailing, have any interest to you?

BUCKLEY: I play a little tennis. Here's the thing . . . I respect baseball enough to feel this about it: that in order to enjoy it, you've got to really study it, become a fan of a club, know something about the players, and it's an enormous investment of time. So it isn't just exposure to a single game that transmutes you into a fan. It's getting into the whole ritual, and that takes a long time.

ROSE: We're now talking about a George Will kind of commitment.

BUCKLEY: That's right . . . exactly right. He would be a marvelous example, George Will, or Bart Giamatti, the late president of Yale. So I don't feel an impulse to give it that kind of time. In fact, take learning Russian. Some people say, "Well, you've got to learn Russian because you can't read Pushkin unless you make the investment."

ROSE: And you say?

BUCKLEY: Sorry, I'm going to have to read it in translation.

ROSE: When you began these wonderful sailing extravaganzas, you would take . . . for example, I think on the first long, cross-Atlantic cruise on a sailboat you took *Moby-Dick*.

BUCKLEY: You have a good memory.

ROSE: But you don't do that much anymore. You're doing other things, aren't you?

BUCKLEY: I don't get to read a lot of novels, but I am a novel reader. I get a great kick out of novels.

ROSE: How about movies? Do you go to movies?

BUCKLEY: No, I get tapes and watch them at home, which is much more comfortable, I think.

ROSE: How about writing for you, writing novels? I mean, it always amazed me that you were able to create [Blackford] Oakes and be successful at it. What does that say about— does it say that you, a former CIA operative, just had a capacity to tell a story and that's what made you successful as a spy novelist?

BUCKLEY: Well, I suppose it probably has to do also with an individual's threshold of boredom. I get bored very easily.

ROSE: So you want to move the pages along for your own—

BUCKLEY: That's right. So you're sitting there clacking away, and some people—that lovely Southern lady can write about the wisteria for seven pages . . .

ROSE: Eudora Welty?

BUCKLEY: Yes, and I love her for it, but I can't do that. I don't have those skills. So therefore, I've got to have action and words.

ROSE: Do you like John le Carré?

BUCKLEY: Yes, I do . . . I haven't read all of his novels, but I think he's a marvelous writer. But he and I have a very interesting quarrel.

ROSE: What's that?

BUCKLEY: Well, he is kind of an egalitarian. His Western spy and the Russian spy are pretty much the same.

ROSE: Same moral/ethical—

BUCKLEY: Yes. And our guy is [always] sort of a paunchy—he gets cuckolded all the time, and he drinks a lot of booze, whereas my guy is just a better human being.

ROSE: Your guy is closer to Tom Clancy's guy.

BUCKLEY: Yes. Or his guy's closer to mine.

ROSE: Since you started earlier.

BUCKLEY: That's right. So I see no reason for this kind of insistence that there isn't really basically any difference between Lyndon Johnson and Khrushchev. There's an enormous difference between them.

ROSE: He also reflects a sense that somehow there was something—even though he also was part of British intelligence, which he acknowledges now, without talking about what he did, as I guess you don't talk about whatever you did during— You acknowledge that you were—

BUCKLEY: I was blown. I didn't know it. I was—

ROSE: How were you blown?

BUCKLEY: By William Sloane Coffin, who . . .

ROSE: Who also was Yale, who went into the CIA. And he blew your cover?

BUCKLEY: Yup. I don't know how he found out about me because if I'd been captured and tortured and spilled everything I knew, I would have been able to identify one human being, who was my boss, Howard Hunt. That was the only person I knew the name of, so I don't know how Coffin found out about me. But he did. . . .

ROSE: What's interesting about this [book] is not only that this is a collection of columns . . . between the years, what, eighty-eight to ninety-two? But there is also an appreciation of some people, of Malcolm Forbes, for example. I mean—speak about Forbes. You still communicate?

BUCKLEY: Oh, sure.

ROSE: He's a good friend? A friend?

BUCKLEY: Yes, he is. Indeed. I went to that crazy party of his in Tunis.

ROSE: Morocco?

BUCKLEY: Yes. And he was given a very hard time. So I wrote a piece where I said this is a guy whose joy in life is very conspicuous consumption, but you can't fault—

ROSE: It's his money, so therefore . . . ?

BUCKLEY: Well, it's his money and there is such good nature in it. Imagine sending a plane over to bring Gorbachev in, an airplane called *Capitalist Tool.* . . . So there's kind of a joyous, utterly unashamed buoyancy about this guy that I thought very captivating.

ROSE: Speaking of Gorbachev, how will history treat him? You reflect on him in this book.

BUCKLEY: I think history will acknowledge with some gratitude that he didn't decide massively to resist change, but I don't think history will necessarily believe that he had the power to do so. . . .

ROSE: What do you think of Mr. Yeltsin?

BUCKLEY: I think Yeltsin's got a hell of a job, and he's doing on the whole well. It's nice to know that he has Gaidar back . . .

ROSE: Right. He brought him back into the government.

BUCKLEY: Yes. You know, very few people remember Gorbachev—I know this intimately because I just finished a novel about him.

ROSE: A spy novel?

BUCKLEY: Coming out in January. But he was a very bad boy for a couple of years. When he first came into power. He came to power in March 1985, and he was absolutely determined to win that war.

ROSE: In Afghanistan?

BUCKLEY: In Afghanistan. And he said about Sakharov that he was a traitor to the sacred cause of communism. Then of course later on he bailed Sakharov out. But I would say this: It's safe to say that half the people who were killed in Afghanistan were killed while he was the Premier of the Soviet Union.

ROSE: You thought Carter did the right thing in refusing, in not going to Russia for the Olympics because of the Afghanistan invasion?

BUCKLEY: Yes. I think that a country that's determined to express its opposition to something but not going to war should use whatever instruments it has that are not military. And the psychological instrument of a sports boycott is huge. South Africa, for instance, felt it enormously. So I was very much in favor of using that particular weapon. And Moscow was terrified by it. They had a great psychological stake in the success of their Moscow games.

ROSE: It would mark them as a member of the world community. And if in fact they were rejected, it would paint them in the world community as the, to use the expression of a friend of yours, "Evil Empire."

BUCKLEY: You're exactly correct. And of course, the invasion of Afghanistan was the great big rupture in the accepted notion that the expansionism of the Soviet Union was done. Arthur Schlesinger and all of our resident pundits had told us that we didn't have to worry about this anymore. [The Soviets] had expanded as far as they wanted to go.

ROSE: They'd lost their expansionist urge? There was no more imperialism in the Soviets?

BUCKLEY: The doctrine of containment had worked. But there we were now with a brand-new aggression, and the implications of it were enormous. I think almost certainly on account of it that we succeeded under Mr. Reagan in deploying those theater weapons in eighty-three and eighty-four.

ROSE: Other than your father, tell me the three or four people that you think have had profound influence, on you, on your own personal and intellectual development.

BUCKLEY: Well, Mark and Paul and Matthew. That's three.

ROSE: By the way, you're writing a new book on Catholicism, aren't you? Have you finished it?

BUCKLEY: No, I've started it.

ROSE: What is it to be? An affirmation? A sort of Malcolm Muggeridge type affirmation of Christianity and Catholicism?

BUCKLEY: Just a little book you can consult when you need to see how much of a sinner you are. When you need a quick reading. [*Both laugh*]

ROSE: What's the church meant to you? And when Pope John the Twenty-third talks about liberation theology, you're right there with him.

BUCKLEY: Oh, John Paul the Second. I'm not only with him, I've anticipated him.

ROSE: You mean he's been reading Buckley?

BUCKLEY: We talked about liberation theology before he got around to it. Liberation theology was an effort to transmute Marxism into a theologically acceptable formula, and as such its principal spokesman was Bishop Arns of Rio de Janeiro. Incidentally, one of the nicest people in the whole world. I had him on my program. He's so damned nice, and he said these absolutely preposterous things, but he says them with such a benign smile.

ROSE: Speaking of this, it reminds me. They just had a big meeting of the Christian Coalition. I think, you know, a lot of people are worried about their influence on American politics. Do you worry about that at all?

BUCKLEY: Charlie, if every single thing that the Christian Coalition wants were done tomorrow, I would not recognize any difference between the society I lived in and the society I grew up in. But I don't think of myself as having been manumitted by the Warren Court. When I was at school, I could do everything that I wanted to. So I wouldn't be able to buy whisky on Sundays or buy pornographic literature as easily. Beyond that, what is it that they want to do that should upset me so?

ROSE: Well, their views on abortion are similar to your views on abortion.

BUCKLEY: Abortion is probably the interesting exception, although as you know, illegal abortions reached up to six or seven hundred thousand per year pre–Roe *v.* Wade. Now they're doubled. So it's inconceivable that in my lifetime or probably in yours, people who want an abortion won't get one pretty easily. But beyond that, what's all the fuss about? *Hustler* magazine?

ROSE: Well, no, I think the fuss is probably the belief among a number of people that there's too much of an intrusion . . . the Christian Coalition . . . notion being intolerant of another group's beliefs and values—

BUCKLEY: But we should be.

ROSE: —and therefore want to impose their values on them.

BUCKLEY: You should.

ROSE: You should be intolerant of another group's values?

BUCKLEY: Absolutely. The principal progress we've made in . . . civil rights is to be intolerant towards people who don't respect other people's rights. So that if somebody is anti-Semitic or if somebody is anti-black to the extent of manifesting it, intolerance of behavior of that kind is the principal force for change. Thomas Jefferson said laws are much less important than opinion because laws merely codify opinion. So to be intolerant of people who have illegitimate children every ten months is something we're very much behind on.

ROSE: But suppose the intolerance is of people who don't have the same religious view you have. Not whether they're anti-Semitic, not whether they're anti-black . . .

BUCKLEY: Name me one . . .

ROSE: —or the same sense of tolerance for— You know where the argument goes.

BUCKLEY: Name me one human being I've heard of who would limit the right of anybody I know of to practice his religion except perhaps to the extent that it implied polygamy or human sacrifice.

ROSE: Okay then, speaking of that, your political hero Barry Goldwater, who you supported early, has been very outspoken in arguing for the right of gays in the military. Do you part company—

BUCKLEY: Now why are you shifting around? I asked you to talk about the subject that you raised, namely the threat to the practice of other people's religion.

ROSE: What I'm doing is going through the engagement of the tolerance of the rights of minorities and tolerance—

BUCKLEY: Well, do me the favor—

ROSE: —and tolerance for minorities.

BUCKLEY: Well, do me the favor of saying, Bill, I retreat on that question because you were right. There is no threat to any other religion posed in the activity of the Christian Coalition.

ROSE: Well, I don't want to say that specifically about the Coalition without knowing everything—I don't know enough about all the things that the Christian Coalition believe and don't believe . . .

BUCKLEY: Don't you think you would have heard about it if one of them said, "We want to close down all synagogues"?

ROSE: Well, of course they're not saying something like that.

BUCKLEY: Well, then what are you talking about?

ROSE: But the point I raised about the tolerance in terms of the tolerance of other people's political—other people's religious views if they're not—it's not part of the Judeo-Christian tradition, that kind of thing.

BUCKLEY: Well, I don't know anybody who proposes the persecution of another denomination. I know some people who think you will go to hell if you don't become a Unitarian or a Catholic or whatever, but as long as this is a private, theological conviction . . .

ROSE: Can I go on to Barry Goldwater? Do you differ with him with respect to gays in the military?

BUCKLEY: Yes. Here's the principal error that he made . . . The people who wanted things to be different in the military in respect of gays had reached an accommodation with people who didn't want it to be different. And that was a formula that says, "Okay, we won't ask them whether they're gay and persecute them if we find out that they are gay; however, if they practice gay activity which we think is inconsistent with the correct deportment of the military, then we will let them out. Honorable discharge, not dishonorable discharge." Now that had been agreed on when Barry came in, Senator Goldwater came in and said, "No. Let's go back and start from scratch." And so he resubmitted in effect the Clinton proposals and in doing so in my judgment polarized the forces. He was speaking at this point not as a diplomat or as a politician, but speaking as a fundamentalist moralist, and he should have made that statement in January, not in June after fourteen agonized weeks of trying to come to a conciliation. . . .

ROSE: Well, you know what I thought about it? I thought, regardless of the issue, I just liked seeing him out there being as outspoken and as frank as he was even when he was going against the grain of what might have been expected.

BUCKLEY: He's one of my favorite people.

ROSE: For that reason. I know.

BUCKLEY: Yes. He came to my concert in Phoenix two or three years ago.

ROSE: Harpsichord concert?

BUCKLEY: Yes. And a reporter stopped him and said, "What'd you think of it?" And he said, "Terrific. Terrific. Of course, this is the first time I've ever been to a concert." Only Barry Goldwater would have the guts to say that at age eighty-two. . . .

—OCTOBER 12, 1993

* * *

One has to be careful when interviewing Buckley; if your questions are good enough, you could get hired. As did this young woman, whose interview ran on August 17, 1979, and not long after, she became a full-time assistant editor of *National Review*. She is now a syndicated columnist.

* * *

Mona Charen, a New Yorker, graduated this spring from Columbia University. While there, she conducted an interview for the yearbook, *The Columbian,* with WFB—from which the following are excerpts:

Q. Lionel Trilling has written in *The Liberal Imagination:* ". . . the conservative impulse and the reactionary impulse do not, with some isolated and some ecclesiastical exceptions, express themselves in ideas but only in action or in irritable mental gestures which seek to resemble ideas." As you survey your colleagues on the Right, how much truth do you find in this assertion?

A. Not much. Trilling is correct only in the sense that conservatives are guided substantially by prescriptive reactions. One can, for example, register a disapproval of the proliferation of pornography without experiencing the necessity to externalize one's thoughts in theoretical parades. The liberals, on the whole, would rather write than think; let alone act.

Q. But if conservatives do not "experience the necessity to externalize [their] thoughts in theoretical parades," a few explanations present themselves. Either conservatives are mostly inarticulate, conservatives are complacent, or conservatives are somehow incapable of abstract theorizing.

A. I think it is correct to say about conservatives as a class that they engage less in abstract theorizing than ideologues or schematizers . . .

Q. Conservatives are distinct from ideologues?

A. I think so. Those conservatives who are ideologues are not conservatives, they're abstractionists. Burke's mistrust of schematism was a conscious preference, a thought that was guided by an accumulation of experience, and a transcendent morality. Now, I don't think anybody would accuse Burke of being inarticulate. A conservative in my judgment is guided less by absolutes than by presumptions. That is to say, there is a presumption against state interference, not an absolute law.

Q. All things considered, do you now regret having introduced Henry Kissinger to Richard Nixon?

A. No. Kissinger was the best of Nixon's advisers. An adviser who would have counseled Nixon to do what I wish he had done would probably have got him impeached before Howard Hunt got out of bed.

Q. Taking into account your temperament, which you have acknowledged to be something other than conservative, if you were an influential pundit in 1776, would you have been a Tory or a rebel?

A. Hard to say. I am easily irritated, and would probably have found His Majesty's interventions intolerable. On the other hand, I'd have looked for organic solutions. I'd have found little in common with Sam Adams, much in common with John.

Q. It is widely believed that three of the thinkers who have most influenced the intellectual life of the twentieth century were Freud, Marx, and Darwin. If you were granted the power retroactively to silence anyone of your choosing, would the work of any of the above troublemakers survive?

A. I am not disturbed by anyone's work. Only by how it is received. The problem is not heresy, but invincible ignorance.

Q. Well, leaving Marx aside, in what sense are Freud and Darwin heretics? From what orthodoxy do they depart?

A. The principal trouble with Freud and Darwin is really the trouble with their exegetes. This is particularly true of Darwin—a little less so of Freud; that is to say, Freud went a long way in constructing theological absolutes centered on himself . . .

Q. Theological?

A. I call it theological in the sense that he really calls upon you to have a faith which is non-empirical. I think "theological" as a metaphor is perfectly suited to Freudians who insist that there is *a* Freudian answer to all those enigmas, even as Ayn Rand believes the same thing about herself. It would be a word which would upset both of them, since they don't consider themselves to be theological about anything.

Q. In what ways would your life have been different if you had been born female?

A. I'd have seduced John Kenneth Galbraith and spared the world much pain.

Q. Who is your most formidable debating opponent?

A. Well, I've been asked that a hundred times as you can imagine, and I can't answer it. Different people have different strengths, and some of the people who are most formidable are very poor debaters.

Q. But they are formidable; why?

A. Because they have a way of appealing to an audience. You know the injunction you should never fence with an amateur because he'll likely kill you? He doesn't know the rules.

Ramsey Clark is really very maladroit as a debater, but almost certainly he would win any debate with me. You know, he puts on that humble-pie business, "I really believe in free speech. I know you-all don't agree with me, but I really respect your right, and gosh, I'm not cocksure. Why I go to bed every night thinkin' maybe I just made a lot of wrong decisions . . ." And you see these Ph.D.s and college students cheering lustily. Nixon, by the way, pulled that at the Oxford Union. He had those people cheering after the most intellectually disreputable performance I've seen in a lifetime of watching people debate.

So all I ask is that people who vote against me in debate have a hangover the next morning.

Q. Nabokov once described the "pen-poised pause." Do you ever stop in midsentence when writing and tap your pen on the desk, searching for the right word?

A. Seldom. Although occasionally I'll have trouble thinking of a word I know exists and it drives me nuts. Just the other day I couldn't recall for the life of me the word "reincarnation."

———

One of the exceptions to the no-interview format of *Firing Line* was when Buckley met Borges. The result was impressive—WFB's restraint and unabashed admiration, Borges's quiet eloquence, accomplishments, and dignity. (This is from WFB's book *On the Firing Line: The Public Lives of Our Public Figures*.)

———

BORGES AND BUCKLEY: A CONVERSATION

And, finally, a gentle titan.

Jorge Luis Borges (1899–1986) was living in Buenos Aires. I had lunched with him a few years earlier in Boston while he was visiting professor at Harvard. . . . Borges was already blind. He did not mind it, he said, because now he could "live his dreams with less distraction."

He took early to his craft, translating at age six from English into Spanish Oscar Wilde's demanding *The Happy Prince*. That translation was thought to have been the work of his father, and was used as a school text. He began to publish in the twenties—poems, essays, short works of fiction. In the late thirties he got his first job, as a menial assistant in a library.

When General Perón, against whom Borges had signed a declaration, was ousted, Borges was made director of the National Library. He traveled and lectured extensively, and was for decades the writer who for some unknown reason had not been awarded the Nobel Prize.

We met in Buenos Aires, in 1977, during the reign of the military junta. He seemed astonishingly frail, but he spoke without hesitation.

I did not interrupt him. The following pages I think of as the fairest ever minted by *Firing Line*.

WFB: You have been compared to both Milton and Homer in terms of a highly illuminated internal vision. Is this a correct judgment, as far as you're concerned?

BORGES: Well, I do my best to think it a correct judgment. At least, I try to put up with blindness. Of course, when you are blind, time flows in a different way. It flows, let's say, on an easy slope. I have sometimes spent sleepless nights—night before last, for example—but I didn't really feel especially unhappy about it, because time was sliding down that— was flowing down that easy slope.

WFB: You mean, you'd have felt more *un*happy if you *had* been able to see?

BORGES: Oh yes, of course I would.

WFB: Why?

BORGES: I can't very well explain it. These are the thoughts of years. When I first went blind—I mean, for reading purposes—I felt very unhappy. But now I feel that being blind is, let's say, part of my world. I suppose that happens. One's heard about it. When one is in jail, one thinks of being in jail as part of one's world; when one is sick, also.

WFB: How do you refresh yourself, as someone who is blind?

BORGES: I'm reading all the time. I'm having books reread to me. I do very little contemporary reading. But I'm only going back to certain writers, and among those writers I would like to mention an American writer. I would like to mention Emerson. I think of Emerson not only as a great prose writer—everybody knows that—but a very fine intellectual poet, as the only intellectual poet who had any *ideas*. Emerson was brimming over with ideas.

WFB: Well, you did a great deal to reintroduce many Americans to many American writers, including Emerson, isn't that correct?

BORGES: Yes, yes. I've done my best. Emerson and also another writer I greatly love.

WFB: Hawthorne?

BORGES: Well, but in Hawthorne—what I dislike about Hawthorne is, he was always writing fables. In the case of Poe, well, you get tales; but there was no moral tagged on to them. But I think of Melville, one of the great writers of the world, no?

WFB: How do you account for the failure of Melville to achieve any recognition during his lifetime, any significant recognition?

BORGES: Because people thought of him as writing travel books. I have the 1911 edition of the Encyclopaedia Britannica. There's an article about Melville, and they speak of him much in the same way as they might speak about Captain [Frederick] Marryat, for example, or other writers. Melville wrote many travel books; people thought of him as writing in that way, so they couldn't see all that *Moby-Dick; or, The Whale,* meant.

WFB: Yes. Well now, you say that you spend most of your time reading the older writers. Is it because you reject the new writers, or because you choose to continue to be unfamiliar with them?

BORGES: I am afraid that I'd find the new writers more or less like myself.

WFB: You won't.

BORGES: I suppose I will. I suppose all contemporaries are more or less alike, no? Since I dislike what I write, I prefer going back to the nineteenth, to the eighteenth century, and then, of course, also going back to the Romans, since I have no Greek, but I had Latin. Of course, my Latin is very rusty. But still, as I once wrote, to have forgotten Latin is already, in itself, a gift. To have known Latin and to have forgotten it is something that sticks to you somehow. I have done most of my reading in English. I read very little in Spanish. I was educated practically in my father's library, and that comprised English books. So that when I think of the Bible, I think of the King James Bible. When I think of the *Arabian Nights,* I think of Lane's translation, or of Captain Burton's translation. When I think of Persian literature, I think in terms of Browne's *Literary History of Persia,* and of course of FitzGerald's. And, frankly, I remember the first book I read on the history of South America was Prescott's [*History of*] *the Conquest of Peru.*

WFB: Is that right?

BORGES: Yes, and then I fell back on Spanish writers, but I have done most of my reading in English. I find English a far finer language than Spanish.

WFB: Why?

BORGES: There are many reasons. Firstly, English is both a Germanic and a Latin language, those two registers. For any idea you take, you have two words. Those words do not mean exactly the same. For example, if I say "regal," it's not exactly the same thing as saying "kingly." Or if I say "fraternal," it's not saying the same as "brotherly"; [then there is] "dark" and "obscure." Those words are different. It would make all the difference—speaking, for example, of the Holy Spirit—it would make all the difference in the world in a poem if I wrote about the Holy Spirit or I wrote "the Holy Ghost," since "ghost" is a fine, dark Saxon word, while "spirit" is a light Latin word.

And then there is another reason. The reason is that I think that of all languages, English is the most *physical* of all languages. You can, for example, say "He loomed over." You can't very well say that in Spanish.

WFB: *Asomo?*

BORGES: No; they're not exactly the same. And then, in English you can do almost anything with verbs and prepositions. For example, to "laugh off," to "dream away." Those things can't be said in Spanish. To "live down" something, to "live up to" something. You can't say those things in Spanish. I suppose they can be said in German, although my German really isn't too good. I taught myself German for the sake of reading Schopenhauer in the [original] text. That was way back in 1916. I had read Schopenhauer in English; I was greatly attracted to Schopenhauer, and then I thought I would try to read him in the text and then I taught myself German. And at long last I read *Die Welt als Wille und Vorstellung* in the text, and *Parerga und Paralipomena* also.

WFB: Do you write your poetry in English or in Spanish?

BORGES: No, I respect English too much. I write it in Spanish.

WFB: . . . Do you personally pass on the translations, or do you simply entrust them to people like Kerrigan or di Giovanni?

BORGES: No, I have people like Alistair Reid, di Giovanni, and Kerrigan, who are greatly better than I am at my texts. And then of course in Spanish words are far too cumbersome. They're far too long. For example, if you take an English adverb, or two English adverbs—you say for instance "quickly," "slowly," and then the stress falls on the significant part of the word. *Quick*-ly. *Slow*-ly. But if you say it in Spanish, you say "lenta*mente*," "rapida*mente*." And then the stress falls on the *non*significant part. And all that makes a very cumbersome language. But still, Spanish is my destiny; it's my *fate,* and I have to do what I can with Spanish.

WFB: Well, does the fact that the Spanish language is less resourceful than the English language necessarily make it less complete as poetry?

BORGES: No. I think that when poetry is achieved, it can be achieved in *any* language. It's more than a fine Spanish verse that could hardly be translated to another language. It would turn to something else. But when *beauty* happens, well, there it is. No?

What Whistler said—people were discussing art in Paris. People spoke about, well, the influence of *heredity, tradition, environment,* and so on. And then Whistler said, in his lazy way, "Art happens." "Art *happens*," he said. And I think that's true. I should say that *beauty* happens.

Sometimes I think that beauty is not something rare. I think beauty is happening *all* the time. *Art* is happening all the time. At some conversation a man may say a very fine thing, not being aware of it. I am hearing fine sentences all the time from the man in the street, for example. From anybody.

WFB: So you consider yourself a transcriber, to a certain extent.

BORGES: Yes, in a sense I do, and I think that I have written some fine lines, of course. *Everybody* has written some fine lines. That's not *my* privilege. If you're a writer you're bound to write something fine, at least now and then, off and on.

WFB: Even Longfellow?

BORGES: Longfellow has some very beautiful lines. I'm very old-fashioned, but I *like* "This is the forest primeval. The murmuring pines and the hemlocks." That's a very fine line. I don't know why people look down on Longfellow.

WFB: Is it in your experience possible to stimulate a love of literature, or is it something that also just happens, or doesn't happen? Is it possible to take twenty people and make them love literature more?

BORGES: Of course. I was a professor of English and American literature during some twenty years, at the University of Buenos Aires.

WFB: That's why I asked you.

BORGES: And I tried to teach my students not literature—that can't be taught—but the *love* of literature. And I have sometimes succeeded, and failed many times over, of course. If the course has to be done in four months, I can do very little. But still I know there are many young men in Buenos Aires—maybe they're not so young now—young men and young women, who have their memories full of English verse. And I have been studying Old English and Old Norse for the last twenty years. And I have also taught many people the love of Old English.

WFB: And so there is a pedagogical art? It isn't simply a matter of—

BORGES: But I think literature is being taught in the wrong way all the time. It's being taught in terms of history and of sociology. And I wouldn't do that. I have seen many teachers who are always falling back on dates, on place names.

WFB: You don't do that?

BORGES: I do my best to avoid it.

WFB: On the grounds that it is distracting?

BORGES: Yes, of course. Yes, I feel that it's irrelevant. For example, if I give you a beautiful line of verse, that verse should be as beautiful today as it was centuries ago. Or had it been written today, it should be beautiful also.

WFB: Well, doesn't the context in which you read it attach a certain meaning to it?

BORGES: Yes, but I suppose if a line is beautiful, the context can be safely forgotten, no? If I say, for example, that "the moon is the mirror of time," that's a fine metaphor, don't you think?

WFB: Yes.

BORGES: A mirror as being something round; it can be easily broken; and yet somehow the moon is as old as time, or half as old as time. Now, were I to add that that comes from Persian poetry, it wouldn't really add to the beauty. Perhaps it might add in a certain way. But still, had that metaphor been invented this morning, it would be a fine metaphor, no? The moon, the mirror of time? It happens to be a Persian metaphor.

WFB: But certain things are accepted as beautiful in part depending on the prevailing style. The kind of enthusiasm, for instance, that was shown for Restoration comedy. Some of that stuff isn't very funny now. Some of the romantic excesses of the nineteenth century aren't—

BORGES: But I suppose all that's rather artificial, no? That's one of the reasons why I'm so fond of Old English poetry. Nobody knows anything whatever about the poets [other than] the century they wrote in, and yet I find something very stirring about Old English poetry.

WFB: It has to stand on its own two feet, you mean?

BORGES: It has to. Or maybe because I like the sound of it. "Maeg ic be me sylfum sothgied wrecan,/Sithas secgan"—now, those sounds have a *ring* to them.

WFB: What does that say? What does that mean in dollars?

BORGES: That would say—in dollars that would be: "I can utter a true song about myself. I can tell of my travels." That sounds like Walt Whitman, no? That was written in the ninth century in Northumberland. "Maeg ic be me sylfum sothgied wrecan,/Sithas secgan"—and Ezra Pound translated it as this (I think it's a rather uncouth translation): "May I for my own sake song's truth reckon, journey's jargon." Well, that's too much of a jargon to *me,* no? Of course, he's translating the sounds. "Maeg ic be me sylfum sothgied wrecan,/Sithas secgan"—"May I for my sake song's truth reckon,"—"sothgied wrecan." He's translating the sounds more than the sense. And then "Sithas secgan"—"tell of my travels"—he translates "journey's jargon," which is rather uncouth, at least to me.

WFB: Whose translation did you say?

BORGES: It's Ezra Pound's translation. From the Anglo-Saxon, yes.

WFB: How would you have translated . . .

BORGES: I would translate it literally. "I can utter, I can say a true song about myself. I can tell my travels." I think that should be enough.

English can receive no higher tribute than that it was so loved by such a man, who used it from time to time to tell of his travels, in the world, and in his mind.

—WFB

Chapter 4

Usage II:
The Great
Who/Whom Wars
& Other
Matters

Herewith, some salvos from ancient, continuing wars, not only on *who/whom* but on the dispensable *the;* on *was/were* and the fading subjunctive; plus a ukase from Editor Bill which produces more than the usual number of demurrers, comma comments, plus a volley on *that/which,* than which there can be no thornier ambush. A welcome note on verbosity ends this short engagement, just in time.

———

Dear Mr. Buckley:
Reverting to James Burnham's objection to the "whom" in the *National Review* poll, "Please list the five men whom—as of right now—you consider the *leaders* contending for the Republican Presidential nomination . . .": I take it that "to be the leaders" is what this would say, expanded. And may I remind Mr. Burnham that the subject of an infinitive is in the accusative case? So you are, as always, right and impeccable.

MARION H. SAMSON

ABILENE, TEX.   DECEMBER 12, 1967

Re The Great Who/Whom Controversy, the subject of an infinitive is in-deed in the accusative case—*except* if the infinitive is copulative. So Mr. Burnham is right. It should be "who," because "to be" is implied.

NEIL MCCAFFREY

PELHAM MANOR, N.Y.

(DECEMBER 26, 1967)

Dear Mr. Buckley:

Re The Great Who/Whom Controversy and Neil McCaffrey's letter [Dec. 26], I doubt many authorities will consider he to be correct.

CHARLES M. BARRACK

BAKERSFIELD, CAL.

. . . Grammatically, Mr. B. is wrong and the editor, right. However, "whom" is fighting a losing battle, especially in spoken English; e.g., *Who* do you mean? *Who* did you speak to? *Who* did you say I should see? All grammatically incorrect but normal in spoken English. So, Mr. B. has spoken usage on his side.

J. P. EGAN

BROOKLYN, N.Y.   JANUARY 30, 1968

Dear Mr. Buckley:

The contributors to, and the editors of, *National Review* all write in a lively, natural, easy style. Why must they be so damn prissy about such trivialities as who *vs* whom? And you are not always impeccable: I re-member that the list of contributors on your cover once ended with "and etc."

RICHARD D. MULLEN

TERRE HAUTE, IND.

Correspondence on this topic is now closed.

—ED. [WFB]

But, of course, it wasn't.

   —Ed. (of this book)

Dear Mr. Buckley:

Since you often seem to be the American Grammar Clearinghouse, I wanted to ask you about this sentence I recently saw. "Who are risking their lives?" This sounds awkward, but I can't figure out why. "Who are they?" and, "They are risking their lives," are both correct as far as I can tell, but combined they sound very bad. Is this a proper, simply unusual, construction, or is there something subtly wrong with it?

Humbly,

BRUCE L. HOLDER

BOULDER, COLO.

Dear Mr. Holder: Why not? "They are risking their lives for world revolution." "*Who* are risking their lives?" "The Marx Brothers." OK? Cordially,

—WFB   JULY 21, 1978

Dear Mr. Buckley:

It has bothered me for years to see or hear people, including real pros like you, using the relative pronoun "that" in place of the personal pronoun "who," when the pronoun is referring to a person as opposed to a thing. An example would be "Henry was the only person that wore black to the funeral." I guess it's perfectly good grammar but it still grates on me. Am I being a silly old perfectionist?

A Faithful Follower,

HARRY BIRCHARD, CPA (RTD.)

WEST CHESTER, PA.

Dear Mr. Birchard: Waal, it's not *that* easy. Herewith a fragment from Evans (Bergen and Cornelia), page 505: "During the seventeenth century *that* almost disappeared from literary English and *who* replaced *which* as a relative referring to persons. But by 1700 *that* was coming into favor again. At first many educated people considered it a vulgar innovation. The *Spectator* of May 30, 1711, published a 'Humble Petition of *Who* and *Which* against the upstart Jack Sprat *That*,' in which *Who* and *Which* say: 'We are descended of ancient Families, and kept up our Dignity and Honor many Years till the Jacksprat *That* supplanted us.' Actually, they were the intruders and eventually *that* regained its old position. In the Authorized Revision of the Bible (published in 1885) we find *Our Father that art in heaven*, the form that had been used in the Wycliffe translation of 1389. Today we make a distinction between *who* and *which*, and use *who* in speaking of persons and *which* in speaking of anything subhuman. *That* is generally preferred to *which* where both words are possible, but many people prefer *who* to *that* when the reference is to a person. Twentieth-century translations of the Bible are likely to read, *Our Father who art in heaven.*" It does go on, does it not? Cordially,

—WFB   NOVEMBER 2, 1992

MEMO TO: C. H. Simonds [assistant editor of *NR*]
FROM: WFB
> *Who had* does not contract to "*who'd.*"
> *He has* does not contract to "*he's.*"

MEMO TO: WFB
FROM: C. H. Simonds
Subject: Lines to the man who succeeded, after sixteen years of education had failed, in teaching me the difference (I forget it just now) between "which" and "that"; and who has just called yet another failing to my horrified attention . . .

> *What'd I do widout Buckley?*
> *He's wonderful—really, he's swell!*
> *If he wasn't here, who'd do that voodoo*
> *(Or voo'd who?) that he do so well?*
> *When I "who'd" where I'd ought to've "who had";*
> *When, seized by the sleazes, I "he's";*
> *A missive descends*
>   *(It never offends);*
>   *I never defend,*
>   *But promise to mend;*
>   *To avoid future howlers*
>   *I brush up on Fowler's—*
> *But way down deep I mourn Bill's actions:*
> *He lacks the courage of my contractions.*

DECEMBER 31, 1971

Dear Sirs:
Re "Notes & Asides," Dec. 31:
> "*Who had* does not contract to '*who'd.*'
> "*He has* does not contract to '*he's.*' "???

If, as I suspect, "Good English" comprises, inter alia, widely accepted locutions that would not cause the linguistically sophisticated instinctively to recoil, and "Bad English" those that would (e.g., "he flaunted all the rules"; "he is one of those people who does . . ."; "Charles' book"; "the spitting image"; "he inferred in his letter that he would arrive next week"; "he said that, very soon, that he would make an announcement . . ."; "he used to always and emphatically say that . . ."; etc.), then I think you are wrong about "he's" and "who'd."

"He has got the whole world in His hands"? No! "He's had too much to drink"—yes; "he has had too much to drink" is awkward and unnatural in conversation. "He's been here for a week"—sorry, I don't recoil. Unless "I've" (as in "I've had enough, thanks"), we've (as in "we've been looking all over for you"), and "you've" (as in "you've changed quite a bit") are not part of our language, then, surely and logically, "he's" is a proper contraction for "he has."

"Who'd ever heard of Pearl Harbor before December 7, 1941?" "He's the man who'd warned us of it long before it happened." OED to the contrary notwithstanding, my not-entirely-insensitive ear is not offended by these sentences.

My failure to cite dozens of additional examples of the proper use of "he's" for "he has" and "who'd" for "who had" should be regarded as merely aposiopetic.

> With best regards,
> ROBERT J. CAHN
> NEW YORK, N.Y.

Dear Mr. Cahn: Correct. I should have said, "Does not *normally* contract to he's."

> —WFB MARCH 3, 1972

––––––

One little misuse of a word by Buckley can provoke hundreds of words by a word-sensitive correspondent. In the following instance, a casual *momentarily* produced reams of the letter writer's unfavorite things.

––––––

Dear Mr. Buckley:

Only one American in five hundred knows the correct meaning of the word "momentarily." I have learned with amazement that you are among the four hundred ninety-nine.

In one of your newspaper columns I have read the statement that "Congress will close momentarily." Well, there is only one way that Congress might close momentarily; its members would have to leave their legislative chambers for just a minute—and then come right back again!

At one time, sleazy blunders in word usage could spread only slowly and sometimes died out before they got very far. But with press, radio and television, such errors are disseminated with the same frightening celerity as the spreading of wheat-rust by the wind. Let a popular columnist or commentator deliver himself of a blooper in New York and the next day his colleagues are inflicting his error upon the multitudes in Chicago, Atlanta, Dallas and LA.

Here is a collection of ghastly locutions which have made me grind my teeth for years.

a) "Senators and congressmen." This absurdity is employed thousands of times a year in print and on the air.

b) "Border-states." When a foreign visitor sees a reference to the "border-states" in one of our papers, he assumes inevitably that it refers to those commonwealths which touch Canada or Mexico. But no, it pertains to a group of states in the *middle* of the country (Delaware, Maryland, West Virginia, Kentucky, Missouri). The bewildered foreigner is bound to ask: Border of *what?* Well, that's what I want to know. It's true, these states touched the Southern Confederacy. But the Confederacy lasted only four years and perished more than a century ago. Apparently to a lot of journalists and editors, American history came to a stop in 1865.

c) "Underprivileged." The origin of this preposterous barbarism is an etymological mystery of the first class. It must have been put together by a genius in a nut-house. In order to appreciate its inanity, try to think of a dialogue between yourself and a friend.

The friend says he feels sorry for slum-dwellers because they are "underprivileged." You reply: "Well, perhaps you'd like them to become 'overprivileged.'" Your friend thinks about it for a moment and says: "No, I don't expect that." You then remark: "Then perhaps you'd like them merely to be privileged." When the impact of that strikes him, he probably can see the absurdity of applying the word "privileged" in any form to slum-dwellers. It's as nonsensical and contradictory as the Marxian slogan "dictatorship of the proletariat." Or the statement that Stalin invented "the cult of personality," an expression which probably means something in Russian but certainly means nothing in English.

d) "Ethnic." This word is a perfectly good adjective which has been turned into a noun by politicians and their dim-witted journalistic attendants. Then to make things worse, this bastard-noun is applied (with patronizing disparagement) to those Americans who belong to cultural and racial minorities. This is another idiocy which must have come straight from an asylum.

e) "Lugshury." One of the most repulsive nuisances of our time is the broadcasting-pitchman who rhapsodizes over the "lugshury" of consuming this or that commodity. Any advertiser who says "lugshury" is a "lug" himself and ought to be met by a necktie-party as he leaves the studio.

I dream of a constitutional amendment which would require the courts to impose a heavy fine upon any politician or publicist who thinks that "momentarily" is a synonym for "soon." . . . Very truly yours,

PATRICK B. HENRICKSON

Aw, lay off, fellas.

—WFB   JANUARY 19, 1973

Dear Mr. Buckley:

On April 15, 1987, an article of yours appeared in the *Los Angeles Daily News,* "Moralist Rooney plays Solomon," in which is this clause: "We would be morally engaged in the question if it was a Tobacco Road situation." The context and your sentence following the clause above make it quite clear that the condition is contrary to fact. Why, then, did you use *was* instead of *were?*

I know of the gradual disappearance of the subjunctive mood but have had no reason to think that the contrary-to-fact condition has joined the demise. At last printings, both Follett and Crews held with *were,* Follett considering the usage to be a dividing line between educated and uneducated speakers.

In short, why did you use *was?*

Sincerely,

DAVID E. JONES

VAN NUYS, CALIF.

Dear Mr. Jones: I don't object to using the subjunctive when its use is both euphonious and realistic. I would say, "If it weren't for Mother, I wouldn't be." But I would say, "If Jane was there, she'd be guilty." To say, "If Jane *were* there, she'd be guilty" comes close to letting form dictate fact. The first clearly implies that you don't think Jane was there; the second, that you're not sure. . . . Subjunctives are dying out, and in part it's a good thing. (You wouldn't go around, Jones, confess it, saying, "If I be wrong, correct me"?) Cordially,

—WFB   SEPTEMBER 3, 1990

Dear Mr. Buckley:

Is it true that you gave orders to your editors that the American Party ticket was not to be mentioned throughout the campaign, in the pages of *National Review?* If so how much did it monetarily profit you personally?

ANON.

Dear Anon.: No, it isn't true. I have only given one order to the editors, see below.

MEMORANDUM

December 18, 1972

TO: Priscilla, JB, Jeff, Linda, Kevin, Alan, Joe, Pat, Carol, Chris, Barbara, and George Will
FROM: WFB

Two things. We are suffering at *NR* from an epidemic of exclamation-itis. Two issues ago, in the review of Garry Wills's book, I was quite certain that Will Herberg would succumb from it, before finishing the review. It is a dreadful way to go. In the current issue, Mrs. Nena Ossa concludes her interesting essay on Chile, "That would be the moment to pack and leave!" "That would be the moment to pack and leave" I submit is a much tenser way of suggesting that that would be the moment to pack and leave. A few pages later, Herr Erik von Kuehnelt-Leddihn, discussing the economic situation in Spain, remarks that "it is significant that workers who had gone abroad are now coming back in large numbers because wages (for the skilled!) have become quite attractive." Why !? (or, if you prefer, Why?!) The reader had nowhere been led to believe that Erik had constructed his argument in order to mock the superstition that unskilled wages were attractive in Spain. So why? I ASK YOU, WHY!

The other thing. A ukase. *Un*-negotiable. The only one I have issued in seventeen years. It goes: "John went to the store and bought some apples, oranges, and bananas." NOT: "John went to the store and bought some apples, oranges and bananas." I am told *National Review*'s Style Book stipulates the omission of the second comma. My comment: *National Review*'s Style Book *used* to stipulate the omission of the second comma. *National Review*'s Style Book, effective immediately, makes the omission of the second comma a capital offense!

MEMO TO: WFB
FROM: PLB
Dec. 20

Lest you think there is insubordination in the ranks when you see the current mag (Jan. 5) and the next (Jan. 19) your Stakhanovite cohorts in Editorial had already sent up the Books and Arts & Manners sections of the Jan. 19 magazine by the time they received the Memo on serial commas and, rather than raise the, sleeping, dragons, of, the, Finance, Committee, for unnecessary Author's Alterations, have suspended the decreed change until the issue of Feb. 2, which, will, look, roughly, like, this.

FEBRUARY 16, 1973

Dear Priscilla:

I have read with dismay WFB's ukase on the serial comma. I can't do it. No way. It's just plain ugly. WFB says this is *un*-negotiable. You're his sister . . . How serious is he? Can I arrange a dispensation?

Look . . . I'll compromise. There should be peace in the family. Instead of "John went to the store and bought some apples, oranges, and bananas . . ." How about if he just buys oranges and bananas? Or a head of non-union lettuce. You see what this sort of restriction leads to. And they ask me why fiction is dying. Erich Segal, I bet, uses the serial comma.

You may tell WFB that, from now on and as ordered, I salute the red and white. Sincerely,

D. KEITH MANO

BLOOMING GROVE, N.Y.

P.S. However, the first ukase on exclamationitis was long overdue. The exclamation point may be used only in dialogue and then only if the person speaking has recently been disemboweled.

Dear Priscilla:

In re the serial comma controversy in the current *NR,* on *this* issue, amusing, as, your, comments, are, I agree 100 per cent with Bill's ukase on this matter. "My coats are green, red, black and white" means something different from "My coats are green, red, black, and white," as a rather silly example. But in my book the serial comma is a *must.*

CORINNA MARSH

NEW YORK, N.Y.

Dear Mr. Buckley:

About your *un*-negotiable Style Book ukase: Fowler says the comma before the "and" is considered otiose (his word). Too many sections.

Seventeen years of silence, then the ukase labored and brought forth a comma, by caesuran section no doubt. That indeed is exclamationitis! Yours,

VOX DICTIONARIUS

c/o GEORGE FOSTER

LOS ANGELES, CALIF.

Dear Vox: Otiose blotiose. *He dreamed of conquering Guatemala, Panama, San Salvador and Nicaragua?* Without the comma, San Salvador and Nicaragua appear positively zygotic. Is that what you want, Vox? Well, count me out!

—WFB

Dear Mr. Buckley:

As a bemused admirer of your continuing love affair with the English language, I am delighted to welcome you to the side of the angels in the matter of serial commas.

Now, if you are still in a ukase-handing-down mood, you might set a few people straight (including yourself, I'm afraid) on the uses of *that* and *which*. Even good writers, in which your stable abounds, fail to recognize the difference. The feeling seems to be, as Fowler points out, that *that* is the colloquial and *which* the literary relative—a feeling that he further suggests results from misreading the evidence.

In the interests of lucid writing, the rule is that *that* should be the pronoun introducing defining clauses, and that *which* should be the pronoun introducing non-defining clauses. Or, putting it another way, if the clause is necessary to the sense of the sentence, *that* is the word; and if the clause can be omitted without destroying the sense of the sentence, then *which* is the word. Further, if the pronoun itself can be omitted, then *that* is the word. And only if the clause can be set off by commas without looking stupid is *which* the word.

The only real problem with following this rule out the window is that one occasionally (frequently?) collides with the related question of prepositions at the ends of sentences, *which* will be the subject of our next lecture.

These examples, I think, show that an insistence on knowing the difference between these two words is more than just pedagogic petulance. (Lord knows I ain't no pedagogue, just an unfortunate with a technical education and a gut feeling for the language.) Their proper use can make a hell of a difference in how the message gets across. On the other hand, if your intent is obfuscation, then you just go on that/whiching the way you've always done it.

I can't think which I approve more, your political economy or your mode of expression. Probably I wouldn't appreciate either one so much if I didn't appreciate the other. Sincerely yours,

GEORGE A. HEINEMANN

PALATINE, ILL.

Dear Mr. Heinemann: You are wrong that the rule is absolute. The preference is absolute. Fowler himself confesses to misgivings on the point, though he knows the rule, and you state it correctly. Remember, you can even get away with saying, Our Father, which art in heaven. Thanks. Cordially,

—WFB MARCH 16, 1973

Dear Kilpo [James J. Kilpatrick]:

A splendid column on Cornell. However, I disagree that a letter cannot be both verbose and redundant. Verbosity need not be redundant. Correct?

But I would write more confidently if it were not that you are Number One, being addressed by your faithful servant,

—BILL

Dear Bill:

I venture no positive pronouncements on this difficult issue. My tentative feeling is that it is quite possible to be redundant without being verbose, but I would think it difficult to be verbose without being redundant.

To say, as so many of our friends in broadcasting so often say, that a meeting will be held "at 10 A.M. in the morning" is to fall headlong into redundancy. But this is not verbosity.

I encounter verbosity (or what strikes me as verbosity) whenever I travel to the Senate press gallery and spend an hour marveling at the butter and marmalade professions on the floor. "Permit me to yield, Mr. President, to my able and distinguished friend, the senior senator from thus-and-so, for whom I entertain the highest regard and the warmest admiration. Indeed, Mr. President, I must say that no member of this deliberative body is held in higher regard, or more justifiably so, than my brilliant and erudite colleague, to whom I deferentially yield such time as he may require." That is verbosity; it is also redundancy.

I am supported in these impressions by the lexicographers of *Webster's*. Under the heading of "redundant," they encourage us to seek amplification under "wordy." At "wordy," we are educated in the subtleties that distinguish *wordy, verbose, prolix, diffuse,* and *redundant.* From these first cousins we are led to a remarkable array of second cousins, great-uncles, step-sisters, and great-aunts once removed: *tedious, garrulous, repetitious, loquacious,* and so forth. From all this I conclude that there are times, alas, when I am both verbose and redundant, while you, my mentor, are merely richly detailed.

Deferentially,

JAMES J. KILPATRICK

Dear Kilpo: We ought to put our act on the road. Herewith a trial balloon. Cordially,

—BILL   NOVEMBER 25, 1977

Chapter 5

Sexist, Anti-Sexist, and Other Foreign Languages

Dear Mr. Buckley:

I have thought long and deep about the problem of HARASS (perh. from O.F.: to set a dog on). Is it har'ass or harass'? Since the word really fills a need in our litigious age (where is the jurist who dares say: *de minimis non curat praetor?*) could not you start a movement to clarify this point?

Sincerely,

G. J. WAGENINGEN
CHICAGO, ILL.

Dear Mr. Wageningen: Want to know our preferences? Accent the first syllable when the construction is passive ("Jane was HAR-assed by Tarzan"), the last syllable when the mood is active ("Tarzan ha-RASSED Jane"). Cordially,

—WFB

Buckley has been responding to the more tortured efforts to de-sex English, usually by torturing back. This seesaw battle has been going on since the 1970s at least, and therefore not as long as he has had to defend himself (and others) against charges of a fulsome or undemocratic vocabulary, but it shows promise for the future. One senses that the battle stays joined partly out of the joy of combat but also because WFB believes himself to be on the side of what he calls Right Reason. His opponents are worthy. The cause is just, even if some of the proposed solutions are singularly lacking in grace or euphony.

DEATH TO TEXTBOOK SEXISM

I had an encounter recently with Ms. Germaine Greer, the anti-sexist sex bomb who has wrangled with lots of people including Norman Mailer, about whom, incidentally, she wrote the most galvanizing polemic in the recent history of the art (*Esquire,* September 1971).

Ms. Greer is a brilliant woman who, however, in the course of making her case against "sexism" exploits the hell out of sex. The kind of attention devoted to her in *Playboy, Evergreen Review,* et al., is inconceivable except that she obligingly spices her remarks with lascivious sexual detail as reliably as the boilerplate pornographers. I think—I am not absolutely certain, but I *suspect* that she is capable of humor, though her use of it is certainly embryonic; and that she will be rescued by humor. Somebody has got to rescue us from the women's liberation movement, and if Ms. Greer gets over her fundamentalist iconoclasm, she might be just the person to do it.

To do what? Well, for instance, to cope with Scott, Foresman & Company. They are the big textbook publishers, and I have here a pamphlet issued by the company called "Guidelines for Improving the Image of Women in Textbooks." How do you define sexism? "Sexism refers to all those attitudes and actions which relegate women to a secondary and inferior status in society . . ." The editors warn against stereotypes. "For example, writers should take care that a joke about a woman who is a bad driver, a shrewish mother-in-law, financially inept, etc., does not present these qualities as typical of women as a group."

Mercifully, the editors do not supply examples, though one can use imagination. Bob Hope has a line that goes something like this: "I bumped into a car today." Straight Man: "Why?" "There was a woman driver and she stuck out her hand for a left turn." S.M.: "What happened?" "She turned left." In the Scott, Foresman Joke Book presumably the line would be added: "The way men sometimes do."

The editors give examples of sexist language, and, opposite, examples of how to correct the abuse.

For instance, "early man." That should be "early humans." "When man invented the wheel . . ." should become "When people invented the wheel . . ." Now of course this is something we might be able to get away with when discussing prehistorical inventions. But Scott, Foresman funk the historical problem, unless they are prepared to recommend: "When the Wright people invented the airplane," or "When the Ford human invented the car." Will no one tell the people at Scott, Foresman about the synecdoche?

"Businessmen" is out: "business people" is in. Presumably the singular is a "business person." What do you want to be when you grow up,

Johnny? A business person. What do you do with "repairmen"? Not even Scott, Foresman dared come up with "repairperson," so they offer: "someone to repair the . . ." which can be spotted as a syntactical cop-out in sexist and non-sexist societies.

The use of the pronoun "he" to do androgynous duty is out. For instance, you can't say, "The motorist should slow down if he is hailed by the police." You have to say: "The motorist should slow down if he or she is hailed by the police" (or policewoman?).

They are so carried away, over at Scott, Foresman, that they appear to have lost all sense of inflection. For instance, the sexist "The ancient Egyptians allowed women considerable control over property" has got to be changed to "Women in ancient Egypt had considerable control over property"—which is, very simply, a totally different statement from the first.

Will they ever make a concession? Yes. "In some cases, it is necessary to refer to a woman's sex, as in the sentence: 'The works of female authors are too often omitted from anthologies.' " I don't know how you could come up with a permissible way of saying: "The works of female authors are too often included in anthologies." I guess you just can't think that. "Galileo was the astronomer who discovered the moons of Jupiter. Marie Curie was the beautiful chemist who discovered radium." *Wrong.* Try: "Galileo was the handsome astronomer who discovered the moons of Jupiter. Marie Curie was the beautiful chemist who discovered radium." But what if Galileo was ugly? Or, heaven forfend, what if Galileo was really handsome and Marie Curie was really ugly (which I happen to know was the case)?

Ms. Greer had better hurry. Her movement is gravely imperiled by the boys at—I mean, the boys and girls at, Scott, Foresman & Company.

NOVEMBER 25, 1972

CAN WE AVOID SEXISM?

Twice in as many days I have been reproached as a sexist, having intended no offense, and I fear that the line I had thought best left undefined needs now a little chiseling, lest things get out of hand. I mean, more out of hand.

I am reviewing a book for the *New York Times*. It is a fine book about the Antarctic, and includes engrossing chapters about the great expeditions of a half century ago. I conclude the review by observing (can any observation I have observed in the past ten years have been more innocent?) that the book would appeal not only to scientists and students of the Arctic but to "boys who love adventure stories."

Two pieces of mail already, the first especially indignant. "Just what makes you think that only boys love adventure stories? I read adventure stories throughout my childhood, and it is typical of male chauvinists to assume that only boys like to read adventure stories."

A day later, in the company of two distinguished journalists, I sought to examine a question going the rounds, namely: "Where are American leaders?" That last is the question explored in the current issue of *Time* magazine, at great and rather resourceful length. A lady panelist raised her hand to ask had we noticed that of the two hundred young potential leaders in America, listed by *Time,* only nineteen were women? "Approximately nine and one half percent," she said, exactly. We were all temporarily nonplussed, and it was then that I found myself saying that, really, the figure was not all that surprising, because it remains a fact that more men than women are attracted to those conspicuous professions from which leaders are taken. I felt a chill in the audience, as if I had said the kind of thing Professor Shockley specializes in saying.

Accordingly, I issue herewith a modest manifesto.

The movement for equality between the sexes will not, at my hands at any rate, issue in a death sentence for the synecdoche.

That there are grown people in the world who go around saying things like "chairperson" is testimony not to bisexual attempts to create equality, but to the tendency of transsexual resolutions to sound stupid. The phrase "will appeal to adventure-loving boys" is not an exclusionary phrase, because the word "boys" in this case means not only boys, but also girls. You cannot maintain the equilibrium of the English language by saying that "man's inhumanity to man" is measured in part by the sexism of that phrase. Is it seriously thought that man's inhumanity to man is to be distinguished from man's inhumanity toward women? Or that "he who laughs last laughs best" means that girls laugh best when they laugh first, whereas boys laugh best when they laugh last?

And as for the business of future leaders: Ten years ago, at the start of the women's lib movement, approximately ten percent of the students in law school were female, and now that figure has risen by approximately fourteen percent. This statistic has been cited in such tones of despair as would be appropriate in saying that over a ten-year period, death from starvation had diminished by only a few percentage points in America.

It is the uniformity of the standards that is wrong, a tiresome point but no less true for the making of it: the notion that the male lawyer is necessarily engaged in more productive or more humane work than the female non-lawyer. This morning's newspaper brings the news that our Secretary of Health, Education and Welfare, Mr. Caspar Weinberger, has solemnly announced that it is not a regulation of his office that boys and girls attend jointly school lectures on sexual hygiene. At the University of Arizona, it has been announced that unless exactly as much money is spent on girls' sports as on boys' sports, the entire federal subsidy will be withdrawn.

What kind of prehensile lengths are we going to? Germaine Greer recently debated with me on the general subject, and asked me to propose a formal resolution. I typed out, "Resolved, Give them an inch and they'll take a mile"—but prudently thought better of it, as one does not play mischievously with metaphors with Germaine Greer. But, you know, it's true.

—WFB   JULY 13, 1974

Dear Mr. Buckley:

The recent discussion in your pages of sexist language prompts me to the following observations.

Among the more egregious of the many verbal insults to sexual equality is the use of "he" to mean both sexes. *Vide* the well known passage from Proverbs:

> *He that is slow to anger is better than the mighty;*
> *And he that ruleth his spirit than he that taketh a city.*

The blatant male chauvinism of this passage would be eliminated by replacing the ubiquitous "he" with "she" alone, viz.:

> *She that is slow to anger is better than the mighty;*
> *And she that ruleth her spirit than she that taketh a city.*

Unfortunately, while this version would be poetic justice, it must be rejected as discrimination in reverse.

Another method would be to substitute for "he" the compound "he or she" (or, in the appropriate context, "his or her"):

> *He or she that is slow to anger is better than the mighty;*
> *And he or she that ruleth his or her spirit than he or she that taketh a city.*

Thus revised the passage is entirely free of sexism, but the gain is offset by the loss of clarity and conciseness.

An unobjectionable solution might lie in a fusion of "he" and "she," for example, "heshe" or "shehe." There is greater precision in these composite words, but regrettably both are phonetically repellent.

I think the most acceptable answer is a compromise:

I propose the words "shim," a composite of "she" and "him," and "shis," from the union of "she" and "his." Although a mixed bag grammatically, these synthetic terms are compact, unambiguous, and wholly without sexual signification. Moreover, "shim" has its analogue in the common English word meaning a thin piece of material wedged into a joint to take up wear or prevent squeaking. The quoted passage from Proverbs would then read:

> *Shim that is slow to anger is better than the mighty;*
> *And shim that ruleth shis spirit than shim that taketh a city.*

The slight loss of elegance in the revision is more than compensated by the passage's utter freedom from sexual invidiousness.

Extensions of the principle will doubtless occur to the thoughtful reader.

Yours very truly,
BERTRAM EDISES
ATTORNEY AT LAW
OAKLAND, CALIF.

Dear Mr. Edises: . . . What worries me, Edises, is the slurs on mightyism, not to say the implicit disparagement of the spirited. So how about:

> *Shim that is slow to anger is betterworse than the mighty;*
> *And shim that ruleth shis spirit than shim that taketh or loseth a city?*

Cordially,
—WFB   MARCH 28, 1975

Dear Bill:

In a recent column in which you recounted a chance meeting in a broadcasting studio with J. K. Galbraith you wrote, quite in passing, that while you and the economist were conversing a "*lady theologian*" was on the air.

Reading that "lady" bit I was instantly reminded of Archie Bunker.

All in the Family, as you know, is the Americanized version of a popular British TV show designed to caricature the Anglo-Saxon bigotries and class prejudices of the lower class Englishman who is the last ditch defender of middle class Victorian attitudes.

Archie, the dock-walloper, like his British counterpart, considers himself a member of the superior race and sex. Archie is especially faithful to the genteel nineteenth-century tradition that a gentleman is a man who refers to any woman who isn't obviously a trollop as a "lady," Archie speaks of "lady cabdrivers," "lady cops," "lady short-order cooks." His gentlemanly mark of respect for the "weaker" sex is, however, not altogether unmixed with disdain and resentment. Archie makes it quite plain—all in the family—that "ladies" who try to do any "man's job" are really "amatoors" who have no business to be in the business.

Even Archie's next door neighbors, the "Eyetalian lady" and the "colored lady," cannot trifle with Archie's masculine sense of racial and sexual superiority without being instantly downgraded into "that female wop," or "that colored female," who are ruining the neighborhood. Archie seldom refers to a woman as a "woman." This is probably because he views women less as persons than as the reproductive and nurturing function of a man-made world, made for men. A "woman" is what goes to bed with a man, has his babies, and gets his food on the table. In Archie's sex lexicon the men are men, but women who are not "ladies" or "females" are "the girls" or "the wives."

Altogether, Archie is a crude but powerful master of what feminists today call "verbal sexism"—the patronizing putup or contemptuous putdown of women *just because they are women.* When Archie speaks of women in any social relation to men, he never puts them on man's level. For example, in Archie's world the women are sometimes permitted to bowl with the men. As Archie might tell it, "Us men give them female bowlers a good licking," or "Us fellers let the lady bowlers win a few offn us."

So permit me, dear Bill, as woman writer, former congresswoman, and former ambassador, to remind you that professional women today view the "lady" bit as a conscious or unconscious masculine putdown. And allow me further to suggest that my favorite man columnist (who is also a gentleman) should leave the use of "lady" as a sex classifier and/or gratuitous social status indicator of professional persons to the Archie Bunkers of the writing profession.

> Affectionately,
> CLARE [BOOTHE LUCE]
> HONOLULU

Dear Clare: Your point is clearly made, and magnificently advocated. Henceforward I shall confine my use of the word to such references as "lady wrestlers," where the oxymoronic imperative clearly prevails.

> Love,
> BILL   NOVEMBER 22, 1974

FEMINISM: UNSEX ME NOW

What do Mary McCarthy, Joyce Carol Oates, Muriel Spark, and Joan Didion have in common?

Ans. They are first-class writers. If you like, you can say they are "first-class women writers." But it must be somewhere along the line communicated that by that you mean that they are first-class writers who are women. Otherwise there is a patronizing residue, as in "he is a first-class junior skier." Ironically, one of the reasons these ladies (patronizing? All right, these women) are first-class writers is that they would shun like the plague such exhortations as are being urged on all writers by the National Council of Teachers of English (NCTE), in the name of eliminating sexism.

As a rather agreeable surprise, the latest bulletin from the anti-sexist league is itself literate. We are told: "The man who cannot cry and the woman who cannot command are equally victims of their socialization." The trouble is that by the time they are through with their recommendations, they make everybody cry who cares for the mother tongue.

Unhappily, there is no way in the English of Shakespeare, Milton, Pope, and Faulkner to get rid of the synecdoche "man," which, as in "mankind," means man and woman. One of the things you cannot do in English is to replace "man" in some situations. Consider the efforts of the NCTE.

The common man becomes *the average person,* or *ordinary people.* Try it out . . . "The century of the average person." No. Why? If you don't know, I can't tell you. Ditto for "The century of ordinary people." Here, at least, you can point out that ordinary has several meanings and that whereas common does too, the conjunction of *common man* instantly excludes all but the Henry Wallace use of the word common; whereas the conjunction *of ordinary man* does not exclude such a sniffy remark as, say, Lucius Beebe might have made about vulgar people. Clarity is one of the objectives of good writers, which is why Mary McCarthy would never write about "the century of ordinary people."

The bulletin offers you a typical sexist slur: *The average student is worried about his grades.* Suggested substitute: *The average student is worried about grades.* There again, you will note a difficulty. The two sentences do not mean exactly the same thing. In the first, the student is worried about his (or her) grades. In the second, the student is worried about grades as a generic concern. Perhaps he is worried about, say, the role that grades play or do not play in getting into graduate school. Anyway, there is a residual indistinction, and English teachers shouldn't be teaching people how to write imprecisely.

The bulletin notes that English does not have a generic singular common-sex pronoun, the convention being to use the male. This will be proscribed . . . *If the student was satisfied with his performance on the pre-test, he took the post-test.* This becomes, *A student who was satisfied with her or his performance on the pre-test took the post-test.* That is called killing two birds with one stone. You eliminate the generic male singular, and reverse the conventional sequence (her and his). The distortions ring in the ear.

At one point, the NCTE wants us to validate improper usage. Here we are asked to rewrite *Anyone who wants to go to the game should bring his money tomorrow* to *Anyone who wants to go to the game should bring their money tomorrow;* and I say anyone who does that kind of thing at this point should not be hired as a professional writer.

So mobilized are these folk that they do not stop at a war far from the cosmopolitan centers, designed to wipe out little pockets of vernacular resistance. *Gal Friday* has to become assistant. A *libber* must become a *feminist* (here I think they have dealt from the bottom of the deck: what's inherently sexist about libber?). A *man-sized job* becomes a *big* or *enormous* job. Question: How do you describe a job that requires physical exertion beyond the biological powers of wopersons?

It is comforting to know that this effort to correct the language will precisely not succeed because the genuine artists among women writers are more concerned for their craft than for fashionable sociological skirmishes. Nothing more persuades the general public of women's inferiority (which doctrine is of course preposterous) than efforts at equality achieved by indicting good prose.

—WFB   APRIL 29, 1976

Stop!

A colleague the other day was aghast at seeing in print, in a piece he had written for a small magazine, the word "chairperson," where my friend in his manuscript had written "chairman." He takes seriously his responsibility for language that appears over his name, and so telephoned to the editor and said in words less than entirely conciliatory, Where do you get off putting "chairperson" where I specified "chairman"? Well, she said, it's just this simple, you were talking about a woman. To which he replied that it was just this simple, namely that "chairman" refers, and has done so for hundreds of years, equally to men as to women, which is so also of the word "man," which in certain formulations ("Man is made in the image of God") is genderless. And anyway, he said to her, what right do you have to impose your preferred forms over mine, given that I am the author of the piece? To which she said, smiling sweetly, to the extent this can be ascertained in the voice of someone coming in over the telephone, that that was the style rule of that magazine. And style rules govern.

Now magazines and newspapers are entitled to have style rules that govern such matters as whether "theatre" can be spelled that way or must appear as "theater." That is plain house editorial privilege. But what happened to my friend, of course, is that he was being inducted into a movement—the feminist movement, as it calls itself, although it must be understood that the feminist movement is not necessarily a movement all good men, or women, should come to the aid of.

There is no end to the lengths to which such impositions can go. Or was the extreme reached by the National Union of Journalists in Great Britain? About a recent experience there, I must inform you.

Most men and women who want to work in journalism need to join the NUJ because most newspapers are closed shops in Great Britain. The story begins when a Mr. Terry Lovell, a newspaperman in Manchester, got into trouble with the NUJ for writing a story in which he passed along the theory that, to quote the paraphrase of the London *Times*'s Bernard Levin, "women tend to concentrate on and encourage the part of them they think the prettiest." For this offense against equality—i.e., he suggested that in some respects women comport themselves differently from men—he was officially rebuked. His colleagues thought this very funny, and decided to punish him, and amuse themselves, by designating him as the Manchester branch "Equality Officer"—charged with hearing complaints alleging bias.

So a few weeks go by, and a complaint is brought against a colleague of Mr. Lovell who, when interviewing a football manager and his lady friend, described the latter as "bra-less."

As far as the complainant was concerned, the case was open and closed. The writer had violated Clause 10 of Rule 18 of the union's disciplinary code, which forbids discrimination on grounds, among others, of gender. How? Because he had not described the man's underwear, even though he had referred to the lady's lack of it.

In his response, Mr. Hughes was an absolute model of docility. He told the NUJ jurors that the reason he had referred to the subject's being bra-less was that indeed she was not wearing a bra. Moreover, he promised— "you may rest assured," he solemnly spoke, that if the football manager *had* been wearing a bra, he'd have made it a point to mention this.

Well, that kind of thing makes very good reading, but humor—spelled humour in England, which is perfectly OK—doesn't work when trafficking with ideologues. All the defendant got for his pains was a portentous reply by the complainant: "I may have my own criticisms of aspects of equality policy, not least the severe problems in their implementation in the face of open contempt from some sections of the membership . . ." snore, snore—and the defendant was put on probation. The Equality Committee will keep its eyes on him, and if ever he should make reference to a woman who had served as "chairman," well, kaput. Exit that writer from the national scene.

Here is an appeal. I direct it to Clare Boothe Luce, because she has been an ardent champion of women's rights throughout her lifetime. But Mrs. Luce is also an artist of refined literary taste. And, add to all this, she knows how to manage causes. I desire her to head up a committee of illustrious women writers to protest the lengths a movement is being taken in their name. The Women's Committee to Protest the Vulgarization of the Women's Rights Movement, how is that for a title?

—WFB   APRIL 30, 1985

Chapter 6

On Latin & Other Lively Languages

Clarification

What in the world is "entrepreneurial ebullience?"

MARJORIE KADERLI
AUSTIN, TEXAS

Ardor negotiorum curatoris, natch.

—WFB   AUGUST 28, 1962

Buckley's use of foreign languages is not affectation. Given his particular, peculiarly belated introduction to English, explained elsewhere,* it is perhaps not surprising. He speaks Spanish fluently; it was his original language; in fact, he later taught it. His feeling for Latin is not defensive; it is a passionate advocacy.

Not surprisingly, then, his mailbag and his writings often are concerned with the use of foreign words and phrases and he enjoys reaching for the right example in French, say, as much as he does the arcane, unusual, or recherché in English.

One column in 1965 began . . .

Pas d'Ennemi à Gauche

The reason writers are given in certain circumstances to using phrases from foreign languages rather than their English translation is not merely that they sometimes have a special piquancy in the original (*vive la différence,* for example) but because they have a special incantatory sound, suggesting a special, sometimes extrarational meaning—an abracadabra-

---

* In chapter 8 on diction, etc.

special magical authority. Such a phrase is *"pas d'ennemi à gauche"* which literally translated means: no enemies on the left. Freely translated it means: any two-bit leftist individual or nation can do whatever he or it desires to an American or America and get away with it. By contrast, a right-winger, or a right-wing nation, is by definition hostile. . . .

Dear Mr. Buckley:
I was more than surprised to see that most offensive term "hocus-pocus" in your editorial, "A Sane Explosion" [February 27].

Says Tillotson (an accepted authority): "Those common juggling words of *hocus-pocus* are nothing else but a corruption of the *hoc est corpus* by way of ridiculous imitation of the priests of the Church of Rome in their trick of transubstantiation." Works, Vol. 1, Sermon 26.

M. J. HOGAN

PHILADELPHIA, PA.

Dear Mr. Hogan: Oxford English Dictionary; *Volume V, p. 320:* "Hocus pocus . . . *17th c . . . the appellation of a juggler (and, apparently, as the assumed name of a particular conjurer) derived from the sham Latin formula employed by him . . . The notion that* hocus pocus *was a parody of the Latin words used in the Eucharist rests merely on a conjecture thrown out by Tillotson . . .*

—WFB   MARCH 12, 1960

Dear Bill:
Can you hum the *Die Meistersinger?*
How about the *Il Trovatore?*
Do you dine at the El Morocco?
Does your column run in the *Le Monde?*
No. Then don't say that Galbraith's theory of redistribution was originally discovered by *the* hoi polloi ("On the Right," July 16, 1972). Even with duplicated articles, I like your articles. Keep up the good work.

Sincerely,

BOB HARDWICK

FT. PIERCE, FLA.

Dear Mr. Hardwick: Nice. Thanks. And now, if I may, from Fowler: "**hoi polloi.** These Greek words for the majority, ordinary people, the man in the street, the common herd etc., meaning literally 'the many,' are equally uncomfortable in English whether the (= hoi) is prefixed to them or not. The best solution is to eschew the phrase altogether." "**Pedantry** may be defined . . . as the saying of things in language so learned or so demonstratively accurate as to imply a slur upon the generality, who are not capable or not desirous of such displays. The term, then, is obviously a relative one; my pedantry is your scholarship, his reasonable accuracy, her irreducible minimum of education, and someone else's ignorance. It is therefore not very profitable to dogmatize . . . on the subject." Cordially,

—WFB   AUGUST 18, 1972

Dear Mr. Buckley:

Greetings! Your country has called upon you at this critical . . . Now that I have your attention, I again call upon you to rectify the grievous' *faux pas* perpetrated upon the theopneustic pages of *National Review.* I must battologize: there is not, nor has there ever been, a language called "Mongolese" ["On the Right," March 1]. Please rectify this grave *lapis linguae . . .*

Unmitigatedly yours,
ERIC S. OLIN
MENDHAM, N.J.

Dear Mr. Olin: Hey. I like that "theopneustic" to describe *NR,* but getting "battologize" out of battologist is, well, a bit much; and it's *lapsus* (as in *calami*) not lapis (as in lazuli). Cordially,

—WFB   MAY 10, 1974

Dr. Mr. Buckley:

I am stranded here without my reference library for a couple of weeks, and have come across a sentence from Terence used as an epigraph of sorts, which I am unable to translate. Would you be so kind as to do so, and let me have it in the enclosed envelope? It is: "*Bono animo es: tu cum illa te intus oblecta interim et lectulos iube sterni nobis et parari cetera.*" Many thanks.

M. PATRICK GLENVILLE
SUN VALLEY, IDAHO

Dear Mr. Glenville: It defeats me, sorry, and also one or two of my colleagues. Normally, I would write to Garry Wills and ask him to translate it for me. However, I am so outraged by his recent stupid, preposterous column on the Shockley debate at Yale, I declared a ninety-day moratorium on any correspondence with him. There are still thirty-two days left. If you can hold out, I'll ask him then, and ship you out the translations to Sun Valley.

Yours cordially,
—WFB   AUGUST 2, 1974

Dear Sirs:

Since Mr. Buckley has placed me under Interdict [August 2] I must translate for Mr. Glenville through your mediation: [*"Bono animo es: tu cum illa te intus oblecta interim et lectulos iube sterni nobis et parari cetera"*] "Relax. Amuse yourself inside, for a while, with her. Order the banquet couches spread and the other things prepared . . . "

Best,

GARRY WILLS

BALTIMORE, MD.

P.S. Bill—I thought you promised to stop reading my column if I promised to stop sending it!

Best,

GARRY

Dear Mr. Buckley:

It just struck me, Mr. Buckley . . . that you might get a chuckle from my commentary, "Tuning Up a Datum." Here's a copy.

Best regards,

WEN SMITH

ASHLAND, ORE.

Tuning Up a Datum

My neighbor Phil is a grease-monkey by trade, but his ear is almost as sensitive to bad grammar as it is to an engine out of tune. Phil came by yesterday with a copy of *National Review.*

"Bill Buckley is one writer who knows his grammar," Phil said. "Who else knows the difference between *datum* and *data?*"

"I do," I said. "I just don't know the difference between a gear box and a transmission."

Phil gave me a pitying look. "They're the same thing," he said.

"So what's new with William F. Buckley, Jr.?" I said.

"It's the precise way he uses grammar," Phil said. He had the magazine open to a Buckley commentary. "Here he's talking about minorities and crime. He says 66 per cent of black children are born to unwed mothers." [*NR*, May 16.]

"That's not a crime," I said.

"Not my point," Phil said. "Buckley goes on to say, 'This is a datum none of the disputants deny.' "

"Well, he used *datum* correctly," I said. "It's the singular, and *data* is the plural."

"Exactly," Phil said. "I took beginning Latin when I was in high school. But these days I hardly ever hear anyone use the word *datum*. And mostly I hear *data* used as singular. You know, 'The data *is* incomplete.' "

"Well," I said. "Nobody speaks Latin any more, except the Pope—and Bill Buckley. What about his English? Read that line again."

Phil read again from Buckley's article. " 'This is a datum none of the disputants deny.' You see? *'Is a datum.'* Perfect grammar."

"Well," I said, "consistency is for little minds. You wouldn't want to hang Bill Buckley with that noose. Anyway, a lot of people use none as a plural today."

"Yeah," Phil said. "I guess none of us are perfect.

"Thanks for the tune-up," he added, and he went home to read the rest of *National Review.*

Dear Mr. Smith: Enjoyable column, nice try, but, alas, no cigar. See below. Cordially,

—WFB   AUGUST 15, 1994

From the New York Public Library Style Book, *1994:*
None

None can be used with either a singular verb or a plural verb, but most grammarians and style manuals prefer the plural. The old belief that none means "not one" is not true in most cases; a closer look will usually show that "not any" is the thought being expressed in almost every instance.

None of the reporters were able to interview the defendant.

Television is the chief way that most of us partake of the larger world, of the information age, and so none of us completely escape its influence.
(*The New Yorker,* March 9, 1992)

Dear Mr. Buckley:

A recent issue of *The Nation* was given over to a sustained polemic against Daniel Patrick Moynihan in which he was indicted for, *inter alia,* being (1) a demagogue, (2) a racist, and (3) an unscrupulous scholar. One article revealed that Moynihan received wide press coverage because of his use of the word "floccipaucinihilipilification."

Now, I consulted three unabridged dictionaries before discovering in the New Oxford Dictionary that this polysyllabic monstrosity means "the act of estimating as unworthy."

Questions: (1) Have you ever heard of this word? (2) Have you ever used it? (3) Why is Moynihan the *bête noire* of the Left? (4) How come you know *everything*?

> Admiringly yours,
> GORDON HANSON
> SEATTLE, WASH.

Dear Mr. Hanson: (1) Yes, have known it for years; it used to be tossed about in the young teen-age set during the thirties as a can-you-match-this-one word. You have it slightly wrong, by the way. It's flocci-nauci-nihili-pilification, and as the Oxford advises you, it is a humorous agglutination of Latinisms from an Eton grammar. Though I can't find authority for it, we used to give out as its meaning, "full of sound and fury signifying nothing." (2) No. (3) Moynihan is a *bête noire* of the Left because he has their number and is brighter than they are. (4) I don't know everything, but I absolutely know why Moynihan is a *bête noire* of the Left. Cordially,

> —WFB   JANUARY 25, 1980

Dear Mr. Buckley:

Your syndicated column "Musings of a Deposed Dictator" [printed in *NR* as "Okay, Okay, I'm Coming," Feb. 5] appears to be in the form of a dramatic monologue, though the identity of the speaker is never given direct enunciation. In the course of the text, the following passage occurs, "I have plenty of plata, nice 24-karat plata."

Not all newspaper stylebooks require the italicization of such unassimilated foreign words as *plata,* for which reason you are not held to account for what may be a copy-editor's lapse. SPELL [Society for the Preservation of English as a Literary Language] does not doubt the utility, sometimes the necessity, of introducing foreign terms into English discourse. We pick bones, not nits.

We do, however, require that such terms be employed with some clear apprehension of the word's lexical meaning, derivation, and common usage on its home turf. It is on these standards that you stand in the dock on a charge of egregious and pretentious solecism.

In Spanish *plata* means silver; *oro* means gold. In the Anglophone world, the purity of gold is expressed in karats, units per 24 parts of absolute purity. The relative purity of silver is sometimes expressed as "sterling" (92.5 per cent pure) or "coin" (90 per cent). In all other formulations the purity of silver is expressed domestically in parts per thousand, as is the purity of both silver and gold internationally.

I am certain that you would never entertain a defense grounded in your ignorance, nor does it seem likely that some editor or gremlin substituted "*plata*" for "*oro*" as your prose proceeded from your teeming brain to my breakfast table. I invite your attention to this matter, with an aim to contrition.

In the hope, not only of contrition, but of amendment, I am,

Sincerely,

JOHN K. METCALFE

FACTOTUM AND ENFORCER

SPELL

PITTSBURGH, PA.

Dear Mr. Metcalfe: The word "plata" is commonly used in Latin America to signify: money; dough; bread. As in, "*Desgraciadamente, estoy sin plata.*" Direct your energies elsewhere. Cordially,

—WFB

ASSISTANT INSTRUCTOR IN SPANISH,

YALE UNIVERSITY, 1947–51

APRIL 1, 1990

Bill Buckley's sadness or anger over the loss of Latin in the Catholic mass is mixed, in the several pieces that follow, with parallel sympathies for his cousins in the Anglican Communion. He sees their fall from linguistic grace as a loss, also.

It might be said that his conservative instincts in matters political find resonance in his attitudes toward matters religious. In neither case are his sentiments . . . well, sentimental.

The End of the Latin Mass

In January of this year my sister died, age forty-nine, eldest of ten children, and mother of ten children, the lot of us catapulted into a dumb grief whence we sought relief by many means, principal among them the conviction, now reified by desire, that our separation from her is impermanent. It was the moment to recall not merely the promises of Christ, but their magical cogency; the moment to remind ourselves as forcefully as we knew how of the depths of the Christian experience, of the Christian mystery, so that when one of us communicated with her priest, we asked if he would consent to a funeral mass in the manner of the days gone by, which request he gladly granted. And so, on January 18, in the subzero weather of a little town in northwestern Connecticut, in the ugly little church we all grew up in, the priest recited the mass of the dead, and the organist accompanied the soloist who sang the Gregorian dirge in words the mourners did not clearly discern, words which had we discerned them we would not have been able exactly to translate, and yet we experienced, not only her family but her friends, not alone the Catholics among us but also the Protestants and the Jews, something akin to that synesthesia which nowadays most spiritually restless folk find it necessary to discover in drugs or from a guru in mysterious India.

Six months later my sister's oldest daughter—the first of the grandchildren—was married. With some hesitation (one must not be overbearing) her father asked the same priest (of noble mien and great heart) whether this happy ritual might also be performed in the Latin. He replied with understanding and grace that that would not be possible, inasmuch as he would be performing on this occasion not in a remote corner of Connecticut, but in West Hartford, practically within earshot of the bishop. We felt very wicked at having attempted anything so audacious within the walls of the episcopacy, and so the wedding took place according to the current cant, with everybody popping up, and kneeling down, and responding, more or less, to the stream of objurgations that issued from the nervous and tone-deaf young commentator, all together now, Who Do We Appreciate? Jesus! Jesus! Jesus! Je-*zus*—it was awful. My beloved wife—to whom I have been beholden for seventeen years, and who has borne with me through countless weddings of my countless relations, who was with me and clutched my hand during the funeral a few months earlier, whom I had not invited to my church since the vulgarizations of 1964, so anxious was I that, as a member of the Anglican Communion, she should continue to remember our services as she had known them, in their inscrutable majesty—turned to me early in the ritual in utter incredulity, wondering whether something was especially awry. Hypersensitive, I rebuked her, muttering something to the effect that she had no right to be so ignorant of what had been going on for three years, and she withdrew in anger. She was right; I was utterly wrong. How could she, an innocent Protestant, begin to conceive of the liturgical disfigurations of the past few years? My own reaction was the protective reaction of the son whose father, the chronic drunkard, is first espied unsteady on his feet by someone from whom one has greatly cared to conceal the fact. Let it be objected that the essential fact of the matter is that the sacrament of matrimony was duly conferred, and what else is it that matters? My sensibilities, that's what.

They do not matter, of course, in any Benthamite reckoning of the success of the new liturgy. Concerning this point, I yield completely, or rather almost completely. It is absolutely right that the vernacular should displace the Latin if by doing so, the rituals of Catholic Christianity bring a greater satisfaction to the laity and a deeper comprehension of their religion. There oughtn't to be any argument on this point, and there certainly isn't any from me. Indeed, when a most learned and attractive young priest from my own parish asked me to serve as a lector in the new mass, I acquiesced, read all the relevant literature, and, to be sure warily, hoped that something was about to unfold before me which would vindicate the progressives.

I hung on doggedly for three years, until a month ago, when I wrote my pastor that I no longer thought it appropriate regularly to serve as lector. During those three years I observed the evolution of the new mass and the reaction to it of the congregation (the largest, by the way, in Connecticut). The church holds 1,000 people, and at first, four hymns were prescribed. They were subsequently reduced to three, even as, in the course of the experiment, the commentator absorbed the duties of the lector, or vice versa, depending on whether you are the ex-commentator or the ex-lector. At our church three years ago perhaps a dozen people out of 1,000 sang the hymn. Now perhaps three dozen out of 1,000 sing the hymn. (It is not much different with the prayers.) That is atypical, to be sure; the church is large and overawing to the uncertain group singer—*i.e.,* to most non-Protestant Americans. In other Catholic churches, I have noted, the congregations tend to join a little bit more firmly in the song. In none that I have been to is there anything like the joyous unison that the bards of the new liturgy thrummed about in the anticipatory literature, the only exception being the highly regimented school my son attends, at which the reverend headmaster has means to induce cooperation in whatever enterprise strikes his fancy. (I have noticed that my son does not join in the hymn singing when he is home, though the reason why is not necessarily indifference, is almost surely not recalcitrance, is most likely a realistic appreciation of his inability to contribute to the musical story line.)

I must, of course, judge primarily on the basis of my own experience; but it is conclusive at my own church, and I venture to say without fear of contradiction that the joint singing and prayers are a fiasco, which is all right, I suppose—the Christian martyrs endured worse exasperations and profited more from them than we endure from or are likely to benefit from the singing of the hymns at St. Mary's Church. What is troublesome is the difficulty one has in dogging one's own spiritual pursuits in the random cacophony. Really, the new liturgists should have offered training in yoga or whatever else Mother Church in her resourcefulness might baptize as a distinctively Catholic means by which we might tune off the Fascistic static of the contemporary mass, during which one is either attempting to sing, totally neglecting the prayers at the foot of the altar which suddenly we are told are irrelevant; or attempting to read the missal at one's own syncopated pace, which we must now do athwart the obtrusive rhythm of the priest or the commentator; or attempting to meditate on this or the other prayer or sentiment or analysis in the ordinary or in the proper of the mass, only to find that such meditation is sheer outlawry, which stands in the way of the liturgical calisthenics devised by the central coach, who apparently judges it an act of neglect if the churchgoer is permitted more than two minutes and forty-six seconds without being made to stand if he was kneeling, or kneel if he was standing, or sit—or sing—or chant—or *anything* if perchance he was praying, from which anarchism he must at all costs be rescued: "LET US NOW RECITE THE INTROIT PRAYER," says the commentator, to which exhortation I find myself aching to reply in that "loud and clear and reverential voice" the manual for lectors prescribes: "LET US NOT!" Must we say the introit prayer together? I have been reading the introit prayer since I was thirteen years old, and I continue unaware that I missed something—*e.g.,* at the Jesuit school in England when at daily mass we read the introit prayers all by our little selves, beginning it perhaps as much as five seconds before, or five seconds after, the priest, who, enjoying the privacy granted him at Trent, pursued his prayers, in his own way, at his own speed, ungoverned by the metronomic discipline of the parishioners or of the commentator.

Ah, but now the parish *understands* the introit prayer! But, my beloved friends, the parish does not understand. Neither does the commentator. Neither does the lector. Neither, if you want the truth of the matter, does the priest—in most cases. If clarity is the purpose of the liturgical reform—the reason for going into English, the reason for going into the vernacular—then the reforms of the liturgy are simply incomplete. If clarity is the desideratum, or however you say the word in English, then the thing to do is to jettison, just to begin with, most of St. Paul, whose epistles are in some respects inscrutable to some of the people some of the time and in most respects inscrutable to most of the people most of the time. The translation of them from archaic grandeur to John-Jane contemporese simply doesn't do the trick, particularly if one is expected to go in unison. Those prayers, which are not exacting or recondite—are even they more galvanizing when spoken in unison? LET US NOW RECITE THE INTROIT PRAYER. *Judge me, O God, and distinguish my cause from the nation that is not holy; deliver me from the unjust and deceitful man.* Judge-me-O-God/And-distinguish-my-cause-from-the-nation-that-is-not-holy/Deliver-me-from-the-unjust-and-deceitful-man/—Why? How come? Whose idea—that such words as these are better spoken, better understood, better appreciated, when rendered metrically in forced marches with the congregation? Who, thinking to read these holy and inspired words reverentially, would submit to the iron rhythm of a joint reading? It is one thing to chant together a refrain—Lord deliver us/Lord save us/Grant us peace.

But the extended prayer in unison is a metallic Procrusteanism which absolutely defies the rationale of the whole business, which is the communication of *meaning*. The rote saying of anything is the enemy of understanding. To reduce to unison prayers whose meaning is unfamiliar is virtually to guarantee that they will mean nothing to the sayer. *"Brethren: Everything that was written in times past was written for our instruction, that through the patience and encouragement afforded by the scriptures we might have hope. I say that Christ exercised his ministry to the circumsised to show God's fidelity in fulfilling his promises to the fathers, whereas the Gentiles glorify God for his mercy, as it is written: 'Therefore will I proclaim you among the nations, and I will sing praise to your name.'"* These were the words with which I first accosted my fellow parishioners from the lector's pulpit. I do not even now understand them well enough to explain them with any confidence. And yet, the instruction manual informs me, I am to communicate their meaning "clearly" and "confidently." And together the congregation will repeat such sentences in the gradual.

Our beloved Mother Church. How sadly, how innocently, how—sometimes—strangely she is sometimes directed by her devoted disciples! *Hail Mary, full of Grace, the Lord is with you . . .* The Lord is with who? *Thee to you, Buster,* I found myself thinking during the retreat when first I learned that it is a part of the current edification to strip the Lord, His Mother, and the saints of the honorific with which the simple Quakers even now address their children and their servants. And the translations! *"Happy the Humble—they shall inherit. . . ."* One cannot read on without the same sense of outrage one would feel on entering the Cathedral of Chartres and finding that the windows had been replaced with pop art figures of Christ sitting in against the slumlords of Milwaukee. One's heart is filled with such passions of resentment and odium as only Hilaire Belloc could adequately have voiced. O God O God O God, why hast thou forsaken us! My faith, I note on their taking from us even the canon of the mass in that mysterious universal which soothed and inspired the low and the mighty, a part of the mass—as Evelyn Waugh recalled—"for whose restoration the Elizabethan martyrs had gone to the scaffold [in which] St. Augustine, St. Thomas à Becket, St. Thomas More, Challoner and Newman would have been perfectly at their ease among us," is secure. I pray the sacrifice will yield a rich harvest of informed Christians. But to suppose that it will is the most difficult act of faith I have ever been called on to make, because it tears against the perceptions of all my senses. My faith is a congeries of dogmatical certitudes, one of which is that the new liturgy is the triumph, yea the resurrection, of the Philistines.

—WFB　　　　　NOVEMBER 10, 1967

ANGLICAN AGONY

As a Catholic, I have abandoned hope for the liturgy, which, in the typical American church, is as ugly and as maladroit as if it had been composed by Ralph Ingersoll and H. L. Mencken for the purpose of driving people away. Incidentally, the modern liturgists are doing a remarkably good job, attendance at Catholic mass on Sunday having dropped sharply in the ten years since a few well-meaning cretins got hold of the power to vernacularize the mass, and the money to scour the earth in search of the most unmusical men and women to preside over the translation.

The next liturgical ceremony conducted primarily for my benefit, since I have no plans to be beatified or remarried, will be my funeral; and it is a source of great consolation to me that, at that event, I shall be quite dead, and will not need to listen to the accepted replacement for the noble old Latin liturgy. Meanwhile, I am practicing yoga so that at church on Sundays I can develop the power to tune out everything I hear, while attempting, athwart the general calisthenics, to commune with my Maker, and ask Him first to forgive me my own sins, and implore him, second, not to forgive the people who ruined the mass.

Now the poor Anglicans are coming in for it. I am not familiar with their service, but I am with their Book of Common Prayer. To be unfamiliar with it is as though one were unfamiliar with *Hamlet,* or the *Iliad,* or the *Divine Comedy.* It has, of course, theological significance for Episcopalians and their fellow travelers. But it has a cultural significance for the entire English-speaking world. It was brought together, for the most part, about four hundred years ago, when for reasons no one has been able to explain, the little island of England produced the greatest literature in history. G. K. Chesterton wrote about it, "It is the one positive possession, and attraction . . . the masterpiece of Protestantism; the one magnet and talisman for people even outside the Anglican Church, as are the great Gothic cathedrals for people outside the Catholic Church."

What are they doing to it? Well, there is one of those commissions. It is sort of retranslating it. As it now stands, for instance, there are the lines, "We have erred, and strayed from thy ways like lost sheep. We have followed too much the devices and desires of our own hearts. We have offended against thy holy laws. We have left undone those things which we ought to have done; and we have done those things which we ought not to have done."

That kind of thing—noble, cadenced, pure as the psalmist's water—becomes, "We have not loved you [get that: *you,* not *thee.* Next time around, one supposes it will be "We haven't loved you, man"] with our whole heart, we have not loved our neighbors as ourselves." "Lead us not into temptation" becomes "Do not bring us to the test."

Well, if the good Lord intends not to bring his Anglican flock into the test, he will not test it on this kind of stuff. As it is, Anglicanism is a little shaky, having experienced about a hundred years earlier than Roman Catholicism some of the same kind of difficulties. I revere my Anglican friends and highly respect their religion, but it is true that it lends itself to such a pasquinade as Auberon Waugh's, who wrote recently, "In England we have a curious institution called the Church of England . . . Its strength has always lain in the fact that on any moral or political issue it can produce such a wide divergence of opinion that nobody—from the Pope to Mao Tse-tung—can say with any confidence that he is not an Anglican. Its weaknesses are that nobody pays much attention to it and very few people attend its functions."

And it is true that in a pathetic attempt to attract attention, the Anglicans, and indeed many other Protestants, and many Catholics, absorb themselves in secular matters. "The first Anglicans," Chesterton once wrote, "asked for peace and happiness, truth and justice; but nothing can stop the latest Anglicans, and many others, from the horrid habit of asking for improvement in international relations." International relations having taken a noticeable turn for the worse in the generation since Chesterton made this observation, one can only hope the Anglicans will reject any further attempt to vitiate their line of communication with our Maker.

—WFB   JULY 16, 1975

HIS NEW PRAYER

Those outsiders (I am not an Anglican) who have been following the agony of that Christian communion oscillate between feelings of sorrow and anger. It is conceivably a part of the Lord's design to torture his institutional representatives on earth, and of course it is generally conceded that the special object of His displeasure in the past decade has been His old favorite, the Roman Catholic Church, which He has treated with stepfatherly neglect. But as if some providential version of equal treatment under the Law were guiding Him, it has been recently the season of torment for the Episcopal Church, which indeed is now riven in factions so resolutely opposed to one another that schism itself has set in.

This last was precipitated by the question whether to ordain women priests. There is an Anglican bishop in New York who is given to extreme formulations in any field whatsoever. About a year ago he was anathematizing businessmen who were driven from New York, having looked at their ledgers and decided that, on the whole, they and their flock would be better off in an area in which the tax overhead was less, as also the incidence of murder, rape, and mugging. Bishop [Paul] Moore would have lectured Moses himself on his lack of civic pride in departing Egypt in search of greener pastures. Well, the bishop not only came out for ordaining women, for which there is at least a coherent argument, he proceeded to ordain a self-professed lesbian, which struck many of his flock as less a gesture of compassion than of defiance.

The other morning, the Church of England issued its rewording of the Lord's Prayer. Now the head of the Church of England, at least titularly, is the Queen of England. One would think that sometime before the British Court worried about anachronisms in dealing with God, they would accost anachronisms in dealing with the Queen of England. But while she continues to be addressed with all the euphuistic pomposity of Plantagenet prose, they are modernizing the form of address appropriate to God. One continues to refer to the Queen as Your Majesty, and as "Ma'am"; but for God, "Thee" and "Thou" are—out. The Lord's head has been placed on the Jacobinical block.

It now goes not, "Our Father, who art in Heaven, hallowed be Thy name"—but "Our Father in Heaven, hallowed be Your Name." Granted, they have left the capital letter in "Your," which must have been done after grave debate in the relevant councils. But clearly it was felt that "Thy" was simply—too much. Who does He think He is? The Queen of England?

It goes on, "Your will be done on earth as in Heaven."

One wonders what has been gained by that formulation over the traditional formulation, which read "Thy will be done on earth as it is in Heaven." There is transparent here something on the order of a Parkinsonian imperative: A venerable passage will be reworded by a rewording commission insofar as a commission to reword possesses the authority to do so.

Is it suggested that more people will understand the phrase in the new formulation? In the first place, we are hip-deep in the aleatory mode when we say, "Thy will be done," since we all know that it is very seldom done; and, indeed, some of us would go so far as to say that it is most unlikely that it is being done by the Royal Committee on the Vulgarization of the Book of Common Prayer when they take such a sentence as "Thy will be done on earth as it is in Heaven" back from the alchemists who worked for the Lord and for King James, and beat it into the leaden substitute which they have now promulgated.

One wishes that were all; but there is no sin of omission for which we might be grateful. "Lead us not into temptation, but deliver us from evil" has been changed to "Do not bring us to the time of trial, but deliver us from evil." Why? For the sake of clarity? (That is the usual answer.) I know, because every sense in my body informs me, and every misinclination of my mind, what is temptation, from which we seek deliverance. But "*the time of trial?*" That sounds as if the Supreme Court is in session.

Perhaps it was ordained that the Episcopalians, like their brothers the Catholics, should suffer. It is a time for weeping, and a time for rage. Do not go kindly into the night. Rage, rage against the dying of the light. That would be the advice of this outsider to my brothers in the Anglican Church. They must rage against those who bring upon Christianity not only indifference, but contempt.

—WFB   NOVEMBER 17, 1977

INTRODUCTION TO *AMO, AMAS, AMAT, AND MORE,* BY EUGENE EHRLICH. HARPER & ROW, 1985.

It is not plain to me why I was asked to write the Introduction to this book. (There are true Latinists around. Not in abundance, but for instance one thinks of Garry Wills, or Ernest Van den Haag, just to mention two noisy, and brilliant, writers.) Nor is it obvious why I accepted the invitation (the little stipend is being forwarded to charity).

I suppose I am asked because the few Latin phrases I am comfortable with I tend to use without apology. For instance, for some reason I find it handier even in idiomatic exchanges to say "*per impossibile*" over against, say, "assuming that the impossible were actually to take place." Nor is the usefulness of *per impossibile* sui generis—if you see the kind of situation one is capable of falling into. And, of course, there are those Latin phrases that have a utilitarian function, as for instance the lawyers' "*nolle prosequi,*" which has become so thoroughly transliterated as to have acquired English conjugational life: thus, "The case against Dr. Arbuthnot was nol-prossed"—the lawyer's vernacular for "The prosecutor decided not to prosecute the case against Dr. Arbuthnot."

So, there are those Latin phrases—and, really, there are not so many of them—that cling to life because they seem to perform useful duties without any challenger rising up to take their place in English. Sometimes these special exemptions from vernacularization in the mother tongue derive from the distinctive inflection that flows in from the Latin. There is no English substitute, really, for "He faced the problem *ad hoc,*" which is much easier than the cumbersome alternative in English ("He faced the problem with exclusive concern given to the circumstances that particularly surrounded it"). Other Latin phrases, the kind against which Fowler inveighed, have the sense of being dragged in. The reader, when he comes across them, will judge on the basis of circumstances whether he is on to a felicitous intonation communicated by the Latin and not by the English. The scholarly Mr. Ehrlich, for instance, includes in this collection *Ab asino lanam,* giving as the English meaning (which is different from the English translation), "blood from a stone." And further elucidating, "Anyone who tries to achieve the impossible is doomed to failure. Thus, an attempt to get *ab asino lanam,* literally, 'wool from an ass,' will inevitably fail." The above is for the scholar, not the practitioner of idiom.

But then why not? Mr. Ehrlich touches on the difficulty of assembling a list meagerly. Inevitably some readers would be dissatisfied. For all one knows, there is someone about who, day in and day out, denounces efforts to reason with the Soviets as ventures *ab asino lanam,* and it would ruin their life if a collection of Latin sayings were published that left out that expression. Better, then, to include *ab asino lanam,* and also the kitchen sink; which Mr. Ehrlich does, and I am very glad that he decided to do so.

Probably the principal Latin-killer this side of the Huns was Vatican II. The other day, sitting alongside a Jesuit college president, I mentioned, by way of indicating the distinctive training of English Jesuits, that my schoolmasters at Beaumont College when engaged in faculty discussions addressed each other in Latin. He replied matter-of-factly that so it had been with him and his classmates. "But now, after fifteen years, I would have a problem with relatively simple Latin."

No doubt about it, the generations of Catholic priests trained in Latin, and the seepage of Latin to parishioners, students, altar boys, will diminish, drying up the spring which for so many centuries watered a general knowledge of Latin and held out almost exclusively, after the virtual desertion of Latin from curricula in which it held, in e.g., English public schools, an absolutely patriarchal position. But it is not likely that the remaining bits and pieces will all be extirpated by the vernacular juggernaut. And even if that should be so, it would happen generations down the line. Meanwhile I know of no book to contend in usefulness with that of Mr. Ehrlich, who has given us a resourceful, voluminous, and appetizing smorgasbord.

—WFB

Memo to: WFB
From: McF [James McFadden, publisher of *National Review*]

Bill: Did you see the review in the *Albuquerque Journal* of Christo's book, *Thank You for Smoking,* by Steve Brewer? I'll pass it along, and will quote just one line from it here: "[Christopher] Buckley, son of William F. Buckley and already twice the writer his old man will ever be, previously wrote [*The White House Mess*] . . ."

Dear Jim: Yes, I did see that. Poor Brewer. Or did you hear? He committed suicide. Left a note, something about atoning for a life of misjudgments. Poor guy. Well, at least he got to read Christo's book before popping off.

> Warmest,
> BILL

Supplementary memo to: McF
From: WFB

Jim: Just as I wrote you the above, I received a translation program for my computer: English-French, French-English. To practice, I followed instructions to translate from the English to the French, and the computer ground out the following:

De: McF

Bill: Vous faisait voit la révision dans *l'Albuquerque Journal* du livre de Christo *Merci pour Fumage,* par Steve Brasseur? Je passerai il, et citera l'on juste ligne de lui ici: "[Christopher] Buckley, fils de William F. Buckley et déjà deux fois l'écrivain son vieil homme jamais soyez, a écrit précédemment [*Le Désordre de la Maison Blanc*]."

Jim: Oui, j'ai vu ce. Brasseur pauvre. Ou vous faisait entend? Il s'a se suicidé. Gauche une note, quelque chose environ expier pour une vie de [misjudgments]. Type pauvre. Eh bien, au moins il a pu lire le livre de Christo auparavant crever teint. Plus chaud, Bill

I then asked the computer to take the French, as given above, and retranslate it into English. The result is utterly captivating. Hotter, Bill . . .

Of: McF

Bill: Did you make see the revision in the *Albuquerque Newspaper* of delivers of Christo *Thank You for Smoking,* by Steve Brewer? I will pass he, and will mention him one right line of him here: "[Christopher] Buckley, son of William F. Buckley and already two times the writer sound old man is ever, has written previously [*The Disorder of the House White*]."

Jim: Yes, I saw this. Poor brewer. Or did you make hear? He has himself killed. Left a note, something about expiate for a life of [misjudgments]. Poor type. Eh well, to the minus him could read the book of Christo before croak complexion. Hotter, Bill

> —WFB   SEPTEMBER 26, 1994

Dear Mr. Buckley:

I agree with conservatives who want to make English the official language of America. But while we're at it, how about making English the official language of *National Review?*

Maybe it was a bad fortnight, but in the December 31 issue, we see *perestroika* (p. 20); *ad nauseam* (p. 26); *vere dignum et justum est* (p. 29); *ad infinitum, cogito ergo sum, Märchen, sum ergo cogito* (all on p. 31); *credo quia absurdum est* and *anima* (p. 32); *nomenklatura* and *glasnost* (p. 40); *magnum opus* (p. 41); *soi-disant* (pp. 41, 42); *de haut en bas* (p. 42); *a fortiori* (p. 44); *Kraft durch Freude, Ordnung,* and *Achtung* (p. 46); *jeu d'esprit* (p. 49); *tour de force* (p. 50); and *billets-doux* (p. 53).

Now, I consider myself reasonably well educated in languages: I have a degree in Russian with minors in German and French, and am fluent in legalese and nineteenth-century American English. But I confess that some of these phrases are Greek to me.

I'm not advocating eliminating foreign words from the lexicon. But if you cannot persuade your erudite writers to use English, could you at least provide translations for your harried readers?

Yours truly,

JOHN BRADEN

FREMONT, MICH.

Dear Mr. Braden: It is an old complaint, the use of foreign words. I would even quote to you from Fowler, except that I can't find anything under "foreign words" in my Fowler here and I am isolated in Switzerland at the moment. However, delicately used, they do bring little piquancies and with them—well, *aperçus* which, because they are extra-idiomatic, give you a fresh view of the subject. As if, in a gallery, you could rise—or descend—ten feet, and look at the picture from that fresh perspective. Don't you think? Or is mine a *fausse idée claire?* . . . By the way, knowing no German, Russian, or Greek, I often experience your frustration; but when I do, I bite my tongue on the grounds that somebody, out there, is getting pleasure. *Noblesse oblige.* Yours cordially,

—WFB   APRIL 29, 1988

Dear Bill:

As one who writes regularly on geopolitical affairs, you may be interested in the attached essay of mine re what I call "semantic black holes" in our language of politics relating to the Soviet Union. The three examples of namelessness examined in this piece, which is pending publication in a major newspaper, are:

a) the absence in our language of a proper antonym for the seductive Russian word *glasnost;*

b) the absence, also, of a proper antonym for the powerful Russian word *perestroika;* and

c) the continued namelessness of the Soviets' SDI equivalent—their "Starsky Warsky," so to speak.

If you agree that these gaps in our language pose a significant problem, please consider ways in which your own excellent Op-Ed writing might help to get *skrytnost* (the Russian word for the closedness, hiddenness, and official silence of the Leninist system), *pokazukha* (the Russian word for what is superficial, temporary, and essentially meaningless), and Soviet Star Wars (SSW) into common usage.

Your insertion of any or all of these terms into your writing would undoubtedly prompt others in journalism and in academia to follow suit with appropriate words and actions of their own.

With continued good wishes, I remain,

Sincerely,

JIM GUIRARD, JR.

WASHINGTON, D.C.

Dear Jim: See your point, but to go around talking about *skrytnost* and *pokazukha* would terminate whatever reputation I have left for writing in English. Cordially,

—WFB   JUNE 2, 1989

Dear Mr. Buckley:

I have noticed that advertisements for your magazine are quite good except for one minor omission. You forget to tell your prospective readers that they must be at least bi-lingual, but preferably multi-lingual in order to read *National Review.*

I am just an average citizen with only the average public school language requirements and I become quite dismayed when I cannot read the poems, quips, endings of articles, beginnings of articles because of the language barrier. I hope to see the Latin, African, Spanish, French, and Sanskrit kept to a minimum, or better yet, perhaps you could put out a special all-English edition.

MRS. E. F. WAKEFIELD

BALBOA ISLAND, CALIF.

FEBRUARY 26, 1963

Mrs. Wakefield's short letter to *National Review* was followed by another, much more graphic. It appears here as it appeared in the magazine, after we located a compositor who was a font of wisdom.

I agree with Mrs. E. F. Wakefield who complained in "Lecteuse Clamat" [Feb. 26] that your writers use foreign languages too much. Even the *English* of writers like Buckley and Rickenbacker is obscure enough.

J. VALENTINE BARTON
CHICAGO, ILL.

—ED.

Puis-je vous éclaircir sur une faute dans le titre d'une lettre? Tandis que "chanteur" se transforme en "chanteuse" la plupart des noms qui terminent en -teur au masculin veulent le suffixe -trice au féminin. Il est de même en ce qui concerne le mot "lecteur." Donc on devrait lire "Lectrice Clamat."*

MAURICE LEIBOWITZ

NEW HAVEN, CONN.

Lectrice, ist das nicht das, was Consolidated Edison hervorbringt?

—WFB   MARCH 26, 1963

---

* May I point out an error in the title of a letter? While *chanteur* does become *chanteuse*, most nouns that end in *-teur* in the masculine take the suffix *-trice* in the feminine. It is the same situation with the word *lecteur*. Therefore it should read "Lectrice Clamat."—Ed.

Chapter 7

On Dirty, Bawdy, Profane, Vulgar, Scatological, Etc., Words: A Short Chapter

Dear Mr. Buckley:
    If it be true that resorting to the use of foul language is the result of a poor vocabulary, what is your excuse?
                                    Sincerely yours,
                                    ELEVRA M. SCORPIO
                                    JOHNSTON, R.I.

Dear Mrs. Scorpio: Knowing just which word to use.
                                    Cordially,
                                    —WFB

Bill Buckley (to keep it colloquial) seldom uses or resorts to profanity, much less vulgarity. His usual signoff—i.e., what used to be called the "complimentary closing," is, as we have seen, "Cordially." But now and then, out of fatigue or boredom or in simple impatience, he becomes a little less than cordial. Ending one exchange, he used the simple word "Crap," thereby producing a torrent of mail. One defender, not surprisingly, cited the well-known attribution to Sir Thomas Crapper, who was knighted, one hopes, for reasons beyond his invention of the flush toilet. After many months, Bill had to call a halt to the correspondence (not reproduced here).

One column of thirty years ago (see next page) Buckley now sees as poor prophecy. But was he so far off?

PORNOGRAPHY: SHOWDOWN AHEAD

The *New York Review of Books,* which is the thing to read nowadays among the high literati, and not without reason, features in the Letters section of the current issue a discussion among its readers over whether it should have published a commonplace obscenity in a recent number. The letters are so angled by the editors—how easy it is, *mea culpa,* for an editor to do this kind of thing—as to present in a more favorable light those who professed themselves as utterly undisturbed at seeing the forbidden word in print. The principal objector presents his views in a long, plodding epistle. It has the effect of satisfying the reader whose judgment on the issue is suspended that those who oppose the obscenity speak out from the depths of Philistia. The editors' own position is of course clear: after all, they published the obscenity in the first place.

It seems to me surprising that taste has become so dead a language. It is not by any means necessary that an avant-garde should be tasteless. But the avant-garde *is* tasteless—passages in Mary McCarthy, the perennial Miss Avant Garde, are a case in point. And taste is not only a natural inclination that flows from the finer nature of man. It is usually explainable in rational terms.

Take the use of the controversial word. Ten years ago Professor John P. Roche (since become head of the Americans for Democratic Action) wrote a telling review of the incumbent lubricity of Norman Mailer and pointed out that the excuse that Realism is only achieved by literal transcriptions of the way people talk is for artistic reasons untrue. In barracks talk, obscenity is so commonplace as to be altogether unremarkable, no more noticeable than the act of breathing. In literature, the convention being against certain obscenities, the appearance of them unbalances the situation the author means to describe. This criticism would, on reflection, appear to be so self-evident as to cause special concern that the editors of a highbrow journal, engaged after all in tastemaking, should appear to be if not ignorant of it, at least unconvinced by it. Moreover, in the disputed case they had not even the excuse of transcribing a colloquy that took place in the men's room. The reviewer simply chose to use the word for his own purpose: it came, explicitly, from his own mouth.

The episode suggests the collision course that has been charted between American society and its intellectual class. The old Comstockian code had to go—no literary convention is defensible that would exclude the circulation of the works of James Joyce. But the liberal intellectuals took their victory in the famous case of *Ulysses* and ran with it—with no idea whatever of any goal line. They are still running with it, having defended such indefensibles as *Candy* and lesser-known works of pornography. "The controversy over obscene literature," the *Wall Street Journal* now observes, "which has raged periodically in this country for about 100 years, seems to be getting hotter than ever." The *Journal* cites various problems that lie before the Supreme Court. The pity is that such problems should end up in the hands of courts of law. As one might expect, the Supreme Court has in effect thrown up its hands in helplessness. On the one hand it is pressured by free speech fundamentalists who maintain that the First Amendment gives a man the right to merchandise his obscenities even as Galileo should have had the right to merchandise his understanding of the order of the universe. On the other hand, practical sense recognizes that a society has the moral right and the intellectual resources to distinguish between the right of dissent and the right to pander to a low voluptuousness. The Supreme Court, besotted by ideology, tends to acquiesce to the former pressures. But the pressure on the other end is mounting for a general showdown. The licentious use of privilege, whether by the demagogue or by the editors of a highbrow magazine, undermines the glory of freedom, and strengthens the hand of those lurking opportunists who are always looking to strengthen the case against it.

—WFB   MARCH 13, 1965

Dear Mr. Buckley: How do you square your "goddams" with your Catholicism? Are you *really* blaspheming (which I tend to doubt), or is there some distinction between "goddam" (*NR*) and "God damn" with which I'm not familiar? If so, I'd be interested to know how one makes this distinction in the *spoken* word; also, to have your definition and understanding of "goddams," not in *my* dictionary.

ANN JONES

NEW YORK HILTON HOTEL

Dear Miss Jones: No, I am not really blaspheming, or in any case, do not mean to be blaspheming, blaspheming being one of those things I am against. "Goddam" is nowadays a simple expletive, an intensifier. It is that by cultural usage. In the most cloistered convent in Catholic Spain, you will hear from the venerable lips of an aged nun, "Jesus Mary and Joseph, I forgot my umbrella!" "I would pray hard to his Maker to save his soule notwithstanding all his God-damnes," a writer is quoted by the Oxford English Dictionary as saying in 1647, back when they were fighting religious wars. Three hundred years later, the American Heritage Dictionary of the English Language lists "God damn" and "goddam" as a profane [i.e., a-religious] oath, once a strong one involving God's curse, now a general exclamation . . . used as an intensive."

—WFB   NOVEMBER 18, 1969

Dear Mr. Buckley: Regarding your polemics on profanity [Nov. 18] I am somewhat comforted to know that you "do not mean to be blaspheming" when you employ the "expletive" God-dam. Further comfort may be derived from Thayer's Greek-English lexicon of the New Testament which ascribes blasphemy to those who by contemptuous speech *intentionally* come short of the reverence due to God or sacred things. Here the comfort ends giving place to a godly concern. For the Word of God which I equate with the Scriptures of the Old and New Testament specifically commands: "Thou shalt not take the name of the Lord thy God in vain" (Ex. 20:7). In the Hebrew the words "in vain" mean "to no good purpose," thus, "thou shalt not take [use] the name of the Lord thy God to no good purpose," which leads me to believe that unless you are willing to argue that your calling upon God to damn an inanimate or animate object is purposive and conscionable, you are guilty of transgressing the law of God, which is no light thing. As one who professes the faith of Roman Catholicism, I would expect you to yield more readily to the "thus saith the Lord" of Exodus 20:7 than to the culturally conditioned value of the *American Heritage Dictionary of the English Language.*

Sincerely,

(REV.) GEORGE MILADIN
Reformed Presbyterian Church
WOODLAND HILLS, CALIFORNIA

Dear Dr. Miladin: The meaning of words is established by their usage, which would suggest that blasphemy is defined by that which is intended, rather than by that which is spoken, at least in such cases as permit of ambiguity. In such cases, one should invoke the transcendent virtue: Charity shall cover the multitude of sins. IPe. 4:8.

—WFB

Despite the damage done to "some Italian guy" in the following letter from column reader Moran and to used-car salesmen in Attwood's letter preceding, the following exchange may be instructive despite the stereotypical slanders:

Dear Bill:

Here's an amusing letter I thought you might like to answer personally.

I didn't realize Nixon had kept those leftover JFK and LBJ fructs in the White House, but what can you expect from a guy who looks like a usu-car salesman?

Yours,

WILLIAM ATTWOOD

Publisher, *Newsday*

enc.

Dear Mr. Buckley:

Now really what the hell kind of word is this to use in a column directed to the average person with the average vocabulary. ["He likes being President. He likes the power, the usufructs of the Presidency . . ." *NR*, March 1.] It annoys me to run across any such ludicrous words that I'm supposed to leave my easy chair and dig out the old Funk—to find out what you are about. I realize you know what it means and probably a couple of other people on this planet like the professors of English at Oxford and a fop like Truman Capote. But I'll tell you this, to the average American "usufructs" sounds like some Italian guy telling another guy what kind of loving he enjoys. Really what a stupid word usage—sometimes you are just too much. Regards anyway.

ROBERT MORAN

WANTAGH, NEW YORK

Dear Mr. Moran:

What then would you do to the nursery rhyme,

> *Could eternal life afford*
> *That tyranny should thus deduct*
> *From this fair land*
> *. . . A year of the sweet usufruct?*

—WFB   MARCH 29, 1974

Dear Mr. Buckley:

Could I ask your view on something that has been bothering me for several years?

Why were Clark Gable, Gary Cooper, John Wayne, Spencer Tracy, Jimmy Stewart, and all of my other movie idols able to make great classic films without once uttering the "F" word on screen?

Several weeks ago I attended a cinema and the "word" was repeated so many times that out at the refreshment stand I absentmindedly asked for a "f—— tub of popcorn, a f—— box of Milk Duds and a f—— medium Coke" and got thrown out of the theater by the manager.

Even cute little Macaulay Culkin gets to say the "word" in his new thriller, *The Good Son,* so what was wrong when I repeated it at the concession counter? Is it realism when an actor declaims it on screen, but a vulgarity when I ask the popcorn girl to "please hold the f—— butter"? Is there some sort of double standard here?

Sincerely,

JOHN BOLAND

GODFREY, ILL.

P.S. You know Charlton Heston and Tom Selleck, so, if by any chance you also know June Allyson, would you tell her I've loved her forever?

Dear Mr. Boland: Hollywood gets away with f—— murder. . . . Sorry, I don't know Miss Allyson, but I understand how you feel about her. Cordially,

—WFB

On the Use of "Dirty" Words

I guess I was seven when I first heard the maxim that only people with a small vocabulary use "dirty" words. I am forty-seven and have just received a communication from a reader delivering that maxim as though he had invented it. The trouble with the cliché is (a) it isn't true; (b) it doesn't take into account the need to use the resources of language; and (c) the kind of people who use it are almost always engaged in irredentist ventures calculated to make "dirty" words and expressions that no longer are, and even some that never were.

The first point is easily disposed of by asking ourselves the question, Did Shakespeare have a good vocabulary? Yes; and he also used, however sparingly, profane and obscene words.

The second point raises the question of whether a certain kind of emotion is readily communicable with the use of other than certain kinds of words. Let us assume the only thing it is safe to assume about the matter, namely, that every emotion is experienced by everyone, from the darkest sinner to the most uplifted saint. The sinner, having no care at all for people's feelings, let alone for propriety abstractly considered, lets loose a profanity not only on occasions when his emotions are acutely taxed, but even when they are mildly stirred. The saint—or so I take it from their published writings—manages to exclude the profane word from his vocabulary, and does not resort to it under any circumstances. It was for the saint that the tushery was invented. "Tush! tush!" the saint will say to his tormentors, as he is eased into the cauldron of boiling oil.

Non-saints, it is my thesis, have a difficult time adopting the manners of saints; and even if they succeed most of the time in suppressing obnoxious words, they will probably not succeed all of the time. Moreover, as suggested above, they are up against a community some of whose members are always seeking to repristinate the world of language back to the point where you could not even say, "Gosh, Babe Ruth was a good baseball player," because Gosh is quite clearly a sneaky way of saying God, the use of which the purists would hold to be impermissible under any circumstances—indeed they, plus the Supreme Court, reduce the permissible use of the word to the innermost tabernacles. . . .

I had reason to reach, a while back, for a word to comment upon a line of argument I considered insufferably sanctimonious. "Crap," I wrote: And the irredentist hordes descended upon me in all their fury. I have replied to them that the word in question is defined in a current dictionary in several ways. That among these are meaning 2: "nonsense; drivel: *Man, don't hand me that crap.* 3. a lie; an exaggeration: *Bah, you don't believe that crap, do you?*" Notwithstanding that the word has these clearly nonscatalogical uses, there is an Anglo-Saxon earthiness to it which performs for the writer a function altogether different from such a retort as, say, "Flapdoodle."

There are those of us who feel very strongly that the cheapest and most indefensible way to give offense is to direct obscenities wantonly, and within the earshot of those who seek protection from that kind of thing. There will always be a certain healthy tension between Billingsgate and the convent, but in the interest of the language, neither side should win the war completely. Better a stalemate, with a DMZ that changes its bed meanderingly, like the Mississippi River.

—WFB   APRIL 14, 1973

Professor (emeritus) Thomas Bergin
Department of Romance Languages
Yale University
New Haven, Conn.

Dear Tom:
    The enclosed letter challenges my scholarship in a most sensitive way. Would you kindly read, and comment?

Dear Mr. Buckley:
    Commenting on the shocking behavior of Dutch Catholics during the Pope's recent visit to the Low Countries, you tried to explain "a term unknown to most nice people," namely "the *fico.*"
    Unfortunately, you did not succeed very well.
    First, the term is not "*fico*" ("*il fico*" being the fig in Italian) but "*fica*" (Italian vulgar term for vulva), and second, it does not mean to "keep all your fingers lowered and raise the middle finger erect," but it consists in thrusting the thumb between two of the closed fingers.
    Surely you remember that, in Canto XXV of *The Inferno,* Vanni Fucci "*le mani alzo' con ambedue le fiche . . .*" (which in the Binyon translation reads, "Raising his hands with both figs on high . . ."). In addition, Villani reported that on a high tower in Carmignano, destroyed by the Florentines in 1228, there were two marmoreal arms making "*le fiche*" toward Florence. "*Le fiche*" is, of course, the plural of "*la fica*" and not of "*il fico.*"
    It would appear that you are not very conversant with terms "unknown to most nice people." You must shape up. The times require it.
                                    Sincerely yours,
                                    PLINIO PRIORESCHI
                                    OMAHA, NEB.

Dear Bill: Mr. Prioreschi has indeed got it right . . . However, I would not urge you to "shape up." Stay as sweet as you are . . .

> *A scholar I knew in Woonsocket*
> *Would for lunch put into his pocket*
> *Tubes of library paste—*
> *It's not everyone's taste,*
> *But till you have tried it don't knock it.*
> *Saluti affettuosi,*
> TOM

Dear Mr. Buckley:

Abolitionists are indeed "hoist by their own petard" ["Notes & Asides," Dec. 17] if the word is used in its seventeenth-century sense: being caught in a trap by a trick of their own contrivance. Applied originally to cheating at cards, or rolling loaded dice, the phrase found favor with dramatists of that era to account for all manner of impudicity. A pox on the French meaning of the term!

> Sincerely,
> KENNETH ROSS
> LOS ANGELES, CALIF.

Dear Mr. Buckley:

. . . The word [*petard*] does basically denote breaking wind in French. Note the similarity in sound to our own vulgarism. Because of this, however, it was also the slang term used by French siege engineers for an improvised black-powder charge, usually on wheels, that could be advanced up to a gate or door to blow it in. We all know how unstable the ignition of such demolitions can be, and not infrequently the sappers would still be messing with the device when it went off, thus being "hoist by their own petard."

It is the curiously apt double entendre that entertains us here. When a man was thus truly "hoist," the occasion could be likened to his drawing unwelcome attention to himself by the unexpected blast of his own exhaust gases—figuratively so, as in Shakespeare.

> Cordially,
> JEFF COOPER
> PAULDEN, ARIZ.

Dear Mr. Buckley:

If recollection from a military-history course thirty-plus years ago serves me well, wasn't a petard a bomb for breaching *mounted on the end of a pole,* which is what differentiated it from a grenade? The pole facilitated placement of the explosive against a wall above the foundation, or against the hinges or bolt of a gate. This all dates back to the seventeenth or eighteenth century and the days of primitive black powder and fuses lit with a tinder or match.

Webster notes the correct usage of "hoist by (or with) one's own petard" but perhaps should add sufficient detail to its definition of the term so that the expression makes sense. The means of hoisting has to be the pole. Being hoist by, with, or on the point of one's own petard would at the very least have an element of surprise, suspense, and contemplation that gives the expression its commonly understood meaning. One could not be hoist with one's own grenade absent some other mechanical agent (a rope and a tree limb?) and, probably, the meddling of a cumbersome judiciary, which is to suggest the procedure would take forever if it ever happened and may explain why we stick with petards in verbal jousts.

> Best regards,
> MARIO E. DE SOLENNI
> CRESCENT CITY, CALIF.

Dear Bill:

The expression "hoist with his own petard" is used by *NR* with sufficient frequency as to approach triteness. Why the hell "hoist," a perfectly useful verb never meant to connote injury?

> Sincerely,
> VICTOR R. MATOUS
> SEATTLE, WASH.

Dear Messrs. Ross, Cooper, and de Solenni: Many thanks for the clarification. I shall feel free, henceforward, to use the phrase with with, or with by.

> —WFB

Dear Vic: Aren't you confusing this with heist? And there is certainly an injury to the victim there, unless he was heisted by his own petard. Cordially,

> —WFB   —JULY 29, 1991

Chapter 8

The Spoken Word: Speech, Students, Diction, Politicians

Words. Many of us in this room [the occasion was *National Review*'s twenty-fifth anniversary] live off them, if not by them. They are useful, dangerous, salvific. "If any man offend not in word," St. James tells us, "the same is perfect man, and able also to bridle the whole body. Behold, we put bits in the horses' mouths, that they may obey us; and we turn about their whole body. Behold also the ships, which though they be so great, and are driven of fierce winds, yet are they turned about with a very small helm, whithersoever the governor listeth. Even so the tongue is a little member, and boasteth great things. Behold, how great a matter a little fire kindleth!"

—WFB   DECEMBER 31, 1980

William F. Buckley, Jr., gives many speeches and formal lectures every year. A lecture by Buckley is never a crowd-pleasing piece out of the old school of Hollow Oratory, attempting to conjure up emotion while causing reason to disappear, though he can on certain occasions be touching. He always pays the audience the ultimate tribute of a prepared talk of substance and style.

Those who think Buckley's distinctive accent an affectation are unaware that Buckley spoke no English until he was seven. Spanish was his first language and French his second. He was schooled in France and England before starting school in the United States. His father, whose business was in Mexico, was a stickler not only about written language but about elocution. (See the first essay in this chapter.)

Given the reasons why he came late to English, Bill could be thought of as a passionate convert to his mother tongue. Coincidences: I am struck by his deep feeling for the uses of English and with that his interest in

Conrad (also a sailor), Brodsky (also an anti-Communist), Nabokov (a friend), and Borges (an idol). The thought of these very different but precise writers could lead to a perspective suggesting that a late start—and/or English as a *second* language—can lead to a high regard for it and in some cases a virtuoso result.

What Did You Say?

I recently spent the better part of a day with a college student who had much on his mind to tell me. I in turn was much interested in what he had to say. But after an hour or so I gave up. It wasn't that his thinking was diffuse, or his sentences badly organized. It was simply that you couldn't understand the words. When they reached your ear they sounded as faint as though they had been forced through the wall of a soundproofed room, and as garbled as though they had been fed through one of those scrambling devices of the Signal Corps.

"Somi iggi prufes tometugo seem thaffernun."

"What was that?"

(*Trying hard*) "So mi IGgi prufes tometugo seem THAaf fernun."

"Sorry, I didn't quite get it."

(*Impatiently*): "So MY ENGLISH PROFESSOR TOLD ME TO GO SEE HIM THAT AFTERNOON." And on with the story. By which time, let us face it, the narrative had become a little constipated, and soon I gave up. My responses became feigned, and I was reduced to harmonizing the expression on my face with the inflection of his rhetoric. It had become not a dialogue but a soliloquy, and the conversation dribbled off.

I remarked on the event later to a friend who works regularly with boys and girls of college age. "Don't you understand?" he said. "*Nobody* at college today opens his mouth to speak. They all mumble. For one thing, they think it's chic. For another, they haven't got very much to say. That's the *real* reason why they are called the Silent Generation. Because nobody has the slightest idea what they are saying when they *do* speak, so they assume they are saying nothing."

It isn't a purely contemporary problem. Two generations ago Professor William Strunk, Jr., of Cornell was advising his student E. B. White to speak clearly—and to speak even more clearly if you did *not* know what you were saying. "He felt it was worse to be irresolute," White reminisces in his introduction to *The Elements of Style*, "than to be wrong. . . . Why compound ignorance with inaudibility?"

I remember when I was growing up, sitting around the dining room table with my brothers and sisters making those animal sounds which are understood only by children of the same age, who communicate primarily through onomatopoeia. One day my father announced after what must have been a singularly trying dinner that exactly four years had gone by since he had been able to understand a *single* word uttered by any one of his ten children, and that the indicated solution was to send us *all* to England—where they *respect* the English language and teach you to OPEN YOUR MOUTHS. We put this down as one of Father's periodic aberrations until six weeks later the entire younger half of the family found itself on an ocean liner headed for English boarding schools.

Mumbling was a lifelong complaint by my father, and he demanded of his children, but never got, unconditional surrender. He once wrote to the headmistress of the Ethel Walker School: "I have intended for some time to write or speak to you about Maureen's speech. She does not speak distinctly and has a tendency, in beginning a sentence, to utter any number of words almost simultaneously. Anything the school can do to improve this condition [the school did not do very much] would be greatly appreciated by us. I have always had a feeling [here Father was really laying it on, for the benefit of his children, all of whom got copies] that there was some physical obstruction that caused this, but doctors say there is not."

Frustrated by the advent of World War II and the necessity of recalling his children from England before they had learned to OPEN THEIR MOUTHS, my father hired an elocution teacher and scheduled two hours of classes every afternoon. She greeted her surly students at the beginning of the initial class with the announcement that her elocution was so precise, and her breathing technique so highly developed, that anyone sitting in the top row of the balcony at Carnegie Hall could easily hear her softest whisper uttered onstage. Like a trained chorus we replied—sitting a few feet away—"What did you say? Speak up!" WE DID NOT GET ON. But after a while, I guess we started to OPEN OUR MOUTHS. (There are those who say we have never since shut them.)

No doubt about it, it is a widespread malady—like a bad hand, only worse, because we cannot carry around with us a little machine that will do for our voices what a typewriter does for our penmanship. The malady is one part laziness, one part a perverted shyness. Perverted because its inarticulated premise is that it is less obtrusive socially to speak your thoughts so as to require the person whom you are addressing to ask you twice or three times what it was you said. A palpable irrationality. If you have to ask someone three times what he said and when you finally decipher it you learn he has just announced that the quality of mercy is not strained, or that he is suffering the slings and arrows of outrageous fortune, you have a glow of pleasure from the reward of a hardy investigation. So let the Shakespeares among us mumble, if they must. But if at the end of the mine shaft you are merely made privy to the intelligence that the English professor set up a meeting for that afternoon, you are entitled to resent that so humdrum a detail got buried in an elocutionary gobbledy-gook which required a pick and shovel to unearth.

I do not know what can be done about it, and don't intend to look for deep philosophical reasons why the problem is especially acute now. . . . I nevertheless suggest the problem be elevated to the status of a National Concern. Meanwhile, the kindergartens should revive the little round we used to sing—or, rather, mumble:

> *Whether you softly speak*
> [crescendo] *Or whether you loudly call.*
> *Distinctly! Distinctly speak*
> *Or do not speak at all.*

WORDWISE, ZILCH

The good news is that there are people around who are trying to discover why it is that American youth, year after year, are having greater and greater difficulty in expressing themselves. There are a lot of wisecracks readily available ("they have nothing to say"), but one tires quickly of them, and then genuine worry sets in.

Professor George Miller, the distinguished psychologist at Princeton University, is studying the problem with heroic resolution, and it occurred to him and a colleague that perhaps two or three professional writers might shed light on the subject, which is how it came that on a Tuesday evening in April I found myself at dinner in a private dining room of a splendid restaurant with Tom Wicker on my left and Tom Wolfe on my right, answering questions, or—better stated—trying to answer them.

Question: Why is it that "Sam"—let us call him—scores well enough on multiple-choice verbal tests to get into Harvard but, having arrived there, it soon transpires that Sam cannot write a lucid, straightforward sentence. More properly, why now, when a generation ago the problem was less than epidemic?

Tom Wicker recalled that the most exciting event of the week when he was a boy was the arrival of the *Saturday Evening Post*, which was read from cover to cover, after which he—and everybody he knew—would re-sume the reading of books. Although Professor Miller advises that no cor-relation can be found between illiteracy and time given over to watching television during one's youth, Wicker remains skeptical—and so do I. You can't simultaneously spend four hours watching television and four hours reading good prose. Correct? Correct: but that does not explain the high literacy of many young writers whose youths in fact were spent watching television instead of reading Sir Walter Scott.

Tom Wolfe tried out a couple of ideas. The first is that learning to write requires application—about twelve years, he reckons. So that if you don't begin to write until you go to college, it isn't likely that you will learn to write competently until some years after you have left college. This generality holds a little water, but not a lot of it, because, of course, it does not account for those classmates of Sam, however few in number, who are writing very competently in their freshman year, but whose background was similar to poor Sam's.

Tom Wolfe then thought it might be worth stressing the social point. Wolfe is too fastidious to use words like "peer pressure," but that is what he meant. What would happen, he wondered out loud, if freshmen were divided in some rather ostentatious way between those who were literate and those who were not? Let us suppose, just to suppose, that those who could write lucidly were given a special card that gave them access to—whatever it is college students tend to desire access to. Some sanctuary for the privileged. Might this cause those left behind to wish to catch up? He then set out to undermine his own thesis by recalling that not long ago he had heard a program during which Dick Cavett had asked taxing questions of such professional wordsmiths as John Simon, William Safire, and Edwin Newman, all of whom were greatly disconcerted at the end when Dick Cavett suddenly asked, "Why does it matter?" Tom Wolfe permitted himself to wonder whether in fact it does matter, so long as communication is actually effected. Everybody then recalled Ike, whose verbal instructions, exhortations, and rhetoric communicated unambiguously. But if you transcribed what he said, you wouldn't know whether he had told you to invade Normandy or Brittany. We chewed on that one a bit.

I wondered whether there was a reason for the deadening of the mimetic faculty. For instance: a generation ago it was widely supposed that before long there would be a deregionalization of speech differences. Everyone would sound like Walter Cronkite. That hasn't, of course, happened: in the Deep South they still speak pre-CBS English. Another thing: Why is it that Mexican illiterates never make grammatical mistakes? The chances in America of going through a whole day without having someone say to you, "Between you and I" are, when I last checked with Lloyd's of London, very small. But no Mexican would ever confuse the objective with the subjective pronoun. Americans are supposed to be a musical people, right? We buy recordings by the hectare—all that time listening to music, but failing to develop any sense of cadence for words. How can that be?

We resolved, at the end of the evening, to put the problem right back in George Miller's lap, but we remembered to thank him for the meal, in impeccable sentences.

—WFB   APRIL 26, 1980

Dear Mr. Buckley:

Several months ago on a Saturday morning I began introducing my (then) eighteen-month-old daughter to various public figures. Prior to that time she was able to identify by name only family and friends she had met. She quickly, and first, mastered your name. Now, whenever she watches *Firing Line,* she points to you and says, "Buckey." (Please excuse her difficulty with the letter "L.") You may be interested in the company you keep. She also identifies, with much zeal, Jesus and Moses; the latter name sometimes being given mistakenly to Robert Bork. Although she will sometimes identify "Kenney" (J. F. Kennedy) for my wife, who is more liberal than I, she does not have a clue as to the identity of Roseanne Barr, Geraldo Rivera, or Oprah Winfrey. I hope her experience with the programs of the aforementioned continues to match your own.

Grace to you and peace,
RICHARD W. BOHANNON
STORRS, CONN.

Dear Mr. Bohannon: Your daughter is doing very nicely. Best you don't let her grow any older. Cordially,

—WFB

———

If Buckley is a man of a thousand speeches, he is also, despite a cherished private life, a man invited to a thousand parties and thus, to an extent, a social creature. He has had to develop exacting standards for how much socializing may precede or follow a lecture. When trapped into a party, or on the less frequent moments when he has happily risen to an occasion, he nevertheless finds himself at times, sophisticated fellow that he is, in the standard party predicament: whom to speak to and about what, and how to escape if it's your own foot you have suddenly discovered, not standing on someone else's but in your own mouth.

The dilemma has led to a splendid instance of finding the right word, one suggested by a writer friend of Buckley's, and a foreign word at that— although we could wish that finding our own *querencia* weren't so foreign to our experience.

———

PARTY POOPER

. . . There is the special problem raised by the party at which you have a social objective. There are difficulties here because it may be necessary, having spotted your mark, to move over to him or her, passing by eleven people with whom, in the normal course, you would feel obliged to dally, even if only for a moment. And then in the pursuit of your quarry you may find yourself guilty of behavior if not exactly boring, certainly boorish.

I have a memory of this. Along with my wife, I arrived at a boat party with Mrs. Dolly Schiff, whom I liked, who was among my employers (she published my syndicated column in the *New York Post,* the newspaper she then owned) and who was an important political presence in New York at a time when my brother James was its junior senator, preparing to run for reelection. Boarding the boat, Mrs. Schiff said to me, "Do you know, I have never even met your brother?" Well, said I, I shall certainly cure that tonight—I knew that my brother was among the invited guests.

Some time later, chatting with my brother on the crowded deck, I spotted at the extreme other end the imperious forehead of Dolly Schiff. I grabbed my brother and told him we must forthwith go to the other end of the deck, past the eighty-odd people sipping champagne, so that he could be introduced to Mrs. Schiff. Ignoring a dozen old friends, we reached her—at a moment when her head was slightly bent down, exchanging conversation with a petite woman whose back was to us. I charged in, "Dolly, this is my brother Jim, whom you wanted to meet. Jim, Dolly Schiff." The little woman we had interrupted turned around slowly to us and smiled.

She was our hostess, the Queen of England, but it was too late to undo the damage, so I proceeded with the introduction to Mrs. Schiff (Jim had sat next to the queen at dinner and needed no introduction to her; the rest of us had been through the receiving line). Jim said he was sorry to interrupt Mrs. Schiff, who smiled down at Her Majesty. I thought I'd break the ice by suggesting that the entire company join me in pleading with Mrs. Schiff to give me a raise. The queen reacted with a half smile and excused herself to greet another of her guests. There can be casualties of a determined mission at a party.

It is, of course, the objective of some guests to mingle with absolutely everybody at the party. I remember at the casual cocktail hour in California talking quietly at the edge of a social congregation with the president-elect of Yale University. I told him that a year earlier the outgoing president, Kingman Brewster, had been at this same affair. "The difference between King and me," Bart Giamatti said, "is that when he walks into a social gathering, his eyes fix instinctively on the center of the densest social activity and he homes right in on it, the true social animal. My own instinct is to look to the farthermost edges of the gathering and head softly in that direction. Where I am standing right now," he said, smiling.

Yes, and that raises the question of one's *querencia,* a favorite word of mine, one that I learned many years ago from Barnaby Conrad and have tirelessly used. The word describes a tiny area in the bullring, maybe fifty square feet, within which the fighting bull fancies himself entirely safe. The difficulty lies in that each bull has his own idea exactly where his *querencia* is, and it is up to the matador to divine, from a ferociously concentrated study of the bull's movements as he charges into the ring, its location; because the matador must, at peril to life and limb, stay well clear of it when executing his critical passes. The bull who finds himself close to his *querencia* and is pained or perplexed will suddenly head for it, and in doing so jerk his horns in an unpredictable direction, at the same spot the matador's groin or abdomen might find itself.

We all have, in any social situation, an undefined querencia, and we instinctively seek it out immediately upon entering the crowded room. Most usually, it is where one's spouse is—but that is a difficult sanctuary to avail yourself of because it is deemed socially backward at a party to glue yourself to your spouse. So you look elsewhere for your querencia. Generally, it is one human being, someone with whom you feel entirely comfortable, whom you can trust to greet you as if your company were the highlight of his day. You have tons to tell him, and he has tons to tell you, all of it of mutual interest. Is he . . . she . . . there? You look around.

No.

Is there an alternative querencia anywhere about?

Well, yes. Somebody told you that Algernon MacNair was going to be there. Not quite the company you most looked forward to attaching yourself to, but quite good enough to avoid the high stilt of tonight's social affair, and there is a specific point of interest. Maybe his Op-Ed piece this morning, in which he took those peculiar positions about taxation. But no. He is not there, nor is anyone else who will fill the bill in the same way.

Ah, but then the querencia can be greatly elastic. You can develop a consuming interest in the appointments of the sumptuous apartment. Every picture deserves close attention, worth at least three minutes of your time, as you look first this way at it, then that way, then examine the artist's signature. And the books! You pick up one from the fourth shelf and open it with delight transfiguring your face. How is it that this neglected volume found its place into this library? How discriminating the taste of our hostess! By the time you have examined that book, perhaps two or three others and a dozen pictures and a score of family photographs—it is time for dinner!

With some apprehension you look down at your card and wonder who will be seated on your right, who on your left; and it is at such moments, as when in a foxhole, or on a sinking boat, that you rediscover God and the need to utter a silent prayer.

———

But enough of niceties. To politics, land of parties—the Grand Old one, the always threatened new Ones, to fund-raisers, and, worse, to hair-raisers, the political speech-makers, recidivist abusers of language. In this arena, more than seldom is heard a discouraging word, but very rare is the right word, the felicitous phrase, or the graceful expression of an idea, whether issuing from Right or from Left.

Buckley, with a jeweler's eye, has been examining these pearls for a long time, starting in this instance with the now-silent voice of Nelson Rockefeller, who liked to greet strangers with "Hi'ya fella!"

———

MYSTIFIER

It must be very discouraging to be a politician. Here is the governor of the most influential state of the union, running hard for the presidential nomination of his party, richer even than Bobby Kennedy, abetted by one of the two or three most expensive speechwriters in the English-speaking world, addressing the editors of just about every newspaper in America, delivering a much-heralded speech in which he managed to spend prospectively 150 billion American dollars—and you know what the headline is the next morning? In one of the nation's most liberal newspapers, devoting maybe second most linage in the country to national and world affairs? "Rockefeller Speech/Heard in Silence."

Surely Mr. Rockefeller envisioned other headlines? "Rockefeller Solves/ Problems of City," might have been one. Or, "Rockefeller Magnetism/ Wows Editors" would have been satisfactory. Or even, "Rockefeller Speech/Brings GOP Raves." But the reporter (David Broder, one of the nation's best) was as uninspired as the general audience, as uninterested in what Mr. Rockefeller ended up saying as the editors who heard him. A total of two sentences from the massive speech was reproduced in the morning paper—way off, toward the end of the first-page story which began: "Governor Nelson A. Rockefeller of New York made his long-heralded debut as a 'non-candidate' yesterday, delivering a thirty-minute speech on urban problems, uninterrupted by applause, to the luncheon meeting of the American Society of Newspaper Editors at the Shoreham Hotel."

What happened?

Well, to begin with, the speech was so heavy with rhetorical pomposity that it would have required a Saturn IV Booster to launch it. Would you like a taste?—"Our time of testing now follows—like a twin heritage of challenge—from both these earlier ages [Lincoln's and Roosevelt's]. The signs of peril—and the chances for leadership—rise as high on both fronts: from within—and from without—our nation. For we are not only struggling to build peace in the world. We are also striving to live at peace with ourselves."

If you believe that I selected the single worst passage, I give you the peroration which, I have a paralyzing suspicion, somebody at Rockefeller's shop actually thought was eloquent . . .

"I believe deeply in such a new government, such a new leadership, and such a new America.

"We as a people, have—right now—a choice to make.

"We must choose between new division or new dedication.

"We can live together as bullies—or as brothers.

"We can practice retribution or reconciliation.

"We can choose a life of the jungle, or a life of justice.

"We cannot have both.

"We cannot live for long with parts and pieces of both.

"We must choose."

We must cut the crap.

Really, we must. And it is an objective indication that such emptinesses are boring that they bored the audience, and bored the reporters, and permanently traumatized the muses. "The audience reaction," says the account in the *Washington Post,* "was noted with concern by some Rockefeller for President sponsors in the room. One of them said afterwards, 'I hope this convinces Emmet Hughes [the Rockefeller adviser and writer whose stylistic touches were evident in the text] that it will take more than the power of *his* words to nominate Rockefeller."

A pity, really. Because Mr. Rockefeller is a very able man. His delivery is first-rate. He has great facility for extempore talk and his ideas, if one excavates them from all that lard, are worth pondering. For instance, the recognition that the private sector is five times more resourceful than the public sector, and that if the cities are to be saved it will have to be largely by private enterprise. For instance, his observation that we are spending five times as much money subsidizing our rich farms as our poor cities. But it takes men of archaeological passion to find Mr. Rockefeller's ideas in Mr. Rockefeller's current prose. Next time he should furnish his audience with a trot.

—WFB   APRIL 23, 1968

THE SIGHTS AND THE SMELLS (OF A POLITICAL CONVENTION)

KANSAS CITY.—What kind of a show is it? A few observations:

After a couple of days, one got the impression that to be a member of the Mississippi delegation is a profession. It is one that requires political skills, high physical stamina, and a theological flair. "What did granddaddy do, Mommy?" "He was a member of the Mississippi delegation" would be an appropriate response. . . .

The level of oratory has not been uniformly high. Howard Baker was very good, though he knoweth not the virtue of brevity. Speaking to that huge auditorium requires that the speaker do a good bit of what Mencken once called "plain hollering." The only way you can get a political convention actually to stop and listen to what you are saying is either to intimate in advance that you are going to do something very dramatic (say, defy the Mississippi delegation); that, or summon the eloquence of a very great speaker. This does not mean that you need to say anything—Barbara Jordan subdued Madison Square Garden as totally as Bob Dylan in concert ever did, and said even less.

Once you have the audience listening to you, your narrative must roll, and you must at all costs avoid telegraphing the huge expanses of wisdom you have left to deliver. Do not, after thirty-five minutes, say such a thing as: "We come now to the field of foreign policy . . ." Those who view these speeches over television should close their eyes if they mean to listen, because inevitably the television director will distract you—by flashing his camera on a ninety-seven-year-old lady with a Carmen Miranda Reagan hat, swigging from a bottle of hooch.

We must be grateful that Brutus delivered his oration away from the television cameras, otherwise at the moment the crowd was finally stirred to action, the cameraman would be showing an urchin scribbling on the wall, *Kilroy hic erat.*

John Connally made the mistake of overadvertising his oration. There is a danger that attaches to a press announcement along the lines of, "At 8:35 P.M., on all networks, the Honorable John Connally will deliver the Gettysburg Address." He is a very eloquent man, but makes the mistake of screwing up his face in a contortion of lapidary concern for the republic at moments that suit less the requirements of the text than the rhythms of the paragraph. He must not look equally gloomy in anticipation of a nuclear war and a rise of one penny in the price of a gallon of gasoline.

Nelson Rockefeller's enemies will no doubt conclude that his speech—which was really quite quite awful—was intended to subvert the ambitions of the Republican Party, now that [as retiring Vice-President] he will not have an official role within it. I don't really believe that, disinclined as

I am to the conspiracy view of history. But I have to confess I can't think of a plausible reason for someone to say about his own unsuccessful pursuit of the presidency that the reason for it was, "Somehow I could never get to the church on time . . ."

—WFB   AUGUST 21, 1976

Few occasions summon the full oratorical resources of William F. Buckley more than the anniversary dinners held to celebrate the continued existence of his magazine. Here is the conclusion of one such speech, as the festive, glittering evening wore down. . . .

. . . Still, the campfires continue to burn, and every now and then you hear the chorus singing—the old songs, free of the tormented, tormenting introspections of the new idiom; ignorant altogether of the litany of reasons why we should hate our own country; axiomatic in their demand for human freedom; and the heart stirs, and the blood begins to run, and each one of us in his own way continues the effort. Those who doubt that the spiritual resources are left have only to read a speech—almost any speech—by Patrick Moynihan in the United Nations. Those who doubt that the analytical resources are left need only read any issue of *National Review*, or of *The Public Interest*. Viewed from the right angle, we suddenly see that: Communism is theoretically and empirically discredited. That all over the world enslaved people continue to dream about freedom. That inroads against poverty are successful in almost exact correspondence to the vitality of the private sector. And—most significant—that there are no signs at all that God is dead; He appears to have survived even Vatican II. "I see it as one of the greatest ironies of this ironical time," Malcolm Muggeridge recently wrote, "that the Christian message should be withdrawn for consideration just when it is most desperately needed to save men's reason, if not their souls. It is as though a Salvation Army band, valiantly and patiently waiting through the long years for judgment day, should, when it comes at last, and the heavens do veritably begin to unfold like a scroll, throw away their instruments and flee in terror."

We have stood together for one-tenth of the life span of this Republic, and we must resolve to stand with it, and its ideals, forever.

DECEMBER 5, 1975

And what follows is part of the author's speech on the occasion of *National Review*'s thirty-fifth anniversary, given at a dinner at the Waldorf-

Astoria in New York on October 5, 1990, when he made a surprise announcement about his future with his beloved magazine.

———

There are too many men and women to whom I am indebted to make it feasible to enumerate them. So I won't even mention my sister Priscilla, nor pause to say that without her my thirty-five years at *National Review* would have been intolerable. . . .

I suppose that if there is a single occasion in which a professional will be indulged for speaking personally, it is the occasion when he retires. (If that isn't the case, then *National Review* will establish yet another precedent.) When my father first saw the offering circular with which in 1954 I traveled about the country attempting to induce American capitalists to invest in our prospective journal, my father spotted only one sentence that disturbed him. I wrote in the offering circular that I pledged to devote ten years of my life to *National Review*. My father, who was very . . . formal about personal commitments, told me he thought this exorbitant: "Ten years is simply too long," he said. "Suppose you decide you want to do something else with your life?"

Well, the warning became moot, because there never was anything else around seriously to tempt me. For the fun of it I divulge that in 1970 I was approached by a very small delegation of what one is trained to call "serious people" whose proposal was that I should run for governor of New York, that I should expect to win the election, and position myself to run for the presidency. I was nicely situated to say two things, the first that anyone who had run for mayor of New York getting only 13 percent of the vote shouldn't be too confident about winning an electoral majority in a general election. And I finally silenced my friends by adding that I didn't see how I could make the time to run for governor, given my obligations to *National Review*. My friends couldn't understand my priorities. But I was very content with these priorities.

Oh yes, I won't cavil on that point. The magazine has been everything the speakers tonight have so kindly said it was—is. It is preposterous to suppose that this is so because of my chancellorship. How gifted do you need to be to publish Whittaker Chambers and Russell Kirk, James Burnham and Keith Mano? But yes, the journal needed to function. Somehow the staff and the writers had to be paid—if an editorial note is reserved for me in the encyclopedias, it will appear under the heading ALCHEMY. But the deficits were met, mostly, by our readers; by you. And, yes, we did as much as anybody with the exception of—himself—to shepherd into the White House the man I am confident will emerge as the principal political figure of this century. And he will be cherished, in the nursery tales told in future generations to young children, as the American President who showed the same innocent audacity as the little boy who insisted that the emperor wasn't wearing any clothes at all, when Ronald Reagan said, at a critical moment in Western history, about the Union of Soviet Socialist Republics that it was an evil empire. It is my judgment that those words acted as a resolution to the three frantic volumes of Solzhenitsyn. *The Gulag Archipelago* told us everything we needed to know about the pathology of Soviet communism. We were missing only the galvanizing summation; and we got it, in the Mosaic code: and I think that the countdown for communism began then.

I owe you all an account of my exercise of my fiduciary authority in handling the journal you have sustained. I am, speaking now the language of corporate America, its owner: The stock of *National Review,* which commercially is about as valuable as Confederate bonds, is mine. My resignation as chief executive officer will give me the opportunity to receive the magazine in the mail, as you do, with no specific knowledge of what I'll encounter between its covers, save for my own continuing editorial contributions in my new role as editor-at-large. It is my plan, at some point in the future, to deed my stock to a successor. The highest tribute I can pay to Wick Allison and to John O'Sullivan is that I am turning over to their management a property to the health and hygiene of which I have devoted practically the whole of my adult lifetime. It is inconceivable to me, having watched them in operation for over a year, that I have made a mistake. Still, I elect not to risk being designated at some point in the future as another King Lear. While I am still intact, I'll be there to judge the continuing performance of *National Review,* conscious that I owe to all the readers who have sustained it an obligation that cannot be lightly discharged, and won't be.

Since you were so kind as to ask about my personal plans, I intend to continue to be active on other fronts. Early this week I performed a harpsichord concerto with the North Carolina Symphony, and resolved, with the full acquiescence, I am certain, of the orchestra and the audience, that I will not devote my remaining years to performing on the keyboard. One month from today I will set out, with my companions, on a small sailboat from Lisbon, headed toward Barbados via Madeira, the Canaries, and Cape Verde, forty-four hundred miles of decompression at sea, the cradle of God; needless to say, a book will come out of this. But on reaching the Caribbean, unlike the Flying Dutchman I will jump ship, to get on with other work. I have not scheduled the discontinuation of my column, or of *Firing Line,* or of public speaking, or of book writing. But these activities by their nature terminate whenever the Reaper moves his supernatural, or for that matter, democratic hand, whereas *National Review,* I like to think, will be here, enlivening right reason, for as long as there is anything left in America to celebrate.

And of course, it will always crowd my own memory. Two thousand seven hundred and fifty fortnightly issues of *National Review.* The hour is late, nearing five in the afternoon of press day, and the printer's messenger is already there waiting, so we move into the boardroom, the only room at *National Review* in which more than four people can fit, and Priscilla [Buckley] reads out the editorial lengths, and I mark them down on the paleolithic calculator I bought in Switzerland in 1955, and Linda [Bridges] checks to see that I have got the right count. We have 1,259 lines of editorial copy but space for only 718. We absolutely need to run something on the subject of Judge Souter's testimony, but I see we can't afford the 78-line editorial I processed earlier in the day. "Rick [Brookhiser], would you shorten this?"

"To what?" he asks, as a tailor might ask what the new waistline is to be.

The copy is spread about the room, occupying every level surface, and you walk about, counterclockwise, turning face down any editorial that can wait a fortnight to appear, and subtracting on your little calculator its line count from the rogue total. I need to cut 541 lines. First your eyes pass by the editorials and paragraphs that deal with domestic issues, Priscilla having grouped them together; then those that deal with foreign countries or foreign policy; then the offbeat material. You look down at the calculator, having made the complete circle of the room, returning to where you began: it shows 854 lines, and so you start the second counterclockwise circuit, the killer instinct necessarily aroused: You have *got* to cut another 136 lines. "Jeff, shrink this one by ten lines, okay?" . . . The editors always say okay when a deadline looms.

So it is done, down to line length. And then you ask yourself: *Which paragraph is just right for the lead?* The rule: It has to be funny, directly or obliquely topical, engaging. I remember one from years and years ago: "The attempted assassination of Sukarno last week had all the earmarks of a CIA operation. Everyone in the room was killed except Sukarno."

And, during the days when we feuded almost full-time, "Gerald Johnson of *The New Republic* wonders what a football would think about football if a football could think. Very interesting, but not as interesting as, What would a *New Republic* reader think of *The New Republic* if a *New Republic* reader could think?" Last week there wasn't anything absolutely, obviously preeminent, but ever since it came up on the dumbwaiter from Tim Wheeler's fortnightly package, this one about colors burrowed in the mind. . . . Time is very short now. Okay, we'll lead with this. It reads,

Iraq and the budget are as nothing compared to the firestorm following the retirement of maize, raw umber, lemon yellow, blue grey, violet blue, green blue, orange red, and orange yellow, and their replacement by vivid tangerine, wild strawberry, fuchsia, teal blue, cerulean, royal purple, jungle green, and dandelion, by the makers of Crayola crayons.

Nice, no? Orson Bean used to say that the most beautiful word combinations in the language were Yucca Flats and Fernando Lamas; though Whittaker Chambers, along with Gertrude Stein, preferred *Toasted Suzie is my ice cream.*

And then you need the bottom eye-catcher, the end paragraph, traditionally very offbeat, usually nonpolitical but not necessarily. You knew which would be the end paragraph the moment you laid eyes on it, early in the day, another by Tim, whose reserves of mischief are reliable, and now you find it and designate it as such. It reads:

> This week's invention is a sort of miniaturized bug zapper, battery-powered, to be inserted in the cervix for contraception and, the inventor hopes, prophylaxis.
>
> If you aren't shocked by this, you will be.

The editorials are now in order, and the line count is confirmed.

Another issue of *National Review* has gone to bed; and you acknowledge, the thought has ever so slowly distilled in your mind, that the time comes for us all to go to bed, and I judge that mine has come, and I leave owing to my staff, my colleagues—my successors—my friends, my muses, my God, an unrequitable debt for having given me so much, for so long. Good night, and thanks.

———

Perhaps no invitation summons up the best in any speaker more than one held in honor of, or in the spirit of, Winston Churchill. Bill's call from the International Churchill Society came, and he complied on October 27, 1995, with a speech that combines personal recall with an analysis of the precise meaning of certain Churchillian utterances, and no attempt to imitate the inimitable. His American eloquence is a fitting salute to a grand master.

———

Ladies and gentlemen:

When I was a boy I came upon the line, *Let us now praise famous men.* In succeeding decades I found myself running its implications through my mind. The evolution of my thinking is of possible interest to you under the auspices of this celebration.

Early on I found myself wondering why exactly it was thought appropriate, let alone necessary, to praise famous men. If such men as were to be praised were already famous, as the biblical injunction presupposes, then would they not disdain as either redundant, or immodest, the solicitation of more praise than they had already? It seemed, in that perspective, just a little *infra dig* to enjoin such praise.

Some time later I bumped into the melancholy conclusion of the historian who wrote that "great men are not often good men." That finding curdled in the memory. Does it require of a famous man to be praised, that he be praiseworthy? And if he is not a good man, merely a successful man who became famous by inventing the wheel or invading Russia or writing *War and Peace,* should not the praise be confined to bringing to the attention of those who are behind in the matter that which the person being praised actually did that merits more vociferous admiration? Or is that obvious? Jack the Ripper was famous, but our praise of him, if such it is to be called, does not focus on his attainments.

And then much later, much, much later, on reading recently a review of the life of Abraham Lincoln justified, or so it seemed, primarily by the author's diligence in bringing to light episodes in Lincoln's life and aspects of his character that serve to diminish the myth, I found myself wondering at what point is it in the interest of civilization to devise a line between research designed to satisfy the curiosity and research bent upon defacement, this last often an instinct of the egalitarian, who really thinks that all men should be equally famous, in the absence of which all men should be equally infamous. As in, If everybody can't be rich, then everybody should be poor. I am at this stage in the development of my thought on that passage from Ecclesiastes more and more inclined to believe that the point comes when it is prudent, unless one's profession is in historical clinics, to accept that which was legendary as legend; that which was mythogenic, as myth—fortifying myth, ennobling myth.

When I was a junior in college and editor of the student newspaper I received an invitation to attend the speech at the Massachusetts Institute of Technology to be given by Winston Churchill, commemorating a mid-century celebration. I drove with a fellow editor to Cambridge and awaited the appearance of the great man with high expectation, made higher by advance notice given by Mr. Churchill to the press, to the effect that the speech he would give at the M.I.T. celebration would be an important historical statement.

Mr. Churchill's preceding visit to the United States had been to Fulton, Missouri, and we wondered whether he would go further in characterizing the Soviet Union and its leader. We watched him with fascination come to the chair—he was shorter than I had envisioned, less rotund. He guided a cane with his right hand, but even so needed help to rise to the lectern. The hypnotizing voice boomed in, and our attention was at tiptoe.

I remember rushing back to New Haven with some trepidation, hoping that the story I would write might feature something Winston Churchill had said that was different from what the *New York Times* and the Associated Press and the United Press agreed was the major news story. In fact Mr. Churchill hadn't said anything different from what he had said before, which was that the discovery of the atom bomb, as we then called it, might prove to be the greatest humanitarian invention in history, making war so awful that wars would never again be fought. That hope did not prove prophetic, in that eighty million people have been killed in warfare since he gave it voice, but then it is true that most of them were killed in battles in which there was no general at hand with the atom bomb in his quiver.

But what mattered in 1949 was the *possession* of the bomb. When Mr. Churchill spoke it was exclusively ours, copyright Los Alamos, U.S.A.; but the pirate paid no attention and within months he would develop his own or, more exactly, succeed in transforming blueprints provided by U.S. and British spies into a nuclear bomb.

Of course the real nightmare had already come, by the time of the mid-century celebration of M.I.T., to Eastern Europe, and had only a year before spread to Czechoslovakia. Mr. Churchill was to some extent on a diplomatic rein that night, because he did not mention the name of Stalin, referring instead to "thirteen men" in the Kremlin. But the image of Stalin was clearly in his mind when he reminded his audience that the Mongol invasion of Europe, well underway seven hundred years earlier, had been interrupted by the death of Genghis Khan. His armies returned seven thousand miles to their base to await a successor, and they never returned. Might such a thing happen again? Churchill wondered.

Four years later, Stalin obliged us all by going, one hopes, to a world even worse than the one he created, assuming such exists; but it was not as when Genghis Khan left the world without a successor: Stalin's successors would keep intact the evil empire for almost forty years. The plight of the captive nations, the dismaying challenges that lay ahead, the struggles in Berlin and Korea and Vietnam, the hydrogen bomb, the Cuban crisis, all unfolded with terrible meaning for those whose statecraft had failed us.

In October of 1938, a despondent Churchill had spoken in Commons about the failed diplomacy of his colleague Neville Chamberlain. He said then, "When I think of the fair hopes of a long peace which still lay before Europe at the beginning of 1933 when Herr Hitler first obtained power, and of all the opportunities of arresting the growth of the Nazi power which have been thrown away; when I think of the immense combinations and resources which have been neglected or squandered, I cannot believe that a parallel exists in the whole course of history." Well, but of course a parallel would come again, in Mr. Churchill's lifetime, and in that parallel he was a major player, if not, alas, the critical player.

In the same speech after the Munich conference in 1938 Mr. Churchill had ruminated on British history. Only an Englishman, surely, is capable of the following commentary except in parody. "In my holiday," he said, "I thought it was a chance to study the reign of King Ethelred the Unready." (What did you study during *your* holiday, Mabel?) "The House"— Mr. Churchill was addressing Parliament—"will remember that that was a period of great misfortune, in which, from the strong position which we had gained under the descendants of King Alfred, we dove swiftly into chaos. It was the period of Danegeld and of foreign pressure. I must say that the rugged words of the Anglo-Saxon Chronicle, written a thousand years ago, seem to me apposite, at least as apposite as those quotations from Shakespeare with which we have been regaled by the last speaker from the Opposition Bench. Here is what the Anglo-Saxon Chronicle said, and I think the words apply very much to our treatment of Germany and our relations with her. 'All these calamities fell upon us because of evil counsel, because tribute was not offered to them at the right time nor yet were they resisted; but when they had done the most evil, then was peace made with them.'

"That," Mr. Churchill said, "is the wisdom of the past, for all wisdom is not new wisdom."

Seven years later, after England's and his finest hour began to tick when England denied to Herr Hitler the right to enslave Poland, Churchill prepared for the Yalta summit meeting in January 1945. He confided to his private secretary, *All the Balkans except Greece are going to be Bolshevised. And there is nothing I can do to prevent it. There is nothing I can do for poor Poland either.* To his cabinet, he reported that he was certain that he could trust Stalin. The same man whose death he so eagerly anticipated at M.I.T. five years later, in 1945 he spoke of as hoping he would live forever. "Poor Neville Chamberlain," he told Mr. Colville, "believed he could trust Hitler. He was wrong. But I don't think I'm wrong about Stalin."

His concluding experience with Stalin came just six months later, at Potsdam, at which Winston Churchill had come upon another historical force, for which he was, this time, substantially unprepared. The first week in June he had gone on BBC to alert the voters against a domestic catastrophe which he was quite certain would never overpower even a country exhausted by the exertions of so fine an hour. "My friends," he spoke, "I must tell you that a socialist policy is abhorrent in the British ideas of freedom. Although it is now put forward in the main by people who have a good grounding in the liberalism and radicalism of the early part of this century, there can be no doubt that socialism is inseparably interwoven with totalitarianism and the abject worship of the state. It is not alone that property, in all its forms, is struck at, but that liberty, in all its forms, is challenged by the fundamental concept of socialism."

But it was the fate of Winston Churchill to return to power in 1951 resolved *not* to fight the socialist encroachments of the postwar years. He, and England, were too tired, and, as with Eastern Europe and Poland, there was nothing to be done. There was no force in Europe that could move back the Soviet legions, no force in Great Britain that would reignite, until twenty-five years later, the vision Mr. Churchill displayed, speaking to the BBC microphones on June 5, 1945, since nobody else was listening.

Mr. Churchill had struggled to diminish totalitarian rule in Europe which, however, increased. He fought to save the empire, which dissolved. He fought socialism, which prevailed. He struggled to defeat Hitler, and he won. It is not, I think, the significance of that victory, mighty and glorious though it was, that causes the name of Churchill to make the blood run a little faster. He spoke diffidently about his role in the war, saying that the lion was the people of England, that he had served merely to provide the roar.

But it is the roar that we hear, when we pronounce his name. It is simply mistaken that battles are necessarily more important than the words that summon men to arms. The battle of Agincourt was long forgotten as a geopolitical event, but the words of Henry V, with Shakespeare to recall them, are imperishable in the mind, even as which side won the battle of Gettysburg will dim from the memory of men and women who will never forget the words spoken about that battle by Abraham Lincoln. The genius of Churchill was his union of affinities of the heart and of the mind. The total fusion of animal and spiritual energy:

"You ask what is our policy? I can say: It is to wage war, by sea, land and air, with all the might and with all the strength that God can give us.

"What is our aim? I can answer in one word: It is victory. It is victory, victory at all costs, victory in spite of all the terror, victory, however long and hard the road may be."

In other days, from other mouths, we would mock the suggestion that extremism in defense of liberty was no vice. Churchill collapsed the equivocators by his total subscription to his cause. "Let 'em have it," he shot back at a critic of area bombing. "Remember this. Never treat the enemy by halves." Looking back in his memoirs on the great presidential decision of August 1945, he wrote, "There was never *a moment's* discussion as to whether the atomic bomb should be used or not." That is decisiveness we correctly deplore when we have time to think about it, but he was telling his countrymen, and indirectly Americans, that any scruple, at that time of peril to the nation itself, was an indefensible and unbearable distraction. He was from time to time given to reductionism in other situations, and Churchill could express frustration in searing vernacular. Working his way through disputatious bureaucracy from separatists in New Delhi he exclaimed to his secretary, "I hate Indians." I don't doubt that the famous gleam came to his eyes when he said this, with mischievous glee—an offense, in modern convention, of genocidal magnitude.

But this was Churchill distracted from his purpose. The little warts Cromwell insisted be preserved; which warts, however, do not deface the memory of Churchill, because of the nobility of his cause and his sense of the British moment. "Hitler knows that he will have to break us in this Island or lose the war. If we can stand up to him, all Europe may be free and the life of the world may move forward into broad, sunlit uplands. But if we fail, then the whole world, including the United States, including all that we have known or cared for, will sink into the abyss of a new Dark Age made more sinister, and perhaps more protracted, by the lights of perverted science. Let us therefore brace ourselves to our duties and so bear ourselves that if the British Empire and its Commonwealth last for a thousand years, men will still say, 'This was their finest hour.' "

It is my proposition that Churchill's words were indispensable to the benediction of that hour, which we hail here tonight, as, gathered together to praise a famous man, we hail the memory of the man who spoke them.

Chapter 9

On
Style & Eloquence,
Dress and
Address

Whatever else he may be taken for, Buckley is a man of style, not all of it a model. Correspondents reproach him, among other things, for his manner of dress. Admittedly, his style in clothing is as far from elegant as his expositions are eloquent. (Speaking of the limits of language—were we?—there seems to be no surplus of synonyms for "rumpled," although "disheveled" comes to mind.) No matter: the style we are considering here is more than a matter of matching socks and color-coded shirts and ties. Perhaps no one has summed up, or served up, a deconstruction of WFB's style better than James J. Kilpatrick in *National Review* ten years ago.

———

UTTER BUTTER

James J. Kilpatrick
Right Reason, by William F. Buckley, Jr. (Doubleday, 454 pp., $19.95)

Is it a chrestomathy? A collection? An anthology? Whatever it is, this latest volume from the genial gentleman who helms this magazine is Buckley at his stylish best.

The master of revels at *National Review* sailed past his sixtieth birthday on November 24. He matches the young Cleopatra. Age cannot wither him nor custom stale his infinite variety. In this omnium-gatherum, edited splendidly by Richard Brookhiser, Buckley looks at Mexico, at Poland, at Spain. He writes about Karl Marx, Pope Paul VI, and Henry Kissinger. He concludes that style in human relations is largely a matter of timing. He offers a paean to peanut butter, as follows:

> *I know that I shall never see*
> *A poem lovely as Skippy's peanut butter.*

This he grandly describes as "a couplet." If he had composed some such rhapsody as "I know that I shall never utter / Two words to rank with peanut butter," he would have had a respectable couplet, but no matter. When Buckley attacks the language, the language had better get the hell out of the way.

Let me turn around on this business of style. I have known and corresponded with the ineffable WFB for twenty-five years and have delighted in his company; I have read twenty of his books and hundreds of his columns, and except when he instructs me in navigation I have understood most of them. Long ago I concluded that style is half of what Buckley has going for him. I am not thinking of his neckties, dummy; everyone knows that Buckley's ties are thirty years old and that he wears the two of them on alternate days. I am thinking of style totally.

Right Reason opens with an essay Buckley wrote in response to critics who attacked his book *Overdrive*. Most readers will recall that *Overdrive,* like the earlier *Cruising Speed,* was a journal of one week in his life. The book stirred up an astonishing response—a response distilled from awe and envy, but mostly from envy. *Kirkus Reviews* called the work "tedious at best, sleekly loathsome at worst." The *San Francisco Chronicle* called it overdone, overwritten, and overblown. Nora Ephron, in the *New York Times,* found parts of it "appalling." Some really mean things also were said about it.

The reaction of these green-eyed critics, if I am not mistaken, was miles removed from the reaction of thousands of persons who bought the book and found it absorbing. Buckley was writing happily and engagingly about his own lifestyle, and in the world of arts and letters this is a lifestyle that few can enjoy with equal gusto. I delighted in the book, but, as Buckley says, the major reviews were terrible.

It is a pleasure to read his response to the critics, for this is pure Bill. If your purpose is to tick someone off, this is how it should be done—stylishly, with grace and civility and an unbuttoned foil. In this same way he disposes of Henry Fairlie: "To the great relief of Great Britain, he is an expatriate." He contemplates a welcoming address by Yale's president A. Bartlett Giamatti to the freshman class of 1981: "To be lectured against the perils of the

Moral Majority on entering Yale is on the order of being lectured on the danger of bedbugs on entering a brothel." He takes on the Reverend Jesse Jackson, a "man of transient fixations." But in the thirteen pieces that Brookhiser has grouped under the heading of "Assailing," you will never see the red eye of anger or hear the coarse voice of rage. This is style.

A second group of twenty-two writings, chosen almost entirely from Buckley's syndicated columns, deals mostly with foreign affairs. In a third section we find nine essays defined as "Commenting." . . . Every one of these hundred-plus passages of English prose is written with—style.

In that observation I am not thinking so much of grace, or manners, or civility, but this time of style in writing. If you were putting Bill's stuff to music, you would score it for harpsichord and cello, two good muscular instruments that sound best only when a virtuoso plays them. The criticism is made—I have made it unavailingly, myself—that my friend employs too many hard words, unfamiliar words. . . . Such objections leave him puzzled: The words, he says, are not unfamiliar to *him.* Let others look them up. It is the Marie Antoinette school of prose composition.

What's the other half? I said that style was half of what makes Buckley's work such a constant pleasure to read. The other half is substance. All of us in our racket, the syndicated-column racket, write thumb-suckers now and then. These are the pieces that wash thinly over a topic and leave no residue of thought behind. We had nothing to say that was worth saying in the first place. Bill writes very few of these. He nearly always has something thoughtful to say, and even his throwaway pieces—such as the column he wrote when he got mad at Varig, the Brazilian airline—are thumb-suckers of a different sort. Buckley reads, listens, experiences, thinks. They say his stuff is infuriating. I find it a joy.

JANUARY 31, 1986

Questions of style inevitably take us from matters of dress to forms of address. In an age when not many people seem to know who William Jefferson Clinton is—the man competing with "Bob" Dole for the presidency—Buckley's "Just Call Me Bill" (1975) bears revisiting.

JUST CALL ME BILL

Very soon I will be fifty, a datum I do not expect will . . . revive the fireworks industry. I reflect on it only because of a personal problem of general concern I had not solved twenty years ago, the nature of which keeps changing as you grow older. It is, of course, the first-name problem.

My inclinations on the matter have always been formal. In part this was a matter of inheritance.

I heard my father, days before his death at seventy-eight, refer to his best friend and associate of forty years as "Montgomery"; who, in deference to the ten-year difference in their ages, referred to him only as "Mr. Buckley."

I grew up "mistering" people, and discovered, after I was fully grown (if indeed that has really happened), that in continuing to do so I was bucking a trend of sorts: the obsessive egalitarian familiarity which approaches a raid on one's privacy.

So on reaching thirty, I made a determined effort to resist. Even now, on the television program *Firing Line,* I refer even to those guests I know intimately as "Mr. Burnham," or "Governor Reagan," or "Senator Goldwater." (This rule I simply had to break on introducing Senator Buckley, but even then the departure from the habit was stylistically troublesome.) The effort, I thought, was worthwhile—a small gesture against the convention that requires you to refer to Professor Mortimer Applegate as "Mort" five minutes after you have met. I suppose a talk show host would have called Socrates "Soc."

I came on two difficulties. The first was the public situation in which mistering somebody was plainly misunderstood. Or, if understood at all, taken as an act of social condescension. For a couple of years I would refer, on his program, to "Mr. Carson." In due course I discovered that the audience thought I was trying to put on an act: Mr. Carson does not exist in America. Only Johnny does.

The second problem, as you grow older, lies in the creeping suspicion of people a little older than you that your use of the surname is intended to accentuate an exiguous difference in age. If you are eighteen and the other man is twenty-eight, you can, for a while, call him Mr. Jones without giving offense. But if you are forty and he is fifty and you call him Mr. Jones, he is likely to think that you are rubbing in the fact of his relative senescence.

The complement of that problem, which I fear more than anything except rattlesnakes and détente, is trying to be One of the Boys. "Just call me Bill," to the roommate of your son at college, is in my judgment an odious effort to efface a chronological interval as palpable as the wrinkles on my face and the maturity of my judgments. On the other hand, one has to struggle to avoid stuffiness: so I arrived, for a while, at the understanding that I was Mister to everyone under the age of twenty-one or thereabouts, and only then, cautiously, Bill. It is a sub-problem, how to break the habit. Here I made a sub-rule: that I would invite younger people to call me "Bill" exactly one time. If thereafter they persisted in using the surname, well that was up to them: a second, redundant gesture on my part could be interpreted as pleading with them to accept me as a biological equal.

My bias, on the whole, continued in the direction of a tendency to formality, so in the last few years I made a determined effort to overcome it, wherein I came across my most recent humiliation. Mrs. Margaret Thatcher was my guest on *Firing Line*. Rather to my surprise, the English being more naturally formal than we are, halfway through the program she suddenly referred to me, once, as "Bill." I declined to break my *Firing Line* rule, and so persisted with "Mrs. Thatcher." However, the next day when we met again at a semi-social function, I braced myself on leaving and said, "Good-bye, Margaret." And a week later, writing her a note congratulating her on her performance, I addressed it: "Dear Margaret."

Today I have from her a most pleasant reply, about this and that. But it is addressed, in her own hand (as is the British habit: only the text is typed): "Dear Mr. Buckley." Shocked, I looked at the transcript of the show—only to discover that, on the program, she was talking about a "Bill" that lay before the House of Commons.

The trauma has set me back by years, and I may even find myself addressing "Mr. Carson" next time around. I suppose, though, that at fifty, the problem becomes easier in respect of the twenty-five-year-olds. At seventy it will be easier still. Well before then, I hope to be able to address Margaret, I mean Mrs. Thatcher, as Madam Prime Minister.

—WFB   OCTOBER 28, 1975

House of Commons
London SWI

Dear Bill,
    Having just read your article in the *Washington Star* of 28th October, I have made my first New Year Resolution. From 1st January, 1976, Mr. Buckley shall be "Bill."
    I shall assume the appropriate reciprocity.

Yours sincerely,
MARGARET THATCHER

Funny, how discussions of style can swing quickly from matters of dignity and privacy to the near-scatological.

Dear Bill:
    I remember a column you wrote a while back in which you clucked about unseemly familiarity in modes of personal address. I agree with you. In fact, I'm rather standoffish myself; I've been at Dartmouth for over a

month now, and I haven't even met Jeffrey Hart. Oh, I've *seen* him, but I haven't actually met him, and when I do I'll certainly call him Mr. Hart, at least to begin with.

But I presume to call you Bill. There are several reasons. I did actually meet you once, years and years ago—you were on the lecture circuit at St. Michael's College in Winooski, Vermont (and you spoke very well). Also, I got a nice little note from you several years back, in which you signed your-self "Bill." I had responded to your annual appeal for funds to keep *NR* afloat by saying that I wished I could kick in a hundred or two but I didn't have any money (I was writing my dissertation at the time and really didn't have any money—still don't). Your reply was a gracious gesture, and it made me feel as though I knew you a little better. In fact, as an almost-charter sub-scriber to *NR* and a regular viewer of *Firing Line* I feel that over the years I have grown to know the contours of your mind excruciatingly well.

Still, I don't think I would be calling you Bill even now if it weren't for the startling familiarity with which you greet me, through your subalterns, every other week when I rush to the mailbox to pick up my copy of *NR*. What do I see?

> M BRWNOOIR OIO 7721 — 3 25 —
> ROBERT E BROWNE
> CLAREMONT ANUS
> I VALIANT WINTER ST
> CLAREMONT NH 03743

Never mind that this perfectly captures my feelings about Claremont, New Hampshire; do you think you could send future issues in a plain brown wrapper with the address on the inside? Or change it to "Arms"? Or talk to Mr. McFadden? Him I shall continue to address with decorous for-mality. Thanks, Bill.

Yours appreciatively,
ROBERT E. "BOB" BROWNE
ENGLISH DEPARTMENT
DARTMOUTH COLLEGE

Dear Bob: I checked with James McFadden, our Associate Publisher. He is awfully busy, and began by muttering something that sounded like "Up Claremont." But he was mollified, the correction will be made, and he says you can call him Jim.

Cordially,
BILL

In the two essays following, Buckley turns to the subject of eloquence, a style so rare as hardly to seem a subject any longer.

In the first, he speaks to a lament by James Reston, a newspaperman who had frequent brushes with eloquence, in the course of composing thousands of columns. That Mr. Reston seems to have been seeking examples of eloquence at the United Nations, a fabled house of talk but little of it memorable, troubles WFB. It involves the question not only of verbal felicities but of truth, and Buckley, himself a veteran of the United States Mission there, has seen both too often lacking.

In the second piece, he speaks to a little-noticed quality in those who have style, a finely tuned sense of timing,

Why No Eloquence?

James Reston, who is a very eloquent man, wonders what has happened to eloquence these days. His reference is to the performance thus far at the United Nations, where the mighty of the world have met to deplore the huge planetary budget for arms. It isn't that Reston expected that anything would come of it; nothing, really, ever does under U.N. sponsorship. But Reston bemoans the absent voices. Men like Roosevelt, and Churchill, and de Gaulle, he said, could by their eloquence affect events. Their successors—Carter, Giscard, Callaghan—speak, and all the birdies stay perched on the trees. Meanwhile the objective situation, as described, is quite awful. He recites the figures.

We are spending four hundred billion dollars per year on arms in the world, which is more than we are spending on education.

The figures rise notwithstanding the nuclear factor. One would think that with the invention of nuclear power, there would be less of a need for the conventional weapons. But of course it doesn't work that way because the success of nuclear technology has precisely the other effect: the weapon is so apocalyptic, it is necessary to rely on lesser weapons, so that the production of airplanes and tanks and machine guns and rifles continues unabated. And the poor nations are buying weapons valued at eight billion dollars per year. Symbolic of the emptiness of the big [U.N.] ritual in New York is that in the opening days, as much time was given over to discussing a border fracas in Zaire as to the problem of armaments.

One hesitates to instruct Mr. Reston, but one does so anyway. True eloquence is based on reality, even mythic reality. Prince Hal, delivering the most famous charge in the history of literature, exceeded even Knute Rockne's to the Notre Dame football team.

What would Shakespeare say about disarmament? He could make almost any cause beguiling, witty, ingenious; he could harness the language wonderfully to the uses of seduction, or ambition, or even treachery, these being great human passions. Indeed, viewed through contemporary prisms, King Harry was up to no good at Agincourt, coveting French territory on flimsy genealogical authority. Still, he stirred what then were accepted as honorable passions: to fight for king and country.

But the problem with attempting eloquence at the United Nations is that that which is affirmed by all the surrounding moral maxims is regularly and systematically flouted. The United Nations is about things like a covenant on human rights; about things like genocide; about self-rule; about the dignity of man. But [most of] the countries that dominate the United Nations have no use for these goals. This does not prevent them from praising them, which they do copiously. A speech by the ambassador from East Germany praising human liberty and democracy is as routine at the U.N. as a water fountain in Central Park.

But how then does a statesman go about appealing to such an assembly for world disarmament? Nations take up arms for reasons good and bad: to defend their liberties—and to wrest from others their liberties. We have not fought an imperialist war in the lifetime of all but American octogenarians. But it was only ten years ago that the Russians used their vast army to douse a flicker of liberalism in Czechoslovakia. The size of our hundred-billion-dollar-per-year budget is a function of the budget of the Soviet Union. If the communists disarmed, we could disarm; if the communists armed purely for the sake of self-protection, even then we could disarm. But the reality is that two great superpowers, the Chinese and the Russians, are bent on world revolution, and every state that opposes them, however tatterdemalion—Shaba Province is their most recent objective—is a nubile target. But how do we address them?

The trouble with the search for eloquence is that eloquence cannot issue except from telling the truth. And in the United Nations one is not permitted to tell the truth, because protocol is higher than the truth. The problem, then, is not so much the deterioration of the gift of eloquence as it is that constipation that must come when we are told to speak untruths, or to build our speeches on untruths. That is why the only great eloquence in the world today is that of Solzhenitsyn and his fellows—and they are not permitted to speak at the United Nations.

—WFB   JUNE 1, 1978

A MATTER OF STYLE

I feel the need to admit that I have not given much explicit thought to the definition of style, notwithstanding that I am said to possess it, by which a compliment is sometimes but not always intended ("style" is widely misread as affectation). But finding myself in the pressure cooker, it came to me after very little ratiocination that style is, really, timing. Let me tell you, by giving you a story, what I mean by this.

It is a story by one of the nineteenth-century Russians . . . Tolstoy, I think; in any event, the story I read sometime during my teens was about a very rich young prince who one evening engaged in a drinking bout of Brobdingnagian dimensions with his fellow bloods, which eventually peaked, as such affairs frequently did in that curious epoch of genius and debauchery, in a philosophical argument over the limits of human self-control. The question was specifically posed: Could someone succeed in voluntarily sequestering himself in a small suite of rooms for a period of twenty years, notwithstanding that he would always be free to open the door, letting himself out, or others in? In a spirit of high and exhibitionistic dogmatism, the prince pronounced such hypothetical discipline preposterous, and announced that he would give one million rubles to anyone who succeeded in proving him wrong.

You will have guessed that a young companion, noble but poor, and himself far gone in wine's litigious imperatives, accepted the challenge. And so with much fanfare, a few days later, the rules having been carefully set (he could ask for, and receive, anything except human company), Peter (we'll call him) was ushered into the little subterranean suite of rooms in the basement of the prince's house.

During the first years, he drank. During the next years, he stared at the ceiling. During the succeeding period, he read—ordering books, more books, and more books. Meanwhile the fortunes of the prince had taken a disastrous turn, and so he schemed actively to seduce Peter to leave his self-imposed confinement, dispatching letters below, describing evocatively the sensual delights Peter would experience by merely opening the door. In desperation, as the deadline neared, he even offered one half the premium.

The night before the twentieth year would finish at midnight, half the town and thousands from all over Russia were outside to celebrate and marvel over the endurance of Peter upon his emergence. One hour before midnight, the startled crowd saw the celebrated door below street level open prematurely. And Peter emerged.

He had, you see, become a philosopher; and in all literature I know of no more eloquent gesture of disdain for money. One hour more, and he'd have earned a million rubles. What *style,* you say; and I concur.

But what is it about that one hour that speaks so stylishly, in a sense that Peter's emergence one year before the deadline would not—lacking, as one year would, in drama; or, at the other end, one minute before midnight, one minute being overfreighted in melodrama?

It is style, surely.

Even so the speed of human responses which, indicating spontaneity, communicate integrity. "Is it all right if I bring Flo's sister and her husband along for the weekend?" demands *instant* assent; the *least* pause is, to the quick ear, lethal. When such a proposition is posed, the man of style will make one of two decisions, and he must here think with great speed. He will either veto the extra guests, going on to give whatever reason he finds most ingenious, or he will accept them *on the spot*. Absolutely nothing in between. In between are many other things defined as lacking in style.

It is so, I think, with language, and with that aspect of language on which its effectiveness so heavily relies, namely rhythm. It matters less what exactly you say at a moment of tension than that you say it at just the right moment. Great speed might be necessary, as above, or such delay as suggests painful meditation as required to ease, console, or inspirit the other person. Style is not a synonym for diplomacy. Style can be infinitely undiplomatic, as in the stylish means selected by John L. Lewis to separate his union from the CIO. "We disaffiliate," he wrote on an envelope, dispatching it to headquarters. It is sometimes stylish to draw attention to oneself, as Lewis was doing. Sometimes the man of style will be all but anonymous. Some men are congenitally incapable of exhibiting a stylish anonymity. Of Theodore Roosevelt it was said that whenever he attended a wedding, he confused himself with the bride. The Queen of England could not feign anonymity, neither could LBJ, or Mr. Micawber. But whichever is sought—being conspicuous or inconspicuous—timing is the principal element. Arrive very early at the funeral and you will be noticed, even as you will be noticed arriving at the very last minute. In between, you glide in, on cat-feet.

In language, rhythm is an act of timing. "Why did you use the word 'irenic' when you say it merely means 'peaceful'?" a talk show host once asked indignantly. To which the answer given was: "I desired the extra syllable." In all circumstances? *No, for God's sake.*

In the peculiar circumstances of the sentence uttered, and these circumstances were set by what had gone just before, what would probably come just after. A matter of style. A matter of timing.

—WFB   JANUARY, 1983

Usage III:
W. H. Fowler
Lives

Even *National Review* columnists—perhaps especially *NR* columnists—write to Buckley, protesting certain interpretations put on words. Here, the formidable and unique Florence King . . .

———

Dear Mr. Buckley:

I am sitting here under a pile of letters from readers about my "Tender Hooks" column (*NR*, June 21). Most of them start out, "Imagine my despair . . ." Several people sent me Xeroxes of the dictionary page containing "tenterhooks," and one man wrote a disquisition on the textile industry, explaining that a "tenter" is the frame on which fabric is stretched to dry, and the "hook" is the nail driven into the frame to hold the fabric while it dries; the fabric is thus in a state of suspended tension, etc. etc.

As I plan to say in my address to Congress as soon as they invite me, the State of the Punnybone is not good. My use of "tender" hooks was deliberate, designed to take a poke at the tender-hearted people who worry constantly about the tender sensitivities of others.

Since you believe in public service, here is your chance. I enclose a flag, hand-sewn by me, containing a coiled snake and the motto, SHE SAID IT

ON PURPOSE. Please fly it from the roof of the *NR* building so I don't have to answer all these letters.

Yours sincerely,
FLORENCE KING
FREDERICKSBURG, VA.

P.S. Keep the flag. I'm sure you'll need it again. In the immortal words of Lizzie Borden: "I have a feeling somebody is going to do something." P.P.S. Stet the "P" in Punnybone.

Dear Miss King: Your flag flutters even as I do, in addressing you. Cordially,

—WFB   JULY 19, 1993

Dear Mr. Buckley:

I feel somewhat like the parent who, as he raises the strap, says, "This is going to hurt me more than it hurts you," for I must assure you that I am a devoted but discreet admirer of yours—and I never thought that I could come to this point: I am about to criticize you for a fairly flagrant mistake in grammar contained at the front of *American Conservative Thought in the Twentieth Century,* headed Acknowledgments.

The offending sentence is, "I wish to record . . . my thanks to Professor Leonard W. Levy for his patience and for the excellence of his advice which, if he had given any more of it, this would have been a book about twenty-first-century American thought."

It can readily be seen that if one takes out the clause "if he had given any more of it," the word "which" is left dangling without a verb.

In view of the thousands of words that you turn out, my criticism may seem niggling so I would be obliged if you would regard it as a gentle reproach. Yours truly,

BARBARA LAMON
(MRS. R. LAMON)
LONDON, ONTARIO

Dear Mrs. Lamon: The grammatical error isn't *fairly* flagrant, it is *very* flagrant. Indeed, it was first called to my attention by Professor Levy himself. The verbal wrench is designed to superordinate the idiomatic over the grammatical, for rhetorical effect. The late Professor Willmoore Kendall, at the time a senior editor of *National Review,* once wrote an editorial paragraph the first sentence of which began, "The weekend conference at Arden House, which by the way why doesn't somebody burn it down, reached several conclusions . . ." Reproached by the (then) managing editor Miss La Follette with a large dictionary in hand, Professor Kendall said, "Suzanne, don't you realize that when people get around to writing dictionaries, they come to people like me to find out what to put in them?" I don't mean that the way it sounds, which by the way isn't so good, is it? Anyway, you are right grammatically. Many thanks. Cordially,

—WFB   JULY 21, 1972

ERRATUM (of sorts): Our esteemed friend and colleague Professor Hugh Kenner writes in to correct a misreference to him in our last issue. An entire line—we say, in our defense—was inadvertently omitted at the printers, resulting in a mad but plausible confusion in giving the biography of Mr. Kenner. But we shall take our punishment like a man, and reproduce Mr. Kenner's letter, as follows: "March 23, 1960, Dear Sir: Reluctant though I am to interfere with the mixture of encomium and fantasy that animates your doubtless eyewitness description of me as 'critic, philosopher, yachtsman' (March 26), I must intervene on behalf of my alma mater when you ascribe to me an academic post at the University of Toronto. The English Department of which I am chairman is located far from native skies, at the University of California, Santa Barbara.

"I must also protest your statement that I recently authored a study of T. S. Eliot. I composed that book, sir, and I typed it, but author it I did not, and author, while a tatter of the English language remains mine to defend, I never shall, Yours faithfully, Hugh Kenner."

We refer Professor Kenner to the words of another Eliot (Sir J.) who wrote (in 1632) of "The divine blessing . . . which authors all the happiness we receive," and confess to digging Warner in his contention (1602) that "A good God may not author noysome things"—not even noisome verbs like author. And finally, appreciating as we do Mr. Kenner's epistles, we devoutly pray, sir, that yours of the 23rd instant will not prove (Chapman, 1596) "the last foul thing Thou ever author'dst." To us, that is.

—WFB   APRIL 9, 1960

Dear Mr. Buckley:

I have just read your thoroughly enjoyable *Marco Polo, If You Can.* As one who had more than a casual connection with the U-2 program, as a Buckley aficionado, and as one who loves the graceful use of the language, I was absorbed and delighted.

But with what dismay did I read the final (excluding epilogue) sentence: "The meeting between the three allies lasted another two hours"! How could the man who serves up such succulents as "adumbrated" and "brummagem" be so lax with "among" and "between"?

If, perish the thought! you are among the Safire-phobes who rebel against grammatical discipline—if this is the sort of pedantic nonsense up with which you will not put—consider that "between" stems from the O.E. roots of "two," an etymological heritage that simply cannot be ignored for the sake of freedom.

I beg you to restore my faith in you. Tell me you made a mistake.

> With great respect,
> JOHN A. WOLFE
> BURLINGTON, MASS.

Dear Mr. Wolfe: Sorry, you lose. See Fowler: "between is a sadly ill-treated word . . . 1. *B.* and *among.* The OED gives a warning against the superstition that *b.* can be used only of the relationship between two things, and that if there are more *among* is the right preposition. 'In all senses *between* has been, from its earliest appearance, extended to more than two. . . . It is still the only word available to express the relation of a thing to many surrounding things severally and individually; *among* expresses a relation to them collectively and vaguely: we should not say *the space lying among the three points* or *a treaty among three Powers.*' " Cordially,

> —WFB   MARCH 22, 1985

———

A Simple Little In-house Memo in Which One William (Rickenbacker) Corrects Another William (Buckley), Forgiving Nothing.

———

Wm—

It is now almost exactly thirty years since I sent you a copy of my long letter to *Modern Age,* in which I gave my comments on several dozen mistakes in the then current issue. *Modern Age* has for many years been produced with care, and I haven't had to crack the whip again in that direction. But, old shoe, what's happening on East 35th Street? I attach a discussion of the mechanical problems in the current issue [March 19] of dear old *NR* and hope you'll tie a bomb to it and place it on the appropriate desk. I couldn't refrain from talking about one or two points that are strictly stylistic; questions of style would have covered twenty pages more, and, besides, that's not my business any more. [Rickenbacker had resigned his position as a senior editor a year earlier.] But I do care very much about *NR* and about my mother tongue, which I need not defend myself for defending. I have in that regard what Ortega so nearly calls *una razón vital.*

> Ever of thee (as AJN* liked to sign off),
> WM

———

* Albert Jay Nock.—Ed.

Dear Wm: Your note is welcome and deserved. Much happened during the fortnight in question, not least the vacation of the managing editor, and in-house experiments of a recondite technological character. We have imposed a *frein vital* on all projected changes that make us vulnerable to your criticisms.

Ever,

WM

[Rickenbacker's] Notes on March 19 *National Review*

p. 12—Second paragraph: Here I find "apparatchiks." The "t" is correct (the noun is *apparat*). However, on p. 29 I find "*apparatchiki,*" the Russian plural transliterated correctly, and the word in italic as befits the foreigner. You offer still another variant on p. 31, where I find *apparatchiks,* i.e., the English plural while the word is in italic. Then on p. 33 I find the "t" missing in both *apparachiki* and *apparachiks.*

p. 13—"What better way," etc., should end with a question mark. What better way to show it's a question?

p. 17—Lefthand column, mid: A "quorum" can't be reduced to a "symbol." A quorum is a body competent to do business. A symbol need be no more than a flag. If we stationed only one soldier in Europe, he would stand as the symbol of our resolve to carry out our policy; but he would not constitute a quorum.

p. 17—Righthand column, top: "As Clemenceau might put it" would be all right if the old boy were still alive. "Might have put it" keeps us properly oriented in history.

p. 20—Middle column, uppish: "Already-existing" is a phrase that exhibits the needless hyphen. "Already" is a fully grown adverb and can modify any damned adjective it takes a shine to.

p. 20—Right, mid: "Because of his curious role the junk bond market." This would be good syntax in Hebrew, but we need a piece of connective tissue between "role" and "market." Probably "in" is the word everyone overlooked.

p. 22—Left, high: It's "Eastern Air Lines" (three words), unless Frank Lorenzo has started stealing capital letters from his unhappy subsidiary.

p. 23—Bottom left: We need a full stop after Tito's death in 1980. Hell, we needed a full stop to him forty years earlier.

p. 24—Left, top: "Drags" should be "drag." The subject is "the crisis . . . and inflation."

p. 24—Tense sequence, that forgotten art, causes trouble at the end of the next paragraph. "With Slovenia gone, . . . would deteriorate . . . , had been getting is diminishing." The idea should be clear, and I'll let you clean up this mess during your own business hours.

p. 24—Right, lowish: A real monster: *dejá vû.* That's a new one to me, certainly the furthest thing from *déjà vu.*

p. 25—Left, lowish: *Verboten* is not a noun and need not take the initial capital. Such gaffes around *NR* were at one time *streng verboten.*

p. 25—Left, bottom: "The only known example of the Germans actually *shortening* a word." The Germans are like all speakers of all languages: they use apocopations when they can. *Der Oberkommandant* becomes *Der Ober,* and so on, and why not?

p. 25—Last paragraph: L.A. is not "the City of Angels." It is La Ciudad de Nuestra Señora, Reina de los Angeles—the City of Our Lady, Queen of the Angels. The name is far too beautiful to be ignored.

p. 28—Lefthand, mid: I see the cheeky hyphen barging into German now. It's not *Mittel-Europaische,* but *Mitteleuropäische,* and don't forget the umlaut over the "a," or my armies move at dawn.

p. 28—Next para: Out, out, damned hyphen! All my life it has been ice floes, and now *NR* has discovered "ice-floes." What *is* it about your fulminating hyphenosis? Did you buy an oversupply of them and are you trying to work off the inventory? They're a drug on the market, I say. Take your losses, throw the bum stuff out, and start with a clean slate.

p. 30—Left, top: *Newshour* should be *NewsHour.* I know it's weird, but so are Jim and Robin sometimes.

p. 30—Five lines down, "doubtlessly" should be "[sic]ced," and sicced good and hard.

p. 31—Left, middle: Who's the worry wart who wrote, and allowed to stand, "an highly decentralized federation"? Must have been some escapee from an herb farm.

p. 31—Left, bottom: "Multicandidate" is much ugliness. Oh, Hyphen, where art thou when we need thee? The little busybody is so bemused by sticking his nose in other people's business that he has neglected his own rightful chores.

p. 32—Right, bottom: "A stem-winding speech." This is what linguists call a "back formation"; starting with a known term ("stem-winder"), someone proceeds by analogy to create its other formations. Trouble is, the ignorant make the wrong assumption. In this case, "stem-winder" is not "someone who stem-winds." In the old days men told time by sundials, water clocks, roosters, the moon. By and by they invented clocks, big ones. Then by and by they made smaller and smaller clocks until they had one so small they could carry it around. It was on its way to becoming a pocket-watch. But it was still wound up by inserting a key in the face, just like the old grandfather clock. Then some genius hit upon the novel idea of rearranging the gears so that the watch could be wound up by working the "stem" at the top (it was the knurled knob at 12 o'clock high). The English unimaginatively called this a keyless watch, but the delighted Yankees called it a stem-winder, and from that moment anything fine, anything first rate, anything that commanded attention and respect, was a real stem-winder. So, in American idiom, a fine speech can be a stem-winder. But you cannot give a stem-winding speech, nor can an audience be stem-wound by it. Sorry! And by the way—is the idiom, as distinguished from grammarbook talk, a dying form of speech?

p. 37—Left, near bottom: "Likely" is not an adverb, at least not yet, at least not in my book, at least not in my neck of the woods. And we don't need it. (There is one special locution in which it is acceptable, but I won't tell you about it; you might misunderstand.)

p. 38—Righthand: We have Smuzynski, and Sumzynski, and I say it's spinach. But his mother would like to have the name treated with some respeck.

p. 42—Middle, uppish: "Thankfully, the debtor nations have . . ." The debtor nations don't know the meaning of thankfulness. Somebody else must be thankful. I wonder who?

p. 56—Right, mid: FDR did not "serve four terms." He was elected four times, and dropped in his tracks shortly after the last election.

p. 59—Left, near bottom: "The *Grief* concerto." It's Grieg, need I say? and no italic is needed. It's not a title. The title is *Piano Concerto in A Minor.* Good "Grief," indeed!

p. 64—Middle, middle: What a nice surprise it would have been if you had had the courage to use an exclamation point after the sentence that starts, "What a nice surprise"! It is the one time, other than in the imperative or the interjection, when the use of the exclam is positively commanded. Seeking to avoid the monster because it has been abused by careless writers, one should not shrink from its ordained use. Hop to it! What a fine chance to hit 'em with a bang!

(WFB's columns not proofed by me.)

For which, thank the Lord!

—WFB   MAY 14, 1990

Chapter 11

A Journalist
on Journalism

It might surprise some that Buckley thinks of himself as a journalist. Not only a journalist, to be sure, but more than a journalist in spirit: a working one, with the curiosity, nose for news, talent for telling stories quickly, and empathy for other journalists that characterize the best of them. He responds promptly to queries from magazine writers and newspaper reporters, believing them to be doing their jobs, as he is doing his. To be sure, he is the owner and was the founder and longtime editor of a journal of opinion; an author, a lecturer, a television host-plus, and a political force in his own right, etc.; but part of his everyday basic work is his syndicated newspaper column, an obligation he takes as seriously as breathing—getting ideas, researching, meeting deadlines, even on occasion suggesting ways for a newspaper editor to shorten his columns. Journalism is part of the rhythm of his busy, peripatetic life. He is friends with journalists of many political colorations and convictions. In his comments on or quarrels with or admiration for other journals and journalists, we see a great deal of how his character expresses itself as well as his continuing passion for the meaning of words.

Oh, yes: and for a man who spent less than a year in the CIA, just out of college, Bill Buckley has had an awful lot of explaining to do for his first job *before* going into journalism.

On Leveling with the Reader

In recent weeks several correspondents, thoughtfully sending me copies, have triumphantly advised editors of newspapers in which this feature appears, that "Mr. Buckley was himself a member of the CIA," and that under the circumstances, that fact should be noted every time a newspaper publishes a comment by Mr. Buckley on the CIA.

Now the *Boston Phoenix,* which is that area's left-complement to the John Birch Society magazine, publishes an editorial on the subject that begins with the ominous sentence, "William F. Buckley, Jr.'s past is catching up with him. In the 50's he served as E. Howard Hunt's assistant in the Mexico City CIA station. . . ." Accordingly, the *Phoenix* has protested to the editor of the *Boston Globe,* and reports to its readers, "Ann Wyman, the new editor of the *Globe*'s editorial pages, is now considering whether to append Buckley's past CIA affiliation to his column, which appears regularly in the *Globe.* Wyman intends to consult with other *Globe* editors. . . . The *Globe* may finally be on to him."

If so, it would indeed have taken the *Globe* a very long time, since it began publishing me in 1962, and my CIA involvement, [and] twenty-five-year-old friendship with Howard Hunt, are, among newspaper readers, as well known as that Coca-Cola is the pause that refreshes. But one pauses to wonder what is the planted axiom in the position taken by the *Boston Phoenix?*

It is true that I was in the CIA. I joined in July 1951, and left in April 1952. Now the assumption, not always stated, is that obviously anybody who was ever a member of an organization defends that organization. But one wonders: Why should this be held to be true? The most prominent critics of the CIA are former members of it.

I attended Yale University for four years. Is it the position of the *Boston Phoenix* that, therefore, everything I write about Yale is presumptively suspect, because as a Yale graduate I am obviously pro-Yale? But it happens that shortly before entering the CIA I wrote a book that was very critical of Yale. And, as a matter of fact, I have in recent years written critically about Yale on a dozen occasions. So consistently, indeed, that Miss Wyman may feel impelled to identify me, at the end of every column I write about Yale, in some such way as: "Mr. Buckley, a graduate of Yale, is, as one would expect, a critic of that university."

I am a Roman Catholic, and have written, oh, twenty columns in the last ten years critical of developments within the Catholic Church. Should I be identified as a Roman Catholic?

I like, roughly, in the order described, (1) God, (2) my family, (3) my country, (4) J. S. Bach, (5) peanut butter, and (6) good English prose.

Should these biases be identified when I write about, say, Satan, divorce, Czechoslovakia, Chopin, marmalade, and *New York Times* editorials?

I wonder if Miss Wyman is being asked, implicitly, to label the religious or ethnic backgrounds of her columnists? "Mr. Joseph Kraft, who writes today on Israel, is a Jew." That would presumably please the editors of the *Boston Phoenix.* Or, "Mr. William Raspberry, who writes today about civil rights in the South, is black." Or how about: "Mr. John Roche, who writes today in favor of federal aid to education, receives a salary from Tufts whose income depends substantially on federal grants."

Pete Hamill, who laughed his head off a few years ago at the hallucinations of Robert Welch, asks in the *Village Voice:* "Is Bill Buckley still a member of CIA? Have any of Buckley's many foreign travels been paid for by CIA?" One columnist recently wrote that *National Review's* defense of the CIA, and my own friendship with Howard Hunt, might suggest that the CIA had indeed put up money for *National Review* over the years, though he conceded that if that were the case, the CIA was indeed a stingy organization—Mr. Garry Wills knows, at first hand, something of the indigence of that journal. Unfortunately Mr. Wills is the exact complement of Mr. Revilo Oliver, who was booted out of the John Birch Society for excessive kookiness some time after he revealed that JFK's funeral had been carefully rehearsed. Both are classics professors by background. Perhaps one should identify anyone who writes about politics and is also a classics professor as such? The *Boston Phoenix* and Miss Wyman should ponder that one.

—WFB   MARCH 11, 1975

THE CIA ON THE DEFENSIVE

The CIA investigation unfolds, mostly in the press—and there is no doubt that the Agency has become the major hobgoblin of the day. The height of the hysteria was voiced at Yale University. Mr. John Lindsay, briefly in residence there to be debriefed on his experiences in municipal affairs, attacked the composition of the Rockefeller panel ("not one of them [the members] has a record of civil liberties"), and added that he himself always knew that "the CIA would become a monster and smite us all." Presumably the CIA is to blame for the bankrupt condition of New York City after eight years of leadership by Mr. Lindsay. Come to think of it, there is no more plausible explanation for the mess in New York than that the enemies of Mr. Lindsay were secretly running the government.

There was seldom a situation in which journalistic semantics played so great a role. Thus, the newspaper sentence, "Mr. Angleton believes that anti-war efforts were backed by foreign agencies" is read by one and all to mean, "Mr. Angleton entertains the obviously absurd notion that anti-war efforts were backed by foreign agencies."

The spokesmen for CIA have not rushed forward to give detailed accounts of the Agency's activities, and that's wrong. Or, as it is usually put, the CIA has "refused to specify the basis of its allegations." But it is okay for Seymour Hersh of the *New York Times* to make unqualified statements on the basis of unspecified "well-placed sources." You will perhaps have observed the technique. One day Mr. Hersh alleges that the CIA has done thus-and-so. The next day he quotes his own report of the day before beginning with the phrase, "Yesterday the *New York Times* revealed . . ."

Then there is the subtle use of quotation marks. "Richard Helms told the Senate Foreign Relations Committee that he could not 'recall' whether the White House had urged the CIA to engage in domestic spying. The *New York Times,* quoting well-placed sources, said that the CIA had violated . . ." Why the quotes around Helms's "recall," where they do not belong? Why *not* quotes around "well-placed sources"—where, according to the rules of punctuation, they *do* belong? Consider, for a moment, how differently these two sentences would read if the placing of the quotation marks had been reversed.

The topsy-turviness progresses. Mr. Miles Copeland, the author who has had considerable experience with and within the CIA, wrote recently a letter to the *London Times* skewering a typical report on the williwaw. The *Times's* reporter had quoted President Ford aboard *U.S. One,* flying to Vail. "The President said he had been assured in a mid-flight telephone call from Mr. William Colby, the CIA Director, that such activities 'did not exist' now." Commented Mr. Copeland: "What Mr. Colby said was that such activities 'do not exist.' The 'now' in the *Times's* story was added by your reporter. 'I do not beat my wife now' conveys a meaning rather different from 'I do not beat my wife.' "

The only fresh air recently was the story in the *Washington Post* quoting the former liaison man between the CIA and the FBI who said that there are "gray areas" in the law, resulting in the CIA's crossing into domestic operations for legitimate reasons. Mr. Sam Papich blamed these murky areas on a statute that "goes from the vague to the ridiculous."

"For example, he said"—I quote the *Post* story—"a CIA training program for local police departments was widely thought to have been aimed at anti-war activists and therefore represented an incursion into the domestic field. In fact, its purpose was to share with local police several devices and methods the CIA had developed in its own work. One device, he said, is engaged in the apprehension of murderers by detecting whether a suspect has held a piece of metal in the last 24 hours."

The charter says that the CIA shall have "no police, subpoena, law enforcement powers, or internal security functions." But, Mr. Papich reminds us, it also says that the CIA Director is "responsible for protecting intelligence sources and methods from unauthorized disclosure."

"A Soviet spy in France out of the blue travels to the U.S.," he said. "You don't just pick up the telephone and tell Hoover. . . ."

Complexities are being lost to the ideological rigidities. One wonders whether the critics of the CIA would really demand that it reveal its files on connections between U.S. protests and foreign money. Or—conceivably—will a thorough investigation reveal that the CIA has not done enough? Does it make sense, in any case, to repeal the law of hot pursuit when the enemy is detected flying into your own territory?

—WFB　　　　　　　　FEBRUARY 4, 1975

———

Well in advance of the Pentagon Papers, the Nixon tapes, Whitewater, Vincent Foster, etc., Buckley raised questions of the right to privacy, or confidentiality, of a public figure or a public official.

———

PUBLIC FIGURES AND THE PRESS

"An indignant Mayor Lindsay arrived at La Guardia Airport from Washington at 5:10 P.M. yesterday"—says the item in the newspaper—"and told waiting reporters he did not have to answer any of their questions. Besieged with queries about City Hall's asserted intrusion in police matters, John Lindsay did say: 'That's ridiculous.' When a radio reporter held a microphone close to his face, the mayor roughly shoved it away and said: 'I'm the mayor of the City of New York and you have an obligation to treat me with respect.' As he left the airport in a small sports car, Lindsay partingly told a reporter, 'I don't have to answer your questions, I don't have to talk to you—I'm the mayor.' "

Well, Mr. Lindsay certainly made *that* clear, i.e., there is no doubting that he *is* the mayor, although it isn't exactly clear what he means by requiring that he be treated with respect on that account. He cannot mean that a reporter must not ask Lindsay questions when he arrives at the airport—it is the duty of the reporter to attempt to appease the public curiosity. On the other hand, it is up to the public official to decide when he desires to speak, and under what auspices; and if he doesn't like to give running interviews while going to, or coming from, an airport, that is a decision for him to make; but Mr. Lindsay should recognize that you don't have to be mayor of New York in order to enjoy that privilege.

Everyone has an obligation to treat everyone else with respect, if by respect is meant a regard for that man's sovereignty over his own affairs. If anything, the public figure is, in this narrow respect, perhaps less entitled than others to respect for the simple reason that the press is indispensable to the achievement of his own ambitions and the press, under the circumstances, comes to expect reciprocal accommodations. When you become, say, President of the United States (I am no longer addressing Mr. Lindsay), all the rules are broken because you are such a hot property that you need grant no interviews, not even to Walter Lippmann, and still you have a hope of surviving. But for lesser public officials, the relationship with the press is a two-way thing.

Now the press can be very bumptious indeed. An airline stewardess told me a few days ago of having been on an airplane with Senator Goldwater and his family in the fall of 1963, en route to the funeral of Mrs. Goldwater's mother. The plane pulled in at Chicago, the door opened, and a reporter fell through it, grabbed Senator Goldwater and said: "President Kennedy has just been shot and killed. How do you figure that affects your chances to become President?" Goldwater turned white, sucked in his breath, brushed the reporter aside and walked quickly down the ramp. He might very easily have hit the reporter. But he would not have said to him, "I am a United States Senator. You have an obligation to treat me with respect."

I remember an occasion in 1952 when President Truman's presidential train stopped at Stamford, Connecticut—the President was making stops along the line from New Haven to New York, campaigning for Adlai Stevenson as his successor. He had a little five-minute speech prepared, half folksy, half don't-let-them-take-it-away anti-Republicanism; and a few minutes after he began, a soprano voice rang out from a boy perched on a tree branch above the tracks: "Tell us about the red herring, Harry!"—an allusion to Truman's unfortunate designation of the Hiss investigation as a red herring. The crowd laughed good-humoredly. Mr. Truman did not laugh. "Young man," he snapped, "have you no respect for the President of the United States?" It was like a sudden cold snap. And Truman knew it, and rushed through the rest of his little talk; the candidates were quickly introduced, and the train pulled out, leaving the crowd nervous, undemonstrative. It is not known how the little boy was handled by his parents, but if he said "Gee, isn't the President stuffy!" he merely echoed his elders' unverbalized reaction.

If a treaty between public officials and press were to be written I should think it would stress one point, namely that the press would agree not physically to obstruct a public official—i.e., to stand directly in his way to where he is going, or to thrust a microphone in his face in such a way as to require him to duck, if he would avoid it. So that a mayor of New York, arriving at an airport, could on the one hand hear the questions directed to him by the press and weigh the desirability of replying to them then and there; on the other hand, be left free, if that is his pleasure, to walk quietly and resolutely out the door, without having to stop to lecture anyone at all on the importance of himself and the unrequited respect owing to his great office.

—WFB   MARCH 15, 1966

EASY DOES IT

MADRID. They didn't give a very big play to the *Washington Post* hoax in Madrid, and this is relevant because evidence of United States degeneracy is on the whole lavishly memorialized. I suspect the reason for it is that, really, Miss Janet Cooke's dishonor* was something that fell in newsrooms considerably on this side of the Donation of Constantine or the Protocols of Zion, but it is being given treatment about that heavy.

Let us, first, attempt a distinction of some importance. Some years ago, I sought to make the point that the Pentagon Papers collected and released with such fanfare by Daniel Ellsberg were tendentious—i.e., that they collected idiocies that could only have been one part of the whole story, unless we were prepared to believe that the people who staffed the Pentagon during the early and mid-sixties were all morons. Accordingly, I assembled three or four artisans and together we sat down and in three days composed, even unto imitating the prose style of generals and admirals and assistant secretaries of defense, memoranda, the difference between our own and the real ones being that ours were intelligent analyses of the deteriorating Indo-Chinese situation under the subversive attrition of the North Vietnam–backed Vietcong.

The *Washington Post* assigned a small platoon of reporters to check out what we had labeled as the "Secret Pentagon Papers." The results were quite extraordinary. A reporter would call, e.g., retired Admiral Arthur Radford, over whose signature we had written several memoranda, and Admiral Radford would say over the telephone, "Gee, fellows, I don't actually remember those exact memoranda—but after all it was eight years ago. But it does sound like me, and it's certainly what I was thinking of saying at the time." Others (for instance Dean Rusk) reacted similarly. Accordingly, the *Washington Post* ran full accounts of the "Secret Pentagon

---

* Ms. Cooke was the *Washington Post* reporter who wrote an account of an eight-year-old heroin addict, won a Pulitzer Prize, and later admitted that the child she wrote about was a fiction, or a composite.—Ed.

Papers." Back in the office we were alarmed that the hoax hadn't been penetrated, and so called a press conference to explain that the documents were forgeries, and to give the motive for their fabrication. To say that the editors of the *Washington Post* (and others) were annoyed with us is on the order of saying that Medea was irritated with Jason or that King Lear fell into a pout.

The similarity is that just as the Pentagon Papers we fabricated probably did and do substantively exist, in other forms to be sure, so the story of an eight-year-old addicted to heroin is, in our wretched times, far from unlikely. In this world, routinely twelve-year-old girls get pregnant, girls even younger—and boys—engage in sex for hire, and get their kicks from drugs. We don't need Pulitzer-quality reporters to tell us what crawls under the stones of our culture, and not only in black Washington, but in white East Hampton.

So that Miss Cooke's dishonorable act was less heinous than what it might have been. She did not violate the commandment against bearing false witness. She was not the woman who took the stand at the murder trial intentionally misidentifying the defendant and then happily watching him swing on the gibbet while she collected the bounty. The distinction between a *malum in se* and a *malum prohibitum*—the distinction between that which is inherently evil and that which is forbidden—is not entirely out of place here. Miss Cooke acted badly, she exposed certain supervisory frailties in the system, the prize was taken from her and she was fired.

But my goodness, the wailing and gnashing of teeth! When a generation ago Professor Charles Van Doren was shown to have been apprised ahead of time of the information that permitted him to gain fame and riches as the omniscient scholar on the $64,000 quiz program, people wrote about how the entire American academy was forever disgraced. The American academy may be disgraced, but hardly because one of its members yielded to the temptation of cupidity.

Ellen Goodman, the columnist, writes as though Miss Cooke had diminished the entire profession of journalism, which is to suggest that the entire profession of journalism enjoys a level of esteem the National Opinion Research Center declines to validate (ninth out of thirteen in institutional esteem as of 1979). And Roger Wilkins, the prominent black journalist who writes for the *Washington Star,* has gone so far as to say that Miss Cooke has set back the entire cause of black journalism because her misrepresentations will cause editors to lower their esteem for black perceptiveness.

As one member of the white majority, I'd prefer the company of a black newspaperwoman who fabricated a story centered on a mythic but entirely plausible little victim of drugs, to the company of the relatively untroubled black (or white) drug pushers who ride around in their Cadillacs sowing their poison. If you wish to know who to get mad at, go back and read Claude Brown's *Manchild in the Promised Land.*

So I say: Forget it. Probably, net, it was a salubrious experience, since some members of the press have got rather bloated notions of their sanctity. Elmer Gantry was, on the whole, a good thing, reminding us of the endemic weakness of the flesh, restoring our perspective.

—WFB   APRIL 25, 1981

REVIVE THE NATIONAL NEWS COUNCIL

The attention given to the Sharon (General) versus *Time* (magazine) trial goes beyond American curiosity on whether the magazine libeled the general. The professionals were interested, of course, in the evolution of the libel law. But the public was interested in the drama.

Drama here is defined as the press at the bar.

The *New York Times*'s version of the verdict: "The jury found an absence of malice, but no shortage of arrogance."

And then the *Times* went on to deliver a lecture worth contemplating. It is time, said the editorial, "for journalists to stop muting their criticism of one another. The best protection of free speech is more free speech, not less. To deserve the extraordinary protections of American law, *Time* and all of journalism needs a stronger tradition of mutual and self-correction. The more influential the medium, the greater the duty to offer a place for rebuttal, complaint, correction and re-examination. Beating the arrogance rap is even more important than escaping one for libel."

Flash back now to the San Francisco Republican Convention in 1964. General Dwight Eisenhower is speaking. He says the usual things, ho-hum, and then suddenly he utters the following sentence: "Let us particularly scorn the divisive efforts of those outside our family, including sensation-seeking columnists and commentators . . ." The crowd rose spontaneously to its feet and cheered as if, single-handed, Dwight Eisenhower had just won the Super Bowl.

Flash forward to November 1969. Vice President Spiro Agnew, speaking in Des Moines, Iowa, denounces the bias of network television, charging that TV's immense power over public opinion was in the hands of "a small and unelected elite" of network producers, commentators and newsmen, "to a man" reflecting the "geographical and intellectual confines of Washington, D.C., or New York City." The result? Practically the whole country hoists Mr. Agnew on its shoulders, and for a brief period he is a popular hero. Something indeed was going on.

In 1973, the Twentieth Century Fund, without acknowledging the Agnew assault on media bias, let alone stressing it, made possible the founding of something called the National News Council. The council was set up as a fifteen-man board composed of responsible citizens, half of them members of the media, half of them so-called "public members." The council had a staff of a half dozen that operated under the presidency of a series of distinguished figures, among them Richard Salant, the eminent former director of news for CBS.

The procedure was as follows. If a person or an institution thought he or it had been wrongly treated by a newspaper, magazine or television station, he could file a complaint with the National News Council. But—listen to this—before the council would agree to look at the complaint, the plaintiff had to agree that whatever the council decided, he would waive a libel action. The council, in short, knew that it could not get the cooperation of the media at large if, in effect, the council was acting as a pre-trial discovery panel.

Members were given staff reports on the alleged unfairness, including—when available—the defense of the alleged tortfeasor. I say when available, because some, indeed a significant number, of media flatly declined to cooperate. And most conspicuous of these was: the *New York Times*.

So here we had an organization begun in 1973 . . . that, in 1982, just plain ran out of steam. It folded for lack of funds. But that lack of funds was the result of the indifference with which its findings were treated in the press. The press, in effect, denied the council the only sanction that could keep it alive: public respect for its findings.

The National News Council was a body that, if beefed up by institutional respect, might have acted as a satisfactory alternative to a jury trial. It could have received the complaint of General Sharon (alongside his promise not to bring legal action), heard the response of *Time* mag, conducted its investigation, and issued its finding. But of course these things don't work unless people pay them some heed. In the relevant case, *Time* would have bound itself to reporting the finding of the National News Council.

Well, the editors of the *New York Times* have aptly phrased what's troubling so many people. It is a pity that when presented the opportunity to do something about it, as recently as in 1973, they were out to lunch.

—WFB   JANUARY 31, 1985

(Excerpt from The New Yorker, *January 31, 1983,*
"A Journal—Overdrive—I" by William F. Buckley, Jr.)

The *Times* called to ask who had taken a photograph of Pat and me on the Orient Express that they will use in the travel section; they want to send the photographer a check (for $75). I tell Frances that the picture in question was taken with my own camera by a waiter, and it would not be feasible to find him. The spread will not be out until next Sunday, and I haven't seen it, but the galleys, corrected over the weekend, amused me, because I had privately gambled that one sentence I wrote would never see the light of day. On learning that the *Times* had, as represented, a strict limit of $500 for any travel piece . . . I had written that aboard the Orient Express "the consumption of [drinks from the bar] is encouraged, by the way, and they are cash-and-carry, and there is no nonsense about special rates. A gin-and-tonic is $4, a liqueur $6. These prices, weighed on the scales of the Old Testament, are not prohibitive, unless you are trying to make a living writing for the travel section of the *New York Times.*"

I won—the third sentence did not survive. It's a funny thing about the *Times:* I don't know anybody who works for it who *doesn't* have a sense of humor. (Big exception: John Oakes. But then he retired as editorial-page director several years ago, and is understandably melancholy about having to live in a world whose shape is substantially of his own making.) A. M. Rosenthal, the working head of the newspaper, is one of the funniest men living. Arthur Ochs Sulzberger, the publisher, is wonderfully amusing, and easily amused. And so on. But there is some corporate something that keeps the *Times* from smiling at itself: don't quite know what.

(Telegram addressed to WILLIAM F. BUCKLEY, JR. NATIONAL REVIEW NEW YORK, *February 2, 1983.)*

YOUR VICIOUS AND TOTALLY UNCALLED-FOR CHARGE THAT THE NEW YORK TIMES HAS NO SENSE OF HUMOR ABOUT ITSELF WAS SIMPLY ANOTHER EXAMPLE OF THE NATIONWIDE ATTACK AGAINST THE FIRST AMENDMENT. WE PLAN TO RESIST THIS CONSPIRACY DIRECTED AT THE FREE PRESS WITH ALL OUR MIGHT.

> A. M. ROSENTHAL
> EXECUTIVE EDITOR
> THE NEW YORK TIMES

TED TURNER'S RUSSIA

If you want to lift your eyes for a tiny moment from events in the Democratic convention center in Atlanta, let them travel to another part of the city that is the headquarters of the Turner Broadcasting Co. This is the outfit that has given us the most innovative (and valuable) TV programming idea of the decade: round-the-clock news. That news is reported evenhandedly. But the strangest transformation since the discovery of the transsexual operation is what has happened to Ted Turner, the founder of CNN. He has become a Soviet apologist. In fact, his stuff is so red it would embarrass the *Daily Worker* to publish it.

But not the Encyclopaedia Britannica, and here lies the story. Last March, Turner Educational Services, which is an arm of the broadcasting company, aired a seven-hour program called "Portrait of the Soviet Union." The next thing we knew, Turner teamed up with the Encyclopaedia Britannica to take those seven hours and run them for the education of schoolchildren. And this notwithstanding the universal panning received when "Portrait" was broadcast on WTBS. The first sentence of *Washington Post* reviewer Tom Shales, who guards the liberal tablets in this world as Fafner guarded the Nibelungs' treasures, was, "Does Ted Turner have a few thousand acres in the Urals that he's trying to unload?" Shales was just warming up. "This is not a 'Letter from the U.S.S.R.' It's more like a postcard from Binky and Biff at Camp Whitewash."

Even so, the E.B. people undertook to make it a seminal instrument for the instruction of America's schoolchildren. How bad is the Turner portrait of the U.S.S.R.?

—The Kremlin used to belong to the czars. "Now, it belongs to the people."

—What did Lenin face when he took over Russia? His party "needed to mold a new kind of citizen, one who would embody all the virtues of the socialist ethic—clean-limbed, right-thinking and dedicated to the state. The kind of model superperson that would be a shining example to all."

—What is the goal of communism? "A highly developed people, giving freely all they can to a society and in return taking back all they need."

—How has the Soviet Union dealt with its artists? "Just outside of Moscow, living in the most amazing grace, is an enclave of top Russian artists. [These] princes of literature have their homes in this Russian Beverly Hills."

—Is there freedom of religion in the Soviet Union? Forgawdsakes. "Atheist though the state may be, freedom to worship as you please is enshrined in the Soviet constitution."

—But haven't the Soviet Union's managers in fact failed to create an advanced society? Horsefeathers. "It's modernization on a grand scale—a great success."

—Didn't a dozen million citizens perish in Siberia as the result of the policy of Gulag? Siberia "used to be a one-way ticket to exile; it's now a chance for young Soviets to do something for their country, make some extra money, maybe even start a whole new life."

—Don't Soviet history books lie about everything? Well, "increasingly, Soviets feel it is essential for the young, indeed everyone, to have an honest account of their own history."

—Could it be that all this time, all these years, our thoughts about Lenin and Stalin and Khrushchev and Brezhnev and Andropov were mistaken? "The longer you're here, the more you discover how many wrong ideas you have about the Soviets."

Ted Turner was accosted about this travesty on his own *Crossfire* feature. Pat Buchanan put it to him that this was the most concentrated pack of lies about the Soviet Union in one package since a broadcast by Goebbels on the Jews. His answer? "I wanted to go over there and paint a beautiful portrait of the Soviet Union." Pressed to explain the distortions, he just said it again. "Well, that's true, that's absolutely true, we went over there to paint a portrait, we painted a portrait, and I'm not going to apologize for it."

The wonderful irony is that when this beautiful portrait of the Soviet Union was exhibited *in* the Soviet Union, the Soviet government ran a disclaimer, criticizing the program for failing to describe the harsh realities of the Soviet Union.

This was all too much for L. Brent Bozell III, chairman of the Media Research Center in Washington, who wrote to the Encyclopaedia Britannica distributors, and got back from Mr. Michael Jirasek, who is "manager, communications services," the dumbest letter of the year. Jirasek's position is that whatever is told inadequately by the movie gets corrected by educational reading matter that accompanies it. So? Make a movie about how wonderful life was under Adolf Hitler in Germany, distribute it to all the schoolchildren, and then expose them to some light reading taking exception to this position. The Kremlin should give Turner the Order of Stalin, except that the Kremlin would be embarrassed to associate Stalin with Turner's ideas of Stalin.

—WFB   JULY 15, 1988

COME UNDRESSED AS YOU ARE

It is axiomatic that the underworlder will by ostentatious public benefactions seek the approval of the same community he systematically despoils. Mafia boss Joe Bananas supporting the local church. Billy Sol Estes hosting a Boy Scout picnic. Louis B. Mayer contributing to an institute of higher learning. No one has practiced the art of civic diversion more prodigiously than Hugh Hefner, founder of *Playboy* magazine and godfather of the sexual revolution. His formula was as straightforward as the advertisements in *Playboy* for sexually stimulating paraphernalia: make a lot of money by pandering to the sexual appetite, elevating it to primacy—then spend part of that money co-seducing critics or potential critics.

Years ago Harvard theologian Harvey Cox wrote an essay on *Playboy*, denominating it the single most brazen assault on the human female as a person in general circulation. What seemed like moments later, the same scholar found himself writing earnest essays for *Playboy*; and before long he forgot all about his mission to identify *Playboy* for what it essentially is: an organ that seeks to justify the superordination of sex over all other considerations—loyalty to family, any principle of self-discipline, any respect for privacy, or for chastity or modesty. *Sex omnia vincit*, Hugh Hefner's magazine told us, issue after issue.

Really, I wonder if anyone in the future can ever again take seriously the Anti-Defamation League. Here is an organization "dedicated to the combating of prejudice and discrimination against Jews and other minorities, and to the protection and extension of our democratic system for the benefit of all Americans." "The League," the brochure continues, "works with the various institutions of our society, public and private, religious and secular, to achieve these ends." And it is celebrating later this month its First Amendment Freedoms Award by giving a dinner-dance in honor of—Hugh M. Hefner.

About the honoree the ADL says, with an apparently straight face, that he "began with little more than a unique idea for a magazine" (nude women, jokes about copulation, and advice on how to seduce young girls) "and a philosophy of social change." (The "philosophy," quite simply, that the gratification of the male sexual impulse is to be achieved without any second thought to the possible effect on (a) the girl, (b) her family, (c) your family, (d) any code of self-restraint.) "The empire he founded has had a far-reaching impact, not only on the publishing industry, but on the mores of American society as well." That is correct. Any serious disciple of Hugh Hefner would not hesitate to purr anti-Semitic lovelies into the ears of his bunny, if that was what was required to effect seduction.

The Anti-Defamation League has, in the past, surrendered to temptations alien to its splendidly commendable purpose, namely to focus public attention on, and bring obloquy to, acts of racial discrimination. It meddled actively in the presidential campaign of 1964, endeavoring to scare its clientele into believing that Senator Goldwater was an ogre of sorts, backed by fanatics. Its current director, Mr. Nathan Perlmutter, is a man of high sensibility, gentle, firm, discriminating, a scholarly man long associated with Brandeis University. One notes that he is charging $250 a plate to guests who seek the privilege of joining with him to honor Hugh Hefner.

The tawdriness of the symbolism is driven home. Even as Hugh Hefner sells pictures of parted pudenda in order to make the dollar, a nickel of which he donates to institutions devoted to the rights of Nazis to march in Skokie, and of fellow pornographers to hawk their wares, the ADL raises money to combat discrimination by honoring the principal agent of the kind of selflessness that deprives racial toleration of the ultimate sanction. This sanction rests on a profound belief in the sanctity of the individual, yes, even that of the nubile girl. Take away from the struggle for racial toleration the profound spiritual commitment to the idea of a higher law, and the code against anti-Semitism becomes a mere matter of social convenience, the kind of upwardly mobile patter one is taught in the pages of *Playboy* to imitate, on the order of wearing Dior handkerchiefs or Gucci loafers.

Racial toleration draws its principal strength from the proposition that we are all brothers, created equal by God. The *Playboy* philosophy measures human worth by bustline and genital energy. The affair will be celebrated, appropriately enough, in Hollywood, at the Century Plaza Hotel. The invitation specifies "black tie." Well, if the guests arrive wearing only a black tie, that will be more than some of the guests wear at Hef's other parties.

—WFB   SEPTEMBER 6, 1980

Exit Mr. Shawn

It shouldn't be hard to understand the two points of view. On the one hand the frenetic undertow of competition, and the feeling that that which must eventually happen (the retirement of Mr. Shawn) should perhaps be accelerated (to accommodate anxious business and editorial pressures). That is the point of view of management, and management's concern for quality of leadership is documented by its choice of a successor, a bookish, imaginative editor, Robert Gottlieb, in some ways not unlike his legendary predecessor. When asked some time ago what were his concerns, he replied that they were his work, his reading, his family, and the ballet. He is not encumbered, in his ascendancy from editor of Knopf to editor of *The New Yorker,* by any shortage of skills or taste. His difficulty, which will probably be short-lived, is his lack of consanguinity. He was not (the objection from the second point of view) a member of the *New Yorker* family.

In a perfect world, Mr. Shawn would have lived forever. Not that there was always satisfaction: Inasmuch as Mr. Shawn's whole world was *The New Yorker*, sometimes *The New Yorker* read as though it was edited only for those whose whole world would be *The New Yorker*. But his traits were for that very reason unique: Caring only for his creature, he gave everything within his power to give, and the creeping asphyxiation of the long, leisurely time for the written arts that is a function of this hectic century was something the century would need to worry about, because Mr. Shawn would not. His ways were his ways, and those who worked with him—worked for him—knew that they had experienced true singularity in a world bent on Procrusteanism.

                    —WFB   FEBRUARY 13, 1987

DEFEAT OF CLAY, AMONG OTHERS

Time magazine's witty headline ("Defeat of Clay") gives the bare-bones story: Clay Felker lost control of *New York* magazine in 1976 . . . vowed it wouldn't happen again . . . bought *Esquire* . . . lost money . . . lost more money . . . began giving up stock for money . . . couldn't finally get more financing. . . . A Swedish conglomerate has combined with an outfit in Tennessee that publishes a giveaway, ad-oriented, ad-soaked journal for young people, is taking over. . . . "I never even *heard* of the [new owners]," wailed *Esquire*'s ace political reporter Richard Reeves. . . . New management is expected to transform the mag into a "service-oriented" journal. . . . Lotsa ads.

And not very much journalism.

One reflects on the magazine which, during the thirties, published Scott Fitzgerald and Ernest Hemingway.

Last December, Editor Clay Felker called in a young writer, one of the Roving Editors thus described on his masthead. FLASH! How about a really good piece on the King of Spain? People don't really *know* much about him. Go to Spain. Interview him. Interview everybody who knows him. Interview *everybody*. Get a *good* piece.

The writer goes to Spain, spends six weeks questioning the whole bloody Spanish establishment—prime ministers, opposition leaders, dukes, bishops, cardinals, rejected pretenders, taxi drivers—finally sees The Man himself, threads his way through a marvelously candid interview given off the record.

The writer uncovers an incredible historical footnote, heretofore unpublished: Franco got it into his head, not so long ago, that the Bourbons never really *understood* Spain, so he communicates secretly with Dr. Otto von Habsburg, who if things had gone differently in World War I would today be the emperor of Austria-Hungary; and Franco says: How would you like to be the king of Spain? Dr. Habsburg says, No thanks, I'm not much for taking other people's crowns, but thanks for asking.

The young man sweats back to New York and in ten days reduces it all to six thousand words. He has spent two months on the story. His expenses come to $2900. His salary is $830 per fortnight. Add it all up and it comes to about a dollar per word. Worth it? Every penny, I say: but *Esquire* lost four million dollars last year, doing that sort of thing; and the new owners are not likely to indulge such extravagant curiosities, let alone cultivate them.

The young writer was hired by *Esquire* six months before Clay Felker bought it. He had made a good impression on the editor-in-chief, and six months after being hired, fresh out of college, he was appointed Managing Editor. He cabled the news of his promotion to his father, who at the time was working his way around the Baltic on a cruise ship as an "enrichment lecturer." The father was very proud, and when he got back to New York, he escorted his son to the most expensive restaurant in New York for a private father-son celebration.

On that occasion, the young man, whose loyalties had clearly been involuted by his new responsibility, brazenly advised his father that the fee *Esquire* had contracted to pay for Old Dad's next scheduled piece—was too high! Old Dad mobilized all his reserves of authority, which by all accounts are formidable, and said to his son, "If you pursue this line of discussion, I shall be required to reduce your allowance." Managing Editors are not often exposed to such definitive intimidations.

Where do the writers go, in the ever-diminishing world of serious journalism? *The New Yorker* is still there, thank God; and *Harper's*, the *Atlantic*. The new *Life* runs some, but not a lot of copy; ditto the born-again *Look*. The skin mags buy some pretty expensive fig leaves. And there are the journals of opinion. A generation ago, *Esquire* apart, there was the *Saturday Evening Post, Collier's, Liberty*, a huge *Life* mag which serialized Churchill, a huge *Look,* which serialized William Manchester.

It may be true that Felker has "feet of Clay." But the bigger point is that there is less and less space in magazines willing to lay out six thousand dollars for a *really* good piece about the king of Spain. Besides, where is my son to go now for a job?

—WFB   MAY 3, 1979

Editor's Footnote

Christopher Buckley went on to other accomplishments beyond reducing WFB's fee. He is editor of *Forbes's* bright publication *FYI;* regularly writes humorous essays for *The New Yorker;* and has published several highly re-garded and popular books.

New Guard, *New York Times*

We do not disguise that beyond the reach of memory, we at *National Review* have used the *New York Times* as our very favorite pincushion. Much of this the paper has earned, particularly in its editorial pages where, especially under the leadership of an editor providentially retired several years ago, the *Times* was militantly, not to say disreputably, tone-deaf, showing an enthusiasm for such disparate calamities as Fidel Castro and John Lindsay.

But the *New York Times* even then was a very great newspaper, with a profound sense of its responsibility to cover the news, even if the temptation, often, was to do so tendentiously, as when Barry Goldwater ran for President. But the news last weekend of a shifting of the guard brings to mind how heavily indebted all readers of the *New York Times,* and all readers of readers of the *New York Times,* are to A. M. Rosenthal for the extraordinary vision he brought to the paper, which he dominated (save only the editorial pages) for almost twenty years. The brightness of the Gray Lady, its appetite for the news, for features, for supplements, the sheer universality of its coverage make it the outstanding newspaper in the world. It is sad that Mr. Rosenthal is retiring, but reassuring to know that the traditions he accepted and reinforced will be maintained by his successors.

Mr. Rosenthal once noted that it is not easy for the editor of the *New York Times* to move through the city with any sense of security, as the *Times* is blamed for everything that goes wrong. (It should be blamed for only about half of what goes wrong.) He cited to the editor of this journal an example: One evening, after a very long day at work, he eased into his bed and pulled out the freshest issue of *National Review,* opened it, and read in the lead editorial, "Abe? Abe Rosenthal! Are you listening, goddammit? That story you published last week about . . ." *Requiescat in pace.* Abe Rosenthal will write two columns per week for the Op-Ed page; Arthur Gelb, his gifted associate, will serve as managing editor; and Max Frankel, from the editorial page he substantially rescued, will be the new boss. Best wishes to them all. Goddammit.

—WFB   NOVEMBER 7, 1986

Dear Mr. Buckley:

A few years ago [the newspaperman] Bob Considine wrote from Nairobi that he "never knew until this trip that 'hippopotamus' means river horse in Latin." We must, however, make allowances for Bob. Being a liberal, he labors under the misapprehension that history began with the French Revolution and is probably totally unaware of the existence of Classical Greek.

However, in your column of today's date in the *San Antonio Light* I read: "An acting President cannot be made to feel like Macbeth's uncle, the successor king, sleeping in incestuous sheets."

Referring you to *Hamlet,* Act I, Scene 2, Lines 156 and 157, I remind you that I have adduced an excuse for Bob, but I would like to hear yours.

Sincerely,

MURL J. MANLOVE

SAN ANTONIO, TEXAS

Dear Mr. Manlove:

Come on. I am perfectly capable of typing out the sentence, "When Washington delivered his Gettysburg address . . ." I mean, that kind of thing happens. When it does, it should be caught (a) by me, when I reread my column; failing that (b) by my office, if the column is on that day traveling to the syndicate via my office; (c) by the syndicate before it sends it out to the newspapers; (d) by the newspaper editor before sending it to be set; (e) by the proofreader on reading proof. It is safer, when a fail-safe mechanism as elaborate as this fails, to assume that all human systems are capable of concerted carelessness, than that the entire editorial structure of American journalism has lapsed into historical or literary amnesia. Cordially,

—WFB   MARCH 1, 1974

What's So Bad About Writing Fast?

If, during spring term at Yale University in 1949 you wandered diagonally across the campus noticing here and there an undergraduate with impacted sleeplessness under his eyes and coarse yellow touches of fear on his cheeks, you were looking at members of a masochistic set who had enrolled in a course called Daily Themes. No Carthusian novitiate embarked on a bout of mortification of the flesh suffered more than the students of Daily Themes, whose single assignment, in addition to attending two lectures per week, was to write a 500-to-600-word piece of descriptive prose every day, and to submit it before midnight (into a large box outside a classroom). Sundays were the only exception (this was before the Warren Court outlawed Sunday).

For anyone graduated from Daily Themes who went on to write, in journalism or in fiction or wherever, the notion that a burden of 500 words per day is the stuff of nightmares is laughable. But caution: 500 words a day is what Graham Greene writes, and Nabokov wrote 180 words per day, devoting to their composition four or five hours. But at that rate, Graham Greene and Nabokov couldn't qualify for a job as reporters on the *New York Times*. Theirs is high-quality stuff, to speak lightly of great writing. But Georges Simenon is also considered a great writer, at least by those who elected him to the French Academy, and he writes books in a week or so. Dr. Johnson wrote *Rasselas,* his philosophical romance, in nine days. And Trollope . . . we'll save Trollope.

I am fired up on the subject because, to use a familiar formulation, they have been kicking me around a lot; it has got out that I write fast, which is qualifiedly true. In this august journal [the *New York Times Book Review*] on January 5, Morton Kondracke of *Newsweek* took it all the way: "He [me—WFB] reportedly knocks out his column in twenty minutes flat—three times a week for 260 newspapers. That is too little time for serious contemplation of difficult subjects."

Now that is a declaration of war, and I respond massively.

To begin with: it is axiomatic, in cognitive science, that there is no necessary correlation between profundity of thought and length of time spent on thought. JFK is reported to have spent fifteen hours per day for six days before deciding exactly how to respond to the missile crisis, but it can still be argued that his initial impulse on being informed that the Soviet Union had deployed nuclear missiles in Cuba (bomb the hell out of the missile sites?) might have been the strategically sounder course. This is not an argument against deliberation, merely against the suggestion that to think longer (endlessly?) about a subject is necessarily to probe it more fruitfully.

Mr. Kondracke, for reasons that would require more than twenty minutes to fathom, refers to composing columns in twenty minutes "flat." Does he mean to suggest that I have a stopwatch which rings on the twentieth minute? Or did he perhaps mean to say that I have been known to write a column in twenty minutes? Very different. He then goes on, in quite another connection, to cite "one of the best columns" in my new book—without thinking to ask: How long did it take him to write that particular column?

The chronological criterion, you see, is without validity. Every few years, I bring out a collection of previously published work, and this of course requires me to reread everything I have done in order to make that season's selections. It transpires that it is impossible to distinguish a column written very quickly from a column written very slowly. Perhaps that is because none is written very slowly. A column that requires two hours to write is one which was interrupted by phone calls or the need to check a fact. I write fast—but not, I'd maintain, remarkably fast. If Mr. Kondracke thinks it intellectually risky to write 750 words in twenty minutes, what must he think about people who speak 750 words in five minutes, as he often does on television?

The subject comes up now so regularly in reviews of my work that I did a little methodical research on my upcoming novel. I began my writing (in Switzerland, removed from routine interruption) at about 5 P.M., and wrote usually for two hours. I did that for forty-five working days (the stretch was interrupted by a week in the United States, catching up on editorial and television obligations). I then devoted the first ten days in July to revising the manuscript. On these days I worked on the manuscript an average of six hours per day, including retyping. We have now a grand total: 90 plus 60, or 150 hours. My novels are about 70,000 words, so that averaged out to roughly 500 words per hour.

Anthony Trollope rose at five every morning, drank his tea, performed his toilette and looked at the work done the preceding day. He would then begin to write at six. He set himself the task of writing 250 words every fifteen minutes for three and one-half hours. Indeed it is somewhere recorded that if he had not, at the end of fifteen minutes, written the required 250 words he would simply "speed up" the next quarter-hour, because he was most emphatic in his insistence on his personally imposed daily quota: 3,500 words.

Now the advantages Trollope enjoys over me are enumerable and nonenumerable. I write only about the former, and oddly enough they are negative advantages. He needed to write by hand, having no alternative. I use a word processor. Before beginning this article, I tested my speed on this instrument and discovered that I type more slowly than I had imagined. Still, it comes out at eighty words per minute. So that if Trollope had had an IBM, he'd have written, in three and one-half hours at my typing speed, not 3,500 words but 16,800 words per day.

Ah, you say, but could anyone think that fast? The answer is, sure people can think that fast. How did you suppose extemporaneous speeches get made? Erle Stanley Gardner dictated his detective novels nonstop to a series of secretaries, having previously pasted about in his studio 3-by-5 cards reminding him at exactly what hour the dog barked, the telephone rang, the murderer coughed. He knew where he was going, the plot was framed in his mind, and it became now only an act of extrusion. Margaret Coit wrote in her biography of John C. Calhoun that his memorable speeches were composed not in his study but while he was outdoors, plowing the fields on his plantation. He would return then to his study and write out what he had framed in his mind. His writing was an act of transcription. I own the holograph of Albert Jay Nock's marvelous book on Jefferson, and there are fewer corrections on an average page than I write into a typical column. Clearly Nock knew exactly what he wished to say and how to say it; prodigious rewriting was, accordingly, unnecessary.

Having said this, I acknowledge that I do not know exactly what I am going to say, or exactly how I am going to say it. And in my novels, I can say flatly, as Mr. Kondracke would have me say it, that I really do not have any idea where they are going—which ought not to surprise anyone familiar with the nonstop exigencies of soap opera writing or of comic strip writing or, for that matter, of regular Sunday sermons. It is not necessary to know how your protagonist will get out of a jam into which you put him. It requires only that you have confidence that you will be able to get him out of that jam. When you begin to write a column on, let us say, the reaction of Western Europe to President Reagan's call for a boycott of Libya, it is not necessary that you should know *exactly* how you will say what you will end up saying. You are, while writing, drawing on huge reserves: of opinion, prejudice, priorities, presumptions, data, ironies, drama, histrionics. And these reserves you enhance during practically the entire course of the day, and it doesn't matter all that much if a particular hour is not devoted to considering problems of foreign policy. You can spend an hour playing the piano and develop your capacity to think, even to create; and certainly you can grasp more keenly, while doing so, your feel for priorities.

The matter of music flushes out an interesting point: Why is it that critics who find it arresting that a column can be written in twenty minutes, a book in 150 hours, do not appear to find it remarkable that a typical graduate of Juilliard can memorize a prelude and fugue from "The Well-Tempered Clavier" in an hour or two? It would take me six months to memorize one of those *números*. And mind, we're not talking here about the *Guinness Book of World Records* types. Isaac Asimov belongs in *Guinness* . . . but surely not an author who averages a mere 500 words per hour, or who occasionally writes a column at one-third his typing speed!

There are phenomenal memories in the world. Claudio Arrau is said to hold in his memory music for forty recitals, two and a half hours each. *That* is phenomenal. Ralph Kirkpatrick, the late harpsichordist, actually told me that he had not played the "Goldberg" Variations for twenty years before playing it to a full house in New Haven in the spring of 1950. *That* is phenomenal. Winston Churchill is said to have memorized all of "Paradise Lost" in a week, and throughout his life he is reported to have been able to memorize his speeches after a couple of readings. (I have a speech I have delivered fifty times, and could not recite one paragraph of it by heart.)

So cut it out, Kondracke. I am, I fully grant, a phenomenon, but not because of any speed in composition. I asked myself the other day, Who else, on so many issues, has been so right so much of the time? I couldn't think of anyone. And I devoted to the exercise twenty minutes. Flat.

—WFB   FEBRUARY 19, 1986

Chapter 12

A Columnist on Column Writing— and on Choosing Carefully Your Words and Your Opponents

At times, the tension between writers dueling in public almost snaps the bonds of friendship that, in many cases, lie beneath. Buckley's jousts with Professor John Kenneth Galbraith over the years—and they *are* friends— reminds one of the desirability of picking worthy adversaries. I have often thought that (as WFB suggested to Kilpatrick) they could take their act on the road. As indeed they have done, or at least in print.

The touchiness and testiness between WFB and another regular opponent—a regular guest on *Firing Line*—threaten to stretch on into the next century.

THE VIOLATION OF ARTHUR

Just after Mr. Kennedy's inauguration, I met with Professor Arthur Schlesinger, Jr., historian and dogmatic theologian for Americans for Democratic Action, in public debate in Boston on the subject of the welfare state. It was on that occasion that Mr. Schlesinger, countering some point or other I had made, announced that the "best defense against communism is the welfare state." Now everybody expects that professors will say foolish things from time to time, but Professor Schlesinger had just then taken leave of Harvard to accept a position as special assistant to the fledgling President of the United States, so that a great deal of publicity was given to that remarkable statement. A decent interval should have elapsed before an egghead academician would presume to press such homeopathic nonsense about how to deal with communism on practical men of exalted station but the assembly was sobered on witnessing the professor's grand entry into the lecture hall, twenty minutes late, escorted by screeching police cars—it obviously hadn't taken long for Mr. Schlesinger to acquire princely habits.

And along with them, it is my sad duty here to report, he seems to have lost—an occupational risk for humble folk who suddenly find themselves supping with the great—whatever sense of humor he once possessed.

Schlesinger had been accustomed to such fawning audiences as he regularly came upon at Harvard and elsewhere in the academic world, where they preach academic freedom and practice liberal indoctrination; and was quite visibly disconcerted on discovering from the audience's reaction that one half of those present were quite adamantly opposed to his views and those of the New Frontiersmen. Under the circumstances, he thought to curry the opposition's favor by handing me, as their spokesman of the evening, a most redolent bouquet. Quoth Arthur: "Mr. Buckley has a facility for rhetoric which I envy, as well as a wit which I seek clumsily and vainly to emulate." The crowd (or my half of it) purred with pleasure. As an old debater, I knew exactly what he was up to, and determined, when my turn came to rebut, to say something equally oleaginous about Arthur. But I had only fifteen minutes before getting up to speak during which to compose a compliment, and I guess my imagination failed me—I forget.

And indeed I forgot about the whole incident until a couple of months ago when I received a letter from a lady in Boston who had been there that night. She cited Mr. Schlesinger's cream puff to illustrate his exemplary "fairness to the opposite political camp." It happened that at just that moment I was supposed to furnish my publishers with some quotations for the jacket of my new book, *Rumbles Left and Right.* I thought it would be mad fun to include the words of Arthur Schlesinger—you know, sort of the literary oxymoron of the year.

Well sir, you'd have thought this was the biggest swindle since the Donation of Constantine. A few weeks ago, while minding my own business, I received a frantic telegram from my publisher announcing that Arthur Schlesinger, having seen the blurb in an advertisement for my book in *National Review,* demanded to know where and when he had said any such thing about me. I wired back: "MY OFFICE HAS COPY OF ORIGINAL TAPE. TELL ARTHUR *THAT'LL* TEACH HIM TO USE UNCTION IN POLITICAL DEBATE BUT NOT TO TAKE IT SO HARD: NO ONE BELIEVES ANYTHING HE SAYS ANYWAY." Needless to say, I sent a copy of the telegram to Mr. Schlesinger, with the postscript: "Dear Arthur: I am at work on a new book which, however, will not be completed until the spring of 1964, giving you plenty of time to compose a new puff for it. Regards." And then, on the upper left-hand corner of the letter, properly addressed to Mr. Schlesinger at his august quarters (The White House, Washington, D.C.), I wrote, "Wm. 'Envy His Rhetoric!' Buckley," with my return address.

That, apparently, did it. Before even Arthur could say "I-believe-in Free-Speech," the firm of Messrs. Greenbaum, Wolff and Ernst let it be known to my publisher and to *National Review* that they would demand an apology—or Schlesinger would sue. Now there is a very good case to be made for everyone apologizing who has ever quoted Arthur Schlesinger; but isn't it droll to be asked to apologize *to* Schlesinger for quoting *from* Schlesinger? Messrs. G., W. & E. have solemnly announced that I have "invaded Mr. Schlesinger's privacy . . ." A most interesting complaint, considering that Mr. Schlesinger's words had been uttered before an audience of fifteen hundred or so, before television and radio, and before members of the press and the wire services. For someone who wants what he says to be kept private . . . that's a strange way to go about it, wouldn't you say? . . .

Ah well, it is a mad world. But I shall certainly put in for next year's Freedom Award. On the grounds that the more time Schlesinger devotes to me, the less time he has left over to devote to public affairs.

—WFB   MARCH 30, 1963

The brouhaha continued, with less haha. An exchange with lawyers and several parting shots followed, though, as often with Buckley, the shots were neither fatal nor intended as such.

Schlesinger *vs.* Buckley *et al.*

Mr. Arthur Schlesinger has told the press he does *not* intend to sue Putnam's or *National Review* or William Buckley for their outrageous decision to quote his sentences on the dust jacket of *Rumbles Left and Right.* So WFB wrote to Messrs. Greenbaum, Wolff and Ernst and asked, Is it all off? To which they replied, in effect, Never mind what Arthur said to the press, we will hold you "fully responsible" for "any further use of the quotation by anyone in conjunction with the promotion, sale or advertising of" *Rumbles Left and Right* . . . Our letter to the lawyers had included a P.S.: "While you are at it, would you be so kind as to ask Mr. Schlesinger to okay the following translation of his quotation into French: '*Monsieur Buckley a une facilité de rhetorique que j'envie de même qu'un bel esprit que je tâche maladroitement d'imiter et sans succés.*'" But the lawyers' reply ignored the request . . . Mr. Schlesinger, by the way, told *Newsweek* he had said the words in "ironic derision." We propose to announce, shortly, the availability of a 45 rpm recording of Mr. Schlesinger saying all those nice things about Mr. Buckley . . . By the way, did you know that Mr. Schlesinger finds *National Review* "entertaining reading"? Well, he does. He said so. Same debate. Context? "I think we are all charmed by the characteristically delightful mixture of fantasy and hyperbole which Mr. Buckley has served us, and which makes his magazine such entertaining reading." Tell your Liberal friends! *Schlesinger finds National Review entertaining reading!* Never mind his pixyish phrase, "mixture of fantasy and hyperbole"—he was just being ironically derisive. . . . Being mustered: National Committee to Secure Privacy for Arthur Schlesinger, Jr. . . . A columnist, Mr. Wm. Hogan of the *San Francisco Chronicle,* reviewed *Rumbles* two weeks ago, before the brawl was made public. . . . Gist of review: Buckley is awful, everybody he disapproves of is wonderful, and everybody he likes is almost as awful as Buckley, though not quite. And then (. . . So help us, we didn't put him up to it), "Even Arthur Schlesinger, Jr., another of Buckley Jr.'s arch enemies, has been quoted on his fellow essayist: 'He has a facility for rhetoric [etc., etc.]' No question about it—he is one of the most suave and challenging writers around." Ho! ho! ho! Er. Harrumph! AttenSHUN GREENbaum! Wolff! Ernst! Sue that man Hogan! (Not to be continued.)

—WFB   APRIL 30, 1963

Exchanges with Schlesinger followed over the years—some funny, some a touch acrimonious—but the historian and sometime political figure continued to be one of Buckley's favorite adversaries. None can claim service in such a long-running dogfight, however, as that between WFB and John Kenneth Galbraith. In the next column, WFB reports on what happens when writers on holiday gather in one small village with a hard-pressed bookstore.

THE GREAT CADONAU WAR

GSTAAD, SWITZERLAND.—Gstaad is a sleepy little town that bustles two or three months per year, when people descend on it in great numbers, most of them to ski or to look at the skiers, or to drink with them. Everyone runs into everyone at Cadonau's, which is where one picks up the daily edition of the *International Herald Tribune,* paint supplies, Scotch tape, stationery—and, occasionally, a book.

Madame Cadonau's window is a showcase for a few recently published books which are there in three languages, available for the occasional tourist in Gstaad who knows how to read. The saga of the past few months has to do with my looking into the showcase to find prominently displayed David Niven's bestseller, *The Moon's a Balloon.* Mr. Niven is a local resident who is very highly regarded. It came as something of a blow to the professional writers in residence when Mr. Niven managed to dash off a superbly written bestseller. The comment of the playwright George Axelrod was dead on: "How dare he write so well? Do I go about playing British colonels?" Fortunately, Mr. Niven is not a professionally qualified skier—otherwise he would be intolerable.

I felt no resentment at all against the display of his book. But just next to it was another book by a famous local resident—*War, Economics, and Laughter,* by John Kenneth Galbraith. Bad enough, I thought, to pollute this unspoiled Alpine retreat by displaying a book by Mr. Galbraith, but altogether intolerable in light of the fact that a chapter in it is devoted to the disparagement of a classic on municipal government written by a third distinguished writer-in-residence of the area, to wit, me.

Added to this slight was the mysterious nonappearance of my own recently published book, a lacuna which Madame Cadonau embarrassedly explained on the grounds that the book, though ordered months ago, had not arrived presumably because of the New York dock strike. I replied that New York's longshoremen are distinctly my kind of people, and I could not imagine their consenting to load the innocent bottoms of Liberian transports with books by Galbraith, and declining to ease their conscience by supplying them with my own. I called New York and had air-expressed six copies to Madame Cadonau, and then went to China.

I returned to find, in the window, all the old entries, plus a paperback of Mr. Galbraith's *Ambassador's Journal.* I thereupon collected from an old trunk a copy of my anthology of conservative writing, and handed it, wordlessly, to Madame Cadonau, who dutifully shoehorned it into her feverish window. The next day, I saw there a copy of *The New Industrial State*—in German, which is the kind of thing that happens when Galbraith decides to pull rank. I wired New York and got hold of the single extant copy, in German, of a book I had a hand in writing eighteen years ago on Senator McCarthy, which desiring not to lose it (there were only eighty-seven copies printed), I priced at a level beyond the reach even of the ski set of Gstaad.

At this point it had become necessary to retire from the window *Everything You Always Wanted to Know About Sex,* by Dr. Reuben, and everything you didn't want to know about sex by Harold Robbins. Everyone has been moved out except of course David Niven, and now the showcase has in it the original doctoral dissertation of Professor Galbraith, written in 1936 and entitled, "Economic Reasons Why the Government of South Vietnam Cannot Last Another Fortnight." That one was hard to beat, but I have written to Buckingham Palace for the original of a letter I dispatched to King George when Mr. Galbraith was a sophomore at college.

Late last night, a tall, lean man with a lock of graying hair was spotted going into the back door of Madame Cadonau's, so I have today written to Dr. Kissinger to ask him please to make a secret visit to Madame Cadonau, who has for days now refused to move from her upstairs apartment, and to promise mutual de-escalation and the repatriation of all American incunabula, as tensions diminish. I believe in taking the initiative, where peace is concerned.

—WFB   MARCH 14, 1972

———

Buckley, the columnist, occasionally makes a mistake or is charged with having made one, and at times his responses make you glad he made the mistake, for the reward of what ensues.

———

Explain *Why* You Get Up in the Morning!

As a columnist myself, I try to keep in mind that as often as not it is as easy to do the natural thing as the unnatural thing, and that therefore it makes sense to be reasonably sure that the man on whom you have trained your sights is in fact acting inexplicably, before closing your finger on the trigger. Drew Pearson types need to operate on a quite different assumption, namely that a public figure will go out of his way in order to betray his trust. Okay. So? So it pays to remember that Drew Pearson types are doing what comes naturally to them when they ascribe venal motives to their victims, venal motives being the gas on which they fuel their engines.

My brothers Evans and Novak are not, by and large, Drew Pearson types, but occasionally they feel the tug, most recently at my expense. They say that Washington is buzzing over my role as "bard" for Frank Shakespeare, the Director of the United States Information Agency, because I have been "singing his praises with the help of the taxpayers' money." Altogether disreputable, they suggest, inasmuch as I am a member of the President's Advisory Commission on Information, charged under the law with "conducting forthright appraisals of USIA policies."

The criticism is in two parts.

One: Money. Yes, I *have* traveled "at the taxpayers' expense," which is how they always phrase it when they want to taint a use of public money.

The three trips in question, one to Vienna, one to Russia, a third to Vietnam, were taken at the instigation of Mr. Shakespeare. After two of those trips, I reported my findings to the President, at his request. After one of those trips, I was called to testify before a congressional committee, to report my findings, which I did, and got from the Democratic chairman of that committee his most effusive thanks.

Mr. Jack Anderson last summer complained that my air travel was paid during these trips even though I wrote columns as I traveled. I advised his assistant, who was kind enough to call me on the telephone, that that was indeed true. But when I am asked by a government agency to go somewhere for purposes prescribed by it, I shall damned well charge the government for fare. My philanthropy is my time. The commission's members are unpaid.

Two: Messrs. Evans and Novak take Jack Anderson's complaint a step further. Their complaint isn't that I write columns when I travel for the USIA (I write columns wherever I am, that being what my contract requires), but that when I travel, I write "glowingly" about the USIA. Consider, those of you who are interested in the uses of rhetoric, the following sentence from E & N: "When Buckley was attacked in the press for using taxpayers' money to travel the world and write encomiums for the head of the agency he oversees . . ." Tricky? (a) The "press" never "attacked" me, Jack Anderson did, and there is, thank God, still a difference. (b) Anderson's attack wasn't that I traveled in order to write encomiums of the agency, but that I wrote anything at all. But never mind, E & N have insinuated their point.

Now, as to the impropriety of writing "encomiums" on the Director of USIA, (a) In fact I never wrote one, (b) I have written two columns about Mr. Shakespeare. The first I wrote while in Vienna. The subject? Shakespeare's wonderful performance in Vienna? The glories of meeting with USIA's choir boys in Vienna? No, the subject was the attack on him by Joe McGinniss in the book *The Selling of the President,* which was published while I was in Vienna, in which Mr. McGinniss suggested that Mr. Shakespeare's views on communism were naïve. Inasmuch as Mr. Shakespeare's views on communism are exactly the same as my own, I tend to the conclusion that they are not naïve. Therefore I defended Shakespeare.

The other column I have written in defense of Mr. Shakespeare was when he was the object of a considerable attack by *Pravda* a few weeks ago. I wrote that column in New York City, and I did not charge the depreciation on my typewriter to the USIA.

All of which is awesomely trivial . . . if there is an effective anti-Communist who has *not* been praised by me, do me the favor, and send me his name. I shall then write about him. And Anderson, Evans and

Novak will construct an evil motivation, so that you may understand why I did as I did.

—WFB   JANUARY 5, 1971

The Ethics of Junketing

My friend Mr. Mike Wallace, a gentleman who is given to protracted concern with scruple, called recently in his diligent way to inquire what are my rules concerning "junkets," by which he means trips paid for by someone else. He proposes to do a television program on the subject, and I am grateful to him for his maieutic inquiry about my own views, which had not crystallized.

1. When a columnist is invited on a trip, he should begin by asking whether the host expects that his guest will write about the trip. Obviously if you are invited, say, to look in at the opening of Disney World, your hosts expect that you will write about Disney World. If you are invited (as I along with 1,000 others were) to travel in great luxury to witness the dedication of a new refining plant in a distant arctic archipelago, your host clearly does not expect that you will write about the plant.

2. In the second case, then, there is obviously no inhibition in accepting the invitation. In the first, you need to say to yourself: if I find that Disney World is a great bust, will I feel altogether free to say so notwithstanding that the trip down was paid for, as also the hotel bill? That question is only coped with by the injunction: to thine own self be true. But here a qualification is appropriate. Going to Florida and back is not a very big deal, in this peripatetic age. So that the indebtedness of the visiting journalist is not really as heavy as, say, a trip to, well, Mozambique, to examine the policies of the Portuguese government there.

3. Here the situation becomes more complex, and more interesting. On the one hand there are newspapers that pridefully insist that no journalist should travel to a foreign country at that country's expense because implicit obligations are incurred. That point of view is defensible.

But there is another point of view. It is a part of a journalist's duty to move about, and to report to his readers on what he sees. Most often he will use his own money to pay the fare. But—and here are more subqualifications—sometimes (a) the trip is too expensive to justify the amount of time the journalist reasons he can devote to the subject (how many columns can one write about Mozambique?); and (b) sometimes the journalist is simply not certain whether the trip will produce anything interesting enough to justify the trip.

It is my opinion that in such circumstances the journalist should feel free to accept the round-trip fare, cutting his potential losses to his own time.

But once again he must know that he will feel free to write as he sees the situation, without any inhibition deriving from the auspices. This is especially difficult because one often tends to lean over backward to establish one's analytical independence, and that is as unjust as to shill. To say the problem is easily solved by simply avoiding the temptation is to take the easy way out.

Some examples, from my personal experience:

I traveled, at the expense of South Africa and the Portuguese Government, eleven years ago, to South Africa and Mozambique. I wrote three columns, and a long essay-piece. Where I came out on the general subject of South African domestic policies is, I suppose, best situated by saying that a pro-South African committee in the United States made reprints of my essay, while the government of South Africa refused to distribute it.

I traveled over one hectic weekend, at the expense of the government of Northern Ireland, to view the situation there just before Orangeman's Day. It was an excruciatingly uncomfortable trip of seventy-two hours. I wrote three columns, in which I find not a hint of servility to my hosts.

I traveled, at the expense of the United States Government, from New Zealand to the Antarctic, and stayed there five days, visiting the South Pole and writing about U.S. operations there. This is one for the naturalists, and though I treasure the experience, I would not undergo it again, even to bring peace with honor to the nations that contend there for scientific advancement.

The general impression is that such jaunts are offered daily to columnists. That has not been my experience. Of course, it is possible that from afar they smell in me that incorruptibility that causes the angels and the saints to chant my name.

—WFB   DECEMBER 25, 1973

[CHRISTMAS]

COLUMNISTS ARE PEOPLE

People who write newspaper columns are also people, and that is a great, but unexpungeable, distraction. It is sometimes useful to be a people, in addition to a newspaper columnist—there is no other way, for instance, to have a family, or to drink good wine, or engage avocationally in other practices than writing a column. But let me, just this one time, share my problems with you as a fellow people, giving four examples.

1. A fortnight ago, a tape was played at the Watergate trial. The voice of President Nixon came in loud and clear, talking to Haldeman, discussing clemency for Howard Hunt. He said: "We'll build, we'll build that son-of-a-bitch up, like nobody's business. We'll have Buckley write a column and say, you know, that he, that he should have clemency . . ."

Within a very few minutes, my office reached me at the airport en route to Boston. The newspapers had begun to call in, asking the obvious question: Was Mr. Buckley approached? Does he have any comment? I dictated over the telephone two sentences that were then given by my office to the *New York Post,* the *New York Times,* and the Associated Press: "At no time did any member of the Nixon Administration approach me. Besides, I don't need to be reminded to write columns urging clemency even for sons-of-bitches, as Mr. Nixon has every reason to know from personal experience."

The next morning, the charge was carried very conspicuously in the *Boston Globe*—together with my retort, which I also saw in the New York papers and in *Time* magazine. Notwithstanding, I have received much mail asking why I was silent on the subject raised at the Watergate trial. And two large newspapers have carried letters by readers suggesting that I have been an appendage of the Nixon Administration—without any comment from the editor bringing to the writer's attention my brief reply. One more example of the difficulty of catching up with a misleading story:

2. A month ago, I wrote a column on the now famous [Arthur] Goldberg book by Victor Lasky, in which I expressed the view—having now read the book—that although it was of course hostile to Justice Goldberg, it was far from being libelous. I remarked that the only distortion in it was Lasky's statement that Mr. Goldberg was the worst public speaker in the State of New York, since in fact he was the worst in the country. I received a letter from a journalist who covered the campaign advising me that it was going the rounds of the boys in the bus toward the end, that "if Goldberg gives one more speech, Rockefeller will carry Canada." Mr. Goldberg called me on the telephone and was extremely amiable, and made no criticism of the book, merely of its provenance.

I did not note, in my column, that I am the chairman of the board of the parent company that owned the company (Arlington House) that published the Goldberg book. I did not do this for two reasons. The first was that when the book was first discussed, my position in the corporate hierarchy was widely identified, so that I proceeded on the happy or, if you prefer, unhappy assumption that most people knew about it. The second reason is that never having heard of the book before, I was in no way implicated in the decision to publish it. But if I had mentioned my corporate affiliation in the column, I'd have had to go on to make the connecting point, and this struck me, on balance, as unnecessarily self-concerned. Result: a big article in *Editor & Publisher* on whether my omission of my connection was ethically correct. You decide.

3. Maybe four or five times a year, I am greatly struck by an article or analysis published in *National Review.* Now I am the editor-in-chief of

National Review, and its sole owner. So when I mention the article, I give the name of the author—but leave out the name of the magazine where the article was published, lest it should appear that I am attempting to advertise my impecunious but magnificent journal (150 East 35th Street, New York 10016—$12 per year). Then I get mail asking me how could I have been so sloppy as to fail to give the name of the journal where the article I wrote about appeared. . . .

Finally, (4), there is no way to avoid writing, occasionally, about the doings and sayings of James Lane Buckley. How should I identify him? As "My brother the senator"? That has the obvious disadvantage of calling attention to myself, and the less obvious disadvantage of snuggling up against the cognate cliché, "my son the doctor." So, I resolved to refer to him as "the sainted junior senator from New York." Hyperbole is a form of self-effacement; but I still get a letter or two, complaining. These I answer by expressing great surprise that the reader is unaware of the beatific character of the junior senator from New York. But there, now, you share my problems this one time, and I shan't ask you soon again to share them. Many thanks.

—WFB   DECEMBER 5, 1974

Dear Mr. B.:

If you wrote the enclosed column, I'll change my religion from Catholic to atheist, my Republican affiliation to liberal—and I'll even eat the goddam newspaper. Well????????

Faithfully,

AL PACETTA

VERO BEACH, FLA.

Dear Mr. Pacetta: I am happy to be the instrument of retaining your religious and political faiths and the good order of your stomach: No, I did not write it. Sometimes newspapers run me under Art Buchwald's logo, and AB under my logo, the cumulative result of which is to make me seem funnier than I am, and him wiser than he is. But I don't even recognize the columnist whose wild meanderings appeared in the *Vero Beach Press-Journal* (Oct. 16) under my name. Cordially,

—WFB   DECEMBER 5, 1986

STUCK?

It is conceivably of interest to the world out there what happens when a columnist gets stuck . . .

You see, poring over a table of figures, I wrote yesterday a careful piece announcing certain conclusions about the nature of economic distribution that I thought astonishing. Indeed they proved to be. Later that day, at a social function, I accosted a very bright gentleman, head of a big banking house in New York, and announced my findings to him. Startled is not quite the word to describe his reaction. He said I was quite simply wrong. Not possible, I said, citing the source of my figures.

Half an hour ago, when my researcher got to the office, I telephoned and told her that, just to be sure, she might check. Ten minutes later she rang to say that the gentleman who had put the chart together intended that it should be read—well, upside down is the best way to put it. The difficulty then—and it happens to columnists every now and then, though I don't remember in twenty years its coming quite so close—is how to write interestingly on no notice whatever, running (in this case) between engagements in Chicago, live appearances, one more or less on top of another, which cannot be put off. The question is whether, in the interstices, I can meet my professional obligations to this newspaper.

Once, two or three years ago, I was doing a program with the amiable Mr. Gene Shalit of NBC. Everything went swimmingly. Too swimmingly. Because he played me like a cobra, undulating hypnotically this way, that way, as I gradually lost any sense of caution. He said then: "How do you know what to write about, when you write a column?" I found myself saying, "Gene, when you have been at the profession for long enough, you can, if in a bind, close your eyes and point to the front page of the *New York Times,* and whatever story you are fingering when you open your eyes—you can write a column on that story."

"Yes"—Shalit struck—"I think I remember that column."

Victor Borge documented the art of improvisation as practiced by a musician. During his great one-man show he neared the end, turned to the audience and asked for volunteers to pronounce any one of the first seven letters of the alphabet. He would point to one and then to another, until he had a series: A G E F B D C. These, of course, correspond to musical notes. He would sit down and tap the notes out in consecutive order. Then he would vest a little rhythm into the sequence, and suddenly a tune emerged. This tune he played out in the style, respectively, of Bach, Mozart, Schumann, Chopin, Brahms, Liszt, Gershwin. A smash exhibition of improvisatory powers.

But a scribbler cannot easily duplicate a musician's powers—though I suppose a poet, or the versifier, could do so. Write a piece, without the opportunity to research, on this morning's stories on the front page of the *Chicago Tribune:* "Embassy Raiders Release Four More." Well, you could go on a bit about international terrorism, but we've done that. "Cut U.S. Deficits/IMF Nations Ask." Not bad, actually. Representatives of the nations of the world meet in Toronto to accuse the United States of economic malpractices, such as deficit spending and inflation. You could play with that, but you would need to dig up the corresponding figures of our critics. It would be fun if one of those were a representative of Mexico. Or Brazil. Or Argentina. Or Great Britain. But you see the problem.

"Israel Demands Security Zone/In Lebanon As Tensions Grow." Oh no! Not another column on Israel and Lebanon. You cannot do that to the American-speaking world. Not after a dozen columns on the subject during the past dozen weeks. And, finally, "Health Hazard Waste Heads for Chicago." No, that won't play even in Peoria, which is near enough to Chicago and probably shares Chicago's concerns.

So you sit—you have max twelve, fourteen minutes, and you think: What on earth can I write about? It is a pickle, and so you sit down and write a column about human nature or the United Nations or John Kenneth Galbraith, all of them, always, live wires.

—WFB   SEPTEMBER 11, 1982

FROM *OVERDRIVE*

George Will once told me how deeply he loves to write. "I wake in the morning," he explained to me, "and I ask myself: 'Is this one of the days I have to write a column?' And if the answer is 'Yes,' I rise a happy man." I, on the other hand, wake neither particularly happy nor unhappy, but to the extent that my mood is affected by the question whether I need to write a column that morning, the impact of Monday-Wednesday-Friday is definitely negative. Because I do not like to write, for the simple reason that writing is extremely hard work, and I do not "like" extremely hard work.

I work for other reasons, about which mostly dull people write, dully. (I have discerned that those who are given to the formulation, "I am one of those people who . . ." would generally be safest concluding the sentence, ". . . bore other people.") Is it some aspect of a sense of duty that I feel? Moral evangelism? A fear of uselessness? A fear that it is wrong to suppress useful, here defined extramorally as merchandisable, talent? I do resist introspection, though I cannot claim to have "guarded" against it, because even to say that would suppose that the temptation to do so was there, which it isn't. Indeed, these very words are prompted by an imperative handed to me by my friend and editor Sam Vaughan, the least imperious of men: but curiosity is, in such circumstances, his professional business. Why do I do so much? I expect that the promptings issue from a subtle dialectical counterpoint. Of what? Well, the call of *recta ratio,* and the fear of boredom. What is *recta ratio?* The appeal of generic Latin terms (*habeas corpus, nihil obstat, malum prohibitum*) derives in part because the language is indeed dead and therefore unmoved by idiomatic fashion. In part, however, it is owing to the complementary character of its tantalizing inscrutability. It is just faintly defenseless; so that one can, for instance, interpret a Latin term—use it metaphorically, even—without any decisive fear of plebiscitarian denial. We know that the term translates to "right (rightly) reason(ed)," and that the Scholastics used it to suggest the intellectual instrument by which men might reason progressively at least to the existence of God, at most to how, under His aegis, they should govern themselves in all major matters, avoiding the major vices, exercising discipline, seeking virtue. The search for virtue is probably best drowned out by *commotion,* and this my life is full of. It is easier to stay up late working for hours than to take one tenth the time to inquire into the question whether the work is worth performing.

And then, as I say, that other, the fear of boredom. Thoreau is known for his compulsion, day by day, to discover more and more things he could be without. But I have enough of everything material, at least measured by ordinary standards. But not the reliance to do without distraction; so that I would not cross the street without a magazine or paperback, lest the traffic should immobilize me for more than ten seconds. The unexamined life may not be worth living, in which case I will concede that mine is not worth living. But excepting my own life, I do seek to examine, and certainly I dilate upon, public questions I deem insufficiently examined.

I was saying that I do not enjoy writing. I envy those who do. John Chamberlain once told me that if he has not written during the day he will not sleep, and it is only when he wonders why he cannot fall asleep that he remembers that he has not written during that day; and so he rises, and writes. John Chamberlain is as incapable of affectation as Muhammad Ali of self-effacement. It is simply the case that some people like to sit down hour after hour and write, and with some of them the disease is so aggravated that it doesn't particularly matter whether what they write will be published. . . .

––––

It is inevitable, even in a book where the focus is on words, that a writer's tools of the trade will come up. Here is Buckley the columnist on such instruments in his (and our) pre-computer phase.

––––

What's Going On?

Aboard a cruising vessel bound for China a few months ago I unpacked an aluminum suitcase in which I had stored my cassettes, player, and portable typewriter. The typewriter was gone! There is no panic to equal that of the journalist caught without his typewriter, and accordingly I rushed back down the gangway, asked a guide where I might buy a typewriter, was directed to a department store nearby. An escalator plotted me through the crowd up to the third floor and there my eyes feasted on a counter-load of typewriters. I grabbed a sturdy-looking red portable, pausing only to establish that the lettering sequence was conventional. Back on board, I tapped out a few lines on it to discover that it was as near to being a totally satisfactory portable as the old Royal on which I was weaned—and my memory was jarred.

I first heard the word "obsolescent" when at school, in England, at age thirteen. A master (he was a Jesuit priest) had informed a class of older boys (age fourteen) that American car manufacturers engaged in "planned obsolescence." I took this as an affront on my homeland and demanded an explanation, and was given a kindly and abstruse explanation, which was the first time I looked up the meaning of the word "jesuitical."

Flash forward thirty years to a taxi driver in Hartford, Connecticut, who, having helped stow my bags at the station, noticed my Olivetti portable. For many years, he said, he had worked at the Royal typewriter factory but, he said, he had given up his job in disgust over the deteriorating standards of workmanship. I told him I had had a most splendid Royal portable for ten years beginning at age fifteen, which had been stolen in Mexico, and that ever since I had wandered like the Flying Dutchman from portable to portable. The Olivetti was nice to handle, but was as fragile as a soufflé, that I had gone through a dozen of them. He clucked his misgivings about American technology, and I thought of the obsolescence I had first heard about in 1938.

A year ago, I stopped at an airline newsstand to buy a copy of *Time* magazine, putting down my Olivetti to reach into my wallet. After pocketing the change, I leaned down to pick up the typewriter—which, however, was not there. It had been stolen, a venture in planned obsolescence perfected in New York City. I was bound for Cambridge, Massachusetts, to do battle with the big dragon Professor Galbraith, whose lovely secretary, a closet Republican, volunteered to help me. But there are no portable Olivettis in Cambridge, and so she came up with a Swiss Hermes, a small machine that requires the finger action of a pneumatic jackhammer, not bad for writing a speech that penetrates Galbraithian goulash, but not quite the right thing for flights of fancy. That was the machine missing in Kobe, Japan, when Providence put me in the hands of the Brother Valiant 413 ($80 FOB Kobe, Japan).

Why is it that what had been so securely American—the fine, reliable, relatively inexpensive machine—is disappearing? The idea behind planned obsolescence in Detroit, if that is what it was, was to cause you to buy another American car every three years or so. But American typewriters that drive you to Japanese typewriters via Italian and Swiss typewriters would seem to be making an economically unconsummated point. Goodness knows it did not used to be that way. The Woodstock typewriter used by Alger Hiss was still functioning ten years after it had been used to transcribe half of America's defense secrets for the benefit of Mr. Hiss's spymasters.

At home I used, for years, serenely and with pleasure, a Royal Standard I bought in my freshman year in college, in 1946. Are we the victims of nefarious economic design? The kind of thing Ralph Nader, or Michael Harrington, or the boys and girls who write for *The Nation* magazine, would like to think about American enterprise? Again, it would not appear to make sense, any more than it would make sense, having eaten one McDonald's hamburger, to resolve to move over to Burger King.

It is very sad, whatever the explanation. At age fifty-seven, I'd have a harder time talking back to that Jesuit priest than I did at age thirteen.

—WFB   JANUARY 1, 1983

Memo to: Bill
From: Priscilla

The *Christian Science Monitor* (March 13) reports you are looking after *NR*'s interests while airborne. See attached: (Headline: "Today's High-Flying Businessman: Have Typewriter, Will Travel." ". . . According to a longtime TWA flight attendant I know, no business traveler is quite so capable of wrapping himself in a six-mile-high cocoon as William F. Buckley Jr. 'I had Mr. Buckley on a transatlantic flight,' she said, 'and he had what looked like a month's worth of work beside him, piled all the way up in his lap. I noticed he didn't speak to the man beside him, he was so totally engrossed. When he got up to stretch his legs, the other man called me over. He said he couldn't find his shoes under the pile of Mr. Buckley's discarded papers. We finally found one and then another, but it wasn't his shoe. Sure enough, when Mr. Buckley came back he was wearing the other man's shoe on one of his feet.' ")

Memo to: Priscilla
From: Bill

Now I know why I was limping when I arrived in Geneva! XXX Bill

     —WFB   MAY 4, 1984

Buckley has long since left the ranks of the typewriter users and has been for years an enthusiastic computer user—and pusher. Years back, he put in my lap when we were working in Switzerland a little jewel of an early Epson laptop, taught me the commands for SAVE and for BACKSPACE, which, as computer nerds know, also means ERASE, but does not say so. (Computer keyboards are still under the influence of engineers whose first language is logarithm—see: they don't even know how to spell *rhythm*—not in English or even Japanese.) I proceeded to type my notes about his manuscript-in-progress. The next day he said, delighted with his computer's ability to count (all right, *compute*), "You wrote eleven thousand words!" He also loves the instant feather touch by which he can summon up his built-in dictionary and thesaurus. I was dazzled properly and still am, especially by Buckley's ability to stay at the cutting edge of word processing, where a new "annual" model is produced every month.*

 Next, he writes of an encounter with a Teletype machine and then of the word processor and those who would criticize its use, making what is, for him, a natural reference to other types of keyboards, the piano's and the harpsichord's, with which he is intimately at home.

Shop Talk

I have been asked over the years, in person and by correspondence, about the mechanics of column writing, and today is a good day to give some details of the craft and its engineering.

 Why today? Because columnists whose material goes to the newspapers by mail are hit by a circumstance, the kind of thing that happens, oh, a half-dozen times every year. On Monday, I wrote a column outlining the problems of the U.S. Government in respect of Libya, and what might usefully be done about them. On Tuesday night, President Reagan came out with his own ideas on the subject, so to speak scooping me. I don't

* Recently, WFB combined two loves by writing the bilingual introduction to a new book, *De DOS a Windows,* an *Introduccion a las computadoras personales*—a basic introduction to personal computers for Spanish-speakers, by Jaime A. Restrepo (Random House, 1996).

suggest that the analysis sent out by this pundit on Monday is useless or even anachronized by the President's press conference, merely that if the columnist had known exactly what the President was going to say, the column would have addressed his remarks, rather than go out self-launched.

You see, there are two flotillas of pundits. The first set is, so to speak, on the scene. These pundits write their columns minutes or at most hours after the event they write about, and their copy goes to client papers by wire. A James Reston, for instance, will appear in Wednesday morning's newspaper reporting on Tuesday night's presidential press conference. Such types have the advantage of instant communication.

The second flotilla moves in a stately gait for massive bombing after the front-line forces have undertaken their initial action. We have the disadvantage of coming in late, but then we have the countervailing advantage of surveying the scene a day or so after the arrival of the shock troops, and selecting our targets more deliberately.

Columns and the paraphernalia that go with them (research, correspondence, etc.) are subject to vicissitudes, common and not so common. In Moscow once I found that the only way I could possibly meet my deadline was to borrow the *New York Times*'s Teletype machine. Having done so, I faced the problem that I did not know how to operate it, or rather that operating it, given my unfamiliarity, was taking me about a half-hour per sentence. Taking pity on me, *New York Times* correspondent Bernard Gwertzman sighed, eased me out of my seat, and in a few minutes dispatched my column to New York. Bernard Gwertzman figures in my last will and testament; and, no doubt, he remembers the high point of his political education while in Moscow.

Getting material from faraway places can be as easy as popping a salted peanut, or it can present quite extraordinary difficulties. Answering two hundred to three hundred letters and dictating notes on a few matters of interest consumed most of three days' working time aboard a sailboat during the Christmas holidays, and a friend in St. Maarten was entrusted with two large plastic sacks, each one with the relevant ninety-minute cassette for transcription in New York. Three days later, a hysterical telephone call from New York advised me that the sacks had arrived, but not the cassettes.

One fumed over wretched pilferers who would steal a two-dollar cassette onto which to pipe one more abomination by Boy George, but lo, three days later it transpired that for reasons known only to God and some officious post office bureaucrat in Miami, the cassettes had been extracted and sent back to St. Maarten, presumably because they were suspected of containing dope, or instructions to Libyan hit men. Never mind, my friend in St. Maarten reassured me over the telephone to the Dominican

Republic, he would see to it that the very next day his houseguest would take the tapes to New York.

But going the next day to fetch his houseguest for their last lunch together before the flight, my friend found the bathroom door locked. Worried, he finally broke it open, and his houseguest was in the tub, quite dead.

Requiescat in pacem, to be sure; but there was also the problem of the cassettes, and his guest (it was Mr. Sam Spiegel, the—late—movie mogul) had already packed his bags, requiring my friend to undertake a morbid search until he discovered the two cassettes, in one of which were notes dictated after an interview with the president of the Dominican Republic, which would serve as background detail for a newspaper column.

Which, for reasons now divulged, appeared a few days later than originally scheduled. That's the way it is.

—WFB   JANUARY 11, 1986

ON SOME OF THE TOOLS OF LEARNING

Since it has become everybody's business to reform education, permit from this corner a word about the mechanics of learning. Many years ago I asked the dean of my alma mater why no credit was given for the mastery of typing or shorthand, and he replied beneficently, "There is no body of knowledge in typing." Quite right: It is not a three-dimensional discipline, on the order of poetry or physics, but it is the principal means by which John communicates with Jane or, for that matter, with the world at large.

Typing reached a new age with the discovery of the chip. It is fashionable to condescend to word processing. Never mind. It is to the writer, whether professional or amateur, what the tractor is to the farmer. And those who rail against it do so for the most practical reason: They have not mastered its use. They strive for metaphysical formulations to justify their hidden little secret (sloth and fear). But those of us with X-ray vision: We know, we know.

Consider the recent denunciation of word processing by the poet Louis Simpson, done for the *New York Times.* When Milton described the obstruction of Lucifer ("Whence and what art thou, execrable shape,/That dar'st, though grim and terrible, advance/Thy miscreated front athwart my way/To yonder gates?") he spoke no less scornfully than Mr. Simpson of the word processor. Listen:

"Poets do have to make changes, but they cannot think so; they must think that the next word and phrase will be perfect. At times, and these are the happiest, they have the feeling that words are being given to them with absolute finality. The word processor works directly against this feeling; it tells you your writing is not final. And it enables you to think you are writing when you are not, when you are only making notes or the outline of a poem you may write at a later time. But then you will feel no need to write it."

To accept Mr. Simpson's thesis is to suppose that writers (and poets) always feel that the language of the moment is lapidary, never mind that, when detoxified, they proceed to make changes. The easiest way to handle Mr. Simpson's miscreated affront is to remind him that words engraved onto a computer's memory are everlastingly there if that is the writer's election, but that they are vaporized instantly and handily if that becomes the writer's election.

If it should happen that someone prefers to compose using a pencil, the proper attitude toward him is simply to look to one side, as one would do if one came upon a writer who could only compose with a teddy bear on his desk. The word processor is very soon discovered by the writer to be something on the order of overdrive in an automobile: like shifting from first gear, into overdrive, that's what it feels like. Like swimming in a pool infinitely long, so that you need never turn around. Aahh!

Just as schools and colleges should encourage students in word processing, they should encourage the mastery of touch-typing, which permits the user to turn his head to one side, reading material he is simultaneously typing, without looking at the keyboard.

The prejudice against learning by heart those thirty little keys is one of the great mysteries of the world. The great Rosalyn Tureck, who can play from memory all the keyboard works of Johann Sebastian Bach, leans over her typewriter and, I kid you not, hunts and pecks. Even though she can sit down and play the 27th Goldberg without missing a note, she never bothered to learn that, on a typewriter, the order is, Q W E R T Y. . . . It is a note of minor historical interest, offered by the fine computer popularizer Peter McWilliams, that the typewriter keyboard reflects the deficient technology of a hundred years ago. When the typewriter was invented, keys could not be got to move as quickly as fingers, so that the configuration of characters was done to slow the typist down.

Let our teachers encourage the use of the tools of learning, and forswear nonsense about how Shakespeare would have written flatly if he had had a word processor. It is likelier that he'd have written eight more masterpieces, one of them at the expense of Luddites.

—WFB   JANUARY 19, 1988

SEE YOU LATER

ST. THOMAS, VIRGIN ISLANDS—Syndicated columnists are given two weeks off every year. And this, I note in passing, is by no means a venerable convention (in my case, the vacation came only after my fifth year in the trade). Moreover, there have been columnists who as a matter of principle never took a vacation, lest their public discover that life was possible, nay even keener, and more joyous, without the columnist's lucubrations.

The late George Sokolsky wrote six columns a week for King Features, and then a seventh for the local Sunday paper. When he learned that he had to have his appendix out, he carefully composed columns ahead based on all the variables in the arts of prognosis: two columns in the event everything went smoothly; four columns in the event of complications; six columns in the event of major complications. I asked him, on hearing the story, whether he wrote a seventh column in the event of terminal complications, but he replied that his interest in his worldly constituency was only coextensive with his life on earth.

Mine isn't: when I go, I intend to hector the Almighty even as, episodically, I do from here, to look after my friends and (most of) my enemies. But I confess to being uncomfortable at taking my two weeks together, instead of separating them as is my practice (one week in the winter, one in the summer). Still, I am setting sail on a splendid racing vessel, from here to Bermuda to the Azores, and to Spain. The second leg of my journey will keep me incommunicado (at sea) for eleven days, in the unusual posture of being only on the receiving end of the world's events. During that period President Carter, Senator Kennedy, the airlines, the people who spend their days profaning the English of King James, may misbehave safely in the knowledge that there will be no reproach from me. It is horrifying to meditate what enormity the White House will execute, I having advertised my isolation. On the other hand, if President Carter is determined to make me one of the boat people, I am splendidly well ahead of the game: I need only to sail on.

But sail on to where? Ah, there's the rub, as the poet intuited four hundred years ago. Where can we go if distress should come to America? There is only Switzerland, but nature so arranged it so that you cannot sail to Switzerland, and this would not be the season to rely on U.S. naval helicopters to pick up my boat and ferry it into Lake Geneva. Accordingly, I adjure my Lords, secular and spiritual, not to be too licentious while I am gone.

What shall I concern myself with? Well, the exact time of day. I really must know—no kidding—exactly what the time is. I wear a chronometer which for several years lost exactly one second per week. Even folk as disorganized as I can cope with such retrogressions, and I happily set it right every Christmas and every Fourth of July, and I always knew what time it was. But in an idiotic fit of hubris, I returned it to the clockmaker reminding him that my watch was guaranteed not to gain or lose more than twelve seconds per year. It has never been quite right since. So—well, I have a computer I navigate with, and it has an inbuilt chronometer. It keeps excellent time. But, you see, excellent time will not do—you need the exact time. So, I also have a little radio (thirty-six dollars at Radio Shack) which is supposed to bring in WWV from Fort Collins, Colorado, which vouchsafes to all the ships at sea the exact time. Mostly the little radio brings in that signal. Every now and then it does not. In which case I ask my sailing companion Danny for the time, and his watch is pretty reliable. Dick Clurman's cheap little Casio keeps disgustingly good time. And I can tell from friend Reggie's sly smile that he believes, in a pinch, he can come up with the time.

I need sun. Not to darken my skin, because in fact the doctor says that sun is the enemy of fair skin and I must now use something called Total Eclipse No. 15. I need the sun, and the time, to discover which way to point in order to effect a rendezvous at the Azores. If in this matter I should fail, the reader may deduce, two weeks hence, that I am absent without leave. The moon is getting lean right now, but will flower again; and when it is half-bright, it gives you a horizon, and on some magical moments you can combine that horizon with the North Star, and before you know it, you have your latitude, even as Columbus had that, and only that, with little idea of the time, and yet managed to discover our wonderful country.

The chances, then, are overwhelming that, like MacArthur, I shall return. In the meantime, the Republic is on probation.

—WFB   JUNE 12, 1980

Chapter 13

Man of
Letters

As is evident throughout this book, WFB is not only a man of letters in the larger sense, but a man who receives a great many missives and does his best to answer them *(missives* and *missiles* are both apt in this case). His mailbag, with his dictating machine and his computer, goes where he goes. Two notices over a long period of time give inadvertent witness to the volume and flow of his correspondence.

Memo to: Unknown, and unknowable, correspondents
   From: WFB
     Re: A missing briefcase

On December 12, a briefcase crammed full with correspondence for the most part as yet unread (I had been traveling) was lost somewhere between La Guardia Airport and Miami International Airport. Heroic efforts at retrieval have been unavailing. The result: 100 to 150 communications addressed to WFB are scheduled to go unacknowledged and, worse, unread. If you chance to be the author of one of these, pray send a copy.

—JANUARY 20, 1978

> STOLEN. From WFB's car, one seabagful of unanswered mail (three to four hundred letters) including a dozen unread manuscripts. Date of theft, December 16. The bag could have contained letters dating back to the first week in November. There is no record of such letters, and WFB greatly regrets any inadvertent failure to reply. There is a record in the office of the mss. and in due course the authors will be advised.

FEBRUARY 8, 1985

These are real letters, not the slippery faxes which seem to demand instant response, or E-mail, which calls for the same, only faster. (My favorite reaction to such "labor-saving" devices was the line uttered by one electronically oppressed man in *New York* magazine, I believe: "The fax has changed my life!" he wrote excitedly. And in more somber voice added: "It's shortened it.")

In any case, letters are part of the sum and substance of Buckley's life and he answers almost all—from children, antagonists, friends, strangers, loved ones, etc.—with virtually the same courtesy and verve.

In earlier collections, he has given glimpses of the traffic, as in this excerpt from *Cruising Speed* (1971).

. . . I have a telegram from a young playwright: "Dear Mr. Buckley. The soul of a secular nation is its theater. Our theater is all but dead. I send you a modern classic tragedy and you are too busy and important to read it. How disgusting." Frances Bronson, my secretary, was very much annoyed by the telegram, because only five days earlier she had sent a letter to Peter Glenville that I had dictated. "I would not normally send along a manuscript, but I am so fetched by the vigor and grace of the letter that accompanied it (I attach it) that I wonder if you could possibly tell me whether you think it has a chance?" Frances heatedly wrote out a telegram which she proposed to send, rebuking the playwright for his impatience. I told her not to send it, because I react against declamatory rudeness that is coercive in intent—obviously the playwright thought that his telegram would get him some action. (The following week Peter told me that the author was talented but the play, in his opinion, was not ready for commercial production. I assume he is a very young man, I said, the telegram in mind. "If he isn't," Peter replied, "then you will have to counsel him to stop writing plays.")

. . . I wrote to a friend in Switzerland: "It occurs to me that you have sought by your silence to communicate your displeasure with me. I find that too bad, particularly since I am by all odds the nicest man I know. However, I do think that in order to save us embarrassment, we ought to know ahead of time whether on my return to Switzerland [where I spend February and March] we are supposed, on happening upon each other, to exchange only Averted Gazes, because my Averted Gaze is a little rusty, and needs some practicing up. Or, we can resume our amiable relationship, wherein you admire my prose, I admire your art, and we agree to leave moot the question of your business acumen. Why don't we leave it this way, that if I do not hear from you in response to this letter, I shall regretfully assume that the former is your election? My love to the girls [his wife, daughter, and dog, who is Rowley's* second cousin]."

There are the routine requests, all of which I regularly resolve to handle with form letters, but how to compose a form letter adequate to the resources of some writers, particularly the very young ones? "Well, here I am again. Yes sir, it takes more than a broken typewriter to keep this kid down. This is my third letter to you . . . But gee-wiz golly-darn Mr. Buckley, when are you going to answer my letters? To totally ignore a seventeen-year-old high school conservative, I must warn you, could prove to be dangerous. We are not only relatively rare but also very sensitive. After all if you keep ignoring my letters I might get the idea you don't want young people in the conservative movement. Wouldn't that be terrible? (The answer is 'yes'). But if you ignore me you are ignoring more than a young conservative. Your [sic] ignoring a young conservative from Indiana. A Cardinal Sin! . . . But Hark! All is not lost. And to prove to you I am not really sore I am going to give you this chance to make-up with me and the state of Indiana (both of whom have been ignored too long). You, Mr. Buckley, are cordially invited to be the guest speaker at our high school's Good Government Day program . . . Please understand that Key Club is a service organization for high school boys and as such we wouldn't be able to pay the high price that I know you normally get . . ."

He gets a non-form letter, the key sentence of which is, "Whenever you are disposed to be sore at me, try to remember that *National Review* is available to you for five or six dollars a year in part because of activities I

---

* One of the Buckleys' dogs.—Ed.

undertake which result in my having to answer rather briefly notes from such pleasant people as yourself, and say no to nonpaying invitations to speak." . . . A form letter suffices for "I am writing a term paper in high school about Communism in America. I would appreciate it if you would send me some information about this subject. My teacher told me that you are a conservative who is probably a strong anti-Communist." *The teacher would not have got a form letter.* . . . The *Notre Dame Lawyer* wants a review of Ramsey Clark's book *Crime in America:* "Upon publication of a review, we would be glad to send you fifty complimentary copies of the review, and a one-year subscription to the *Lawyer.*" I have always thought that the most genial of all form letters is the one that suggests that the correspondent did not get through, so that he won't therefore feel that his persuasiveness was met and resisted. Whence, "Mr. Buckley has asked me to interdict all requests for interviews, articles, reviews, etc., for the next period—probably about six months, as he is drastically in arrears on commitments he has already made. I hope you will understand that to take on any further commitments at this point simply means failing to keep those he has already made. Thank you for writing. Very truly yours, Frances Bronson." . . . Then, what is about as hard a sell as I ever get, from the student government head of DePauw an elaborate wind-up: "Surely this letter will rank among the very oddest of the wide and weird assortment which no doubt floats your way each week. I am writing to attempt to persuade you to accept a speaking engagement here. Please hear me out—if it's of any consequence, I've shown you the same courtesy countless times in your columns and books, in spite of profound philosophical disagreements." Then about DePauw, and how important it is. But, however good the education at DePauw, there is "one glaring defect: the absence of an even reasonable articulate conservative spokesman." The letter goes on. "It is entirely possible—nay, probable—that the overwhelming majority of DePauw students graduating in the last decade have *never heard* so much as a syllable from an intelligent conservative." And a little guarded flattery. "Do not think me a flatterer [the word "flatterer" comes out charmingly home-typed, which I always like: something like "flatterer"]; *you* know you are intelligent—why should I peetend [sic] *I* don't? To these people the term conservatism (please forgive this unavoidable use of labels) conjures up images of Hoosier anti-communist hysteria or (worse) the editorial pages of the *Chicago Tribune* and *Indianapolis Star,* intimately connected with this institution—on both of which many students here have been spoon-fed from infancy.

"The deleterious effects of this homogenized diet are several: slow-witted conservative students here are imbued with the fuziest sorts of ideas about American society and are rendered utterly incapable of defending themselves intellectually against even a mediocre liberal spokesman. (Let us face facts: it does not require overwhelming philosophical utensils to make intellectual puree out of the grade triple-Z grist cranked out by the *Tribune* and *Star.*) Perceptive conservative students become either bored with or nauseated by such drivel and abandon the conservative cause for the better articulated, more sophisticated, and more popular liberal theses available in abundance through the media and other sources (e.g., university faculty). Liberal students all along the intelligence gradient acquire a sense of smugness and self-righteousness, and grow intellectually paunchy due to a dearth of skillful conservative sparring partners.

"We are not a wealthy organization. We can afford very little beyond your travel and associated expenses, plus perhaps a small honorarium (no doubt a pittance compared to what you could usually command). However we can promise a capacity turn-out, excellent coverage by the mass media, and unlimited flexibility—you can pick any date you wish. *Please,* give this a moment's consideration." . . . I did, of course, and decided not to take on the student body president of DePauw University on the question of the triple-Z incapacity of the chief editorial writers of the *Chicago Tribune* and the *Indianapolis Star,* both of them Phi Beta Kappas from rather exacting universities; that kind of argument one simply hasn't time for. "Your letter touched me," I wrote. "I say that quite sincerely. But you must consider my situation. I work overtime so as to be able to send *National Review* to anybody who wants it for approximately $12.00 per year. [The disparity in the cited cost is because, for students, we have a crazy-rate system, which reduces the subscription price by a couple of dollars.] It costs us approximately $20 a year to produce it. The difference is made up by fund appeals and my own activities as a lecturer. The obvious answer to your generic question is: If your fellow students have any intellectual curiosity at all, they will pick up *National Review* at a very small cost to them. If they want me personally, what they want is theater. [A deucedly good point, what?] For theater, I charge—and remit my earnings to *National Review.* I don't like to say it because it sounds self-serving, but there are over five hundred applications from colleges willing to pay the full fee [I exaggerate. More like two hundred], and it would not be fair to penalize *National Review* by patronizing DePauw, however much I am inclined to do so as a result of your own eloquence. It is not the same thing, but I would be very happy if you would lunch with me next time you come to New York."

No answer would ever come to my answer; that often happens. The kids are, a lot of them, first-rate at turning on the charm when they want something. And then, win or lose, they deploy their charm elsewhere. I believe in thank-you letters, and I have a tickler-system that reminds me when a delinquent institution writes to me for a speech, or article. The all-time offenders are the graduate students, who manage to get free speeches from you as you succumb to their sycophantic embraces, and then you never hear from them again, like the girl in any de Maupassant story. Ah, but I have learned, have I learned. The Dean of the Graduate School at Princeton, an irresistible liberal of charming habits, now calls in the student lecture head, or that is my impression, and dictates to him the thank-you letter he is to send me after my dutiful appearances there, free gratis, every couple of years, a murderous habit I fell into in the fifties, before I got around to composing my super-form letters. *I am waiting to be asked back by a certain organization at Harvard . . .*

———

At times, letters arrive which are deeply touching:

———

Dear Mr. Buckley:

In the fall of 1986, Captain Paul J. Weaver and I arrived at Hurlburt Field, Florida, prepared to learn how to operate our new aircraft, the AC-130H Spectre Gunship. Aviators rarely discuss anything other than flying, but Paul was unique in his interests and breadth of knowledge. Our conversations quickly moved to politics.

Paul was passionately conservative, and as our conversations progressed, I realized he was extremely well read on the issues of the day, and I was not. He suggested a subscription to *National Review* and I shall forever be in his debt.

Paul was equally passionate in his respect and love for your magazine, your columns, and most of all *Firing Line*. He was one of your greatest unknown admirers.

On January 31, 1991, Major Weaver was the aircraft commander of a gunship, Spirit 03, engaged with enemy forces during the battle of Khafji. He and his crew of thirteen were desperately searching for an Iraqi surface-to-surface missile site that was threatening U.S. Marines in the area. Numerous anti-aircraft-artillery sites were reported to the crew by two gunships exiting the area, but they elected to stay and support the Marines.

Spirit 03 was shot down that morning and all fourteen aboard were lost. I don't know if you knew any of America's casualties personally, but one of them knew you very well. In Paul Weaver, America has lost a great patriot and warrior, and you, a faithful follower.

I thought you should know.

Sincerely,
CHARLES G. MCMILLAN
CAPTAIN
USAF
EDWARDS AFB, CALIF.

Dear Captain McMillan: I am profoundly moved; and I extend you, his friend, our condolences, even as we share your pride in our friend. Gratefully,

—WFB   MAY 27, 1991

———

But if someone really wants to take Buckley on by letter or column or book, he can expect a polite barrage back. And he should be prepared to stay the course—or face the most serious response of all: silence.

———

Memo to: Bill
From: Priscilla
Did you catch Herb Caen's latest?

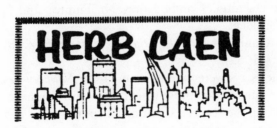

How Little We Know

SLICE OF WRY: Maxwell Arnold suggests that William Buckley Jr., fairest flower of the right wing, is an odd choice to act as host of the TV series based on Evelyn Waugh's classic English novel, "Brideshead Revisited" (tonight's installment is on KQED at 9). On Page 543 of "The Letters of Evelyn Waugh," we find the author writing to Tom Driberg on June 6, 1960. After congratulating him on a magazine article about right-wing movements, Waugh asks Driberg, "Can you tell me: did you in your researches come across the name of Wm. F. Buckley Jr., editor of a New York, neo-McCarthy magazine named *National Review?* He has been showing me great & unsought attention lately & your article made me curious. Has he been supernally 'guided' to bore me? It would explain him" . . . If anything can.

★   ★   ★

Herb Caen
San Francisco Chronicle
Dear Herbert:

The item on Brideshead, Waugh, and me was understandable fun. Though perhaps a little skepticism would have been in order, even as I'd have shown skepticism toward any writer who pronounced that "Herb Caen is a bore." We are other things. The letter, Waugh to Driberg, was an inside joke. Waugh had just finished reading a book by me the last chapter of which is an attack on Driberg. Following the letter you quoted were several not listed by the anthologist, Mr. Amory, for reasons unknown. Mr. Waugh also went on to submit a piece to *National Review* and write a book review for us. His last letter to me I quote:

Combe Florey House, Combe Florey, Nr. Taunton 2nd April 63
Dear Mr. Buckley:

Very many thanks for *Rumbles.* [*Rumbles Left and Right* by WFB, New York, Putnam's, 1962].

Some of the essays were familiar to me from *National Review.* I reread them with the same zest as those which were new. You have the very rare gift of captivating the reader's attention in controversies in which he has no direct concern. I congratulate you on the collection. At your best you remind me of Belloc; at your second best of Randolph Churchill.

. . . Please accept my greetings for Easter (which I shall be spending in Rome).

Yours sincerely,
EVELYN WAUGH

Herb, I thought the world of Evelyn Waugh, but sometimes when I think of what he wrote about me, I blush. Yours cordially,

BILL   —MARCH 5, 1982

Mr. Mark Amory
Ticknor & Fields
London

Dear Mr. Amory:

I'm not sure why I put off writing to you for so long. Perhaps it was my general admiration for the job you did in editing the letters of Mr. Evelyn Waugh [*The Letters of Evelyn Waugh,* edited by Mark Amory, Ticknor & Fields, 1980].

But now, with yet another smirking allusion [see "Notes & Asides," March 5] to the low opinion Waugh had of me, my magazine, and my abilities (this one in New York, following similar references in Los Angeles and San Francisco), I must ask you for an explanation.

1. I enclose a copy of the San Francisco column by Mr. Herb Caen. I enclose a copy of the letter I then addressed to Mr. Caen.

2. I enclose a copy of the feature "Notes & Asides" from *National Review,* November 14, 1980. I should have addressed a copy of that feature to you at the time, so that I'd have had access to your explanation for the missing letters, EW to WFB.

3. My confusion is reinforced by the acknowledgments in your book. Apparently I gave you permission to enter my files and to take from them copies of letters from EW to me. When the book came out, I asked the Yale University Library, which keeps my papers, to give me in turn copies of letters from EW to WFB. I instantly received the entire set published in the *National Review* feature. It is, I should think, logical to conclude that you were in possession of the identical set. Why then did you not, even if you elected not to publish any of his subsequent letters to me, mention in a footnote that Mr. Waugh was friendly to me, and to my journal? I am most anxious for your explanation, as it will facilitate my handling of my critics, who are greatly enjoying themselves on this point.

I am sending a copy of this letter and enclosures to Auberon Waugh, not in the spirit of intimidation, but because, as an old personal friend, I would not want him to be surprised that there was contention, so to speak, in the family.

Yours faithfully,
WM. F. BUCKLEY, JR.

Combe Florey House
Somerset, England

Dear Bill:

Thank you for sending me your correspondence with Mark Amory. I am sorry that he seems to be making cheap capital from the few rude references to you in my Father's correspondence. If he had known you better there would probably have been more of them, but that would not mean that he held you in anything but the greatest esteem. He always spoke of you with admiration, as I remember, and was delighted when I started writing for you many years ago.

The problem with opening anyone's letters or diaries is that one is bound to find unkind references to friends, relations, and even strangers which the writer would never have intended to see published. It was a difficulty which I met particularly in the Diaries, by a blanket policy of publishing everything. There were many extraordinarily rude references to myself and other members of the family, both in the Diaries and in the Letters. My policy was to hide nothing simply on the grounds that it would have been rather a despicable thing to discriminate. We all write unkind jokes and even deeply wounding remarks about our best friends in circumstances where we do not expect them to read them. One just has to learn not to take offense. But I am sorry that people are using these references to embarrass you. The only policy in my experience is to rise above it all. One of the joys of journalism is that everybody forgets it within a week or two.

Mark Amory is a very old friend of mine, but of course he is a Liberal. His mother decided to stand as Liberal candidate while he was at Oxford, and the result is to be found in a little-read novel of mine called *Path of Dalliance* where she appears as Mrs. Sligger. I am sure that no malice is intended, merely the impulsive journalistic urge to make jokes.

Have you ever been to Combe Florey? I hope we may tempt you down here one day. I practically never move nowadays except for twice-yearly pilgrimages to the Far East, but it would be lovely to see you again, when you are in England. I was in Cuba two weeks ago and brooded on the terrible struggle in your breast between patriotism and appreciation of good cigars which you somehow solved by leaving a box of Cuban cigars in my house in Wiltshire. There is a fast train service from London if ever you are tempted.

All the best.

> Yours ever,
> BRON
> [AUBERON WAUGH]

Dear Mr. Buckley:

When I asked for letters from Evelyn Waugh, I was indeed sent the complete set and I am sorry to have returned evil for good. I edited ruthlessly on grounds of interest or amusement, fairness coming a poor third.

Certainly your relationship with Waugh was distorted as a result. His rudeness about you was clearly meant to cheer up Driberg, an old friend whose book you had criticized. My explanation will not seem strong to you but was for me: to put in corrective footnotes throughout would have been laborious, dull to read, and lead into the tricky, almost impossible, area of deciding how much of what Waugh said he meant.

You have my sympathy and my apologies for the resulting annoyance but I see that they are not much good to you.

Yours sincerely,

MARK AMORY

Dear Auberon:

I attach this note to my letter [not here reproduced] to you, as I have just seen Mark Amory's letter, a copy of which I enclose. I have decided it doesn't require an answer.

As ever,

BILL   —NOVEMBER 23, 1982

———

O\ne wonderful letter-writer appreciates another, for a regular exchange of letters is like a continuing conversation.

———

EVELYN WAUGH AND LADY DIANA COOPER, CORRESPONDENTS

Everybody knows who Evelyn Waugh was. Not so Diana Cooper, to whom Waugh wrote about three hundred letters from 1932 until he died in 1966, twenty years before her own death at a very advanced age. One way to begin to situate her is to note the wedding presents she received in 1919 when, as the beautiful young daughter of the Duchess of Rutland, she married the penniless, untitled Duff Cooper: "The King and Queen gave a blue enamel and diamond brooch bearing their own initials; Queen Alexandra a diamond-and-ruby pendant; the French Ambassador a gold ewer for incense-burning; the Princess of Monaco a diamond ring; Lord Wimborne a William and Mary gold dressing-case; King Manuel a gold sugar-sifter; Lord Beaverbrook a motor car; Dame Nellie Melba a writing-table." (The list of wedding gifts, as Philip Ziegler reports in his biography *Diana Cooper*, occupied eighty-eight pages of a large notebook.)

Lady Diana Cooper was, then, socially noticeable. By the time Waugh met her, she had been a screen actress and also played on the stage. In the late 1950s she turned to writing, producing three volumes of memoirs; Waugh wrote that he thought them "a single work of art, one of the great autobiographies of the century." Lady Diana's granddaughter, Artemis Cooper, provides samples of these expressive skills in *The Letters of Evelyn Waugh and Diana Cooper*, as when Lady Diana addressed Waugh severely (she often did so) following Duff Cooper's death, just after the midnight that brought in the new year, 1954:

> You have never, I think, known real Grief—panic, melancholia, madness, night-sweats, we've all known for most of our lives—you and me particularly. I'm not sure you know human love in the way I do. You have faith and mysticism—intense inner interests—a diverting, virile mind—gusto for vengeance and destruction if necessary, a fancy—a gospel.
>
> What you can't imagine is a creature with a certain iridescent aura and nothing within but a beating frightened heart built round and for Duff. . . . For two days I am quite alone—in these empty rooms with one thought one prayer—'let it end now'—an absurd feminine desire to die in the same way exactly as Duff. [I have now a] fearlessness of death—so let it come now before custom of living disinclines me for dying.

But such grief was not characteristic. Diana Cooper loved people and traveling and adventures and fun—and she loved Evelyn Waugh, though one surmises that they were happier when planning to see each other than when in each other's company. The dour Waugh ("I am an insensitive lout") was relentlessly adoring. Among Lady Diana's attractions were her blue blood and her tendency to move about "grand architecture"—bringing him "delight. . . . Still more the aesthetic joy of seeing you in your proper setting of luxury and splendour. Still more, and incomparably more, the happiness to know that you have kept a warm place for me in your heart all through my ice age. I love you."

But she didn't *always* bring him delight. "Baby" (as he called her) could irritate Waugh by what she said or by her occasional bouts of silence or by misinterpreting his catechisms. "You know perfectly well," she reassured him after one such misunderstanding, "you have no Baby as loyal as this Baby and that if you believe anything else you are very foolish. I thought, if you want to know, that you did it to irritate—or rather from Irritability's possession. It's an unexorcisable demon. . . . O dear how sad it all is."

In the big 1980 volume of his letters edited by Mark Amory it was made clear, as only Waugh could make things clear, that he considered it the burden—the very function, the *raison d'être*—of the correspondent *to inform and to entertain.* He was lavish in discharge of this duty. Thus he tells Lady Diana of a visit to Hilaire Belloc: "Two civil and pretty grandsons received us. Sherry in the hall. Then a long wait for Belloc. Shuffling and stumping. Then an awful smell like the wolves at the zoo, then entry. A tramp, covered in garbage. A sweet, wise, mad face. An awful black growth like a truffle under one eye. First words: 'Old age is a curious thing. It leaves a man crawling like a beetle while his mind is as strong and young as ever.' Second words (rather disconcerting, because I have met him twenty times or more since you first introduced us . . .): 'It is a pleasure to make your acquaintance, sir.' "

Belloc was very nearly unique in eliciting something like awe. Mostly Waugh's world was populated by lesser creatures, such as those he came upon in his travels. During a cruise of the Mediterranean in the fall of 1933 he undertook, one by one, to describe his traveling companions. Miss Marjorie Glasgow was, for example, "a very rich young lady whom I had met before on account of her mother giving parties I used to go to before I became fastidious. She was the leader of the left-wing nudists. She was attended by three naked Counts, one Polish, one Belgian and one Italian, one carried her gramophone, another her backgammon board and the third her sunbathing mattress."

He was especially fine when transmitting hilarities in the matter-of-fact tones of the schoolteacher: "I wish you had come to Goa. It is really a very singular place. . . . At the moment it is full of pilgrims from all over India and Ceylon—the descendants of people Francis Xavier preached to without knowing their language. . . . Did you know that when F.X. went to Japan he asked the word for God and they told him the Japanese for [penis] so he spent weeks preaching phallic worship without knowing it."

Evelyn Waugh depended on his friends, especially when traveling—which was much of the time—for news of the kind he most wanted. "Please keep writing and tell me about the general election and who is sleeping with whom and so on." He spoke of vacations, but never seemed to let up. It isn't widely recognized how very much he worked, how copiously he produced. He proffered as the reason for writing the sheer need for the income to care for his wife and six children, athwart the predatory hands of a socialist government. "I cannot with the utmost economy live on less than £5,000 a year and I have to earn £62,000 to spend that and I am getting too old and downcast to earn it," he wrote in December 1951, surveying his crowded household. His children were all very well, but children were very simply "defective adults." He was "glad to possess" his own, but got "little pleasure from their use—like first editions." He found it comfortable to be comprehensive in his dislikes—"Hate everyone except you and Maimie"—even if he knew that was somehow wrong, and could make himself write: "I am full of regret for failures in gratitude and patience and service and that has made me think of my failures towards all I love. . . . Please . . . believe always in my love."

It is well known that Evelyn Waugh rejoiced in the upper class, in particular the titled nobility, however ironic his oblique references to this fixation ("After I left you I went to play dominoes with the poor"). Anyone wishing to document this affinity will lean heavily on the comprehensive footnotes appended to these letters by Artemis Cooper, the talented and industrious editor of this intricate volume. Here one runs into—or else that is the sensation—just about every titled person in Britain; somehow they all manage to figure in Waugh-Cooper colloquies. The footnote for Waugh's mother-in-law reads: "She was born the Hon. Mary Vesey, and married Aubrey Herbert M.P. (1880–1923) in 1910. Aubrey Herbert, who was twice offered the throne of Albania, was a half brother of the fifth Earl of Carnarvon (the patron of Howard Carter, who discovered the tomb of Tutankhamun)."

Lady Diana does not disappoint this appetite or conceal its mannerisms. "Will it be soon" that Waugh pays another visit? she wonders. "I fear the hols are over and you are happy at home. The house is warm and there are no guests for bed or board. You could do your [diet] here—no cook, no maître d'hotel, no one who can read or write. Pierro who puts 'CRI' for gruyère. Jacqueline—my life, my memory—is off with a garagiste to be knocked about by a frog husband, her place is taken by a Czech child—utterly unlearned. Antoinette, the Polish milker, is in command—she can't even make herself plain—but cooks with originality and charm. . . . Louise has had her lung out and is like a roebuck in spring. Phyllis, and my dearest sister Marjorie, to say nothing of Viola Tree and Clarissa's mother, might all have been saved most hideous deaths [from lung cancer]." There is nothing to do, nobody to go out with that one would care to go out with. "There is no sap in Nature—nor in me. Spiritless, not in pain or acute melancholy I languish chilly—not happily resigned."

It has long been my own reading of Waugh that his delight in the festoonery of the titled class was merely a perverse aspect of his resentful co-optation by a populist history-on-the-march that disregarded the forms he revered: in religion, the old Roman Catholic Church; in society, the standards of decorum and behavior that marked, if not so much the separation of classes, the acknowledgment of the idea of class. That the upper classes had long since lost any meritocratic credentials he seldom paused to notice. What Waugh bothered with was the loss of his privacy. "The only human relationships I abide are intimacy, formality and servility. What is horrible here [England] and in America is familiarity. That doesn't exist in Asia." And again, "I live in a world which seems to me to deteriorate daily before my eyes." But his problem, he knew, was also personal: "How right you are about not losing friends. . . . I lose mine fast. . . . You find something agreeable in almost everyone. I am put off by anything not wholly agreeable."

Diana Cooper was one exception. Not that she was always reliably agreeable. ("If only you could treat friends," he chided, "as something to be enjoyed in themselves not as companions in adventure.") But she was a lifelong source of joy for Waugh, the quality of which is transmitted by these letters to readers who knew neither of them, and presumably care little for their workaday concerns. Waugh wrote that "it ought always to be disappointing to meet an artist; if his work is not something otherwise invisible in him he can't have the real motive for work. Artists to be heard and not seen." But in his triumphantly readable letters Waugh tells us otherwise—though, granted, we experience him in the written word with the kind of safety that would not have protected us when experiencing him in person.

I have jocularly ventured for some years now that a dispositive proof of the existence of the Holy Spirit is that Evelyn Waugh died just after attending church on Easter Sunday in 1966, immediately after which the convention was introduced in the Catholic Mass of the sign of peace, a moment when worshipers are bid to shake hands with fellow worshipers to their right, to their left, in the pew ahead and in the pew behind. Such an exercise could not have coexisted with Evelyn Waugh, defender of the faith. Either he had to go, or else the ritual had to be postponed. The Holy Spirit made His choice. Waugh went, but not before having a certain satisfaction at the expense of the Cardinal most responsible for the "reforms" of the Second Vatican Council:

Combe Florey
7 February 1965

Darling
 . . . Nice to go to Rome. They are destroying all that was superficially attractive about my Church. It is a great sorrow to me and for once undeserved.

If you see Cardinal Bea spit in his eye.
All love
BO

To which Lady Diana replied:

> 10 Warwick Avenue
> [postmarked March 7, 1965]
> Can you imagine the luck—I went up in a tiny lift with Cardinal Bea in full canonicals preceded by two candles—so with a spluttered greeting I was able to spit in his eye for you. . . .
>
> PUG

These letters are a great exotic flower in modern literature.

—WFB

Chapter 14

Usage IV: Oh, What's the Usage?

Buckley and one of his discoveries, a young writer who became the formidable author, teacher, and syndicated columnist Garry Wills, no longer make beautiful music together, but they still correspond. Wills, for example, wrote a complaining letter to protest someone's substitution in a piece he wrote of *mesocephalic* for *mesomphalic,* feeling no need to apologize for having used the word in the first place.

In the exchange that follows, WFB, after a passing reference to Wills, picks up a criticism of something Buckley has written from a respected critic and friend—and thereby triggers a flood of exegesis, response, and counter-response.

———

One Sentence

Inasmuch as I am encouraged by my colleagues to fill this space as I please, I take liberties. Or do I? What follows is primarily of interest to syntacticians. How many of them are there? Not many. But—ah!—how many voyeurs? What follows is interesting, also, to students of friendship, nothing less than an assiduous case of which could have prompted the redoubtable Professor Hugh Kenner to such heroic efforts to demonstrate the demerits of a single English sentence. . . .

HK to WFB Sept. 19, 1968

. . . Garry [Wills] under pressure tends to deliquescent metaphor (vide his Miami piece, *NR*), as does WFB to filigree syntax (vide current *Esquire*, first sentence, which while it parses . . . resembles less a tensioned intricacy in the mode of M. Eiffel than it does a toddler's first efforts with Tinkertoy). . . .

WFB to HK Oct. 1

. . . You are surely wrong about that lead sentence? I re-read it, found it springy and tight.

HK to WFB Oct. 15

. . . about that *Esquire* lead: it reads in my copy:

"Robert F. Kennedy had a way of saying things loosely, and it may be that that is among the reasons why so many people invested so much idealism in him, it being in the idealistic (as distinguished from the analytical) mode to make large and good-sounding generalities, like the generality he spoke on April 5 after the assassination of Martin Luther King, two months exactly before his own assassination."

"Springy and tight" my foot. Those aren't springs, they're bits of Scotch tape. Have your syntactic DNA checked for mutations; it just isn't governing the wild forces of growth as of yore.

WFB to HK Oct. 17

Come on now, you are a goddam professor of English, so stop name-calling and get to work. . . .

HK to WFB Oct. 25

. . . Okay, that sentence:

One way of putting the problem is that it's not discernibly heading anywhere; it ambles along, stuffing more and more odds & ends into its elastic bag, until it simply decides to sit down. Mr. Niemeyer has ridiculed my interest in syntactic energy, countering my regret that Johann Sebastian Bach should be taking out the garbage with his pleasure that it's being taken out, whazzamatter, don't I want a tidy house? Yet I revert to the concept: something, something corresponding to tension and relaxation, to the turn of the key and the swing of the door, to departure from and return to the tonic, makes us willing to accept the necessity of a long sentence being one sentence and not three spliced by mispunctuation. Back to the exhibit: if there were a period after "loosely" no one would feel that a flight had been arrested in mid-course. Or after "him," or after "generalities." I think one test of the long sentence is that if it's stopped before it's over the reader should sense the incompleteness. This is sometimes a matter of formal grammar: if we start with "because" the reader won't accept a full stop until he's been accorded a principal clause. It's sometimes just a matter of promising in the opening words or by the opening cadence (a device of Gibbon's) some amplitude of concern the reader expects to see implemented. But here the offer to develop the proposition that RFK had a way of saying things loosely creates no syntactic expectation because it's capable of standing as a sentence by itself; nor does it retrospectively command the rest of the sentence, because the sentence has managed to end not with an amplification of RFK's looseness but with a triplicated irrelevancy about the date.

"Robert F. Kennedy had a way of saying things loosely: large and good-sounding generalities which being in the idealistic (as distinguished from the analytical) mode help explain why so many people invested so much idealism in him: generalities like the one Martin Luther King's assassination prompted him to utter on April 5, just two months, as it happened, before he was assassinated himself."

A possible improvement, if one *must* include all those components. The main difference is that by putting the colon after "loosely" one gives notice that the opening clause will preside over the remainder, not simply join to the next section of track. Then repeat of "generalities" to hitch the peroration to the second member. And rearrangement of terminal items keeps the mention of King and *l'affaire* Sirhan from sounding like doodles irrelevantly prompted by "April 5." I do not offer the improved version as anything but an exercise; I wasn't writing the article and haven't in my blood the points you anticipated making, so all I can manage is a piece of engineering.

I do not fuss about your occasional sentences to preserve a professorial edge. I merely call attention to dangers when I chance to see them. You revise carefully, I know, and it never hurts to have a few explicit criteria of revision. One is the rationale of the long sentence, as above (and failing that rationale, or failing time to adequate one's drafts to the rationale, vita being brevis and deadlines being yesterday, one ought, I think, to cut spaghetti into shorter sentences where natural stopping places occur). Another is that grammatical lint is best picked: in my suggested version I've avoided "that that," "reasons why" (your ear had told you to eschew yet a third "that"), and "it being." These all have rhetorical uses, as colloquialisms bounced off girders, but strung along in a row like old peanut shells they suggest WFB just plain improvising while he awaits a glimpse of daylight, and suggest to *les* Dwight Macdonalds that the Scrambled Egghead Method is to talk till one figures out what one is saying. This method is of course frequently necessary, and inoffensive, *viva voce,* say on TV, but its appearance should be avoided in print.

WFB to HK Nov. 4

. . . I worry about that confounded sentence, as one worries upon failing to appreciate something which one is prepared to postulate as good, to wit your criticism of it. I shan't even apologize for belaboring the point, because I know that you will know that by talking back, I am proving that I have not put you to such inconvenience merely for my own amusement.

"Robert Kennedy had a way of saying things loosely" followed by the colon you suggest means to me that I am about to demonstrate my allegation, or give an example of it. Followed by a period, the lilt of the sentence is, it seems to me, self-consciously dramatic, as in "John F. Kennedy had a way of seducing women." Followed by a comma, I thought it to be leading rather gradually to a point I did not want for a while yet, until the mood set in, to crystallize: whence, *", and it may be that that is among the reasons why so many people invested so much idealism in him"*—again, if the period had come here, I'd have attempted, or so it strikes me, a stolen base, and the reader would have been annoyed by the intimation that I have proved my point; or that I infer that the reader will merely permit me to asseverate it. When, i.e. by way of further explanation, begging the reader's indulgence so to speak, *", it being in the idealistic (as distinguished from the analytical) mode to make large and good-sounding generalities"*—department of amplification, not without—yet—the example I am about to furnish, and spend several hundred words confuting, *", like the generality he spoke on April 5, after the assassination of Martin Luther King"* surely writing about what Kennedy said about another man's assassination a few days after Kennedy's own assassination (which is when I wrote this article), gives a certain spooky suspense, which is ratified, Robert-Louis-Stevenson-wise, with the adverbial clause *", two months exactly before his own assassination."* That last I take to be a fair substitute for "two months exactly, as it happened, be-

fore his own assassination." Seems to me that, although the sentence is long it is not impossibly long, and that although the commas appear somehow to be loose and thoughtless linkages they are justified by their meiotic contribution to the plot I am contriving. Hell, it merely disturbs me that while I *understand* your generic points, my ear does not grant them a preemptive relevance in this instance; and I repeat, that I worry because undoubtedly you are right and I wrong. Anyway, I shall remember the generic advice. Believe. Me. Pal.

HK to WFB Nov. 7

. . . Not to wrangle, I'd make a final suggestion: that your inability to relate my comments, which you follow, to the sentence, the intentions of which you expound convincingly, is perhaps based on this, that you're not reading the printed sentence but hearing yourself speak it. By pause, by suspension, by inflection, by variation of tone and pace, you could make the "little plot" you speak of sing. The written language provides no notation for such controls, and your intention as graphed by printed words leaves the reader too much to supply, and too many options for supplying the wrong tacit commentary, e.g., that WFB is standing in an open space scattering peanut shells.

We have no such public style as Pope could posit, and vary from minutely, in an aesthetic of microscopic inappropriatenesses. We have instead the convention that the writer creates his operating conventions *de novo.* "Robert Kennedy had a way of saying things loosely."—followed by a hypothetical period, you say, its lilt is self-consciously dramatic. Yes, but those are the very first words of a long essay; we are just tuning in to station WFB; his eschewal of the self-consciously dramatic is not yet an operative principle; and one of the options open to us is to suppose that a dramatic opening was intended but muffed by a fault of punctuation. I think your rebuttal to my statement that the sentence could be terminated by a period at several points without creating a sense of incompleteness consists in an appeal to nuances of taste: it would make nuanced differences to cut it off here or here. So it would. But the reader hasn't yet a feel for the governing structure of taste in the piece before him. *Especially* in an opening, the reader would be well served by a syntactic tension, as inevitable as gravitation on an inclined plane, which makes it essential that the sentence incorporate, as it proceeds, the members it does, or else fall down. . . . *Mais passons.*

WFB *urbi et orbe,* Jan. 1, 1969: Who's right?

Kenner v. Buckley

Herewith my response to the well-aimed point from Professor Kenner ["Notes & Asides," Jan. 14]:

> *Syntactic energy is drained*
> *While pondering a thought.*
> *It's more important to have gained*
> *In logic than been caught*
> *By cadence, which could well ensnare*
> *The ruminating process.*
> *Professor, Sir, I couldn't care:*
> *Less.*

POLLY WILLIAMS
MOUNTAINSIDE, N.J.

Professor Kenner offers Mr. Buckley an "out" through his remark that the written language contains no notation for the subtle controls of pause, suspension, inflection, variation of tone and pace, which WFB would have required to make his *Esquire* lead "sing." Certainly I must agree with him that the sentence as WFB has written it and punctuated it does not sing; in fact, I had to reread it a couple of times to pin down its proposition. Unfortunately, Professor Kenner's edition singeth not itself, though it burns with a cold, gem-like flame.

There is an alternative course, though I'm sure the editors of *Esquire* might have been more than a little startled to see it adopted by WFB. It is, to utilize *all* the flexibility, all the nuances, of modern notation . . . to adapt and adopt the conventions of punctuation displayed by Cummings, Pound (particularly Pound—ain't he loverly?), and others in poetry, by Tennessee Williams in his plays and by William Faulkner in his prose, plays, and poetry.

RALPH D. COPELAND
LOCK HAVEN, PA.

The lamentable fact is that Wm. F., like the late Robt. F., has a way of saying things loosely, especially when he is writing about the late Robt. F., there being something contagious even in the recollection of the hard little Boston moptop who declaimed in the same flat accents for the brotherhood of man and the bugging of Jimmy Hoffa, whose enmity Kennedy craved as a crocodile feeds on barracuda steak.

It was a bum sentence, Bill. But you are still the greatest editor in the world.

JAMES JACKSON KILPATRICK
ALEXANDRIA, VA.

Dear Mr. Buckley:

At first I couldn't believe. Then, others confirmed. Our usually precise hero had slipped. On *Firing Line* he had lapsed into saying: *a number of.*

Thus, I'm impelled to point out—as I've done to Presidents, *N.Y. Times* editors, TV anchorpersons & others—that this three-word combination has been defined as "a meaningless phrase used by lazy writers & speakers" . . . has a variety of alternatives such as few, many, dozens, scores, etc. . . . & frequently can be eliminated without effect on a message's import.

Ban this inanity from publishing & politics & there'd be a vast saving of natural resources—forests, oil, coal & energy—currently wasted on its reproduction & dissemination. There also would be ancillary benefits including smaller newspapers (fewer hernias from handling Sunday editions), briefer newscasts &, conceivably, an occasional political speech that makes sense.

Of greater significance would be the spread of the addiction to literature:

> *Think of the poetry lost*
> *Had the phrase been used by Robert Frost,*
> *Lord Tennyson & Mr. Browning,*
> *Or in songs we enjoy singing.*
> *People would think Tennyson mad*
> *For: ". . . rode a number of lads."*
> *And Browning, feet of clay*
> *For: ". . . I love thee a number of ways."*
> *Plus, what of the cost to Frost*
> *For: ". . . I have a number of promises to keep & a*
> *   number of miles to go before I sleep"?*
> *And who'd want to dance with one's love*
> *To "Tea for a Number Of"*
> *Or join a singalong*
> *Of "A Number of Frenchmen Can't Be Wrong"?*
> *But all would wish a whammy*
> *On both Al Jolson & his "Mammy"*
> *For: "I'd walk a number of miles for a number of*
> *   your smiles."*

Please, kind sir, seek to provide a better example.

Sincerely,

ALEX W. BURGER

NEW ROCHELLE, N.Y.

Dear Mr. Burger: How do you handle the need to communicate, "A number of the odd-numbered series was revealed as the key to the missing formula?" Or should one simply abandon the search for the formula? Many thanks,

—WFB　　　　　　OCTOBER 19, 1984

To the Editor:

In a recent issue of *National Review*, a reader takes Mr. Buckley to task for using the phrase "a number of," calling it strictly meaningless. It is the critic himself who is at fault for not knowing an idiom when he sees one. As far back as 1380, Wyclif wrote: "In the Church above in heaven is a number of great saints." Bacon in 1626 says that water lilies have roots in the ground "and so do a number of other herbs that grow in ponds." The phrase has the clear meaning of *several*, a word that in our day tends to sound formal—hence the frequent and unambiguous recourse to "a number of."

To require logic of an idiom is waste of time—the critic might as well have said that "a good number" is a foolish expression because numbers are neither good nor bad. Yet "a number of" is not entirely unexplainable. It clearly implies that the thing described is not absent or even unique: a number*ing* is possible. Note that the adjective *numerous*, which is literally the same as "a number of," goes idiomatically in the other direction and means "a great many."

JACQUES BARZUN

NEW YORK, N.Y.　　　　JANUARY 11, 1985

The Editor
The Baltimore Sun
Baltimore, Md.

Dear Sir:

I have two objections to your editorial, "Buckley, *ex Cathedra*" (September 24).

You write of my calling Reagan's refusal to lay down tariffs to protect U.S. steel "the correct Christian decision," and you ask, "We trust that Jewish, Moslem, Hindu, and Buddhist teachings on the religious aspects of international commerce in steel were considered and dismissed as 'incorrect.' "

If you will consult Webster III, you will find that under "syn." for the adjective *Christian* is given, "decent, civilized." The example cited is, "act in a Christian fashion."

And then you write, "William F. Buckley, Jr., whose elegant arrogance and affectation of a British accent has won him fame and fortune . . ." You should have written, "William F. Buckley, Jr., whose elegant arrogance and affectation of a British accent *have* won him fame and fortune . . ." You see, arrogance and affectation being separate modifiers, they require the use of the plural verb.

Yours faithfully,

WM. F. BUCKLEY, JR.   FEBRUARY 8, 1985

Dear Mr. Buckley:

I enjoyed reading your response to the editor of the *Baltimore Sun* ["Notes & Asides," Feb. 8]. In pointing out his egregious grammatical error, however, you happened to commit one slight faux pas yourself. In the sentence "William F. Buckley, Jr., whose elegant arrogance and affectation of a British accent have won him fame and fortune . . ." arrogance and affectation are not modifiers; they are subjects (abstract nouns) of a modifying clause. Indeed they give the appearance of acting as modifiers (much, so my liberal colleagues assure me, the way Ed Meese can give the appearance of acting improperly). Furthermore, in your sentence "You see, arrogance and affectation being separate modifiers, they require the use of a plural verb," the word *they* is a redundant subject—though I find the usage stylistically apropos, considering its intended affectation.

Forgive me, Bill. This is what's become of the mind of an associate professor of English who has been forced to teach rudimentary grammar to his college students.

Sincerely,

RICHARD ORODENKER

PEIRCE JUNIOR COLLEGE

PHILADELPHIA, PA.

Dear Professor Orodenker: That's quite all right, quite all right, I understand the pedantic imperative. By the way, the device used above is called an anacoluthon. Cordially,

—WFB   MAY 17, 1985

Dear Mr. Buckley:

I recently read, with great interest, your article appearing in *Harper's* on "Giving Yale to Connecticut."

In that article you said: "if mind and conscience led them to the conclusion, they would be not only free, but compelled to decide . . ."

I assume that your use of the construction "not only . . . but . . ." is a form of "not only . . . but *also* . . ." If so, how can someone who is free also be compelled? If not, what did you intend to say?

Otherwise keep up the good work.

> Sincerely yours,
> SCOTT BREWER
> SUNY AT STONYBROOK, N.Y.

Dear Mr. Brewer: What I wrote is a contraction of "not only free, but [assuming your mind and conscience are in working order] compelled to [etc.]." Any time. And thanks very much. Cordially,

> —WFB   APRIL 16, 1982

Dear Mr. Buckley:
Some years ago, in correspondence, a gentleman prominent in the "peace" movement made one point on which I had to agree he was absolutely correct. I pass the lesson on to you, since the Dec. 1 *NR* (e.g., the editorial "Peking Duck") contains the same mistake in your own ordinarily impeccable prose. The fact is, words such as "escapee" and "attendee" should never be used in their vulgar senses. The ending "-ee" strictly means that the subject is acted on, not acting. Thus, in a jailbreak, the convicts getting away are escapers, the jailers are escapees. If a person has fleas, they are his attenders, he is their attendee.

I need not point out to you the importance of conserving precision in language. But I might say that, on occasion, the deft interjection of this particular point in debate can be useful in confounding the ungodly, including those in the "peace" movement.

> POUL ANDERSON
> ORINDA, CALIF.

Dear Mr. Buckley:
Re the first sentence of one of M. Stanton Evans's "Lawmakers" columns, which began: "Lincoln said it: . . . 'When you see eye-beams hoisted . . .' "???

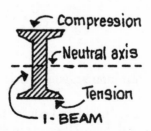

I am familiar with "I" beams (but I don't think Lincoln was)—first in cast iron and then steel, and rarely used in wood houses. Lincoln saw beams, girders, rafters, etc., but what the hell is an eye-beam except that which you fix on some blonde in a bikini? Elucidate for a very ancient architect.

FRANK ROEHR

WILSONVILLE, ORE.

Dear Mr. Roehr: The use of "eye" for "I" is common in telegraphic communications, as in: "Please ship me four eye-beams before eye go nuts." Cordially,

—WFB   JULY 24, 1981

Dear Mr. Buckley:

I have stumbled too long over the clumsy locutions journalists use for the way bureaucrats speak, e.g., *bureauspeak, bureaucratese.* I propose the following as euphonious and descriptive:

> **bureaulalia 1.** speech, esp. of functionaries, connoting progress while concealing its lack; **2.** mental disorder of one claiming to aid the commonweal, while feeding on it, often ravenously (*from* bureau: any government rathole, + lalia [Greek]: defective speech)

Are you able to give this word your endorsement? If so, a plug in the magazine would make our public discourse more sonorous.

Sincerely yours,

DENNIS R. KELLEY

GLENVIEW, ILL.

Dear Mr. Kelley: I can give your word exposure, but not my endorsement; sorry. It's pedantic, and wouldn't flow into the vocabulary, leaning as it does on a Greek word that no one is familiar with—except, presumably, Greeks. Cordially,

—WFB

Dear Mr. Buckley:

Although I no longer subscribe to your journal, every Christmas I would give a subscription to Hazel Overland, my grandmother. Although she did not always agree with your politics, she enjoyed your writing and loved your God. I recall how she raved about your pilgrimage to Lourdes. My grandmother died on Easter Sunday. They said it was peaceful. I'm glad. I'm also thankful for all the enjoyable moments you gave my grandmother during her last years on Earth.

Sincerely,

JOSEPH HOLPER

DEKALB, ILL.

Dear Mr. Holper: Many thanks, and may your grandmother R.I.P. By the way, it's *our* God, you know. Cordially,

—WFB   JUNE 13, 1994

Dear Mr. Buckley:

You have a maddening habit of using the words "England" and "Britain" interchangeably; most recently in the column based on your interview of Mr. Kinnock. You present a scenario in which the Soviets "take out Cardiff," and the U.S. President asks whether he should issue an ultimatum to the Soviet Union to "leave England alone"—as if Cardiff were part of England.

Listen: England is England. England plus Scotland and Wales is Britain (Great Britain, if you prefer). Britain plus Northern Ireland is the United Kingdom.

It would be wrong to go to Cardiff or to Glasgow and remark to the locals, "It's nice to be in England." Moreover, it would be most inadvisable.

Sincerely,
RICHARD R. DOBSON
EDITOR OF THE EDITORIAL PAGE
MINOT DAILY NEWS
MINOT, N.D.

Dear Mr. Dobson: Does that mean I can't say anymore, Oh, to be in Cardiff, now that April's here? Cordially,

—WFB   AUGUST 20, 1982

Dear Mr. Buckley:

Am a bit annoyed because two, maybe three, times in *NR* I have seen "transpired" used as a synonym for happened. I almost swear I saw it so used in one of your columns. Possible? Naw!

I still use the essay on language you did for the American Heritage Dictionary* and would by inference swear that you would rub the bugger out on every occasion. Do I infer too much?

Sincerely,
(MR.) CONNIE MACK REA
ENGLISH DEPARTMENT
CALIFORNIA UNIVERSITY OF PENNSYLVANIA
CALIFORNIA, PA.

* See chapter 16, "Passing in Review."

Dear Mr. Rea: Thanks for your act of faith, which is by the way justified. I'd as soon slit my throat as misuse *transpire*. If it was misused by others in these sacred glades, let's hope that this way of telling them satisfies all relevant diplomatic requirements. Cordially,

—WFB   JULY 20, 1992

Chapter 15

On
Fiction

Buckley—at an age when many men are thinking of consolidating their gains, taking no new risks, and settling for doing well what they already know how to do—turned to fiction. In this introduction to *The Blackford Oakes Reader* (Andrews and McMeel, 1995), he gives his version of how the novels came about.

––––––

BLACKFORD OAKES: AN INTRODUCTION

I take the opportunity to answer some of the questions most often put to me as the author of the ten novels featuring Blackford Oakes. A question that continues to intrigue is: What is it that, at age fifty, beckoned me to write fiction?

It's a brief story, rather mundane, but it has its charm. I had for many years been in touch with Samuel Vaughan, then of Doubleday, a gentle, bright, shrewd man of letters who suggested we lunch and said he'd bring along two friends. It developed that they too were associates of Doubleday. The agenda for the lunch never materialized formally, though at some point, Sam asked if I had recently read any action thriller I thought especially well of and I said, Yes, I read *Day of the Jackal* last week and thought it tremendous. "Why don't you try writing a novel?" he said. I answered, as I remember, "Sam, why don't you play a trumpet concerto?" The conversation proceeded, pleasantly and aimlessly, and the next morning I found on my desk a proposed contract to write a novel for Doubleday.

I was titillated by the entrepreneurial initiative of my friend Sam, but it happened that that very day, the newspapers carried the story of William Safire. He had turned in, to Morrow, his volume on Richard Nixon, for which an advance commitment had been made to pay him $250,000. What the news story told us was that William Morrow had rejected his manuscript on the grounds that it was not "satisfactory."

Now what everybody who knows anything knew, indeed knows, is that Bill Safire does not submit "unsatisfactory" manuscripts. What was "unsatisfactory," in the summer of 1975, was Richard Nixon. He had a year before left office, the first American President to be run out of town so to speak with wet towels. The publishing company was taking an unseemly advantage of that little phrase in the publisher's contract that specifies that the writer's manuscript has to be "satisfactory" and that the publisher is the sole judge of whether that criterion has been met.

Accordingly I wrote to Sam Vaughan and said, Well sure, I'll try to write a novel, but how about this: You pay me up front one third of the advance and I write one hundred pages. I send these to you, and you then say after reading them: "Go ahead"—in which case you are committed to paying me the balance of the advance. Or else you say, "It was a fun idea, but kindly abort immediately"—in which case I'll have become an ex-novelist before ever becoming a novelist. . . . As it turned out, it was all very good news. *Saving the Queen* appeared on the best-seller list one week before its official publication date, and stayed there for thirteen weeks.

What was the novel about? Well, it featured one Blackford Oakes.

I am occasionally asked about the genesis of Blackford Oakes, the protagonist of my novels.

He was a kind of distillate. I arrived in Switzerland with only a single idea in mind, and that idea was to commit literary iconoclasm: I would write a book in which the good guys and the bad guys were actually distinguishable from one another. I took a deep breath and further resolved that the good guys would be—the Americans!

I had recently seen a movie called *Three Days of the Condor.* Perhaps you will remember that Robert Redford, a CIA agent of Restless Intelligence, working in a CIA front in New York City called the American Literary Historical Society, goes out one day to buy a hamburger, and returns to the CIA brownstone to find all nine of his colleagues quite dead. Murdered. By pistols firing ice pellets. In due course we discover that the Mr. Big who ordered the killings isn't a robber or a member of the Mafia or of the KGB. He is very high up in the government of the United States. Indeed, if the movie had endured another half hour, by the law of compound interest the viewer would have been satisfied only on discovering that the evil spirit behind the killing of Robert Redford's CIA colleagues was the President of the United States; or, to be really dramatic and reach all the way up to the highest vault in the national pantheon, maybe Ralph Nader.

Thus the movie went, deep in suspense. Mr. Big, who had ordered the mass killings, might have been exposed, finally, as a conventional double agent: posing as an American patriot, but actually a spy working for the Soviet Union. It transpired, however, that the man who ordered the slaughter was a one hundred percent American, period. And there was nothing at all unusual about him in the movie. His decision to eliminate all those nice people at the American Literary Historical Society was entirely routine. He did so because they were about to stumble on a secret, contingent CIA operation—by following a lead turned up by Robert Redford's Restless Intelligence.

So finally, in a dramatic sidewalk confrontation, Mr. Big's deputy—on instructions from Mr. Big—explains to Redford that the unfortunate killings were motivated by high patriotism: they were a necessary safeguard against the discovery of a top secret plan to protect America against a contingent shortage of oil. Stressing the importance of keeping Redford's knowledge secret, the deputy invites Redford to come back into the Agency, no hard feelings, and simply accept the imperatives of real life . . . of an intelligence agent in the modern world.

But Redford, taking off his glasses in anticipation of heady thought, says, "No, *never*. This very day, I have disclosed everything to . . ." The camera slithers up to a marquee above the two men and you see the logo of . . . *The New York Times*. The director of *Three Days of the Condor* neglected only to emblazon on it, "Daniel Ellsberg Slept Here."

The deputy reacts like the witch come in contact with water. He snarls and shivers and slinks away after muttering half-desperately: *"Maybe they won't print it!"* But Redford has by now seeded the audience with his Restless Intelligence, and we all know that *The New York Times will* print it, and thus we shall all be free.

The film's production notes stated, "Over a year ago, Stanley Schneider, Robert Redford, Sidney Pollack, and Dino de Laurentiis decided to create a film that would reflect the climate of America in the aftermath of the Watergate crisis."

"The climate of America" is a pretty broad term. They really meant, "the climate of America" as seen by Jane Fonda, the Institute for Policy Studies, and *The Nation* magazine. One recalls Will Rogers returning, in 1927, from the Soviet Union, where he had witnessed a communal bath at which the bathers were nude.

"Did you see all of Russia?" a reporter asked.

"No," Rogers said, weighing his answer carefully. "But I saw all of parts of Russia."

Redford-Pollack-de Laurentiis had shown us the climate in all of parts of America. It was very cold out there.

And so I thought to attempt to write a book in which it was never left in doubt that the CIA, for all the complaints about its performance, is, when all is said and done, not persuasively likened to the KGB.

I was myself an agent of the CIA, for nine months beginning in 1951 when I left college. I do not confuse my admiration for the mission of the CIA with its overall effectiveness. A few years after leaving the CIA I published [as noted earlier] in *National Review* an editorial paragraph that read, "The attempted assassination of Sukarno in Jakarta last week had all the earmarks of a CIA operation. Everyone in the room was killed except Sukarno."

The point I sought to make, and continued to do so in subsequent novels, is that the CIA, whatever its failures, sought, during those long years in the struggle for the world, to advance the honorable alternative. When I wrote, it wasn't only Robert Redford who was however obliquely traducing the work of our central intelligence agency. He had starred in a movie the point of which was that the CIA is a corrupt and bloody-minded secret instrument of an amoral government, and that it routinely embarks on stratagems that beggar moral justification. Many others were making similar points in every branch of the media: in novels of the recent past, novels by Graham Greene, and John le Carré,* and Len Deighton, for instance. The point, really, was that there wasn't all that much to choose from in a contest between the KGB and the CIA. Both organizations, it was fashionable to believe, were defined by their practices. I said to Johnny Carson, when on his program he raised just that question, that to say that the CIA and the KGB engage in similar practices is the equivalent of saying that the man who pushes an old lady into the path of a hurtling bus is not to be distinguished from the man who pushes an old lady out of the way of a hurtling bus, on the grounds that, after all, in both cases someone is pushing an old lady around.

The novelistic urge of the great ideological egalitarians who wrote books under such titles as *The Ugly American* had been to invest in their Western protagonists appropriately disfiguring personal characteristics. So that the American (or British) spy had become, conglomerately, a

---

* See review of le Carré in chapter 16, "Passing in Review."

paunchy, alcoholic, late-middle-aged cuckold—moreover, an agent who late at night, well along in booze, ruminates to the effect that, when all is said and done, who really was to judge so indecipherable a question as whether the United States was all that much better than the Soviet Union? The KGB and the CIA really engage in the same kind of thing, and what they do defines them, not why they do it, right?

When I sat down, a yellow sheet of paper in my typewriter, to begin writing that first novel, it suddenly occurred to me that it would need a protagonist. By the end of the afternoon I had created Blackford Oakes, the principal character in *Saving the Queen.*

A year later, the editor of *Vogue* magazine wrote to me to say that many reviewers had denominated Blackford Oakes as being "quintessentially" American. She invited me to explain, explicitly, what was the "American look." I thought to reject the invitation, because I resist the very notion of quintessentiality, as here invoked. It seems to me an image that runs into its inherent incredibility. You will remember that F. P. Adams once said that the average American is a little above average.

The reason you cannot have the quintessential American is the very same reason you cannot have a quintessential apple pie, or indeed a quintessential anything that is composed of so many ingredients. In all composites there has got to be an arrangement of attributes, and no such arrangement can project one quality to the point of distorting others. This is true even in the matter of physical beauty. An absolutely perfect nose has the effect of satellizing the other features of a human face; a beautiful face is a comprehensive achievement.

So anyway, Blackford Oakes is not the quintessential American, but I fancy he is *distinctively* American, and the first feature of the distinctively American male is, I think, spontaneity, a freshness of sorts born of curiosity and enterprise and native wit.

Would you believe that three days after meeting her, Blackford Oakes was in bed with the queen of England? (Not, I hasten to elucidate, the incumbent queen. Blackford Oakes, as the distinctive American, is a young man of taste, who sleeps only with fictitious queens, thereby avoiding international incidents.) There was something yes, distinctively, wonderfully American, it struck me, about bedding down a British queen: a kind of arrant yet lovable presumption. But always on the understanding that it be done decorously, and that there was no aftertaste of the gigolo in the encounter. Moreover, in my novel the queen was the seducer, Blackford the seduced.

I remember with some trepidation—even now, almost twenty years later—the day that my novel came out in London. The first questioner at the televised exchange was, no less, the editor of *The Economist,* Andrew

Knight, and he asked me a question I thought quite un-English in its lack of circumspection: "Mr. Buckley, would you like to sleep with the queen?"

Now such a question poses quite awful responsibilities. Just to begin with, I am a married man. And then, there being a most conspicuous incumbent queen, one could hardly wrinkle up one's nose as if the question evoked the vision of an evening with Queen Victoria on her diamond jubilee. The American with taste has to guard against any lack of gallantry, so that the first order of business became the assertion of an emancipating perspective, which would escort Queen Elizabeth II gently out of the room, lest she be embarrassed. This I hoped to accomplish by saying, just a little sleepily, as Blackford Oakes might have done, "*Which* queen?"— and then quickly, before the interrogator could lug his incumbent monarch back into the smoker—"Judging from historical experience, I would need to consult my lawyer before risking an affair with *any* British queen."

The American male must be tactful, and tact is most generally accomplished by changing the subject without its appearing that you have done so as a rebuke. It worked, and another aspect of my novel came before the house, the character of Blackford Oakes.

He appears on the scene at age twenty-two, a veteran of the war. So I stuck him in Yale, which gave me the advantage of being able to write about a familiar few acres. It has been observed by several critics that Blackford Oakes emerged with characteristics associated, in the literature, with Yale men.

Like what?

Principally, I suppose, self-confidence; a certain worldliness that is neither bookish nor in any sense of the word anti-intellectual. Blackford Oakes is an engineer by training, the kind of engineer who learns how to build bridges, and his nonroyal girlfriend is studying for her Ph.D. and doing her doctorate on Jane Austen. *She* is not expected to dwell in conversation on her own specialty, let alone show any curiosity about how to build bridges. The American look wears quite offhandedly its special proficiencies: If one is a lawyer, one does not go about talking like Oliver Wendell Holmes, any more than Charles Lindbergh went about sounding like Charles Lindbergh. Though Blackford quite rightly shows a qualified, if not extensive, curiosity about Jane Austen, and probably has read (actually, reread: one never reads Jane Austen, one only *rereads* her) *Pride and Prejudice,* and his girlfriend has no objection to the profession of engineering.

Now Blackford Oakes is physically handsome, in a sense a metaphor for his ideals. Here I took something of a chance. I decided not only to make him routinely good looking, but to make him startlingly so. I don't mean startling in the sense that, let us say, Elizabeth Taylor is startlingly beautiful. It is hard to imagine a male counterpart for what we understand as pulchritude. An extremely handsome man is not the *equivalent* of an extremely beautiful woman, he is her complement, and that is very important to bear in mind in probing the American look—which is not, for example, the same thing as the Italian look. When Schopenhauer exclaimed that a sixteen-year-old girl is the "smash triumph of nature," he made a cosmic statement that could only have been made about the female sex.

So that when I decided that Blackford Oakes should be startlingly handsome, it was required that he be that in a distinctively American way, and what does *that* mean? Well it doesn't mean you look like Mickey Rooney, obviously. But it doesn't mean you have to look like Tyrone Power, either. I think the startlingly handsome American male is not made so by the regularity of his features, however necessary that regularity may be, but by the special quality of his expression. It has to be for this reason that, flipping past the male models exhibited in the advertising sections of the local newspaper or of *Esquire* magazine, one seldom finds oneself pausing to think: That man is startlingly handsome. But such an impression *is* taken away, from time to time, from a personal encounter, or even from a candid photograph. Because the American look, in the startlingly handsome man, requires animation, but tempered by a certain shyness; a reserve.

I thought of Billy Budd. I have long since forgotten just how Melville actually described him, but Melville communicated that Billy Budd was startlingly handsome. But looks aside, his distinctiveness was not that of Blackford Oakes. Billy Budd is practically an eponym for innocence, purity. Oakes, though far removed from jadedness, is worldly. And then, and then . . .

Billy Budd, alas, is humorless. Correction: not *alas*. "Do not go about as a demagogue, urging a triangle to break out of the prison of its three sides," G. K. Chesterton warned us, "because if you succeed, its life will come to a lamentable end." Give Billy Budd a sense of humor and he shatters in front of you into thousands of little pieces, which you can never reconstruct. Blackford Oakes doesn't go about like Wilfrid Sheed's protagonist in *Transatlantic Blues,* or John Gregory Dunne's in *True Confessions,* being hilariously mordant. The American look here is a leavened sarcasm. But careful, now: Escalate sarcasm and you break through the clouds into the ice-cold of nihilism. The American must *believe.* However discreetly or understatedly. Blackford Oakes believed. He tended to divulge his beliefs in a kind of slouchy, oblique way. But at the margin he was, well—an American, with Judeo-Christian predilections; and he knew, as with the clothes he wore so casually, that he was snug as such; that, like his easygoing sweater and trousers, they—fitted him. As did the ideals, and even most of the practices, of his country.

I remember with delight reading a review of that first novel, published in *The Kansas City Star,* written by a professor of English from the University of Missouri, I think it was. I had never heard of the gentleman, but he made it quite clear that he had spent a considerable part of his adult life abominating me and my works and my opinions. He was manifestly distressed at not quite disliking my first novel, which he proceeded to describe. He salved his conscience by concluding, "The hero of *Saving the Queen,* Mr. Blackford Oakes, is tall, handsome, witty, agreeable, compassionate and likable, from which at least we can take comfort in knowing that the book is not autobiographical."

There arose, as a practical matter, the responsibility of recreating in fiction men who have been very much alive in recent history, and investing in them conspicuous attributes for which they were well known.

Consider, for instance, the proud, patrician, sarcastic Dean Acheson, Secretary of State under Harry Truman. He is an adamant critic of the Republican Party, the party of his old friend Allen Dulles, the Director of the Central Intelligence Agency who, one afternoon in 1953, soon after Truman was replaced by President Eisenhower, comes to call on him to confer about a looming crisis in West Germany:

> Allen Dulles had missed the day-to-day analysis of international events—mordant, clairvoyant—of this infuriating man, with whom he had been officially associated, until the last election, in the administration of President Truman. Now Mr. Acheson had just published a book, called *A Democrat Looks at His Party,* in which he had calmly announced that the principal distinction between a Republican and a Democrat is that Democrats tend to be bright, and Republicans tend to be stupid.
>
> "It's just that easy," he now teased his guest while tea was being poured. "You mustn't be offended by this, Allen. Besides, you must find it consoling that your people will stay in power a good long time."

There was a special tone of mock resignation in Acheson's observation.

> "In some discursive reading the other day I found interesting corroboration for this thesis. It is from a speech by John Stuart Mill delivered, I believe, in the British parliament."

With his left hand, Acheson extends his teacup to the maid who refilled it as he adjusted his glasses with his right hand.

"Mill said"—Acheson reads now from a book—" 'I never meant to say that the Conservatives are generally stupid. I meant to say that stupid people are generally Conservative. I believe that is so obviously and universally admitted a principle' "—the Secretary raised his eyebrows in tribute to the majesty of First Principles—" 'that I hardly think any gentleman will deny it. Suppose any party, in addition to whatever share it may possess of the ability of the community, had nearly the whole of its stupidity, that party must'—take heart, Allen—'by the laws of its constitution be the stupidest party; and I do not see why honorable gentlemen should see that position as at all offensive to them, for it ensures their being always an extremely powerful party.' " Dean Acheson smiled with great satisfaction, and looked up again, as if to acknowledge, reverently, yet another providential insight.

Here, then, was an attempt to recreate theoretically, if you like, a dominant impulse in a dominating American character of the fifties. I would write a dozen such vignettes in the novels that lay ahead. I needed, for instance, to cope with John Fitzgerald Kennedy. How to do so? I elected the device of the soliloquy. Talking to himself. He is all alone in the Oval Office, at the end of a day, a few minutes before he is summoned upstairs to prepare for a state dinner. Listen. . . .

I've got just one hour before I need to go upstairs to dress for the state dinner for what's-his-name, the little hypocrite. Allen Dulles told me he's stolen maybe forty, maybe fifty million bucks, and he is always poor-mouthing about his people. Damn right they're poor. He stays in power another ten years, what's-his-name (I must make it a serious point to get his name straight before the state dinner—why aren't they all called Gonzalez? I mean, most of them are as it is)—ten more years and his "people" will have nothing at all left.

Ah, but if only the worst problems were Latin American. Latin America. Chiquita Banana, da-da-da da-da. How does it go?

. . . But I'm putting off what I need to concentrate on. More hard thought on Khrushchev, the bastard, and Berlin. I can't remember whether Dad told me that all Communist chiefs of state, like all American businessmen, were s.o.b.'s. Maybe he thought I'd simply take that for granted.

Two weeks from now I'll have met with Khrushchev . . . Is it possible to count the number of hours I've spent studying Khrushchev? With Dean Acheson, for instance? Good old Dean, he wants just one little world war before he dies . . . What do they say about Khrushchev? Pretty much the same thing. I've studied the minutes of: God! Geneva summit, 1955. Camp David summit, 1959. And Paris summit, 1960. Khrushchev aborted the damned thing on account of our U-2 flight! That was vintage Khrushchev, right? Complaining about espionage! Especially the press conference he gave when he stopped over in Vienna. Said maybe Ike was just a little cuckoo . . .

Brings up an interesting point. One of the things I have to ask myself is: How far do I let him go? I mean, if he starts to scream and yell, what do I do in the cause of Peace with Honor? God, I wish that phrase had never been coined. Fact is, you don't often get both at the same time.

Okay, so what's he up to? Seriously, what is he up to? Jack old boy, I mean, Mr. President old boy, let's start that at the other end. What's he *not* up to?

Well, he's not up to beginning a nuclear war. Among other things, Poppa Marx wouldn't like that. A nuclear war with maybe only Patagonians left over isn't going to do much to validate the Marxist theory of class struggle. Okay, at what point do we start dropping nuclear bombs? A hell of a question to ask, but I'm the one who's going to decide.

Khrushchev is sort of unique, they all say. But so are all Soviet chiefs of state. That's the way they talk, the way they behave.

Well by God, that's not the way they're going to talk to me! Screw summit conferences.

No, that's the wrong word. Don't want to say anything unfriendly about screwing.

To hell with summit conferences.

If Khrushchev is just being Khrushchev, then the boys have got to weigh whether just being Khrushchev is the best way to advance their cause. And the only means they have to measure that is me. How do I react? That's the question. How does John Fitzgerald Kennedy, President of the United States, maximum leader of the imperialist powers, react? And what will I come up with, in my search for something we can give them, that we can do without?

The special telephone on his desk rang, to which, at the other end, only one person had access.

"I'm coming, dear."

. . . The second book confronted a dilemma. What to do about the inspiring young West German nobleman who in 1953 was emerging as the probable victor of impending national elections on a platform of reuniting Germany at any cost? Stalin had communicated to Eisenhower: Get rid of that man, or—prepare for a Russian invasion of Germany.

What to do?

Stained Glass, I happily recall, went on to win the American Book Award as the best mystery story of the year. I like to think it was not the narrative suspense that overwhelmed the judges. What the book did was to pose the central question of counterintelligence and espionage as conducted by a free society.

The decision had finally been reached, in Washington, to accede to the demands of the Kremlin and to assassinate my fictional West German, Count Axel Wintergrin, whose startling rise to power threatened a world war.

And so the execution—rigged as an electrical accident, at the count's old Gothic castle—was arranged. Blackford Oakes supervised the plan (even though, at the end, he refused to take a personal hand in its consummation). And so the gallant and idealistic young German politician, who might seriously have challenged the Russian hegemony, was dead. And a devoted legend about him was born, so that every year, around the reconstructed thirteenth-century family chapel, larger and larger crowds gathered to commemorate the anniversary of his death. On the tenth anniversary, Blackford Oakes, the count's executioner, was discreetly present in the chapel and he spotted, traveling incognito, the man who, by coded telegraph ten years ago, had given him that awful, terminal command to proceed with the execution: It was retired CIA chief Allen Dulles.

By now—ten years later—it was retrospectively clear that Stalin would not have reacted to a political victory by Wintergrin by moving into Europe. So that the execution, in hindsight, had been a most gruesome mistake strategically, its moral hideousness quite apart.

Walking back to his car in the parking lot, after the memorial services, Blackford Oakes espied the man, the head of the agency for which he worked, but a man he had never laid eyes on before today. Inflamed by the memories evoked during the ceremony mourning the young man he had put to death, Oakes suddenly—impulsively—approaches the car of Allen Dulles. The text reads . . .

He waited until the old man had unlocked the door at the driver's side and entered. He knocked on the window opposite. Surprised, but without hesitation the old man reached over and tripped open the door handle. Blackford opened the door, got in, and closed it. Sitting with his hands on the steering wheel, Dulles turned his head. Blackford did not extend his hand. He said simply,

"I am Blackford Oakes."

"I see." Allen Dulles did not go through the formality of introducing himself.

There was a pause.

"Well, Mr. Dulles, did we do the right thing in 1952?"

"Mr. Oakes, the question you asked, I do not permit myself to explore, not under any circumstances."

"Why not?"

"Because in this world, if you let them, the ambiguists will kill you."

"The ambiguists, as you call them, were dead right about Count Wintergrin."

"You are asking me to break my rule."

Blackford replied: "Excuse me, sir, but is your goddamn rule more important than Wintergrin and his cause?"

"Actually," said Dulles, "it is. Or, if you prefer, put it this way, Oakes: I have no alternative than to believe it is more important. And I hope you will understand, because if you do it will be easier. If you do not, you are still too inexperienced to discuss these matters with me."

"I don't want it to be easier for me." Oakes turned now to look directly at the man whose will had governed Blackford's own for ten years. He found himself raising his voice, something he never did. "Wintergrin was the great hope for the West. The great opportunity. The incarnation of western idealism. You made me . . ."

He stopped. Already ashamed of a formulation that stripped him of his manhood. Nobody had forced Blackford to lead Axel Wintergrin to the execution chamber.

He changed, as quickly as possible, the arrangement of his thought. "You lost a great chance."

Dulles was now aroused. He lit his pipe with jagged movements of his hands.

"I believe you are right. I believe Wintergrin was right. The Russians, I believe, would not in fact have moved. But do you want to know something I don't believe?" His voice was strained.

Blackford was silent.

"I don't believe the lesson to draw is that we must not act because, in acting, we may prove to be wrong. And I know"—his eyes turned to meet Blackford's—"that you know that Axel Wintergrin thought so too."

There was nothing more to say. Impulsively, Blackford extended his hand, and Dulles took it.

When I finished that book, and before I had given it a title, I wrote to an old friend—we had met in 1954—to say, "Henry, I have written a book, the narrative of which is set forth in the accompanying blurb written by the publisher. I should like to dedicate it to you, and perhaps to call the book *Détente*. But I would not want to do this if it would cause you any embarrassment."

Henry Kissinger wrote back, "Dear Bill: Many thanks, but I think the book, which I look forward to reading, would best be inscribed to someone else while I am Secretary of State. If you wish to dedicate your next novel to me, I would be very grateful. Provided it isn't on the subject of Cyprus."

Well, Blackford Oakes has not visited Cyprus. After his terrible mission in Germany he was in Paris, in *Who's On First*, where he faced a moral dilemma that got him fired.

He was next seen (*Marco Polo, If You Can*) in the Lubyanka Prison in Moscow, condemned to death after his U-2 plane was shot down over southwest Asia, a constituent episode in a great master plot designed to accelerate crystallizing differences between Khrushchev's Soviet Union and Mao's China.

He went then, in *The Story of Henri Tod,* to Berlin, where he immobilized himself, rather than abort a patriotic attempt by West German patriots to frustrate the Soviet creation of the Berlin Wall.

In *See You Later Alligator,* Blackford Oakes was in Cuba, negotiating, at the direction of President Kennedy, with Che Guevera a possible détente. At one point in the story he declines to obey abrupt orders from Washington to abort his mission and return home.

In *High Jinx* he was in London, on assignment to penetrate the leak of highly secret documents which foretold the slaughter of the men sent out to liberate Albania.

In *Mongoose, R.I.P.,* we learned that the Russians, retreating from Cuba after the missile crisis, had left one missile secretly in place, programmed to land in Dallas. Fidel Castro had planned for the missile to be fired at Dallas—on November 22, 1963, when President Kennedy would be there.

In *Tucker's Last Stand,* the protagonist—yes, an American intelligence officer—turns over our critical plans on how to block the Ho Chi Minh trail to his girlfriend, even after he learns that she is an agent, working for the enemy. Blackford Oakes finds himself powerless to intervene.

And in *A Very Private Plot,* Blackford Oakes has to report to President Reagan that there is an entirely native plot afoot in Moscow to assassinate Gorbachev. And how does Reagan react? With excruciating difficulty.

In the first novel I guess it is correct to say that I intuitively got the idea that the novel should frame a single person (primarily). That person's character and experiences should illuminate the story. In *Saving the Queen* it was Blackford himself, at school in England, developing a character and a knowledge of Britain and its institutions that he would come to lean on only six years later.

In *Stained Glass* I sought to portray a young, aristocratic German idealist, to tell what he did when Hitler took Germany to war, how he comported himself during the war years and immediately after, as the dream consolidated in his mind: that his mission would be to deliver his country from the post-Hitler tyranny.

In *Who's On First* I felt the need to convey something of the feeling of life in Gulag. I had read Solzhenitsyn and sought to explore what life was like for two dissenting scientists during the last few years of Stalin, and what it was like to emerge from Gulag and confront the challenge of servitude to the new Soviet masters.

In *The Story of Henri Tod* I focused on a young Jewish boy, in hiding with his family from Hitler, spirited away to Great Britain, cut off from a younger sister with whom he had been inseparable, and the hardening of a resolve, like that of the aristocratic young count in *Stained Glass*, to lift the iron curtain that divided Berlin.

In the two Cuban-set novels I focused on a young Spaniard, lured to the Communists after the civil war. He was the object of a quixotic effort to rob a bank which resulted in years of imprisonment, followed by a devoted apprenticeship to the Party—which dispatched him to Mexico to take part in the assassination of Leon Trotsky. He found himself a party to the (historically correct) assassination of Soviet ambassador Oumansky—and his own wife.

And *A Very Private Plot* gives us a portrait of a young Ukrainian growing up under the Communist lash, a prodigy at school, sent to the Afghanistan front where, viewing the carnage, a slow resolve within him consolidates. He decides, quietly, that he will assassinate Gorbachev.

Some of the portraits lean directly on history. They are the kernel of the ten novels, and are here set down for the first time unencumbered.

Well, the Cold War ended. Blackford Oakes, in a few flash-forward scenes in *Plot*, is seventy years old. The time had come to pack it in. The novels will, it is my judgment, survive, for reasons I leave it to others to indite. The purpose of this volume is to extract from each one of them one portrait, perhaps memorable.

I have taken care to isolate the portraits in this volume so that they stand on their own two legs. No reader need know anything that happened before in that novel or, for that matter, anything that happened subsequently. . . .

I pray that the reader will enjoy even languorously the animations here collected. . . .

Entertainment and distraction are the objective. The educational objective in the novels has been to make the point, so difficult for so many Westerners to comprehend, that counterintelligence and espionage, conducted under Western auspices, weren't exercises in conventional political geometry. They were—they are—a moral art.

Consider one hypothetical dilemma and reason backward, from the particular to the generality. I give you a question and ask that you wrestle with it, confining yourself, if you can, within the maxims of the conventional morality.

Is it wrong to effect the execution of a chief of a state with which you are not at war?

Yes, it is wrong to do so.

Is it wrong to countenance a destructive event of such magnitude as conceivably to trigger a world war?

Yes, it is wrong.

What then do you call it when it appears to rational men that the second injunction cannot be observed save by defying the first?

Scene: Uganda. Colonel Idi Amin has got possession of a nuclear bomb and plans at midnight to dispatch a low-flying plane to drop that bomb on Jerusalem. A CIA agent in the field communicates to Washington that Idi Amin will lie between the crosshairs of the agent's rifle at the airport before the bomber is dispatched. Should he squeeze the trigger?

There are those, and Blackford Oakes was one of them, who would address that morally wrenching point by saying two things: (1) As to the particular question, yes, authorize the agent to shoot, in order to abort the destruction of Jerusalem and all that might then follow. But (2), do not then require as a condition of this decision that laws or rules be set down that embody the distinction. It isn't possible to write such judgments into law, no more than to specify to the artist the exact arrangement of circumstances that call for a daub of Prussian blue or, to the composer, the exact harmonic situation that benefits from rules that admit the striking of an A-augmented eleventh chord.

Blackford Oakes lived in an age when what mattered most was the survival of one of two systems. Us and Them—that was the difference that mattered. The failure by beneficiaries of life in the free world to recognize what it was that we had here, over against what it would have been had our lives been transformed so that we too might live under totalitarianism, amounted to moral and intellectual nihilism. This was far more incriminating of our culture than any transgression against eristic scruples of the kind that preoccupied so many of our moralists who inveighed against the protocols of the CIA and MI-6.

Blackford Oakes had weaknesses spiritual and corporeal. But a basic assumption guided him. It was that the survival of everything we cherish depended on the survival of the culture of liberty; and that this hung on our willingness to defend this extraordinary country of ours, so awfully mixed up so much of the time, so schizophrenic in our understanding of ourselves and our purposes, so crazily indulgent in our legion of wildly ungovernable miscreants. Yet, without ever saying so in so many words, Oakes thought this country the finest bloom of nationhood in all recorded time, worth the risk, which he so often took, of life and limb.

He did all that, but he recognized also that a vital part of America's singularity is its capacity to give pleasure, which it is the primary aim of the Oakes novels to do.

—WFB   JULY 15, 1994

The resulting novel sequence was a phenomenon. Blackford Oakes entered the language as a well-known (if not well-understood) character, and almost every one of the novels was a best-seller, until WFB ended the series of novels at ten. The following is a sample of the kind of expanded attention Buckley awards to at least one new major character in each novel.

Erika Chadinoff

The parents of her friends in America would make references to her "privileged" upbringing and now and then would imply, not without admiration, and not without envy, that she had been spoiled. Sometimes over a weekend visit or vacation, Erika's hosts, in the effusive style of the forties, would push Erika forward to exhibit one of her accomplishments, even as they might ask an older brother to show off a card trick. Erika went through the usual stages: she would be shy, she would be recalcitrant, she would use evasive tactics, but after her third year at the Ethel Walker School in Simsbury, Connecticut, she surprised everybody who knew her. Her fat friend Alice begged her after dinner one night to play on the piano excerpts from the first movement of the Grieg A-Minor Concerto, which Erika had played before the entire school at the annual concert only the week before—accompanied by the school piano teacher, who knew very little about music, but that didn't matter because it was recorded and rerecorded that in her youth she had actually studied under Clara Schumann. Erika surprised Alice, and rather dismayed Alice's parents, who went once every summer to the Lewisohn Stadium when Alexander Smallens did *Porgy and Bess* and thought themselves thereby to have acquitted a full year's responsibility to music, by getting up without demurral and proceeding through twenty-two minutes of music, stopping only to sing at the top of her husky voice the parts written by Grieg for the missing orchestra.

"You certainly are a privileged young girl," Alice's mother said admiringly while the father, fearful that his daughter would suggest that Erika play an encore—had Grieg written another concerto? he worried . . . everyone knew that Mozart had written over, was it four hundred concertos?—clapped loudly, looked at his watch, and said as a treat he would drive them all to the late movie with Bob Hope and Bing Crosby off and away on the Road to Morocco. The girls went happily to get their coats and Erika had time in the car to muse over her privileged upbringing, in

Germany and England, before coming to the United States three years before at age thirteen.

Of course, being the daughter of Dimitri and Anna Chadinoff *was* a privilege, this she did not deny, though she wondered—she truly wondered—what her parents would have done about her if she had not been . . . clever. She had picked up that word in England and thereafter used it—there being no satisfactory American substitute, as she told Alice. Her friends supposed that her early memories of Germany were of intellectuals and artists coming to her parents' elegant apartment to eat stuffed goose and read aloud each other's poems and short stories and argue long into the night the meaning of a fable by Pushkin. What Erika in fact remembered was the awful physical discomforts and the utter indifference of her father to them. She was very young when she learned that something called "money" was terribly important. When her mother looked into her handbag, either there was money in it or there was not money in it. In the former event Erika would eat dinner, in the latter event she would not. Beginning in midafternoon, Erika would find that her attention was substantially given over to the question, Would there be money that night when her mother opened her handbag? Her mother, though not as stoical as her father, was twice as vague. If, on opening her handbag, she had pulled out a diamond necklace, she'd have said, "Dimitri, dear, I apparently have a diamond necklace here I hadn't reckoned on." Dimitri would have said, "That's fine, my dear," which he would also have said if his wife had announced that she had found an armadillo in her handbag.

Her mother did concern herself for Erika, and in the especially cold winter of 1936, washed dishes at the corner restaurant in return for bread and potatoes left over at the end of the evening's meal. Sometimes Erika had her dinner at one in the morning on her mother's return. Sometimes there was food left over from the night before. But sometimes there was no food at all. During these daily struggles her father was always reading or writing. He had access to the public library and spent much of his time there, often taking Erika because that way she could be warm. It was troublesome to do this at first because the guard at the door announced that the library was not a nursery in which to keep little girls. Dimitri Chadinoff asked just when could children be brought into the library, and the answer was: When they are old enough to read. Dimitri turned around, took Erika home, and was with her for three days, interrupted only when Erika could no longer stay awake. On the fourth day, triumphantly, he led her back and was stopped at the same entrance by the same guard. Calmly, Dimitri made his announcement. The guard leaned over from his high desk, put a newspaper into the girl's hands and, pointing to the headline, said: "Read this, little girl." Her face solemn, Erika read, haltingly, but without error: "Roosevelt Sweeps Country/Dems Control Both Houses." She was three years old.

Her father showed no particular pride in his daughter, then or later when, at age seven, she earned a few pennies by drilling two dull teen-age boys, sons of a noble family, in English; or when Anna's friend Valerian Bibikoff, a fellow expatriate from Russia who taught piano and gave lessons to Erika, reported that the girl was singularly talented. Her father was as surprised as if he had been informed that his daughter was remarkable because she had ten fingers. He showed displeasure as rarely as he showed pleasure. When, freshly arrived in England, Erika returned to their flat to say she had made friends at school with the daughter of the Soviet military attaché, Dimitri looked down at her from his desk and told her that he would just as soon she did not associate with the children of barbarians.

"Why are they barbarians?" Erika asked in French, that being the only language spoken at the Chadinoff household on Thursdays (Monday, German; Tuesday, English; Wednesday, Italian; Thursday, French; Friday, Saturday, and Sunday any language save the language spoken in the country being inhabited).

"They are barbarians," said Dimitri Chadinoff, "because they wish to obliterate everything important that human beings have learned about how to treat each other in three thousand years."

"Why do they want to obliterate it?"—Erika had no difficulty with unusual words. Her problem, at school, was in learning that some words *were* unusual: she had to study them attentively and learn to use them with great discretion, or preferably not at all, since at home they were used as nonchalantly as kitchen utensils. She got off to a bad start her first day at Blessed Sir Thomas More's School in Cadogan Square by asking a girl whether the policies of the school were "latitudinarian." It was years before she could explain to anyone—the solemn Paul, at the Sorbonne—that she had been guilty of affectation throughout much of her youth only by searching out simple substitute words for those that occurred to her naturally.

"They want to obliterate it," said her father, "because they are bewitched by the secular superstition of communism, which is a huge enterprise that will settle for nothing less than bringing misery to all the people of the world."

"Why should they want to bring misery to all the people of the world?" Erika repeated her father's formulation piously.

"It isn't that they want to bring misery, though some do. They strut up and down in their baggy clothes swinging golden chains from their vests as if the keys to happiness were attached. All they have succeeded in doing is killing and torturing people and promising to do as much to people fortunate enough not to live in Russia during this period. To think that they have done it to Russia, the most beautiful land in the world," said Dimitri Chadinoff, and Anna agreed, recalling how the weather would be now in their native hills outside St. Petersburg.

"Did they take away all your money?" Erika wanted to know.

"Yes, they took away all our money."

Such an indifference as Dimitri Chadinoff's to money had not been seen since the natives begged St. Francis to accept a copper if only to have the pleasure of giving it away. But he did not deign to express from where, in the hierarchy of Soviet offenses, the loss of the family money had come. *Infra dignitate.* Erika, a thoughtful girl, assumed that her father was correct but promised herself one day to think the matter over more exhaustively, and turned to her homework in mathematics, which she was always pleased to express her concern with because she knew it was the single subject in which neither her father nor her mother could help her.

"What exactly is an integer? I don't understand."

"Ask your teacher. He's getting well paid," said her father.

Well, not so well paid by modern standards, but the school was well staffed and now Dimitri was making five pounds per week translating for a London publisher on a piecemeal basis, and that same publisher had sent out Chadinoff's fresh translation of Pushkin to be assessed by scholars at Oxford and Cambridge. "I could advise you," Chadinoff wrote to his editor, "which of the scholars at Cambridge and Oxford are competent to evaluate my work, but I suppose that if you agreed to accept my judgment in the matter the entire enterprise would be circular. Anyway, for the record the only man at either university who has the necessary background is Adam Sokolin at Cambridge. He studied under my old tutor, who beat some sense into him thirty years ago. Sokolin has done good work on Pushkin, from which we may safely conclude that he will not get very far in Cambridge." The editor took the letter by the corner, his fingers raised as if carrying a dead rat by the tail, walked into the office of his superior, dropped it on his desk and asked: "Have I your permission to tell this egomaniac to go and peddle his Pushkin elsewhere?"

The next day, manuscript back in hand, Chadinoff sent it to the Harvard University Press. The following day, the London publisher dropped him as a part-time editor and then, after Erika had gone to sleep, Anna took Dimitri aside and, even though it was Tuesday, spoke to him in Russian and said that they had to do something to bring in some money, that all their friends and relatives were equally impoverished, that there was no money for the next week's rent, nor for the next month's school bills for Erika.

Well, said Dimitri—ever so slightly disposed to point out, by twiddling his fingers on the open page of his book, that Anna had interrupted his reading—did she have any suggestions?

Yes, she said, she had recently been talking to her friend Selnikov (former colonel in the Czar's prime equestrian unit). Poor Sergei Babevich had not only himself and his wife to look after but three daughters and a son. He had taken a position as a maître d'hôtel at a medium-priced restaurant where a knowledge of several languages was useful. "The trouble with you, dear Dimitri, is that your knowledge of food is really not very refined. You could write a scholarly book about the feasts of Lucullus, but you would not be able to distinguish the actual food from fish and chips at Lyons. So I have another idea."

Dimitri had sat without any show of emotion thus far. "Well?"

Anna couldn't, at first, remember what her other idea was, and Dimitri waited. Finally the newspaper caught her eye.

"Ah yes. There is an advertisement in the paper for a concierge. He must be presentable—here." She reached for the paper, shuffling through to the marked section. "Presentable, must be fluent in French and German. Some Italian and Spanish desirable. References."

Dimitri took the job. His hours were from one until midnight. He would sleep until six and then resume his own work. Erika was not permitted to see her father at the hotel during working hours. Once she decided mischievously to do so. She was small for twelve years, so that her head only just reached the counter. She had on a friend's hat, and her light-brown hair was knotted under it. She put on spectacles and, carrying a handbag, she said in a little girl's voice, imitating her father's own imperious accent and speaking in German: "Concierge, please get me a sleeper to the Finland Station!" Dimitri permitted himself a smile, and then in Russian said to her: "Get yourself out of here, Rikushka, before I invite the manager to paddle your behind." She went out roaring, and told her mother, who laughed, and then said not, ever, to do such a thing again. The following morning, when she went off to school, she found tucked into her notebook, in her father's unmistakable hand, a fable dedicated to her. It was called "The Little Girl Who Took the Train to the Finland Station, and Woke Up Lenin." That day, she thought, she was closer to her father than she had ever been before.

When the letter came from the Harvard University Press, Chadinoff was pleased, but not particularly surprised. He knew his Pushkin was superior. But he was surprised a month later to be invited by the Department of Slavic and Romance Languages to go to Harvard to lecture during the spring term. Chadinoff replied that, thanks very much, he would be happy to do so, and able to do so inasmuch as his job as concierge at the

Basil Street Hotel required him to give only three weeks' notice, and February was still three months away.

They made reservations for the tenth of December on the S.S. *Mount Vernon,* and it was well that they did, because after the seventh of December, which was the day of Pearl Harbor, no reservations were accepted save for returning residents of the United States. Chadinoff and his family carried Nansen passports, and his excited wife and daughter were apprehensive, up until the moment the gangplank was lifted, about having to yield their room to returning U.S. residents.

During the commotion Erika, snugly dressed in a white skirt, peasant blouse, and tweed jacket, excitedly accosted a tall, handsome blond boy—at least two years older, she judged—wearing an English public-school blazer, chewing an apple, and affecting the ways of the cosmopolitan traveler.

"Do you think we will pull out on time?" she began the conversation.

"Oh, sure," he said. She was surprised his accent was American. "They always pull out on time. Especially when there are submarines."

"Why should a ship be punctual for the sake of the submarines?"

Blackford Oakes looked at her pert face, and frank, inquisitive eyes accented by her austerely coiled braids. "Because"—he spoke just a little less casually than before—"there are escort vessels, and it is quite a muddle if every boat decides for itself when to start out."

She did not answer, but looked at her lumpy watch. She would wait—for what, later at Smith College, the philosophy professor would tell her is called "empirical verification." And, in fact, at exactly one forty-five in the afternoon the gangplank was pulled, the whistles and horns blew, the crowd at the pier interrupted its waving and yelling, and her parents rejoined her. Before skipping off she turned to the boy, munching a fresh apple and looking very self-satisfied.

"You were right."

He smiled—it was a splendid smile, warm, animated. He reached into the brown paper bag and said, "Here, have an apple." She looked up at her mother, who nodded her head, so she took it and said, "Thank you," and then with her free hand grabbed her straw hat, which almost blew away as the great steamship slid out of the lee of the quay.

By the time Erika was sixteen her father was well known in the academic world and now held down a chair at Brown University, delivering learned, acidulous, witty lectures that would become famous. There was now money enough to pay the tuitions at the Ethel Walker School and, later, Smith College, and in her senior year her father gave her a secondhand car which Erika rejoiced in, traveling about New England tirelessly, to celebrate the end of gas rationing. She took on every challenge, competing for the classics prize, the philosophy prize, winning one, placing second in the other. In her junior year the dean had called her in to ask whether she would consider *not* competing for the Russian, German, French, and Italian prizes. She had won them all in her freshman and sophomore years, and now the teachers were finding it hard to persuade anyone to compete against so certain a winner. Erika said she would have to consult with her father, whose instructions to her had been to enter every competition. He wrote back and told his daughter that, noblesse oblige, she should allow other girls a chance at the prizes, but if she wanted to compete for the big Prix Giscard she might focus her energies on winning it. This prize went annually to four girls selected from applicants throughout the country to study in Paris, all expenses paid, and its renewal, now that the war was over, had recently been advertised.

Erika competed and won without much difficulty, and without causing resentment. Though serious by nature, she could participate in gaiety and do so convincingly. Her friends now accepted matter-of-factly her prolix virtuosity and had long since ceased to think anything about it. She was like the boy or girl at graduation whose name recurs and recurs and who has to walk up to the headmaster fifteen times before he is done collecting the silver: Best Athlete, Best Student Leader, Best Scholar—Best Prig, often as not. But Erika got on well with her friends, all of whom assumed that she would either go on to become a professor of almost anything, or else that a very gallant and very rich man, desiring a beautiful girl of exotic manner and prodigious attainments, would take her off and make her duchess of something where she would preside over salons for a couple of generations of Princes of Wales. At home the night before leaving, in the comfortable house in Providence exploding with books and order, she actually managed to catch her mother's and father's attention at dinner by saying, "Are you glad we won the war, Father?"

Chadinoff, dressed in his velvet smoking jacket, finished chewing what he had in his mouth.

"I am glad we won. I am sorry *they* won. I am sorry that they now occupy Eastern Europe. I predict they will still occupy Eastern Europe one, maybe two years from now."

Erika remembered the night her father so greatly embarrassed her during her last year at Ethel Walker, before two friends spending the weekend in Providence. It was the critical weekend when at first Stalingrad was reported captured by the Germans, and then the Russians were reported holding out. As the radio reports came in the girls cheered on all the news of Russian advances and hissed all the news of German advances. It soon became uncomfortably clear that their host, Professor Dimitri Chadinoff, was unmistakably cheering the other side. Alice, who was well known for her ingenuous candor, looked up during the late morning and said, "Professor Chadinoff, are you pro-Nazi?"

"No, Alice," said Chadinoff. "Permit me, are you pro-Communist?"

"Why, no," said Alice.

"Very well, then?" Chadinoff's eyebrows lifted, and he was evidently prepared to change the subject.

"But we are at war with the Nazis."

"Who is 'We'?" Chadinoff replied.

"Well, Americans . . ." Then she gasped. She hadn't thought about it before. She turned to Erika, hoping for help. But Erika's father was in charge.

"We carry Nansen passports, Alice. They are a kind of diplomatic Man-Without-a-Country passports. We are grateful to the United States for its hospitality and express our gratitude by paying exactly the same taxes we would be paying if we had been born and raised in Topeka, Kansas. We have not taken any oath to support America's foreign policy and, my dear Alice, if truth were told, no one's reputation for intelligence could survive the taking of such an oath."

Alice was a fair student of biology, a little backward in languages, including English, so she thought at least she could charm the famous linguist by trotting up a phrase from her Ethel Walker School French: "Well, Professor, *chacun à son goût.*"

"*Chacun à sa bêtise,*" Professor Chadinoff retorted and returned to his reading.

That afternoon, when her guests were dressing for the Brown-Yale football game, Erika pleaded illness, sending her date off alone to the game. She then turned to her father as she had never done before and, fire in her eyes and a great ball of resentment in her stomach, she blurted out: "I think what you did to Alice was disgusting! Doesn't it matter to you that one million—*one million*—Russians have died in the last two months defending Stalingrad? They can't be as mad as you are at communism for having taken away *their* landed estates!" She flung the door shut, went up to her room, locked the door, and wept. She wept fitfully through the afternoon and her intelligence alerted her, after a while, that her discomposure was deeply rooted. She did not know exactly what was the cause or causes of it, and now, three years later, she still did not know. Characteristically, neither her father nor her mother had ever again alluded to the incident.

This time she said, "Father, do you believe in God?"

"No. But I believe in some of the things attributed to God."

"Like what?"

"Like the Ten Commandments. Most of the Ten Commandments. One or two are arguable, explained by Jewish cultural idiosyncrasies."

"What do you believe in?"

"I believe in the life of the mind, and in human fancy, and in the everlasting struggle against vulgarity."

"What do you mean, you believe in *the struggle against vulgarity*? Does that mean you believe that that struggle is going to happen, or does that mean that you believe that that struggle is worth winning?"

"It is obviously worth winning. But it will never be won. That is why I qualify it by calling it an everlasting struggle."

"The Communists believe more than you do."

"That is certainly correct. So do African witch doctors."

Her mother was following the argument, but was now distracted by something, and she could not remember what it was. She had mistakenly begun the meal by serving the chocolate soufflé because she had found that, by misreckoning, it was done when they sat down, and obviously would not wait, whereas the lamb would.

"As a matter of fact," broke in Anna Chadinoff, her points of reference not immediately clear either to her husband or to her daughter, "lamb will wait very nearly indefinitely."

"What did you say, Anna?"

"I said that lamb would wait very nearly indefinitely."

"Do you mean, like the everlasting struggle?"

"What do you mean by that, dear?"

Chadinoff, knowing when the door was finally closed on any possibility of nexus, pronounced the chocolate soufflé quite excellent, and wondered whether they would now be served kippered herring.

No, Anna said. Now there would be lamb. And Chadinoff then understood. Erika understood. God, if he existed, now understood. Erika thought that, really, her parents were quite splendid, but how wonderful it would be to be gone from them for a while: for a long while, she thought that night.

Erika arrived in Paris in the awful, depressed postwar season three years after the war. She was loaded down with letters from her father and mother commending her to the attentions of their numerous friends in the expatriate world. She began dutifully with the first names on the list: Mr. and Mrs. Valerian Sverdlov. Mme. Sverdlov was a niece of Tolstoy; her husband had commanded a czarist cavalry regiment; both had known Erika's parents since childhood and both greeted her warmly once communication was effected.

This proved difficult because although Erika rang the telephone number her father had given her and, after a few days during which there was never an answer, checked it against the telephone book to find it correct, *still* there was no answer. So she sent a letter and got back a prompt invitation to come to tea, which the following day she did. Mr. Sverdlov, quite bald, with a mustache, bad teeth, pink cheeks and twinkling eyes, was always laughing, and he rejoiced at seeing his beloved Chadinoff's daughter, rejoiced at being able to speak in Russian to her, and several times emptied his glass of vodka to celebrate the general celebration. His wife, though more reserved, was also warm. She worked as a tutor in Russian and found now in the postwar world a considerably increased demand for her services. Beginning the following week, Valerian would return to his job as driver of an American Express tourist bus. Erika was faintly surprised to learn this, but then reminded herself that, until a few years ago, her father worked as a concierge and her mother as a dishwasher.

When she alluded to the difficulty in getting through to the Sverdlovs on the telephone, he laughed and laughed and said several times that the French were the *silliest* people in the *whole* world. You see—he adopted a conspiratorial voice—I was a *collaborator*! Yes! I worked for the Germans! One day I traveled with the German Army as far as St. Petersburg. Not *into* St. Petersburg, but as *far* as St. Petersburg—and there—he stood theatrically, and waved his arm forward, "there from the hilltop I could see— my house. My father's house. My grandfather's house. Where your father played with me when we were boys."

But, he said, that was as far as they had got. Russian resistance proved effective and the retreat began. He returned to Paris and resumed his clerical work as translator of Russian war documents and radio communications—it was understood he would work only against the Soviets.

"Now," he said with delight to Erika, who struggled to conceal her chagrin at her father's friend's collaborationist activity but little by little was caught up by his ebullience—"now," he said, "the French know that I was a collaborator. And *they* know that *I* know that *they* know that I was a collaborator. But!"—he stood again and howled with glee, his mustache high over his white, crooked teeth, his wispy hair tousled, cheeks pink with mirth and stimulation—"they cannot prove it. And the reason they cannot prove it is that before the Germans left, I said to Colonel Strassbourg: 'My dear Colonel, you can have very little use for my file in Berlin, so be a good chicken and let me have it.' And he did, and I burned it, right there"—he pointed to the shabby little fireplace with the four pieces of coal warming, or trying to warm, the whole apartment.

"So what do these silly Frenchmen do? They take away my telephone! They do not tell me: 'Mr. Sverdlov, you are a traitor, and we cannot send you to jail, and we cannot send you to the firing squad, so we are going to take away your telephone.' No. They just disconnect it. Everything else is the same. And when I ask about it they just shrug their shoulders and say I must wait!" He laughed at this trivialization of treason, although of course he too, Erika knew, would have used the same arguments her father used about the Nansen passport, so she did not catechize him. She enjoyed him most unabashedly, and he offered to take her the next Monday to Chartres; and, on the bus, where he wore a chauffeur's cap without any apparent self-consciousness, he buoyantly situated her in the seat directly across from him and they chatted as he drove.

When, like her parents, he had run out of money, he had applied to American Express for a job as a bus driver, stressing his knowledge of French (perfect), German (excellent), English (shaky), and then he qualified his application by saying he would be interested in only a single route: to Chartres. His employer was puzzled until Sverdlov explained that the cathedral at Chartres was the most beautiful sight in the world, more beautiful even than any sight in Russia, and if he was destined to drive a bus every day he might as well drive it to the most beautiful sight in the world.

"Why not?" he exclaimed, his whole face and shoulders rising in interrogation. When after a month the dispatcher told him that that day he would have to drive the bus to the cathedral at Rheims, Sverdlov said that under no circumstances would he go to Rheims—the cathedral there, for all its reputation and pretensions, being simply inadequate. American Express tried suggesting that he was, in fact, under no obligation to join the tourists in the cathedral, but Sverdlov was so affronted by the implied mechanization of his role, American Express quickly retreated, undisposed to discipline the driver who was the favorite of the tourists. By now, even after the war's long interruption, his title to Chartres was secure and no one would question it, he said happily. Later, in a whisper, he told Erika that after seeing the cathedral, he would take her to a little Russian delicatessen where they would have some vodka and some cheese and sausage while the other tourists had their regular lunch.

Erika's reaction, on seeing the cathedral, gratified Sverdlov: she found it was everything Henry Adams said it was—in the book she was assigned to read by one of her art professors at Smith—and other things that Henry Adams had failed to say it was. She asked Sverdlov, whom now she was told to call Valerian Babeyevich, whether he had read Adams's book on Mont St. Michel and Chartres, and he replied that he had not, that he did not want to read about the cathedral, only look at it. Erika mused that her father, who would much prefer reading about a cathedral to seeing it, would scarcely approve of Valerian's attitude: and in the course of the afternoon she discovered that Valerian really knew nothing about her father's career except, vaguely, that he had become a success of sorts in America.

"When he writes me letters"—Valerian laughed, as he tipped his fifth jigger glass of vodka down his throat—"he writes about obscure poets or writers he has discovered, and always he forgets to tell me about Anna and his darling and beautiful daughter."

He looked at his watch and said that they must go back to the bus now, the tourists would be assembling as instructed. He insisted to Erika on paying the bill, which proved painless when the old Russian shopkeeper in turn insisted on refusing payment from his old friend, who had brought that day such an "elegant"—he bowed to Erika—"and beautiful daughter of an old friend."

From the American Express bus terminal it was a short walk to the apartment Erika rented at Rue Montalembert: a bedroom, study/living room/dining room, kitchen, and bath—for thirty-five U.S. dollars per month, on the Left Bank almost but not quite overlooking the river. From there she could walk to the Sorbonne, and did now regularly, even though the weather had turned cold, attending classes in philosophy and the history of art. The classrooms were cold and dirty, the students poorly dressed, and on the faces of many of the boys there was a premature gauntness of expression. Erika noticed a sharp divergence in the attitude of the students. Half, perhaps more than half, diligently took notes on what the instructor said, particularly in the class taught by Jean-Paul Sartre, who when he spoke did so with a precisionist nonchalance, a quiet and perfect engine of volubility whose words, transcribed, could have formed completed chapters of books, indeed regularly did so. But other students, though they might make a note occasionally, were studiedly skeptical, as if to communicate to the instructor that no presumptive respect was owed either to him or to the words he spoke. During the exchanges these students, when they said anything at all, tended to challenge this or that generality of the teacher, or ask whether, by this inflection, he had meant to say such and such. M. Argoud, who had written a history of art, answered questions, however provocative, neither with indignation nor with servility. If the question was barbed he would ignore those parts of it that were provocative, giving unadorned answers to whatever was left. "Would you not say, M. Argoud, that you slip into confusion when you suggest there are similarities between the theoretical defenses of abstractionism and of primitivism?"

"The similarities to which I alluded are listed in the chapter on Braque in my book."

Next question.

M. Argoud did not care for his students, and did not care if his students cared for him. But he would do what he had contracted to do so that as quickly as possible he might get back to his own work. He broke his rhythm on one occasion to notice Erika, with her tweed skirt, blouse, and sweater, her full bosom—perhaps she reminded him of something Braque had said, or painted, or loved? Erika looked at the teacher, still young but utterly unconcerned. If he could look ten years younger by snapping his fingers, she thought, he would probably not take the trouble. But to inquire into the authenticity of a Del Sarto in a museum, he had devoted seven months—and came up calmly with the pronouncement that it was a forgery. Erika guessed that, on the whole, M. Argoud would probably prefer coming up with a forgery than with an original: the whole exercise would somehow reinforce his misanthropic inclinations.

Except, of course, for Paul. M. Argoud obviously cared for Paul. Paul's (infrequent) questions were answered in a tone of voice distinctly different. M. Argoud was even seen, on at least one occasion, talking casually with Paul in the cold, high-ceilinged corridor. Since Paul was young and beautiful and intense, Erika wondered whether the relationship was unnatural, but when Paul sat next to her in the cafeteria one day at lunch and they fell to talking she discovered that Paul Massot was François Argoud's stepbrother and that they had belonged to the same guerrilla unit during the resistance. Both had been tortured in the same cellar at the same time, she would learn weeks later when she and Paul were lovers, and Paul whispered to her early one morning, stroking her breasts with his chin, that if he had known her then, he'd have probably told them everything, done anything, espoused any creed, incurred any risk, performed any treachery, lest they deprive him of her—his—Erika, no one else's, ever, ever—his rhythms were matching now the words, and her responses were elatedly fused to his own, as he repeated the word, ever, ever, ever, ever, ever, more excitedly, more quickly, almost shouting now, as she closed her eyes and moaned, then opened them to observe her beautiful Paul, EVER!

Whenever he left her apartment, whether to fetch a book in the library or perform an errand or check the mailbox, there was prolonged discussion. Exactly how long would he be gone?

Twelve minutes?

That was too long, Erika said, and Paul would agree. And he would say that perhaps if he ran both ways he could manage it in eleven minutes. As often as not, Erika would suggest that the safest way to handle the problem would be for both of them to leave together. His solemn young face would light up with pleasure and, taking her hand, he would open the door, pausing on the stairway, now for a passionate, now for a tender kiss.

Paul Massot's stepfather, the elder Argoud, had died during the war. Since he wasn't shot by the Nazis and did not die in a military prison, he didn't qualify for the Vermork; but he was listed officially as a "casualty" of the war because, suffering from diabetes, he was medically undernourished owing to scarcities that were an undisputed result of the war; so that his impoverished widow, Paul's mother, received a little pension on which Paul now drew a few francs every month to finish the studies interrupted when, at seventeen, he withdrew from the university to devote himself to the resistance.

He had gone then, instinctively, to his austere, normally unapproachable half-brother, older by eight years, with whom he associated during the nearly three years before the American troops, General Leclerc heading the procession, entered Paris. There were long, tedious hours of joint activity. On one occasion, Argoud and Paul were responsible for checking the movements of a Gestapo official. They huddled in a single room across the street with their stopwatches and notebooks, clocking the monster's goings and comings for nearly three months. In the long stretches of inactivity Argoud undertook two missions, the first to teach his half-brother something about the esthetic history of the world: it would prove, before long, a substantial history of the Renaissance. And the second, to convince Paul that the only hope for humanity lay in acknowledging the truths of Marxist analysis and historiography and in backing the Soviet Union's lonely, and acknowledgedly often brutal, efforts to export to the world that which only Russia was experiencing.

Paul knew about Erika's background and had even read some of the works by Chadinoff, whose fame had come to France. Neither he nor she was perturbed by Chadinoff's reactionary politics. Why should one expect Chadinoff to feel or reason otherwise? Paul said. How natural! If it were *easy* for the world to accept communism, it would have done so by now. The forces aligned in opposition to communism aren't merely those specifically identified by Marx. There are all those other accretions of man: his nostalgia, his fear of the unknown, his conservative temptation to resist change.

"But, Paul, there *are* other things." They were at dinner, in their favorite restaurant where, unless instructed otherwise, the waiter brought them the same appetizer, the same entrées, the same house wine, and the same bill, but no longer any cigarettes (Paul having told Erika she must give up smoking), which came to seventy-five U.S. cents apiece. "There's the suffering in Russia."

"There has been suffering everywhere. Look at the suffering in Germany and Italy. Even in the United States, one hundred years advanced over Russia industrially, they could not manage their Depression. Stalin is not a gentle man, and he has made many mistakes, and will make other mistakes. But unlike the Catholic Church, the Marxists do not claim infallibility for their leader. We claim only that history has imposed a responsibility on him, and we must help him discharge that responsibility. There is no way of getting around the fact, Erika, that millions of Russians fought for Stalin and for their country: and no one disguised from them that they were fighting for communism. Of course it has been bitter and hard. And it will be harder and more bitter if we are to prevent the forces in opposition from gainsaying the effort of all those years, all those lives, because"—he dug into his meatloaf with his knife; he never used a fork—"that is exactly what will happen if, just because the formal fighting is over, we think of ourselves as other than at war."

Erika heard the arguments but could not say, really, that she had listened to them. All through her life she had resisted only that one intellectual challenge, an examination of the ideology that had banished and impoverished her father. She did not, really, want to go into the arguments now, though she would if Paul wanted her to. She would do anything Paul wanted her to. She could not imagine that it was possible to know such joy as she knew, whether at the table listening to him, seeing his straight dark hair fallen over his brow, his sad brown eyes, his pointed and delicate mouth deftly retrieving the morsels of food from the knife, his long, tapered fingers, explaining his position to her, sensitive to every sound, every inflection, or in bed during those long bouts of ardor and tranquillity. Or sitting next to him, listening to his unprepossessing but acknowledgedly brilliant half-brother. She could admire her father, but she could not ever really *believe* in him. In Paul she believed—entirely. And she knew that she would never betray him. If it should happen, in a final philosophical revelation, that his ideology was wrong, and the contrary of it right, it would matter far less that she had taken the wrong course, than that she had followed him. He was her ideology, her idyll, her lover, her friend, her counselor, her Paul, forever forever forever.

"Do you understand what I'm talking about?"

"I understand what I need to understand. If you want me to study Marxism, of course I'll study Marxism. And"—she smiled at him—"I'll even win the Marxist Prize if you want me to."

No, he did not want her to study Marxism, he said. He would like it if she read Marx, but that didn't matter so much; he, Paul, would tell her everything she needed to know about politics. What he did not want was for her to associate openly with Marxists, because that would put her in the way of unnecessary harassments. The anti-Communist French were mobilizing against the French Communists, and there were divisions already even among men and women who had worked together during the resistance. The Croix de Feu, which drew from the militant wing of the anti-Communist coalition, were talking violence. The forces of American fascism were everywhere. There was no need to alert anyone, save his own special friends, to her new political allegiance. He himself had been careful not to enroll in the Party, and not to attend any of its official functions—François, though himself an active Party member, had so counseled him.

And thus it was left, during that golden autumn. One day every week he was away, by himself, pursuing duties which, he told her, he could neither neglect nor explain. One other evening per week he required her to share with his political intimates, who, after the briefest experience with her, were all of them happy that Paul, whose star was so manifestly ascendant, had found so accomplished and lovely a companion. She liked especially Gerard, and when one day he actually stopped smoking long enough to make it possible to see through the smoke to his wry face, she was surprised to notice how much he looked like her own father, though younger of course. He presided over the meetings, which is what they really were, and there was a worldliness but also a spirituality in his analysis of the French contemporary scene that touched Erika, which she found wanting in her own father. Gerard was especially kind to Erika and one day surprised her by addressing her in a Russian which, though clearly not native, betrayed a convincing knowledge of Russia, a knowledge the details of which Erika did not feel free to probe; these were, after all, clandestine meetings. She did not know Gerard's surname, nor where he lived.

It had proved difficult to locate Gerard, but finally Erika succeeded in doing so, exactly one week after the day when, groceries in hand, she had opened the door, exhilarated at the prospect of seeing Paul lying there as she so regularly came on him, dressed only in his undershorts, reading easily in the dim light. He was there exactly as she had anticipated, but the book rested flat on his olive-skinned chest and his head was slightly turned, by a bullet that had entered his brain.

Erika was released from the hospital just in time to attend the funeral three days later. Scant attention was given to the extraordinary shooting—execution?—of young Paul Massot. Paris was inured to death and terror, after five years of it. The detectives came, but eventually they left, without formal findings. Still white when she tapped the doorknob of Gerard's apartment, she waited, and Gerard came and, on opening the door, beheld a grown woman ten days after knowing her as a university schoolgirl.

"Who did it?" she asked.

"I don't know," he said.

"You do know"—she looked him in the eyes, and the psychic pressure was greater than the torturer's that nightmare night in 1944. He yielded.

"It was almost certainly the work of the Croix de Feu. Paul was assigned to penetrate the organization." Gerard held out his arms to her but she was past tears, and simply took his extended hand in hers and said good-bye, and told him that if ever he needed her services, he might have them.

In 1988 the editor of the *Paris Review,* George Plimpton, asked Buckley to sit for the sort of lengthy author interview for which that literary journal has become well known. Buckley agreed, on condition that I conduct the questioning.

We did the interview—actually several interviews, done several ways—with, after a long period, several additional questions by Plimpton, and turned it in. After eight years, the interview has just appeared in the *Paris Review.*

The prefatory biography and scene-setting are by the editor of this book.

William F. Buckley, Jr.
The Art of Fiction

William Frank Buckley, Jr., founder, editor, and now editor-at-large of the *National Review*; author, lecturer, and host of Public Television's *Firing Line,* the longest-running serious TV talk show, was born in New York City on November 24, 1925. His early schooling was in England and France. He graduated from the Millbrook School in N.Y., studied at the University of Mexico, and took a B.A. with honors at Yale in 1950, where he had fenced, debated, was Class Day Orator, and chairman of the *Yale Daily News.*

Drafted into the Army as an infantry private in 1944, he was discharged as a 2nd Lieutenant in 1946. From 1947 to 1951, Buckley taught Spanish at Yale and in 1952 became associate editor of the *American Mercury.* Then he resigned to do freelance writing. In 1955, he started his own magazine and is generally held to be responsible for assembling a coherent, responsible, modern Conservative movement in the United States. In 1962, he began a syndicated weekly column, which continues; in 1965 ran for Mayor of New York; in 1966 began hosting his weekly television show.

He was Lecturer at the New School, was a member of a Presidential Advisory Commission on the USIA, and in 1973 was appointed by the president as a public delegate to the UN.

He has received 36 honorary degrees and sixteen awards in journalism, literature, television (an Emmy). His latest, the Presidential Medal of Freedom, was awarded in 1991.

From his first, *God and Man at Yale*, in 1951, to his most recent, the novel *Brothers No More* (1995), he has written 36 books and contributed to nine others, including volumes on intellectuals, Catholicism, the Beatles, etc. It was at fifty that he first turned to fiction, producing *Saving the Queen* (1976) and in 1980 won the American Book Award for Best Mystery (*Stained Glass*). After ten novels featuring his hero, CIA agent Blackford Oakes, he produced his eleventh novel, *Brothers No More*, taking a new tack.

Any attempt to catch William F. Buckley, Jr., in one place at one time must fail to catch the essence of a man in motion. Interviewing Buckley at his most characteristic offers several choices; the interviewer took them all. He can be caught on the move, which means most of the time; or in repose, which usually means at work in other ways. This "interview" is the result of a series of exchanges over a period of time. The settings were as varied as Buckley's interests and attachments.

His weekdays are crowded with traveling, writing, lecturing, etc., and his weekends are reserved for Pat (Mrs. Buckley), family, and friends, and yet always and everywhere, some form of creative work. The cars are parked outside, including a middle-aging Volvo, and a stretch limo, which he has recommended for its efficiency to others (in *Overdrive*), attracting considerable criticism. It serves as a rolling office, complete with phone (he had one early), computer, etc., and is frequently completed as well with Mrs. Buckley, three King Charles spaniels, and household staff, and is driven by a large, protective man called Jerry.

The family's main house, in Stamford, Connecticut, is a large, comfortable old establishment with a stucco exterior, painted a surprising purple, surrounded by flower and herb gardens, tended carefully by Mrs. Buckley, and it is a house filled with flowered cushions and eccentric bathrooms. Books and framed photographs are everywhere. Part of the talks took place in the music room, which houses a harpsichord, bookshelves, a projection screen television set, and audio equipment. A Bosendorfer piano is visible within the house, used over the years for concerts by Buckley's friends like Rosalyn Tureck, the virtuoso harpsichordist; Dick Wellstood, the jazz pianist; and Buckley himself. Outside the big glass windows, beyond a sloping lawn, is Long Island Sound, one of Buckley's favorite sailing grounds.

Buckley's office is in the capacious garage, and overflows with papers, computer equipment, books. Over the garage is a small apartment where the Buckleys' son, Christopher, the novelist, humorist, and editor, has done some of his own writing.

The principal setting for our talks was in the Buckleys' pied-à-terre, off Park Avenue in Manhattan, an elegant place, with most of the conversations conducted in the Red Room. This serves as Pat Buckley's city office—she is a formidable fund-raiser for good causes, most of them in the arts—and as library, small sitting room, bar, etc. Outside, in the foyer, is a harpsichord at which arriving visitors are likely to find the master of the house practicing or playing for his own enjoyment.

It is a true Buckley place, handsome but not staid, warmly hospitable. Evidences of their enthusiasms are everywhere: again, photographs, books, as well as paintings, picked out by small spotlights; a candlelit dining room; and a long salon for entertaining, with the aid of the Buckleys' largely Hispanic staff. Much of the daily small talk in the house is in Spanish, with English almost a second language.

Other exchanges took place by telephone, from his car, by letters, faxes, and E-mail, some from the Buckleys' winter place near Gstaad, Switzerland, . . . and once from the Concorde on the way to Sri Lanka, on which plane he was leading a round-the-world tour group and which had recently suffered "the humiliating loss of one-third of its tail after takeoff from Sydney."

Despite his peripatetic existence, Buckley, an unfailingly gracious man, with a wry smile and a quick laugh, gives full attention to questions, as if he had all the time in the world. He just uses well all the time in his world.

The first two interviews took place in the afternoons of December 12 and 14, 1988.

INTERVIEWER: What sort of things had you been writing before the novels? You tend to group your previous books into categories, yes?

BUCKLEY: The most obvious, I suppose, are the collections of columns, articles and essays, four or five of those before my first novel. There were two or three offbeat books: a book on the United Nations and the term I served there. A book on running for mayor of New York. A book on crossing the Atlantic, which has the ocean as *mise-en-scène*, and then a sort of autobiographical book on a week in my life, *Cruising Speed.* So when you suggested that I write a novel, I had at that point published twelve or fifteen nonfiction books.

INTERVIEWER: I remember your saying you might like to try a novel one day. The word "Forsythe" came up and I thought your reference was to the *Forsyte Saga,* which was then on television . . . as well as in the literature. You said, No, like *Frederick* Forsyth.

BUCKLEY: Well, my memory of it was that I had just read *The Day of the Jackal* and admired it hugely. That the reader should know exactly how it ended and nevertheless still pant his way with excitement through three hundred pages—I thought that was really a splendid accomplishment. I remember saying something along the lines of, If I were to write a book of fiction, I'd like to have a whack at something of that nature.

INTERVIEWER: So you liked the challenge of writing about an occurrence in contemporary history where the reader knew the outcome and . . .

BUCKLEY: Yes, although I proceeded not to do so. That is, *Saving the Queen* did not have a predictable and well-known outcome, though some of the succeeding novels did. However, I have this problem—perhaps some people would think my problem is greater than that—which is that I have never succeeded in pre-structuring a book. I've never started a novel knowing what the end is going to be. When I get about halfway through—and I go into this only because I assume it's of some technical interest to other writers—I then need to stop and force myself to figure out how the Gordian knot is going to be severed, because at this point there are a lot of characters and dramatic questions that need to be consummated. Some people feel that a book comes out better written that way—i.e., if the author himself doesn't know what's going to be in Chapter Two when he writes Chapter One, Chapter Two might then be more freshly minted and read that way. I'm skeptical. It seems to me that a thoroughly competent operator would sit down and think of what's going to be in Chapter One through Chapter Forty, and simply move ahead. What I do at the end of an afternoon's work is write two or three lines on what I think is the direction of the narrative, and where we might logically go the next day.

INTERVIEWER: If you stop yourself halfway through—almost as "Ellery Queen" used to stop three quarters of the way through and say, Now that you have all the clues necessary for a solution, what is the solution?—is there a tendency then to load too much resolution into the end of a book?

BUCKLEY: I think that's a danger. It's what I hope I've avoided, in part because I'm very easily bored, and therefore if I can keep myself awake from chapter to chapter, I assume I can keep other people awake. That is why I don't reserve all the dynamite for the end. This may be the moment to say that in all of my novels, to the extent that I have a rule, it is to devote a very long chapter, close to the beginning, to the development of a single character. In Book One it's Blackford Oakes, which is natural. In Book Two, *Stained Glass,* it was Erika, a Soviet agent. I lifted her as though Vladimir Nabokov had a daughter, not his son, Dimitri. I confided my invention to Nabokov which perhaps precipitated his death. He didn't live to read the book, but he was very enthusiastic, as you remember, about the first book, and his widow liked *Stained Glass.* In any event, I've always felt that the extensive development of one character gives the book a kind of beef that it doesn't otherwise have. That's the only regimen to which I willingly subscribe and towards which I naturally drift.

INTERVIEWER: One of the questions about your novels is: How much is true, and how much is invented?

BUCKLEY: Well, I poach on history to the extent that I can. For instance, when I was in the CIA it was reported to me that the evidence was overwhelming that the destruction of Constantin Oumansky's airplane—he was the Soviet ambassador to Mexico—was an act of sabotage, ordered by Stalin. Stalin was killing people capriciously anyway in those days, so it was inherently believable. On the other hand, as I remember, Oumansky lived for a few hours after the plane came down, so the explosion wasn't very efficient. Thus there's a school of thought that sees it as a genuine accident. But for a novel I don't trouble myself about matters of that kind. That is to say, if something was in fact a coincidence, but might have been an act of treachery, I don't hesitate to decide which is more convenient for the purpose of the narrative. The books are, after all, introduced as works of fiction. Everybody knew that Charles de Gaulle was going to survive the OAS, and everybody knows that Kennedy is not going to survive the twenty-second of November, 1963, and everybody knows that the Berlin Wall is going to rise. Even so, I attempt to create suspense around such episodes.

And manifestly, succeed. The books get heavy criticism, positive and negative, but no one says, Why read a book in which you know what's going to happen?

INTERVIEWER: Still, it's a nice challenge of art to put yourself up against that.

BUCKLEY: Sure. And I owe that idea to Forsyth.

INTERVIEWER: In the patterns you've developed, one of them is the unspoken premise: This is the way it *might* have been behind that great event that we all know about.

BUCKLEY: That's right. I found myself attracted to this idea of exploring historical data and visiting my own imagination on them. The very successful book on the death of Kennedy written by Don DeLillo—*Libra*—does, of course, that. In a sense overcomplicated and ineffectively ambitious in some of its sections, it's a magnificent piece of work, in my judgment. As long as the reader isn't persuaded that you are trying, via fiction, an act of historical revisionism, I don't think you meet any hard resistance.

INTERVIEWER: So the reader will go with you in a combination of invention and known history, but won't accept so cheerfully an editorial.

BUCKLEY: Yes. Of course, I think it probably depends also on how contentious the theme is. For about twenty-five years, dozens of books were published to the effect that Roosevelt was responsible for Pearl Harbor. Never mind whether he *was,* in a sense, or was not, I think that if during that period a novel pressing his guilt had been written, there would have been a certain amount of polemical resentment. If one were to write today a novel about a senator from Massachusetts and a young woman in Chappaquiddick, and how he drowned her or deserted her or whatever—readers would tend, under those circumstances, to think of it as more effort to make the case against Teddy Kennedy, rather than as a work of fiction.

INTERVIEWER: There seems to be a period that has to elapse before you can safely . . .

BUCKLEY: I think so. At this point I think you can speculate about the death of JFK and not get into trouble. Like Sacco and Vanzetti.

INTERVIEWER: You consciously stayed away from that event for a long time.

BUCKLEY: Until novel Number Eight. *Mongoose, R.I.P.* flatly says that although Oswald took the initiative in suggesting that he intended to try to assassinate the President, Castro, without acting specifically as an accomplice, urged him to proceed.

INTERVIEWER: To go back for a moment to the one character you chose to develop at length, do you decide as you're writing your way into the novel which character you will give a full history, or do you decide that before you write?

BUCKLEY: Again, I sometimes don't know who the character is going to be until I've launched the book, but I'm consciously looking for a target of opportunity. For instance, in *Stained Glass* I decided that the Soviet woman spy, who is acting as a translator and interpreter for Count Wintergrin, the protagonist, was the logical person to have a complex background. So I made up the daughter of Nabokov and went through her whole childhood and love life and her apostasy from the West.

INTERVIEWER: The Cold War is an essential handicap . . .

BUCKLEY: I hate to use the word in this context, but I must—these are novels that *celebrate* the Cold War. I don't think that's a paradox that affronts, any more than, say, a novelist who celebrates a world war. But my novels "celebrate" the Cold War, and therefore the passions awakened by this titanic struggle are really a narrative obligation. The fact of the matter is that in our time—in my adult lifetime—somewhere between fifty and sixty million people were killed by *other* causes than as a result of war or pestilence. And most cases—the great exception being the victims of Hitler—were the victims of the Communists. Now that struggle is sometimes made to look like a microcosmic difference, say some slight difference of opinion between Alger Hiss and Whittaker Chambers. In fact, it was a typhoon that roared across the land—across bureaucracies, academia, laboratories, chancelleries. One week after Gorbachev was here in New York, I find myself using the past tense about the Cold War, which shows you how easily co-opted I am. But the Cold War is the great political drama of the twentieth century, and there is extraordinarily little literature about it written in the novel form. There are great exposés—*The God That Failed, The Gulag Archipelago.* But if you think about the American scene, there isn't really an abundant literature, is there?

INTERVIEWER: Why do you think this is so?

BUCKLEY: I think that there's a sort of feeling that much of the conflict has been an *alien* experience. Of course, there are those New York intellectuals who are exceptions. I remember one middle-aged man who came to *National Review* a couple of weeks ago and said that when he was growing up he thought the two political parties in the United States were the Communist Party and the Trotskyist! That was all his mother and father ever talked about. Irving Kristol will tell you that the fights at CCNY were always on this or that modality of communism. But on the whole it has not been a national experience. When you think of Updike or Bellow or Walker Percy, and the tangentiality of their involvement in the Cold War, there isn't really a hot concern for it. It must be because our novelists disdain such arguments as grubby, or because they think that it's an ideological quarrel with no genuine intellectual interest for the mature person. But of course it has been the great struggle of our time. For that reason I think of my novels as entertainment but also designed to illustrate important problems in that setting. It means a lot to me to say this: when I set out to explore the scene, I was determined to avoid one thing, and that is the kind of ambiguity for which Graham Greene and to a certain extent Le Carré became famous. There you will find that the agent of the West is, in the first place, almost necessarily unappealing physically. He drinks too much, he screws too much and he's always being cuckolded. Then, at some dramatic moment there is the conversation or the moment of reflection in which the reader is asked to contemplate the difficulty in asserting that there *is* a qualitative difference between Them and Us. This I wanted to avoid. So I was searching, really, for a little bit of the purity of Melville's Billy Budd in Blackford Oakes. Billy Budd has no sense of humor, and without a sense of humor you can't be genuinely American . . . I made him almost spectacularly good-looking in defiant reaction to these semi-disfigured characters that Greene and Le Carré and Len Deighton specialize in. I got a little tired of that after Novel Three or Four, so I didn't belabor the point as much.

INTERVIEWER: Your reference to Graham Greene. Does he matter to you, or figure in your . . . ?

BUCKLEY: Graham Greene has always struck me as being at war with himself. He has impulses which he sometimes examines with a compulsive sense to dissect them, as though only an autopsy would do to dissect their nature. He is a Christian more or less *malgré soi.* He is a Christian because he can't quite prevent it. And therefore he spends most of his time belittling Christianity and Christians. He *hates* the United States, and his hatred is in part I suppose a reaction by some finely calibrated people to American vulgarity. But with him it's so compulsive it drives him almost to like people who are professional enemies of the United States. And since the most conspicuous critic of the United States in this part of the world during the last twenty-five years has been Fidel Castro, he ends up being, God help us, pro-Castro. He once gave the answer—it might have been in the *Paris Review,* I forget—to the question, "What is the word you least like in English?" "America." And he set out to prove it. Given the refinement of his mind, it's always been a mystery to me that he should be so besotted in his opposition to that towards which he naturally inclines— Christianity and all that Christianity bespeaks—in order to identify himself with those he sees as the little man? Okay, but when the little man is such a person as Fidel Castro or Daniel Ortega? It all defies analysis.

INTERVIEWER: Who else among the people practicing this kind of fiction do you pay attention to?

BUCKLEY: Well, I'm not a systematic reader. I read a little bit of everything. I've never studied the achievement of any particular author seeking to inform myself comprehensively of his technique or of his point. I occasionally run into stuff that deeply impresses me. For instance, Updike's *The Coup,* which I reviewed for *New York* magazine.* It astonishes me that it is so little recognized. It's *the* brilliant put-down of

* See chapter 16, "Passing in Review."

Marxist Third World nativism. It truly is. And hilarious. It's a successor to *Black Mischief,* but done in that distinctively Gothic style of Updike's—very different from the opéra bouffe with which Evelyn Waugh went at that subject fifty years ago. And then I think that Walker Percy's *Love in the Ruins* is another *1984.* An exquisite extrapolation of what life might be like if we don't dominate technology, and yield to totalitarian imperatives. He combined in it humor with a deep and often conscious explanation of human psychology via this vinous character—the doctor—who dominates the novel so convincingly.

INTERVIEWER: Somehow, for some unannounced reason, we are talking about Christian novelists. I'm struck by this only because the much-remarked phenomenon of the nineteen-fifties, sixties and seventies has been—certainly in America—the Jewish novel, or the novelist who writes from background in Jewry.

BUCKLEY: That reminds me that along about nineteen fifty-one or two—whenever it was that Graham Greene wrote *The Love Affair* [*The End of the Affair*]—one critic said, "If Mr. Greene continues . . . if he writes one more book like this, he must thereafter be evaluated as a "*Catholic* novelist." He didn't say "Christian novelist." And indeed Greene's succeeding book was a rather sharp departure. It occurs to me that the point you really make is more nearly about *Christians* who write novels, not Christian novelists. Chesterton, Belloc, and Morris *were* Christian novelists. But Updike is a Christian who writes novels. A reading of his work wouldn't permit you to decoct from it, with any sense of certainty, that the author was a professing Christian. I don't think from *Love in the Ruins* you could guess Walker Percy was a Catholic.

INTERVIEWER: I was thinking about your own deep religious faith.

BUCKLEY: Well, yes. I'm a professing Christian, and every now and then I take pains to let the reader in on the fact that so is Blackford Oakes. On the other hand, it would be hard, I think, to pronounce my books as "Christian novels" unless you were to go so far as to say that any novel that acknowledges epistemological self-assurance to the point of permitting us to say, *They're wrong and you're right,* has got to trace to that sense of certitude that is distinctively Christian.

INTERVIEWER: Yes, you're certainly not *preaching* in the novels. Blackford Oakes occasionally prays, which is just as natural to him as breathing, but his Christianity doesn't color everything. I was just wondering whether the Christians who write novels have become an underground sect, as Christians were at the outset.

BUCKLEY: I think to a significant extent they have. Raymond Williams—the late British novelist—was the last novelist I can think of offhand who was a flat-out Christian novelist. Am I wrong?

INTERVIEWER: Frederick Buechner has been plying his trade as a Christian novelist. George Garrett—his big novels are set in the Elizabethan era, but they're written with Christianity very much alive and at issue. And, at times, include spies. I wonder if spying and religion are in some way natural literary bedmates.

BUCKLEY: Well, isn't it safe to say that people who pursue the Communist objective—certainly early on—were motivated by ideological convictions which were almost religious in nature? Religious in the sense that they called for sacrifice and for the acceptance of historicism. That became less and less so as fewer and fewer people of moral intelligence actually believed in Leninism and communism. What they then believed in was Russian expansionism, and they became mere agents of the Soviet Union . . .

INTERVIEWER: So it began with religious fervor which supplanted what traditional religion might have been for some.

BUCKLEY: I think so. These days it would be hard to find somebody in his twenties comparable to Whittaker Chambers in his twenties. This doesn't mean that there aren't still Communists—Angela Davis is a very noisy Communist, but she's shallow. But there isn't really a sense of life in the catacombs, the kind of thing you had in the twenties and thirties, when people like Malcolm Muggeridge (until his early epiphany) were, temporarily, in thrall to the idea of the collectivist state.

INTERVIEWER: Do you think that in a time when the visible attachment of many people to formal religious institutions has been waning that there has been a corresponding attraction to other causes?

BUCKLEY: Yes, I do. And for that reason it is not easy to command a large public. Most writers want a large public, and tend for that reason not to write religious novels. And explicitly religious—God, it's been so long since I've read one!—an explicitly religious novel would be looked on merely as a period piece.

INTERVIEWER: How do you handle the technical stuff in the novel? Do you do your own research?

BUCKLEY: I am very unmechanical. I remember once, halfway through writing *Stained Glass,* I had to fly back to New York from Switzerland to do two or three episodes of *Firing Line* to catch up. I called my electrician in Stamford and I didn't have a lot of time; so I just said, "Could you please tell me how to execute somebody with electricity?" Well, he was sort of dumbfounded.

INTERVIEWER: He doesn't make house calls of that kind?

BUCKLEY: That's right. And he hadn't really given it much thought. He sort of muttered a couple of utterly unusable things like, "Put him in a bathtub and have him fix electricity." So I mentioned this in a letter to a historian at the University of San Jose. He wrote back and said, I must introduce you to my friend, Alfred Aya. Aya turned out to be a bachelor, aged then about fifty-five, who worked for the telephone company. As my historian described him, at heart a physicist—and more. When he was six years old and traveled with his parents, he would inevitably disappear for four or five minutes in the hotel, and from that moment on anybody who pushed "UP" on the elevator went down, and anybody who pushed "DOWN" went up. Aya loves challenges. So I wrote him a letter and said: Look, I've got this problem. . . . He gave me the idea of executing him via this device—what I call Chromoscope—which was entirely plausible. Later, he gave me all the information I needed to write satellite scenes in the novel that dealt with the U-2, including how to make the thing appear to be coming down, and how to destroy it, etc., etc. I remember when I came to the nuclear missile question—at this point we communicated with each other via MCI because he's an MCI nut, as am I—so I shot him a message via computer. Here's the problem: there's one nuclear weapon left in Cuba, and I have to know what it looks like. I must know what is needed to fire it, what is needed to redirect it to a target other than the one prescribed for it. And twenty-four hours later, I had a twenty-nine-thousand-word reply from him. Absolutely astonishing. Which made me—temporarily—one of the world's foremost authorities on how to handle a single nuclear bomb.

INTERVIEWER: Does he give you any credit for helping him work off aggressions?

BUCKLEY: He's absolutely delighted to help.

INTERVIEWER: What else is your system of research, since there is so much fact?

BUCKLEY: Wherever there is something concerning which I have a factual doubt, I put in a double parenthesis, which is a code to the librarian at *National Review,* who moonlights on my books, to check that, so she often will find five or six or seven hundred of those in the course of a novel. And she then copes.

INTERVIEWER: Are you aware of the category they now call the techno-thriller, like the novels of Tom Clancy and so on?

BUCKLEY: Well, I know Tom Clancy.

INTERVIEWER: I just wondered whether these writers who make a fetish out of hardware have influenced you?

BUCKLEY: No, except that I admire when it's done skillfully. For instance, Frederick Forsyth, in the book mentioned earlier, describes the assembly of the rifle with which he's going to attempt the assassination; I like the neatness with which he names the various parts. I have a book called *What's What,* in which you can look up "shoe" and find out exactly what you call this part of one, or that, etc.

INTERVIEWER: Now, famously, you write, *everywhere.* You write in New York at *National Review;* you write in New York in your home; you write in Connecticut in your home; you write in the car, you write in planes, you write presumably in hotels. Is it only your novel-writing that is done in Switzerland?

BUCKLEY: In order not to break the rhythm, I almost always write a chapter on the airplane from Switzerland to here when I come back for my television work. Working on a novel, I like to write every day so as not to break it up. There are two nights when I cannot do it. Those are the nights when I am preparing for the television the following day. But I try not to miss more than two nights.

INTERVIEWER: Do you think when a novelist begins a novel, he has to live the novel . . . that you have begun to become one or more of the characters, and you don't want to be interrupted playing those roles any more than an actor wants to be interrupted . . .

BUCKLEY: Oh, I am *feverishly* opposed to that idea. I've seen people wreck their lives trying to do it. I know the MacDowell Colony and Breadloaf and such are pretty successful, but I also know that some people seclude themselves to write and become alcoholics precisely because they have nothing else to do. I have a close friend who has that problem, because when he sets out to write a novel, he wants to clear the decks. Nothing would drive me battier than to do *just* a novel over the course of an entire month. I have only x ergs of purely creative energy, and when I'm out of those, what in the hell do I do then?

When one sets out to write a book, I do believe one should attack it two or three hours a day, every day, without fail. You mustn't interrupt it to do a week's lecture tour or whatever. On the other hand, don't ever devote the entire day to doing just that, or the chances are you'll get bored with it, or simply run out of energy. But I'm glad you asked me that question, because I feel so strongly about it. I'd like to see more novels *not* written by people who have all the time in the world to write them.

INTERVIEWER: As an editor I spend half of my life trying to persuade people who think they should write books that they don't have to give up careers and certainly not family in order to write a book. They do have to find time—they have to make time—but they don't necessarily have to jump ship.

BUCKLEY: It seems so marvelous when you realize that and can say, Look, fifteen hundred words a day and you've got a book in six weeks.

INTERVIEWER: Now when you wrote your first novel, I found it a surprise—an agreeable surprise because I somehow thought it would be in homage to writers you liked . . .

BUCKLEY: Imitative? I don't have the skill to imitate. For instance, I admire people who can come up with a touch of a foreign accent. I just don't know how. There may be a school somewhere—Cornell?—that teaches you how to do that. And if I thought I could go somewhere for a half-day and learn how to make a character sound like a Spaniard, I would. My son has that skill, marvelously developed. I can't do it. And I can't in speaking either. I sometimes call somebody and don't want to be recognized, but I don't know how to do it. And I don't know how to write like anybody else.

INTERVIEWER: As your editor, I didn't think you'd write a page-turner. I thought, as I've said, that you would write a clever novel, an intelligent novel, maybe ideologically weighted. What I didn't see coming was the novel that moves ahead. I wondered if that comes at least in part from the fact that you write fast?

BUCKLEY: Well, perhaps in part. But mostly, it's my terribly overdeveloped faculty against boredom. I was introduced into the White House Fellows annual lunch affair by a man who had done some research on my books and he picked up a line I had forgotten. "Mr. Buckley," he said, "has written that he gets bored winding his watch." True, I was greatly relieved when they developed the quartz. I never *just* brush my teeth—I'm reading and brushing my teeth at the same time—so, if something bores me, then it's certainly going to bore somebody else.

I live a hectic life. Someone once asked me if I ever could lay aside my Christian scruples so as to have a mistress, and I said, "I really don't have the time."

INTERVIEWER: You once said to me that you are not particularly reflective, or thoughtful, and you said, I think, it is perhaps because you're so compulsively busy. How can you write a novel with as many parts and qualities, as many components, as many subplots and themes as you do, and still say that you're not thoughtful, not reflective?

BUCKLEY: Well, what that takes is hard concentration. I don't think that people who are very busy are for that reason diluting the attention that they give to what they are doing when they are doing it. For instance Churchill in his wonderful essay on painting said when he's painting that's *all* he's thinking about. When I'm painting, that's *all* I'm thinking about. I happen to be a lousy painter, I should admit instantly, but I enjoy it, and I concentrate on it. Sometimes, going up in the lift with, say, Doris Brynner, a ski-mate, who's a wonderful listener, I'll say, Now I've got to the point where I've got this problem, and this girl has to come out alive. On the other hand, she's going to be in the Lubyanka . . . that kind of thing, and just saying it helps. I only really think when I'm writing or talking. I suppose it's a gift of extemporaneity. But also, added to that method, I think is the usual one. When you reach a knotty problem in your novel, you sometimes have to sit back in your chair and think, What am I going to do next? I don't want to give the impression that I simply keep using my fingers.

INTERVIEWER: Reviewers have noticed, and it has always intrigued me, that you write your enemies so well that it sometimes seems as if you characterize them better than *our* guys—the good guys. Your portraits of Castro, of Che Guevara, of Khrushchev, Beria, and so on, are all close, pores and all . . .

BUCKLEY: Nobody can possibly like the Beria that I depicted.

INTERVIEWER: No, I don't mean it's necessary to *like* them, but you give them so much color. Blackford sometimes pales—and I suspect this is your intention—by comparison to the roster of heavies.

BUCKLEY: Well, exposure to these historical characters is almost always limited. In the first book in which Khrushchev appears, he makes, I think, two appearances. Therefore you take the essence of Khrushchev and give it to the reader and the reader is grateful, because it *is* the essence of what we know or can imagine about him. If you had to write four hundred and fifty pages about Khrushchev, you'd run the danger of etiolation. I think I've read enough about these characters to have some idea of what they're like. I depended heavily on Carlos Franke when I wrote about Castro and Che Guevara. Guevara was a very magnetic human being. Cruel, and entirely obsessed, but nevertheless attractive. Fidel Castro is more attractive to ten thousand people than he is to ten people, whereas Che Guevara was the other way around. I think I captured Castro well, but I'm equally pleased with the portraits I've drawn of Americans. The Dulles brothers, and Dean Acheson . . .

INTERVIEWER: Let's speak for a moment of the amount you write and the presumed speed at which you write, novels and everything else. Do you have any models or inspirations who helped you to this sustained burst of intellectual and creative activity?

BUCKLEY: I'm not sure I'm all that fast or all that productive. Take, for example, Trollope. He'd rise at five-thirty, do his toilette, and have his breakfast, all by six. He would then begin writing, and he had a notepad which had been indexed to indicate intervals of two hundred and fifty words. He would force himself to write two hundred and fifty words per fifteen minutes. Now, if at the end of fifteen minutes he hadn't reached one of those little marks on his page, he would write faster. And if he passed the goal in fifteen minutes he would write more slowly! And he wrote that way for three hours—three thousand words a day.

INTERVIEWER: Do you approve?

BUCKLEY: If you were told to write a cantata every Sunday, and you got what Bach got out of it, how could you disapprove of it?

INTERVIEWER: Do you keep to a particular standard with your work?

BUCKLEY: It's true about everybody, that some stuff is better than other stuff. But I don't release anything that isn't roughly speaking—I say roughly speaking—as good as it can be. If I reread, say, my column, a third time, I probably would make a couple of changes. I'm aware of people who create both, so to speak, the "quality stuff," and the "non-quality stuff," who think nothing of writing two or three pulp novels per year. Bernard De Voto was that way. I don't do that and I'm not sure I could. What I write—especially the books—needs a lot of work. So I always resent critics who find themselves saying, "Mr. Buckley's novels look as though they were written with one eye on the in-flight movie."

INTERVIEWER: Nobody's been clever enough to say that.

BUCKLEY: Sheppard in *Time* magazine did. Who, by the way, has often praised my books. So it would be odd, I think, for someone who has reached age sixty-three, which I have, writing as much as I do without being able to discipline himself.

INTERVIEWER: Although you don't measure it out like Trollope, nevertheless you know you have so many days and weeks in February and March in which to write a novel.

BUCKLEY: Well, I'm much slower than Trollope . . . and never mind the differences in quality. If Trollope had given himself, say, six hours instead of three, would his novels have been that much better? I don't know that anybody could reach that conclusion. But then he took three hours to write three thousand words, which is very fast writing when using a pencil, but not fast at all when you're using a word processor.

INTERVIEWER: It should change the statistics.

BUCKLEY: When I sit down to start writing every day in Switzerland—which is usually about a quarter to five to about seven fifteen, two and a half hours—it's inconceivable to me that I would write less than fifteen hundred words during that time. That's much slower than Trollope, even though I have faster tools. So although I write fast, I'm not a phenomenally fast writer.

Speechwriters get told by the President that he's going to declare war the next day and please draft an appropriate speech. And they do it. Or, Tom Wicker. I've seen him write ten thousand words following one day's trial proceedings, and all that stuff will appear in the *New York Times*. Now it's not belletrism, but it's good journalistic craftsmanship.

INTERVIEWER: There's no automatic merit in being fast or slow. Whatever works, works. Georges Simenon, who was a phenomenon of production, always got himself in shape to write each novel. I hate to mention this in your presence, but he usually wrote his novels in seven or eight days. He had a physical beforehand—I think perhaps particularly for blood pressure—and then went into a kind of trance and wrote the novel, and then was ordered by his doctor to go off and take a vacation.

BUCKLEY: I'll go you one better. Rotzan Isogner, who does not go to sleep until he has finished the book.

INTERVIEWER: You've said more than once that you find writing is hard work . . .

BUCKLEY: But how would the reader know? That doesn't solve it at all. Writing, if it's done at all, has got to yield net satisfaction. But that satisfaction is long after the foreplay. I'm not saying that I wish I were otherwise engaged professionally. I'm simply saying that writing is terribly hard work. But it doesn't follow at all that because it's hard work, it's odd that it's done so quickly. I think that's quite natural. If writing is pain, which it is to me, it should follow that the more painful the exercise is, the more quickly you want to get on with it. The obvious analogy, I suppose, would be an execution. For years they've been trying to figure out how to execute a person more quickly, so that he feels less protracted pain.

That's a *reductio ad absurdum,* but in any event, if your living depends on writing a piece of journalism every day, and you find writing painful work, you're obviously much better off developing the facility to execute it in an hour rather than ten hours.

INTERVIEWER: Your workroom in Switzerland. What is that like?

BUCKLEY: Well, it's a converted children's playroom. I have my desk and my reference library at one end; there's the harpsichord and gramophone, and there's a Ping-Pong table . . . on which all the paints are . . .

INTERVIEWER: Do you play music while you're writing? Do you write to Scarlatti, or to Bach, or—

BUCKLEY: Do I play? . . . Oh, my goodness! Heavens, yes! I thought you meant, did I play myself? Occasionally, I get up and— you know, in a moment of boredom or whatever—and hit a few notes. But the answer is, Yes, I have the record player on most of the time. Also, in Switzerland, one of the better socialized institutions—but I love it—is that you can, for a few francs per month, attach to your telephone a little music-box device which gives you six channels, one of them a good music channel.

INTERVIEWER: Is there any link between what you're writing and what you're listening to?

BUCKLEY:	No, none whatever.
INTERVIEWER:	So you could play Fats Waller one time and Beethoven another?
BUCKLEY:	I don't play jazz when I write. I don't know why but I just plain don't. But I do when I paint.
INTERVIEWER:	What about revising?
BUCKLEY:	Of all the work I do, it's the work I look forward to most—rewriting. I genuinely, *genuinely* enjoy that—especially with the invention of the word processor, which makes it mechanically so neat.
INTERVIEWER:	So partly it's the technological joy of working with these instruments?
BUCKLEY:	Yes.
INTERVIEWER:	You're a computer maven, you've been through all the known stages of man with regard to writing and its instruments. You presumably started writing by hand or, as some people would insist, with a quill pen, yes?
BUCKLEY:	Well, I did in this sense: until I was writing every day for the *Yale Daily News,* as its editor, I would write by hand and then type, so the typewritten copy would be draft number two. It happens that my handwriting is sort of malformed. In fact, my father, when I was fifteen years old, sent me a typewriter with the instructions: (a) learn to use it, and (b) never write to him in longhand again. So I learned the touch-type system, and by the time I was, I guess twenty-three, it wouldn't occur to me to write anything by hand. In fact, I was so unhappy doing so that I would ask my professors' permission, on the honor system, to type an exam instead of writing it. And with one exception, they all said, Sure. I'd take one of those blue books into the next room and type away.
INTERVIEWER:	About vocabulary: you get criticized, or satirized, for your use of arcane words. Are you conscious of reining in your vocabulary when you're writing a novel?
BUCKLEY:	No, I don't think I am. In the novels, there's less obvious analysis than in nonfiction work. I'm attached to the convic-

tion that sometimes the word that you want has an in-built rhythm that's useful. And there are some words that are ono-matopoeic, and when they are, they too can be very useful. Let me give you a concrete example. This morning, I wrote about Arafat's speech, and the coverage of the speech, which consumed most of the television news last night. This had to do with the question, Did he or did he not live up to the de-mands of the State Department that he denounce violence absolutely, agree to abide by the relevant resolutions of the United Nations Security Council, and acknowledge the ex-istence of Israel? Now all the commentators said, Well he skirted the subject; his language was sometimes ambiguous. I concluded that he had more nearly consummated his in-herent pledge—"however *anfractuous* the language." Now the word came to me not only as a useful word but also as a *necessary* word. I first ran into that word in a review by Dwight Macdonald of Norman Mailer's book on the Penta-gon *(Armies of the Night)*, and I didn't know what it meant; I couldn't figure it out by internal inspection, so I looked it up. And that's *exactly* the word to describe Arafat's discussion of Israel's existence. There is an example of where one could use the word "ambiguous," but that extra syllable makes it sound just a little bit more "windy."

I remember once in a debate with Gore Vidal at which [TV talk show host] David Susskind was deriding me in San Francisco, 1964. I used the word "irenic," which didn't disturb Vidal, of course. So after it was over, Susskind said, "What's irenic?" I said, "Well, you know, sort of serene, sort of peaceful." "Well, why didn't you say serene or peaceful?" And I said, "Because the other word is a better fit." At this point believe it or not, Vidal, who was on Susskind's side a hundred percent during the exchange, said, "You know the trouble with you, David, is that you don't learn anything, ever."

INTERVIEWER: Irenic is a nice word.

BUCKLEY: And again onomatopoeic. So, in defending the use of these words, I begin by asking the question: Why were they in-vented? They must have been invented because there was, as the economist put it, "a felt need" for them. That is to say, there came a moment at which a writer felt that the ex-isting inventory didn't quite do what he wanted it to do.

These words were originally used because somebody with a sensitive ear felt the need for them. . . .

INTERVIEWER: "Anfractuous" is a more vigorous, almost violent word.

BUCKLEY: Yes. It suggests a little hint of the serpentine, a little bit the impenetrable going around and around. So therefore why not use it? Years ago, the review of *God and Man at Yale,* again by *Time* magazine, referred to my "apopemtic" book on leaving Yale. So, of course I looked it up, because I didn't know what it meant, and it's different from "valedic-torian," because an "apopemptic" speech, if memory serves, is usually what the ruler gives to the pilgrims en route somewhere. His sort of final message and advice. So the writer on *Time,* whoever he was in 1951, was making a very shrewd difference between "valedictory"—I'm leaving Yale—and giving Yale my parting advice; in effect, *Time* set me up as if I were the ruler of Yale, giving my subjects my advice. Very nice. So occasionally I use "apopemtic," and when I use it, it's strictly when I want that tiny little differ-ence in inflection, which is worth making.

INTERVIEWER: You once said you used the words you know.

BUCKLEY: A good point. Everybody knows words that other people don't know. Reading *The Coup,* I found twenty-six words in it I didn't know. I listed them in a column, and there were great hoots in my office because everybody knew quite a lot of them. . . .

INTERVIEWER: So words are put into your vocabulary by other writers?

BUCKLEY: Yes. I'm offended by people who suggest—and some have—that I spend my evenings with dictionaries . . . There are certain words that I couldn't bring myself to use, not because they aren't instrumentally useful, but because they just look too inventionistic. How they got there, one never quite knows. A lot of them are sort of medical.

INTERVIEWER: So, for those who might have thought your use of language elitist, you have quite the reverse view. You trust your reader either to know it or look it up, or go over it like a smooth ski jump.

BUCKLEY: The reader can say, I don't care, it's not worth my time. But there's no reason why he should deprive other people grateful for that augmented chord, which gives them pleasure. Did you know that forty percent of the words used by Shakespeare were by him used only once? I've never read a satisfactory explanation of the seventeenth-century capacity to understand the stuff we hear with some sense of strain. Shakespeare used a total of twenty-eight thousand words; most of them were within reach of the audience. And when you consider that books by Newman were serialized as recently as a hundred years ago. The *Apologia* was serialized and upped the circulation of a London daily. Imagine serializing the *Apologia* today. Or take the difference between a Lincoln-Douglas debate and a Kennedy-Nixon debate. . . . Lincoln, in that rich, biblical vocabulary of his, was not at all self-conscious about using a wide vocabulary.

I've never seen a test, though I'd like to see it done, that would scan, say, three or four pages of the current issue of the *New York Times,* and three or four pages of a hundred years ago of, say, the *Tribune,* and find out what the so-called Fry Index reveals.

INTERVIEWER: The Fry Index?

BUCKLEY: The Fry Index is the average number of syllables per word and the average number of words per sentence.

INTERVIEWER: In writing fiction, your vocabulary is nevertheless somewhat constrained by the fact that you are limited to the words that your characters would use?

BUCKLEY: Absolutely. Except that one of my characters is a Ph.D., and I remember on one occasion she used the word "syllepsis." Christopher Lehmann-Haupt wrote, "Mr. Buckley's character doesn't even know how correctly to use the word 'syllepsis,' she really meant . . . " Anyway, he gave me a wonderful opportunity, since a second printing was coming out right away, to go back and rewrite the dialogue to have her say, "syllepsis—a word the correct meaning of which is not even acknowledged by the *New York Times* critics."

INTERVIEWER: To shift a bit, in a conversation with Louis Auchincloss you asked, Why do people take less satisfaction from novels than they used to do?

BUCKLEY: Well, I mentioned television as the principal time consumer, and it just plain is. It's established statistically that the average American has the television set turned on between thirty-five and thirty-nine hours per week.

INTERVIEWER: If people derive fewer rewards from novels than they used to, does this reflect something about the novels themselves, rather than the competition for time?

BUCKLEY: Well, it certainly can. It can also suggest that the passive intelligence is less resourceful than it used to be. My favorite book at age nine was called *The Magic of Oz.* If you could correctly pronounce a string of consonants, you could turn yourself into a giraffe. I can't imagine a nine-year-old today being engrossed—being *diverted,* let alone being engrossed by that because he would want to see it happening on the screen.

INTERVIEWER: He'd want to see dancing consonants.

BUCKLEY: That's right.

INTERVIEWER: People have traditionally turned to novels, at least some, for a way to get a grip on the world; a way to see the order in the chaos. Have we gone past that period; is it that many novels are not so avidly consumed because they provide small delights, they don't provide epiphanies, or grand epiphanies?

BUCKLEY: Well, I have to reflect on that. We spoke about the scarcity of, say, the Christian novel, and to that extent one is probably justified in talking about the absence of great spiritual themes. By the same notion there isn't the eschatological novel in which one has a sense of achieving order, as for instance *A Tale of Two Cities* did, i.e., persuade the reader that what he had read and vicariously experienced was a narrative *beneath* the order of things—the gods. Now, all experiences tend to become more individuated. But then of course all larger experiences are solipsistic. And for that reason I think reading the many contemporary novels you get some of that feeling of, Where in the hell have I been that it was worthwhile going to?

INTERVIEWER: People either accuse you, or are interested in the Blackford Oakes novels, because they think you're writing about yourself.

BUCKLEY: Of course, it becomes very easy if one takes the obvious profile. You begin with the fact that we were both born the same year and went to Yale at approximately the same time. Now, I made him a Yale graduate—I think it was the class of 1951—for sheer reasons of personal sloth. I was in the class of 1950, so that I knew that I could coast on my knowledge of the scene without having to go and visit a fresh college and see how things happened there. Then, for the same reason, i.e., sloth, I made him an undercover agent of the CIA, so that I could give the identical training I had received and know that it was absolutely legitimate. So that much was, if you like, autobiographical . . . if you can say it's autobiographical that two different people went to Yale and to the CIA. . . . But beyond that, people who want to sustain the parallel have a tough time. In the first place he's an engineer, a Protestant. He has a sweetheart whom he has yet to marry—I married when I was twenty-four years old. He's a pilot which I was not. He signed up in the CIA as a *profession* which I didn't. I knew I was only going to be temporary and I'd quit after nine months. He's not a writer. There's a little touch of James Bond in his experiences, which there never was in mine, which were very sedentary. To be sure, it is quite true that he's conservative. In fact for the fun of it, I have him read *National Review* and occasionally read stuff of mine and Whittaker Chambers and so on. And he's also pro-American. And we're both bright, sure.

INTERVIEWER: And you're both admirers of Bill Buckley.

BUCKLEY: Exactly! Though sometimes he kind of lags behind a little bit.

INTERVIEWER: About Blackford Oakes again: there are some sort of serious disagreements about your style. Just running barefoot through some of these critical notices, I see: "Oakes is as bloodless as well-done English roast beef"—that's a reviewer in Florida—versus Broyard in the *New York Times:* "In every respect he is a welcome relief from the unromantic superiority and disengagement of a James Bond. Beneath this Cold War there beats a warm heart." Then we get from another reviewer: "Blackie has a distinctive personality"—and from another lines like: "A flat character and an annoying name dropper." You attract lines like: "A

Rambo with a Yale degree" and all sorts of things. This character of yours seems to be capable of stirring up a lot of confusing and conflicting opinions. Maybe that's biographical.

BUCKLEY: Well, yes, I have a feeling—I hate to say it, but I have a feeling this is mostly a confusing of things about me. I simply decline to believe that two or three of those things said about Blackford Oakes would have been said if the books had been written by Mary Gordon, say. They just wouldn't have said it—and they wouldn't have *thought* it. Now, whether they convinced themselves that this was so, or whether they feel the stereotypical compulsion to say it must be so because I wrote it, I don't know. I've never asked anybody. I'd like to think that Anatole Broyard is not easily seduced—at least not by me!—and I like to think that Blackford Oakes is an interesting human being. True, in certain of the novels he plays a relatively minor and flat role. But never quite as minor as people have sometimes charged.

INTERVIEWER: You seem to attract reviews which don't have much to do with the book at hand.

BUCKLEY: My son Christopher thinks I suffer from overexposure, and I'm sure he's right. I'd like to think some of my books would have done better if they had been published under an assumed name, so that people wouldn't feel they had to do the Buckley bit before talking about the book. It's especially true in England, by the way, although I'm underexposed in England in the sense that I'm not all over the place. Some aspects of my situation as a novelist are probably unique. Gore Vidal is very public in his experiences, but he's episodic. He goes away for a year and a half—thank God!—and then he writes his books and then he comes back and publicizes them. Norman Mailer, during his *Village Voice* period, and right after, was almost always in the news, not for something he said or for a position he had taken, about which people ceased caring, but about something he had done. You know, urinated in the Pentagon, or married his seventh wife, or got drunk at his fiftieth birthday, that kind of thing. But I assault the public three times a week in the column, and once a week on television, and every fortnight if they elect to read the *National Review.* So that's kind of a hard battering ram for people disposed to be impatient, either as critics or as consumers, of a novel written by me.

INTERVIEWER: That puts your critics to a particular test—that is, to detach themselves.

BUCKLEY: Anatole Broyard has been very attentive and receptive, and so has Lehmann-Haupt. Between them they've reviewed almost everything I've written.

INTERVIEWER: Did you say once that when you decided to write a novel, John Braine sent you a book on how to write a novel?

BUCKLEY: We were friends. John Braine was born again, politically. This was along around 1957 or '58 when he ceased to be an angry young man, and became an early deplorer of the excesses with which we became familiar in the sixties and seventies. So he used to write me regularly, and I had lunch with him once or twice in London; he was on my television program, along with Kingsley Amis. But then he—he was a little bit moody, and then he sort of stopped writing his letters. There wasn't any implicit act of hostility—I just had the feeling he wasn't writing his twenty-five people per week, that kind of thing. But when I sent him a letter saying that I was going to write a novel, he said, Well, I wrote a book on how to write a novel, and here it is. So I read it.

INTERVIEWER: Was it helpful?

BUCKLEY: I remember only one thing—which doesn't mean that I wasn't influenced by a hundred things in it—but he said that the reading public expects one coincidence, and is cheated if it isn't given one, but scorns two.

INTERVIEWER: Is there anyone or anything you would never write about?

BUCKLEY: I wouldn't write anything that I was simply not at home with. I wouldn't write a Western novel, for instance. I'm not sure I'd want to write *Advise and Consent*—the inside-the-Senate type of novel . . .

INTERVIEWER: Why don't you think about writing a novel like Tom Wolfe's—the novel of manners, of certain strata of society, of the mixture of social and political and business life. You have the keen observer's eye, and maybe not quite the same rapier instinct that Tom has for the false note, and—

BUCKLEY: And certainly not his descriptive powers, or his talent for caricature. Because those are indispensable weapons. For the first few chapters of *Bonfire,* I underlined just his descriptions of people's clothes, and in a million years I couldn't achieve that.

INTERVIEWER: It's true, there are no caricatures in your novels that I can think of. Tempting as it must have been to do so with some of the darker figures in those novels.

BUCKLEY: Well, some people thought the Queen was. I didn't think so. I thought she was a somewhat Dickensian, original creation. I'm really quite serious. The fact that she's terribly sharp-tongued, and terribly sarcastic; terribly aware of the fact that she's nominally sovereign, and actually powerless, I think adds to the credibility of her character. I would love to see her on the stage. As would have been done by Bette Davis.

INTERVIEWER: It's amusing to think back on how difficult it was for your agents to find publication in England for *Saving the Queen* because of your sacrilege in having Blackford Oakes bed down with her, even though a fictional queen.

BUCKLEY: And I have no doubt that not only killed that book in England, but probably inhibited its successors also.

INTERVIEWER: Have the novels been any kind of turning point? What have they meant to you? I have a feeling you took on the first one as a challenge—you wanted to test yourself against the form, and have some fun, which you certainly did—and then?

BUCKLEY: I did find that there were reserves of creative energy that I was simply unaware of. Obviously, as a nonfiction analyst, one has to think resourcefully, but if, let's say in the novel I'm depicting a Soviet prison train going from Moscow to Siberia, I've got to create something that can hold the reader's attention during that journey. The answer became: You can do that. And it's kind of nice to figure out that you *can* do that . . . create a story that carries you from there.

O f Buckley's eleven novels to date—ten of them concerned with Blackford Oakes, the CIA and the Cold War—the second, *Stained Glass,* occupies a special place. For years, it was *the* best-seller among his best-selling novels. More serious, less a jape than his debut novel, *Saving the Queen,* though all his novels are at bottom serious entertainments, it seems to convey a special feeling for its tragic hero—a German count, not Oakes— and for the unavoidable, undeclared human predicaments of that war in the shadows.

Invited by the Actors Theatre of Louisville, Kentucky, to contribute to their new playwrights program, the Humana Festival of new American plays—a commendable effort to get writers accomplished in other forms to try writing for the theater—WFB's play was produced in March–April 1989. Here is how their bulletin described the novel and introduced their interview.

Among his many books are eight novels which follow the adventures of the dashing Blackford Oakes, American secret agent, through an array of international intrigues and political hotbeds. Buckley has adapted his play from the second work in the series, *Stained Glass* . . .

In *Stained Glass,* Oakes is undercover in 1953 West Germany, as an engineer rebuilding a chapel. There, his assignment is to keep tabs on Count Alex Wintergrin, a charismatic leader seeking to reunite East and West Germany and quickly gaining popular support, to the dismay of both Washington and Moscow. Oakes soon becomes caught in the middle of Cold War détente and faces a moral dilemma: whether to obey his CIA orders and eliminate Wintergrin, or to follow his personal allegiance to a leader he respects as "the most admirable man alive." In a conversation with his Soviet espionage counterpart, Oakes expresses the confusion of his predicament: "Our people agreed to his 'elimination'—what a Sunday-suited word, his elimination—because *you* gave us no alternative. *That's* the official view of it. God knows it isn't my view of it."

An Interview with the Playwright

Why did you accept a commission from Actors Theatre to write a play?
Well, I hadn't done one before, and I thought it would be interesting to try it.

Had you thought about writing one before?
No, I hadn't . . . though my son had produced a play the summer before, at Williamstown, and he thought it was an exhilarating experience. So I thought, well, I'll try it.

And how did you find it, writing a play?
Writing a play was very difficult, very novel, in the sense that after a day's work I had no idea if I had done anything particularly good. Obviously, if you are a professional playwright, you develop enough experience to coach you on whether you are moving in a right direction or in a bad direction. I can do that in a novel or in nonfiction, but not yet in a play. It was very il-luminating to me to have the thing read professionally. Then I got some idea of what it was that I had performed. It made a tremendous difference.

From your various novels why did you choose to adapt Stained Glass?
It seemed to me to have a high dramatic potential, and also one that didn't require visits to six planets in two acts; most of the action is concentrated right there. To the extent that it isn't, you can *make* it happen there. Now, I had a wildly permissive letter which said in effect that anything you write we can produce, but my son warned me against excesses of that kind.

The Blackford Oakes character and the series of novels he appears in certainly make for some dramatic material. I'm surprised that we haven't seen any movies. Has Hollywood ever been interested in making films of your novels?
Yes, they dart in and out, they're doing that right now. There was a big hia-tus as a result of the financial failure of Robert Redford's CIA film, *The Day of the Condor,* some years ago. They lost their shirt on that, so no one would touch a spy film. Anyway, this will be the first venture in non-book form. Several screenplays have been written, not by me, but by others of various of the novels, but none of them have been produced.

You're known as a very prolific writer, and you seem to move quite easily from political essays to books on sailing and novels. At the end of the process of writ-ing Stained Glass, *did you find yourself more comfortable with playwriting?*
Yes, by the time I sat down with the script a couple of months later to look at it again and rewrite it, I found I had achieved a perspective that I didn't have the very first night I started in. That may have been simply the pas-sage of time, also comments on draft one from one or two people, espe-cially my son, who had had some dramatic experiences. So it's fair to say the missing perspective began to crystallize—the idea of communicating with an audience exclusively through spoken words, without the reliance on nonspoken words which novelists rely on very heavily.

Do you find that it's easier to make a political point in writing a play instead of an editorial or novel?
The availability of another voice—so to speak, a Greek chorus sitting in your pocket to be trotted out anytime you want—can't be discounted. It's obviously advantageous. On the other hand, the stage has the overwhelming advantage of the utterly direct experience with a listener who is engrossed, or who is supposed to be engrossed—he is a captive audience for a couple of hours—so *that* obviously gives you a dramatic purchase on the stage that you don't have in the passive material. What I'm trying to say is the advantage of the novelist is the one I've exploited, having written eight novels and only one play.

In the play we get a sense that the U.S. is buckling under, giving in to pressure from Stalin. Do you feel that the U.S. allowed itself to be intimidated, and could have more strongly opposed the Soviet occupation of Eastern Europe?
Absolutely. In that respect a lot of renowned strategists agree that from Yalta on, until we started to wake up, we did really nothing. The Marshall plan was an important economic step, and NATO was an important economic step, but we in effect sat around while the Soviet Union developed hydrogen bombs and crystallized its hold on Eastern Europe. It's of course wildly ironic when you consider the reason we went to war was to save Poland's freedom in 1939.

In the play we get the sense that the reason for the Americans' intimidation is fear. Why did we sit around letting the Soviets develop hydrogen bombs?
The big example is 1956 when the Soviets moved into Hungary and Eisenhower had an opportunity to do something or not do something. He opted to do nothing. In doing that he more or less documented the fact that as long as they stayed behind their own frontiers they were absolutely safe. *Stained Glass* foresees the fear felt by Western leaders every time an ultimatum was handed down by Stalin.

East-West relations have changed since 1952 and since 1978, when you wrote Stained Glass. *In the age of Gorbachev and* glasnost, *what point does* Stained Glass *make about East-West relations?*
In *Stained Glass,* set in 1953, Stalin was still head of the Soviet Union. He was succeeded by a troika, which became Khrushchev; the violence of Khrushchev was documented in his oppression of running tanks over students in Czechoslovakia. Khrushchev denounced Stalin and then Brezhnev came in. He denounced Khrushchev. And now Gorbachev just denounced Brezhnev. But none of them denounced Lenin, and we're still dealing with a country whose huge, huge overhead is inexplicable except in terms of wanting to dominate the politics of the world. We've had all

these ups and downs of détente and friendship and summit conferences, but the substantive causes of antagonism have not dissipated and won't dissipate until they renounce that part of Lenin that says, 'Go out and make the world a huge socialist state, which you will serve as a motherland.' They've got a lot of problems that distract them from doing that right now, of course, but none of the elements of the drama of *Stained Glass* is in any way affected by what's happened since.

What about the reunification of the two Germanys, is that a dead issue?
It's pretty dead, and it's not really an issue concerning which there's even German solidarity. The East Germans are afraid of the West Germans, and the West Germans are not absolutely sure that East Germany can be assimilated, and all the surrounding countries who twice in this century have been mauled by united Germany are in no particular hurry to patch them up. Clemenceau uttered a great line at Versailles. He said, "I love Germany so much I think there should be more of them."

In the play, Rufus makes a point that the end can at times be justified by the means. That reminded me of Darkness at Noon, *in which the excesses under Stalinist oppression could be justified by referring to its historical goals. What's the difference, with Rufus talking about U.S. covert action—*
Rufus was saying, Don't use the cliché "The end does not justify the means" because the end *very often* justifies the means. The correct statement is, "The end does not justify *any* means." We had a first-strike potential against the Soviet Union in 1953—we didn't use it, we didn't think of using it, quite correctly. If there is a single lesson to be learned from the eight novels I've written it is that there is a world of difference between *their* doing something and *our* doing something because the motives in both cases are entirely different. They want to maintain their slave state, we want to defend free people from being enslaved by them.

So when the U.S. plays dirty in terms of manipulating a nation's elections (as in Stained Glass*) and that sort of thing, it's because the Russians play dirty—?*
No, it's to save them from the Russians. Italy would have gone Communist in 1948 if we hadn't gone in there and spent millions of dollars and, as you put it, manipulated the vote. I wish to hell we'd manipulated the vote in Germany before Hitler got in, but the answer is what are we trying to accomplish? We're not trying to enslave somebody, we're trying to keep them free. We haven't dominated Italian politics since then, we left them on their own, but meanwhile they were free to act on their own rather than free to act as their Communist boss would have told them to do—as Stalin would've told them to do. . . .

This is a central point in your play; what place does personal morality have in government service?
We were reminded at Nuremberg that personal morality *at some point* transcends any loyalty to the state so that if the state were to say, you, I give you instructions to kill all Jews, or all Catholics or all blacks, you say just, I'm not going to do it. So there is always a surviving role for the conscience in any state, notwithstanding a presumptive obligation to obey orders.

Is that the case in Stained Glass*?*
Yes, Blackford Oakes reserves for himself a tiny little area of independent action and he says Okay, I work for the CIA, I acknowledge that the commander in chief thinks there's a danger of a world war, and under the circumstances I don't consider this a Nuremberg type of event, but let someone else do the actual pulling of the trigger. Now I don't necessarily defend that . . .

What is the significance of the chapel to you in the play?
It was a metaphor in the novel as it is in the play: the desire by Count Wintergrin to reconstitute the chapel fused in his spirit and his imagination with his desire to reintegrate Germany. They were part of the same dream. . . .

—THOMAS AUGST

Chapter 16

Passing in Review

All authors, perhaps especially those few who profess not to read their reviews, would like to talk (scream?) back at some of those who review their latest works. Prudence, caution, and publishers suggest otherwise. Bill Buckley more than once has dared to review his reviewers. This is either a bold and courageous maneuver or a kamikaze impulse. Asked to write an introduction to the paperback edition of the nonfiction book, *Overdrive* (Little, Brown & Company, Boston and Toronto, 1984), he wrote what follows, slightly abridged. WFB suggested that the reader could read the "Introductory Epilogue" before reading the book or after reading the book, or skip it entirely (he has suggested skipping when writing the inevitable chapter on navigation that adorns, or afflicts, each of his sailing narratives, sensitive to the fact that not every reader will be as enthralled by the techniques of navigation as he).

He gives more space to quoting the attacks on his book (and him personally) than to his ripostes or to his favorable reviews, most of them summed up in a footnote. Once again, he charges when he sees red and he most enjoys those negative reviewers who are clever—see the splendid parody in the following—not those who would merely tear him limb from limo.

INTRODUCTORY EPILOGUE

When Ray Roberts, who is my editor for a paperback edition of *Overdrive,* asked if I would write an introduction to it I agreed right away . . . I thought the reviews of it worth going over with some thought, hoping that such a study would interest readers, and knowing that it would interest me. There are over a hundred of these (*Overdrive* was handled intensively by the critical press) and they say something about the book but also about the culture in which they cropped up.

I begin, in search of focus, with a chronology. I reveal in the text of *Overdrive* when exactly it occurred to me (quite suddenly) to write this book, a journal of that particular week in my life. I had done such a book ten years earlier. It was here and there suggested by some critics that I had dreamed up a way to discharge an obligation to my publisher. In fact, the contrary is the case because when I decided to write this book I needed to get my publisher's agreement to postpone a commitment I had already made. . . .

It took me as many weeks to complete, almost exactly, as any of my other books, including my novels. It was suggested by one critic (you will see) that I more or less dictated scraps of this and that into a machine, presumably while skiing in February. Other critics, however, did not challenge that the book was written with care.

When I returned to New York, the manuscript complete except for the fine-tuning I do in July, I sent a letter to the editor of *The New Yorker,* Mr. William Shawn. I told him I thought it unlikely he would want to see my new book, given that I used exactly the same formula I had used ten years before in writing *Cruising Speed,* which *The New Yorker* had excerpted. Mr. Shawn replied that he would like to read *Overdrive,* which he subsequently bought.

It happened that the task of editing *Cruising Speed*'s excerpts fell to Mr. Shawn, if it can be said that anything at *The New Yorker* "falls" to Mr. Shawn. In any event, I had the extraordinary experience of working with him, he going over every sentence. When we lunched together one day I remember that a substantial part of our meeting was concerned with my habit of placing commas in unconventional places. This finally drew from Mr. Shawn, over the telephone, what I take it must be the sharpest kind of reproach the gentleman ever permits himself: "I am afraid, Mr. Buckley, that you do not really know the proper use of the comma." If St. Peter had declared me unfit to enter the Kingdom of God, I could not have felt more searingly the reproach, delivered in Mr. Shawn's inimitable manner. I hardly intend to suggest that he is otherwise permissive, though he sticks firmly, after *The New Yorker* makes the first-draft selection, to his determination to let authors whose works are being excerpted signify what they wish included, what excluded. Merely that he is meticulous. "I want *you* to be pleased with what we publish," he said to me. I have had a wonderful relationship with *The New Yorker,* having submitted five book manuscripts to Mr. Shawn, and received five acceptances.

I did not again work directly with Mr. Shawn. My next editor, William Whitworth, also demanding, and thorough, and civil, is now the editor of the *Atlantic Monthly.* The succeeding editor was Patrick Crow, a genial, surefooted, relaxed and amusing man who does not for a moment attempt to conceal that Mr. Shawn is *the* editor of *The New Yorker,* who reviews every controversial decision made during the many hours spent between the author and his *New Yorker* editor. When the author especially pleads for inclusion of a passage to which Mr. Shawn unwaveringly objects, what happens is that Mr. Shawn calls the author up and patiently explains why he is opposed to the inclusion of that passage. This author always relented. I would do anything for Mr. Shawn save join the Communist Party, and I am happy that it is unlikely he will ever ask me to do so.

All of this is by way of background, given that some critics (a) concluded that I expanded by force-feeding into a book (about 75,000 words long) what I had written for *The New Yorker* (the *New Yorker*'s version ran about 45,000 words); while others (b) pretended to flirt with the idea that Mr. Shawn had coaxed me into writing a self-parody, that he had acted as an editorial *agent provocateur*—a reading of Mr. Shawn wildly ignorant of the kind of person he is; leaving also (c) a few critics who, though reviewing my book, obviously had not read it, having clearly read only the excerpts published in *The New Yorker.* One critic especially comes to mind, who warned, "Readers seeking the tart side of Mr. Buckley will be disappointed." The tart side of Mr. Buckley is well represented in the book, less so in *The New Yorker* excerpts because Mr. Shawn explained to me over the telephone, after I had pitched for the inclusion of one very tart episode, that *The New Yorker* does not have a letters column in which editorial targets can fire back, and that therefore he feels it morally important to avoid anything that might be thought as hit-and-run.

In due course (January, February 1983), the *New Yorker* excerpts were published, and the reaction to them was, well, out of the ordinary. The *Washington Post*'s Curt Suplee reported joyously in his column, "That incessant scrunching noise you keep hearing to the north is Wm. F. Buckley Jr. attempting to squeeze his ego between the covers of the *New Yorker.* The behemoth first half of his two-part personal journal makes Proust look positively laconic. Buckley maunders along like Macaulay on Quaaludes about his house, limo, kids and friends, gloating and quoting his snappiest ripostes . . . *And yet you can't put the damn thing down!* Odd anecdotes bob up in the verbal spew (e.g., the time a typo in his column made it seem as if Pat Boone and his wife were wild about porno movies). The rhythm becomes hypnotic and . . . is there such a thing as smug-o-lepsy?"

I think I can only describe the reaction of *Newsweek* as hysterical. Before the *New Yorker's* ink was dry, Mr. Gene Lyons published an excoriation in high tushery of indignation ("So who is this preposterous snob?"). Not satisfied with this, *Newsweek* then published letters from readers for whom the mere mention of my name is obviously emetic. And not content with *that*, *Newsweek* then published a piece speculating on who might be the successor to William Shawn when he retires as editor of *The New Yorker*, including reference to unnamed critics' concern over Mr. Shawn's wilting powers, as witness that he had published the "self-indulgent" journals of Mr. Buckley. (The three assaults prompted me to write to *Newsweek* to observe that I hoped their obsessive concern over my self-indulgent journals had not got in the way of their enjoyment of the two-million-dollar party *Newsweek* had given itself in New York to celebrate its fiftieth anniversary. The letter was published, but in bowdlerized form.)

Now, leading up to publication of the book and fired by *The New Yorker*, came the parody-makers. There was one by Jon Carroll of the *San Francisco Chronicle* which was quite funny, burlesquing among other things my occasional use of Latin phrases. He had me referring to "Nihil Obstat, our Cuban-American cook," summoning my "Honduran-American driver, Pari Passu," sailing my "71-foot sloop, Malum In Sea," and using the services of my "ever efficient secretary, Gloria Mundi." There was another treatment by Richard Cohen of the *Washington Post*, good-natured and clever. Another in the *New York Review of Books*, some of it very funny, and still another in the *New Republic*.

I have elected to publish here in full the parody I thought funniest. It was written for the University of Chicago daily, the *Chicago Maroon*, by an undergraduate, David Brooks, the week before I went there as a visiting fellow. I put it all here in part because it is exuberantly readable but also because it communicates the nature of the irritation felt by some of the readers of the *New Yorker* articles. He touches, in the manner of the parodist, on themes that would be sustained by many of the critics when the book came out in August.

The Greatest Story Ever Told

William Freemarket Buckley was born on December 25, 1935 in a little town called Bethlehem. He was baptized an Episcopalian on December 28 and admitted to Yale University on the 30th.

Buckley spent most of his infancy working on his memoirs. By the time he had learned how to talk he had finished three volumes: *The World Before*

Buckley, which traced the history of the world prior to his conception; *The Seeds of Utopia,* which outlined his effect on world events during the nine months of his gestation; and *The Glorious Dawn,* which described the profound ramifications of his birth on the social order.

Buckley attended nursery school at the School of Soft Knocks, majoring in Art History. His thesis, "A Comparison of Michelangelo's David and My Own Mirror," won the Arthur C. Clarke award for Precocious Criticism and brought him to the attention of world luminaries.

His next bit of schooling was done at Exeter, where he majored in Pre-Yale.

Buckley's education was interrupted by World War II, during which he became the only six-year-old to fight in Guadalcanal and to land on the beaches of Normandy. Combat occupied much of his time during the period, but in between battles he was able to help out on the Manhattan Project, offer advice at Yalta, and design the Marshall Plan. His account of the war, *Buckley Versus Germany,* perched atop the *New York Times* Best Seller List for three years.

Upon his return to Exeter, Buckley found that schoolwork no longer challenged him. He transferred his energies to track, crew, polo, golf, tennis, mountain climbing, debate, stock brokerage, learning the world's languages, playing his harpsichord and, of course, writing his memoirs. By this time he had finished his ninth volume, *The Politics of Puberty,* which analyzed angst in the international arena and gave advice on how to pick up women. A friend at the time, Percy Rockefeller-Vanderbilt III, remembered, "Everybody liked Bill at Exeter. His ability to change water into wine added to his popularity."

The years at Exeter were followed by the climax of his life, the Yale years. While at Yale he majored in everything and wrote the bestseller, *God and Me at Yale,* which was followed by *God and Me at Home,* and finally, *God and Me at the Movies.*

His extracurricular activities at Yale included editing the *Yale Daily News,* serving as President of the University, and chairing the committee to have Yale moved from New Haven to Mount Olympus. He also proved the existence of God by uttering the Cartesian formula, "I think, therefore I am."

While a senior, Buckley founded the publications which would become his life's work: one was a journal of politics entitled *The National Buckley,* and the other was a literary magazine called *The Buckley Review.* Later, he would merge the two publications into what is now known as *The Buckley Buckley.*

On the day of graduation, Buckley married Miss Honoria Haight-Ashbury and fathered a son and a daughter (Honoria helped) both of whom would be named Yale.

As any of you who read *The New Yorker* know, life for Mr. Buckley since then has been anything but dull. On any given morning he will consult with a handful of national leaders and the Pope, write another novel in the adventure series, "Bill Buckley, Private Eye," chat with a bevy of Academy Award winners, write a few syndicated columns, and tape an edition of his TV show, "Firing Pin." He also tames a wild horse, chops down trees to reduce U.S. oil imports, and descrambles some top secret Soviet spy transmissions.

In the afternoons he is in the habit of going into crowded rooms and making everybody else feel inferior. The evenings are reserved for extended bouts of name-dropping.

Last year, needing a break from his hectic fast-lane life, Buckley sailed across the Atlantic in his yacht, the HMS *Armsrace,* and wrote a book entitled *Atlantic High.* In one particularly riveting scene, the *Armsrace* runs out of gas in the middle of the ocean and Buckley is forced to walk the rest of the way.

Buckley has received numerous honorary degrees, including an M.B.A., an Ll.D., a Ph.D., an M.D. and an L.H.D., all of them from Yale, of course.

During his two days at this University, Mr. Buckley will meet with students, attend classes, deliver a lecture and write four books.

So that as the countdown approached for the publication of *Overdrive,* one had the feeling that pens were being taken to the smithies to be sharpened. My son Christopher has a sensitive ear for these matters and advised me to batten down the hatches: I had seriously provoked, he warned me, substantial members of the critical community. And sure enough, his Farmer's Almanac proved reliable because the flak from the most conspicuous critical quarters (the *New York Times,* the *Washington Post,* the *New York Review of Books,* the *New Republic, The Nation, Atlantic,* and *Harper's*) was instantaneous, and heavy. These critics were uniformly . . . upset, might be the generic word to describe their emotions. They expressed themselves differently and at different lengths, ranging from the four-thousand-word review by John Gregory Dunne in the *New York Review of Books,* to the two-sentence review in the *Atlantic Monthly.* They found the book variously boring, boorish, presumptuous, vain, arrogant, illiterate, solipsistic, and other things.

The Virginia Kirkus Service, a prepublication bulletin designed for bookstores and libraries, summarized that "most readers will probably find this [book] tedious at best, sleekly loathsome at worst." The writing is "sloppy." An example of the kind of thing one finds in it is that at one point I ask myself why I labor, and answer, " 'the call of *recta ratio,*' and 'the fear of boredom.' He then goes on, patronizingly, to explain what *recta ratio* means." I think this means either that everybody already knows what *recta ratio* means, or that if not everybody knows what it means, an author should not explain the meaning, as to do so is patronizing. Writing for the *New York Times,* novelist Nora Ephron was oh so scornful. "He has written a book about money," was her principal finding. She imputed anti-Semitism (ever so deftly, but more readers would catch that than the meaning of *recta ratio*) and insensitivity to the suffering of my friends all in a single sentence: (". . . it's appalling that Mr. Buckley should mention Shylock when discussing *National Review*'s landlord or discourse so blithely on the physical infirmities of his friends"). And closed by suggesting that my affectations might best be understood by using a little ethnic imagination ("The English used to say, give an Irishman a horse and he'll vote Tory, but never mind").

So certain was Miss Ephron that much would be made of the fact that I get about in a chauffeur-driven limousine that she led off with it, . . . to wit:

> I cannot imagine that anyone who reviews this book will fail to mention the part about the limousine, so I may as well begin with it. Only a few pages into *Overdrive,* WFB gets into his limousine . . . and the occasion inspires him to reveal the circumstances under which he had the car custom-built. "What happened," he writes, "was that three years ago when it came time to turn in my previous car, which had done over 150,000 miles, the Cadillac people had come up with an austerity-model limousine, fit for two short people, preferably to ride to a funeral in. The dividing glass between the driver and driven was not automatic, there was no separate control for heat or air conditioning in the back, and the jump seats admitted only two. . . . This simply would not do: I use the car constantly, require the room, privacy, and my own temperature gauge. . . . There was, as usual, a market solution. You go out (this was in 1978) and buy a plain old Cadillac. You deliver it to a gentleman in Texarkana [I should have said Ft. Smith, Arkansas]. He chops it in two, and installs whatever you want. Cost? Interesting: within one thousand dollars of the regular limousine, and I actually don't remember which side."

Don't you see, Miss Ephron asks, "the story of the limousine is *emblematic*"? (My italics.)

My colleague Joe Sobran, on seeing Miss Ephron's review, sent me a memorandum: "Dear Bill, The critical reaction is interesting: Nora Ephron calls it 'a book about money,' when it's her *review* that's about money. I can't imagine you dwelling on the subject as she does; for that matter, I can't imagine you writing about your worst enemy as she writes about her ex-husband. Wonderful to hear such a woman lecture on poor taste, vulgarity, the nouveau riche. . . . My impression was that you can only be nouveau riche for the short-term; she seems to want to make you out as *second-generation* nouveau riche. She sees bigotry in a Shake-spearean tag, then proceeds to make a crack about the Irish which the *Times* wouldn't tolerate about just *any* ethnic group."

Grace Lichtenstein, writing for the *Washington Post,* leaned heavily on the tease that William Shawn was pulling a fast one. "When parts of this book first appeared in *The New Yorker,* I thought it was a joke, a Buckley parody of how some leftist might view Buckley's preoccupation with material possessions and his aristocratic lifestyle. Alas, it is not an inten-tional parody, although there are, swimming in this sea of trivia, some amusing anecdotes. . . ." Again, the business about my obsession with wealth, the slouchiness of my writing style; and then, to preserve her cre-dentials as an even-minded critic, "Now let me tell you the most awful part of *Overdrive.* After plowing through a third of it I realized . . . I was also (deep breath here) [her deep breath] quite envious. I mean, who wouldn't want a stretch limo in which to dictate one's letters? [etc., ex-tending to a cook and a chauffeur]—plebeian clod that I am," said Miss Lichtenstein, teasing us, because we are all supposed to know she is not *really* a plebeian clod.

Harper's took pretty much the same line, done by Rhoda Koenig, and the *Atlantic Monthly* saved space with a two-line review. "Mr. Buckley has assumed that a move by move record of one week in his bustling life, to-gether with such recollections, reflections, and droppable names as occur to him en route, will be of benefit to the public. Ah, well, to err is human, and Mr. Buckley is not divine." . . .

The *San Francisco Chronicle* also elected a short dismissal, by Patricia Holt. "Buckley has produced an overdone, overwritten, overblown 'per-sonal documentary' whose preview in *The New Yorker* earlier this year pro-voked a brilliant sendup by Jon Carroll in these pages. Better to read that column than waste your time with this book." The revelation to the citi-zens of San Francisco that an editor of the *San Francisco Chronicle* was ac-tually concerned about wasting their time was apparently met with such exuberant skepticism that *Overdrive* became, in that city, a modest best-seller.

The attack in the *New York Review of Books* was hefty and unexpected, this because its author, John Gregory Dunne, an acquaintance of long standing, had written to me after the *New Yorker* articles had been pub-lished to say in a pleasant context that he had "inhaled" the *New Yorker* pieces and looked forward to the book treatment. Usually, if you hear that something you created had been "inhaled," you are likely to conclude something other than that your friend had been bowled over by a mephitic encounter. In any event, when Mr. Dunne's attack was pub-lished, the editor Robert Silvers punctiliously offered me space to reply.

The gravamen of Mr. Dunne's objections was, really, my technicolored view of life. Unhappily, the descriptions he gave of episodes touched on in the book justified his criticisms of them. If I were to write that Hamlet was a man who never could make up his mind and therefore manages to bore us to death I am, as a reviewer, fully protected—except against anybody who proceeds to read *Hamlet*. In my reply to the *New York Review of Books* I was concrete in the matter, excerpting exactly Dunne's description of one episode in the book (my quarrel with the *Boston Globe*) and then describing the episode itself. Mr. Dunne's version will live as a locus classicus of distortion. (Locus Classicus, I should say for the benefit of Jon Carroll, is my Shangri-la.)

A week after seeing Dunne's review I received a letter: "If they ever listen [to what you wrote] (which must be a question) you will teach them not to take the sacred elixir of life and splash it all over the roadside, as they are too prone to do." That was the comment on *Overdrive* by Louis Auchincloss. Lance Morrow (I anticipate my narrative) wrote, "I was just thinking about your book again, and about several exceptionally stupid reviews of it that I read. It seems to me that there was some massive point-missing going on there, but I can't quite account for it. Well, maybe I can at that."

Not easy. *People* magazine said of it, "Less self-confident men would be embarrassed to flaunt themselves so openly, but Buckley is obviously never shy." By contrast, Mr. Dunne was complaining: "[Buckley] is really not very giving of himself." *People* magazine would shrink to four pages if the editors suddenly found it "embarrassing" to express a curiosity about People ten times more inquisitive than any I would consent to satisfy. But Dunne was relentless in at once protesting the lack of profundity, while trivializing or ignoring what is there. Thus (in pursuit of the general vision of my hedonism), "[Buckley] spends every February and March skiing in Switzerland." That was on the order of my reporting, "Mr. Dunne spends every morning brushing his teeth." (My skiing occupies as much of my day in Switzerland as Mr. Dunne's stair-climbing does his days in Los Angeles.)

But oh how he worries about me! . . . I closed my letter to the *New York Review of Books* by quoting Dunne's final strictures . . . :

"The show has been on the road too long," Dunne pronounced. "Mr. Buckley has spread himself so thin that he has begun to repeat himself, repeatedly. *Overdrive* is *Cruising Speed* redux as last year's *Atlantic High* is *Airborne* redux. As might be expected, Mr. Buckley is unrepentant." I answered, "As well complain that I edit a 28-year-old magazine which will celebrate the fourth of July again on the fourth of July. I have written a dozen non-fiction books, six novels, and a few books that are not routinely classified, though they are, by some, glibly dismissed. In 1985, I shall write a book called *Pacific High,* patterned after the first two. The literary technique explored in *Cruising Speed* . . . is so majestically successful I intend to repeat it ten years hence, and ten years after that. At which point I shall be happy to review John Gregory Dunne's *True Confessions IV,* inasmuch as I am certain there will be great wit in it, as there was in its progenitor; as also in *True Confessions Redux,* published last year. [My reference was to his novel *Dutch Shea Jr.*] I promise in my next book to scratch up a friend about whom I can say something truly unpleasant if Greg Dunne promises in *his* next book to come up with a murdered woman who doesn't have a votive candle [as he had written] protruding from her vagina."

But others viewed *Overdrive* very differently. Take, for instance, the question of snobbery. A number of critics came gleefully to the conclusion that *Overdrive* was the work of a snob. Mr. Charlie Slack of the *Chattanooga Times* said it quaintly: "To call William F. Buckley Jr. a snob is to call the U.S.S. Nimitz a boat, the Sahara Desert a sandbox." The charge, widely if less picturesquely framed, struck the sensitive ear of *Time* essayist Lance Morrow. Now Morrow was himself disturbed by what he apparently deemed an unnecessary elongation in this book of hedonistic passages . . . "Buckley luxuriates in his amenities a bit too much, and one hears . . . in his prose the happy sigh of a man sinking into a hot bath." But he scotches conclusively, in a striking passage, the correlations so widely drawn about people who luxuriate in soapsuds. "So his enemies [note the *mot juste*] try to dismiss him as Marie Antoinette in a pimpmobile. They portray him as, among other things, a terrible, terminal snob. To make the accusation is to misunderstand both William F. Buckley, Jr., and the nature of snobbery. Buckley is an expansive character who is almost indiscriminately democratic in the range of his friends and interests. He glows with intimidating self-assurance. The true snob sometimes has an air of pugnacious, overbearing self-satisfaction, but it is usually mere front. The snob is frequently a grand porch with no mansion attached, a Potemkin affair. The essence of snobbery is not real self-assurance but its opposite, a deep apprehension that the jungles of vulgarity are too close, that they will creep up and reclaim the soul and drag it back down into its native squalor, back to the Velveeta and the doubleknits."

Closely related to the charge of snobbishness was that of arrogance (egotism, vanity, what you will). The reporter for *Palm Beach Life,* who should be familiar with the phenomenon, wrote, "His book is outrageous in its egotism," he concluded, "but amusing withal. Treat yourself to it."

Phillip Seib, writing in the *Dallas Morning News,* took arrogance for granted but ventured an explanation: "A certain arrogance is essential if one is to publish what Buckley calls 'a personal documentary.' " The trouble with that extenuation, as far as an author is concerned, is that it gives such comfort as you would get from reading, "Mr. Joseph Blackburn, who traverses Niagara Falls on a tightrope, is said to be a damned fool. But who else but a damned fool would be expected to traverse Niagara Falls on a tightrope?"

Thomas Fox of the *Memphis Commercial Appeal* evidently thought he caught it all when he pronounced *Overdrive* "nothing more than the product of a smug exhibitionist who likes to wave his ego in public," while Peter Richmond, writing for the *Miami Herald,* gritted his teeth: *Overdrive* "may be the most egregious example of the abuse of literary license since Jack Kerouac, well into fame, actually published 250 pages of his dreams." The publisher of *The New Republic,* James Glassman, wrote in *USA Today* that *Overdrive* was "an act of sheer gall" but he quickly gave an individuated explanation for it. "My theory is that Buckley wrote *Overdrive* as proof of his own security in social and literary matters. He must have known that the literati would make fun of the book, but he wrote it anyway, just to flout them." That is an interesting insight, but it fails to explain why I should go out of my way to slight so many critics in this special way, since I tend to do so routinely in so many other ways. And it is incorrect to say that I expected anything like the reaction *Overdrive* got. . . .

Pamela Marsh of *The Christian Science Monitor* said that, really, it was worse than sheer arrogance. "Add to that his obvious relish in what seems an overwhelming arrogance—he is in fact proud of his pride." That tends to ask for more thought than one is routinely prepared to give to such facile statements, unless they come in from philosophers. (Let's see: John is proud to be an American. John is proud of his pride in being an American. How about: John is proud of his pride in his pride in being an American. I wonder if Miss Marsh ever thought of that? Ever *worried* about that?)

Doug Fellman, a student writing for *The Hopkins Newsletter,* tried to be reasonable about the whole thing: "Naturally, some persons will complain that Buckley, in recording his life in such a journal, is committing an act of great egotism and conceit. Yet the autobiography is a common and accepted form of biography, and Buckley simply chooses to record his life in the present and as an excerpt." But untuned objections were everywhere. *Booklist* said comprehensively that, for some readers, *Overdrive* would prove "a cross section of everything that is wrong with America, from elitism to Reaganomics." The *Cleveland Plain Dealer* found "the private Buckley who appears in this book . . . laced with pride, unflinchingly materialistic and self-centered—all in all, a popinjay."

I (happen to) prefer temperamental reactions to the lorgnetted sort of thing *Overdrive* drew from what one might call The Social Justice Set. I especially preferred Miss (Ms. would here be safer, I suppose) Carolyn See of the *Los Angeles Times,* who saw the author of *Overdrive* as "an American institution . . . lounging elegantly in his talk-show chair, driving Norman Mailer into a conniption fit, teasing and torturing Gore Vidal until he just can't take any more, driving at least 49 percent of the viewing audience into a state of mind that can't really be described in words, but it involves lurching up out of your chair, burying your hands in your hair and shrieking 'Yuuggh! Turn it off! Make him go away!' " There's no quiche in Ms. See's diet, 100 percent All Bran.*

The refrain on the matter of wealth was widespread, the popular corollary of which was to [comment on] insouciance with respect to poverty, as (Ann Morrissett Davidson, *Philadelphia Inquirer*) for instance: "But there is something rather beguiling and even enviable about this over-driven patrician and his way of life. Perhaps it is his apparently blithe blindness to most of the world's miseries." The patronizing explanation is both sweet and deadly. Jack the Ripper just didn't know it was wrong to strangle ladies, don't you see?

Two weighty voices, however distinct, came in from the Big Leagues.†

One of them Eliot Fremont-Smith of the *Village Voice,* the other Norman Podhoretz, the editor of *Commentary.* Fremont-Smith, in voicing qualified approval of the book and its author, is a prominent liberal who found himself teeming with things to say.‡

He began with the novel point that those who harp on the theme of the privileged life of the author of *Overdrive* tend to neglect a not insignificant point. "I think of *his* dilemma. No public figure I know of has been so chided by people he likes or is willing to admire or takes it with such aplomb." He insisted that *Overdrive* was ultimately a book about friendship. "Friends are more important, indeed all important. *Overdrive* is a record and celebration of connection, of how association (memories, locales, daily working intercourse, surprise, pleasure) improves the soul and

---

* Sometimes such wholesome antagonists go on to blush. Ms. See concluded her colorful review, "Buckley shows us a brittle, acerbic, duty-bound, 'silly,' 'conservative' semi-fudd, with a heart as vast and varicolored and wonderful to watch as a 1930s jukebox."

† I am grateful to a score of critics whose reviews, appearing in newspapers and magazines that seldom penetrate the Eastern Seaboard Establishment's switchboard, were understanding in every case, in some cases even encouraging, in a few even affectionate.

‡ His task was concededly complicated by a personal friendship, recently formed.

perhaps the cause of civilization and bestows grace on all and sundry, by no means least of all" on the author. Fremont-Smith, unlike the automatons who approached the book with floodlights in search of Social Justice and a hemorrhaging psyche, had eyes for *detail* (of which, in many reviews, there was a total absence). "He . . . discourses on Bach and Scarlatti with the likes of . . . Fernando Valenti and Rosalyn Tureck, and also mediates between them (the sections on music and the ego requirements of great performers are among the funniest, most scrupulous, and moving in the book)."

F-S becomes concrete, and it is interesting to reflect here on observations by one critic, alongside observations by two others.

On what I wrote in *Overdrive* about homosexuality, Fremont-Smith: "His riff on homosexuality, for notorious example [of my occasional waywardness], seems deliberately blind to all sorts of subtleties he should, at his age, with his antennae, be less innocent of."

On my treatment of homosexuality, Franz Oppenheimer in the *American Spectator:* "Another pernicious myth touched upon in *Overdrive* is the supposed biological and hereditary nature of homosexuality. . . . My father, who practiced psychiatry, first in Germany and after his emigration in San Francisco, collected substantial evidence in support of Buckley's impression that homosexuality is a disease that can be cured. During my father's entire professional life he endeavored to find a true 'biological,' i.e., an incurable homosexual. He never did."

And then at a personal, more evaluative level, referring to a eulogy and a testimonial I gave in my book, Fremont-Smith:

"[In *Overdrive*,] love is couched in courtly encomiums that are heartfelt but nevertheless embarrass."

Norman Podhoretz: "He is so good at delivering tributes that one would choose him above all others (well, perhaps not above Daniel P. Moynihan) to deliver the eulogy at one's own funeral, or better still, the speech in one's honor on some appropriate occasion. There are samples of both kinds of speeches in *Overdrive* and they are, without exception, masterpieces of the extremely difficult art of praise." Some say tomayto; which of course is to be preferred.

Fremont-Smith, finally, declines to accept my implied proposition that the literary form I adopted (one week in the life of X) is generally viable. He rejects the notion that the form is widely useful. Rather, he insists that it must be taken as a singular phenomenon. "Two questions [in fact] arise: a) How is all this activity possible? b) Can we stand it? Particularly, can we stand Buckley's glorying in it? . . . basically *Overdrive* is a log—not a how-to-do-it but how-has-it-been-done in a particular frame of time by one particular energy."

Norman Podhoretz... in November led the Book Review section of *Commentary* with an answer to the critics of *Overdrive,* interrupting a long silence as an active book reviewer. I am moved by the self-pride abundantly so designated in quotes already cited—but above all by feelings of gratitude most readers in my position would, I think, understand—to quote from this review. Podhoretz began, no less:

"The first thing to say about *Overdrive* is that it is a dazzling book. The second thing to say is that it has generally been greeted with extreme hostility."

Podhoretz went on to examine the causes of such hostility, discarding routine ideological antagonism as a satisfactory answer. "I do not believe that the injustice done to *Overdrive* can be explained in strictly political terms. Something deeper and more interesting is at work here." What that is is not easily distilled, though I will have a few thoughts on the subject at the end of this essay.

To those who declaimed first against the insubstantiality of *Overdrive* and then against the craftsmanship, like the woman who thought it should have been subtitled "Dictated but not read," Podhoretz replied: "The material is fascinating in itself and all Buckley's virtues as a writer are called forth in the recording of it. The prose flows smoothly and elegantly, its formality tempered with colloquial touches that somehow never jar, its mischievous wit coexisting in surprisingly comfortable congruence with its high rhetorical solemnities, its narrative pace sure-footed enough to accommodate detours and flashbacks without losing the necessary forward momentum." (Compare Grace Lichtenstein in the *Washington Post:* "What Buckley needed was a snappy rewrite by an experienced *People* hand. . . .") Podhoretz, who does not like to give ground, dealt defiantly with the matter of Money: "I for one do not doubt that the delight Buckley takes in his privileges is an exemplary spiritual virtue. If I do have a doubt, it concerns the extent of this delight. I mean, is he always so cheerful? Does he never suffer from anxiety?" (Eliot Fremont-Smith was more direct on this point: "In the book, Buckley has exquisite sandwiches but never takes a pee.") I wrote to Mr. F-S that I had trained myself never to pee, but he has not answered this letter, nor publicly celebrated my achievement.

("... What I was most struck by were the parts in which you tell us what you have to be sober about," my colleague Richard Brookhiser wrote me.)

To Mr. Podhoretz, I take the opportunity to say that I thought the shadows were there, in *Overdrive,* and that if they were not discernible to him, I do not know what is the appropriate reaction. Angst, in this volume, would not work.

Well, then. I have before me page after page of excerpts from reviews that make interesting observations. But economy requires that I put aside these notes and conclude. I do so by probing two questions, one concrete, and in its own way heuristic, the second general and critical.

The first is the matter of the limousine and the prominence it was given.

There was remarkably less fuss about my limousine when it figured in *Cruising Speed*. What, then, was the provocative difference between my *1970* limousine and my *1981* limousine? Hard scrutiny of the reviews suggests that the second *having been "custom-made"* caused it to be marginally insufferable. This is very interesting, especially so since the offended reviewers did not (many of them) hesitate to quote my narrative, in which, as Miss Ephron has reminded us, I revealed that, in 1978, buying a limousine with roughly the same features as the traditional, i.e., pre-austerity, limousine, cost approximately the same as the regular commercial limousine now being offered by the Cadillac company.

What then was it about the customizing that so inflamed?—that caused the *New York Times Book Review* critic to begin her review by concluding that *everyone* would focus on the limousine, whereafter she proceeded to devote almost one-third of her review to it?

Is it—I explore the question again—simply, the economic point? That a limousine is expensive? If so, isn't it odd to weigh in so heavily on this, given that a limousine costs only about twice what a Ford sedan costs? It does not require that one belittle the figure to ask: Why is it, when other finery of affluence is there to choose from, that a limousine is so conspicuous? I explain, in *Overdrive*, how I spend my days; and it quickly becomes obvious that it would no more be feasible to spend my days as they are spent in the absence of a car and driver than it would be to run a taxi service without taxis. Without going over a time sheet, in the week I recorded I would guess that eight hours of work resulted from being driven rather than driving. What is it that especially affects so many about this particular auxiliary to one's commercial life? The cost of it?

But that is hardly rational. Well then, is it the point that one ought not to expect rationality in a review of how one American (this American) leads his life if his *modus vivendi* is judged obnoxious? I say it is irrational because hardly anyone bothered, in reviewing *Overdrive,* to dilate on his objections to extravagances even when clearly unrelated to productivity. E.g., owning and maintaining a 36-foot sailing auxiliary which (by the way) costs three times what a limousine costs (ask any of the hundred thousand Americans who have one). I own a grand piano worth more than my limo; used less, and mutilated more. Or consider articles of un-questioned and unmitigated professional uselessness, like a thirty-three-year accumulation of one's wife's jewelry. . . . What *is* it about a limousine?

Sometime after the first dozen reviews appeared, I lunched with Sam Vaughan of Doubleday and told him I was astonished by the intensity of the concentration on the matter of my limousine, which at this point I was tempted to paint khaki. Sam observed that typical luxuries go largely unobserved, but that a chauffeur-driven car is the single most provocative possession of the modern urban American. "Everyone," he expanded, "no matter who, has been caught on a street corner in the rain, waiting for a bus, or trying to hail a taxi. And inevitably they will see a limousine slide by, with the lumpen-bourgeois figure in the back seat, maybe smoking a cigar; maybe even reading *The Wall Street Journal.* That is the generically offensive act in the big cities."* A good point, if the idea is to explain the spastic hostility toward limousine owners. Not, I think, a sufficient point to understand the peculiar emphasis put on the limo in some of the reviews.

I think that of the several points raised in opposing the book, this concrete point puzzled me the most. I dwell on it because American culture has tended to be guided—not finally, but substantially—by utilitarian criteria. Does John Appleseed produce more using a tractor than a horse-drawn plow? Does Tom Wicker perform more efficiently using a typewriter, and going on to a word processor, than with a pencil? Why isn't the utilitarian coefficient dispositive in the matter of a limousine? Is it because the critic cannot distinguish between the limousine *qua* limousine, i.e., a luxury ve-hicle associated with inaugurations, weddings, and funerals, and the lim-ousine as mobile office? If so, there are two problems, the first the failure of the critical intelligence. The second, whether the envious view, trans-formed to resentment on that rainy day, on the sidewalks of New York, of the man comfortable in his limousine isn't, to use Miss Ephron's freighted word, "emblematic" of a public, rather than a private, disorder.

The second point touches on the corrosive use of the word "gleeful" to describe a reaction to one's material situation. I have especially in mind, because it was so frequently adduced by reviewers, my reference to a swim-ming pool. What I said about it parenthetically—words (if I may say so, gleefully reproduced)—was that it is "the most beautiful indoor swim-ming pool this side of Pompeii."

---

* After lunch, Buckley, ever generous, offered me a lift in his limo back to my office. "Are you crazy?" I said, ever paranoid, waving him off.—Ed.

Now I found it odd that several reviewers of obvious intelligence bridled at this. . . . In doing so it seems to me, on hard reflection, that they must have understood me to be saying something different from what I intended to say, so that the fault is either mine or theirs, and it is worth inquiring: Whose?

My indoor swimming pool is of modest dimensions (I give them, in *Overdrive*). In the book, as a matter of course, I acknowledge the architect who designed the pool, and the artist I engaged to give me a mosaic pattern to decorate it. My delight, therefore, was clearly not with my own doing, but with theirs. I cannot imagine resenting any expression of pleasure uttered by the man who, having, say, commissioned the Parthenon, goes on to describe it in his diary (presciently) as "the most beautiful pre-Christian temple ever constructed." What would he have been saying that a rational, self-respecting critic could object to? Mine was the voice of acclamation: a celebration of the architect, and of the artist: hardly of the author who accumulated the money with which to pay them.

But how odd, so widespread a reaction at an expression of delight at others' competence and artistry (many made as much of my reference to an "exquisite" sandwich made by our cook). Isn't it the job of the critic to distinguish between a compliment slyly paid ostensibly to someone else, actually to oneself, and a genuine compliment? Or are the critics reading self-congratulations by the man who had the wit to commission the pool, and the taste to appreciate the singularly well-made sandwich? That surely is reaching, isn't it? Would a reviewer single out a diarist's encomium on the performance of a visiting artist as an effort to draw attention to the author's piano? Or to his leverage on the artist?

I focus, finally, on what appears to have been a highly provocative literary proposition, namely my contention that a scrupulous journal of a week in an individual's life is at least a literary form worth thinking about, at best a literary idea worth celebrating. Many years ago the editor of the humor quarterly *Monocle* (it was Victor Navasky, now editor of *The Nation*) asked me to do a review of the work of the columnist Murray Kempton. I replied that he was asking me for the equivalent of a review of the work of Walter Lippmann, never mind that it would be more fun. Was I supposed to go back and read, or rather reread, fifteen years of Murray Kempton in order to write three thousand words?

I came up with a formula that satisfied Navasky, satisfied me, and planted, I think, the idea that blossomed, if that word is not too tendentious, in *Cruising Speed* and, now, *Overdrive*. Why not take a week of columns by Murray Kempton—next week's columns, say—and talk your way through them? He was writing five times a week back then, so that the chances were on your side that you would catch Murray Kempton reacting to a satisfactory range of challenges, phenomena, provocations, scandals, whatever. Enough to acquaint the reader with the moods (penetrating), style (incomparable), and thought (unreliable) of Murray Kempton.

It worked, in my judgment.

And so does it work, again in my judgment, on a larger scale in *Overdrive*.

To ask and quickly answer the most sensitive question, let me simply blurt it out:

Not everyone can write such a book. . . .

William Murchison, the columnist from Dallas, Texas, wrote, "Few indeed are the authors who could bring off such an enterprise as this. A week, literally speaking, with Ralph Nader; or Walter Mondale; or Phil Donahue; or General Westmoreland! To think of it is to weep."

Now Mr. Murchison has a point here, but not of the kind that should cause the egalitarian furies to howl.

We seem to concede, without any problem, that only people who are technically qualified can satisfactorily perform on the piano before an audience. So we concede, again without any apparent problem, that unless one deftly uses paint and canvas, one ought not to expect to be able to merchandise one's art. I do not see why there should be so much difficulty in applying the same implicit criteria in order to distinguish what one might call the "performing writer." Perhaps the problem exists at all only because very few people without the technique to bring it off would undertake to play the "Flight of the Bumblebee" on the piano. Not many weekend painters would expect to sell their canvases even to the very little galleries.

By contrast, everybody—writes. And, in writing, there is progressive fluency that approaches artistry. No one can say exactly where the line is, but it is to comply with the requirements of the full disclosure laws to admit: it would probably separate those who, using this standard, could, and could not, publish their journals, only the former being "performing writers." Okay. So why should it be difficult to accept the proposition that, from a writer, one expects work of a distinctive quality, even as one would from a painter or musician or plumber? If one managed that problem, one would cope with the preliminary objection to a journal based on a single week in a person's life: The person needs to be a writer.

But if the writer *is* qualified, what besides that does the reader, in order to be satisfied, require?

The reader would want an interesting sensibility. What is in process, in such an undertaking, is a literary self-portrait. I say "literary" only because the author's reactions are sometimes limned with operative emphasis on *the way* in which the reactions are expressed: and what then happens is that you collect, one by one, the little colored dots which, when they are, however chaotically, assembled, leave you with a mosaic, at best a pointillist portrait of—one human being.

Why should you care to have a self-portrait, as done, for instance, by William F. Buckley, Jr.—or by Groucho Marx? Or by Kay Graham?

Because, I think, self-portraits of many people can be interesting. If they work, they amuse. Enlighten. Explain. They provoke. And—I cling to the point—although the formal autobiography lets the actor stage his life and thought with more regard for conventional architectural prominences, the week's journal has complementary advantages. If I were offered today the alternative of reading an autobiography of Walter Lippmann, tracking his career, with which I am routinely familiar, or another comprehending his activity and his thought hour by hour during a single week, I *think*—I'm not sure—I might not lose by choosing the former. Remember that the supplementary alternative isn't necessarily excluded.

A book like *Overdrive* written by Ralph Nader? Well—who knows? He has not, true, achieved his reputation as a writer. . . . On the other hand, if he had the training to carry it off, would I be interested in reading a journal of a week in Ralph Nader's life? My own answer is, Yes: I would. So would I—I mean it—a week in the life of Phil Donahue. In fact, I would sleep outside the bookstore, waiting to put my hands on such a book, if it were such a book. It would take only one or two other explorers to set the form in concrete. Murray Kempton comes to mind as ideal. Or Patrick Moynihan. Or how about Jesse Jackson? If he would speak Honest Injun, as I do.

I regret many things about the reception of *Overdrive,* though I am obliged to record here two qualifiers. The first is that the book has been a solid, if not spectacular, entrepreneurial success. The second is that the book has generated an extraordinary amount of mail from strangers, strangers who, after reading it, thought to write to me, their motives varied. The volume of that mail I was unprepared for—the reach of *The New Yorker* always astonishes me; I think no book I have written (with one exception) has got such a response—but overwhelmingly grateful, for what I take to be the sense communicated of a common and joyful search for serenity, in which the readers appear to have been helped. (One wrote, "Rambling, idiosyncratic, amused, cranky, occasionally flamboyant— your observations and recollections were most enjoyable testaments to a vital life. You actually believe *something:* Something old, something blue, with flecks of tweed, patches on the elbows, old Nantucket and Martha's Vineyard before everyone else came, in short: the right way of doing things." Another: "In a confusing world, I must express my gratitude . . .") For that reason, among others already given, I regret the facile dismissal of the literary form by some reviewers (there were exceptions: *Time*'s Roger Rosenblatt wrote, "I think you've invented a genre. Pepys on speed, but better") who, in their haste to disparage, did not give sufficient thought to the potential uses of such a form by people whose thought and careers they would read about with less resistance. I hope, before I die, to see others using this form. I said airily that in ten years I intended to write a sequel to *Cruising Speed* and *Overdrive,* and ten years after *that,* a fourth journal. The prospect of this will cause a disturbing number of people to wish me . . . retired sooner, rather than later. But I caution them against strategic optimism in these matters. My limousine has miles to go before I sleep.

———

A critic who is also a friend has particular potency. Here, excerpts as "Kilpo" tries to get Buckley to cease and desist from breaking the Seventh Rule, which might be defined as the "you'all" commandment:

———

How Not to Write Dialect
by James J. Kilpatrick

In his hilarious essay on the literary offenses of James Fenimore Cooper—an essay that every novelist should read—Mark Twain laid down eighteen rules that govern the writing of romantic fiction. This was Rule No. 7:

"It requires that when a personage talks like an illustrated, gilt-edged, tree-calf, hand-tooled, seven-dollar Friendship's Offering in the beginning of a paragraph, he shall not talk like a Negro minstrel in the end of it."

I was reminded of Rule 7 the other day in reading William F. Buckley's new novel, *Tucker's Last Stand.* It is the ninth in his series starring CIA agent Blackford Oakes, and it is Buckley at his best. Believe me, his best is very good indeed.

But—you could feel the "but" coming—but my beloved friend neglected Rule 7. One of his principal characters is President Lyndon Johnson. Buckley undertook to capture the President's speech. He might with equal success have attempted to catch a soap bubble in a butterfly net.

Thus we observe that sometimes Lyndon says "I," and sometimes Lyndon says "Ah." On Page 147 the President is thinking of sending a note to Hanoi: "Ah know we never done it before. That's one of the reasons I want to do it now." Over the course of two pages, Lyndon says "Ah" six times and "I" nine times.

In Buckley's dialectal spelling, Johnson sometimes says "an" and then inexplicably reverts to "and." The President drops a *g* in "talkin' " and "confusin' " but sounds the consonant in "telling" and "going." In the same fashion, Barry Goldwater sometimes says "them" and sometimes says " 'em." All the other characters speak like Oxford dons.

The trouble is that the rendering of speech is a fearfully difficult task, in part because most of us vary our speech patterns to the occasion at hand. Lyndon Johnson was no exception. When he was in his molasses mode, seeking to cajole a waffling senator, he spoke as if he had a ripe plum in his mouth. On other occasions, when the cactus juice was flowing, he spoke Texan. I would not attempt to reproduce Lyndon's nasalities. He had a large nose, packed with resonant cavities, and the sound chambers did odd things to his speech.

Let it be said that Bill Buckley, as always, is in distinguished company. Not long ago I had occasion to reread Robert Louis Stevenson's *Kidnapped.* It remains a great yarn. Early in the novel David Balfour befriends Alan Breck. Alas, Stevenson could not decide whether Alan says "you" or "ye." Sometimes Alan speaks in "hoot, mon" Scottish, and sometimes not.

Owen Wister also neglected Rule 7. Off and on throughout *The Virginian,* Wister spelled "you" as "yu." It is not clear why he used this peculiar orthography, for 99 percent of English-speaking people pronounce "you" as "yu." On one page the hero says "an'." On the same page he says "and." . . .

A few writers have looked at the challenge of dialect and brought it off. Twain himself had a fine record of consistency. Huck Finn speaks in the same voice, and in the same spelling, throughout the novel. William Faulkner accurately caught the cadence and verbal structure of much black speech.

Dialectal writing demands more than an ear for individual words. There are regional vocabularies as well as regional accents. In some parts of the country the hour of 9:45 is a quarter to ten, in others it is a quarter of ten. Many Southerners carry groceries in a tote bag; Midwesterners carry groceries in a sack . . . Mastering these nuances is the work of a lifetime.

Sometimes, I know, the impulse to write dialect is overwhelming. Let me offer a word of sound advice: When the impulse strikes you, lie down until it goes away.

—MAY 12, 1991

To the Editor
American Spectator
Bloomington, Indiana

Your reviewer, Mr. Joseph Shattan, writes about me (*Who's On First,* by William F. Buckley, Jr.; June 1980), "The Yale-educated Mr. Oakes is no mere fop. On the contrary, he was trained as a nuclear physicist, he gained renown as a fighter-pilot during World War II, and he reads the geopolitical works of James Burnham for relaxation. Fluent in many tongues and related to—among other luminaries—the Queen of England, the young Oakes is at once effortlessly cosmopolitan and deeply patriotic." Elsewhere, Mr. Shattan advises us that he read Mr. Buckley's book about me in a single sitting. Could that have been the trouble?

You see, I took my degree at Yale in mechanical engineering, not nuclear physics. It is true that I fought in the war and knocked down two Nazi planes, but I took sick, and didn't therefore have the opportunity to gain renown, though I appreciate Mr. Shattan's assumption that, had my health stood up, I'd have shortened the war. It is true that I have read the works of James Burnham, hardly true that I read them "for relaxation." It is more nearly true that they are to be read as realistic substitutes for horror stories. And, then, unhappily, I am not a polyglot. I made a considerable effort in the spring and summer of 1952 to achieve a limited fluency in German. But my French, as Mr. Buckley pointed out, is at the level of *savez-vous-planter-les-choux.* I am mystified at the news that I am related to the Queen of England. It is correct that Mr. Buckley penetrated my penetration, but he never suggested that I am related to the Queen, though perhaps he knows something about me I don't know, not surprisingly since he is a very clever fellow.

Mr. Shattan shouldn't feel too bad, however. The reviewer for the *New York Times,* Newgate Callendar, pronounced me a "devout Catholic," which certainly qualifies him as a sleuth inasmuch as my mother is Episcopalian, my father Presbyterian, and I am somewhere in between. To be sure, I have a great admiration for Catholics, some of whom are among my closest friends; but I am mystified at how this datum was derived from anything Mr. Buckley, a careful writer though given, I think, occasionally, to euphuism, wrote. My regards to Mr. Shattan.

BLACKFORD OAKES

LANGLEY, VA.   OCTOBER 3, 1980

Perhaps one of the most effective ways to stretch one's neck out in search of a chopping block is for a novelist to review other novelists, a wordsmith to review a dictionary, etc. Naturally, Bill Buckley sails into such situations, chin jutting, eyes gleaming, a strange half-smile playing around his lips. This is from *The New York Times Book Review,* December 19, 1971.

The Oxford English Dictionary
The Compact Edition of the Oxford English Dictionary. Complete Text Reproduced Micrographically. 4,116 pp. New York: Oxford University Press. Two Vols., boxed. $75.

The Oxford English Dictionary was the moon-landing project of the English people, and if Sidney Webb, who was born the year the project was conceived and reached seventy the year it was completed, did not denounce it as a dreadful extravagance in an age when poverty was abundant in the groaning industrial areas of England, it can only have been because he forgot to do so. The enterprise resulted—to use the words of its publishers in connection with the new edition—in "the most prestigious book ever published," even as the moon landing is almost indisputably the most prestigious scientific enterprise ever consummated. Of course, scientific achievement, like an athletic one, is obsolescent in a sense quite different from a cultural achievement. The man who ran the four-minute mile knew that he was not being given tenure as a world record holder. The men who contributed to the O.E.D. achieved a more certain satisfaction.

Not exactly like the individual artist, who defies "improvement" in any measurable sense. But halfway there; far enough to raise the question, on which I shall touch in due course: Why isn't the O.E.D. a *continuing* masterpiece?

It could only have been a sense of historical excitement that kept successive lexicographers working over a period of seventy years to achieve this dictionary, that kept at least one compositor busy during the whole of his working life setting type for this dictionary which was printed in sections that sold for twelve shillings and sixpence each, beginning twenty-five years after the project was conceived, on into 1928. Each of the twelve volumes required anywhere from three to ten years to complete, depending on such variables as whether an editor (at the peak there were three working simultaneously) died, or whether England was fighting a particularly engrossing war, or whatever.

There were moments of doubt and even of panic, as when the whole of it was offered to Cambridge University, which sniffed it away, even as Yale disdained Mr. Harkness's colleges only to discover that Harvard instantly and greedily accepted them. But eventually the thing was done, and a set of the volumes was presented one each to the chiefs of state of the great English-speaking powers, King George V and President Calvin Coolidge, that they should know better their common philological patrimony.

Incidentally, there were American scholars involved in the project, and generous acknowledgment is made of their contributions. Indeed, the principal editor, Dr. James Murray, adjourned the meiotic tradition of his countrymen to say, as early as 1880, that he had discovered in Americans "an ideal love for the English language as a glorious heritage and a pride in being intimate with its grand memories, such as . . . is rare indeed in Englishmen toward their own tongue; and from this I draw the most certain inferences as to the lead which Americans must at no distant date take in English scholarship." Dr. Murray was, of course, correct: The study of linguistics is all but a protected American industry.

And it was the idea of an American, Mr. Albert Boni, head of the Readex Microprint Corporation, to take the entire O.E.D. and bring it out in two volumes. This involved shrinking thirteen volumes, not twelve. The editors brought out the supplemental volume in 1928 to deal with words that had come into being too late to be included in the previous volumes—it was too expensive to collate the new words typographically. And, as lagniappe, they threw in a list of "spurious words" the scholars had come upon in dictionaries dead and extant, which impostors had got into them as the result of typographical or other errors (sample: "*Depectible, a.* Error in Johnson's Dict. and some later Dicts. for *Depertible*") and finally, the Supplement gives the long list of books cited in the great dictionary.

The principal motive for bringing out the new edition is of course to reduce the cost of the dictionary to the reader. The original costs three hundred dollars, so that the current edition of two volumes is if not quite two-thirteenths of the price of the entire set, a large step (at seventy-five dollars) in that direction. Most human eyes will need a little help, and that is tactfully furnished—a magnifying glass mounted on a wooden rectangle a few inches by a few inches, along the base of which lies a groove whose purpose is nowhere explained. If it is intended somehow to permit the reader to manipulate the glass, as a periscope, by remote control, I must report that the motor, or drive shaft, or whatever, was missing from my set. No matter, there are other and better magnifying glasses on the market, and very strong eyeglasses will do.

The economy apart, there is the advantage of space saved, and the general feeling of accessibility that comes from dealing with two instead of thirteen volumes. I am surprised that the publishers neglected to provide a lettered thumb index, but I installed my own without much trouble. The books are well bound and the pages fall open easily, without crowding—four of the original appearing in each page of the miniaturized volumes, which total 4,116 pages. I cannot imagine that anyone who has the money will put off the purchase of a set; or that anyone who hasn't the money will put off borrowing to buy the set. That is the way I feel about it, and if you are a doubter, stay with me for just a moment.

The dictionary is best described by its own editors. They explain, for instance, that they did not include words that had become obsolete by 1150 A.D., giving the reasons why. Beyond that, ". . . it is the aim of the Dictionary to deal with all the common words of speech and literature, and with all words which approach these in character; the limits being extended farther in the domain of science and philosophy, which naturally passes into that of literature than in that of slang or cant, which touches the colloquial. In scientific and technical terminology, the aim has been to include *all words English in form* . . . except those of which an explanation would be unintelligible to any but the specialist; and such words, not English in form, as either are in general use, like *Hippopotamus, Geranium, Aluminium, Focus, Stratum, Bronchitis,* or belong to the more familiar language of science, as *Mammalia, Lepidoptera, Invertebrata.*"

The thought given to the arrangement of the words bore exotic fruit, beyond anything for which mere catalogues are useful. The richness of the work is suggested in the passage that gives the thinking of the editors on how to deal with *Combinations:*

"Under this term are included all collocations of simple words in which the separate spelling of each word is retained, whether they are formally connected by the hyphen, or virtually by the unity of their signification. The formal union and the actual by no means coincide; not only is the use of the hyphen a matter of indifference in an immense number of cases, but in many where it is habitually used, the combination implies no unity of signification; while others, in which there is a distinct unity or special-ization of meaning, are not hyphened. The primary use of the hyphen is *grammatical:* it implies either that the syntactic relation between two words is closer than if they stood side by side without it, or that the rela-tion is a *less usual* one than that which would at first sight suggest itself to us, if we saw the two words standing unconnected. Thus, in the three sen-tences, 'After consideration had been given to the proposal, it was duly ac-cepted,' 'After consideration the proposal was accepted,' 'After-consideration had shown him his mistake,' we have *first* no immediate syntactic relation between *after* (conjunctive adverb) and *consideration; secondly,* the relation of preposition and object; *thirdly,* the relation of attribute and substantive, closer than the first, less usual than the second, (since *after* is more com-monly a preposition than an adjective). But *after-consideration* is not really a single word, any more than *subsequent consideration, fuller consideration;* the hyphen being merely a convenient help to the sense, which would be clearly expressed in speech by the different phrase-accentuation of *a'fter consideration* and *a'fter considera"tion.* And as this 'help to the sense' is not always equally necessary, nor its need equally appreciated in the same place, it is impossible that its use should be uniform. Nevertheless *after-consideration,* as used above, is on the way to become a single word, which *reconsideration* (chiefly because *re-* is not a separate word, but also because we have *reconsider*) is reckoned to be; and indeed *close grammatical relation* constantly accompanies close union of sense, so that in many combina-tions the hyphen becomes an expression of this unification of sense. When this unification and specialization has [?] proceeded so far that we no longer analyze the combination into its elements, but take it in as a whole, as in *blackberry, postman, newspaper,* pronouncing it in speech with a sin-gle accent, the hyphen is usually omitted, and the fully developed com-pound is written as a single word."

Is that not beautiful? One can read it again and again, once for the analysis, again as philosophy, twice more for the music; and there isn't an entry in the dictionary that does not present itself as manifestly the object of the lovingcare (note, no hyphen) these grave, and lively, and penetrat-ing craftsmen gave us; and, no doubt, when the volumes were received by the critics, and for years after, workmen sat as nervously as Mission Con-trol in Houston, lest error be found, or the tiniest miscalibration, such as might propel a future statesman towards war instead of peace. As far as I know, their principal humiliation lay in having omitted the word APPEN-DIX, which had to wait to debut in the Supplementary Volume. It is rumored that, buried deep in the dictionary, is a SPURIOUS WORD of the editors' super-secret devising, so that their grandchildren might know the contemporary estate of plagiarism. If it is true, the identity of the word is a well-kept secret.

The limitations of the O.E.D. are I should think unavoidable. There are a great many words one needs to know about which simply aren't there, so that one always has to have another dictionary—a more contemporary dictionary—at hand. And then, here and there one comes across anti-metaphorical rigidity. For instance, ENTROPY is not permitted, in the O.E.D., to stray out of its thermodynamic cage, so that one gets no hint of Webster's 4th meaning, "The ultimate state reached in the degradation of the matter and energy of the universe. . . ."

The Compact Edition, now that it is done, strikes one as so obviously a useful idea, one cannot imagine why it wasn't done before. So, now, a proposal for the next edition. Probably two stout volumes of supplementary words could be listed, if the successors to the editors who laid down their burden in 1928 were to address themselves to the word explosion of the succeeding four decades. No doubt the enterprise hasn't been revived because the economic cost of typographical collation is discouraging. But—but—these days we have the computer printout! Why not an edition of the O.E.D., made current say every ten years, in which the new words are fed alphabetically into place on the master tape. The user would buy the tape, which would come in a unit that would look like a portable typewriter, a small screen perched on top of the carriage. Whereupon— you guessed it—you would need merely to type out the word you wished to explore, and there you'd have it, illuminated on the screen. The O.E.D., as a continuing masterpiece. The O.E.D. needs updating even as the census does, and the Encyclopaedia Britannica, and the ingenuity of the publishers in bringing out the current Compact Edition ought not to be terminal (lest we reach ENTROPY). But even now, there is no literary excitement quite like the ownership of these volumes, the experiencing of which is like having been out there in the early morning at Cape Kennedy, and seeing the missile stagger up, knowing that it will travel all the way to the moon.

Dear Mr. Buckley:

Some scabrous lout has written me a postcard from Israel without providing a return address and thus unfairly avoiding counterattack.

This is the message, in its entirety, the writer a stranger to me:

"Dear John:

"First of course 'Shalom!', huh? Next, darn, darn, darn but my new 'The Concise Oxford Dictionary' doesn't carry (perhaps among others) such words as 'yare,' 'pica' (as used by you), 'pygal,' 'porpentine.' 'Glistering,' yes—but hell, you could have used glistening, huh?"

John, one Bill Buckley is enough.

"Shalom!

—S. W. HARRIS"

I would have begun my reply with the observation that the new Concise Oxford must be very new and indeed concise and gone on from there to some dizzying height of sarcasm. Instead, I am drunk with frustration and in such condition have before me two Buckleys.

Shalom!

JOHN MCPHEE
The New Yorker

Dear Mr. McPhee:
Dear Mr. McPhee: Drunk with *what?*
        Drunk with *what?*

WFB

WFB   JANUARY 20, 1978

———

Asked to debate in print another member of the American Heritage Usage Panel, WFB takes the negative side on the question of permissiveness.*

———

What is it that brings verbal "acceptability"? It is suggested that usage should be the "chief" determinant. It occurs to me that the two sentences just now composed could not communicate what they now do save that precision in definition and inflection is still possible; and precision is still possible precisely because mere usage, however prolonged, does not baptize. Providence in due course sometimes accepts into its bosom sinners, but usually only after time served in the antechambers. And how will we know just when that dispensation is granted? Well, to answer that only in part in jest: by asking me.

Why me?

* Re: *American Heritage Dictionary,* Second College Edition, 1982.

[As noted earlier,] I had a colleague at *National Review,* a professor of political science at Yale University given to rather endearing narcissism, and another colleague, a lady of scrupulous editorial rigor, the kind who would write "If it be true that . . ." Suzanne La Follette was always approaching Willmoore Kendall, open dictionary in hand, spectacles perched over the end of her nose, to substantiate the illegitimacy of a particular usage by Kendall. After a half dozen of these encounters Kendall, exasperated, commented: "Don't you *see,* Suzanne, when people get around to writing dictionaries, they come to people like *me* to find out what to put *in* them."

I don't know a better penetration of the point. *"People like me."* At once, in Kendall's statement, one discerns the statesmanship of lexicography, which is on the one hand to authorize change, on the other to deny change's plebiscitary presumptions. Or, more exactly, to confine the constituency of change; to insist that only such as Kendall are consulted. It doesn't matter if 99 percent of the American people say "spokesperson." Only if Kendall—and I—agree will it become "acceptable."

That word is in quotation marks to emphasize that it does not automatically convey exactly what it is that actually *happens* when acceptability is achieved. There is a sense in which a great many things become "acceptable" by the fact of their high incidence—for instance, lying and adultery. But the words manage to retain a pejorative impact because the deeds they denote are defined outside a purely democratic sociology. The *presumption* is against lying, as it is against adultery, which is less than to pronounce that lying and adultery are absolutely in all circumstances forbidden (though Immanuel Kant, for instance, always rejects the lie, and strict-constructionist Christianity, adultery). What is implied by the surviving pejorative is that *dispensations* are especially granted—ad hoc, ad personam. If the pejorative were bled out of the acts of lying and adultery, then the words would lose their moral dimension; the prevailing practices of society's citizens would determine the acceptability of the terms *lying* and *adultery.* That the pejorative survives surely tells us that intuitively people, recognizing their own weaknesses as such, do not wish the moral criteria to change. In short, acceptability is by no means routinely achieved merely by democratic affirmation.

And then I ask, What exactly is meant by the "chief" determinant of "acceptability"? What is it intended that the qualifier "chief" should convey? How is "chief" here defined? Is it intended to be conclusive? Or is it merely intended to invert the presumptions? Does it intend to convey that if the majority use "spokesperson," it becomes "acceptable" practice to do so? Or merely that if the majority indeed do so, objectors need to shoulder the burden of making a case for continuing illegitimacy? The resolution, we can see, hedges, both in the use of "acceptability" and in the use of the qualifier "chief." And understandably so, because although the Miss La Follettes of this world cannot be permitted to freeze a language in its tracks, when changes are authorized they must be authorized by the Kendalls of this world. The remaining question, then, is: Why?

Because, as is frequently pointed out by science, human progress is achieved by the taking of exact measurements. Language is inherently inexact, but even though the objective is asymptotically approached, it remains the objective; and such exactitude as language *is* capable of is a casualty of careless usage. But if carelessness is to be deplored, by whom will it be deplored? By those who judge it to be careless. And what are they to consult, in their anxiety, if not a dictionary? That dictionary may, in certain of its declarations, be held to be obsolete. But make sure that it is the Kendalls of this world who judge it so, because they are expertly trained and congenitally gifted. They know how to take careful measurements, and they use the language to do this.

How else?

Language is an aesthetic as well as an analytical tool. And to slur language is as painful to the well-tempered ear as to slur music. In music the individualist seeks to introduce a new modality. He may emerge as a great artist, or he may be held to be witless; juries will judge. Usually, in serious music, a genuinely new style requires fifty years to win acceptance. In language some words have been paying court to the admissions committee for centuries, while thousands upon thousands have simply given up. Some win almost immediate acceptance. But the question is always, acceptance by whom?

Vulgar, Slang, Regional, Nonstandard, Informal: most new meanings or uses need to work their way against that upstream drag; and resistance should be formal, i.e., embodied in a dictionary prepared to accept but also prepared to deny.

Lexicographers are sufficiently conversant with their craft to make judgments, yea, even unto designating a word, or a usage, *illiterate.* The other way is mobocratic, undifferentiated. And what is the purpose of a *guide* to usage if not—as required—to exclude? The negative function of a dictionary is a part of its function. It is not a sign of arrogance for the king to rule. That is what he is there for.

1982

———

Other panelists weigh in on other issues. One such deals with the acceptability of individuals and their redefinitions, at times of a brevity approaching scandal.

———

Dear Mr. Buckley:

You will, I know, be interested, as a member of the Usage Panel of the American Heritage Dictionary, in a copy of my letter to the editor of that dictionary. I reproduced its definitions of "dictator," "leader," "statesman," and "premier." And then: "I think you'll agree, especially in the light of definition 1.b. [a tyrant] that the term 'dictator' has a pejorative connotation . . . the terms 'leader,' 'statesman,' and 'premier,' on the other hand, are not at all pejorative. Quite the reverse.

"Keeping all this in mind, contrast the two biographical descriptions:

> *Mussolini, Benito.* 'Il Duce.' 1883–1945. Italian Fascist dictator (1922–45); assassinated.
> *Hitler, Adolf.* 1889–1945. Austrian-born German Nazi dictator.

with the five biographical descriptions:

> *Stalin, Joseph.* 1879–1953. Soviet Communist revolutionary leader.
> *Trotsky, Leon.* 1879–1940. Russian revolutionary and Soviet statesman; assassinated.
> *Mao Zedong* also *Tse-tung.* 1893–1976. Chinese Communist leader.
> *Castro, Fidel.* b. 1927. Cuban revolutionary premier (since 1959).
> *Pol Pot.* b. 1928. Cambodian political leader.

I would appreciate hearing from you on this subject."

Sincerely yours,

DAVID R. JEFFRIES

SAN FRANCISCO, CALIF.

Dear Mr. Jeffries: Nice going. Let me know what the people at American Heritage say. Cordially,

—WFB   FEBRUARY 5, 1990

Permissive or not, it is just a short hop for Buckley from debating the contents of a dictionary to praising its accessibility. *Home Office Computing* magazine billed this short essay with the line "An Electronic Dictionary Fuels a Well-Known Writer's Love of Language." In it, the author speaks of two pleasures: (1) word processing, which, as I've said, for the computer-happy Buckley is perhaps *the* greatest invention, exceeding even sliced bread; and (2) dictionaries.

MINCING WORDS

Ever since computers entered—and in some respects came to dominate—my life, I have from time to time, quite accidentally, tripped upon a program that caused a glint in the eye of the possessor. I also found that he or she wasn't always all that eager to communicate the discovery. It can be that way with a special joke: Some people just don't want to toss it around indiscriminately, perhaps on the grounds that a universal knowledge of it would cause it to lose its flavor.

It was through such experiences, plus the comprehensive generosity of one or two experts, that I came upon programs that had the effect on me I'd have expected if I were in sixteenth-century Peru and someone suddenly said: "Here, why don't you try this when you move all those rocks around? It's called a wheel."

About two years ago someone casually mentioned the American Heritage Dictionary. Years before I had bought the Oxford English Dictionary on one CD and paid an appalling nine hundred bucks for it. But it isn't that often that you build up the etymological hunger that absolutely requires you to know when, under the scrutiny of lexicographers, was the first use of *bacterial* (1872). And to check it out meant a considerable interruption in your work, or at least in my work, because I can't simultaneously view my screen and my CD. What happened is that I neglected the OED, and indeed sometimes went to the volumes, rather than bother with the CD version.

Along came this retiring soul who said to me that, really, I should get the AHD. What he was talking about, he said, was fifteen floppy disks that you could enter as a subdirectory in your hard drive and instruct your working program to stand by to access it. What then happens, he said, is that you can with one (or two) keystrokes stare at the dictionary meaning of the word you have just finished typing.

"How long does that take?" I wanted to know.

"How fast is your computer?"

"I have a 486."

"It will take about a tenth of a second."

I got the AHD but, even as I installed it, I found myself wondering whether it would be a kid's version of a dictionary. . . .

You will have guessed it is nothing of the sort. There are 361,000 entries in this magical device. If you choose, you can call in the thesaurus. You spelled it *thesorus*? A column of fifteen words on the right gives you the nearest thing to what you were looking for. The AHD is also a mini-encyclopedia. When was Xerxes? 519–465 B.C.

I was so struck by the AHD's effective displacement in my life of the major dictionaries (OED, Webster III), I began to record the words I asked the meaning of which it did not have. Here is the fruit of two years' labor: *seakindly, apopemptic, outrance, angelism, jesuitry, roadkill, ipsedixitism, potvaliant,* and *instantiate.* Two years' search!

My opinion for years has been that the nonusers of word processing simply have to be abandoned. . . . But then I think of my AHD. It changes your habits by enticing you to look up quite ordinary words, to reflect on their etymologies, or usages, or whatever. I mean, I don't have idle hours to spare, but I can give you a tenth of a second any time—just try me. And don't think you can dismiss me as flushed with wedding-night enthusiasm. I remind you, it was a full two years ago I found this, the greatest clerical blessing of my lifetime, excepting only Word Processing, the King of Kings.

The other day, I was in a radio exchange with the senior U.S. liberal, Professor Arthur Schlesinger, Jr., who in a casual survey of technology stunned me by saying that, in his judgment, "word processing is the greatest invention in modern history." Suddenly I was face-to-face with the flip side of Paradise. That means, doesn't it, that Professor Schlesinger will write more than he would do otherwise?

—WFB   APRIL, 1996

———

Now Buckley takes on other writers, including Mailer and Le Carré, Henry James and Updike, with sometimes surprising results. The first column goes back thirty-plus years.

———

NAKED AND HALF ALIVE

Do you know who Norman Mailer is? He complains bitterly because he supposes you do not, and the right *not* to know Norman Mailer is *not* an American right, however free is this land of the brave. Gore Vidal (do you know who he is? Surely. He's been on television) wrote a couple of years ago that the lack of public response is "at the center of Mailer's desperation, [for] he is a public writer, not a private artist; he wants to influence those who are alive at this time, but they will not notice him even when he is good."

With the result, suggests Vidal, that Mailer has become a teensy-weensy bit of an exhibitionist, striking garish public poses with the aim of luring people into his tent, where, where . . . "Mailer is forever shouting at us that he is about to tell us something we must know or has just told us something revelatory and we failed to hear him or that he will, God grant his poor abused brain and body just one more chance, get through to us so that we will *know*. . . . *Anything* to get (the public's) attention, and finally (and this could be his tragedy) so much energy is spent in getting the indifferent ear to listen that when the time comes for him to speak there may be not enough strength or creative imagination left him to say what he *knows*."

Now this sounds like a first-class literary feud, does it not, and in a way it is, Mailer having previously written that, alas, his competitor Vidal has yet to write "a single novel which is more successful than not." Yet they are friends, and, on balance, admire each other's work, but these literary cats are that way when they talk about each other, which is not to say we must dismiss what they have to say. Vidal is quite right about Mailer—he doesn't know what it is he wants to say, but his desperate anxiety to say it, fired by his incandescent moral energy, makes him very much worth watching, if only he could come up with something to say.

If you have not yet placed him, Mailer is the celebrated author of *The Naked and the Dead, The Deer Park,* and *Barbary Shore,* and crowned king of the philosophy of hipsterism, which is the philosophy of a sort of rhythmic detachment from an agonized and agonizing world. The hip are a brotherhood of nonproductive sensual self-seekers, a brotherhood in the same sense of Ayn Rand's brotherhood who take over the world in *Atlas Shrugged*—except that the latter are producers, men of iron will and fist, who bring the world to heel; while Mailer's hipsters construct a world of their own, refusing to live in this grisly world on its own terms.

One of the remarkable things about the modern age is the number of sensitive men who march forward determined to resynthesize all of human experience and give to us a wholly new worldview. Such people sometimes have difficulty being heard, in which case they do not do too much mischief; sometimes they are heard, like Karl Marx, and there is hell to pay. These neoterics begin on the flat assumption that the philosophical patrimony of the Western world is useless, and square. God is dead! Nietzsche announced. God is dying! Mailer corrects him. It is of course the duty of creative men to add to our store of knowledge and accommodate new experience and contingencies. But the boys to worry about are those who want to start completely afresh—who want, in the words of the disgusted back-bencher, to "send a man to the guillotine to do away with a case of dandruff." "How shall I go about founding a new religion?" the young man asked Voltaire. "Go and get yourself crucified," Voltaire answered, "then rise again on the third day." On reading Mailer one has no doubt he might be prepared to do just that, save possibly for fear that during those three days our Maker might persuade him to stay around and stew awhile. But Norman Mailer will never cease trying.

The American conservative is often accused of being complacent in his essential philosophy, and the fact of the matter is that is true, he is. He believes that the cluster of truths which are loosely referred to as our "Judeo-Christian tradition" are—well, are truths, and that while our age must ingeniously improvise on them to meet such apocalyptic demands as face us, there is no need to start afresh, and chase about wildly through hipsterism and existentialism and humanism and Freudianism and communism and fascism and objectivism and what have you, just to say you've got the blackboard clean. What the tormented Mr. Mailer needs so sorely is the grace that hit the young Chesterton with such force early in his lifetime, making him a fountainhead of wisdom and joy. "I am the man," he recalled, "who with the utmost daring discovered what had been discovered before. I did try to found a heresy of my own; and when I had put the last touches to it, I discovered that it was orthodoxy."

—WFB   SEPTEMBER 23, 1962

W hich leads, three years later, to a form of appreciation.

LIFE GOES TO NORMAN MAILER

The life and art of Mr. Norman Mailer are discussed all over the pages of *Life* magazine this week by an intelligent and gifted writer, Mr. Brock Brower, who had the sense to acknowledge even before setting out on his twelve-page journey that he doesn't know (and neither does Mr. Mailer) what in fact is the goal of Mr. Mailer's "reckless quest." The heavy recognition of Mr. Mailer by the editors of *Life* is final confirmation that he is big on the literary scene—and more: that he is big on the American scene, for reasons that most critics do not know how to explain but, by their friendly activity in trying, go so far as to acknowledge that the Quest to Explain Norman Mailer is itself worthwhile.

And indeed it is. He is probably the single best known living American writer, only second to John Dos Passos. It doesn't mean his books have sold as well as Erskine Caldwell's or John Steinbeck's, merely that far more of the people who read Mailer's books wonder about who he is, and what he is trying to get at, than ever have on reading Caldwell or Steinbeck.

Mailer is interesting in two respects. The first—and here is why I love him as an artist—is that he makes the most beautiful metaphors in the business, as many as a dozen of them on a single page worth anthologizing.

The second reason why he is interesting is that to many who read him hungrily (and perhaps too seriously) he represents present-day America. He expresses their feelings that America today is shivering in desolation and hopelessness, is looking for her identity after a period of self-alienation marked by a couple of world wars, a depression and a cyclonic advance through technology and automation.

It was Mailer who developed the cult of the hipster—the truly modern American who lets the bleary world go by doing whatever it bloody well likes, because nothing it does can upset the hipsters' inexhaustible cool. It isn't that Mr. Mailer's characters are without passion; on the contrary they tend to be so highly strung that no matter how gently you stroke them, they emit twangy sharp tones. It is that the workaday pressures of civilization don't affect them. They aren't influenced very much by tradition, or by the venerable arguments for continence and moderation, or by the recognition that other people's existences and hopes abut against our own ambitions and self-concern.

In every categorical sense, Norman Mailer is an utter and hopeless mess. If there is an intellectual in the United States who talks more predictable nonsense on the subject of foreign policy, I will pay a week's wages not to have to hear him.

On the domestic scene, he is a so-so socialist. So-so because even though he finds he can float only in the cool waters of the left, he is transparently unhappy, really, as a socialist, although he is more docile toward that barren religion than toward any other. As a citizen, he is wild, defying not only those starched conventions that are there primarily to stick out your tongue at, but the other conventions, the real McCoys: those that are there to increase the small chance we have, whether as children or as adults, for a little domestic tranquillity.

As a philosopher, however, Mailer is—dare I say it?—in his own fashion, a conservative. Wrestling in the twentieth century with the hegemonies of government and ideology, the conservative tends to side with the individualist. In his savage novels, Mailer's titanic struggles are sustained by the resources of his own spirit (plus booze). In his most recent novel, *An American Dream,* a hero as screwy as Mr. Mailer lurches from Gomorrah to hell and back, but always depends on himself to get out of the jam.

Mr. Mailer is properly denounced by philosophical taxonomists as a solipsist—a man for whom reality is confined to himself and his own experience. Still, it is a relief—sort of a halfway house to the proper blend of the individual and tradition—to read a novel in which the protagonist doesn't depend for his salvation on life rafts cast out into the sea of hope by Marx, Freud, or U Thant.

I confess that Mr. Mailer's tours through the nightspots of hell are not my idea of recreation, even with pad and pencil in hand to jot down what one has learned about Things. I do not enjoy spelunking in human depravity, nor do I wish my machine around to tape-record the emunctory noises of psychic or physical human excesses. Even so, there is hope in Norman Mailer's turbulent motions.

—WFB   SEPTEMBER 25, 1965

The King Must Die, by Mary Renault (Pantheon, $4.50), is the story of the legendary Theseus, who, though heir to the nascent kingdom of Athens, went off to Crete with the fifteen young Athenians who every year were tearfully yielded up to die a bloody death, to sate the bloodlust of the Minotaur. Miss Renault on Greece has been compared to Robert Graves on Rome. But she is even better, more light-footed, self-effacing; and she writes about the most innocent, the most enchanting age in history. Mary Renault is as much a part of ancient Greece as Helen Waddell is a part of the Middle Ages, and she evokes her period with equal skill. She has the total sensual perception to distinguish, and the poetic skill to make readily distinguishable, the generative matrix of everything in Grecian life— the religion, the sport, the love, the wine, the discourse, the battle; and clearly she loves beauty as the Greeks did, with all her heart and mind. Miss Renault accepts the discipline proper to one who writes a historical novel. Her imagery is that of the period: in this case confined to the rudimentary properties of taste and smell that were Homer's only tools. And look what she has done! In the mountain of work of the sprawling, uninhibited writers of what Clifton Fadiman aptly calls the Unedited Generation there is not the evocative power of one of Mary Renault's finished paragraphs.

W. F. BUCKLEY, JR.   OCTOBER 11, 1958

————

And embedded in this appreciation of Tom Wolfe is WFB on what would come to be called political correctness—back in 1970.

————

MAU-MAUING WOLFE

Those of you who are not aware of Tom Wolfe should—really—do your best to acquaint yourselves with him. For one thing, he is probably the most skillful writer in America. I mean by that that he can do more things with words than anyone else: a greater variety of things. He is like the pianist Henry Scott, who can play the "Flight of the Bumblebee" while wearing mittens. That is of course stunt stuff, but Wolfe, the virtuoso, does not depend alone on his flashy cadenzas. He can do anything. Meanwhile he is a leading figure in the New Journalism, which weds the craft of the novelist to the obligations of the journalist. And on top of that, he has written a very very controversial book, for which he has been publicly excommunicated from the company of the orthodox by the bishops who preside over the *New York Review of Books.*

Mr. Wolfe was born in Richmond, Virginia, in 1931, and took his B.A. at Washington and Lee University. His principal enthusiasm at college was baseball, in which he hoped to become a professional. He failed and, dropping out, went to Yale, taking there a doctorate in American Studies. He worked briefly as a copyboy for the *New York Daily News,* principally because an editor there desired the experience of having a Ph.D. bring him his Coca-Colas. Then the *Washington Post,* then the *Herald Tribune,* and now he is an editor of *New York* magazine. His articles, published there and in *Esquire,* are regularly compiled into books with crazy titles. The first was *The Kandy-Kolored Tangerine-Flake Streamline Baby;* then there was *The Pump House Gang* and *The Electric Kool-Aid Acid Test.* And, now, *Radical Chic and Mau-Mauing the Flak Catchers,* the first part of which is about the famous party that Leonard Bernstein threw to raise money for the Black Panthers who had been indicted for conspiring to bomb a few department stores, presumably racist department stores, in New York City, during Eastertide.

Well sir, what happened shouldn't happen to an honest hangman, let alone an artist. What Mr. Wolfe did in his book was *make fun* of Bernstein et al., and if you have never been told, you *must not make fun* of Bernstein et al. when what hangs in the balance is Bernstein's moral prestige plus the integrity of Black Protest; learn the lesson now. Tom Wolfe, although thoroughly apolitical, focused on the paradoxes involved in the spilling of Black Rage over the extra-porous sensibilities of an antimacassar liberal, who has been trained to salivate over the plight of any Negro, even one whose cause is the absolute right of Black Panthers to commit revolution, bomb department-store buildings, and rage against the Jews while they are at it.

Anyway . . . Tom Wolfe is an unfortunate victim of ideological ire. His wit attracts the witless among the critics. For instance? Well, here is Wolfe, talking about how some of the black militants in San Francisco succeeded in terrorizing Poverty Program types into giving them money, namely by frightening them. "There was one genius in the art of confrontation who had mau-mauing down to what you could term a laboratory science. He had it figured out so he didn't even have to bring his boys downtown in person. He would just show up with a crocus sack full of revolvers, ice picks, fish knives, switchblades, hatchets, blackjacks, gravity knives, straight razors, hand grenades, blow guns, bazookas, Molotov cocktails, tank rippers, unbelievable stuff, and he'd dump it all out on somebody's shiny walnut conference table. He'd say, 'These are some of the things I took off my boys last night . . .' "

This is the kind of thing that is met (by Mr. Jason Epstein of the *New York Review of Books*) with such embarrassing moral pith-and-moment phrases as that Mr. Wolfe is "cruel and shallow," that his "sin is a lack of compassion," that his is an "intellectual weakness" because he "finds himself beyond his depth, frailties that commonly accompany moments of great personal or public stress," and so on and so forth: Cotton Mather reviewing Peter Pan.

Tom Wolfe will survive the humorless of this world—that or else the world will not, should not, survive. If he feels down, after such reviews as Mr. Epstein's, he can go back and reread Karl Shapiro's that appeared in *Book World* after his previous book: "Let us . . . pay homage to Tom Wolfe right off the bat. He has given us the finest mug shots of the soi-disant revolutionaries we shall see in a long time. He has pinned their little wriggling personae to the bulletin board for all to gape upon. He has performed necessary acts of vilification with a superb aristocratic cool. He is a master of intonation and an extrapolator who can put to shame the regnant sociologists of guilt and hedonism. . . . Tom Wolfe is more than brilliant . . . Tom Wolfe is a goddam joy."

Read his book, and see if you don't agree.

—WFB   DECEMBER 24, 1970

TERROR AND A WOMAN

The Little Drummer Girl. By John le Carré. Alfred A. Knopf.

The beginning of John le Carré's new book is, for a spy thriller, entirely orthodox: There is a bombing, a bombing by a terrorist. Where? Near Bonn, but the location does not matter. There have been so many others, in Zurich, in Leyden, here and there. It matters only that the victim was an Israeli. Although the reader spends time in Bonn and in Tel Aviv and in Vienna, Munich, Mykonos, London, it matters hardly at all, except that the ambiance of these places is an invitation for Mr. Le Carré to use his palette. The places are simply where the terrorist strikes, or where the antiterrorists are collected.

It becomes instantly apparent that we are in the hands of a writer of great powers. In the very first paragraph of *The Little Drummer Girl* he reveals the skill with which he can write in shorthand: "It was the Bad Godesberg incident that gave the proof. . . . Before Bad Godesberg, there had been growing suspicion; a lot of it. But the high quality of the planning, as against the poor quality of the bomb, turned the suspicion into certainty. Sooner or later, they say in the trade, a man will sign his name."

And then Mr. Le Carré informs the reader that he is in no hurry at all; he has all the time in the world. So he gives us a little belletrism, and that also works. He describes the residential diplomatic area in which the bombing took place: "The fronts of some of the houses were already half obscured by dense plantations of conifers, which, if they ever grow to proper size, will presumably one day plunge the whole area into a Grimm's fairy-tale blackout." There is the "patently nationalistic" look of some of the dwellings. "The Norwegian Ambassador's residence, for example, just around the corner from the Drosselstrasse, is an austere, redbricked farmhouse lifted straight from the stockbroker hinterlands of Oslo. The Egyptian consulate, up the other end, has the forlorn air of an Alexandrian villa fallen on hard times. Mournful Arab music issues from it, and its windows are permanently shuttered against the skirmishing North African heat."

We are very quickly aware that we are reading not Dashiell Hammett but someone much more like Lawrence Durrell. The author does not forget his duty. There is sleuthing galore ahead of the reader; and, in the end, the Palestinian terrorist is emphatically dead. But the momentum of the story is not ended with his death. There is left—the girl. The instrument of the Israeli antiterrorists. An English actress named Charlie, she is permanently changed by the complex role imposed on her—to be faithful at once to the Israeli and the Palestinian causes. And she is in love with the most mysterious character to have appeared in recent fiction, whose flesh-and-blood reification Mr. Le Carré flatly refuses to give us. His name is Joseph, and other than the Israeli superspy Schulmann, the English actress Charlie and, however briefly, the Palestinian superterrorist Khalil, there is only Joseph seriously to ponder. At first he is merely a will-o'-the-wisp, and one is not entirely certain that he actually exists. Then he is incorporated formally into the plot, his persona on the one hand central, on the other hand continuingly elusive. And when finally only he exists for Charlie, after the entrapment, after Khalil is gone, the magnetism is enormous. The emotional tension of the postlude elevates it into a full fourth act. A wonderful achievement.

Mr. Le Carré's novel is certainly the most mature, inventive and powerful book about terrorists-come-to-life this reader has experienced. It transcends the genre by reason of the will and the interests of the author. The story line interests him but does not dominate him. He is interested in writing interestingly about things interesting and not interesting. Terrorism and counterterrorism, intelligence work and espionage are, then, merely the vehicle for a book about love, anomie, cruelty, determination and love of country. *The Little Drummer Girl* is about spies as *Madame Bovary* is about adultery or *Crime and Punishment* about crime. Mr. Le Carré easily establishes that he is not beholden to the form he elects to use. This book will permanently raise him out of the espionage league, narrowly viewed.

I venture this judgment even though I am not familiar with all of his preceding books. Indeed I remember discarding one of them as too steep, in my cursory scouting of its first couple of chapters, to be worth climbing, pending the judgment of others I had confidence in that the view would be worth the effort. *Drummer Girl* has here and there passages that demand diligent reading. And sometimes Mr. Le Carré is drawn, annoyingly, to nondeclarative narrative. Disdain for narrative rigidity is probably closer. There is something of John Fowles in his style, in the liberties he gives himself to wander about as he likes, to dwell at any length that grips him or amuses him, serenely confident as he is that we will be, respectively, gripped and amused—and if not, we should go read other people's books. But he succeeds, almost always, because he is naturally expressive, dominant and in turn dominating in his use of language. And so the liberties he takes tend to be accepted as a part of his tapestry—even if, looked at discretely, they can be, as I say, annoying and even logically dissonant.

Here is an example. The Israeli Schulmann, determined to track down the Palestinian Khalil, has decided (most implausibly) on the attractive instrument for the entrapment—the touring actress, half-gypsy, half flower child, Charlie. And so he kidnaps her and begins a brain-washing operation that in most circumstances would cause the reader to smile with condescending incredulity. Consider the girl being interrogated thoroughly so that the supersleuth can learn literally all he can about her, the better to manipulate the penetration of the terrorist network.

It is known that Charlie's childhood home was taken by creditors when her father was caught up in embezzlement, and the supersleuth presses her for details of the episode: "Charlie, we recognize that this is very painful for you, but we ask you to continue in your own words. We have the van. We see your possessions leaving the house. What else do we see?"

"My pony."

"They took that too?"

"I told you already."

"With the furniture? In the same van?"

"No, a separate one. Don't be bloody silly."

"So there were two vans. Both at the same time? Or one after the other?"

"I don't remember."

Charlie was quite right. The questioner was being bloody silly. But wait.

About the same man who could ask bloody silly questions, Mr. Le Carré can write, "When Schulmann smiled, the wrinkles that flew into his face had been made by centuries of water flowing down the same rock paths and his eyes clamped narrow like a Chinaman's. Then, long after him, his sidekick smiled, echoing some twisted inner meaning. . . . When Schulmann talked, he fired off conflicting ideas like a spread of bullets, then waited to see which ones went home and which came back at him. The sidekick's voice followed like a stretcher party, softly collecting the dead." People who merit such description can be forgiven occasional silliness.

Is there a message in *Drummer Girl*? Yes. A quite earnest one. It is that the intensity with which the Israelis defend what they have got can only be understood if one understands the intensity with which the Palestinians resent what it is that they have lost. The Israelis triumph in the novel, even as they do in life. But Mr. Le Carré is careful to even up the moral odds. I have in the past been discomfited by trendy ventures in ideological egalitarianism, such that the reader ends by finding the Communist spy and the Western spy equally weak, equally heroic; and perhaps the ambiguist in Mr. Le Carré would overcome him in any exercise in which the alternative was moral polarization. But having acknowledged that this may be in John le Carré a temperamental weakness, reflecting the clutch of ambiguity rather than any ultimate fear of moral fine-tuning, one must go on to acknowledge that he permits the Palestinian point to be made with rare and convincing eloquence.

He is a very powerful writer. His entertainment is of a high order. He gives pleasure in his use of language. And his moral focus is interesting and provocative.

—WFB   MARCH 13, 1983

Now and then, Buckley does a movie review—and once again is way out ahead in predicting the tastelessness to which some moviemakers will eventually sink, well after this view of *The Right Stuff.*

The Almost Right Stuff

A few things should be said about the movie *The Right Stuff,* which is coming in with the biggest bang since *Gone With the Wind.*

The first is that seeing it is not an experience comparable to reading Tom Wolfe's book. This is a point especially relevant given that the producers tried very hard, spared no expense and were wonderfully ingenious. The best example of their relative failure is the reception for the astronauts given at the Houston Astrodome. In the book, four or five of the most hilarious pages in modern social commentary describe an event that is at once vulgar, boisterous and poignant. In the movie all the humor is gone, and we are exposed merely to the celebration of vulgarity, which, next to the conquest of space, is what the movie mostly focuses on. Tom Wolfe's genius brings to the study of almost every situation the leavening humor that makes tolerable—well, makes America tolerable.

And speaking of America, *The Right Stuff* is oddly unaware of it. It is always possible, if you are willing to put all collective human ventures under a microscope, to see only discrete personal acts. The movie gives us men who are merely brave, ambitious and competitive. The notion that they were in any way animated by national pride would have struck the director as quaint. Indeed, wherever it becomes necessary to bring in the good old U.S.A., there is a smell of chauvinism and sleaziness.

There can't have been a more obnoxious human being than *The Right Stuff*'s Lyndon Johnson since, well, the real Lyndon Johnson. Jack Kennedy makes boilerplate talks about the challenge to America, various senators are depicted worrying about the political implications of it all—America, in the movie, is a sideshow. In the book, however lightly done, America is, really, the main event. The astronauts were up to something different from Evel Knievel's flamboyant assaults on gravity.

Mind you, it is a wonderful spectacular, with superb acting and direction, and memorable characterizations. You begin with the impact of the loneliness of a remote air base (Edwards, in California) where, out of eyesight, great feats are accomplished. Chuck Yeager, the legendary test pilot, is wonderfully depicted by actor-author Sam Shepard. It is routine, at Edwards, to ride horses wildly (nice juxtaposition, the frontiersmen, old and new), drink up a vat of beer, pursue your woman (all of them marvelously drawn), perhaps break a rib or two because of your earthly recklessness. And then—the next day—you get into the cockpit, chew your gum, get dropped from the mother ship, and break the sound barrier.

A couple of weeks later, the other man at the bar has gone Mach 1.3, so you know that, maybe tomorrow, maybe in a week or two, you will have to go for Mach 1.4. Let's drink to that. And an important point to stress: In those days there were no parades, no publicity, no big contracts with *Life* magazine, because all this was, you see, secret stuff. Shh, get away from that telephone, boy, freedom of the press is one thing, national security is one thing better.

But then we discover the need for great funding. And that spigot can only be turned on by capturing the public imagination. So the flyboys—a brand new set—go public. And when the astronauts went public, they went all the way. It was much harder on them than merely reaching the moon.

But here, again, a complaint. There is one scene—it is in the sequence of physical ordeals to which the astronauts were subjected by the medical examiners before being certified—so glaringly unnecessary as to bring forth from the audience only that nervous laughter that conceals embarrassment. The sheer tastelessness of it defies understanding. Perhaps cinema verité is going to require tomorrow's cameras to depict human beings in the act of excretion.

It is sad to reflect that these are the tastemakers; that what individual directors of individual movies do is said to dictate today's folkways, tomorrow's mores. I have not studied the circuitry of audience resentment, and do not therefore know how a general disgust is communicated. The scene is hardly enough to bring on a substantial rejection of an otherwise entertaining and engrossing narrative. But it is a great blotch in the memory.

Go see it. And then, to remind yourself of the unique power of the written word, read, or reread, Tom Wolfe's book. There is no substitute for that wonderful experience.

—WFB   OCTOBER 10, 1983

Hollywood Piety

Let me be done with it and say that the movie *True Confessions* is (in an opinion with which men may with impunity differ) awful; whereas the book of the same title from which it is taken is (in an opinion with which no man may safely differ) rich as Rabelais, haunting, evocative, synaesthetically sensational. In the movie, Robert De Niro is badly miscast. He is never entirely convincing, and words are put in his mouth ("I've packed up my bags," when he announces he has cancer) that one wouldn't have thought wild horses could have dragged from the typewriters of the talented screenwriters. The scenes are one cliché mounted joylessly on another, so that the unfolding of each reminds you progressively of the weakness of the predecessor. But I am not here to criticize the movie—rather to remark the ease with which Hollywood now handles the theme of the thoroughly disreputable priest, though the priest in *True Confessions* isn't actually all that hateful, no more is his boss the cardinal; nor, for that matter, is his brother Tom, the driven, cynical policeman.

Monsignor Desmond Spellacy is ambitious. In his dealings with the cardinal he is somewhere between docile and servile. He is bright enough to know what's really going on, and that what's really going on shouldn't really go on, because Mother Church in Los Angeles has no business giving one of those annual medals ("Catholic Citizen of the Year," or whatever) to a big, beefy, repulsive character, no matter how much money he has given for the construction of parochial schools, if it is known among the cognoscenti (1949 was before Vatican II outlawed Latin) that said character had got rich by pimping, is probably still connected with organized crime, and regularly devotes himself to the easier part of that biblical injunction to go out and multiply. What fascinates—or is supposed to do so—is the cultural departure in protocol.

It used to be that Hollywood priests were Bing Crosby, going his way, and making ours lighter; or Spencer Tracy, telling the dead-end kid he was a good boy after all, with transmutational effect; or Hollywood nuns were Ingrid Bergman, raising money for the bells of St. Mary's and, while at it, tingling the chimes within the human spirit. Most people, I should think, knew that this was romance; that in real life Bing Crosby neglected his children, Spencer Tracy kept a mistress, etc.

But the theatrical convention was there: that all priests behave in such a way as to dare emulation. Between the Fifties and the Seventies no professional class (save possibly investigative journalists) was presumptively supposed to be engaged in altruistic activity. Ben Stein wrote a book (*The View from Sunset Boulevard*) about a year in Hollywood during which he had come upon not a single "good" businessman, or "good" military officer in the pulp-forests he had seen produced for television and the movies. If John Gregory Dunne had sat down to write a book about a priest who behaved like Mother Teresa, not even with the aid of his talented wife, Joan Didion, would he have been invited to make a movie based on his discovery. The priestly calling is a theatrical victim of an age of skepticism; and it isn't entirely unreasonable that the theatergoer should take this in stride. For one thing there are all those thousands of priests and nuns who have been "laicized," a desertion no man may judge harshly whose own faith, whether in God, marriage, country, or politics, has ever been shaken. But desertion it was: i.e., one pledged one's life to a calling, most spiritual in aspect—and after a while the public recognized you as the fellow drinking beer with the wife or girlfriend while watching Monday night football, waiting your turn at the bowling alley. The stereotype of tenacious Franciscan asceticism is irretrievably gone.

And then, too, there was the ideologization of religion. It's easier, among Catholic clergy, to pick a fight over whether to send arms to the rebels in Nicaragua than whether the Shroud of Turin bears the marks of an extra-worldly implosion.

So that John Gregory Dunne's colorful story about priests who have one eye on ambition, and cardinals who leave it to God to forgive the means by which the local philanthropists accumulated their money in the first place, isn't likely to disrupt the rhythm of the movie audience munching its popcorn. The book, by the way, is infinitely more shocking than the movie: but this was so not because the clergy were proved human, but because the language, particularly of the cop and his sidekick, is textured with a blend of profanity and obscenity which almost everywhere (I think of one or two lapses) transports the imagination to a delight unsullied by the ultimate moral corruption. True corruption is what happens when you are asked to believe that as between right and wrong, there really aren't any differences. It is one thing to discover that the pious priest was really Elmer Gantry all over again. Something else to read in the *Playboy* philosophy that philandering is good because anything that *feels* good *is* good— except maybe lynching uppity niggers. (*Playboy*—and Hollywood—feel they have to draw the line somewhere.) The book *True Confessions* shocks by color and an irreverence that knows itself to be that. You could fit every Christian martyr in the chasm between *True Confessions* and *Last Exit from Brooklyn*.

The cultural difference is worth noting, however. Thirty years ago there was plenty of sin going on. In the Eurasian continent more people were killed probably than in three millennia of recorded history. However, for a period, however brief, in popular culture benign presumptions were indulged. Just as rabbis were "wise," priests were "benevolent." Drank a little too much, like Barry Fitzgerald maybe, but good fellows, professionally devoted to philanthropy of sorts. The viewer was only occasionally teased into examining the underlying dogmatic solemnity of it all.

The Spanish, twenty-five years ago, brought out a discreet little venture in evangelism, as charming as *The Hobbit*. A little orphan boy, living in the monastery, whisked away bread and an occasional apple to feed the disconsolate crucifix in the attic, where, at mealtime, before the dazed stare of the child, the incarnation was reenacted, day after day at 6 P.M.— till the monks, counting lost apples, broke the reverie (*Marcelino, Pan y Vino*).

At the hot end of the electric theological prod, the viewer could see a dazzling blend of faith triumphant over sacrilege (*Le Défroqué*). Without faith there cannot, of course, be sacrilege: and here we had the sometime priest, become agnostic professor of philosophy, dining with his young protégé, who had stayed true to their once-common faith and was now, freshly ordained, in the priesthood. In the noisy, bibulous tavern crowded with hedonists three violinists carry about the huge five-liter tankard of wine, playing noisily and accelerando gypsy-rhythmed catalysts to frenzy, while one at a time guests chug-a-lug, the leader so far having emptied only a fifth of the seemingly bottomless barrel.

It is now routinely refilled, and the violinists place it on the next table down, where the earnest young priest is talking affectionately with his apostate mentor. The audience is distracted—and at just that moment the ex-priest, driven to black-mass exhibitionism, quietly intones, within the hearing only of his young, freshly consecrated friend, the transubstantiating incantation: *Hic est enim Calix Sanguinis mei . . . For this is the Chalice of my Blood . . .* The violinists, unaware, resume the routine. The young priest, dazed by his knowledge that apostate priests are not shorn of their sacramental powers, lifts the tankard—the blood of Christ—to his lips. He begins to drink . . . the crowd goes wilder . . . the violinists sweat . . . the professor is alarmed . . . Now he has emptied the tankard; the crowd is delirious with admiration. . . . The young priest, stumbling outdoors to the cheers of the crowd, succumbs and dies. Flash forward to the funeral. It is being conducted by the professor. Dressed in clerical garb. Returned to the faith. Nobody who saw *Le Défroqué* will forget it.

True Confessions (the movie, not the book) is unlikely to be denounced even by the Legion of Decency. Catholics don't have an Anti-Defamation League, for one thing; for another, there isn't anything there that is truly sacrilegious. Some priests will visit brothels as long as lust is given a fighting chance on earth, and it is the organizing Christian proposition that even Christ was tempted. The Catholic Church is the inspiration for great utterances, even as it has provoked resonant denunciations. G. K. Chesterton, face to face with his time's version of Hollywood agnosticism, concluded a major book by writing that "there are an infinity of angles at which one falls, only one at which one stands. . . . To have avoided them all has been one whirling adventure; and in my vision, the heavenly chariot flies thundering through the ages, the dull heresies sprawling and prostrate, the wild truth reeling but erect."

Those who will be shocked by *True Confessions* may—or may not—achieve perspective by reminding themselves that a century ago Charles Kingsley was writing such witty stuff as, "The Roman religion . . . for some time past, [has] been making men not better men, but worse. We must face, we must conceive honestly for ourselves, the deep demoralization which had been brought on in Europe by the dogma that the Pope of Rome had the power of creating right and wrong; that not only truth and falsehood, but morality and immorality, depended on his setting his seal to a bit of parchment."

Now that's the kind of anti-Papist stuff that makes Hollywood's *True Confessions* taste like no-cal Popsicle. But—a note to all those who seek to offend, or to be offended: Caution! Kingsley, above, brought forth Newman's *Apologia pro Vita Sua,* the crushing masterpiece that British news-paper readers lined up to buy when it was serialized, a book that devastated Kingsley, leaving that urbane, witty skeptic to sound like the village atheist. Impiety breeds piety. I don't know what the movie version of *True Confessions* will bring on, but pending that dreadnaught, you are vouchsafed these little words, good for just enough life-sufficiency to keep you afloat until the genuine article comes along.

—SEPTEMBER 18, 1981

On one occasion, Mr. Buckley, just as he has done self-interviews, did a self-review (in his own magazine), a temptation every novelist, budding or other, will understand.

Saving the Queen. By William F. Buckley, Jr. Doubleday.

Mr. Buckley's first novel features an attractive hero (American, young, handsome, patriotic, sassy); an irresistible Queen (of England; never, in the novel, confused with the incumbent); a great crisis of state (American hydrogen-bomb development secrets are being leaked to Stalin); a super-secret mission (the hero has to find out who the leak is, the suspects having narrowed to the Prime Minister of England and the Queen of England); a dalliance with the Queen (she is described by the *Washington Post* reviewer: "If you will try to imagine a woman who looks like a young Grace Kelly, has the mischievousness of an Alice Roosevelt Longworth, the wit of an early Dorothy Parker, the sweetness of Dorothy in the *Wizard of Oz,* and the breeding of, well, the Queen of England, you will get the picture [of the fictional Queen Caroline]."); a theatrical duel with the traitor (fought over the skies of England, the Queen and the military no-bility innocently looking on); an ironic eulogy delivered at St. George's Chapel, Windsor Castle (by the killer, in praise of the traitor); and, in an epilogue, the frustration of the Rockefeller Commission investigating the CIA (by the hero, invoking a privilege not enumerated in the Bill of Rights; a common-law privilege, so to speak). Since the book's appear-ance, the author has repeatedly been asked whether the novel is autobio-graphical. His answers have sometimes appeared evasive, although he readily admits to having served briefly as a deep-cover agent in the CIA after leaving college. Asked if, like his hero, he was treated sadistically at a British public school, he has answered that no, while at school in England as a boy he was beloved, then as now, of everyone. Asked to reply to the charge that everyone in his novel speaks like himself, he has remarked that this is a weakness he has in common with Jane Austen. Criticized in the *New York Times* for a scene that "reads like the Hardy Boys at a brothel," he replied that, speaking for himself, he would be delighted to read a chapter depicting the behavior of the Hardy Boys at a brothel. Asked why his hero, however amusing, departs so abruptly from the stereotype of Greene, Le Carré, et al., the author observed that not all American spies wear dirty underwear, or toss and turn at night wondering whether maybe Stalin wasn't right after all. Asked whether he has in mind a plot for a future novel, he was—once again—evasive, admitting only that he had mused on the theme of a novel based on a great novelist who consumed his talent worrying about mundane world affairs.

WILLIAM F. BUCKLEY, JR.   FEBRUARY 20, 1976

———

A self-review was called for many times when a reviewer reviewed Buckley rather than the book at hand and what was in it. The steady success of the Blackford Oakes novels was often dampened when splashed or spat on by a reviewer who could not free himself or herself from a political agenda or when a reviewer ignorantly confused Oakes with the author. Even the sailing books called forth reviews, which meant that sometimes, a fella needed a friend.

———

To the Editor
The Washington Post
Washington, D.C.

The review of William F. Buckley Jr.'s *WindFall* was not criticism but a kind of street crime, gratuitously violent, filled with envy and something like hatred. Buckley wrote a wonderful book about friendship, sailing, fatherhood, and getting on in years. Why did you publish such strange, disgraceful ranting about it?

Sincerely,

LANCE MORROW

(SENIOR EDITOR, *TIME* MAGAZINE)

Dear Lance:

Many thanks for sending along your letter reproaching the *Washington Post* for the sick-unpleasant review of my *WindFall*. But if you want to see a *real* killer review, get a load of this!

Planning to Read *WindFall*?

Mr. Buckley has written another of those autobiographical day-by-day books, if you can stand it, which I can't. The vehicle this time is a trans-Atlantic sailing trip (westbound) in which he does everything he can to liken himself to Christopher Columbus whom (come to think of it) he somewhat resembles, both gentlemen being vain, arrogant, and imperious. Those readers who have labored through his other sailing books (*Airborne, Atlantic High, Racing Through Paradise*) will recognize the usual sights and smells. Elaborate cuisine, a boatful of indentured servants/mates/captains, enough to keep Mr. Buckley out of serious trouble. (He goes through one storm which he all but likens to the 1938 hurricane, and after having done everything a good sailor shouldn't do, delivers a lecture at the end of the chapter about what he ought to have done about the storm, which ought to have included not to write about it.)

The book is an attempt to weave great meaning out of quotidian events. Thus his subtitle is "The End of the Affair." Ho ho, are we going to get from Buckley, the chauvinist Christian, some sort of an envoi to a departed mistress? Not at all; his "affair" has been with his magazine (*National Review*), which by everyone's reckoning has vastly improved since his departure as Editor-in-Chief; with ocean crossing (this is his fourth voyage, hence Ocean Four); and with his son, who to the evident surprise of Mr. Buckley actually outgrew, at something like age thirty-five, filial servitude to the Mahster.

One hopes, reading along, to find safe passage from the overweening concern of the author with himself. One is best off abandoning hope at the beginning of "Book One," since in that way one can shield oneself from frustration. Mr. Buckley is bedeviled (*mot juste?*—as he might put it?) by himself. Whatever concerns him, he is determined to inflict upon his audience. Do you care how close Altair and Vega are together, in degrees and minutes measured from the horizon, in mid-November? Well, you had better care, because if you do not, you are going to be wasting more time than most people have available to read trivial books.

Or—this is my favorite in Mr. Buckley's inventory of effronteries—are you interested in how he prepared in his youth for his hilariously unsuccessful avocation as an amateur musician? Well, there are pages and *pages* on this subject, including detailed accounts of several appearances with symphony orchestras evidently broke enough to bring him in for benefit concerts, satisfied that Mr. Buckley will attract idolatrous crowds, which he will, except if there happens to be among them anyone who knows anything about music. We go through a Q&A previously published in the *New York Times* about why he consented to play with the Phoenix Symphony Orchestra in 1989, which is inexplicable enough, alongside which the only thing more inexplicable is his evident conviction that his reasons are of public interest.

The first of the three "books" is simply a compilation of material Mr. Buckley has placed in yacht journals over recent years. They have in common only that the author is the hero in every situation, ranging from the decision to shut down one engine on a power yacht so that he can be heard more easily by his guests, to his decision to settle for smaller and smaller boats as the years go by. At this point one wishes he would settle for a boat he could blow about in his bathtub, the trouble being that he would almost certainly write a book about it: *Ocean Five: The Art of Traversing a Truly Large Bathtub in a Tiny, Frail Boat,* by Horatio Selfhornblower Buckley.

Pretty tough stuff, no? But rather witty in its savagery, I like to think—since I composed the above review, as a lark, one year ago, and sent it to my editor as warning that this is the direction The Enemy would take. . . .

Most cordial regards,

BILL   AUGUST 3, 1992

———

Interesting reviewing results when one prolific writer, intoxicated with language—and a self-reviewer, too—reviews another.

———

YOU'VE HAD YOUR TIME

The Second Part of the Confessions. By Anthony Burgess. Grove Weidenfeld.

Anthony Burgess is an insistent literary presence who comes at us from every direction and who has just now published the second volume in an autobiography that is scheduled to go to a third volume—on the assumption that he will die sometime soon, say before the millennium (he thinks this likely: "I cannot keep myself healthy—too many bad habits deeply ingrained, cardiac bronchitis like the orchestra of death tuning up under water"). Otherwise, there is sure to be a fourth, so compulsive is his productive energy.

Those whose ear responds only faintly to the mention of Anthony Burgess will recognize him as the author of *A Clockwork Orange,* a book that achieved immortality when Stanley Kubrick made a movie of it. (On that novel, Mr. Burgess quotes a critic who wrote of it, and him: "Anthony Burgess is a literary smart aleck whose novel *A Clockwork Orange* last year achieved a *succès d'estime* with critics like William Burroughs, who mistook his muddle of sadism, teddyboyism, jive talk and Berlitz Russian for social philosophy.")

Better-informed readers know that Mr. Burgess has written many books, including nonfiction. A few know that he is also professionally concerned with music and phonetics, and that he is a lapsed Roman Catholic who wrote the screenplay for Franco Zeffirelli's *Jesus of Nazareth.*

It helps, in reading *You've Had Your Time,* to prepare yourself for Mr. Burgess's level of candor, which is pronounced without being exhibitionistic. And, one adds hastily, the documentation of his sexual biography is perfunctory, in contrast to Volume One (*Little Wilson and Big God*), although he is not engaged in concealing anything that interests him. Moreover, he is chronically broke, and he is hardly unaware of the nexus between sexual candor and sales. ("When book-buyers buy books, they look for sex, violence and hard information. They get these from Arthur Hailey, whose characters discuss problems of hotel management while committing adultery before being beaten up.")

Accordingly, the reader must not be put off by casual reference to his polymathic pursuits, which as they come in at us, chapter after chapter, sometimes page after page, yield up finally a pointillist portrait of the man whose autobiography we are reading: "I assessed works on anthropology and sociology and structuralism in a variety of languages . . . and was paid a guinea per report." "By the end of 1961 I had published seven novels and a history of English literature." "I was paid . . . £3,000 for writing the history of a great metropolitan real property corporation." "In 1964, I tried to celebrate the quatercentenary by publicly reciting Shakespeare in Elizabethan phonemes." "Like Dr. Johnson, I would write on anything. I even became an abortive lexicographer." "I was able to write a long article on Shakespeare and music for the *Musical Times* and to give a talk on the same subject, with musical illustrations, in the BBC's *Music Magazine.*"

"Verse is for learning by heart, and that is what a literary education should mostly consist of. I know the whole of Hopkins by heart, a good deal of Marvell, many of Pound's Cantos and most of Eliot. Also the lyrics of Lorenz Hart and Cole Porter." "I proposed some day to write a novel from the viewpoint of a homosexual and achieved this in 1980." "Giuseppe Gioacchino Belli was the great master of the dialect and a scholarly recorder of the filth and blasphemy. He wrote 2,279 sonnets in Romanesco, and one of my tasks became the translation of some of these into Lancashire English." "I had for some time past toyed with the notion of writing a Regency novel, a kind of Jane Austen parody, which should follow the pattern of a Mozart symphony." "After the success of *Cyrano de Bergerac,* he [the director of the play] wanted another new translation of a classic play, and he first proposed *Peer Gynt* . . . I began to work on my Norwegian." "Later we [Mr. Burgess and the composer Stanley Silverman] were to work together on a production of *Oedipus Tyrannus* in my translation."

"I had a novel in mind, one based on the structuralist theories of Claude Lévi-Strauss, but [his publisher] grew gloomy when I gave him an outline. It is unwise ever to give a publisher an outline, unless that outline is a catalogue of modes of fornication: it is like playing the proposed themes of a symphony with one finger." "I could take over [he had been offered] the chair of the retiring Lionel Trilling at Columbia." "I then started drafting a musical version of *Ulysses*. I had no piano at the time . . . and had to rely on my inner ear to assess its tonalities." "The Russian translation [of *A Clockwork Orange*] I read with interest." "I took the New Testament [to the film site of *Jesus of Nazareth*] in Greek, in order to get a fresh or original look at it." "I have started to read Hebrew." "This was in connection with the performance of a work of mine in Geneva, a twenty-five-minute composition for two flutes, two oboes, two clarinets, two bassoons, one horn, one trumpet, timpani, piano, vibraphone, xylophone and glockenspiel."

In the book's last page he resolves to "dig myself deeper into Europe with an opera based on the life of Sigmund Freud." Do not suppose that such challenges are glibly met. For instance, on the Freud opera there is the problem of the baritone's libretto, which will be set in Viennese German. *But*—"I do not know whether this can be done. It will be hard to find a baritone willing to stop singing halfway through because Freud's voice has been stilled by cancer of the jaw. Anna Freud, soprano, takes over from him, and, in a final fantasy before death, he recovers the tones of a denouncing prophet to smash the tables of the law upon cowering Jung, Adler, Rank and Ferenczi. It seems to me that here we have a golden opportunity to use atonality and profound dissonance to represent the workings of the unconscious, while conscious action can be conveyed through the tonalism of Mahlerian music, café waltzes, bands in the park."

Now if the above has bored you, you were not meant to read *You've Had Your Time*. But I am reminded that I was once required ever so gently to tell a lady on my left that she ought to consider the possibility that if indeed Bach bores her, it is her problem, not his. The reader is, however, entitled to ask: is there a human narrative under this truckload of cultural petit point? Not a whole lot, to tell the truth, but some.

At the beginning, a doctor tells Mr. Burgess (at the age of forty-one) that he has one year to live, and so he resolves to write two thousand words per day to accumulate a little money for his imminent widow. That many words a day "means a yearly total of 730,000. Step up the rate and, without undue effort, you can reach a million. This ought to mean ten novels of 100,000 words each." He didn't meet his goal: "I was not able to achieve more than five and a half novels of very moderate size." Later he adds: "I do not boast about the quality of my work, but I may be permitted to pride myself on the gift of steady application." He can do a lot more than that, by my standards. In talking about the Roman *scippatori,* those youthful bandits on Vespas who career by you and snatch purses and briefcases, he records that one summer "I wrote a book on the language of James Joyce, I carried it in its Gucci case towards a Xerox shop to be copied, but it was *scippato* on the way. The typescript was presumably fluttered into the Tiber or Tevere and the case sold for a few thousand lire." Causing him to do what? Go off to a monastery for the rest of his life? Commit suicide? Not at all. "I had to write the book again, not with too much resentment: it was probably better the second time." Mr. Burgess is not like ordinary people. Not even like ordinary writers.

He does not die, but his wife (who never reads his books and is never boring) mostly drinks gin and dies for having overdone it, and he is more shocked than pained. But lo, a one-night stand with an Italian academician, it transpires, bore hidden fruit, and she appears on the scene with their four-year-old son. The author is taken by the woman, for which reason, and also to save the boy from bastardy, they are married. The ensuing chapters take us to Malta, Italy and New York.

Everywhere they go Mr. Burgess has experiences worth recording—if the recorder is as observant and as gifted as Mr. Burgess . . . as a writer, [he] is not universally admired. He quotes liberally his critical detractors: "A viscous verbiage . . . which is the swag-bellied offspring of decay," or (my favorite) "It would be helpful if Mr. Burgess would indicate whether these poems are meant to be good or bad." He amuses himself by reviewing one of his own novels under a pseudonym, from which review he quotes: "This is, in many ways, a dirty book. It is full of bowel-blasts and flatulent borborygmus, emetic meals . . . and halitosis." On the whole he is at war with the critical community, primarily because critics do not help the author cure his own weaknesses, primarily because they (we) cannot spot these weaknesses, or if we can, cannot prescribe for them.

Anthony Burgess flees England eventually, in part because the cultural implications of the class system there forbid him access to readers who might otherwise celebrate his achievements, and partly because he finds life under socialism asphyxiative. He is accused by a tabloid of behaving like the rat who leaves a sinking ship, to which he comments that "rats are wise to leave sinking ships." And he succeeds, imperfectly, in putting England out of mind; but, one is here and there reminded ("I was always ready to call on my abandoned faith when I lacked the courage to make my own moral decisions") he has not succeeded altogether as a lapsed

Catholic. He continues to wonder about hell and about purgatory and though he is oppressed by many problems, he has the satisfaction of knowing what they are, and fights, to quote the phrase, "against the dying of the light," because his mortality means not only "works never to be written, it is a matter of things unlearned."

Is he happy? One would think it impudent to ask Mr. Burgess so private a question. He surprises us by asking it of himself: "Am I happy? Probably not." But he has certainly earned his keep, and the reader's time.

—APRIL 28, 1991

NEW YORK TIMES BOOK REVIEW

Two inspired, practically perfect matchups of book to reviewer were commissioned by the editors of *The New York Times Book Review*. The first, an assignment for WFB to review the massive two-volume work of Henry James on the subject of travel; the other a book by two unknown authors on sailing, about which more later.

HENRY JAMES: COLLECTED TRAVEL WRITINGS

Great Britain and America: English Hours, The American Scene, Other Travels. By Henry James. Edited by Richard Howard. The Library of America.

HENRY JAMES: COLLECTED TRAVEL WRITINGS

The Continent: A Little Tour in France, Italian Hours, Other Travels. By Henry James. Edited by Richard Howard. The Library of America.

It fair takes your breath away. Page after page, chapter after chapter; cities, towns, villages, churches, monuments, in country after country, described and probed by a belletrist with a mighty, enchanted caduceus in hand. He uses it to crown in elaborate liturgical ceremony the glories of man and nature, but also to squirt ice water on those aspects of the world and its inhabitants that are not, well, not according to Henry James. And, manifestly, he has all the time in the world at his disposal.

But then what accumulates is more than most readers have time for, even though we must all marvel at what we read. In 1897, when in his mid-fifties, Henry James complained of soreness in his wrist. This can hardly surprise us. (He thenceforward dictated to a secretary.) In 1909, he burned forty years' worth of letters and papers, and one can't seriously suppose that he found the time to reread them before burning them—not at the pace at which he wrote and in the hours left over from his work. A year later, he spoke of having had "a sort of nervous breakdown." Might this have been a reaction to the consuming demands of his creative curiosity? Five years after that, he decided to make his expatriation official and so became a British subject. The following year, in 1916, he was dead, at seventy-two. A prodigious talent, and a most industrious artisan. Perhaps his biographer, Leon Edel, has calculated the size of his total output. The Library of America's two tightly formatted volumes of his *Collected Travel Writings* (*Great Britain and America* and *The Continent*) I estimate at about three quarters of a million words. Approximately the size of a nine-hundred-page issue of *Time* magazine, back when *Time* printed mostly text.

He was very famous, though not very rich. (Edith Wharton sneaked a few thousand pounds into his bank account.) He was the gregarious bachelor, fiercely conventional, who recorded that he had dined out 105 times in one London social season. During the Civil War, when he was studying law at Harvard, he grew a beard. When he was fifty-seven, he got rid of it, because it had turned white. He was close to his siblings; his brother William, the preeminent philosopher, was as famous as he. He spent time with Flaubert, Zola, Stevenson, Maupassant, Conrad, Browning, Kipling, Shaw and Wells, and wrote enduring novels, including *The Wings of the Dove, The Portrait of a Lady* and *The Ambassadors.* As a gift to celebrate his seventieth birthday, his friends gave him his portrait, done by Sargent. King George V gave him the Order of Merit, an award reserved for the very few, the mightiest in talent and achievement. His novels transformed the model, with their stream of consciousness and their literary hauteur— as much so as, a generation later, Hemingway's would do, in a very different mode.

What runs through the mind, then, of the reader of these travel pieces? Two things. The first is that nobody, except for Eagle Scouts in graduate schools, is going to read the entire text. The second? You can close your eyes and open either volume at any page and find yourself reading prose so resplendent it will sweep you off your feet. Yet after a while, after a long while, you will recognize that, really, you have to come down to earth because there are so many other things to do. And besides, if you stay with him for too long, in that engrossing, scented, colored, brilliant, absorbing world, you feel strung out, feel something like hanging moss.

For instance? In his incessant travels, one day he leaves Italy to go to Germany. Henry James does not gad about the world with his mind shut or his pen locked in his drawer. As he once put it, "I have it on my conscience to make a note of my excursion." So how does one square things with one's conscience upon traveling to Germany from Italy? One ruminates on the differences between the two countries. Read how Henry James does it, and abandon any hope of competing with him:

"A few weeks ago I left Italy in that really demoralized condition into which Italy throws those confiding spirits who give her unlimited leave to please them. Beauty, I had come to believe, was an exclusively Italian possession, the human face was not worth looking at unless redeemed by an Italian smile, nor the human voice worth listening to unless attuned to Italian vowels. A landscape was no landscape without vines festooned to fig-trees swaying in a hot wind—a mountain a hideous excrescence unless melting off into a Tuscan haze. But now that I have absolutely exchanged vines and figs for corn and cabbages, and violet Apennines for the homely plain of Frankfurt, and liquids for gutturals, and the Italian smile for the German grin, I am much better contented than I could have ventured to expect. I have shifted my standard of beauty, but it still commands a glimpse of the divine idea."

As one might put it today, "*That's* what I call being transported!"

James's little paeans are not easily duplicated, even those that are, so to speak, given *en passant*. Walking through the streets of Eton one summer in the 1880s his mind turns to Winchester, the home of another great public school. He recalls "the courts of the old college, empty and silent in the eventide; the mellow light on the battered walls; the great green meadows, where the little clear-voiced boys made gigantic shadows; the neighborhood of the old cathedral city, with its admirable church, where early kings are buried—all this seemed to make a charming background for boyish lives, and to offer a provision of tender, picturesque memories to the grown man who has passed through it." This little recollection, mind you, only for the purpose of reassuring us that "Eton, of a clear June evening, must be quite as good, or indeed a great deal better."

The contrasts are sharply drawn. There is the other face of England, as seen aboard a steamer cruising the "sordid river-front" in London. "For miles and miles you see nothing but the sooty backs of warehouses, or perhaps they are the sooty faces: in buildings so utterly expressionless it is impossible to distinguish. They stand massed together on the banks of the wide turbid stream, which is fortunately of too opaque a quality to reflect the dismal image. . . . The river is almost black, and is covered with black barges; above the black housetops, from among the far-stretching docks and basins, rises a dusky wilderness of masts. The little puffing steamer is dingy and gritty—it belches a sable cloud that keeps you company as you go. In this carboniferous shower your companions, who belong chiefly, indeed, to the classes bereft of luster, assume an harmonious grayness; and the whole picture, glazed over with the glutinous London mist, becomes a masterly composition."

———

In 1904, Henry James had been away from America for twenty years. The death of his parents in 1882 was one reason for not returning; then, too, "the Atlantic voyage" could be counted "even with the ocean in a fairly good humor, an emphatic zero in the sum of one's better experience." And so he gave us extensive impressions of what he saw ("If one is bent upon observation nothing . . . is trivial"). James is now acknowledged as an expatriate. He is a little bit disoriented: "It is of extreme interest to be reminded . . . that it takes an endless amount of history to make even a little tradition, and an endless amount of tradition to make even a little taste, and an endless amount of taste, by the same token, to make even a little tranquillity. Tranquillity results largely from taste tactfully applied, taste lighted above all by experience and possessed of a clue for its labyrinth."

Yet James's fondness for England, though vividly expressed, is not, I concluded after reading his tributes to New England, Italy, France and Germany, by any means exclusive. But, then, wherever he travels, the critical eye is alert: "I had just come in, and, having attended to the distribution of my luggage, sat down to consider my habitation." And so there is, almost always, perspective, so often leavening. And he can be severe. About Geneva he writes that its "moral tone" is "epigrammatically, but on the whole justly, indicated by the fact, recently related to me by a discriminating friend, that, meeting one day in the street a placard of the theater, superscribed *Bouffes-Genevois,* he burst into irrepressible laughter. To appreciate the irony of the phrase one must have lived long enough in Geneva to suffer from the want of humor in the local atmosphere, and the absence, as well, of that esthetic character which is begotten of a generous view of life."

O.K. But what about the Swiss in general? They have, we are informed, "apparently, an insensibility to comeliness or purity of form—a partiality to the clumsy, coarse, and prosaic, which one might almost interpret as a calculated offset to their great treasure of natural beauty, or at least as an instinctive protest of the national genius for frugality."

About the English, James was hardly the sycophant. In these travel writings he trains his eyes on national characteristics. He thinks it supremely a British endowment that they are a people disposed to let people alone. (Seventy-five years later, Anthony Burgess would leave England because, under socialism, he complained that they no longer left people alone.) James observes a political demonstration of a kind that, in countries of volatile temperament, would very likely have caused some consternation. Not so in England, because of this "practice of letting people alone," of "the frank good sense and the frank good humor and even the frank good taste of it."

He will permit himself in specific circumstances to be adulatory. In respect of the ancient rivalry between Oxford and Cambridge, Henry James might have instructed Solomon: "If Oxford were not the finest thing in England the case would be clearer for Cambridge. . . . Oxford lends sweetness to labor and dignity to leisure. When I say Oxford I mean Cambridge, for a stray savage is not the least obliged to know the difference, and it suddenly strikes me as being both very pedantic and very good-natured in him to pretend to know it."

Since his formal mandate in these pieces, many of them written for *The Nation,* was to talk of travel, he talks of the people the traveler comes upon. He compares the Brit to the Yankee in what are, strictly speaking, sociological asides:

"The English have more time than we, they have more money, and they have a much higher relish for active leisure. . . . A large appetite for holidays, the ability not only to take them but to know what to do with them when taken, is the sign of a robust people, and judged by this measure we Americans are sadly inexpert. Such holidays as we take are taken very often in Europe, where it is sometimes noticeable that our privilege is rather heavy on our hands."

Concerning the deportment of travelers, of "tourists," as we would now describe them, James is not unaffected by class prejudices, which is not to say that he should have been. On the one hand, he is easygoingly tolerant about young-blood licentiousness at the races at Epsom, commenting on "a coach drawn up beside the one on which I had a place," in which "a party of opulent young men were passing from stage to stage of the higher beatitude with a zeal which excited my admiration." However, on British women of another class than those who sat in coaches at Epsom getting drunk, he hands down opinions that achieve credibility by the authority with which they are stated. The reader doesn't think of James as motivated by snobbishness, and he is not condescending or in any way bent on inducing contempt. He is pronouncing on how people are. "She is useful, robust, prolific, excellently fitted to play the somewhat arduous part allotted to her in the great scheme of English civilization," he says of the working-class British woman, "but she has not those graces which enable her to lend herself easily to the decoration of life."

Elsewhere, he is, by his standards, blunt on the matter of some habits of the British on holiday: "You must give up the idea of going to sit somewhere in the open air, to eat an ice and listen to a band of music. You will find neither the seat, the ice, nor the band; but on the other hand, faithful at once to your interest and your detachment, you may supply the place of these delights by a little private meditation on the deep-lying causes of the English indifference to them." Why? Well, he says, just think about it. "In such reflections nothing is idle—every grain of testimony counts; and one need therefore not be accused of jumping too suddenly from small things to great if one traces a connection between the absence of ices and music and the essentially hierarchical plan of English society. This hierarchical plan of English society is the great and ever-present fact to the mind of a stranger: there is hardly a detail of life that does not in some degree betray it."

James acknowledges his own preferences, his tastes, but he is not an epicurean or a snob, and in any case he was writing well before the age when tastes were transformed into social prejudices. But he unhesitatingly acknowledges a concern over human behavior and the implications of its neglect. Thus on British tourists visiting Westminster Abbey: "When I reached the Abbey I found a dense group of people about the entrance, but I squeezed my way through them and succeeded in reaching the threshold. Beyond this it was impossible to advance, and I may add that it was not desirable. I put my nose into the church and promptly withdrew it. The crowd was terribly compact, and beneath the Gothic arches the odor was not that of incense."

Did this reaction disturb him? "You feel yourself at times in danger of thinking meanly of the human personality; numerosity, as it were, swallows up quality, and the perpetual sense of other elbows and knees begets a yearning for the desert."

But in one essay Henry James, the great doctor of social manners, makes the definitive point. "It was, I think, the element of gentility that most impressed me. I know that the word I have just ventured to use is under the ban of contemporary taste; so I may as well say outright that I regard it as indispensable in almost any attempt at portraiture of English manners."

On his return to America, James isolated the special difficulty of American women of the affluent class in constituting a link in a social hierarchy. He observes that this is in part because they themselves lack truly institutional caste but also because there is a void in the next station up. American "ladies of the tiaras," lacking any access to royal courts, might instead settle for appearances at operas, "these occasions offering the only approach to the implication of the tiara known, so to speak, to the American law. Yet even here there would have been no one for them, in congruity and consistency, to curtsey to—their only possible course becoming thus, it would seem, to make obeisance, clingingly, to each other. This truth points again the effect of a picture poor in the male presence; for to what male presence of native growth is it thinkable that the wearer of an American tiara *should* curtsey?"

James is particularly rewarding in these copious travel writings when he engages his empirical strengths as an observer with his metaphysical imagination. He is, for instance, unable to discern the reason that affluent Americans at the turn of the century simply ignored the capacity of their clubs to accommodate that which clubs were so especially useful for, a neglect the clubs tended to share with the mansions of the wealthy:

"The American club struck me everywhere, oddly, considering the busy people who employ it, as much less an institution for attending to one's correspondence than others I had had knowledge of; generally destitute, in fact, of copious and various appliances for that purpose. There is such a thing as the imagination of the writing-table, and I nowhere, save in a few private houses, came upon its fruits; to which I must add that this is the one connection in which the provision for ease has not an extraordinary amplitude, an amplitude unequaled anywhere else." The American house, "with almost no one of its indoor parts distinguishable from any other is an affliction against which he has to learn betimes to brace himself."

Would he have said as much about contemporary arrangements? But, to begin with, there is very little club life in modern America, and the typical American who sets out to burn forty years of correspondence will not cause flame enough to heat a cup of tea.

Sometimes, whether plodding or coasting along these journals—and which of the two you find yourself reading can be a reflection as much of your own mood as of the caliber of James's performance—you might screech with impatience. As when you come upon constructions so periphrastic as to approach caricature:

"As for the author of that great chronicle which never is but always to be read"—it is not clear from the context whose journal James is referring to—"you may take your coffee of a morning in the little garden in which he wrote *finis* to his immortal work—and if the coffee is good enough to administer a fillip to your fancy, perhaps you may yet hear the faint reverberation among the trees of the long, long breath with which he must have laid down his pen."

Though one admires the filigree of it, if you wrap yourself in it too massively, you run the risk of choking. As in: "And what shall I say of the color of Wroxton Abbey, which we visited last in order and which in the thickening twilight, as we approached its great ivy-muffled face, laid on the mind the burden of its felicity?"

What we will say, Mr. James, is that you are a bloody genius, but sometimes you are too much. Too much in *this* day and age. Henry James's *Collected Travel Writings* are for long ocean trips and for monasteries, and for those happy to feel the great velveted halls of another, more deliberative age.

—WFB   DECEMBER 12, 1993

The other bit of casting now seems perfectly obvious: a book on sailing? Get Buckley, super-literate, a zealot on the sport, witty, etc. But the irony was that *The New York Times* had just decided to give up cover reviews in its book supplement and to give over the covers to art and a preview of what was within. So Buckley's review of an unheralded little book was the last front-page review in what the book trade refers to as the TBR.

Few knew the *Times*'s motive in eliminating the cover review—to get people to look inside, for example? Anyhow, there was in the air in other quarters some suspicion that print had lost its punch, that "position" didn't matter much anymore. Time was when the cover of *Time* meant virtually certain best-sellerdom, if devoted to a book or author; when a review in the daily *New York Times* was among the most potent forces attracting attention, pro or con, to a new book; when the cover of the *TBR* was akin to the Book-of-the-Week Award. But these and similar sources weren't causing the phone to ring as much as it did in the past.

Then, Buckley, almost anachronistically, wrote his review.

My Old Man and the Sea: A Father and Son Sail Around Cape Horn. By David Hays and Daniel Hays. Algonquin Books of Chapel Hill.

The story is of a voyage done ten years ago on a sailboat by a father (David, as he is everywhere designated, was fifty-four) and his son (Dan, twenty-four). *Sparrow* is 25 feet long. Dan sailed it mostly single-handed from New London, Connecticut, to Jamaica (seventy-eight days), where his father joined him. Together they sailed through the Panama Canal and on to the Galápagos Islands, then Easter Island—and then around the Horn to the Falkland Islands. From there David flew home and Dan soloed *Sparrow* back to New London, putting in at Montevideo, Rio de

Janeiro and Antigua. The entire passage took 317 days, during which the boat traveled 17,000 miles. The account of the passage, related in alternating sections by father and son, will be read with delight one hundred years from now.

What prompted it all? "The voyage was my idea," David writes. " 'Let's do the big one, Dan,' I said. 'The Horn.'

" 'Where's that, Dad?' he asked.

" 'What had I wrought?' "

Answer: a captivatingly unusual and gifted son, as *My Old Man and the Sea* makes clear. Daniel Hays knew very well what and where the Horn is and what it signifies. But he was only twenty back then, a nonchalant college student, breezy, a little cheeky. David Hays served as artistic director of the National Theater of the Deaf (and continues to do so) and is an obsessive sailor. He had taken Dan out for his first sail at the age of three.

"Why Cape Horn?" David asked himself. "Maybe because I grew up sailing with my father and brother and with salts who whispered the great name the way elderly aunts whisper *cancer.* 'The Horn can be tranquil,' one sailor said, but 'The Horn' was whispered."

It took them two years, nights, weekends, hours before breakfast, all summer long, to prepare the 25-foot *Sparrow.* Why so small a boat? "Because this is as big a boat as we could afford to perfect, as we understood that inexact word," David writes. "Dan and I shared a desire for a boat that one of us could strip of canvas in less than a minute in suddenly bad winds."

On arriving in Jamaica, Dan passed judgment on *Sparrow*—"this perfect boat, which I made and sailed." ("She feels big below without an engine," David notes. "There's something perversely snug about being that tight to the water, to every wrinkle in its skin, like a chip of wood or a corked bottle.") "Everything below," Dan noted in his journal, "that is not attached is encased. . . . My theory is that *Sparrow* will be rolled over completely and since I hate mess, I didn't want to clean up afterward as well as prevent her from sinking. Actually Dad and I disagree about messes. . . . But we agree about wanting to sink neatly."

Dan had an unexpected companion: Tiger, a red-and-white kitten all but dumped on board, at the moment of leaving, by a friend. It would become a great romance, Dan and Tiger: "Tiger steps off the cabin top onto my shoulder, nestles into my jacket and settles right on my chest. He looks up. 'Whatcha doing?'

" 'Writing about this very moment,' I say.

" 'Am I in it?' he says, chewing the edge of my notebook."

Yes, Dan says, and threatens to edit the cat out if a certain misbehavior is repeated. "He closes his eyes and smiles, knowing he can and I won't."

The boat is of course self-steering, and Dan's skills as a celestial navigator are highly developed. But without an engine, without radar, the responsibilities of piloting heighten. "I fall asleep on deck for a couple of hours," Dan notes. "I wake as *Sparrow* lifts and a loud roar—not from any direction but all around—fills my ears. I jerk up and see a beach and house looming directly ahead. Waves are breaking *on the beach* only 50 yards from *Sparrow*'s bow! . . . I envision *Sparrow* as she would have been: lying on her side, waves and sand crashing on us. My home, on a beach."

He can see the headline: "BOY WRECKS FATHER'S YACHT ON CALM NIGHT, DRINKING SUSPECTED."

Dan is resourceful. "I love being self-sufficient. To me that has always meant having the right *stuff* for any emergency." He lists the contents of his car back home, approximately 200 items, including 200 feet of parachute cord and a copy of *Winnie the Pooh*: "I mean, you could drop me in the middle of Africa with my car and I'd either drive out or set up an entire new Western civilization based on consumption."

Page after page the observations, of father as well as son, engross the reader by what they choose to observe and by how they do so, always letting us hear the music of the sea and of their company. "After dinner we swim," Dan writes, "making ourselves seem angels of glow light with the phosphorescent creatures—water fireflies—that our arms and legs disturb."

They spend a full week in Panama, going over every square inch of *Sparrow* with a fine-tooth comb. Many miles out, flying fish plop into the cockpit. "We've had a few, and they were good," Dan writes. "I thought briefly of how right it is—even natural—to gather protein from the sea, how insignificant this creature is—so abundant in the ocean that he randomly flew into my boat—out where the word 'vast' does not describe— does not even begin to pull the strings of thought into existence of how big the sea is. I let him go. Maybe to atone for past murders, injuries to life, or maybe because I want to later on justify what I will do, as if there were a karma currency. I feel happy."

He woke two mornings later to a vision of big waves: "During the night there were many squalls and the seas built to over 12 feet. They are long slow rollers like passionate sex and locomotives. I can see the horizon only for a moment when we balance at the crest—then we slide into a blue valley."

The father admires his son's skills. "Dan had hardly ever steered by tiller, but his skill was marvelous, undoubtedly honed by hours of handling the joystick in video-game parlors. He looked possessed. Horsemen have their centaurs, why don't we sailors have a name for the half-man, half-boat that Dan was at that moment?"

David had wondered what it would be like to spend one hundred days "rarely more than three feet apart" from his son in such circumstances. When Dan went off to Washington State to college, David wrote to him every day. "I needed it," David recalls. "He didn't." He spotted now in his athletic son "for the first time, in just a flicker across his face, his distress that I was becoming old." And occasionally Dan squirms: "We're balancing on a tightrope. On one side is our love as father and son, on the other is the way we work as a grown-up team. And the tightrope, woven from a web of all the things that have happened, holds us up."

There was no problem of boredom. "We always had chatter," David writes, "a lifetime of shared projects, as much to talk about as an old married couple, and no awe." And Tiger was an unending joy for Dan: "Tiger and I are so cool—he'll jump in from the hatch, landing expertly on the foul-weather-gear bin. I'm leaning against it, writing and wearing headphones, and I feel him thump land. I immediately turn to touch noses with him. 'Getting any?' he asks. 'Yah, as much as you!' He turns and goes off to cat fantasy."

Sparrow makes ready to leave Galápagos for Easter Island, where wife/mother Leonora will be with them for a week before they set out for Cape Horn. Dan evidently thinks the moment appropriate to send his mother a letter, sort of balancing the books. David had recalled one scene between mother and son, years ago. "Dan, even at eleven, hated to see that self-destruction," David writes of his wife's smoking and Dan's complaint about it one night at supper. " 'My son,' said Leonora. . . . 'I smoke. That's the way I am, Dan, that's the real me, and you just have to live with it.' Dan thought for a moment, then reached over and snatched the cigarette out of her mouth and dropped it into her glass of wine. She started to yell and he said, calmly, 'I just put out your cigarette in your wine. That's me. That's the way I am, the real me, your son.' "

So now the son writes to his mother. "Dear Mom, Did I ever ask you to forgive me for being such a jerk . . . for so many years?" he says in a joyful mix of conceit and submission. "I would like to be forgiven. I want you to know that I forgive you for all the things that I thought/think you did to me. I do. You are hereby forgiven and O.K. as you are. I still have trouble there—I always want people to be how I think they should be to be happier. . . . You're O.K. with me and I love you very much. Love, Dan." Father and son arrive at Easter Island twenty-seven days later, and when they meet the plane bringing in Leonora, "Mom comes bounding off the plane, with the instinct gear set at high, immediately tucking in my shirt," Dan writes. As usual I'm a little embarrassed as she introduces me to half the people on the plane as 'the most beautiful child ever.' I'm eight years old, again."

Now only Cape Horn matters. "One day," David records, "I sewed for fourteen hours to make a canvas envelope to hold our life ring." At sea, he surveyed the scene and drew from it a kind of heroic satisfaction: "My cup of chocolate would be wedged into the corner of the fence that rims the stove, which also swung with the lamp and the shadows. Forward, in the peak of the boat, a string hammock that held rolls of paper towels, spare line, and the spare paddle to the Navik [steering gear] would also be moving, barely seen except as its extended shadow, and the whole side of the boat seemed to breathe as we moved. It was never quiet, but the whooshes, the thumps, and even the thuds were mellow."

He recalls voyages past: "We would hover a moment and then fall forward in slow motion into troughs too deep and dark to see their bottoms, troughs that brought to mind nightmares of bared rocks at the bottom of black waterless pits. You could imagine plunging down and being shattered into a million bits of wood and steel and bone. We fell and splintered the water into a thousand white birds that burst like ducks from the water."

They spy the Horn. Dan: "Day 178. . . . I'm too excited to sleep. To see land after twenty-four days at sea. I'd planned to put on my wet suit and swim away to get a picture of *Sparrow* in front of the Horn, but when we are actually there the thought raises the hairs on my teeth. Dad agrees. He had thought of going up to it—I guess for forty years—and now he's too awed and wants to leave it to itself."

But they had made the passage, survived.

The ride to the Falklands was rough and cold. David had written that his abiding terror was of rising to see his son gone, swept out to sea (the rule was always to be tethered to the lifeline). That didn't happen to Dan (though he came close), but on Day 200 he rose and looked about the tiny boat: "I can't find Tiger: he's not on board."

He writes Leonora: "Dear Mom, Gloomy day—last night, Tiger fell overboard and all day my head's been full of images of him—there's this vacuum where he was—there's no meowing, purring, cuddling or playing. So many things in that sweet fur. He's been on for ten thousand miles exactly, so I guess he was a ten-thousand-mile cat—one thousand miles for each life and one extra because he was so loving. Dismal." He usually finds a good side in bad events, he writes. "But here, not much comes up. Mortality sucks. Love, Dan." That elegy is enduringly beautiful.

What happened, along the way to the Horn, was that the father recognized the earned seniority of the son and got out of the way, to the extent that's possible in a boat the size of *Sparrow.* He made Dan captain. "What changed? A year after the voyage, my wife, Leonora, asked me who my ideal person was. 'You know,' she said, 'a hero, growing up.' The faces flickered in front of my eyes—Abraham Lincoln, my father, Judge Brandeis, Lou Gehrig, Franklin Delano Roosevelt, Arturo Toscanini, my older brother, my father.

" 'My son,' I blurted out and started to cry."

My Old Man and the Sea will do that to everyone who reads it, will make you cry and smile and exult, even. It is an engrossingly beautiful tale of adventure of the spirit, aboard a little boat that dared great deeds.

JULY 23, 1995

———

WFB had called Algonquin, ordered copies of the book as gifts, said he would review it. Christopher Lehmann-Haupt also praised the book in the daily *New York Times*, as did the reviewers for *Sail*, and *Eco Traveller*, and *Yankee*. By August 1995 the book had been through nine printings, by November had some 117,500 copies in print, was on *The New York Times* best-seller list, and stayed there for three months. It had become the first best-seller (but not the first good book) from Algonquin in Chapel Hill.

———

As with Le Carré, with whom he has political differences, Buckley finds much to praise in the work of John Updike, who has powers of description that WFB claims not to have, meanwhile sacrificing sheer narrative drive, which to Buckley, as with more overtly popular novelists, is a major goal. In the case of Le Carré and Updike, it is the marvelous play of language itself which animates Buckley's admiration. A subtle, perhaps, but nice distinction in a field where novelist-reviewers are apt to praise only the kind of books they themselves write.

This review appeared in *New York* magazine.

———

The Coup. By John Updike. Knopf.

The piano people have taken to letting down a gauze curtain to prevent the judges from being influenced by the persona of the contestant. That way, you simply sit and listen, oblivious of musically extrinsic factors. If one did not know, and went through *The Coup,* it would I think drive the reader mad guessing the name of its author. Except that geniuses collaborate only on behalf of Medici, and they are dead, one would think that this novel was written by Antoine de Saint-Exupéry, to whom descriptions of the wind, the sand, and the stars were assigned; Lawrence Durrell (smells, sensuality); Gabriel García Márquez (tribal life); Mary Renault (exotic evocation); and Vladimir Nabokov (philological radiance). If one goes on to ask the question, Would one want to read a single novel composed by these writers, the answer is: John Updike proves that the answer is yes, *God* yes.

The Coup is not to be missed, and it doesn't terribly matter whether you read it from the beginning, or backward, or every other page, though there are no bad pages in it, provided you go in recognizing that John Updike would rather describe than narrate. The muzzle velocity of some of the action in this novel validates the law of Zeno that an arrow shot at the wall opposite will never reach there for having forever to cut the intervening distance in halves. But one does not mind, because every verbal distraction is felicitous ("After the loss of Sheba [the girl], such a fall [the coup] followed as one segment of a telescope brings with it another, slightly smaller. No one to blow me, no one to bow to me. *Takbir!*"). Well, sometimes there is an admixture of verbal virtuosity and leg-pull, as when the protagonist, the mad black superliterate colonel, determined that his vast parched country shall perish from starvation rather than admit U.S. bubble gum, reproaches his lieutenant for not having shot up a bunch of vaguely irksome black and Arab tourists. He threatens the lieutenant with imperialism: "You will be Xed out by Exxon, engulfed by Gulf, crushed by the U.S., disenfranchised by France. . . ." Hmm.

In this book *everybody* is fluent, poetic. Styron's Nat Turner was illiterate by contrast with Updike's corporals. But there is rhythmic wit everywhere. The black attendant at the drugstore of the border town where Western technology is insinuated behind the colonel's back replies to the disguised dictator (the colonel travels everywhere anonymously) when asked if there is a soda fountain,

> "Such frills went out of modern use years ago when the minimum wage for soda jerks went sky high. You are living in the past, it seems. A machine that vends cans of soft drinks purrs in the rear of the store, next to the rack of plastic eggs holding gossamer panty hose. Take care, my friend, not to drop the pull-tab, once removed, back into the can. Several customers of mine have choked to death in that manner. We call it the Death of the Last Drop."

John Updike once said, on being reproached for having given up a formula so successful when he wrote *The Centaur,* that there is no point in reiterating a success (even as Thoreau abandoned his factory after consummating the definitive pencil). And so he rolls on with his experiments, playing this time with Africa, ideologues, racism. Does he harbor strategic political designs? On occasion he sounds as though he were Malcolm X avenging Evelyn Waugh's *Black Mischief.* Thus, attending a college in the

Middle West before returning to Africa to take power, the protagonist lunches with his girl friend's father, who slugs a little whiskey and decides patronizingly to talk to the black foreigner as though he were fully grown . . .

> "Feelicks, if I'm not being too personal, what's your major going to be at McCarthy [College]?"
> "Freshmen are not required to declare, but I had thought Government, with a minor in French Literature."
> "French Literature, what the hell use would that be to your people? . . ."
> "In the strange climate of my native land, Mr. Cunningham, the literature the French brought us may transplant better than the political institutions. There is a dryness in Racine, a harshness in Villon, that suits our case."

There *is* a narrative—of a fanatic brought down by forces not so different from those he so eloquently and ingeniously despises, but forces which have a peculiar faculty for finding ways to feed people who would otherwise starve; and therefore, not altogether bad. What happens to the fictitious country of Kush after they get rid of the colonel is a vulgar fecundity, not to be confused with John Updike's, which is all mead.

—WFB   DECEMBER 18, 1978

Chapter 17

On Saying Good-bye (or) The Art of the Obituary & the Eulogy

Said *Time:* "A good obituary is always hard to write. Celebrating well-lived lives, marking the passage of exemplary men and women—this is a journalistic task with a whiff of the sacred about it." (*Time* magazine, October 2, 1995)

In WFB's case the task is not just journalistic, but a final act of friendship and in some cases love. Even the deaths of his antagonists bring out the courtesies of the man. He never disguises their differences but buries them with the deceased.

Buckley's usually brief obits are as much a feature of his magazine, his writing, and his character as the "Notes & Asides" columns. In finding the right language with which to say farewell, he puts words to a noble purpose.

These examples are limited to only those persons whose lives were, at least in part, remarkable for their writing. WFB does not write most of them as mini-biographical sketches, preferring instead to strive for essence rather than comprehensive treatment—with notable exceptions.

E. E. CUMMINGS, R.I.P.

As in the case of so many artists, what first brought e. e. cummings to public attention was a novel outward trait that over the years proved to have only minor inward meaning: the decapitalizations, especially of the first person singular pronoun and his own name. His oddities of punctuation, syntax and word-splitting were more serious, for through them he aimed at, and sometimes achieved, a kind of verbal analogue of the multi-dimensional simultaneity of certain paintings of Picasso and other twentieth-century artists—an effect which, curiously enough, Cummings never sought in his own rather straightforward paintings. Cummings's eccentricities, in life and in art, were never trivial because they were among the means that he found to define himself as a free individual in a society that makes this so difficult and continuous a task. Like William Faulkner, Cummings never succumbed to any of the political ideologies that periodically swept the intellectuals; and, though he knew and was known by everyone in literature and the arts, he stayed remarkably clear even of the changing literary cliques and fashions. He hated despotism and war—his splendid novel, *The Enormous Room,* written after his experience as ambulance driver and internee in World War I, was a breathtaking commentary on both—but he was not afraid of them. He was a true poet and a true man, and we honor his memory.

      —WFB   SEPTEMBER 25, 1962

Truman Capote, R.I.P.

In Cold Blood, a nonfiction "novel" about two murderers, was probably Truman Capote's best book. Here he was able to apply his literary talents to the presentation of material derived from the external world, which excused him from having to imagine it. He did not have a powerful novelistic imagination, and in this, at least, he resembled Norman Mailer, whose *In Cold Blood* was *The Executioner's Song,* Mailer's best book.

Capote emerged at twenty-three with *Other Voices, Other Rooms,* emerged as a writer and as a personality. The photograph on the dust jacket, depicting a tiny androgynous dandy, reclining, with a blond doe's stare, established the identity. His prose style, which some admired and for which he himself claimed a great deal, reinforced that idea. It was off-beat in its focus on odd details, consistently alienated, and "fragrant"—music for chameleons indeed.

In his later years he had calamitous drug and alcohol problems, not so unusual for writers, and it is useless to try to diagnose his state of mind. Perhaps he had stretched his minor talent as far as it could go; perhaps, in his social life, he was, in Barbara Gordon's phrase, dancing as fast as he could. He died last week in Los Angeles, at the age of fifty-nine.

      —WFB   SEPTEMBER 21, 1984

STEWART ALSOP, R.I.P.

"A dying man needs to die, as a sleepy man needs to sleep, and there comes a time when it is wrong, as well as useless, to resist." These words—from Stewart Alsop's account of his own fatal illness, *Stay of Execution*—have been quoted endlessly in the days since he died, and their simple eloquence is of that kind that affects the hearer immediately and permanently. That is typical of his writing: gently penetrating, frank and critical, yet somehow comforting and even—despite his professed agnosticism—pious. Describing himself as a New Deal liberal, he took his subsequent positions cautiously, never drawn into partisan or ideological wars, his acuity and wide sympathies giving him an uncommon instinct for the political crux of an issue. If he usually wound up defending the status quo, it was because he knew how necessary to social harmony a status quo is, and because he never descried a more humane one on the horizon. Nobody spoke better for the liberal establishment, or better embodied what virtues it has.

—WFB   JUNE 21, 1974

In writing of his mother, Bill backs off from brevity, understandably.

ALOISE STEINER BUCKLEY, R.I.P.

She bore ten children, nine of whom have written for this journal, or worked for it, or both, and that earns her, I think, this half-acre of space normally devoted to those whose contributions are in the public mode. Hers were not. If ever she wrote a letter to a newspaper, we don't remember it, and if she wrote to a congressman or senator, it was probably to say that she wished him well, and would pray for him as she did regularly for her country. If she had lived one day more, she'd have reached her ninetieth birthday. Perhaps somewhere else one woman has walked through so many years charming so many people by her warmth and diffidence and humor and faith. I wish I might have known her, too.

ASB was born in New Orleans, her ancestors having come there from Switzerland some time before the Civil War. She attended Sophie Newcomb College but left after her second year in order to become a nurse, her intention being to go spiritedly to the front, Over there, Over there. But when the young aspiring nurses were given a test to ascertain whether they could cope with the sight of blood and mayhem, she fainted, and was disqualified. A year later she married a prominent thirty-six-year-old Texas-born attorney who lived and practiced in Mexico City, with which she had had ties because her aunt lived there.

She never lived again in New Orleans, her husband taking her, after his exile from Mexico (for backing an unsuccessful revolution that sought to restore religious liberty), to Europe, where his business led him. They had bought a house in Sharon, Connecticut, and in due course returned there. The great house where she brought us up still stands, condominiums now. But the call of the South was strong, and in the mid-thirties they restored an ante-bellum house in Camden, South Carolina. There she was wonderfully content, making others happy by her vivacity, her delicate beauty, her habit of seeing the best in everyone, the humorous spark in her eye. She never lost a Southern innocence in which her sisters even more conspicuously shared. One of her daughters was delighted on overhearing an exchange between her and her freshly widowed sister who had for fifty years been married to a New Orleans doctor and was this morning, seated on the porch, completing a medical questionnaire, checking this query, exxing the other. She turned to Mother and asked, "Darling, as girls did we have gonorrhea?"

Her cosmopolitanism was unmistakably Made-in-America. She spoke fluent French and Spanish with undiluted inaccuracy. My father, who loved her more even than he loved to tease her, and whose knowledge of Spanish was faultless, once remarked that in forty years she had never once placed a masculine article in front of a masculine noun, or a feminine article in front of a feminine noun, except on one occasion when she accidentally stumbled on the correct sequence, whereupon she stopped—unheard of in her case, so fluently did she aggress against the language—and corrected herself by changing the article: the result being that she spoke, in Spanish, of the latest encyclical of Pius XII, the Potato of Rome (*"Pio XII, la Papa de Roma"*). She would smile, and laugh compassionately, as though the joke had been at someone else's expense, and perhaps play a little with her pearls, just above the piece of lace she always wore in the V of the soft dresses that covered her diminutive frame.

There were rules she lived by, chief among them those she understood God to have specified, though she outdid Him in her accent on good cheer. And although Father was the unchallenged source of authority at home, she was unchallengeably in charge of arrangements in a house crowded with ten children and as many tutors, servants, and assistants. In the very late thirties her children ranged in age from one to twenty-one, and an in-built sense of the appropriate parietal arrangements governed the hour at which each of us should be back from wherever we were—away at the movies, or at a dance, or hearing Frank Sinatra sing in Pawling. The convention was inflexible. On returning, each of us would push, on one of the house's intercoms, the button that said, "ASB." The conversation, whether at ten when she was still awake, or at two when she had been two hours asleep, was always the same: "It's me, Mother." "Good night, darling." If—as hardly ever happened—it became truly late, and her mind had not recorded the repatriation of all ten of us, she would rise, and walk to the room of the missing child. If there, she would return to sleep, and remonstrate the next day on the forgotten telephone call. If not there, she would wait up, and demand an explanation.

Her anxiety to do the will of God was more than ritual. I wrote to her once early in 1963. Much of our youth had been spent in South Carolina, and the cultural coordinates of our household were Southern. But the times required that we look Southern conventions like Jim Crow hard in the face, and so I asked her how she could reconcile Christian fraternity with the separation of the races, a convention as natural in the South for a hundred years after the Civil War as women's suffrage became natural after their emancipation, and she wrote, "My darling Bill: This is not an answer to your letter, for I cannot answer it too quickly. It came this morning, and, of course, I went as soon as possible to the Blessed Sacrament in our quiet, beautiful little church here. And, dear Bill, I prayed *so* hard for *humility* and for wisdom and for guidance from the Holy Spirit. I know He will help me to answer your questions as He thinks they should be answered. I must pray longer before I do this."

A few years earlier she had raised her glass on my father's seventy-fifth birthday, to say: "Darling, here's to fifteen more years together, and then we'll both go." But my father died three years later. Her grief was profound, and she emerged from it through the solvent of prayer, her belief in submission to a divine order, and her irrepressible delight in her family, and friends. A few years later her daughter Maureen died at age thirty-one, and she struggled to fight her desolation, though not with complete success. Her oldest daughter, Aloïse, died three years later. And then, three months ago, her son John.

She was by then in a comfortable retirement home, totally absent-minded; she knew us all, but was vague about when last she had seen us, or where, and was given to making references, every now and then, to her husband, "Will," and the trip they planned next week to Paris, or Mexico.

But she sensed what had happened, and instructed her nurse (she was endearingly under the impression that she owned the establishment in which she had a suite) to drive her to the cemetery, and there, unknown to us until later that afternoon, she saw from her car, at the edge of an assembly of cars, her oldest son lowered into the earth. He had been visiting her every day, often taking her to a local restaurant for lunch, and her grief was, by her standards, convulsive; but she did not break her record—she never broke it—which was never, ever to complain, because, she explained, she could never repay God the favors He had done her, no matter what tribulations she might need to suffer.

Ten years ago, my wife and I arrived in Sharon from New York much later than we had expected, and Mother had given up waiting for us, so we went directly up to the guest room. There was a little slip of blue paper on the bed lamp, another on the door to the bathroom, a third on the mirror. They were: love notes, on her 3 × 5 notepaper, inscribed "Mrs. William F. Buckley." Little valentines of welcome, as though we had circled the globe. There was no sensation to match the timbre of her pleasure on hearing from you when you called her on the telephone, or the vibration of her embrace when she laid eyes on you. Some things truly are unique.

Five days before she died—one week having gone by without her having said anything, though she clutched the hands of her children and grandchildren as they came to visit, came to say good-bye—the nurse brought her from the bathroom to the armchair and—inflexible rule— put on her lipstick, and the touch of rouge, and the pearls. Suddenly, and for the first time since the terminal descent began a fortnight earlier, she reached out for her mirror. With effort she raised it in front of her face, and then said, a teasing smile on her face as she turned to the nurse, "Isn't it amazing that anyone so old can be so beautiful?" The answer, clearly, was, Yes, it was amazing that anyone could be so beautiful.

—WFB   APRIL 19, 1985

V.N.—R.I.P.

The cover of this magazine had gone to press when word came in that Vladimir Nabokov was dead. I am sorry—not for the impiety; sorry that VN will not see the cover . . . , which he'd have enjoyed. He'd have seen this issue days ahead of most Americans, because he received *National Review* by airmail, and had done so for several years. And when we would meet, which was every year, for lunch or dinner, he never failed to express pleasure with the magazine. In February, when I last saw him, he came down in the elevator, big, hunched, with his cane, carefully observed by Vera, white-haired, with the ivory skin and delicate features and beautiful face. VN was carrying a book, which he tendered me with some embarrassment—because it was inscribed. In one of his books, a collection of interviews and random fare, given over not insubstantially to the celebration of his favorite crotchets, he had said that one of the things he *never* did was inscribe books.

Last year, called back unexpectedly to New York, I missed our annual reunion. Since then I had sent him my two most recent books, and about these he now expressed hospitable enthusiasm as we sat down at his table in the corner of the elegant dining room of the most adamantly unchanged hotel in Europe: I cannot imagine, for all its recent architectural modernization, that the Montreux-Palace was any different before the Russian revolution.

He had been very ill, he said, and was saved by the dogged intervention of his son, Dmitri, who at the hospital ordered ministrations the poor doctors had not thought of—isn't that right, Vera? Almost right—Vera is a stickler for precision. But he was writing again, back to the old schedule. What was that schedule? (I knew, but knew he liked to tell it.) Up in the morning about six, read the papers and a few journals, then cook breakfast for Vera in the warren of little rooms where they had lived for seventeen years. After that he would begin writing, and would write all morning long, usually standing, on the cards he had specially cut to a size that suited him (he wrote on both sides, and collated them finally into books). Then a light lunch, then a walk, then a nap, and, in nimbler days, a little butterfly-chasing or tennis, then back to his writing until dinner time. Seven hours of writing, and he would produce 175 words. [What words!] Then dinner, and book reading, perhaps a game of Scrabble in Russian. A very dull life, he said chortling with pleasure, and then asking questions about America, deploring the infelicitous Russian prose of Solzhenitsyn, assuring me that I was wrong in saying he had attended the inaugural meeting of the Congress for Cultural Freedom—he had never attended *any* organizational meeting of anything—isn't that right, Vera? This time she nods her head and tells him to get on with the business of ordering from the menu. He describes with a fluent synoptic virtuosity the literary scene, the political scene, inflation, bad French, cupiditous publishers, the exciting breakthrough in his son's operatic career, and what am I working on now?

A novel, and you're in it.

What was that?

You and Vera are in it. You have a daughter, and she becomes a Communist agent.

He is more amused by this than Vera, but not all *that* amused. Of course I'll send it to you, I beam. He laughs—much of the time he is laughing. How long will it take you to drive to the airport in Geneva?

My taxi told me it takes "un petit heure."

Une petite heure [he is the professor]: that means fifty minutes. We shall have to eat quickly. He reminisces about his declination of my bid to go on *Firing Line*. It would have taken me *two weeks* of preparation, he says almost proudly, reminding me of his well-known rule against improvising.

Every word he ever spoke before an audience had been written out and memorized, he assured me—isn't that right, Vera? Well no, he would answer questions in class extemporaneously. Well *obviously!* He laughed. He could hardly program his students to ask questions to which he had the answers prepared! I demur: his extemporaneous style is fine, just fine; ah, he says, but before an audience, or before one of those . . . television . . . cameras, he would freeze. He ordered a brandy, and in a few minutes we rose, and he and Vera and I walked ever so slowly to the door. "As long as Western civilization survives," Christopher Lehmann-Haupt wrote in the *Times* last Tuesday, "his reputation is safe. Indeed, he will probably emerge as one of the greatest artists our century has produced." I said goodbye warmly, embracing Vera, taking his hand, knowing that probably I would never see again—never mind the artist—this wonderful human being.

—WFB   JULY 22, 1977

CLARE BOOTHE LUCE, R.I.P.

I first laid eyes on her in 1948. She was delivering the Keynote Address to the Republican Convention, and she said of Henry Wallace, who was running for President on the Progressive ticket, that he was "Joe Stalin's Mortimer Snerd."* They all rocked with laughter, and the critics, of course, bit her again.

I first met her at her quarters, on Fifth Avenue. She had telephoned and asked if I could come by to discuss the worsening crisis under President Diem in South Vietnam. I was there at four and she opened the door with paint brushes in one hand. I told her by all means to finish what she was doing before we got down to the problems of Southeast Asia, and so she led me happily to her atelier, but instead of herself painting, she undertook to teach me there and then how to use acrylics, launching me in a mute inglorious career. Two months later there came in the mail at my office a big manuscript pulsating with scorn and indignation over the treatment of President Diem by Washington, with special focus on Diem's sister-in-law, Madame Nhu. She called it "The Lady's Not for Burning." I put the article on the cover of the next issue of *National Review* and had a startled call from the press editor of *Newsweek*. He wished to know how it came about that . . . Clare Boothe Luce . . . was writing for . . . *National Review.* I told him solemnly (I could manage a hidden smile, since we were speaking by telephone): *tous les beaux esprits se rencontrent*—roughly translated, that beautiful spirits seek each other out. The following day, Presi-

---

* A corn-fed dummy, used by the ventriloquist Edgar Bergen.—Ed.

dent Diem and his brother, the Dragon Lady's husband, were murdered. The only happy result of that Byzantine mess, for me, was that I was never again out of touch with Clare Boothe Luce, for whom, months ago, my wife and I scheduled a dinner—at her request—to be held here, in New York, on September twenty-ninth, two weeks before she died.

I have thought a lot about her in the past few days and weeks. The last time we stayed with her in Honolulu we were met at the airport by her gardener, Tom. There were twelve of us for dinner. We were seated in her lanai, being served cocktails, while Tom was quietly lighting the outdoor gas lamps. Suddenly he fell. In minutes the ambulance arrived. Surrounded by Clare's anxious, silent guests, Tom was given artificial respiration. Clare gripped my hand and whispered to me: "Tom is going to die." There was dumb grief in her voice; and absolute finality. Two hours later, the hospital confirmed that Tom was dead. Clare said goodnight to her guests, and departed to keep the widow company.

Clare knew when an act was done. In so many respects, she was always a woman resigned.

I think back on her career . . . Look, you are a young, beautiful woman. Pearl Harbor was only yesterday, and you have spent several months poking about disconsolate Allied fronts in Asia and the Mideast. You have written a long analysis, cruelly objective, about Allied disorder, infinitely embarrassing to the Allies and correspondingly useful to the Axis powers. On the last leg of your journey, a sharp-eyed British customs officer in Trinidad insists on examining your papers. His eyes pass over your journal, he reads in it, snaps it shut, and calls in British security, which packs you off under house arrest. What do you do?

Well, if you are Clare Boothe Luce, you get in touch with the American consulate, and the American consulate gets a message through to your husband, Henry Luce. Mr. Luce calls General Donovan, the head of U.S. Intelligence. General Donovan arranges to appoint you *retroactively* an intelligence official of the United States Government. The British agree to let you fly to New York, and there they turn your report over to the British ambassador. He is so shaken by it that he instantly advises Winston Churchill of its contents. Churchill pauses from the war effort to cable back his regards to Clare, who meanwhile has been asked by the Joint Chiefs of Staff to brief them on her analyses, which, suitably bowdlerized, appear in successive issues of *Life* magazine and are a journalistic sensation.

Thus passeth a week in the life of the deceased.

The excitement and the glamour, the distinctions and the awards, a range of successes unequaled by any other American woman. But ten years later she was writing not about tanks and planes, but about the saints. She began coquettishly by quoting Ambrose Bierce, who had defined a saint as a "dead sinner, revised and edited."

But quickly, Clare Luce's tone of voice altered. She wrote that perspectives are very changed now. "Augustine," she said, "came into a pagan world turning to Christianity, as we have come into a Christian world turning towards paganism."

St. Augustine fascinated her. She wrote that "he explored his interior sufferings with the same passionate zeal with which he had explored exterior pleasures, and he quailed to the depths of his being at the [projected] cost of reforming himself. 'These petty toys of toys,'"—she quoted him—"'these vanities of vanities, my long-time fascinations, still held me. They plucked at the garment of my flesh, and murmured caressingly: Dost thou cast us off? From this moment shall this delight or that be no more lawful for thee forever?' Habit," Clare Luce commented, "whispered insistently in his ear: 'Dost thou think that thou canst live without these things?' And Augustine, haunted by Truth, hounded by Love, harried by Grace, 'had nothing at all to answer but those dull and dreary words: Anon, anon; or Presently, or, Leave me alone but a little while. . . .'"

Clare Luce knew that it was truly miserable to fail to enjoy some of life's pleasures. When asked which priest she wished to confess to on entering the Catholic Church, she had said, "Just bring me someone who has seen the rise and fall of empires." But some years later, told by someone how utterly admirable were the characters of Clare's play, *The Women,* she replied in writing, "The women who inspired this play deserved to be smacked across the head with a meat axe and that, I flatter myself, is exactly what I smacked them with. They are vulgar and dirty-minded and alien to grace, and I would not, if I could, which I hasten to say I cannot, cross their obscenities with a wit which is foreign to them and gild their futilities with the glamour which by birth and breeding and performance they do not possess." So much for the beautiful people.

"Stooping a dozen times a day quietly"—Clare Luce was writing now about another saint, St. Thérèse of Lisieux—"she picked up and carried the splinters of the cross that strewed her path as they strew ours. And when she had gathered them all up, she had the material of a cross of no inconsiderable weight. The 'little way of the Cross' is not 'the way of a little cross.'"

One of Clare's biographers, a friend since childhood, wrote five years ago about a trip with her, visiting first the Citadel in Charleston, and then

Mepkin—"which used to be the Luces' southern retreat. . . . Here," Wilfrid Sheed wrote, "the welcome is very effusive, in the manner of priests in old movies . . . and it looks for an uneasy moment as if they are buttering up the patron.

"But Trappists are tricky. Being released from almost perpetual silence by guests, the talk bubbles out gratefully like fizz from a bottle. As this subsides, they turn out to be quite urbane and judicious talkers. . . . They genuinely seem to love Clare," and "she considered them her last family. I have never seen her more relaxed."

". . . After her daughter's death," Sheed continued, "Clare could no longer bear to go [to Mepkin] for pleasure, and [giving the estate away to a religious order] was an ingenious way of keeping it and letting it go at the same time. The expansionist abbot of Gethsemani, Kentucky, . . . was only too happy to take it, and I dimly remember the Luces' ironic discussion of this back in 1949 while the deal was being completed. They were onto the abbot's game but did not think less of a priest for being a shrewd businessman. And what better way to retire the place that her daughter, Ann Brokaw, had loved more than any other in the world?

"Clare immediately moved both her daughter's and her mother's remains to Mepkin, where they now share adjoining graves. And then, to everybody's surprise, it turned out sometime later that Presbyterian Harry had decided to join them, and he was buried in the middle, after a nervous ecumenical service. The cost-conscious abbot of the moment suggested a double tombstone with Clare's name on it too, cutting off, as she noted, all possibilities of future husbands or new religions"—at this point she must have given off that wonderful, wry nasal laugh.

Last Wednesday, in Washington, Clare's doctor confided to the White House that Clare would not live out the week, and that no doubt she would be pleased by a telephone call. The President called that night. Her attendant announced to her who it was who was calling. Clare Boothe Luce shook her head. You see, she would not speak to anyone she could not simultaneously entertain, and she could no longer do this. The call was diplomatically turned aside. The performer knew she had given her last performance, but at least she had never failed.

And then last Sunday, her tombstone at Mepkin no longer sat over an empty grave. She is there with Harry. Over the grave is—"a shady tree sculpted above the names, and to either side her mother, Ann Clare, and her daughter, Ann Clare, in a grove of oak and cypress and Spanish moss running down to the Cooper River."

When Bill Sheed wrote those lines, five years ago, he quoted Abbot Anthony telling him quietly as they walked away, "She's taking it pretty well this year. She's usually very disturbed by this."

Clare Luce, now at Mepkin finally, is no longer disturbed. It is only we who are disturbed, Hank Luce above all, and her friends: disconsolate, and sad, so sad without her, yet happy for her, embarked finally, after stooping so many times, to pick up so many splinters, on her way to the Cross.

—WFB   SEPTEMBER 6, 1987

ALAN PATON, R.I.P.

"In 1948 a book was published with a bewildering title, by an unknown author, on a theme alien to American concerns. The book became the central cultural document of South Africa, where it sold more copies than any other volume save the Bible. *Cry, the Beloved Country* is free of bitterness, telling the story of a fraternal bond between a black minister tormented by the sins of his son and his sister, and a white man."

With these words, in May 1977, I began my introduction of Alan Paton, on *Firing Line*. It struck me, after the hour was done, that a great fatigue was on him: that he had grown old, as some of the prophets grew old, under the pressures of a noncompliant world. Alan Paton stayed active in politics, as head of the Liberal Party (which favored the universal franchise). When he left the party, he also left politics, confining himself to criticism of his country's policies, as also criticism of nostrums favored by other foes of apartheid (Paton consistently opposed economic sanctions).

Last week's *Time* magazine published an incomplete essay by Paton, incomplete because he was taken to the hospital before finishing it. But *Time* gives us what he did write, and Paton began by saying, "I have lost my surefootedness. . . . I do not now feel happy walking among the coarse hummocks of a grassy hill. . . . When I was a young student of seventeen or eighteen, I remember crossing the Umsindusi River . . . on the stepping-stones. I didn't walk, I ran. Today I would fall into the river at the first stone. I have grown very lethargic." And then he quoted four lyrical sentences from one of his books, introducing them with the sigh, "I shall never again write such words as these."

Twenty years ago Bennett Cerf, the founder and publisher of Random House, told me that he kept two young women busy reading fiction books sent to Random House over the transom. "In thirty years, we've only published two titles that came in that way." Why don't you cancel the operation? I asked. "Because one of those books was *Cry, the Beloved Country.*" About the author of that book one could only say that he had reason to be fatigued, and that he had earned eternal rest.

—WFB   MAY 13, 1988

R.I.P. Reginald Stoops, 1925–1988

The following eulogy by WFB was one of three delivered at Trinity Episcopal Church in Newport, R.I., on September 16, 1988. Reginald Stoops served informally as a scientific adviser to NR.

"But how otherwise did you enjoy the evening, Mrs. Lincoln?" has become gallows humor. Even so, it was the line that came to mind on Wednesday morning when Christo* called me and gave me the news. His second sentence—perhaps his training as a journalist prompted it—was, "It happened at 11:22." My eyes turned to a gaudy new chronometer sitting on my desk, guaranteed not to lose more than seven-tenths of one second in one year. The exact time was 11:45.

Ten days ago I told Reggie that our navigational worries at sea over the exact time were ended, that whenever we set out to cross Long Island Sound—or Narragansett Bay—or the Atlantic Ocean—we would never again have to worry about exactly what time it was in Greenwich, England. He said that he longed to see the new clock—our studied fantasy about the months and years we would sail together after his freak illness never flagged in our thirty brief conversations during the past two months. I commented that no doubt he would insist on taking my chronometer apart and ridding it of that seven-tenths of one second annual problematic. I went on to ask him what his weight was today, and he said 137 pounds, which permitted me to say that we would have no further excuse for singling out Danny Merritt to go up to the masthead; and he laughed his gentle laugh, and said with that little hoarseness I was becoming used to, "I guess you're right. On the other hand"—his voice registered now a trace of curiosity—"they're giving me something to make me fatter, so don't count on it." I didn't count on it, because of course I knew; he by then knew it, and he knew that I knew it, and so it goes.

I knew it even back on the eve of his marriage, in June, as a few others did, who managed more successfully than I to internalize that knowledge. But on Wednesday, thinking back to Mrs. Lincoln, I forced myself to think not about what had happened at 11:22 on that morning, but about what happened during all the years I had known him. Was it one hundred nights or was it one thousand and one nights that we shared, in fine and awful circumstances, the cockpit of a boat, and I experienced the soft delights of his understated company? Oh yes, he could drive grown men to tears with the deliberateness of his reactions. Rehearsing an emergency drill, the second night of our Pacific crossing, Dick Clurman asked him

* Christopher Buckley.

where the lifesavers were stored. He reacted as if he had been asked to give a brief definition of the Fourth Dimension. The pause, the slight clearing of the throat, the innocent look of a man accosted by an angular question: but followed by the exhilarating frankness of his innocent reply ("I'm not quite sure at this point"). In the book from which that passage comes, I quoted from Christopher's journal. He had written, a few days before we landed in New Guinea, "You find out on a trip like this who you can *absolutely* depend on. And really, the answer is, Pup and I agreed, that the person who is absolutely dependable in every situation is Reggie."

"We didn't mean"—I added in my book—"that anyone on board had ever broken the inflexible rule of interpersonal courtesy, merely that Reg is a critical mass of intelligence, good nature, and composure. He has never complained about anything." A year later, at a reunion of the crew, he presented us all with T-shirts on which the entire paragraph I have quoted was reproduced in DRINK COCA-COLA sized type.

"*He has never complained about anything,*" I reminded myself on Wednesday, thinking back first on the pleasures he had got from life, and then of the pleasure he had given to everyone who experienced him.

But the climax was ahead of him, when those words were written, co-inciding—providence can be that way: providence has its elfin ways—coinciding with the beginning of the last stages of his illness. Given the human predicament, one can only with dumb hesitation rail against the God Who, at one and the same time, took his life, but also gave him the supreme gift, the woman he married, who did more than all of science's opiates to make those three months endurable; to make that, paradoxically, a period of unparalleled happiness.

When finally I brought myself to visit him other than on the telephone, face to face, it was just before midnight Monday, and we embraced, after his very best friend, my son Christopher, had kissed him on the forehead. He pronounced my name and managed a smile. I looked at his fine face and thought back this time to another moment of great strain. It was mid-March in 1957. The little dinghy in which we had set out to retrieve a duck blind a mile in front of my house on Long Island Sound had upset, and we realized, suddenly, that our lives hung on our ability to swim, in our heavy winter clothing, in freezing water, to a promontory a half mile away. For a full minute we could not judge whether we were making head-way against the northerly wind, but we were. Gradually, painfully, we made progress. Fifty yards from land he looked at me and said, "Go ahead. I can't make it." I could not help him with my frozen hands, but I sang raucously to him, and I prayed with unfeigned imperiousness, ordering him to continue to beat his arms, however limply, against the waves. In five more minutes we were there, crawling on our stomachs to shelter.

What brought this to mind was the infinite dignity on his frozen countenance that afternoon, thirty-one years ago, which I saw again, on Monday night, on his pallid, skeletal face: struggling to live almost as a matter of good manners, but resigned to die; determined only that he would never complain, never let go that fierce dignity which he carried in good times and bad times, drunk or sober, exhausted or animated, in sickness and in health.

I had a bouncy friend who once managed a witticism. "When I get to St. Peter," he said, "I'm going to ask him to take me to the man who invented the dry martini. Because I just want to say, 'Thanks.' "

I am a Christian who, believing that our Redeemer lives, knows that one day I'll be once again in his company, on that endless journey in the peace he now enjoys. When that time comes for me, as for others here, I shan't forget to say, as in my prayers I have said so often during the last days, Thanks. Thanks for the long play that came before that fatal bullet struck him down. Thanks, everlastingly, for the memory, everlasting.

—WFB

Alec Waugh, R.I.P.

When this journal was very young we approached Alec Waugh to serve as travel editor, a position he immediately accepted. We were flattered by this act of recognition, and our admiration of Mr. Waugh was only slightly diminished when we came to learn that his practice was never, ever to turn down a literary commission from anyone, at any time. Whence his copious production—fifty books, and fifty times fifty times fifty (if that is technically possible) articles. Six days out of seven spent in writing, which however never got in the way of his unimpeachable good manners, good humor, and good taste. Unlike his brother, he sought primarily to please, and with one or two exceptions (e.g., his very first book, *The Loom of Youth,* written at age nineteen, in which he revealed the homosexual element in British public-school life) succeeded in doing so. He pleased us greatly, personally and professionally, and so we join in mourning his death, at eighty-three, in Tampa.

—WFB   OCTOBER 2, 1981

Raymond Aron, R.I.P.

Before the *nouveaux philosophes,* before the French intelligentsia discovered Solzhenitsyn and, through him, that strange and thitherto-uncharted country, the Soviet Union, Raymond Aron knew the score. *The Opium of the Intellectuals,* a front-and-center assault on Marxism, appeared twenty-eight years ago. Aron was already fifty. He had been a schoolmate of Jean-Paul Sartre. But unlike Sartre and most other French intellectuals of this century, he did not cleave to any ideological sect, whether of the far right or the Communist left. He remained that increasingly rare thing, a classical European liberal, defending freedom against its totalitarian enemies. Among his last public pronouncements was a call for the deployment of the Pershing and cruise missiles. His memoirs—oh, say, his fortieth book—top the best-seller lists. French scholarship and journalism lose a keen and steady voice.

—WFB   NOVEMBER 11, 1983

The following is WFB's remembrance of another Aloise, his sister. We reproduce both, partly because of this Aloise's wonderful way with words—her own and of those around her. (This is written with his sister, Priscilla.)

ALOISE B. HEATH, R.I.P.

"For her," an august and worldly professor of the social sciences called in when the word leaked out that she was in coma, "I have to confess I have said a prayer, for the first time in many years even though I never met her." His prayer, and others, were unavailing. Aloise Buckley Heath died on Monday January 16, ten days after an unsuccessful operation which was performed a few hours after she had complained of a bad headache and was driven, by her husband, to the hospital in Hartford. Unconsciousness and partial paralysis gradually set in and when the doctor did operate it was only because, as he put it, he would have done so on his own wife under similar circumstances—he gave her only one or two chances out of one hundred. And then a few minutes later when he actually observed the damage done by the cerebral hemorrhage, he simply stitched her back together and waited, as the family did—her husband, her ten children, her mother, her eight brothers and sisters—for the inevitable end. It came later than the young doctors had predicted. "They don't realize," said one doctor, "that at forty-eight the heart is strong. It goes right on beating, for a while, a good while.

"What happened to her brain is the kind of thing that usually happens to people in their late sixties or seventies. That's why she isn't dead—yet. But there won't be any pain, any consciousness." She was buried at St. Bernard's Cemetery, in Sharon, Connecticut, on Wednesday, January 18, alongside two of her sisters, who had died at age three days, and thirty-one years. At the service, said as she would have wanted, in Latin, a memorial card was distributed, a small photograph, the dates of birth and death on one side, and on the other a passage from François Mauriac's *Ce Que Je Crois* that she had seen and expressed admiration for—as a young girl she had been schooled in France, and she knew the language as a native—only a month before. Mauriac wrote: "*Faites, Mon Dieu, que je me recueille dans la paix de votre présence, afin que quand mon heure sera venue, je passe par une transition presque insensible, de vous à vous, de vous, pain vivant, pain des hommes, à vous amour vivant déjà possédé par ceux de mes biens-aimés qui se sont endormis avant moi dans votre amour.*"—"Grant, O Lord, that I might commune in the peace of Your presence, so that when my hour is come, I shall pass through a transition all but insensible, from You to You; from You, the Living Bread, the Bread of Man, to you, the Living Love, already possessed by those of my beloved ones who, in that love, have gone before me to sleep."

"Though I never met her," one reader wrote, "I felt along with thousands of *National Review* readers, I'm sure, the force of her personality; her vibrant, joyous spirit sang out of her seasonal articles for *National Review*." "Of all the writers on your magazine, over the past eleven years," an attorney wrote, "she must surely have been the most lovable." And from a minister: "My wife, my children, and I feel something of a personal loss in the death. . . . As she has on several occasions in the past, she added to the joy of our Christmas celebration with her most recent article, [giving us] that sense of thankful and lighthearted appreciation of the mercies of God which we are trying to nurture in those whom He has given us to love."

Aloise Heath wrote for the very first issue of *National Review,* and had an article in the issue that was on the stands when she took sick. She did not, however, write frequently. There was of course the handicap of her motherhood of ten children, and the very special care she took of them. Besides that she was notoriously disorganized, so much so that generations of editors clamored, unsuccessfully, for her articles, and when she died, she had on her desk, as usual unanswered, a letter from the editor of a prominent monthly, begging for her copy. She had excited, at Smith College, the admiring attention of the academicians, as sharply distinguished from the administrators who at one point got so fed up with her dilatory habits as to suspend her for a year (she graduated with the class of 1941, instead of 1940)—a lever against her which unfortunately no editor inherited. But the professors gave her all the ritual honors of a very bright young writer. She was married in 1942 and got around to writing an article about her first child five years later. It was published in the *Ladies' Home Journal,* and with her check for five hundred dollars she bought expensive presents for all her brothers and sisters, resolved to write regularly, and didn't, not even when the agent for Somerset Maugham—who thus announced himself—offered to handle her material. She was always acquiescent; she would agree to write anything in the world any editor asked her to write, and simply did not do so—she was too busy with her growing family. She did produce a piece for *NR* at Christmastime, the ordeal of whose parturition was an annual agony—bits and pieces would come in by notepaper, telegram, telephone. But they were the most applauded pieces we ever published, even though they seldom touched on politics (one reader suggested we get Aloise Heath to write *all* of *every* issue). Seldom, but not never . . .

She complained in one of them that her children had been over-politicized. For instance "the kindergartner of unshakable opinion—what we can't shake in Janet is her firm opinion announced thirty seconds after she heard of the President's assassination last year that Senator Goldwater shot him. 'Janet, you *mustn't* say that!' her horrified older brothers and sisters exclaim when the subject comes up from time to time. 'I won't. I won't tell *anyone*,' she reassures them. 'Shall it be our two's secret?' "

Janet wasn't the only problem. A year later there was Timothy, with his paraplegic leg: "Six-year-old Timothy, who has been standing aloofly in the background watching you with great concentration, has apparently now accepted you. He whispers in my ear that he has something important to tell you. I transmit the message and Timothy stands before you shortly and informs you somberly that his message is about Communism. The Communists, he thinks you ought to know, are against us and we are against Communists, and they plan to beat us up but, man, are they going to be surprised, because they don't even *know* about Timothy Heath yet! And with modest pride, Terrible Timothy sticks one skinny little leg in the air and shows you his heavy brace and boot. 'One kick with *that* foot,' he grits from clenched teeth; and while you ponder the appalling fate in store for the Communists, Tim smiles and the serious little face breaks into whole galaxies of twinkles and dimples. . . ."

And there was always, in the household, the problem of distinguishing politics and theology. Sometimes, she admitted, she was herself responsible for the confusion. Let her speak for herself on the matter of Mrs. Major and her eternal soul. . . . "Did I really tell Timothy that Tommy Major's mother was going to Hell because she voted for Johnson? No. *I did not.* Once and for all.

"What happened was this. One day Timothy said: 'Would you go to Hell if you voted for Johnson?'

"I said: 'Do you mean me or do you mean people? If you mean me, the answer is yes because I'm an educated voter and I'd be committing a mortal sin if I voted for him. If you mean "people," no, because they are not as smart as your dear, dear, mother, you lucky boy.' Tim looked at me gravely. 'Will Tommy's mother go to Hell? She's going to vote for Johnson.'

" 'Oh, I don't think so, Tim,' I said, not terribly interested in the whole subject. 'She doesn't know enough to know what she's voting for. But wouldn't she be surprised if she *did* go to Hell!'

"It was then that I made my big mistake. You remember those lovely warm days last fall. Well, they affect me very badly. They increase my euphoria to the point of mania. I was near the piano while I talked to Tim and I sat down and played and sang, '*Tommy's mother went to Hell/On the Donkey ticket/Now she knows a Johnson vote/Is very, very wicked.*' Timothy thought it was charming and rushed out to collect his friends Brian and Billy to hear it. Billy called in his sister Beth who was playing with Pammy Shepherd from the next street over. In about ten minutes there were over a dozen children in the house bawling out at the top of their lungs the news that 'Tommy's Mother went to Hell.' And what was I doing? Big fat fool that I am. I was sitting there at the piano bawling it out with them and playing different versions of the piano accompaniment and setting up duets and interesting arrangements and in general behaving not at all like a woman whose living room windows face onto the Major driveway. And that's absolutely all there is to it.

"I don't blame her for thinking it was a rehearsal. I don't even blame the children for telephoning her the next few days and nights to sing it. I drummed it into their heads so hard, they probably still can't think of another tune. And that I swear is the whole story. It is absolutely what happened. And don't believe any other version."

But her madcap problems were not usually political. She was sharply observant and therefore sharply critical; the curse of the whole class of the pretentious, because she had a jeweler's eye for cant, for silliness (which, however, if it was unaffected, she loved), for hokum, political and nonpolitical. One of her weapons was literalness. She wrote several times with vast amusement about some of the practical problems posed by writers in ladies' magazines. There was the article warning the wife against "Becoming Less Appealing," which cautioned against making long social telephone calls, or "talking more loudly than her husband." "In certain isolated circumstances," she mused, "doing so would be justified; chronic laryngitis on the part of the husband, for instance; or the case of a man who might be worried about *his* Becoming Less Appealing, and therefore refusing to talk more loudly than his wife at the very same identical moment that his wife refused to talk more loudly than her husband. We can all see where *this* sort of situation would end, I am sure."

And there was the article that caught her eye, instructing wives on how to be more romantic with their husbands: "There was a *very* moving love scene (in the article) in the course of which a woman stood 'with her hands clasped on Loren's neck, her red hair pressed against his chin, her lips ardently uplifted.' The trouble is, when *I* clasp *my* hands on my husband's neck, press my interestingly graying hair against his chin and ardently uplift *my* lips, all I get is a mouthful of Adam's apple."

She was as amused by all aspects of language. Traveling in France with her sister Priscilla she found herself stuck in the elevator. "I cried: 'To the help!', which is what you cry when you are trapped in an Alpine pass in a blizzard at midnight and wolves are attacking you; and Priscilla shouted: 'The ascendor does not march!', which means that the elevator isn't working. After a while, pausing for a cigarette, we noticed the sign on the door. 'By means of a telephonic apparatus which finds itself at the interior of the ascendor, *ladies* and *gentlemen*,' the sign said pointedly, 'may inform the concierge with all calm that a mechanical anomaly has passed itself.' There is more to this message than meets the eye, we found. And you will find, if you try to say '*Anomalie mécanique*' *without* all calm."

Her strength was the children she loved—to the extent, she always made clear, that that was possible for anyone who truly understands children. One time she received a letter from an irrepressibly attractive and utterly impossible thirteen-year-old boy, friend of one of her sons, asking her whether she would recommend him to a school into which he sought admittance. (The entire, hilarious correspondence caught the eye of the *Reader's Digest*, which published it in its entirety.) She wrote, copy to the applicant, to the headmaster: ". . . [Peter] is more sophisticated today than three years ago, when, at the age of ten, he frequently urged me not to get my liver in a quiver. Today, when Peter and I have what he refers to as 'a difference of opinion,' he retires with complete equanimity to his own back yard until such time as my ill-humor subsides. My change of mood is apparently picked up by Peter's extrasensory perception within the hour, for whenever I decide that the time has come for forgiving and forgetting, he appears at my front door within fifteen minutes, to assure me *he* has forgiven and forgotten. By way of proof (penance?) he then resumes without rancor his status as our daily visitor. . . ."

She knew children, and knew the duty of the parent to try to dominate children, but knew also the limits of any such ambition, children being— children. "If they start throwing books at each other," she wrote in a piece about carpools, "it is best to park the car on the side of the road and exhibit emotional stability until they've stopped. Even this is unnecessary if the books are being thrown by Fourth, Fifth, or Sixth Form boys. Their aim is invariably excellent, and you are in no danger whatsoever. Occasionally there may be stationed on one of your carpool routes a policeman who does not like it when a child sticks his head out of the car and shouts:

'What's old pennies made of?' and all the others shriek, '*Dirty Copper!*' At least he doesn't like it twice a day for nine months of the year, which is when the children like it. If this should be the case, humor him. I myself find that the easiest thing to do is to work out a detour around him, though I understand some mothers make the children stop it."

But she always found her own children (and everyone else's), whatever the generic menace, individually fascinating, individually challenging, individually superior. "Timothy is five years old. He is small, handsome, stern, rather conceited, we suspect; and he has the kind of passion for accuracy which so unduly prolongs even the simplest of bedtime stories. When he comes home from kindergarten, we meet; we do not reune, as did his poor be-momméd eldest brother and I twelve years ago. Nor do I ask for a detailed accounting of Timothy's morning; I say 'Have fun?' and then I say 'That's good!' before he answers . . ."

". . . Timothy was home from school with a cold, and we were glad to see each other, so to speak. We sat alone together in the kitchen, over a plateful of plums, and I said as a gesture of friendship: 'Tim, what's two and two?' Between Heaths, this is not a question; it is the opening gambit of an old routine which ends in 'What's twelve and twelve?' to which the (always) killingly funny answer is, 'Twenty-four. Shut your mouth and say no more.' Furthermore, it is Timothy's absolutely favorite joke: so I felt a little rebuffed when he asked gravely: 'What's two?' "

And thus was his mother introduced to the New Math, in which numbers are second-class citizens, and it all depends on colored rods ("Spare Me the Rods," Dec. 31, 1963).

Always she insisted on the realisms. There was the Christmas when she announced to her children that they would attempt a Trapp Family Christmas, the distinguishing feature of which was that each child would select another child (by ballot) as his special protégé (*Christkindl*), and proceed to shower (anonymously) special favors upon him or her until Christmas day when the *Christkindl*'s benefactor would identify himself. The idea was heroically launched. But her children didn't appear to be exactly Trapp-minded. . . .

"That afternoon they were all in the coat closet (well they *were*, that's all. They *like* the coat closet) making out their Christmas lists. Pam, who can spell, was helping the ones who can't write; and Alison, who is magic, was helping the ones who can't talk. I had my ear at the crack, listening, because I'm still trying to hear one of those childhood conversations whose innocent candor tears at your heartstrings. You've read about them, I'm sure. What I heard was my dear little ones calculating how much more each of them would get for Christmas if they didn't have so many brothers and sisters. They named, giving reasons therefor, their choice—those they would gladly do without. They catalogued the children they would trade for hockey skates or an electric organ with four octaves, or seven Betsey-Wetsies with seven different-colored hairs. From what I could hear through the crack, *nobody* kept Buckley and Timothy, which is understandable, but not nice. . . ."

Undaunted, she went on with her resolute plans for a Trapp Family Christmas.

"I didn't see how the *Christkindl* custom could go wrong, though. I *still* don't. In the Trapp family, everyone writes his name on a piece of paper and the papers are put in a basket which is passed around as soon as the children have finished singing: '*Ye heavens, dew drop from above.*' Everybody picks a name from the basket, and the pickee, if you follow me, becomes the picker's secret *Christkindl,* and the idea is, you do your *Christkindl* a good turn every day until Christmas without ever letting him know who you are. . . ." But at her house it was, as usual, chaotic . . . the children found themselves picking themselves, or prematurely divulging their identities, or whatever. Finally, she contrived a means by which the children would pick out their *Christkindl,* and be picked out. It was not altogether democratic, and by no means left to chance. She reserved a *droit de mère:* All the children were *given* a specified piece of paper. "The baby ate her paper; but it was all right, because I knew whose name she had eaten. I had arranged for us to draw each other, because we're in love. Everybody was getting pretty tense, not to mention bloody, until one of them—I haven't asked which—found a solution: every Sunday now, they each buy seven penny lollipops, and every night they slip a lollipop under their *Christkindl*'s pillow. Well, I *know* that doesn't sound so terribly spiritual, but it's better than what they used to do. What they used to do was steal each other's lollipops. I wouldn't want anybody to think that the baby and I have sunk to such a mundane relationship, though. We haven't had to change our routine at all. Every morning my *Christkindl* allows me to rock her a little; and every evening I rock my *Christkindl* a little."

The last Christmas, never daunted, she had experimented with group singing which meant the children as a body, rather than as individuals; and that, as ever, was something else again, and, as ever, she wrote about it hypnotically . . .

"Gay my children unquestionably are. They rollick into the house from school, burst into paroxysms of laughter at the extraordinary coincidence of their reunion from various carpools, plan their far-flung wickednesses in gales of muffled giggles, are scolded with eyes twinkling above insufficiently suppressed grins, and fall asleep in the midst of a choked chuckle at 8, 9 or 10 P.M., according to whether their bedtime was at 7, 8, or 9. . . .

"One of the reasons—I say one of the reasons because I could easily think of another if I put my mind to it—that I kept on having babies for years after all my classmates had worked up to president of the state *PTA* was that I always thought a big family would be such fun at Christmas. Which who doesn't, including people like me, who know? I know why my husband Ben has the Spirit of Christmas around Thanksgiving and the Spirit of Ash Wednesday around Christmas. I keep telling him I know. 'I know,' I say. 'I know. I know. I know.'

"I know we always get more glitter and glue on the floor than on the candles and that I never remember to wipe it up until the dining-room carpet is permanently (though interestingly) spangled. I know I look absolutely insane, crawling around in the snow for weeks before Christmas, putting candy canes on window sills and then galloping madly off into the dark, jingling sleighbells and shouting 'Ho! Ho! Ho!' I know the newsboy would rather have two dollar bills than a $1.95 flashlight wrapped in green paper and silver ribbon, with 'MERVYN' spelled out in red Scotch tape. I know no one can eat those Cut'n'Bake cookies after the children have decorated them with green sugar and cinnamon hearts (Christmas tree) and then with more cinnamon hearts and melted marshmallow (Santa Claus) and then with more melted marshmallow and pink crayon (angel). I know it's un-Gesell and not even altogether Spock to look a ten-year-old square in the eye and say: 'But Sweetie, how should *I* know why Polly's Santa Claus is really her father? Maybe her father *has* to be her Santa Claus, poor little thing! Maybe Santa Claus just doesn't *like* Polly. Did you ever think of that?' . . ."

Stuff and nonsense? Well . . . "Some day,"—she wrote on Christmas, 1964, taking off with her striking literary skill on the ladies'-type magazines that tell you how to be a perfect wife, promising, in her own caricature, to be "even more emetic"—but somehow accomplishing something quite different. She wrote: "Some day, though, I will have a fling at becoming a perfect woman, nobly planned, which, the way I dope it out, means spending absolute hours making love your whole existence, and keeping silent in the churches, and weeping while men work, and trying to be a better smoke than a good cigar, and constantly widening the gap between your price and rubies', and being good and letting who will be clever, and while your babes around you cling, showing Wordsworth how divine a thing a woman may be made.

"In my case, though, it will have to be while my grandbabies around me cling, because right now, and for the next fourteen and a quarter years, I'm going to be too busy. . . ." Celebrating Christmas in the usual way.

On Christmas Eve last, with only twelve and one half years to go, she was busy, at the apogee of her yearly cycle, stuffing the stockings of her children with candies and puzzles and games and toys, when she stretched out under the tree and slept. This was not totally unusual for her. But the difference was when she woke an hour later. She did not resume her duty, her joy—though there were still four stockings left to fill. She went, without saying a word, to bed; and so her husband and oldest child, astonished, worried, finished the work of the Christmas-maker extraordinary. She didn't know what it was that had happened, and the doctors didn't seem to know, and two weeks later the Christmases were, for her, forever ended. And little Janet, her *Christkindl* of the year of the Trapps, when she got the news, responded that "Nothing will ever be fun again"; which is exactly how others felt, who knew her when we were all children together.

—WFB JR.

—PLB   FEBRUARY 7, 1967

A special place is reserved in Bill Buckley's affection for those who helped him start, develop, and refine his magazine.

WILLIAM F. RICKENBACKER, R.I.P.

He first surfaced for us at *National Review* when he challenged the government of the United States. The Census Bureau had gone to work collecting its data in 1960, and Bill Rickenbacker received what they called the Long Form, designed to elicit detailed information, the better to complete the decennial inquiry into how many Americans were living where, earning what, doing what, living how. Bill looked at the form, put it in his wastebasket, and addressed one of his inimitable letters to the secretary of commerce, whom he addressed as Dear Snoopchief, denouncing the long form as an invasion of his privacy. C. Dickerman Williams, *National Review*'s distinguished lawyer, undertook his defense. He lost, was fined $100, and put on one day's probation: and at the end of the succeeding decade, tasted finally the fruit of his struggle when the Commerce Department announced that the long form would be completed only by those U.S. citizens who wished to complete it.

Rickenbacker came then to *National Review* as a senior editor, and life was wonderful in his company. He retreated after eight years or so, went into business for himself, wrote eight books, and continued his studies of music, of languages, and of the canon of Western thought.

But he never lost touch with us, and in 1991, with Linda Bridges, he published the book *The Art of Persuasion*. A few years ago, responding to a rebuke for his failure to visit New York more often, he wrote me, "I too wish I could move around a bit more, but I seem to have simplified my life a good deal in recent years. Three or four hours a day at the old piano will nail a fellow down good and hard. But I have dreams, dreams in full color, not to mention aroma, of lunch at Paone's [the reference is to the restaurant around the corner, heavily patronized by *National Review*], which, by the way, why doesn't somebody burn it down and rebuild it up here in God's country?"

. . . Bill, in his letter, went on about his schedule. "Now I'm moving steadily through the fifteen volumes of the collected utterance and effusions of Edmund Burke, and the more I see of him the less I trust him. He keeps reminding me of Everett Dirksen—not that Dirksen ever reminded me of Burke."

Bill was a professionally qualified pianist. "I've recorded," he wrote me, "to my satisfaction, four short pieces of our great teacher, the Bach of Bachs, Schubert comes next, and then a dollop of Chopin. I find this project far more difficult than it was twenty-five years ago. Two trends have been in play: my standards have risen, and my physical capacity has fallen. When I piled up my airplane and broke a dozen bones including my right wrist, I didn't advance the cause; my right hand, if I don't pay good attention, is still in danger of being shouted down by the unruly Bolshevik in my left—a faction that gathered its preternatural strength during ten years of intensive club-gripping on the golf course." He had been captain of the golf team at Harvard. And, like his father, Captain Eddie, he flew, until glaucoma stopped him.

His curiosity was boundless. "Did you see my Unamuno in the current *Modern Age*?" The reference was to an essay he had just published. "Next comes Ortega y Gasset. I've read twenty-one volumes of his and am now organizing my notes. I'll probably have sixty pages of notes in preparation for an eight-page piece. I don't think the name for that is scholarship; more like idle dithering."

It seemed endless, his curiosity. "I've been studying Hebrew *very* hard and loving it all the way. A wonderful language. Since college days I've wanted to read the Psalms in Hebrew; now I shall."

He was not altogether a recluse. A couple of years ago he consented to address my brother Reid's public-speaking school in South Carolina. Reid asked how he should introduce Bill's speech. He sent me a copy of Bill's suggested titles:

—How I Spent My Summer
—What the North Wind Said
—Counselor Said I Couldn't Eat Dinner Till I Wrote Home
—Why I Hate My Sis

—Legalization of Crime: Pros & Cons

—Was Mozart Queer?

—The Bartender's Guide to the Upstairs Maid

—Merde! Golfing Decorum in Postwar France

—Are Lasers Protected under the Fourth Amendment?

—Public Speaking Minus One: A Tape Cassette of Wild but Intermittent Applause, with Stretches of Silence to Be Filled with Remarks by the Apprentice Orator

—Sexual Repression in Emily Dickinson's Punctuation

—Why I Am Running for President (applause)

—Why Dead White Males Don't Laugh

—Do Hydrogen and Oxygen Look like Water? I Ask You!: Chemistry Disrobed and Shown to Be the Fraud It Is

He kept in touch with his friends. When *National Review*'s ex-publisher Bill Rusher had his bypass operation, Rickenbacker wrote to me, "I heard from Claire [Bill Rusher's secretary] on Monday that his bypass was sextuple, which I thought pretty damned good for a bachelor, and look forward to sending him something cheerful as soon as they take the chopsticks out of his nostrils."

And his concern for public affairs was alive as ever. "There has been some talk of flying the flag at half mast," he wrote me, "until the Court's decision [permitting the burning of the flag] is nullified, but I don't think a gesture of mourning is in order when the battle has hardly begun. Instead, I'm flying my own flag at full mast, but upside down, in the international signal of distress. A flag that has been abandoned by its own country is certainly in distress, and I intend to fly mine upside down until the Court turns right side up."

He enjoyed always the exuberant flash of muscle that interrupted, and gave perspective to, his serenity. "I have been a grandfather for five days now and I am growing crotchety. I have told both my boys and both my stepsons that the first one calls me gramps gets a knee in the groin but I doubt if I'll be safe much longer."

Though that was in 1990, he was right—not much longer. It was last fall that the cancer came. But after the operation, he wrote to soothe me. ". . . my moribundity is no more serious than anyone else's of similar time in grade. The so-called treatment, which is in reality, as I need not tell you, . . . a form of Florentine poisoning, offers the advective cruelty of the absence of wine. Anyway I now have two Sanskrit grammars, a matched pair, and will present one copy to [his doctor] when next I see her, which I fear will be on Monday. My hope is that she with her wise Velázquez-brown eyes will find a way to administer my Sanskrit intravenously, with a dash of curry and the faintest after-aroma of popadams. (Do you remember when our mothers could buy popadams in large flat tins from India, the cakes packed between green tobacco leaves?)"

And, only a week later, a letter describing his doctor, whom he much admired. But half way down the page, "EGGS ON FACE DEPT. When I sent you the copy of her letter, I failed to proofread her copy with care, and discovered only later that when she says she may extend a certain life span by two or three months, she means *years*. I double-checked her on this. So relax, mon vieux: it will be longer than you think before your life and property shall be safe."

The doctor was right the first time. But Bill went on with his work. "I've been having fun writing my study of three-letter words. Since the emphasis is on their history and not their definition or use, I have elbow room in the definitions. 'Gun' for instance, which has a very peculiar etymology, I define as 'A metallic pipe through which missiles, which have been excited by chemical explosions in their fundaments, are hurled airmail to their recipients.' For the kind of people who like that sort of thing that's the sort of thing those people will like. . . .

Bill had for a while been reading religious literature, and now he wrote, "I'm reading the Pope's book. I bought a copy for each of my boys, gave one to Tommy, and held one back to read myself before giving it to Jamie. I should buy a third, because I want the book at my elbow always. It's so drenched in wisdom and experience and devotion that I can't take it in in one reading. I read sentence after sentence two or three times. What a man! Among the great souls of history, I say."

A month later I spoke with Nancy on the telephone. She had difficulty in speaking, but told me Bill had been given three or four days more to live. I asked whether I should write to him. Yes, she said, giving me the fax number. I had never before written or spoken to someone on his deathbed, to whom circumspection was no longer possible. So I wrote to my dear and gifted friend,

"Wm, [This was our protocol, dating back three decades: All letters from one to the other would begin, Wm, and be signed, Wm]

"This is not the season to be jolly. Miracles do happen, Evelyn Waugh wrote in *National Review*, 'but it is presumptuous to anticipate them.' It will happen to us all, I brightly observe, but you should feel first the satisfaction of knowing that soon you will be in God's hand, with perhaps just a taste of Purgatory for the editorial you wrote when Bobby was killed, though I here and now vouchsafe you the indulgence I merited on declining to publish it. Second, the satisfaction of being with that wonderful Nancy in your tribulation, and third, the knowledge that those who have known you count it a singular blessing to have experienced you. I send my prayers, and my eternal affection. Wm."

In fact he lived three weeks more and, before losing the use of his writing hand, indited his own obituary, two paragraphs of biographical data, and the closing sentences, "A bug or two showed up last fall and began to do what a bug does best, namely, to make a joke out of life's spruce intentions, and to provide a daily wage or two for journalists, whose business it is not my duty as a Christian to inquire into. Sometime between when this ink and mine go dry the bugs will have had their day. He leaves behind him his wife and two devoted sons, two daughters-in-law, three grandchildren, a beloved sister, an unfinished manuscript or two, and a heart filled with blessings."

May he rest in peace.

—WFB   APRIL 17, 1995

JOHN CHAMBERLAIN, R.I.P.

Late one afternoon in the fall of 1955, on the eve of the appearance of the first issue of *National Review,* something people more loftily situated would have called a "summit conference" was set in New York City, for which purpose a tiny suite in the Commodore Hotel was engaged. Tensions—ideological and personal—had arisen, and the fleeting presence in New York of Whittaker Chambers, who had dangled before us in an altogether self-effacing way the prospect that he might come out of retirement to join the fledgling enterprise, prompted me to bring the principals together for a meeting which had no specific agenda, being designed primarily to reaffirm the common purpose. As I think back on it, two of the five people present were born troublemakers. To say this about someone is not to dismiss him as merely that: Socrates was a troublemaker, so was Thomas Edison. But troublemaking was not what was primarily needed to distill unity, and so, one half hour after the meeting began, things were not going smoothly.

And then, when it was nearly six o'clock and I thought I detected in Chambers a look of terminal exasperation, John Chamberlain showed up, briefcase in one hand, a pair of figure skates in the other. He mumbled (he almost always mumbled) his apology . . . He had booked the practice time at the ice rink for himself and his daughters . . . The early afternoon editorial meeting had been protracted, the traffic difficult . . . No thanks, he didn't want anything to drink—was there any iced tea? He stole a second or two to catch up on Whittaker's family, and then sat back to participate in a conference—which had been transformed by his presence at it.

When a few days later Chambers wrote, he remarked the sheer "goodness" of John Chamberlain, a quality that no man or woman, living or dead, has ever to my knowledge disputed.

At the time a sharp difference had arisen, not between me and John Chamberlain, but between Willi Schlamm and John's wife, Peggy (R.I.P.). Schlamm viewed the projected magazine as a magnetic field, professional affiliation with which could no more be denied by the few to whom the call was tendered than a call to serve as one of the Twelve Apostles. Poor Peggy would not stand for it: John was then serving as an editor of *Barron's* magazine and as a writer for *The Wall Street Journal.* Before that he had been with *The Freeman,* before that with *Life,* before that *Fortune,* before that the *New York Times.* In each of these enterprises he had achieved singularity. He had two daughters not yet grown up. How could anyone reasonably ask that now, in middle age, he detach himself from a secure position to throw in with *National Review*—an enterprise whose working capital would not have seen *Life* magazine through a single issue, or *Barron's* through a dozen, and whose editor-in-chief was not long out of school?

I like to remind myself that I did not figure even indirectly in the protracted negotiation, respecting, as I did, not only the eminence of John Chamberlain, but also the altogether understandable desire of his wife for just a little economic security. But Willi was very nearly (nothing ever proved so conclusively shocking to Willi) struck dumb with shock, the thought that *National Review* might be created without John Chamberlain as a senior editor. That was one of the clouds that hung over that late-afternoon discussion, in which Willmoore Kendall exploited every opportunity to add fuel to the fire, principally by the device of suggesting that for *some* people security means *everything;* the kind of thing John did not wish to hear, among other reasons because it so inexactly reflected his own priorities—he was concerned not with security, but with domestic tranquillity.

So it went, and in one form or another the tensions continued, though they never proved crippling. John settled the problem by moonlighting—as lead reviewer for *National Review.* But I learned then, during that tense afternoon, the joy of a definitively pacific presence. Ours might have been a meeting to discuss whether to dump the bomb on Hiroshima; and John Chamberlain's presence would have brought to such a meeting, whatever its outcome, a sense of inner peace, manliness, and self-confidence.

There are stories John never told, even in his memoirs published a dozen years ago. That was characteristic. Bertrand de Jouvenel once told me, at a luncheon devoted to discussing our common friend Willmoore Kendall, that any subject at all is more interesting than oneself. I am not absolutely convinced that this is so—because some people know no other subject so thoroughly as themselves. But with John Chamberlain self-neglect was an attribute not of manners, but of personality. When *National Review* started up, six weeks after our Commodore summit, he would come in to the office every week (the magazine was then a weekly), sit down at whatever typewriter was free, and type out the lead book review with that quiet confidence exhibited by sea captains when they extricate their huge liners from their hectic municipal ships to begin an ocean voyage. After forty-five minutes or so a definitive book review was done; and John would, quietly, leave, lest he disrupt the office.

In those days "the office" consisted of six or seven cubicles, each one with desk and typewriter. Most of *NR*'s top editorial staffers—James Burnham, Willi Schlamm, Willmoore Kendall, Whittaker Chambers, Frank Meyer—from the beginning on, served only part time, so that at any given moment at least one cubicle was unoccupied, though seldom the same one. Four or five months into the magazine's life a young graduate of Smith, age twenty-four, serving in the circulation department, complained to her classmate, my sister Maureen, that the repairman who came once a week to check the typewriters had not once serviced her own. We couldn't wait to tell John Chamberlain, the delinquent typewriter repairman, when he came in the following Tuesday. He laughed heartily, then sat down to write an illuminating review of the entire fictional work of Mary McCarthy.

I never saw him, during the 1930s, slide into his chair at the *New York Times* to write his daily book reviews, many of them masterpieces of the form. Nor at *Fortune,* where he would return from two weeks on the road to write what he called a "long piece," which would prove the definitive article on this or that intricate problem of management or labor. Nor at *Life,* where he presided over the editorial page that was Henry Luce's personal cockpit, from which he spoke out, through John, to God and man in authoritative, not to say authoritarian, accents. But I decline to believe that in any of these roles, or in any of the myriad others he filled—as professor at Columbia, as dean of journalism at Troy State University in Alabama, as a book writer or a columnist—John Chamberlain ever did anything more disruptive than merely greet whoever stood in the way, and amble over to wherever the nearest typewriter was, there to execute his craft: maintaining standards as high as any set by any critical contemporary.

Because John Chamberlain could not sing off key. And the combination of a gentle nature and a hard Yankee mind brought forth prose pure and lasting. His was a voice of reason, from an affable man, unacquainted with affectation, deeply committed to the cause of his country and to liberty. He believed the fate of his country co-extensive with that of civilization; and, certainly, with that of his two daughters from his first marriage, and of his son—a young poet—from his second, to the enchanting Ernestine, to whom he went soon after Peggy's untimely death.

John Chamberlain's memoirs were surely the most soft-throated in the literature of men who took passionate political positions. As a young man who had demonstrated his prowess as a critic (William Lyon Phelps called him the "finest critic of his generation"), and as a political thinker manifestly addicted to progress, he wrote his book *A Farewell to Reform,* in which he seemed to give up on organic change, suggesting the advantages of radical alternatives. But his idealism was never superordinated to his intelligence, and in the balance of that decade of the thirties, and then in that of the forties, Chamberlain never ceased to look at the data, which carefully he integrated in his productive mind. Along the line (he tells us) he read three books, so to speak at one gulp—and the refractory little tumblers closed, after which he became what is now denominated a "conservative." The books in question, by the three furies of modern libertarianism—Isabel Paterson, Rose Wilder Lane, Ayn Rand—provided the needed cement. After that, he ceased to be surprised by evidence, now become redundant, evidence that the marketplace really works, really performs social functions, really helps live human beings with live problems.

His writings told the story of his journey through this century. His calmness and lucidity, his acquiescent handling of experience, free of ideological entanglement, provoked in the reader the kind of confidence that John Chamberlain throughout his long life provoked in his friends. But his friendships would never run any risk of corrupting the purity of his ongoing search, through poetry, fiction, economic texts, corporate reports, and—yes—seed catalogues, for just the right formulation of what may be acknowledged as the American proposition. He sought an equilibrium of forces that would foster the best that could be got out of the jealous, contentious, self-indulgent, uproarious breed of men and women that have made so exciting a world here, giving issue, in one of America's finest moments, to a splendid man.

I last saw him at a little party given in a noisy New York hotel to celebrate his ninetieth birthday. My sister Priscilla sat next to him, and I was with the proud and lovely Ernestine. I reflected on my first meeting with him. He came to the little house in which I had written *God and Man at Yale,* the manuscript of which had been sent him by the publisher Henry Regnery. It was inconceivable to me that he would consent to write an introduction to a book so disruptive in the circles in which he lived. The purpose of his call—he was the editorial-page editor of *Life*—was to say, Yes, he would write the introduction. We were friends for forty-five years, during all of which we knew his goodness. The staff of *National Review* joins in extending our sympathy to his wife and family.

—WFB

MAY 1, 1995

———

And on a final note of friendship—eternal friendship, which underlies so much of Buckley's choice of words—these words were spoken at the memorial service for Richard M. Clurman, journalist, public servant, master of the genuinely curious, genuinely helpful gesture, at Temple Emanu-El on May 20, 1996, in New York City.

———

RICHARD M. CLURMAN, R.I.P.

Three years ago, one evening in July, he asked whether I'd cross the ocean again in 1995, what would have been the fifth such venture, done at five-year intervals beginning in 1975. "I'm prepared to go," he told me. I suppose I smiled; it was dark on the veranda when he spoke. I told him I doubted my crew could be mobilized for one more such trip, and just the right crew was indispensable. He had done with me two Atlantic crossings, one Pacific crossing. He was an instant celebrity for his ineptitudes at sea, done in high spirit with a wonderful, persistent incomprehension of what was the job at hand. He was the object of hilarious ridicule in my son's published journal—and he loved it all, even as Christopher loved him; even when, while discoursing concentratedly on matters of state, he would drop his cigarette ash into Christopher's wine glass, or very nearly set fire in the galley when trying to light the stove. He thrived on the cheerful raillery of his companions, but on one occasion thought to say to me, in a voice unaccustomedly low: "I'm good at other things."

He hardly needed to remind me. Yes, and from everything he was good at he drew lessons, little maxims of professional and extra-professional life of great cumulative impact, instantly imparted to all his friends, at the least suggestion from them, or from their situation, that they needed help, or instruction. It is awesome to extrapolate from one's own experience of his goodness the sum of what he did for others.

When Osborn Elliott, on Shirley's [Mrs. Clurman] behalf, asked me to say something today I went right to my desk, but I found it impossible to imagine his absence from the scene. Was it true that there would be no message from him tomorrow on our E-mail circuit? That we would not be dining together during the week, or sharing a tenth Christmas together? In the strangest sense, the answer is, No, it isn't impossible that we will continue as companions, because his companionship left indelible traces: how to work, how to read, how to love.

It came to me last Thursday when just after midnight my son reached me at the hotel, that I have always subconsciously looked out for the total Christian, and when I found him, he turned out to be a non-practicing Jew. It will require the balance of my own lifetime to requite what he gave to me.

—WFB

A Buckley Lexicon

For some years, the author, at a publisher's request, has been drawing up his own word lists, defined by him and illustrated with examples drawn from his published works, somewhat like a one-man French Academy writing his own dictionary.

They were initiated by the ingenious firm of Andrews and McMeel, which each year publishes a calendar titled *William F. Buckley, Jr.'s 365 Words You'd Like to Know*. Perhaps you would like to know them too, or, more likely, perhaps you know them already and would like to confirm or contest WFB's definitions or usage.

This is a decidedly informal compendium (one section ends with words starting with the letter *i*, for reasons we can't explain), but they all are part of WFB's working vocabulary.

LEXICON I—1991

The following words are taken from *Mongoose, R.I.P.*, by William F. Buckley, Jr., Random House, 1987:

affect (verb) *To pretend; to give the impression of; to feign.*
When Larry Fillmore told his superior in the Agency that he had become engaged, he was told that on no account could he reveal to his fiancée what his actual affiliation was, that he must continue to **affect** to be a Foreign Service trainee. (p. 149)

anomalous (adjective) *Unusual in context; abnormal.*

A U-2 flight, doing its twice-a-week run over Cuba, had yielded an **anomalous** picture taken over San Cristóbal. (p. 267)

arcane (adjective) *Very unusual; the kind of thing generally known only to scholars.*

There were some difficulties, mostly revolving about Spanish translations for **arcane** Russian terminology. Happily most nuclear language relies heavily on Greek and Latin roots and it never proved impossible finally to communicate everything Pushkin wanted to communicate. (p. 274)

ascetic (adjective) *Disposed to do without luxuries; austere.*

Faith Partridge was an **ascetic** woman, in part by nature, in part by necessity; she needed to hold together a household headed by a free-lance writer whose work was mostly rejected, which rejections drove him to despondent drink, even as his occasional acceptances drove him to festive drink. (p. 90)

attenuate (verb) *To stretch out; prolong.*

That was the rumor that caught Cubela's attention and that led, after two months' excruciatingly **attenuated** probing of contacts, to the first communication between Rolando Cubela and Rufus. (p. 160)

auspices (noun) *The umbrella under which you operate; the patronage.*

No questions. No nothing. But perhaps all that would happen in Havana?

Indeed it did, although the **auspices** were unexpected. (p. 198)

avuncular (adjective) *The kind of thing you'd expect of an uncle; benevolent.*

"I was class of 1918." He smiled his warm, **avuncular** smile. "It's hard for old fogies like me to think of women at Yale, though I know they've always been in the graduate school." (p. 96)

badinage (noun) *Light conversation; banter.*

Anthony said something or other, lapsing into **badinage,** and they signed off. (p. 75)

beatific (adjective) *Exalting; radiant; suggesting a special blessedness.*

Her smile was **beatific,** and now she took the glass of sherry, but before she had finished it, her eyes closed. Maria took it from her hand, and Doña Leonarda slept. (p. 126)

bursary (noun) *The arrangement by which students do work for the school or college in return for a remission of a part of their tuition or room and board.*

Sally worked at Vassar ten hours every week as a **bursary** student. (p. 92)

caudillo (noun) *A Latin American dictator, usually self-installed.*

The Americans still thought Castro a banana-republic **caudillo.** (p. 242)

chimera (noun) *An imagined idea, person, or fancy, unusually impractical, romantic.*

Turning his head abeam, the constellation his eyes fixed on had splashes of starry hair that shimmered, and eyes to steer by, and lips set in a pensive, seductive mode. He felt a luff in the sail, snapped his head forward to the mast, and quickly located his navigational star. He had wandered high on his course, while looking back at that **chimera** over Mexico. (p. 81)

communization (noun) *The transformation of a person or movement into complicity with communism, sometimes voluntary, sometimes forced.*

Dr. Alvaro Nueces had turned against Castro in 1960, protesting the **communization** of the 26th of July Movement. (p. 132)

construe (verb) *To put a certain meaning on something; to understand something in a particular way.*

Tamayo might be given an opening to **construe** a conversational jog in an unexpected way. (p. 207)

contiguous (adjective) *Immediately adjacent, in time or location.*
Lindsay Bradford was now engaged in conversation with a **contiguous** beer drinker. (p. 100)

coterie (noun) *A small group of people bound together by common interests or loyalties.*
Lieutenant Gallardo was in charge of the little **coterie** of bodyguards that surrounded Castro wherever he went. (p. 229)

cryptic (adjective) *Having a hidden meaning, perhaps even impenetrable.*
Consuelo stood by the window of his office in downtown Mexico City after receiving the **cryptic** telegram from Miami. The assignment he had received from Rolando Cubela was startling. (p. 172)

diapasonal (adjective) *A musical term which suggests fully orchestrated; full; harmonious.*
The documents they were given to read were in many respects lurid, melodramatic—preposterous even, so their exchanges were not always in the **diapasonal** mode when one of the young CIA agents would interrupt his reading to make a comment or ask a question. (p. 4)

didactic (adjective) *Characteristic of the teacher, whether in manner, or arrangement, or posture.*
"I am glad to hear your Spanish is so good, Blacky. And I, Professor Sally Partridge, am competent to test how good it is." She appeared briefly in the doorway in her dressing gown, affecting her **didactic** posture at the lectern. (p. 30)

dreadnought (noun) *A heavily armed battleship, connoting that nothing can stop it (or you).*
With my Kaypro 386, plus Path-Minder, plus Desq View, plus SideKick, plus Daniel Shurman of Humanware to make sense of it all, I am something of a **dreadnought** on a word processor. (p. 321)

epiphany (noun) *The illuminating meaning of an experience; the sudden penetration of a heretofore elusive truth.*
As he tapped out his message, the **epiphany** crystallized. His redemptive mission was incandescently clear. He, Rolando Cubela, would kill Fidel Castro. (pp. 137–38)

epochal (adjective) *Extremely important, likely to affect future events or the understanding of them.*
During the tumultuous month since being told he would be returning to Cuba on an important mission, he had been given intensive training. And then had come the **epochal** briefing the day before his departure, delivered by Malinovsky himself. (p. 253)

expiate (verb) *To make up for; atone for.*
During those ninety days he came to terms with himself. He decided that he could not **expiate** the sin he had committed against an innocent man until he had undertaken a great and heroic task of redemption. (p. 131)

expostulate (verb) *To plead earnestly in an effort to persuade or correct.*
That afternoon, Nicolai Pushkin shouted himself hoarse and spent himself to the point of exhaustion. His thickly built guard did nothing while Pushkin **expostulated**, except to read, seated at his desk, his comic book. (p. 270)

extrinsic (adjective) *Unrelated to the person or matter or idea at hand; extraneous.*
Maria later realized that she reached maturity only that day, at that moment: she felt a concern entirely **extrinsic** to her own interests. (p. 126)

extrude (verb) *To disgorge; push out; thrust out.*
She looked up at a young, bearded man who, **extruding** the envelope from her hand, said to her politely but firmly, "*Seguridad, Señorita.*" (p. 198)

fastidious (adjective) *Fussy about details; meticulous.*
Among other assets, Maria Raja had a second passport. Her mother, a refugee from Hitler's Hungary, was above all things **fastidious** about security arrangements. (p. 120)

furtive (adjective) *Stealthy; surreptitious; hidden.*

Fidel Castro had got out of the habit of **furtive** midnight meetings, far removed from the handy personal and political apparatus he had got so used to which, with the push of a button, would get him a world leader on the telephone. (p. 239)

hector (verb) *To fuss over insistently, intending to press a point.*

Blackford had made a passing effort to detoxify Sally during senior year at Yale, but hadn't since **hectored** her (or anybody else) on the subject of smoking. (p. 186)

hew (verb) *To cling; to adhere; to hold tightly to.*

As often as not Anthony would take the opportunity to **hew** to the lewd, low road. (p. 74)

hirsute (adjective) *Hairy; covered with hair.*

Fidel was of course **hirsute,** while Rolando had only the trace of a shadow. He wondered whether to shave, as he would do if he were going to a social engagement, or to leave his chin as it was. (p. 19)

histrionic (adjective) *Theatrical; stagey.*

Usually the two men were alone when Tamayo reported his commission had been completed. When that was so, they would both break out into raucous laughter after their **histrionic** exchange. (p. 161)

honorific (noun) *Titles or other forms designed to suggest titles or honors earned or received.*

There were those who believed that no one in memory would ever outshine the brilliant young Luís Miguel, dressed now like an Italian movie star, with a tiny palette of colors below his handkerchief pocket, the flora and fauna of Latin American **honorifics.** (p. 86)

husbandry (noun) *The careful, non-spendthrift management of your money.*

Faith Partridge's **husbandry** did not make her lose all perspective. (p. 90)

ideologize (verb) *To absorb within a system, so as to make it a part of that system, even if the fit isn't very good.*

Che Guevara's concern with medicine was by now almost totally **ideologized.** He cared less how to cure someone suffering from a burst appendix than that the treatment should be the responsibility of the state. (p. 129)

idiomatic (adjective) *Verbally informal.*

"The principal liquid asset is the ten thousand dollars paid by the government when your brother was killed. Faith—your mother—managed to get your father's signature on that check"—Cam Beckett was a family friend as well as attorney, and Sally did not resent his **idiomatic** references to the family situation. (p. 95)

imperturbable (adjective) *Resolutely calm; unshakable; collected.*

The official Castro of tonight, Che reflected, bore little resemblance to the **imperturbable** private Castro of Sierra Maestra. (p. 233)

indigent (adjective) *Poor; impoverished.*

Señora Cubela begged him to stay and eat something, quietly convinced that so distinguished a visitor would not share a meal in such **indigent** surroundings. (p. 175)

internecine (adjective) *Mutually damaging; wounding.*

Stalin had singular historical problems to confront, from the **internecine** question of succession after the death of Lenin, to the dogged resistance of the kulak class, to the war by Hitler. (p. 205)

inveigh (verb) *To protest, in a dogged way; to make vehement, protracted objection.*

One day Castro stormed into a radio station, seizing the microphone and **inveighing** against Batista and praising freedom and democracy and social justice and anti-imperialism for a full ten minutes while his companions kept watch for the police. (p. 18)

jocularity (noun) *Sense of fun; mirthfulness.*

Pano took the rest of his beer slowly. All the usual **jocularity** faded from his face. (p. 171)

limn (verb) *To become visible, traceable, detectable as to features or form.*

Young Jesús Ferrer, with his cosmopolitan background, his derring-do in the mountains, gradually **limned** into the consciousness of the press. (p. 213)

lubricity (noun) *Tendency to sexual stimulation; salacious.*

Blackford remonstrated every now and then when Anthony's **lubricity** got out of hand. "You are like a lot of Englishmen," Blackford once told Anthony. "They learn about sex later than we do and freeze into a Freudian first gear whenever anything remotely suggestive comes up."

lurid (adjective) *Gruesome; horrifying; causing shock or horror.*

The documents they were given to read were in many respects **lurid**, melodramatic— preposterous even, so their exchanges were not always in the diapasonal mode when one of the young CIA agents would interrupt his reading to make a comment or ask a question. (p. 4)

manifestly (adverb) *Obviously; self-revealingly.*

Sally looked at the party-dressed, self-assured, animated young lawyer, like Antonio in his early thirties; probably—no, **manifestly**—more than a lawyer to Antonio. (p. 85)

manifold (adjective) *Various; multiple; of many kinds.*

The following day Olga Kirov walked into the Cuban Embassy, explained that the Señorita Rincona was expecting her, and was admitted into the special reception area, heavily armed because of the **manifold** requirements associated with Fidel Castro's visit. (p. 181)

miff (verb) *To offend; annoy.*

"Is it your guess," Ruth probed, "that Castro would shrug his shoulders if she got **miffed**?" (p. 152)

monitory (adjective) *Warning; admonitory.*

When the censor, at the special request of the Russian-Cuban interpreter, promised a quick reading of the letter to Major Kirov from his wife, he checked his files routinely, and spotted the **monitory** marking. (p. 182)

moribund (adjective) *Deathly; about to die; having to do with death.*

When there was someone else in the room on unrelated business, Castro and Tamayo would satisfy themselves, after the **moribund** dialogue, with an oblique cross-glance, an exchanged wink. (p. 161)

multifarious (adjective) *Many and various; diverse.*

Castro liked it when his intimates joined him in exploring the **multifarious** reefs around Cuba. (p. 225)

nomenclature (noun) *A vocabulary associated with an art, or science, or discipline.*

Rolando had not got used to the brevity of revolutionary **nomenclature** and found it difficult to say "*Buenas noches, Paco*" to a man twice his age. (p. 20)

obtrude (verb) *To thrust out; push forward.*

"Your husband is at San Cristóbal," the interpreter said, a smile **obtruding** her creased face. (p. 180)

officious (adjective) *Showing bureaucratic attention; offering unnecessary and perhaps unwanted advice and services.*

She was surprised when, at the airport in Mexico, a middle-aged man, portly and **officious** (he bellowed out instructions to the porter who accompanied him), approached her at the gate of her flight, his diplomatic badge, pinned conspicuously above his breast pocket, permitting him into the inspection compound. (p. 197)

oleaginous (adjective) *Unctuous; oily; affected.*

On the second evening of his state visit in Moscow, Fidel Castro had been carried away by an **oleaginous** toast in his honor delivered by Soviet President Leonid Brezhnev. (p. 177)

palpably (adverb) *Obviously; transparently; perceptibly.*

She moved, for the first year or so, **palpably** under a shadow and it wasn't until the end of the spring term that her irrepressibly buoyant roommate unearthed the cause of Sally's melancholy and set out to do something about it. (p. 92)

patently (adverb) *Obviously; manifestly; plainly.*

Kirov plied Tamayo with questions of theoretical concern to students of Marxism-Leninism and, **patently,** of immediate concern to him. (p. 204)

penumbral (adjective) *Shadowy; done under the cover of darkness; concealed.*

Consuelo had engaged in interesting enterprises, most of them concerning Mexicans, often Mexicans seeking ways, legal and **penumbral,** of taking out of Mexico sums of money accumulated by political activity. (p. 172)

peroration (noun) *The closing part of a speech.*

The effect of Fidel's **peroration** was slightly marred by Che's aside, directed not so much at Castro directly as to the assembly. "Well, our independence would perhaps be more convincing if we relied less completely than we are forced to do on Soviet economic and military favors." (p. 141)

perquisites (noun) *Those advantages in a job or in a position that aren't a part of your formal contract.*

Perhaps she was simply doing a job, a job that not only paid well but gave her important **perquisites** in Castro's Cuba—access, for instance, to Diplotiendas, where the select few could buy coffee and extra-conventional luxuries, such as a bar of scented soap imported from Canada, or a chocolate bar. (p. 130)

piquancy (noun) *Something attractively offbeat; provocative.*

M'Lou could always make Sally laugh—that had never been a problem. Sally reacted instantly to humor, as to **piquancy.** (p. 92)

precocity (noun) *Early intellectual or artistic development.*

She walked over to her slender neighbor, whose lined face suggested an age greater than the sixty-one she acknowledged when making one of her frequent references to the **precocity** of her important son. (p. 125)

preternaturally (adverb) *Extremely; more than one would think natural.*

In less than fifteen minutes, Blackford felt **preternaturally** at home with the young Cuban designated by Rufus to be his right hand. (p. 34)

promulgate (verb) *To issue a new law or regulation.*

When Rolando Cubela concluded that he had the mandate—to execute Fidel Castro—he was prepared to be ever so cautious in his plans. Nothing reckless. After a month's deliberation, Cubela had it down on paper—in his mind:

1) Castro's death—it must be absolutely assured.

2) A plausible new Cuban government—instantly **promulgated.** (p. 156)

punctilio (noun) *Highly formal observance of formalities.*

"You wonder about me, Pano?" Blackford said.

"I need to wonder about *todo el mundo,* the whole world. My professional *puntillo*—how do you say that, my friend?"

"**Punctilio.** Okay, Pano, but it is only right, then, that we should wonder about each other. Whom do you want to hear from about me?" (p. 41)

putatively (adverb) *Supposedly; ostensibly; reputedly.*

It didn't surprise Sally that Art was talking not to old friends, **putatively** interested in Art Shaeffer, football tactician, but to undergraduates he had never met before. (p. 99)

quixotic (adjective) *Idealistic and impractical. The word comes from Don Quixote, who tilted at windmills, fancying them an enemy overcome.*

Haydee Santamaria was the sister of the brave man tortured to death during the Moncado fiasco of 1953, when Castro led the **quixotic** charge against the well-fortified barracks at Santiago de Cuba. (p. 132)

refectory (noun) *Eating quarters, usually of religious orders.*

The room across the courtyard from the entrance, on the second floor, above what used to be the chapel and was now the printing office from which Castro's instructions flowed out to his subjects, had been the monks' **refectory**. (p. 226)

remonstrate (verb) *To argue rebukingly.*

Blackford knew better than to **remonstrate** on the theme of the Elusive Distinction. (p. 171)

riposte (noun) *A bouncy reply; usually provocative.*

Blackford thought back on the agonies of the Bruderschaft, and for a moment said, reverently, nothing by way of **riposte**. This quickly communicated a hint of resistance to her. He got back into his customary role, the succubus of her taunts. (p. 31)

robustly (adverb) *Unapologetically frank, open, vigorous.*

On entering the **robustly** Victorian Fence Club, to which he had been elected as an undergraduate at about the time of Pearl Harbor, Art's spirits quickly revived. (p. 98)

sagacity (noun) *Wisdom; soundness of judgment.*

Pedrito nodded his head vigorously, in extravagant recognition of her **sagacity**, and they strolled back toward the little knots of Mexican family friends. (pp. 85–86)

sectarian (adjective) *Divisively attached to one faction within a church, ideology, or political party.*

"Khrushchev, we are admiring of the Soviet Union, we are grateful for the aid you are giving us to realize our own socialist revolution, but we cannot be conscripted into the ranks of your **sectarian** wars against Mao," Castro declaimed. (p. 140)

solecism (noun) *A breach of the formal rules, usually of syntax.*

When lunch was served, the rabbinically disguised Oakes, rather than commit any inadvertent dietary **solecism**, ate nothing, and so emerged from the plane, with his false passport, hungry. (p. 211)

somnambulist (noun) *A sleepwalker.*

To the left and right were cell doors with small apertures at eye level. The only sounds were the occasional moans and what sounded like **somnambulists'** soliloquies. (pp. 134–35)

squalid (adjective) *Squat, dirty, or wretched in appearance.*

The elm trees were budding on Vassar's neat green campus in the **squalid** city on the day the envelope arrived. (p. 94)

subterfuge (noun) *A deception.*

"It is inconceivable that Khrushchev should have authorized any such **subterfuge** without—well, without my authorization," Castro said. (p. 143)

surreptitious (adjective) *Hidden; out of sight; clandestine.*

Ingenio Tamayo was a mean-spirited man—who very much enjoyed performing Fidel Castro's highly **surreptitious** commissions primarily because they called for the discreet elimination of someone Castro did not wish officially to detain and execute. (p. 161)

sycophantic (adjective) *The manner of someone who seeks to gain favor by flattery.*

Castro laughed. He laughed uproariously. Such a laugh as demands of subordinates **sycophantic** acquiescence. (p. 22)

tumultuous (adjective) *Violently agitated; uproarious.*

During the **tumultuous** month since being told he would be returning to Cuba on an important mission, he had been given intensive training. (p. 253)

valedictory (noun) *Farewell; that which is said in the course of ending a speech or bidding good-bye.*

Fidel Castro had never succeeded in expunging from his own or others' use the traditional Cuban **valedictory** that one should go forward with God. (p. 146)

verisimilitude (noun) *Authenticity; the appearance of being the genuine article.*

Fidel explained, his voice now conversational, "The repetition? 'A most terrible, a most horrible accident?' As a writer, I would not engage in such crude repetitions. But here, it gives **verisimilitude** to the heat with which I am speaking." (p. 295)

vernacular (noun) *The language spoken in the informal idiom of a trade or profession; informal idiom.*

He reiterated—it had to be a native Soviet. No Cuban, never mind his training in Russian, could master the kind of **vernacular** the Kremlin would expect to receive in telexes from the field, the bureaucratic accretions, the idiomatic twists and turns. (p. 275)

volubly (adverb) *Talkatively.*

Betancourt, who had early on sided enthusiastically with Castro and his insurgency, was by now **volubly** disgusted with what Castro had done to his country. (p. 157)

voluptuarian (adjective) *Lustful; sensuous.*

Anthony leaned forward, got up to stir the log fire, and sat down again, his face radiant in what, under entirely different circumstances, Blackford had once referred to as "your lewd, **voluptuarian** smile." (p. 5)

williwaw (noun) *A gust of cold wind; a mini-gale.*

When the anti-Semitic williwaw of the mid-thirties suddenly threatened to grow to Typhonic force, young Astra led her widowed mother to meet her river friend, the elderly policeman with a fondness for the children who played along the river's verdant banks. (p. 121)

The following words are taken from Mr. Buckley's syndicated column, "On the Right":

---

aberration (noun) *Deviation from the truth or a moral standard, from the natural state, or from a normal type.*

Now Jeane Kirkpatrick is my sister and Pat Buchanan my brother, and if I have ever differed from their foreign policy analyses it can only have been in a moment of **aberration**. (5/4/89)

abortifacient (noun) *A drug or any agent that induces abortion.*

The choicers are now saying that the Griswold decision must be understood as permitting not merely physical barriers to impregnation, but also **abortifacients**. (4/28/89)

abrogate (verb) *To rescind; abolish by official action.*

It would be quite mistaken to **abrogate** the treaty in reaction to these infractions: Nothing would more quickly propel the three quarters of the Panamanian community that dislikes Noriega to return to his fold. (5/16/89)

accretion (noun) *Something that has been added that doesn't necessarily belong.*

The minimum wage is an **accretion** of the New Deal that is not publicly defended by any serious economist. (6/15/89)

aegis (noun) *The direction, control, supervision.*

The key to stopping the erosion of Eastern's assets under the **aegis** of the judge who seems to have the power to conduct either an autopsy or a revivification is, of course, the unions. (6/16/89)

albescent (adjective) *Becoming white, i.e., shining out more conspicuously.*

Nobody knows how Congress is going to leave Social Security and the other entitlement programs untouched and come up with $50 billion or so to save the savings and loans, which we are informed need to be saved because the alternative—letting them fail—is more costly in the long run because Congress has insured the depositors against harm. And there is the **albescent** matter of a United States with (a) no nuclear weapons facilities, and (b) a lot of unmanageable toxic nuclear waste material. (1/6/89)

analogue (noun) *Something similar; another version of the same thing.*

They speak of Sen. Joseph McCarthy paralyzing the Foreign Service: Will history give us any **analogue** more indicative of the power of superstition than that of the antinuclear lobbyists over the development of nuclear power? (7/25/89)

angst (noun) *A kind of perpetual, even neurotic state of anxiety.*

One artist sought to explain his **angst** by sticking a crucifix in a jar of urine. That this exhibit should be financed by taxpayers is a proposition Senator Helms had no difficulty taking on. (7/28/89)

animadversion (noun) *An unfriendly reference, statement, criticism.*

The machinists of Eastern Airlines tend to slur off into **animadversions** on the management of Frank Lorenzo, whose personality poses no threat to Perry Como's. (3/9/89)

anneal (verb) *To strengthen; toughen.*

The myth of Napoleon suffered mortal wounds. It required three more years to put him away permanently, but the resolve to do so was **annealed**. This time they'll probably award Gorbachev not a lifetime on St. Helena, but a Nobel Peace Prize. Machiavelli can be taken too far. (2/9/89)

arbiter elegantiae (noun) *The person who rules on matters of fashion, protocol, taste.*

Professor Arthur Schlesinger, who is the **arbiter elegantiae** of liberal fashion, wrote a few months ago that only bigots would vote against Jesse Jackson. (1/20/89)

arrant (adjective) *Naked, unmitigated.*

Soviet television is showing only pictures of Chinese students attacking Chinese soldiers. And the Soviet press quote only Chinese officials' statements in which the student protesters emerge as "counterrevolutionaries" guilty of sadistic killing of patriotic soldiers.

Any excuses for this kind of behavior are **arrant** Bolshevism of the old school. (6/8/89)

asseveration (noun) *An assertion made in very positive form; a solemn assertion.*

Dr. Robert DuPont gave the impression that he had disposed of any question (as to whether drugs ought to be legalized) before the house by his initial **asseveration**. To wit, "Name me one politician in the United States who has run successfully for political office who believes in legalizing drugs." (2/23/89)

Attican (adjective) *Athenian in its classical simplicity, elegance.*

We should all be in favor of short speeches. But if we're going to set up an **Attican** theatrical background to commemorate the moment of the Soviet departure from Afghanistan, why doesn't General Gromov use up his one minute and seven seconds to fire a bullet into his head? (2/9/89)

avatar (noun) *A high priest; a semi-god; an incarnate authority.*

There was talk by the **avatars** of a free press charging cowardice and betrayal of common responsibilities to defend the First Amendment. (2/28/89)

banality (noun) *Something obvious; repetitious; lacking in originality.*

In Warsaw President Bush told the press, "There are times in diplomacy when a certain delicacy is called for." Putting that on the front page [in *The New York Times*] could have been the work of a sly reporter whose only defense against **banality** is to print it. (7/11/89)

bellicose (adjective) *Characterized by military hostility; provocatively warlike.*

The closeness of de Gaulle and Adenauer was a historical monument to the possibilities of trans-**bellicose** life. (2/24/89)

bellwether (noun) *The guide by which one measures other data.*

The current airline industry load factor (i.e., the percentage of filled seats) is between 65 percent and 75 percent. And the **bellwether** price of a ticket (economy class, non-super saver) is greatly inflated. (6/30/89)

beneficently (adverb) *Kindly; charitably.*

Many years ago I asked the dean of my alma mater why no credit was given for the mastery of typing or shorthand and he replied **beneficently,** "There is no body of knowledge in typing." (1/19/89)

Brobdingnagian (adjective) *Huge. The word is from Jonathan Swift's imaginary country, inhabited by giants, in* Gulliver's Travels.

Finally the Khomeini cried uncle, and, at age eighty-eight, set out to attempt to bring to Iran a small measure of the growing prosperity it was experiencing even while feeding the Peacock Throne the gold, frankincense and the myrrh it had taken to consuming with such **Brobdingnagian** appetite. (2/22/89)

bull (noun) *An authoritative declaration or statement.*

Adult men and women, staring hard at a clause in the Constitution of the United States that forbids an establishment of religion and recognizing no reasonable nexus between that prohibition and the recital at their local public school of a public prayer jointly formulated by rabbis, ministers, and priests, receive on Monday what might be called a juridical **bull** from the Supreme Court, and on Tuesday there is compliance. (6/29/89)

burden (noun) *The central theme; the principal idea.*

The front-page story (the *New York Times,* July 24) is headlined, "H.U.D. Approved Rent Subsidies/After Coors Wrote the Secretary." From the headline alone, the **burden** of the story is communicated. (7/27/89)

Cartesian (adjective) *Relating to the philosopher Descartes, who specified direct and logical forms of thought and analysis.*

In an idle moment during a holiday, I searched the wave band of a portable radio in quest of something to listen to. None of the twenty or so options relayed classical music. It required only a little **Cartesian** *gelandesprung* to alight at the conclusion that it is the responsibility of the government to maintain monuments that are man-made, as well as those given us by nature. (2/7/89)

catechizing (verb) *Severe questioning designed to illuminate moral guilt.*

Tony Coelho, who has spent much of his adult life **catechizing** Republicans, fled office rather than submit to a public study of whether he has himself been submitting to the standards he has preached. (6/2/89)

cavil (noun) *A quibble; a frivolous objection.*

The **cavil** that Beethoven doesn't need looking after since his records sell by the trainload isn't at all satisfying to someone spelunking through radio channels in search of Beethoven. (2/7/89)

chiliastic (adjective) *Relating to the Second Coming; having to do with the reappearance of Christ on earth.*

That the existence of the Congress of People's Deputies, or of the Supreme Soviet, should have meaning at all is positively **chiliastic** in its implications. (6/1/89)

cloying (adjective) *The special taste you get when something is repeated, or heard, or seen so often that it loses its original flavor and becomes simply boring.*

The lawyers are of course active, as also the anti–capital punishment organizations; but lawyers and generic opponents of capital punishment have a way of **cloying**—they sometimes leave the impression they'd have freed Jack the Ripper—and indeed they kept Ted Bundy alive for ten years. (8/11/89)

commonweal (noun) *The common interest; the good-better society.*

The idea of a vote governed by an ethos of the **commonweal**—a voter's fiduciary obligation to vote not alone for his narrow best interest, but for the public interest—is substantially lost sight of as candidates gather together money from the lobbyists and settle down to lifetimes in the House of Representatives. (6/22/89)

contumely (noun) *Disdain; expression of contempt, dislike, hatred.*

Has Michael Milken, in his revolutionary lifetime, re-situated the ethical norms of business conduct in such a way as to earn universal **contumely**? (9/28/89)

credenda (noun) *The constituent elements of what forms your belief, in religion, politics, whatever.*

Imagine a reformist pope who questions the authenticity of the Bible, and you have some idea of the philosophical and spiritual problems that Gorbachev faces. He cannot deny the **credenda** of the Soviet state without denying at the same time his own legitimacy. (5/4/89)

danseur (noun) *The male dancer in a ballet group; often used to suggest said dancer's exhibitionistic impulses.*

George Bush was in Brussels deciding that he would, for once, take the arms control show away from the world's premier **danseur,** Mikhail Gorbachev. (6/1/89)

decoct (verb) *To figure out by deduction what the true meaning is of a statement, a symbol, an oblique communication.*

It isn't easy to **decoct** the machinists' message from the picket signs or from public pronouncements. (3/9/89)

demagogue (noun) *Someone who appeals for public support by saying, or promising, that which most appeals to the crowd, or mob, he is addressing.*

Noriega is an effective **demagogue**. And—always a winner in Latin America—he has defied the United States of America and got away with it. (5/9/89)

deracination (noun) *Cutting off cultural and institutional and ethnic ties, leaving the individual, or tribe, or nation without its traditional support system.*

A European figure so august that ladies curtsy when they are presented to him was telling the table at which we all sat about the great mischief being done by the missionaries in Venezuela who move in on native tribes and totally break down their cultural order, resulting in **deracination** and chaos. (3/14/89)

disingenuous (adjective) *You know what is true, but you argue as though you didn't know it, because you want to make a point that serves your interests.*

Congressional retaliation is based on attempting to fix in the public mind that the President anticipated revenues of ABC, a growth rate of XYZ, and interest rates of GHI—and that these were defective as predictions and **disingenuous** in conception. (2/21/89)

disinterested (adjective) *A position taken—political, moral, analytical—which has no bearing on the position that would suit your own personal interests, because your interests are simply not involved.*

They seek to dramatize a point that choicers should force themselves to acknowledge is entirely **disinterested,** even as demonstrators for civil rights were fighting not for themselves, but for others. (7/20/89)

dithyrambic (adjective) *A truly exaggerated exercise in praising something or somebody.*
In recent weeks we found ourselves interrupted in our **dithyrambic** praise for democracy when the guy in El Salvador whom we did not like won. (5/9/89)

dulcet (adjective) *Done in quiet, sweet, soft tones.*
The question arises of the fear of a united Germany, a fear widely expressed, if mostly in **dulcet** tones, by Europeans east and west of Berlin. (8/10/89)

ecumenical (adjective) *A position that has the backing of more than one faction, political, theological, or scientific.*
Two ideas are current, neither of them the property of conservatives or of liberals. It is an **ecumenical** mix, with some conservatives arguing that the show is up for world communism, some liberals arguing that it is much too early to tell. (6/8/89)

egregious (adjective) *Flagrant; distinctively presumptuous, horrible.*
Recent amendments to the Constitution have merely codified popular passions. But (save for the largely irrelevant exception) there has been no constitutional amendment the purpose of which was to revise the interpretations of a Supreme Court, notwithstanding **egregious** provocations by the Court, most recently during the '50s and '60s when it became commonplace to refer to the "Warren Revolution." (6/29/89)

envoi (noun) *The final communication; valedictory; send-off.*
The portrait of Ronald and Nancy Reagan done by Mike Wallace for *60 Minutes* was their **envoi** to the republic on their presidency. (1/17/89)

epigoni (noun) *Close followers, given to imitating, or being bound by, the star they become the creatures of.*
William Winpisinger, the president of the striking (Eastern Airlines) machinists, is a socialist and is quick to put a class struggle aspect on any labor-management division, and indeed Mr. Winpisinger lost no chance to do this. And the **epigoni** jumped in. Sure enough, there was Jesse Jackson joining the picketers. (3/9/89)

eremitical (adjective) *Characteristic of the hermit; far removed from ordinary life and considerations.*
To say that Mrs. Jones is unbiased in the matter of Colonel North because she was unaware of him, notwithstanding that Colonel North dominated the news in the press, on radio, and on television for about three weeks two springs ago, isn't to come up with a fine mind that missed the entire episode because she was absorbed in **eremitical** pursuits. (2/3/89)

eschatological (adjective) *Pertaining to the ultimate ends of life, existence.*
It became clear—years ago, for the perceptive; only recently, for the true believers—that communism does not work, i.e., communism does not bring on the redemptive **eschatological** paradise predicted by Marx, does not ease the burden of the worker, and does not reduce the power of the state. (3/2/89)

eschew (verb) *To turn down; ignore; disdain; do without.*
The United States has two sovereign responsibilities at this point. The first is to maintain our guard. The second is to **eschew** any invitations to finance the economic rehabilitation of the Soviet Union. (6/1/89)

estop (verb) *To put an end to; bar; prohibit.*
Is it suggested that a defense secretary who had been to a cocktail party, or even one who had gone to bed drunk, would **estop** the flow of instructions from the President? (3/7/89)

evanesce (verb) *Gradually to disappear.*
Marx and Engels promulgated the view that if you eliminate private property, all derivative vices **evanesce**. (3/30/89)

excogitation (noun) *Something thought up and said or written or pronounced. There is an implication of derision, or contempt, when the word is used.*
Roe *v.* Wade was a lousy decision, perhaps even an indefensible act of constitutional **excogitation,** and the choicers know that they are safest by not asking the Court to look again at this century's version of the Dred Scott decision. (1/19/89)

ex officio (adverb) *"In virtue of the office" is the literal translation. What it designates is the power of the pope, in Catholic dogma, to pronounce finally on questions of religion and morals.*
About a year ago, Senator Nunn suddenly announced that the stricter of two plausible versions of the ABM ban on testing was the correct one, and I swear it was like the pope pronouncing **ex officio** on a question of dogma. (2/16/89)

fatuous (adjective) *Silly; thoughtless; inane.*
So much for Tom Wicker's **fatuous** attempt to make his frantic point that the fate of Owen Lattimore is now being visited on Tom Foley by the ass in the Republican National Committee who wrote a silly memo from which only silly people would conclude that the charge was made that Tom Foley is gay. (6/9/89)

ferula (noun) *A cane, or rod, used as an instrument of punishment. Usually a flat piece of wood, sometimes encased in leather.*
Since it is pre-decided that the Bush Administration will not advocate the legalization of drugs, the Bennett basket is going to have to be chock-full of **ferula** with which to beat offenders. (6/27/89)

flaunt (verb) *To exhibit with the view to attracting attention.*
Successful men are not necessarily ascetic men, and although a public is within its rights in declining to elevate to the presidency a candidate who **flaunts** his immorality, it is simply mistaken to suppose that failed marriages and occasional draughts of good spirits ruin the night of our kindly and gentle nation any more than they ruined the wedding at Cana. (2/16/89)

fons et origo (noun) *The source. Literally, the fountain and origin.*
Mikhail Gorbachev can criticize Constantin Chernenko and Leonid Brezhnev—and Brezhnev can criticize Nikita Khrushchev, who criticized Stalin; but no one will criticize the **fons et origo** of all that poison, Lenin. (5/26/89)

fungible (adjective) *Two things that are fungible will intermix without difficulty. Some things are not fungible, e.g., oil and water.*
Although the age of computers and satellites and television dishes has done much to circulate ideas hitherto pockmarked in totalitarian cavities, in fact knowledge isn't all that **fungible.** (6/8/89)

fusilier (noun) *Rifleman; soldier armed with a fusil (musket).*
Deng Xiaoping is seized, in Karl Wittfogel's phrase, with the megalomania of the aging despot, and rather than acknowledge the right of his citizens peaceably to assemble in order to petition the government for a redress of grievances, he shoots them; and, tomorrow, may hang those his **fusiliers** missed. (6/6/89)

fustian (adjective) *Overblown; pompous; wordy.*
The only thing we can reasonably do isn't, at this point, **fustian** retaliation. (6/6/89)

gerrymander (noun) *An electoral district carved up without regard to demographic symmetry, intending to fortify a particular political party at the expense of another political party. The word is also used as a (transitive) verb.*
The fat and rich Democratic **gerrymanders** are going to find a dragon waiting for them when they rev up for the decennial hanky-panky. Those interested in self-government should side with the dragon, Newt Gingrich. (3/24/89)

gravitas (noun) *The kind of solemnity one associates with kings, bishops, and wise men. The word in Latin was used in Rome to designate the mien of thoughtful, civic-minded, wise men.*

The key figure, of course, is Senator Nunn, around whose judgments **gravitas** closes in like clouds gathering around a prophet. (2/16/89)

hegemonic (adjective) *Preponderant influence and authority, to the point of excluding other influence.*

In order to maintain the pressure that orients the Soviet Union and China toward reform in the first instance, we need to continue to roam those quarters of the world where the Soviet Union continues to exercise **hegemonic** influence. (8/1/89)

hegemony (noun) *Preponderant influence or authority; leadership; dominance.*

Since Moscow is still willing to pay $14 million per day to continue to support Fidel Castro, Daniel Ortega reasonably hopes to hang on to that incremental Soviet subvention necessary to eliminate any possibility that the tatterdemalion contras will ever seriously challenge the Marxist **hegemony** in Nicaragua. (2/14/89)

impute (verb) *To attribute accusingly, often unjustly.*

I assume that a communist is a pro-communist, though Tom Wicker sometimes acts as though it would be an act of McCarthyism to **impute** pro-communism to Joseph Stalin, let alone Mikhail Gorbachev. (7/13/89)

The following words are taken from *On the Firing Line: The Public Life of Our Public Figures*, by William F. Buckley, Jr., Random House, 1989:

---

abominate (verb) *To loath; detest.*

I had never heard of the gentleman, a professor of English from the University of Missouri, who wrote a review of *Saving the Queen* for the *Kansas City Star*. He made it quite clear that he had spent a considerable part of his adult life **abominating** me and my works and my opinions. He was manifestly distressed at not quite disliking my first novel. (p. 420)

abstruse (adjective) *Difficult; difficult to understand, to penetrate the meaning of.*

Here is a man [Cardinal Arns of São Paulo] who studied literature at the Sorbonne, where he achieved his doctorate; who taught petrology and didactics at highly respected universities; who has written twenty-five books, including **abstruse** treatises on medieval literature. (p. 34)

accretion (noun) *An addition to the original law, idea, concept, institution, which is not necessarily a legitimate part of the original.*

WFB: You say that the rights of lawyers and priests should extend to journalists.

ABRAMS: As a general matter, yes. There are some differences, but as a general matter, yes, I—

WFB: That's sort of a revolutionary **accretion** and yet, in asserting that point, you tend to do so as an exegete of the Constitution rather than as somebody who wants to amend it. (p. 198)

afflatus (noun) *A creative impulse; a divine warrant or inspiration.*

As Muhammad Ali explained, "I was the onliest boxer in history people asked questions like a senator." But then he was touched by the **afflatus** of Elijah Mohammed. . . . (p. 94)

altruistic (adjective) *An act motivated by concern for others, rather than for oneself.*
 WFB: *(addressing a question to George Gilder)* I am determined to build a cheaper mousetrap in order to get your patronage and to line my pocket. But since in the course of creating a cheaper mousetrap I have made it possible for you to purchase one, I have committed an objectively **altruistic** act for selfish motives. Now, why do you assume there is an incompatibility between those two concepts? (p. 297)

ameliorate (verb) *To improve; make better.*
 To suggest that politics is not the solution is to endanger political careers. It is not a subject directly addressed by Jean-François Revel—the difficulty in achieving the desired circulation of thought, for the purpose of **ameliorating** such problems as race relations in such a country as the United States. (p. 325)

animadversion (noun) *An unkind, critical remark.*
 It seems to me that if you are going to take legendary auspices for current attitudes, you will find ten **animadversions** on man for every one on woman in literature. (p. 440)

animadvert (verb) *To remark or comment critically, usually with strong disapproval or censure.*
 John Kenneth Galbraith asked me just when major corporations had lost 85 percent of their value: and I evaded an answer (I did not have the data in the front of my memory; and in any event, I had exaggerated the effect of the Dow Jones dip of 1969–70 by **animadverting** one of JKG's books, suggesting that its collapse had coincided with that of the market). Manifestly, I did not get away with this, and ought not to have done. (p. 22)

anomaly (noun) *Deviation from the normal or common order, form, or rule; abnormality.*
 The "conservatives" in the Kremlin are those who desire a return of Stalinism. Sometimes the **anomalies** bite back. *The New York Times* ran a sober account from Moscow about a crackdown by "Kremlin conservatives" against the importation of foreign books. One of the proscribed titles was *The Conscience of a Conservative* by Barry Goldwater. (p. 168)

antinomian (adjective) *Opposed to, defiant of, or rejecting moral law.*
 William Kunstler was probably the best-known of the lawyers who identified themselves with dissent, and who sought a kind of **antinomian** liberty for dissenters. (p. 97)

apostasy (noun) *Defection from one's faith, political or religious.*
 I was left to infer that while serving as a courier, Whittaker Chambers was proving to his case officer his utter reliability (subject, of course, to **apostasy** from the Communist movement). (p. 405)

asceticism (noun) *Rigorous self-discipline, severe abstinence, austerity.*
 Bauhaus was the name given to a compound of architects gathered together after the First World War in Germany to remark the general desolation, which they sought to shrive by a kind of architectural **asceticism** noted for a cleanness of line, an absence of ornamentation, the blandness of color, and the "honesty" of generic building materials. (p. 263)

banausic (adjective) *Of purely mechanical interest or purpose.*
 Al Lowenstein was the original activist, such was his impatience with the sluggishness of justice, so that his rhythms were more often than not disharmonious with those that govern the practical, **banausic** councils of this world. (p. 433)

bowdlerized (verb) *Shrunk, with the purpose of expurgating titillating bits. After Thomas Bowdler (1754–1824. R.I.P.)*
 Churchill pauses from the war effort to cable back his regards to Mrs. Luce, who meanwhile has been asked by the Joint Chiefs of Staff to brief them on her analyses, which, suitably **bowdlerized**, appear in successive issues of *Life* magazine and are a journalistic sensation. (p. 444)

cognate (adjective) *Related to each other; analogous.*

Freedom of the press, freedom of speech—these **cognate** liberties are, of course, routinely construed to extend not only to journalism but also to expression of a more subtle kind, namely, artistic expression. (p. 201)

condign (adjective) *Deserved; appropriate; adequate.*

ABRAMS: A reporter, Paul Branzburg, was called to testify in front of a grand jury, and he took the position that he should not have to testify about material he had learned in confidence. The Supreme Court held five to four that he did have to testify. Mr. Branzburg subsequently left the state, and so far as I know has not returned to Kentucky.

WFB: Is that **condign** punishment? (p. 196)

congeries (noun) *A collection; accumulation; aggregation.*

I have seen only two political firestorms that resulted in sharp and immediate political response. The first was the sentencing of William Calley, the anti-hero of My Lai. The crowd simply insisted his penalty was inordinate, insisted on this for a **congeries** of reasons, primarily a frustration with the length and conduct of the Vietnam war. (p. 152)

contumacious (adjective) *Obstinately disobedient; rebellious; challenging the law.*

Francis Plimpton wrote to me, I replied, and toward the end of our correspondence he asked me to make publicly plain his own feeling about **contumacious** lawyers. (p. 102)

cosmology (noun) *A view of the origin, structure, and (often) purposes of the universe.*

Jeff Greenfield wrote a withering piece for the *Yale Alumni Magazine* about an appearance I made at Yale which had begun with a press conference and went on to a formal speech. His piece was a stretch of arrant scorn for my thought, logic, diction, and **cosmology.** (p. 171)

coterminously (adverb) *Contained within the same period; coextensive.*

Allen Dulles was head of the CIA for nine years. During that period, and as a matter of fact since then, he and the CIA are criticized more or less **coterminously:** Allen Dulles was the CIA incarnate. (p. 411)

defi (noun) *A challenge; rejection of.*

Tom Wolfe had published *The Painted Word,* a **defi** hurled in the face of the art critics, challenging their taste, questioning their originality, and lamenting their power. (p. 262)

derogation (noun) *Disparagement; belittling.*

(*WFB posing a question to Allen Dulles*) What is your opinion of the continued **derogation** of the intelligence function? Why should the CIA be made a—a sort of general laughing stock? (p. 412)

desideratum (noun) *That which is desired; the better, or even perfect, state.*

Jesse Jackson began by saying that for a black, his blackness is forever the supreme fact of life. In saying so, without suggesting that he lamented this priority, he moved very far from Martin Luther King's Dream, in which color made no difference: color-blindness isn't a **desideratum** for Jackson. (p. 313)

dialectical (adjective) *The interactive action between one view and a contradictory view.*

You cannot argue effectively with anyone whose position is removed from your own by more than one **dialectical** unit. (p. 365)

dilate (verb) *To write, or speak about, at great or greater, length.*

(*WFB speaking to Mortimer Adler*) You begin by reaching a very interesting conclusion which I would like to hear you **dilate** on, namely that it doesn't really matter whether there was a prime mover [i.e., a force that created the first earthly thing]. (p. 451)

dyspeptic (adjective) *Bitter; morose; spastic.*

George Gilder was working for the *New Leader* magazine, having graduated from Harvard a few years earlier. In **dyspeptic** protest against the Republican Party's nomination of Barry Goldwater, he and a friend had written a book called *The Party That Lost Its Head*—i.e., the GOP, by nominating Goldwater. (p. 299)

egalitarian (noun) *Equalist; one who believes in the doctrine of equalizing the political and economic condition of everyone.*

The novelistic urge of the great ideological **egalitarians** who write books with such titles as *The Ugly American* has been to invest in their protagonist in the CIA appropriately disfiguring personal characteristics. (p. 418)

epicene (adjective) *Sexless; lacking in vigor, virility.*

To spend one hour with a principal British political figure without any critical attention being given to the leaders of the Labour Party or to his critics within the Conservative Party would make for an **epicene** hour. (p. 282)

epistemological (adjective) *The philosophical discipline that has to do with learning; how we learn.*

Is it correct or incorrect to view the adversary process as an **epistemological** process? Will it lead us to the truth, or is it more likely to be described as something which leads us to the only bearable means by which we will agree to proceed in deciding whether to put this guy in jail or not? (p. 232)

eponym (noun) *A person whose name gave meaning to a word that became common. In the case of Billy Budd—as cited.*

Billy Budd is practically an **eponym** for—innocence; purity. (p. 419)

eristic (adjective) *Finely argumentative; taking logic and argument to extreme lengths.*

Any failure by beneficiaries of the free world to recognize what it is that we have here, over against what it is that they (the Communist world) would impose on us, amounts to a moral and intellectual nihilism: far more incriminating of our culture than any transgression against **eristic** scruples of the kind that preoccupy so many of our moralists. (p. 420)

exiguous (adjective) *Scant; meager.*

Five years later, the general prosperity of commercial television edged *Firing Line* over toward public broadcasting (commercial television could not afford to give up the revenue a program like *Firing Line*, with its **exiguous** ratings, displaced). (p. xxxii)

extirpate (verb) *To wrench out; destroy; exterminate; remove any traces of.*

In his late crazy days, as distinguished from his early crazy days, Mao Tse-tung decided that Mozart and Beethoven were great public enemies of the revolution and sought to **extirpate** them and others from the inventory of music the Chinese were permitted to listen to. (p. 327)

gainsay (verb) *To deny; ignore; overlook.*

It was not true that the liberal element within the Republican Party was willing to hand the party over to the right. There was no **gainsaying** the political influence of such prominent Republican liberals as Senator Charles Mathias. (p. 159)

gravamen (noun) *The central point of a complaint; the heart of an accusation or objection.*

The **gravamen** of James Baldwin's complaint was that the *Times*'s publication had aborted the publication by *Playboy* magazine of Baldwin's speech, imposing a financial sacrifice on him of the $10,000 he had been told *Playboy* would pay him. (p. 54)

gregarious (adjective) *Seeking and enjoying the company of others.*

[Clare Boothe Luce] became ill. She was alternately reclusive and **gregarious** in the six months that were left. (p. 442)

homiletic (adjective) *Of the nature of a sermon; having the intention of edifying morally.*

REAGAN: Do you mean, bad as Congress has been all this time with praying, they want us to take it now without praying?

WFB: I think that what you said is so **homiletic** it might itself be unconstitutional. (p. 190)

imposture (noun) *A fake; a substitute of an unreal for the real; an act of deception.*

At the U.N., you regularly hear the totalitarians proclaim that genuine freedom is social and economic security. For that reason, there is "freedom" in East Germany, but not in West Germany. The argument is philosophically an **imposture**—just to begin with—because "freedom" is properly defined as an absence of constraint from man-made impediments. (p. 361)

ineffaceably (adverb) *Impossible to deny or erase.*

It becomes relevant here to bear in mind that [Clare Boothe Luce] was always, necessarily, **ineffaceably**, a very attractive woman, no matter how hard she strove to make a theoretical cultural case forbidding any distinction between men and women. (p. 436)

inimical (adjective) *Injurious; unfriendly to; harmful.*

The resistance to private-sector enterprise as **inimical** to abstract democracy is thoroughly ingrained in many who think themselves especially sensitive in their understanding. (p. 135)

interstitial (adjective) *Coming in the small narrow spaces between the principal parts.*

Professor Donald MacKay is a physicist and a Christian. The remarkable exchange between him and Professor B. F. Skinner I present here with **interstitial** comment because what both men say repays more reflection than the pace of their spoken exchange permits. (p. 82)

invidiously (adverb) *Intending to be critical; at the expense of.*

(*WFB speaking of Roy Cohn*) He shows his adamant loyalty to the FBI, well-sheltered contempt for the character of Martin Luther King, and scorn for hypocritical comparative judgments, he accuses the accuser, and he ends with a mom-and-pop defense of a favorite government agency. I say this, by the way, **invidiously**. (p. 409)

irredentist (adjective) *Having to do with the claim by a nation to lands that once belonged to it.*

While formally going along with Peking in its insistence of sovereignty, we maintained, in effect, diplomatic representation in Taiwan. Meanwhile, the graduated liberal reforms of Chiang Ching-kuo combined with the industry and energy of the people of Taiwan to nurture an evolutionized super-minipower. And direct **irredentist** pressure from the mainland lessened. (p. 336)

laconically (adverb) *With the use of few, rather than many, words; succinctly.*

Professor Galbraith, I'd be most grateful if you would answer my questions directly and **laconically**. (p. 72)

latitudinarianism (noun) *Broadmindedness; permissiveness.*

The feds shrewdly decided to try Harry Reems in Memphis, Tennessee, a venue not given to **latitudinarianism** in matters of obscenity. (p. 204)

licentiousness (noun) *The disregard of accepted standards of meaning, behavior, analysis.*

The terminological **licentiousness** of the day is very striking. In his book Paul Johnson quotes Castro as saying, "Of course we're a democratic society. We have a democracy every day, inasmuch as we're expressing the will of the people." It's that kind of word-play which is the essence, as Orwell told us in another connection, of totalitarianism. (p. 389)

millenarian (noun) *The person who believes that perfection is coming for us down the line, for reasons biological, political, or theological.*

PAUL JOHNSON: Broadly speaking, there are two types of people. One is the person who believes in God. The other is the type who says, "I don't believe in God. I don't believe in an afterlife. It's all nonsense. This life is the only one we've got, and we have to try to improve it, and I don't believe that human—"

WFB: The **millenarian**?

JOHNSON: Yes. "—I don't accept that human nature is permanently imperfect. It can be perfected." (p. 449)

mimetic (adjective) *Imitative.*

WOLFE: In domestic architecture there was constant guerrilla warfare and rebellions and so forth. But not in great public structures.

WFB: What does that tell us about the response of public men—this sort of **mimetic** response as against the relative individualism of the consumer?

WOLFE: In this country, in the midst of what could certainly be called the American Century, we remain the most obedient in matters of the arts—we remain the most obedient little colonial subjects of Europe. (p. 265)

mollify (verb) *To quiet; soothe; lessen.*

Do I understand you, Mr. Reagan, to say that the actual role attempted by, say, President Johnson during the riots of his administration might have exacerbated the situation rather than helped to **mollify** it? (p. 181)

morphology (noun) *The study of the nature of a word, thought, movement, including its causes and its composition.*

Firing Line continued to deal with much else, but, inevitably, spent time in the sixties on The Sixties: on its culture, its **morphology**, and its implications. (p. 3)

nascent (adjective) *Aborning; about to be.*

I had persuaded Steve Allen in the course of a discursive afternoon that the logic of his adamant stand against nuclear weapons committed him to backing a preemptive strike against the **nascent** nuclear-bomb facilities of Red China (as we used to call it). (p. 235)

nuanced (adjective) *Given to slight, delicate, subtle degrees of meaning, explanation, analysis.*

Firing Line is a **nuanced** program, and a thorough knowledge of English is required to do justice to subtle thought. (p. 334)

nugatory (adjective) *Trifling; of little importance.*

It has always seemed to me that the correct balance of police power and individual rights should reflect the crime rate. The interdiction by the airlines of terrorist weapons, conducted at the expense of every American who steps foot on an airplane, can be demonstrated statistically to be **nugatory** in its accomplishments. (p. 230)

obloquy (noun) *Hatred; loathing; discrimination; ostracism.*

The Scarlet Letter was designed to stimulate public **obloquy**. The AIDS tattoo is designed for private protection. If our society is generally threatened, then in order to fight AIDS we need the civil equivalent of universal military training. (p. 212)

oligopolistically (adverb) *In the manner of a small group of agents who control the market.*

(*Speaking of OPEC*) Thirteen governments **oligopolistically** took hold of a great reservoir of the supply of oil and quadrupled its prices overnight. (p. 70)

penchant (noun) *Tendency; inclination; liking for.*

George McGovern is a formidable opponent, a crowd-pleaser with a populist-analytical **penchant** that has carried him a long way, though when he ran for President, he was rejected by forty-nine states. (p. 139)

peroration (noun) *The closing part of a speech.*

After the debate was over I shook McGovern's hand and whispered to him, "George, that **peroration** is as good as when I first heard you use it at Dartmouth in 1957." "Yes," he agreed. "Very effective, isn't it?" (p. 58)

petrology (noun) *The study of the source of a discipline, most commonly, the fathers of the Christian faith.*

Here is a man [Cardinal Arns of São Paulo] who studied literature at the Sorbonne, where he achieved his doctorate; who taught **petrology** and didactics at highly respected universities; who has written twenty-five books, including abstruse treatises on medieval literature. (p. 34)

phlogistonic (adjective) *Heat-producing; combustible.*

Far from demanding with increasing truculence the diplomatic reincorporation of Taiwan, the government of Deng simply let the **phlogistonic** question cool. (p. 336)

piquant (adjective) *Something attractively offbeat; provocative.*

I was amused that Alan Dershowitz revealed on the program that he himself had never seen the movie *Deep Throat*. That was a **piquant** touch: it enabled him to say, in effect, "I am defending a man for taking part in a movie. What is in that movie is so irrelevant to the defense I shall not even bother to view it." (p. 205)

polemical (adjective) *Argumentative; intending to make a point at variance with that of your opponent.*

[Clare Boothe Luce] always had an answer to any question at the tip of her tongue. Though this, I came to know, was **polemical** training; she was often dissatisfied, after consulting her private intellectual conscience, with the answer she gave. (p. 157)

prescind (verb) *To pull out; abstract; disengage.*

(*Speaking to* The New York Times's *super-journalist Fox Butterfield*) On this matter of the economic improvement of the average Chinese life, may I ask, have you found that there is a considerable tendency to **prescind** from the passage of time improvements in literacy or in health or in food consumption? (p. 329)

proclivity (noun) *An inclination; propensity; leaning.*

One thinks again of Jean-François Revel and his indictment—the **proclivity** of democracies to dissipate energies out of a sense of guilt. (p. 407)

Procrusteanize (verb) *To produce conformity by ruthless means. After Procrustes, a mythical Greek giant, who stretched or shortened captives to make them fit his beds exactly.*

Firing Line does not **Procrusteanize** a guest's formal vocabulary. (p. 82)

proximate (adjective) *The nearest cause; the most direct agent of change.*

Mr. Al Lowenstein is generally regarded as the **proximate** agent of the whole [Eugene] McCarthy phenomenon. (p. 425)

prurient (adjective) *That which seeks out sexual stimulation.*

In 1972, when Harry Reems made *Deep Throat*, the courts were being guided by the Roth standard. That decision, handed down by Justice Brennan in 1957, held that something was obscene if it appealed exclusively to the **prurient** interest and had no "redeeming social importance." (p. 204)

puerile (adjective) *Childish.*

A young man was once a guest of *Firing Line* for the sole reason that he had become, at age twenty-seven or thereabouts, the de facto manager of the mind and body of Bertrand Russell. Here was this **puerile** ideologue sending out invitations in Lord Russell's name to statesmen and scholars the world over to attend a War Crimes Trial of Americans for pursuing an objective in Vietnam, quoting Lord Russell to the effect that there were no differences between the United States and the Nazis. (p. 278)

quietus (noun) *An end; the death of.*

The ABM treaty put a **quietus** on U.S. defensive technology: We even dismantled a protective ring of antinuclear defense missiles planted in the area of Wyoming, and did not trouble to avail ourselves of the option to construct a ring of defensive weapons around Washington, D.C. (p. 388)

quintessence (noun) *The essence of; a pure, typical form of.*

The editor of *Vogue* invited me to explain, explicitly, the "American look" since so many reviewers had denominated Blackford Oakes as being "quintessentially" American. I thought to reject the invitation, because I reject the very notion of **quintessence** as here applied. (p. 419)

quotidian (adjective) *Recurring daily.*

I introduced candidate Ronald Reagan in January 1980 with a view to provoking his critics. And I toyed, with the advocate's delight, with the **quotidian** criticisms of Mr. Reagan. (p. 180)

rapacious (adjective) *Greedy; ravenous.*

Tom Wolfe records the **rapacious** success of the Bauhaus school, which within a generation had captured almost the whole of the American architectural academy, bequeathing us such megatonnage as, say, the World Trade Center. (p. 263)

ratiocination (noun) *Systematic thought.*

It has occurred to me (after modest **ratiocination**) that style is, really, a matter of timing. (p. 279)

recidivist (adjective) *Of the kind committed before; back to the old business.*

Prisons are bursting at the seams, with over 200,000 more criminals inhabiting quarters than our prisons were designed for, resulting in a gruesome intensification of the awful experience in prison and a resulting increase in **recidivist** crime. (p. 249)

rectitude (noun) *Uprightness (here used sarcastically); righteousness.*

Taiwan was even denied its athletes' participation in the Olympics in Canada, a seizure of diplomatic **rectitude** that did not affect Prime Minister Pierre Trudeau at the expense of any Soviet satellite, though Russia's de facto rule over the Baltic states is at least as questionable—or at least as offensive—as Taiwan's dream of ruling over China. (p. 335)

regnant (adjective) *The predominating meaning, figure, concept.*

"Are you against labor unions?" an indignant Harriet Pilpel asked Professor Thomas Sowell on *Firing Line.*

Professor Sowell replied, "You asked what were some of the factors that stood in the way of black economic progress and I said that one of them was the labor union. That is a fact, and I'm simply reporting facts, not prejudices." How do you handle such a man, if your political career is staked out on the **regnant** cliché? (p. 319)

reticulation (noun) *Networking, i.e., figuring out diagrammatically where everything is, or should be—so many paces to the right, so many paces up, down, etc.*

Hoffa appeared to believe that the proper organizing principle for [prison] reform was segregation. [Inmates] should be carefully segregated according to age, the nature of the offense, and temperament. One got the feeling that all these **reticulations**, finely drawn, would have isolated James Hoffa as the sole occupant of one federal prison. (p. 243)

rubric (noun) *The governing license; the sponsoring idea, concept, protocol.*

The **rubric** that year of [Jesse Jackson's] PUSH convention was "Black America: An Economic Common Market." (p. 313)

ruminate (verb) *To let the mind dwell on and develop; disport with.*

One **ruminates** on the analysis, the idealism, the inventiveness, the disillusion, the demoralization expressed by Professor Thomas Sowell. (p. 325)

solipsism (noun) *The idea that, actually, only you exist. (From "just oneself")*

Doesn't it strike you as possibly the case that the twentieth century, where the intellectual and romantic odysseys usually begin from yourself and end up with yourself, becomes therefore the age of **solipsism**? (p. 262)

stentorian (adjective) *Loud; declaratory; emphatic.*

I can hear even now the vibrancy of [Norman Thomas's] voice and the **stentorian** tones of the preacher denouncing the sinner. . . . His then current crusade was to save Vietnam and the United States Marines from each other. (p. 4)

synecdoche (noun) *The single example, in place of the whole. The one, for the many.*

LUCE: The Old Testament myth of the Garden of Eden has aroused the ire of women feminists for generations. God creates heaven and earth in this legend in Genesis. He then creates man; man shares in the spirit of God.

WFB: Man the male or man the **synecdoche** for human beings? (p. 439)

tautology (noun) *The statement of that which is obvious, and therefore does not need restating; redundant.*

Now, the fact that six times as many shootings occur in houses that have guns as don't have guns seems to me—well, the **tautology** is, you obviously can't have a shooting where you don't have guns. (p. 215)

tendentiously (adverb) *Stated in such a way as to promote a cause; not impartial.*

In his opening statement, John Kenneth Galbraith got about as much as one can possibly hope to get from twelve minutes: rapport with the audience; a broad statement of his position, **tendentiously** given; a sense of wisdom and of realism; and a bite or two to show the audience that the speaker has plenty of ginger, and knows just where, as required, to stick it. (p. 65)

tocsin (noun) *A bell used to sound an alarm or a general summons.*

Michael Harrington published a book, *The Other America.* The book described a portion of the American population beset by tormenting poverty. Its thesis was brought to the attention of President Kennedy on November 19, 1963. The book sounded the **tocsin** for massive federal action to "make war" on poverty. (p. 306)

trenchant (adjective) *Forceful; tightly constructed.*

Norman Podhoretz was associated with the left in American politics until some time in the late sixties, when he gradually, but with that **trenchant** willpower which even his critics acknowledge, changed his mind. Since then he has been a penetrating critic of disorderly thought and romantic views of the Soviet Union. (p. 112)

truculent (adjective) *Combative; vitriolic.*

Firing Line programs have almost always been governed, temperamentally, by the attitude and behavior of the guest. Norman Thomas was a highly **truculent** debater (a running distemper was a part of his public persona). (p. 10)

vaticination (noun) *A prediction; prophecy.*

(*WFB speaking on* Firing Line *with Norman Thomas*) Because in point of fact, if you don't mind, rather than simply—automatically—accept your **vaticinations**, I'd like to point out that in Korea, we did actually stop the aggressor. (p. 5)

Weltanschauung (noun) *The German word, widely used, to denote one's world-philosophy, the sum of one's essential views (on politics, theology).*

People are curious about the Impossible Guest. I could name but won't the guest whose entire knowledge of life filled eight minutes, so that when the ninth came along, he simply recycled his *Weltanschauung* for the next eight minutes. (p. 43)

—

The following are *more* words taken from Mr. Buckley's syndicated column, "On the Right":

—

auto da fé (noun) *The ritual accompanying the execution of a heretic, used especially in connection with the Inquisition.*

Here was a modern **auto da fé:** not for countenancing heresy, but for denouncing it. (9/21/89)

booboisie (noun) *The dumb class. The term is H. L. Mencken's, and he self-evidently took pleasure in suggesting that the dumb class was composed substantially of the bourgeoisie, normally thought of as the hardworking middle class.*

The critics of those who joined Senator Jesse Helms in protesting the use of public money to finance the "art" of Robert Mapplethorpe and Andres Serrano did a hell of a job of caterwauling about the provincialism of the **booboisie** who protested the exhibitions. (9/21/89)

candor (noun) *Directness of expression.*

It appears that Mayor Koch's most ingratiating quality, an unquenchable thirst for **candor,** was what finally did him in. (9/14/89)

covenant (noun) *A rather solemn agreement, designed as binding.*

There is one aspect to the tax turmoil that asks for reflection. It is the unfortunate breach of the 1986 **covenant** at which time it was generally agreed that the tax committees of Congress would simply let things alone for a while and see how it all worked out. (9/22/89)

dysgenically (adverb) *Genetic profusion of a kind thought inimical to public interests. Thus Dr. William Shockley spoke of the "dysgenic" effect of the greater rate of black population growth.*

Israel does not like the fact that most Russian Jews express a wish to settle down not in Israel but in the United States because it needs a Jewish population to guard against being **dysgenically** overwhelmed by Arabs who procreate with the speed of light. (10/3/89)

indolence (noun) *Laziness; a failure to accept responsibility.*

Children need to feel at a very early age the whiplash of **indolence:** long dull lives washing dishes and seeing television movies of non–Third World countries such as Japan and West Germany with thriving populations. (9/26/89)

inimical (adjective) *Unfriendly; hostile.*

We should be careful when we say we do not "claim the right to order the politics of Nicaragua." The politics of Nicaragua are very much our concern when they are co-opted by a foreign power **inimical** to the best interests of the United States and the Nicaraguan people. (3/28/89)

iniquitous (adjective) *Sinful; evil; wrongful.*

There were those who, reviewing the work of Owen Lattimore, which included eleven days of interrogation by the chief counsel of a Senate committee, came to certain conclusions about him that Tom Wicker suggests were surrealistic at best, **iniquitous** at worst. (7/13/89)

internecine (adjective) *Mutually destructive; harmful.*

It is gradually dawning on the population that the war against Iraq was won by Iraq, if it can be said that there are winners of encounters so **internecine.**

interstice (noun) *A space, usually little, that intervenes between solid matter.*

Under Stalin, a list long but not indefinitely long was drawn up of prohibited activities. Anything not prohibited could be engaged in. That left little **interstices** within which to maneuver. (3/30/89)

intractable (adjective) *Unmovable; inflexible; difficult to lead.*

Is the Brezhnev doctrine really dead if the retreat from Afghanistan is nothing more than an unprofitable collision with a major and **intractable** force? (5/12/89)

junket (verb and noun) *To travel as a congressman or public official at public expense, ostensibly on business, actually on a pleasure trip.*

Members of the judiciary do not send a million letters without postage, do not **junket** around the world, do not get free massages or whatever in the exercise room of the House of Representatives. (2/10/89)

lacuna (noun) *The missing item, datum; the hole in someone's learning.*

Ten years ago a longtime friend of Sidney Hook confided in me the most wonderfully humanizing story of the **lacuna** in Hook's knowledge. (7/21/89)

laggard (adjective) *Slow to act, to respond, to react.*

We are **laggard** on that [deterrent] front and we face a concrete problem in Europe given the tergiversation of Helmut Kohl on the modernizing of the remaining nuclear missiles in West Germany. (2/22/89)

lagniappe (noun) *A gratuitous little gift, in any form, e.g., a free liqueur at a restaurant after dinner.*

Drugstore cowboys walk out into the street, hail the mob, and tell them to come in for free ice cream cones. That is how the Bush administration clearly understands Gorbachev's **lagniappe** when he offered to destroy 500 missiles, 2.5 percent of his inventory, reducing the threat to export glasnostian Bolshevism by a factor of nothing, these missiles having been redundant for years. (5/18/89)

lèse majesté (noun) *An offense against the sovereign; whence an indignity at the expense of the reigning authority.*

When Newt Gingrich took time off to insist that evasion of the reelection finance laws ought to apply not only to lowly congressmen but also to the speaker of the House, he faced a barrage of shocked fraternity brothers unaccustomed to violations of the law of **lèse majesté**. (3/24/89)

libertarian (adjective) *The political philosophy that stresses the absolute right of the individual to make his own decisions, unobstructed by the state.*

Conservatives raised on **libertarian** principles have long since remarked that any invasion of the sacred No Trespassing sign puts you on the slippery slope toward collectivist capitulation. (2/7/89)

literati (noun, plural) *The literate, educated class.*

What proved most curious is that there was a substantial lobby that night, among the **literati** of Louisville, for every position concerning the drug problem. (3/23/89)

lodestar (noun) *The guiding force, star; the focus of attention, inspiration.*

Kissinger Associates would almost certainly not succeed as a partnership of 100 retired Foreign Service officers: The relationship to the **lodestar** becomes too attenuated. (3/17/89)

lotus (noun) *The mythical Greek fruit, the eating of which induced torpid satisfaction, pleasure, forgetfulness of duty.*

The mood is out there, and we are tasting the **lotus** in the green pastures of peace. (9/29/89)

Luddite (adjective) *Pertaining to the nineteenth-century movement that disapproved of labor-saving devices. Hence, opposed to technological progress.*

We, the government, will protect you—even as we protect bank depositors—against lawsuits the effect of which is to enrich the legal participants, protect nobody against a threat not yet perceived, and wrench the United States into a **Luddite** gear which, had such a thing happened two generations ago, would have been the equivalent of forbidding the flight of airplanes on the grounds that one of them would lose its wings and fall on Aunt Minnie. (7/25/89)

manifestly (adverb) *Made obvious by its own appearance; self-evidently.*

We are invited to believe that if John Tower participates in any of the activities engaged in by Alexander the Great, Napoleon and General Grant, he is **manifestly** unfit to serve. (2/16/89)

metaphysical (adjective) *Beyond measurement; transcendent; supersensible.*

Those who rail against it do so for the most practical reason: They have not mastered its use. They strive for **metaphysical** formulations to justify their hidden little secret (sloth and fear). (1/19/88)

miscegenetic (adjective) *Having to do with the mixture of the races; here used as suggesting a mixture of East and West.*

The new policy would say to the Soviet Union: Look, the big dream—the ideological conquest of the world—isn't going to happen. Not only is it not going to happen, other things aren't going to happen—namely a permanent, **miscegenetic** annexation of Eastern Europe by you. So let's make a deal. (8/10/89)

moot (adjective) *Rendered irrelevant by circumstances; no longer of practical significance.*

Suddenly we discover that the FBI knows somebody or some people who have seen John Tower under the influence; but, in any event, the whole question became **moot** when he made his public pledge to give up drinking altogether, if confirmed. (3/10/89)

nabob (noun) *An important character, whether by reason of heredity, power, or wealth.*

Henry Kissinger has an inclination to know who are the movers and shakers. To suggest that this is on the order of a movie starlet wanting to know the industry's **nabobs** is entirely to misunderstand the point. (3/17/89)

nefarious (adjective) *Disreputable; unethical; detestable.*

The feds charge insider trading and a number of other activities, some of them **nefarious,** some of them—well, that is one of the reasons so many people are interested in Mr. Milken. (9/28/89)

obsequious (adjective) *Fawning; servile; sycophantic.*

Even if one accepted Castro's figures, the progress in his country cannot match the progress in other Caribbean nations, so what is there to celebrate, save the hope that the day will come when the mere mention of Castro's name calls to mind not only massive torture, political prisoners and a docile, **obsequious** press, but also a lifeless society, fallen behind in general welfare. (1/3/89)

obverse (noun) *The other, opposite side (in a coin, the obverse of tails is heads).*

The business of finding twelve jurors in Washington, D.C., who so to speak never heard of Colonel Oliver North assumes ludicrous proportions, something like the **obverse** of Diogenes' search for an honest man. (2/3/89)

pander (verb) *To truckle to someone's desires, usually disreputable—e.g., lust, greed, power hunger.*

Would it be possible to institute death as the penalty for drug merchants? Would the court prohibit the execution of drug merchants who had **pandered** to minors? (6/27/89)

peregrination (noun) *A voyage from place to place to place; voyaging about, especially including foreign countries.*

Conceivably one could find life on Mars—nice old ladies and gentlemen who could tell us that Jesus Christ was a planetary figure of parochial dimension, and by doing so spare the Christian world the awful overhead of all those priests, and nuns, and papal **peregrinations,** and missions, and cemeteries. (7/25/89)

perfervid (adjective) *Excessively, unbalancedly ardent.*

If what the optimists are saying is that a wave of reason is sweeping over the world, how do we account for the **perfervid** worship of the Ayatollah Khomeini the day he was buried? (6/8/89)

perfidy (noun) *Deceit; treachery.*

Any effort to pursue an investigation into allegations that the plane that brought down in flames Pakistan leader Zia was sabotaged by sophisticated Soviet chemical explosives was blocked. By the Soviets? No no no, you don't understand. By the United States. Why expose Soviet **perfidy** when détente is at an exhilarating boil? (2/9/89)

periphrastic (adjective) *Ornately long-winded; given to profuse formulations.*

Three cheers for Senator Jesse Helms. As ever, he tends to get to the point of a difficult question with carrier-pigeon directness, leaving many of his sophisticated critics lost in **periphrastic** meaninglessness. (7/28/89)

perspicacious (adjective) *Analytically or visually acute.*

Up until a few years ago, Paris did not permit anyone to publish or to sell the works of the Marquis de Sade. Simone de Beauvoir wrote a book on de Sade in which she stressed the historical and **perspicacious** passages in de Sade, to which the appropriate comment is, "Aha." (7/28/89)

pettifoggery (noun) *Little-mindedness; bureaucratic absorption with silly little details.*

To tell the members of the federal judiciary that they cannot get a raise even sufficient to cope with inflation is **pettifoggery** of an ignoble sort. (2/10/89)

phantasmagoria (noun) *An ongoing vision, nightmare, fantasy.*

The Chinese communists are not likely to renounce their **phantasmagoria** explicitly, nor to sacrifice what they call socialist centrism. (3/21/89)

platonic (adjective) *Otherworldly.*

The **platonic** ideal of the unbiased juror presumes a quarrel in which there hasn't been significant national involvement. (2/3/89)

plebiscite (noun) *A submission of a proposed new law, or whatever, for a vote by the people.*

It was a very splashy and moving open letter, signed by 170 writers, actors and artists, urging Fidel Castro to hold a **plebiscite** on his rule. (1/3/89)

polemical (adjective) *An argument designed to damage someone else's position; disputation, as hand-to-hand combat.*

M.I.T. Professor Lawrence Lidsky predicts that inherently safe nuclear plants that can produce electricity at less than one-half the cost of current reactors are unlikely to come along for twenty years or so, because existing forces stand by their **polemical** guns. (1/12/89)

prescience (noun) *The faculty of being able to see ahead.*

We are talking on the eve of near-universal access to the atom bomb. There is little doubt but that the Iraqis would now have it, save for the boldness and **prescience** of the Israelis. (2/22/89)

prodigality (noun) *Extravagance; reckless spending.*

Newt Gingrich had warmed up on Tip O'Neill, whose genial **prodigality** with the people's purse was accepted as the good-old-boy way of doing things. (3/24/89)

propitiate (verb) *To appease, conciliate.*

Last Sunday's (London) *Times* reveals that the publishers Viking Penguin, who bought Mr. Rushdie's novel, are negotiating with Britain's Moslem leaders. The objective is to **propitiate** them, and to get from them some sort of peace offering that can be waved across the Mediterranean to the Moslem world. (2/28/89)

provincialism (noun) *A narrow, usually uneducated, concern for what lies immediately about you, as distinguished from farseeing, urban, cosmopolitan.*

It isn't a sign of **provincialism** to say that it makes more sense to spend excess dollars on developing domestic fuel options than on inquiring into the flora and fauna of Mars. (7/25/89)

proximate (adjective) *Pertaining to the immediately preceding event, or push, or causative factor.*

It is not to give in to economic determinism to reflect on the **proximate** pressures bringing about these reforms [in South Africa]. (2/21/89)

punctilio (noun) *The concern for form, manners, appearance.*

The story of the Bay of Pigs is told again and again. But always in the telling of it, by modern chroniclers, one tends to lose sight of the bloody landscape, so distracted are we by democratic **punctilio.** (1/24/89)

pundit (noun) *A wise man, but often used sarcastically. Columnists, for instance, are regularly referred to as "pundits" who "opine"—usually by people who disagree with their punditry.*

Now while George Bush is President, no subordinate is going to come out in favor of legalizing the sale of drugs, the culture shock being as it is. Such proposals are here and there made by a **pundit,** or a mad libertarian, or a fatalist. (3/3/89)

putative (adjective) *Supposed; ostensible; reputed.*

Much will happen in the weeks and months ahead in conference between the Senate and the House of Representatives, and Senator Helms would be well counseled to exclude from his proscription any **putative** work of art more than fifty years old. This would distinguish the Rodins from the Mapplethorpes. (7/28/89)

renascent (adjective) *Born again; recrudescent.*

Effective leadership needs to be shown by the bankruptcy judge, who if properly guided buys the long-term prospects for creditors, which are improved by a **renascent** airline rather than by the sale of its nuts and bolts. (6/16/89)

revivification (noun) *The rebirth; the invigoration of; the injection of life into.*

The key to stopping the erosion of Eastern's assets under the aegis of the judge who seems to have the power to conduct either an autopsy or a **revivification** is, of course, the unions. (6/16/89)

rubric (noun) *The governing license; the sponsoring idea, concept, protocol.*

The business of being tried by your peers, which is the governing **rubric** in these matters, makes you begin to wonder whether there isn't a bearing between finding Colonel North's "peer" and deciding what it is that he is being tried for. (2/3/89)

salient (noun) *The cutting point; the apex of the military formation, or of an argument.*

President Bush has not confronted the massed will of the Soviet government in any crisis. This doesn't mean that such a will won't materialize, and won't present a crisis. The most obvious **salient** here is West Germany. (5/2/89)

sate (verb) *To overfill to the point of glutting; cloying.*

What is it that tempers the appetite of Mikhail Gorbachev for bloody expansionism? Answer: There is no evidence that his appetite is tempered, but much evidence that his appetite cannot be **sated** because of what George Bush might call "the economic thing." (3/21/89)

satyagraha (noun) *The pressing of a political or moral position through the doctrine of passive disobedience. Associated with Gandhi.*

Of course, China is the great melodramatic event of the political decade, practicing the **satyagraha** of Gandhi on a massive scale, with tanks being deployed, not in unison to march against the masses, but pointing at each other, on the eve of what became a great civil war. (6/8/89)

schismatic (noun) *A deviant (usually religious); unlike the heretic, the schismatic still belongs to the old communion, but is separated from its core authority.*

Is Swaggert's deviant lechery characteristic of evangelical Protestantism? Is Khomeini's genocidal search for **schismatics** and blasphemers a correct transcription of the word of Allah? Is an excommunicated Mormon paradoxically an example of the practicing Mormon? (2/16/89)

sclerosis (noun) *Hardening of the tissue owing to neglect or overburdening. The metaphor suggests inactivity to the point of sluggishness, owing to years of inattention or bureaucratic overhead.*

Gorbachev hasn't repealed all those accretions of state socialism. To do so would pit him against every Comrade Ulanov who clings to his position of authority. Besides which, the market needs a little time to extrude three generations of compacted **sclerosis.** (5/4/89)

sclerotic (adjective) *The adjectival form to express "sclerosis," above.*

When you meet with Mr. Milken, you meet at the same time with his lawyer and with a couple of aides. The situation is not for that reason **sclerotic.** (9/28/89)

sinologist (noun) *A student of Chinese history, culture, language.*

Novelist and **sinologist** Robert Elegant writes: "Regarding the recent controversy about the emperor of Japan, I should like to quote from an interview that he gave to Bernard Krisher of *Newsweek.*" (2/24/89)

strictures (noun, plural) *The demands, restrictions, requirements of.*

Mr. Bush disappoints his American supporters by failing, once he had left China and was unbound by the **strictures** of diplomacy, to remark sadly on the continuing low estate of human rights in China. (3/2/89)

stultification (noun) *The act or process of invalidation; immobilization; being rendered useless.*

In Brazil, inflation brings unemployment, **stultification** and grinding poverty. (3/21/89)

superannuation (noun) *Becoming useless, because of age.*

I have mentioned that a study last summer reveals that there is a greater turnover in the House of Lords (from **superannuation**) than there is in the House of Representatives (where 99 percent of the incumbents who ran for office were returned to office last November). (3/24/89)

suppurating (adjective) *Generating pus; giving out poison.*

In Leningrad the successor to Romanov was defeated—even though he ran unopposed—thus documenting the failure of communism to transform human nature. Now that is an official part of the Soviet record. And nothing *Pravda* can do to bury the results of the vote can hide the **suppurating** sore: Marxist man is a human badly clothed and underfed. (3/30/89)

symbiosis (noun) *The profitable coexistence of two organisms, to their mutal advantage.*

The counsel to President Truman began by advising him that the president had no authority to engage in secret intelligence work in peacetime, but later, under pressure, revised this opinion to the effect that if a president OKs a secret enterprise and Congress provides the funds for carrying it out, the **symbiosis** between these two acts breeds a little constitutional baby, through artificial insemination. (1/24/89)

tabula rasa (noun) *(From the Latin, "clean slate.") The condition of the mind before it is exposed to anything; total innocence, blankness.*

What Judge Gerhard Gesell and the defendants appear to be looking for is Seven Truly Ignorant Washingtonians, who will approach the question of Colonel North, guilty or innocent, **tabula rasa**—with absolutely unformed opinions. (2/3/89)

tendentious (adjective) *Stated in such a way as to promote a cause; not impartial.*

I pause here to remark that the series is politically **tendentious.** It is a plain matter of record that Bobby Kennedy was the man who authorized the taping of Dr. King. (1/24/89)

tergiversation (noun) *Reversal of opinion; backsliding.*

We are laggard on that [deterrent] front and we face a concrete problem in Europe given the **tergiversation** of Helmut Kohl on the modernizing of the remaining nuclear missiles in West Germany. (5/12/89)

transubstantiate (verb) *To change into another substance; transform; transmute.*

Surely a society that has the power to conscript, and in many cases send [men] to their deaths in defense of that flag and its citizens, has also the right to guard against desecrating the flag that symbolizes, even it if does not **transubstantiate**, their ideals. (6/23/89)

trinitarian (adjective) *Having three parts; threefold; usually referring to the Christian belief in the Trinity. Opposite of Unitarian.*

Now the intricacies of the alleged crime of Salman Rushdie are read for the most part by Westerners for whom discussion of whether the word "prostitute" can conceivably characterize the prophet's wives, or whether the term "Mahmoud" can ever be used to refer to the prophet is about as engaging to Christians and Jews as discussions of the **trinitarian** God of the Christians engage the Moslem world. (2/22/89)

troth (noun) *One's pledged word.*

We should not have been surprised when the spokesman for Castro carefully explained to us that the **troth** had been plighted by the Cuban people thirty years ago once and for all: In the Marxist world there is no retreat from history. (1/3/89)

turpitude (noun) *Corruption; evildoing; iniquity.*

Neither Ronald Brown nor other victims of Republican **turpitude** specify what it is that Republicans did to Wright that Democrats didn't also do to Wright, given the ethics panel's bipartisan vote. (6/2/89)

unshirted (adjective) *Undiluted; unsparing; undisguised.*

Charles Murray, Manhattan Institute author of *Losing Ground,* urges President Bush to give **unshirted** hell to the critics of private education. (1/27/89)

usurpation (noun) *The wrongful assumption of power.*

A constitutional amendment, done athwart the will of the Court for the first time in modern history, would accomplish more than simply bringing relief to the majority who consider themselves victims of judicial **usurpation**. (6/29/89)

velleity (noun) *A slight, i.e., nonfervent wish, much as one might have a velleity for a Popsicle.*

People get annoyed when you use words that do not come trippingly off the tongue of Oprah Winfrey, but how else than to designate it as a **velleity** would you describe President Bush's fair-weather call for landing some people on Mars? (7/25/89)

venal (adjective) *Corrupt; susceptible of being bought.*

Here is what the *New York Times* invites the reader to think. Joe Coors is a wealthy brewer from Colorado and is known to be a hot conservative. It is especially ironic under the circumstances that he should be the **venal** influence peddlar. (7/27/89)

vermiform (adjective) *By derivation, "wormlike"; used almost exclusively to suggest "useless," even as some human organs are thought of as vermiform appendices, e.g., the appendix.*

The other day, historian Arthur Schlesinger, Jr., was lamenting the very institution of vice president, on the grounds that he was not really elected by the people; rather, he is a **vermiform** appendix of the presidential nominee, who comes to life only when the president dies or is shot. (1/6/89)

vulgarian (noun and adjective) *A person of vulgar habits, mind, manners, dress, or behavior.*

All of this adulation, which reaches even into the demonstrators' square, was for a man (Mao Tse-tung) at once the total **vulgarian;** and the Brobdingnagian dictator, a kind of King Kong poet. (5/26/89)

winnow (verb) *To separate, seeking the better, or the best; to analyze, with the same purpose in mind.*

When the anti-federalists mobilized during the days the Constitution was being discussed, they enunciated what was to become the Bill of Rights. This list of rights included Provision No. 7 which was both more wordy and more absolute than what **winnowed** down into the Second Amendment. (7/18/89)

xenophobia (noun) *A hatred, fear, or suspicion of that which is foreign, or of foreigners.*

A factor not to be dismissed is the **xenophobia** of a great power (China) that for a century and a half was a plaything of the younger sons of European noblemen. (5/23/89)

Lexicon II—1992

ab initio (Latin) *From the beginning.*

He had begun Latin, last year, at Greyburn, and had been trained *ab initio* in the English sequence. (From *Saving the Queen,* p. 63, Doubleday & Company, 1976)

ad hominem (adjective) *Marked by an attack on an opponent's character rather than by answer to his contention.*

Beame was so clearly above that kind of suspicion that an insinuation to that effect was never even raised, not even in a campaign desperate for issues and gluttonous for *ad hominem* argument. (From *The Unmaking of a Mayor,* p. 282, The Viking Press, 1966)

ad libitum (adverb) *In accordance with one's wishes; ad lib.*

To have proposed abortions *ad libitum* was, quite simply, unthinkable for a politician. (From *Cruising Speed,* p. 234, G. P. Putnam's Sons, 1971)

abattoir (noun) *Slaughterhouse.*

I wondered amusedly and intensively, what could J. K. Galbraith be up to, revealing these thoughts as we approached the **abattoir,** the Cambridge Union? (From *Cruising Speed,* p. 155, G. P. Putnam's Sons, 1971)

aberrant (noun) *A person whose behavior departs substantially from the standards for behavior in his group.*

It is not unlikely that this book, upon its appearance, will be branded as the product of an **aberrant** who takes the Wrong Side, i.e., the side that disagrees with the "liberals." (From *God and Man at Yale,* p. 140, Regnery Books, 1986)

ablutions (noun) *The washing of one's body or part of it.*

Several witnesses noted the license number, and the California authorities had it within minutes, leaving it a mystery why there was no one there at his apartment to greet Edgar Smith when he drove in to perform the identical **ablutions** of nineteen years earlier—an effort to remove the blood from his person and clothing. (From *Right Reason,* p. 197, Doubleday & Company, 1985)

accession (noun) *Something added, as to a collection or formal group.*

Abbie Hoffman is not the King of England, but the point of course is that he seeks a kind of metaphorical **accession** to the throne by the use of any means. (From *Cruising Speed,* p. 208, G. P. Putnam's Sons, 1971)

acerbic (adjective) *Sharply or bitingly ironic.*

His only apparent extracurricular involvements were an occasional letter to the *Yale Daily News,* **acerbic,** polished, and conclusive in the sense of unfailingly suggesting that any contrary opinion should not presume to expect from him any rebuttal. (From *Saving the Queen,* p. 11, Doubleday & Company, 1976)

acidulous (adjective) *Biting, caustic, harsh.*
By May 14, 1981, Edgar Smith had become, in the **acidulous** words used by one commentator, "the most honored murderer of his generation." (From *Right Reason,* p. 189, Doubleday & Company, 1985)

adjudication (noun) *A formal ruling by a tribunal.*
So how do we make the final **adjudication**? Why not use a Democratic measurement of the Misery Index? Under Mr. Carter, the Misery Index stood at 19.8. Under Mr. Reagan, at this moment, it is 15.8. (From *Right Reason,* p. 94, Doubleday & Company, 1985)

affectation (noun) *A manner of speech or behavior not natural to one's actual personality or capabilities.*
He had intended to ask Anthony whether "10:36" was an **affectation,** but forgot, and accordingly took pains to be punctual. (From *Saving the Queen,* p. 18, Doubleday & Company, 1976)

a fortiori (adverb) *All the more convincingly; with greater reason; with still more convincing force.*
A mother, while obviously exercising de facto authority over the survival of the fetus, is nevertheless legally and **a fortiori** morally nothing more than the custodian of the fetus whose insulation against abuse ought to be guaranteed by the state. (From *Cruising Speed,* p. 241, G. P. Putnam's Sons, 1971)

agglomeration (noun) *An indiscriminately formed mass.*
Yale's mission is not articulate except in so far as an **agglomeration** of words about enlightened thought and action, freedom and democracy, serve to define the mission of Yale. (From *God and Man at Yale,* p. 223, Regnery Books, 1986)

agglutinate (verb) *To unite or combine into a group or mass.*
The clerk uttered the workaday incantation in the humdrum cadences of the professional waterboy at court. The procedure is everywhere the same. The speed must be routinized, and accelerated, like liturgical responses, the phrases **agglutinated,** yet somehow audible. (From *Saving the Queen,* p. 245, Doubleday & Company, 1976)

altruistic (adjective) *A disinterested consideration of, regard for, or devotion to others' interests.*
It could in fairness be said that all the money thus solicited goes straight to the student in one form or another. In the last analysis, it is being solicited for **altruistic** purposes. (From *God and Man at Yale,* p. 134, Regnery Books, 1986)

anarchic (adjective) *Tending toward anarchy; lawless, rebellious.*
The policeman was relieved when the young man suddenly strode off, because his build, though slim, was pronouncedly athletic, and deep in his eyes there was an **anarchic** stubbornness, which policemen detailed to guarding the Soviet legation were experienced enough to spot. (From *Saving the Queen,* p. 17, Doubleday & Company, 1976)

anathema (noun) *A vigorous denunciation.*
I ask reasonable observers to look out for evasive and irrelevant answers, for rebuttal by epithet, for flowery **anathemas.** (From *God and Man at Yale,* p. 140, Regnery Books, 1986)

Anglophilia (noun) *A particularly unreasoned admiration of or partiality for England or English ways.*
Helen had long since become accustomed to Blackford's desire to meet everyone, which she attributed to natural gregariousness, and a galloping **Anglophilia.** (From *Saving the Queen,* p. 128, Doubleday & Company, 1976)

animus (noun) *Ill will, antagonism, or hostility, usually controlled, but deep-seated and sometimes virulent.*
The anti-American **animus** was not really all that transparent until just before the punishment began, and on through the ferocity of it and the hideously redundant final blows. (From *Saving the Queen,* p. 79, Doubleday & Company, 1976)

anomie (noun) *A state of rootlessness in which normative standards of conduct and belief have weakened or disappeared; a similar condition in an individual, commonly characterized by personal disorientation, anxiety, and social isolation.*

Edgar Smith had walked out of Trenton into the more incapacitating bonds of **anomie**. (From *Right Reason,* p. 195, Doubleday & Company, 1985)

antipodal (adjective) *Opposed; widely different.*

More academic and philosophical attention has been devoted in the last fifty years to the flowering of Marxist thought and life under Marxism. Still, it is astonishing how little thought is given to the great residual paradox expressed in the **antipodal** manifestos of our time. (From *Right Reason,* p. 228, Doubleday & Company, 1985)

aperçu (noun) *A brief glimpse or immediate impression, especially an intuitive insight.*

Professor Edward Luttwak came up several years ago with a hauntingly bright **aperçu** calculated to distinguish between Mao man and Soviet man. (From *Right Reason,* p. 275, Doubleday & Company, 1985)

apodictically (adverb) *Expressing necessary truth; with absolute certainty.*

The prediction (mine) that the two major candidates would differ from one another only in the appoggiaturas was, it turned out, correct. The *New York Times* made the point **apodictically**. (From *The Unmaking of a Mayor,* p. 169, The Viking Press, 1966)

a posteriori (adjective) *Arriving at a principled conclusion as a result of an examination of the facts; reasoning from the particular to the generality.*

Will the historians trained in **a posteriori** sleuthing say to us one day, "Kennedy got this insight from the history of Walpole that Galbraith gave him to read"? Did JFK read it? (From *Cruising Speed,* p. 94, G. P. Putnam's Sons, 1971)

appoggiatura (noun) *An accessory embellishing note or notes preceding an essential melodic note or tone.*

He knew not to expect any explanation of how the mission had been accomplished— these romantic **appoggiaturas** on the mechanics of the spy business were peculiarly the anxiety of the Americans and the British. (From *Saving the Queen,* p. 237, Doubleday & Company, 1976)

apriorism (noun) *Reasoning from principles to particulars; thus, if free speech is right, the person who exercises it is right.*

Nothing is more futile—or, for that matter, more anticonservative—than to indulge the heresy of extreme **apriorism**. (From *The Unmaking of a Mayor,* p. 261, The Viking Press, 1966)

arcana (noun) *Secret or mysterious knowledge or information known only to the initiate.*

Truman Capote was something of a lay criminologist, appearing on talk shows, explaining such terms as "sociopath," "psychopath," and other **arcana** of penological psychology. (From *Right Reason,* p. 186, Doubleday & Company, 1985)

artifice (noun) *A wily or artful stratagem; guile.*

Oakes flushed, doodling on his pad, conscious that everyone was looking at him, unlearned in the **artifices** of appearing indifferent. (From *Saving the Queen,* p. 63, Doubleday & Company, 1976)

aspersion (noun) *The act of calumniating; defamation.*

I mention Robert Kennedy without **aspersion** of any kind—on the contrary; because his foes and his friends agree that he felt deeply, and it is at least the public understanding that he was not merely a practicing Catholic but a believing Christian. (From *Cruising Speed,* p. 160, G. P. Putnam's Sons, 1971)

aspirant (noun) *One who is ambitious of advancement or attainment.*

Quite possibly the **aspirant** mayor, in order to get himself elected, would need to make precisely those commitments to the old order which preclude the very actions needed to overcome those crises. (From *The Unmaking of a Mayor,* p. 29, The Viking Press, 1966)

asseveratively (adverb) *With positive or emphatic affirmation.*

I am going to devote my time today to setting forth one or two propositions, some of which I tender **asseveratively,** others—well, inquisitively. (From *Right Reason,* p. 112, Doubleday & Company, 1985)

assiduously (adverb) *Marked by constant, unremitting attention or by persistent, energetic application.*

Robert Price resisted, his contention being that Lindsay's candidacy was best served by flatly ignoring his Conservative opponent, which Lindsay proceeded **assiduously** to do. (From *The Unmaking of a Mayor,* p. 160, The Viking Press, 1966)

assonant (adjective) *Marked by resemblance of sound in words or syllables; resemblance.*

In Garry Trudeau's "Doonesbury," the reader is well nourished, all the more so since there is all that wonderful **assonant** humor and derision in midstrip: indeed, not infrequently the true climaxes come in the penultimate panel, and the rest is lagniappe. (From *Right Reason,* p. 385, Doubleday & Company, 1985)

asymptotically (adverb) *Getting closer and closer to a goal, but never quite reaching it.*

The ceremony reaches cyclical heights of debauchery every few years as the management struggles, **asymptotically,** towards the goal of fully anesthetizing the losers' pain. (From *Cruising Speed,* p. 221, G. P. Putnam's Sons, 1971)

banal (adjective) *Lacking originality, freshness, or novelty; failing to stimulate, appeal, or arrest attention.*

He begins to recount his misgivings about American society, the war, the draft, the profit system, the educational establishment. My answers are diffuse, **banal,** and repetitious. (From *Cruising Speed,* p. 224, G. P. Putnam's Sons, 1971)

bawdy (adjective) *Obscene, lewd, indecent, smutty.*

In undermining religion through **bawdy** and slapstick humor, through circumspect allusions and emotive innuendos, Professor Kennedy is guilty of an injustice to and an imposition upon his students and the University. (From *God and Man at Yale,* p. 15, Regnery Books, 1986)

beleaguered (adjective) *Hemmed in; bottled up: subjected to oppressive or grievous forces; harassed.*

What power did the Mayor of New York, or the **beleaguered** publishers, have to come to the aid of the public—in the wake of a generation's legislation granting special immunities to the labor unions who are free to conspire together in restraint of free trade? (From *The Unmaking of a Mayor,* p. 106, The Viking Press, 1966)

belletristic (adjective) *Relating to the writing of* belles lettres; *speech or writing that consciously or unconsciously is more concerned with literary quality than with meaning.*

The special idealism of the youth who went to college or completed college during the postwar years seized on collective fancies. When these fell apart, they fell back to the paunch liberalism of the fifties, dressed up by the **belletristic** politics of Adlai Stevenson. The end came in Dallas. (From *Cruising Speed,* p. 92, G. P. Putnam's Sons, 1971)

Benthamite (noun) *After Jeremy Bentham, principal architect of utilitarian philosophy: one who adheres to the theory that the morality of any act is determined by its utility, and that pleasure and pain are the ultimate standards of right and wrong.*

The problem is to weigh the voting strength of all the categories and formulate a program that least dissatisfies the least crowded and least powerful categories: and the victory is supposed to go to the most successful **Benthamite** in the race. (From *The Unmaking of a Mayor,* p. 4, The Viking Press, 1966)

bestir (verb) *To stir up; rouse into brisk, vigorous action.*

If the alumni wish secular and collectivist influences to prevail at Yale, that is their privilege. What is more, if that is what they want, they need **bestir** themselves very little. (From *God and Man at Yale,* p. 114, Regnery Books, 1986)

bifurcate (verb) *To branch or separate into two parts.*

Yale shouldn't be turned over to the state because there are great historical presumptions that from time to time the interests of the state and those of civilization will **bifurcate**, and unless there is independence, the cause of civilization is neglected. (From *God and Man at Yale,* p. 1, Regnery Books, 1986)

blasé (adjective) *Apathetic to pleasure or life; indifferent as a result of excessive indulgence or enjoyment.*

I was asked whether I would consent to a public demonstration staged outside my office urging me to run. I was flabbergasted, but sought to act **blasé** about the whole thing. (From *The Unmaking of a Mayor,* p. 103, The Viking Press, 1966)

boiserie (noun) *Carved wood paneling.*

The dinner, discreetly served in the Queen's Drawing Room, in the candlelight with the crystal **boiserie** effect and, always, the soft light, its Fauvist colors standing out in the mortuary of regal ancestors. (From *Saving the Queen,* p. 189, Doubleday & Company, 1976)

bombastic (adjective) *Pretentious, inflated.*

Anthony was incapable of pomposity. He cared more about effective relief for those who suffered than about **bombastic** relief for those who formed committees. (From *Saving the Queen,* p. 10, Doubleday & Company, 1976)

breviary (noun) *An ecclesiastical book containing the daily prayers or canonical prayers for the canonical hours.*

St. James's was dark except for candles on both sides of the sanctuary, the four dim lights overhead for tracing the aisles and the pews, the light inadequate for reading one's missal or **breviary.** (From *Saving the Queen,* p. 209, Doubleday & Company, 1976)

bugaboo (noun) *A source of concern, especially something that causes fear or distress often out of proportion to its actual importance.*

As for the **bugaboo** that an element of internal debt is being passed on to future generations, it is "unmistakably false." (From *God and Man at Yale,* p. 70, Regnery Books, 1986)

bumptiousness (noun) *The quality of one who is presumptuously, obtusely, and often noisily self-assertive.*

After it was all over, the student body president approached me with a wonderful combination of diffidence and **bumptiousness,** to say that he disapproved of the pig-bit, but that I was not to mistake this for approval of anything I had said, presumably not even the passage in my speech in which I deplored race prejudice. (From *Cruising Speed,* p. 71, G. P. Putnam's Sons, 1971)

cacoëthes (noun) *An uncontrollable desire.*

I wink noisily at Rosalyn (Tureck) and suggest that WHO KNOWS, the liquor might just conceivably give her a case of **cacoëthes** piano-itis. (From *Cruising Speed,* p. 143, G. P. Putnam's Sons, 1971)

caliper (verb) *To measure by or as if by calipers, an instrument having two legs or jaws that can be adjusted to determine thickness, diameter, etc.*

Granted that the frame of the Cardinal's letter was melodramatic, and that the melodrama is inhospitable to distinction: even so—call it feticide and **caliper** as you will the differences exquisite between feticide and murder on the moral scale. (From *Cruising Speed,* p. 240, G. P. Putnam's Sons, 1971)

callow (adjective) *Lacking in adult sophistication, experience, perception, or judgment.*

Trust influenced Blackford from the time they were at school together in England just before the war, and Trust was in the fifth form and Blackford a **callow** third-former. (From *Saving the Queen,* p. 10, Doubleday & Company, 1976)

cant (adjective) *The expression or repetition of conventional, trite, or unconsidered ideas or sentiments.*

Boris old boy, although I am entirely committed to our cause, I find the repetition of the **cant** phrases of communism altogether depressing. (From *Saving the Queen,* p. 153, Doubleday & Company, 1976)

caravanserai (noun) *An inn in Near or Far Eastern countries where caravans rest at night; usually a large bare building surrounding a court.*

Although Tito was prepared to spend cold nights in the trenches with his troops, he was manifestly happier in the **caravanserai** of the mighty. (From *Right Reason,* p. 392, Doubleday & Company, 1985)

Catonically (adverb) *In connection to Marcus Porcius Cato (149 B.C.), Roman statesman, or Marcus Porcius Cato (46 B.C.), Roman Stoic philosopher, both celebrated for austerity: repeated injunctions, or warnings, or predictions (e.g., "Delada Carthago est," Marcus Porcius Cato's "Carthage must be destroyed.").*

I haughtily, and indeed just a little sadly, remind Pat that Horrible Foo has, as, **Catonically,** I had always warned her he would, proved to be a wicked, wicked dog. (From *Cruising Speed,* p. 145, G. P. Putnam's Sons, 1971)

centripetalization (noun) *The process by which things proceed in a direction toward a center axis.*

It was obvious to the conservatives who grouped together after the Second World War that the **centripetalization** of power simply had to be arrested. (From *Cruising Speed,* p. 91, G. P. Putnam's Sons, 1971)

chiding (noun) *Reproof, rebuke.*

Johnny turned to Blackford. "You and your goddam . . . continence." . . . [He] got orotund when he was tight, and Blackford smiled at the familiar **chiding**. (From *Saving the Queen,* p. 7, Doubleday & Company, 1976)

chivalrous (adjective) *Marked by honor, fairness, generosity, and kindliness especially to foes, the weak and lowly, and the vanquished according to knightly tradition.*

Let us move towards a **chivalrous** candor, based on a respect for the essential equality of human beings, which recognizes reality, and speaks to reality. (From *The Unmaking of a Mayor,* p. 156, The Viking Press, 1966)

circumlocutory (adjective) *Marked by or exhibiting the use of an unnecessarily large number of words to express an idea; using indirect or roundabout expression.*

Smith was recalling to himself that he had taken great, **circumlocutory** pains never actually to deny his guilt directly to those who had most intimately befriended him. (From *Right Reason,* p. 202, Doubleday & Company, 1985)

clerisy (noun) *The well-educated or learned class; intelligentsia.*

The impact of the scientific developments that have absorbed the moral energies of our bishops and of the American **clerisy** in general prompts questions more basic than the question of selective conscientious objection. (From *Right Reason,* p. 117, Doubleday & Company, 1985)

coadjutor (noun) *A helper, assistant.*

"The Republican party," said Nelson Rockefeller—Lindsay's **coadjutor** in New York modern Republicanism—in the summer of 1963, "is the party of Lincoln." (From *The Unmaking of a Mayor,* p. 80, The Viking Press, 1966)

coda (noun) *A concluding portion of a musical, literary, or dramatic work, usually a portion or scene that rounds off or integrates preceding themes or ideas; anything that serves to round out, conclude, or summarize yet has an interest of its own.*

Ah, the ideological **coda**, how it afflicts us all! And how paralyzingly sad that someone who can muse over the desirability of converting New York into an independent state should, having climbed to such a peak, schuss down the same old slope, when the mountains beckon him on to new, exhilarating runs. (From *The Unmaking of a Mayor*, p. 39, The Viking Press, 1966)

codicil (noun) *A provision, as of a document, made subsequently to and appended to the original.*

"Do you mean, m-m-ma'am," the Prime Minister said to Queen Caroline, "those held in Great Britain by the United States, pursuant to the **codicils** of the NATO Treaty? Or d-d-do you mean those bombs over which we have total authority?" (From *Saving the Queen*, p. 99, Doubleday & Company, 1976)

cogency (noun) *The quality or state of appealing persuasively to the mind or reason.*

A young man cannot automatically be condemned for having acted frivolously if he sets out to weigh the demands of loyalty to this country's government against the **cogency** of the military objective he is being conscripted to risk his life for. (From *Right Reason*, p. 117, Doubleday & Company, 1985)

colloquy (noun) *A high-level, serious discussion.*

The Liberal Party's deliberations—which are a **colloquy** between Mr. David Dubinsky and Mr. Alex Rose—are copiously reported; and Adlai Stevenson, John Kennedy, and Lyndon Johnson all appeared in person to accept the Party's endorsement at great big to-dos. (From *The Unmaking of a Mayor*, p. 51, The Viking Press, 1966)

colonic (adjective) *Having to do with the colon. [A high-colonic medical examination reaches up into the large intestine.]*

"I never went to Yale, Blacky, so I can't answer those high-**colonic** questions." (From *Saving the Queen*, p. 218, Doubleday & Company, 1976)

comity (noun) *Friendly civility, mutual consideration.*

The American President, the British Prime Minister and the Soviet despot make dispositions involving millions of people for the sake of temporary geopolitical **comity**. (From *Saving the Queen*, p. 198, Doubleday & Company, 1976)

complaisant (adjective) *Marked by an inclination to please or oblige or by courteous agreeability.*

Thorton Wilder had first to step over the body; he smiled at me as if he had negotiated a mud-puddle. The Master who followed Mr. Wilder smiled as well. His was less **complaisant**. (From *Cruising Speed*, p. 223, G. P. Putnam's Sons, 1971)

complementary (adjective) *Suggestive of completing or perfecting; mutually dependent: supplementing and being supplemented in return.*

Lindsay emphasized certain themes, foremost among them his own liberalism and his aloofness from the Republican Party. He developed a **complementary** theme, namely the necessity of saving New York City from the curse of reaction. (From *The Unmaking of a Mayor*, p. 286, The Viking Press, 1966)

concatenation (noun) *A series or order of things depending on each other as if linked together.*

José López Portillo, the people's friend who left Mexico with a foreign debt of $90 billion, before he left office built, in addition to houses for himself and each of his children, an astronomical observatory, useful for tracing friendly astrological **concatenations**, if indeed Sr. Portillo acquired all the money with which he built his houses by speculation. (From *Right Reason*, p. 297, Doubleday & Company, 1985)

concupiscent (adjective) *Lustful.*

The Protestant theologian Dean Fitch reminds us that we have recently entered upon the most acutely degenerate of the stages of civilization: The Age of Love of Self. For a period we loved God; then we loved rationalism; then we loved humanity; then science; now we love ourselves, and in that **concupiscent** love all else has ceased to exist. (From *Cruising Speed,* p. 179, G. P. Putnam's Sons, 1971)

confutation (noun) *The act or process of overwhelming by argument.*

It is necessary in making one's complaints against the society we intend to replace, to be vague and even disjointed. To be specific, or to be orderly, is once again to run the risk of orderly **confutation.** (From *Cruising Speed,* p. 213, G. P. Putnam's Sons, 1971)

consanguinity (noun) *The state of being related by blood or descended from a common ancestor; (thus) a close relationship or connection; affinity.*

John Lindsay might have waited until 1965 to oppose Jacob Javits in the primary, but such a move was out of the question by reason not only of political prudence but of ideological **consanguinity.** (From *The Unmaking of a Mayor,* p. 63, The Viking Press, 1966)

contemn (verb) *To view or treat with contempt as mean and despicable; reject with disdain.*

Samuelson would have us not only **contemn** the treatment of economics of such men as Jewkes, F. A. Hayek, Ropke, Anderson, Watt, and von Mises, we are also to doubt their motives. (From *God and Man at Yale,* p. 81, Regnery Books, 1986)

continence (noun) *Self-restraint from yielding to impulse or desire.*

Johnny, opening the window to reach for another can of beer, discovered with horror that there were none left; and reaching into the cigarette box, discovered that he had simultaneously run out of cigarettes. He turned to Blackford. "You and your goddam . . . **continence.**" (From *Saving the Queen,* p. 7, Doubleday & Company, 1976)

contravene (verb) *To go or act contrary to; obstruct the operation of; infringe, disregard; oppose in argument; contradict, dispute.*

It does not take political courage to **contravene** one's own religion, it takes moral infidelity, of which I do not propose to be guilty inasmuch as I put the moral order above the political order. (From *The Unmaking of a Mayor,* p. 180, The Viking Press, 1966)

controvert (verb) *To dispute or oppose by reasoning.*

I find it continuingly relevant, in a book on contemporary politics, to attempt to **controvert** controvertible misrepresentations. (From *The Unmaking of a Mayor,* p. 10, The Viking Press, 1966)

cordon sanitaire (noun) *A line designed to act as a buffer between two territories actually or potentially hostile to each other.*

We arrive [at Fillmore East to hear Virgil Fox, the organist, play Bach], and there are hippies and non-hippies trying to get in, a sellout. One young man ventures forward, do I have an extra ticket? I give him one of the two tickets, thinking to keep the second, under the circumstances, as **cordon sanitaire.** (From *Cruising Speed,* p. 51, G. P. Putnam's Sons, 1971)

Coventry (noun) *A state of ostracism or exclusion from the society of one's fellows.*

The irrepressible and irrational right-crackpot who advances an inanity—say that "Eisenhower and Kennedy have brought us to the brink of surrender"—is instantly identified as what he is, and the forces of opprobrium, social and intellectual, quickly maneuver to consign him to **Coventry.** (From *The Unmaking of a Mayor,* p. 307, The Viking Press, 1966)

cozen (verb) *(1) To deceive by artful wheedling or tricky dishonesty; (2) to beguile craftily: victimize by chicanery; (3) to act with artful deceit.*

It is easy to say that ideally you should stand still and be polite and attentive when addressed and **cozened** by the same man who that same morning berated you as a racist and hater. (From *The Unmaking of a Mayor,* p. 236, The Viking Press, 1966)

credo (noun) *A strongly held or frequently affirmed belief or conviction.*

The term "professionally competent," as used by the academic freedomites to describe a legitimate criterion of employment, can, under their **credo,** be meaningfully applied only to the "fact" aspect of teaching. (From *God and Man at Yale,* p. 146, Regnery Books, 1986)

credulous (adjective) *Ready or inclined to believe, especially on slight or uncertain evidence.*

I have no quarrel with Mr. Seymour, although I should be perhaps less categorical— enough so, for example, to allow me to express preference for a **credulous** Democrat over a profoundly convinced Communist. (From *God and Man at Yale,* p. 178, Regnery Books, 1986)

cudgels (noun) *"To take up the cudgels" is to enter into a vigorous contest.*

He says that he is not even sure whether, when his father dies, he will take up the **cudgels** of the House of Lords. (From *Saving the Queen,* p. 188, Doubleday & Company, 1976)

cursory (adjective) *Rapidly, often superficially, performed with scant attention to detail.*

His introduction in that subject at Maxwell Field ("How to be useful if shot down and incorporated in the resistance movement") was **cursory.** (From *Saving the Queen,* p. 32, Doubleday & Company, 1976)

cynosure (noun) *A center of attraction or interest.*

Blackford's classmates were already dribbling into the classroom and, alerted to the cause of the excitement, looked instantly at the **cynosure** on the blackboard and exploded in squeals of delight and ribaldry. (From *Saving the Queen,* p. 70, Doubleday & Company, 1976)

decorous (adjective) *Marked by propriety and good taste, especially in conduct, manners, or appearance.*

And how long are the professors willing to wait before a **decorous** opportunity presents itself for exposing the steady drive in the direction of collectivism that has gathered so much momentum at Yale over the past dozen years? (From *God and Man at Yale,* p. 104, Regnery Books, 1986)

deify (verb) *To glorify or exalt as of supreme worth or excellence.*

The Department of Economics is not alone in **deifying** collectivism. (From *God and Man at Yale,* p. 99, Regnery Books, 1986)

demurral (noun) *The act of taking exception.*

He permitted himself a smile as he shot out his trigger finger to the door, which was the director's way of saying, "Out"—to which there was no known **demurral.** (From *Saving the Queen,* p. 4, Doubleday & Company, 1976)

denouement (noun) *The final outcome, result, or unraveling of the main dramatic complication in a play.*

Blackford gave Joe the plot, but not the **denouement,** and as they were driving home Joe expressed himself as genuinely indignant at Iago, and Blackford told him that was a really good sign. (From *Saving the Queen,* p. 216, Doubleday & Company, 1976)

derogate (verb) *To make to seem lesser in esteem; disparage, decry.*

Salesmanship is nowadays **derogated,** the assumption being that a salesman is somebody who persuades you to do something you do not want to do. (From *Cruising Speed,* p. 129, G. P. Putnam's Sons, 1971)

desultorily (adverb) *Lacking steadiness, fixity, regularity, or continuity.*

However **desultorily**, his father always kept in touch with him, and the more easily as his son grew older, and the two, though apart, did not grow apart. (From *Saving the Queen*, p. 55, Doubleday & Company, 1976)

de trop (adjective) *Too much or too many; in the way; superfluous; unwanted.*

The swanks at PBS are pretty proud of their audiences, but an exchange in Latin would probably be thought **de trop.** (From *Right Reason*, p. 217, Doubleday & Company, 1985)

detumescence (noun) *The collapse of what was heretofore stiff, as in a penis.*

Surely it was with malice aforethought that he permitted the ash on his burning cigarette to grow to advanced **detumescence.** (From *Right Reason*, p. 435, Doubleday & Company, 1985)

devolve (verb) *(1) To cause to pass down, descend, be transferred, or changed; (2) to transfer from one person to another: hand down; (3) to pass by transmission or succession.*

John Lindsay was to stress repeatedly the nonpartisan nature of his own candidacy, assiduously cultivating the air of transcendence that **devolves** to a candidate too big for any single party. (From *The Unmaking of a Mayor*, p. 45, The Viking Press, 1966)

dialectic (noun) *Any systematic reasoning, exposition, or argument that juxtaposes opposed or contradictory ideas and seeks to resolve their conflict; play of ideas; cunning or hairsplitting disputation.*

It may be in fact that to bring up a particular subject before a particular audience results in a **dialectic** whose meaning is a function of time and place. (From *The Unmaking of a Mayor*, p. 25, The Viking Press, 1966)

dilettante (noun) *A person who cultivates an art or branch of knowledge as a pastime without pursuing it professionally.*

Professor Kirkland does not believe that academic freedom ought to protect the pedant, the **dilettante,** or the exhibitionist. (From *God and Man at Yale*, p. 143, Regnery Books, 1986)

discountenance (verb) *To put to shame; reject; abash, disconcert; refuse to look upon with favor.*

It is an interesting conjecture that the effect of the Republicans' closed shop is not only to **discountenance** a useful bloc of Republican voters but to discourage a potential flow of voters whose background is Democratic, and who might well view the Conservative Party as a way-station to a remodeled Republican Party. (From *The Unmaking of a Mayor*, p. 60, The Viking Press, 1966)

disjunction (noun) *The action of disjoining or condition of being disjoined; separation, disconnection, disunion.*

He [Jesse Jackson] is given to the most grating verbal rhetorical **disjunctions** in contemporary language. ("We're going from the outhouse to the White House." "They've got dope in the veins rather than hope in their brains.") (From *Right Reason*, p. 66, Doubleday & Company, 1985)

dislocation (noun) *A disruption of the established order.*

My host lightly probed me. I told him the truth, that I had heard the not so sotto voce impoliteness on the part of the student. He apologized for the social **dislocation**, and explained that the young man's father was a legislator who reversed himself and cast a deciding vote to relax the abortion law, in punishment for which he had failed of reelection, and that son was overwrought, particularly against conservative Catholics. (From *Cruising Speed*, p. 72, G. P. Putnam's Sons, 1971)

disquietude (noun) *Lack of peace or tranquillity.*

A man formally aligned on the other side of the political fence endorsing all your major platforms has the effect of relieving you of the **disquietude** that the existence of alternative approaches to government necessarily poses. (From *The Unmaking of a Mayor,* p. 99, The Viking Press, 1966)

dissimulation (noun) *Deception; hiding under a false appearance.*

Then there is someone who oscillates from sarcasm to **dissimulation.** You would think he had tipped his hand conclusively by beginning his letter, "Dear Mr. Pukely." (From *Cruising Speed,* p. 81, G. P. Putnam's Sons, 1971)

dissipation (noun) *Wasteful expenditures and intemperate living.*

What he is, is an undisciplined Catherine's wheel, whose columns read like angry and disordered reflections of the previous night's **dissipations.** (From *Right Reason,* p. 39, Doubleday & Company, 1985)

dittify (verb) *To turn into a ditty—a song or short poem, especially one of simple, unaffected character.*

"Remember: *Qui cogitat quod debet facere, solet conficere quod debet facere.*" Mr. Simon beamed as he attempted to **dittify** his maxim in English: "Those who think about their duty/Are those who end by doing their duty!" (From *Saving the Queen,* p. 64, Doubleday & Company, 1976)

doctrinaire (adjective) *Stubbornly devoted to some particular doctrine or theory without regard to practical considerations.*

Mr. Lindblom dislikes a **doctrinaire** attitude toward anything. He incessantly encourages the pragmatic approach to economics. It naturally follows that any reliance on absolutes, or any reference to indefeasible "rights" is unwarranted and anachronistic. (From *God and Man at Yale,* p. 91, Regnery Books, 1986)

dour (adjective) *Marked by sternness or severity.*

Georgianna opened the door, black and **dour** as ever, but instantly docile when Blackford said, "Georgy, lend me a dollar quickly." (From *Saving the Queen,* p. 53, Doubleday & Company, 1976)

dowdy (adjective) *Not modern in style; staid, shabby.*

She would never have got that **dowdy** kind of life with me, but that's what she wanted. (From *Saving the Queen,* p. 158, Doubleday & Company, 1976)

doxology (noun) *Praise to the Deity; thanksgiving for divine protection rendered anaphorically, i.e., repetitious in formulation. E.g., "Blessed be God/Blessed be His holy name/Blessed be His son Jesus."*

I would not expect in a serious conversation with a Cardinal about great affairs that he would punctuate his message with bits and pieces of Christian **doxology.** (From *Saving the Queen,* p. 153, Doubleday & Company, 1976)

dudgeon (noun) *A sullen, angry, or indignant humor.*

The Most Reverend Ernest Trevor Huddleston arrived at the makeshift studio at the nave of St. James's Church in Piccadilly in full Episcopal regalia, and in very high **dudgeon.** (From *On the Firing Line: The Public Life of Our Public Figures,* p. 345, Random House, 1989)

duplicity (noun) *Deception by pretending to entertain one set of feelings and acting under the influence of another.*

I have charged Yale with **duplicity** in her treatment of her alumni. (From *God and Man at Yale,* p. 134, Regnery Books, 1986)

dysphasia (noun) *Loss of or deficiency in the power to use or understand language caused by injury to or disease of the brain.*

REPORTER: But Mr. Lindsay said today that he never knew you at Yale at all—

WFB: Well, I'm surprised he said that because it's not true. If he is suffering from some sort of **dysphasia**, that would make a whole lot of his recent behavior understandable. (From *The Unmaking of a Mayor*, p. 262, The Viking Press, 1966)

eclectic (adjective) *Varied; reflecting different styles, doctrines, methods.*

Knowing Mr. Kennedy's appetite for **eclectic** reading matter, he gave him J. H. Plumb's *Sir Robert Walpole* and a volume of Betjeman's poems. (From *Cruising Speed*, p. 94, G. P. Putnam's Sons, 1971)

efface (verb) *To eliminate clear evidence of; to remove from cognizance, consideration, or memory.*

On those occasions when the Republican Party of New York has won municipal elections it has done so precisely by **effacing** any distinguishable characteristics of the Republican Party. (From *The Unmaking of a Mayor*, p. 42, The Viking Press, 1966)

efficacious (adjective) *Qualities that give power to bring about an intended result.*

I find it continuingly relevant, in a book on contemporary politics, to attempt to controvert controvertible misrepresentations because it is especially interesting to inquire whether they tend to be **efficacious** or not. (From *The Unmaking of a Mayor*, p. 10, The Viking Press, 1966)

effrontery (noun) *Act of shameless audacity and unblushing insolence.*

What they ought to be condemning is what I once called the special **effronteries** of the twentieth century. One of these—eastern seaboard liberalism—substituted ideology for metaphysics, causing the great void which the sensitive of whatever age feel so keenly. (From *Cruising Speed*, p. 93, G. P. Putnam's Sons, 1971)

egalitarianism (noun) *A belief that all men are equal in intrinsic worth and are entitled to equal access to the rights and privileges of their society; specifically, a social philosophy advocating the leveling of social, political, and economic inequalities.*

The adjacent fraternities are far gone in desuetude, for reasons nobody entirely understands, though everybody agrees they have something to do with the affluence-cum-**egalitarianism** paradox. (From *Cruising Speed*, p. 220, G. P. Putnam's Sons, 1971)

eleemosynary (adjective) *Of or relating to charity.*

I intended to probe the question whether an inverted kind of subsidy, to middle and big business, was going on under our **eleemosynary** noses—by encouraging, with social welfare schemes, a cheap labor market. (From *The Unmaking of a Mayor*, p. 36, The Viking Press, 1966)

elide (verb) *To suppress or alter at intermediate stages.*

When a politician has got so given to thinking of himself as a collectivity that he is capable of writing in his diary, "At 8 A.M., we got up and took a shower," he has **elided** from modesty to something else. (From *The Unmaking of a Mayor*, p. 85, The Viking Press, 1966)

elixir (noun) *A concoction held to be capable of prolonging life indefinitely; something that acts potently upon one, invigorating or filling with exuberant energy or cheer.*

The first course was an omelet of sour cream and tomatoes and **elixir**, unlike anything Black had ever tasted, and better. (From *Saving the Queen*, p. 114, Doubleday & Company, 1976)

empirical (adjective) *Originating in or based on observation.*

The **empirical** spirit is interesting both because it is organically American ("if it works, it's good"; "nothing succeeds like success") and because pride is a hugely important factor in the operation of governments, which after all are run by human beings. (From *Right Reason*, p. 80, Doubleday & Company, 1985)

enjambement (noun) *Continuation in prosody of the sense in a phrase beyond the end of a verse or couplet; the running over of a sentence from one line into another so that closely related words fall in different lines.*

" 'Against welfare,' says a woman supporter in a tall magenta hat, 'and not making New York a haven for . . . well . . .' She says no more." So writes *The New Yorker*. Now, great big grown-up people can effect the **enjambement** without strain. The lady in the magenta hat was anti-Black! (From *The Unmaking of a Mayor*, p. 236, The Viking Press, 1966)

enjoin (verb) *To direct, prescribe, or impose by order, typically authoritatively and compellingly.*

Assuming that the Yale graduate, a potential entrepreneur, is an inveterate, dauntless gambler and decides to run all these risks and launch his business, there are further considerations that his economists have **enjoined** him to keep in mind. (From *God and Man at Yale*, p. 84, Regnery Books, 1986)

enumerate (verb) *To relate one after another.*

The Declaration of Independence goes on to **enumerate** the grievances of the colonies. It is a stirring catalogue, but it finally reduces to the matter of the source of power, i.e., who should rule? (From *Cruising Speed*, p. 206, G. P. Putnam's Sons, 1971)

ephemera (noun) *Of transitory existence, interest, or importance.*

The whole thing [Mike Wallace's farewell interview with President and Mrs. Reagan on *60 Minutes*] seems a cheerful mix of nostalgia and **ephemera**, but the portrait was genuine and will be studied (or should be) by future biographers. (From Mr. Buckley's syndicated column, "On the Right")

equerry (noun) *One of the officers of the British royal household in the department of the master of the horse in regular attendance on the sovereign or another member of the royal family.*

An **equerry**, introducing himself genially, supervised turning the car over to a chauffeur, and Blackford's luggage to a footman. (From *Saving the Queen*, p. 165, Doubleday & Company, 1976)

eructation (noun) *A violent belching out or emitting.*

He knew that the center of their earth was heaving and fuming and causing great **eructations** of human misery in its writhing frustration over the failure of Soviet scientists to develop the hydrogen bomb at the same rate as the Americans. (From *Saving the Queen*, p. 104, Doubleday & Company, 1976)

erudite (adjective) *Possessing an extensive, often profound or recondite knowledge.*

"If you are not aware of it," said the Queen, "I am sure there are several members of this **erudite** company who will explain it to you." (From *Saving the Queen*, p. 168, Doubleday & Company, 1976)

espousal (noun) *A taking up or adopting as a cause or belief.*

Despite protestations that Professor Davis had failed to qualify for promotion, it was plain for all to see that he had been eased out because of his outspoken criticism of capitalism, his **espousal** of numerous left-wing causes, and his attacks on several large financial trusts and holding companies with which various members of the Yale Corporation were affiliated. (From *God and Man at Yale*, p. 149, Regnery Books, 1986)

eudaemonia (noun) *Happiness derived through a lifetime devoted to fulfilling moral obligations.*

Her doubts are of course shared by many who are discouraged by the failure of general education to achieve **eudaemonia**. (From *Cruising Speed*, p. 110, G. P. Putnam's Sons, 1971)

evocation (noun) *The act or fact of calling forth, out, or up; summoning, citation.*

Mr. Lindsay first discovered that the idea of taking positive action to relieve New York City of the curse of drug addiction can best be summed up in the haunting **evocation** of "concentration camps." (From *The Unmaking of a Mayor*, p. 164, The Viking Press, 1966)

ex cathedra (adverb) *Authoritative by virtue of or in the exercise of one's office, as with papal authority.*

The public is being trained, as regards the Supreme Court of the United States when it is interpreting the Constitution, to accept its ruling as if rendered **ex cathedra**, on questions of faith and morals. (From Mr. Buckley's syndicated column, "On the Right")

excretion (noun) *The process of eliminating useless, superfluous, or harmful matter.*

The conservative rejection of the John Birch Society, of the anarchists and other fanatics, was an act of **excretion** essential to political and intellectual hygiene. (From *Right Reason*, p. 220, Doubleday & Company, 1985)

execration (noun) *The act of cursing or denouncing.*

The Iranians, after they have done with the rituals of **execration**, are going to want that which is universally popular. Cars, rock music, Bloomingdale's. (From *Right Reason*, p. 72, Doubleday & Company, 1985)

exegete (noun) *A person skilled in critical explanation or analysis, especially of a text.*

WFB: You say that the rights of lawyers and priests should extend to journalists.

ABRAMS: As a general matter, yes. There are some differences, but as a general matter, yes, I—

WFB: That's a sort of a revolutionary accretion and yet, in asserting that point, you tend to do so as an **exegete** of the Constitution rather than as a somebody who wants to amend it. (From *On the Firing Line: The Public Life of Our Public Figures*, p. 198, Random House, 1989)

exigency (noun) *The hard requirements of a situation.*

We must bear in mind that the scholar has has not one but two functions. These pursuits are (1) scholarship, and (2) teaching. They are related solely by convenience, by tradition, and by economic **exigency**. (From *God and Man at Yale*, p. 182, Regnery Books, 1986)

exorcise (verb) *To get rid of the evil content of something.*

President Seymour had made a clarion call for a return to Christian values in 1937, but that did not **exorcise** the extreme secularism that characterized Yale at least during the last four years of his administration. (From *God and Man at Yale*, p. 43, Regnery Books, 1986)

expedient (noun) *Something that is suitable, practical, and efficient in achieving a particular end; fit, proper, or advantageous under the circumstances.*

I herewith request Mr. Charles Buckley to do me, and the voters of New York, the favor of ending the confusion by the simple **expedient** of changing his name. (From *The Unmaking of a Mayor*, p. 253, The Viking Press, 1966)

expunge (verb) *To obliterate completely; annihilate.*

"You, Comandante Fidel Castro," Kirov said, "are my sovereign. You, by your example in Cuba, will illuminate the Marxist movement throughout the world, and perhaps even **expunge** the cruel and barbaric Marxism being practiced in the Homeland of Lenin." (From *Mongoose, R.I.P.*, p. 243, Random House, 1987)

extirpate (verb) *To eradicate; destroy totally; wipe out; kill off; make extinct; exterminate.*

Teaching is not, for most of those who go into it, a priestly calling, a pledge made before God and Man to go out and **extirpate** ignorance from the globe. (From *The Unmaking of a Mayor*, p. 201, The Viking Press, 1966)

extuberance (noun) *Protuberance.*

Seville—At a little kiosk near the park is a child's mechanical rocking horse. You insert 25 pesetas, and for ten minutes your little boy or girl rocks around the clock, gasping with pleasure while holding on hard to the little wood **extuberances** that serve as bridles. (From *Right Reason*, p. 249, Doubleday & Company, 1985)

eyrie (noun) *A room or a dwelling placed high up; remote; isolated.*

Blackford was struck by the ornamental splendor of the scene, with the huge chandeliers, the gilt-red balcony, the steps behind him ascending to the regal **eyrie** whence Queen Caroline had descended. (From *Saving the Queen,* p. 131, Doubleday & Company, 1976)

fallacious (adjective) *Embodying or presenting a false or erroneous idea.*

The administration of Yale, and the president in particular, dwell from time to time on the merits of laissez-faire education, hinting that there exist some alumni with contrary notions—notions which are, of course, demonstrably **fallacious.** (From *God and Man at Yale,* p. 139, Regnery Books, 1986)

fasces (noun) *(1) A bundle of rods having among them an ax with the blade projecting, borne before Roman magistrates as a badge of authority in ancient Rome; (2) the authority symbolized by the fasces.*

Jimmy Jones had his **fasces,** and from all accounts they were liberally used to keep in line those whose restive intelligence or natural hedonism questioned the ideals or resisted the spartan regimen. (From *Right Reason,* p. 217, Doubleday & Company, 1985)

Fauvist (adjective) *Markedly vivid.*

A single early Picasso was lit by a shaft of soft light, its **Fauvist** colors standing out in the mortuary of regal ancestors. (From *Saving the Queen,* p. 189, Doubleday & Company, 1976)

fealty (noun) *The fidelity of a vassal or feudal tenant to his lord; faithfulness, allegiance.*

Congressman Lindsay voted with the Democrats a total of thirty-one times. As such, he was runner-up among liberal Republicans in the frequency of his **fealty** to Democrats-in-a-jam. (From *The Unmaking of a Mayor,* p. 70, The Viking Press, 1966)

fecundity (noun) *Fruitfulness; fertility.*

The story quotes me directly: "We do have similarities to the Kennedys," says Bill. "Our wealth, our **fecundity,** our Catholicism. Other than that, the comparison is engaging but misleading." (From *Cruising Speed,* p. 34, G. P. Putnam's Sons, 1971)

fetid (adjective) *Smelly, rotten.*

The Republican candidate for President should devote himself absolutely to making the atomization of the Marxist myth an official crusade, one to which we will attach ourselves as vigorously as if we were spreading the word of how to extirpate smallpox from the **fetid** corners of the world. (From *Right Reason,* p. 229, Doubleday & Company, 1985)

filigreed (adjective) *Adorned with a pattern or design resembling ornamental work of fine wire of gold, silver, or copper.*

"My dear Mr. Oakes," he read in a **filigreed** but authoritative hand that tilted sharply to the right. "I leave you to your researches during the morning and early afternoon." (From *Saving the Queen,* p. 181, Doubleday & Company, 1976)

flippant (adjective) *Treating or tending to treat with unsuitable levity that which is serious or to which respect is owing.*

References to genitalia are as effective in the classroom as they are at a bachelor party, and **flippant** allusions to sacrosanct subjects are as delightful from the podium as from the soapboxes of Hyde Park. (From *God and Man at Yale,* p. 15, Regnery Books, 1986)

flout (verb) *To treat with contempt; defile; mock.*

The problem with attempting eloquence at the United Nations is that that which is affirmed by all the surrounding moral maxims is regularly and systematically **flouted.** (From *Right Reason,* p. 214, Doubleday & Company, 1985)

forensic (adjective) *Rhetoric used to plead a point.*

There has been some dissatisfaction over the President's speech. Hardly surprising. It was a magnificent **forensic** performance. (From *Right Reason,* p. 100, Doubleday & Company, 1985)

fractious (adjective) *Tending to cause trouble (as by disobedience to an established order); hard to manage or unmanageable; refractory; unruly.*

Teenagers caught and convicted of felonies will be either put in jail or released in the recognizance of their parents. Said parents would have the right to surrender authority over **fractious** children by invoking probationary sentences. (From *The Unmaking of a Mayor,* p. 91, The Viking Press, 1966)

fulminator (noun) *One who denounces, sends forth censures or invectives.*

The 1,267 members of the freshman class of Yale University have been warned against the Moral Majority by President A. Bartlett Giamatti. And what a speech it was: Jerry Falwell, head of the Moral Majority, is said to be quite a **fulminator** himself. (From *Right Reason,* p. 48, Doubleday & Company, 1985)

fulsomeness (noun) *Copiousness, abundance so great as to become offensive.*

John Kennedy so oversold some of his own apostles on the general subject of his being the best qualified to serve as President of the United States that some of them went on to commit sins of **fulsomeness** which, one hopes, deeply embarrassed him. (From *The Unmaking of a Mayor,* p. 84, The Viking Press, 1966)

gambol (verb) *To bound or spring about as in dancing or play; skip about; frisk, cavort.*

"Not tomorrow," said Caroline. "Wouldn't do for me to **gambol** about the woods on my horse while they are lowering Queen Benedicta into the sod." (From *Saving the Queen,* p. 128, Doubleday & Company, 1976)

Gemütlichkeit (noun) (German) *Coziness; good nature, kindliness, cordiality.*

The loneliness of flight is not entirely overwhelmed by cabin movies, the drinks, the food, the ***Gemütlichkeit*** of shoulder-to-shoulder life. (From *Right Reason,* p. 95, Doubleday & Company, 1985)

Goo-gooism (noun) *(from the initials of* good government*) A reform movement in politics, especially in the era of Theodore Roosevelt—usually used disparagingly.*

If John Lindsay won, Republicans in Ohio and California would not be permitted to pass off his victory as meaningless, as merely a triumph of **Goo-gooism** in a jaded municipal situation. (From *The Unmaking of a Mayor,* p. 68, The Viking Press, 1966)

grandiloquence (noun) *Lofty, extravagantly colorful, pompous, or bombastic in style, manner, or language.*

Ramsey Clark is now and then just a little grandiose, e.g., "Dissent has been the principal catalyst in the alchemy of truth," which, substituting as it does "in the alchemy of" for the simpler "of," suffers not only from straitened **grandiloquence,** but from an edgy syntactical ineptitude. (From *Cruising Speed,* p. 121, G. P. Putnam's Sons, 1971)

guilelessly (adverb) *Innocently; naïvely; unsophisticated in manner.*

Professor Kennedy subverted the faith of numbers of students who, **guilelessly,** entered his course hoping to learn sociology and left with the impression that faith in God and the scientific approach to human problems are mutually exclusive. (From *God and Man at Yale,* p. 17, Regnery Books, 1986)

hagiographer (noun) *A writer of biography of an idealizing or idolizing character.*

"For John Lindsay, the device of playing up 'the candidate' rather than 'the party' has been startlingly successful." But as if to guard against the perils of an untoward de-Republicanization, the **hagiographer** cautiously adds: "He identified himself with Senator Javits, former Mayor La Guardia and others." (From *The Unmaking of a Mayor,* p. 72, The Viking Press, 1966)

hauteur (noun) *An assumption of superiority; an arrogant or condescending manner.*

Very soon after, we were back in Connecticut, and I strained to speak like Mortimer Snerd, so as to disguise from my friends the ignominy of my foreign experiences. The fashion is to comment on the **hauteur** of my diction. (From *Cruising Speed,* pp. 151–52, G. P. Putnam's Sons, 1971)

hebdomadal (adjective) *Meeting or appearing once a week; weekly.*

Sometime after Adlai Stevenson announced his candidacy for President in 1952, he telephoned his former wife and told her to prepare the "boys" to be picked up on Sunday. Sure enough, photographers were there to record the **hebdomadal** piety of Adlai Stevenson. (From *Right Reason,* p. 315, Doubleday & Company, 1985)

hegira (noun) *A journey or trip, especially when undertaken as a means of escaping from an undesirable or dangerous environment or as a means of arriving at a highly desirable destination.*

All of New York was wired to trip him up—local police, FBI, California sheriffs. In the interval, Edgar Smith undertook a **hegira**. He went deep into Pennsylvania, in search of a cemetery, he said later, at which he could meditate. (From *Right Reason,* p. 199, Doubleday & Company, 1985)

heterodoxy (noun) *An unorthodox opinion or doctrine.*

The president of the Conservative Book Club assigned *Message from Moscow* to readers, who reported back against it, on the grounds that the author's own prejudices were in favor of socialism; and such **heterodoxy** a small minority of CBC readers would not tolerate even as they would not have tolerated the distribution of *Animal Farm* in the light of Orwell's persistent inclination toward socialism. (From *Cruising Speed,* p. 48, G. P. Putnam's Sons, 1971)

heuristic (adjective) *(1) Providing aid or direction in the solution of a problem but otherwise unjustified or incapable of justification; (2) heightening curiosity about further scholarly or scientific exploration.*

Conservatives know that some human beings, as Albert Jay Nock stressed in his **heuristic** lectures at the University of Virginia, are educable, others only trainable. (From *The Unmaking of a Mayor,* p. 173, The Viking Press, 1966)

holographic (adjective) *Written in the hand of the person from whom it proceeds.*

A dotted line from the lips of the master led to a balloon, within which Blackford, imitating the **holographic** style of his teacher, who a few days earlier had explained the English evolution ("micturate") of Caesar's word to describe his soldiers' careless habits when emptying their bladders, indited the words: "Mingo, Mingere, Minxi, Mictum." (From *Saving the Queen,* p. 70, Doubleday & Company, 1976)

homily (noun) *A lecture or discussion on a moral theme.*

Senator Moynihan and Anthony Lewis charge that Ambassador Jeane Kirkpatrick and her legal adviser, Allan Gerson, are ignorant of the law. Moynihan added the **homily** that even though the Soviet Union does not abide by the law, that doesn't mean we shouldn't. (From *Right Reason,* p. 127, Doubleday & Company, 1985)

hortatory (adjective) *Using language intended to incite or to mobilize.*

The police reached the man, who had moments before jumped onto the stage and danced there naked, but poor Ken Galbraith, although he plowed a straight furrow through his **hortatory** address to the effect that the earth would open up and swallow us all if Nixon was reelected, was not able to engage the distracted audience. (From *Cruising Speed,* p. 58, G. P. Putnam's Sons, 1971)

hurly-burly (noun) *Confusion, turmoil, tumult, uproar.*

I never got around to it, in part because of the lack of time, in part because, of course, it would not, in the **hurly-burly,** have been publicly pondered. (From *The Unmaking of a Mayor,* p. 36, The Viking Press, 1966)

ignominious (adjective) *Marked by, full of, or characterized by disgrace or shame; dishonorable; deserving of shame.*

Mr. Leonard Hall added his voice to the chorus of breast-beaters after the **ignominious** defeat of Senator Goldwater. (From *The Unmaking of a Mayor,* p. 41, The Viking Press, 1966)

ignoratio elenchi (noun) *A fallacy in logic of supposing that the point at issue is proved or disproved by an argument which proves or disproves something not at issue.*

Lindsay ignored the challenge a half-dozen times, and finally replied to it by saying: "I don't know why you ask me to renounce Adam Clayton Powell, Jr., since Powell has come out for Mr. Beame." A classic example of what the logicians call **ignoratio elenchi.** (From *The Unmaking of a Mayor,* p. 271, The Viking Press, 1966)

impalpable (adjective) *Incapable of being felt by the touch.*

Boris knew to take the nearest church exit, keeping his eyes down, under no circumstances looking about him, lest his eyes fall on the intangible, **impalpable** Robinson. (From *Saving the Queen,* p. 208, Doubleday & Company, 1976)

impetuosity (noun) *Undisciplined thought or action.*

He has the faculty, where legal problems are concerned, of releasing, say every fifteen minutes or so, a gossamer blanket over your **impetuosities.** (From *Cruising Speed,* p. 116, G. P. Putnam's Sons, 1971)

implacable (adjective) *Incapable of appeasement or mitigation; inexorable.*

Castro kept both radio sets on, but after a while turned them down. There was the faint monotonic sound of people talking, from the one set and, from the other, the muted beat of the rock music, **implacable** in its cacophony. (From *Mongoose, R.I.P.,* p. 293, Random House, 1987)

importune (verb) *To press or urge with frequent or unreasonable requests or troublesome persistence.*

He wondered whether he would ever again feel so close a kinship as he had felt for the two men he had just now got killed. With morbid shame he recalled **importuning** them to request a transfer, after V-E Day, so that they could serve out the balance of their terms with him. (From *Saving the Queen,* p. 142, Doubleday & Company, 1976)

imputation (noun) *The act of laying the responsibility or blame for something falsely or unjustly.*

Blackford knew all about Meachey. He had led the Oxford Committee to protest the **imputation** of guilt to Stalin during the show trials in the late thirties. (From *Saving the Queen,* p. 92, Doubleday & Company, 1976)

incertitude (noun) *Absence of assurance or confidence.*

Either the Supreme Court will more or less laze up to different specific cases in different ways, leaving the question of what are and what aren't the rights of parties in dispute, in boundless **incertitude,** or else basic laws will have to be rewritten. (From *The Unmaking of a Mayor,* p. 198, The Viking Press, 1966)

inchoate (adjective) *Imperfectly formed or formulated.*

At Berkeley, that corporate sense of mission is as diffuse and **inchoate** as the resolute pluralism of California society. (From *God and Man at Yale,* p. 1, Regnery Books, 1986)

indefeasible (adjective) *Not capable of or not liable to being annulled or voided or undone.*

Mr. Lindblom dislikes a doctrinaire attitude toward anything. He incessantly encourages the pragmatic approach to economics. It naturally follows that any reliance on absolutes, or any reference to **indefeasible** "rights" is unwarranted and anachronistic. (From *God and Man at Yale,* p. 91, Regnery Books, 1986)

individuation (noun) *The process by which individuals in society become differentiated from one another.*

The kind of community Nisbet told us we all needed, and the kind that now Reich enjoins upon us, is inconceivable in the absence of **individuation;** and the individual is what happens when the state ceases to be taken for granted as the necessary instrument for human progress. (From *Cruising Speed,* p. 93, G. P. Putnam's Sons, 1971)

ineluctable (adjective) *Not to be avoided, changed, or resisted.*

The loose-jointedness of their mode leaves the revolutionists in a frame of mind at once romantic and diffuse, and the rest of us without the great weapon available to King Canute, who was able to contrive what would nowadays be called a Confrontation between—the **ineluctable** laws of nature and the superstitions of his subjects. (From *Cruising Speed,* p. 213, G. P. Putnam's Sons, 1971)

inept (adjective) *Lacking skill or aptitude for a particular role or task.*

A man gifted in research is not thereby gifted in the art of transmitting to the pupil his knowledge. This is periodically brought to mind in widespread student resentment at the retention by many universities of scholars who, while often distinguished in research, are miserably **inept** in teaching. (From *God and Man at Yale,* p. 182, Regnery Books, 1986)

inertia (noun) *Indisposition to motion, exertion, or action; inertness.*

For many teachers the prospect of commuting to disagreeable sections of the city, to grapple with **inertia,** indiscipline, and hostility, is not what they had in mind at all when deciding to teach. (From *The Unmaking of a Mayor,* p. 201, The Viking Press, 1966)

inexorable (adjective) *Not to be persuaded or moved by entreaty or prayer.*

The wisdom and indispensability of government action to regulate economy becomes the **inexorable** next step. (From *God and Man at Yale,* p. 67, Regnery Books, 1986)

inhere (verb) *To be a fixed element or attribute of; belong.*

States are amoral institutions. In a "state" **inheres** the authority to preserve itself. (From *Right Reason,* p. 247, Doubleday & Company, 1985)

in medias res (Latin) *Into the thick of it.*

Even then, blissfully distracted, he found himself wondering, **in medias res:** Would his future duties require him to . . . seduce women routinely? (From *Saving the Queen,* p. 14, Doubleday & Company, 1976)

insouciance (noun) *Lighthearted unconcern; nonchalance.*

The refrain on the matter of wealth was widespread, the popular corollary of which was to reason on to **insouciance** with respect to poverty as (Ann Davidon, *Philadelphia Inquirer*) for instance: "But there is something rather beguiling and even enviable about this overdriven patrician and his way of life. Perhaps it is his apparently blithe blindness to most of the world's miseries." (From *Right Reason,* p. 16, Doubleday & Company, 1985)

interloper (noun) *An unlawful intruder on a property or sphere of action; one that interferes or thrusts himself in wrongfully or officiously.*

I do not deny, and do not regret, that the general tendency of an opinion journal is to be particularly critical of any politician one considers as an **interloper** in one's own party. (From *The Unmaking of a Mayor,* p. 95, The Viking Press, 1966)

interposition (noun) *The actions of a state whereby its sovereignty is placed between its citizens and the federal government.*

I have a dream that one day the state of Alabama, whose governor's lips are presently dripping with the words of **interposition** and nullification, will be transformed. (From *Right Reason,* p. 63, Doubleday & Company, 1985)

intone (verb) *To utter in musical or prolonged tones; recite in singing tones or in a monotone.*
Black sternly discoursed on the illogic and immorality of the United States getting involved in a European war, recapitulating the phrases and paragraphs he had so often heard his father so earnestly **intone.** (From *Saving the Queen,* p. 52, Doubleday & Company, 1976)

intrinsically (adverb) *Inherently; having to do with its own nature, property. Thus, charity is intrinsically good.*
Now the idea of reinstating the IRA for everybody is **intrinsically** appealing. Any tax modification that reduces taxes on savings is appealing. (From Mr. Buckley's syndicated column, "On the Right")

intuit (verb) *To know or apprehend directly.*
Prosecutor Neely at this point **intuited** what Smith's strategy was. (From *Right Reason,* p. 201, Doubleday & Company, 1985)

inure (verb) *To reside in, be inherent in.*
What rights, then, **inure** to the country whose responsibility it is to safeguard the lives of its citizens? (From *Right Reason,* p. 78, Doubleday & Company, 1985)

invidious (adjective) *Detrimental to reputation, designed to denigrate.*
It is not intended as ethnically **invidious** to remark that history shows a propensity for violence in Latin America. (From *Right Reason,* p. 255, Doubleday & Company, 1985)

involuted (adjective) *Of an involved or complicated nature; abstruse, intricate.*
Recently Mr. Sargent Shriver said, "I am delighted to be in any cathedral where Mr. Adam Clayton Powell, Jr., is in the pulpit." Here is an **involuted** form of racism. It is short for: "Even though I know that Adam Clayton Powell, Jr., is a demagogue, whose power and reputation have been built on hatred between the races, I recognize he is a Black leader, and must treat him as though he were a qualified object of universal admiration." (From *The Unmaking of a Mayor,* p. 156, The Viking Press, 1966)

ipso facto (adverb) *By the very nature of the case.*
I do not mean to imply that simply because my viewpoint was not energetically circularized, the Council proved itself **ipso facto** ineffective. (From *God and Man at Yale,* p. 132, Regnery Books, 1986)

Jacobinical (adjective) *Of or relating to violent or revolutionary political extremism.*
At Columbia, Mr. Allard Lowenstein was hooted down and literally silenced for defending the right of Professor Herman Kahn to speak unmolested, and faculty members in that audience countenanced and even egged on the **Jacobinical** furies that ruled the crowd. (From *Cruising Speed,* p. 209, G. P. Putnam's Sons, 1971)

jape (noun) *Something designed to arouse amusement or laughter.*
"Oh," said Blacky, "so it was here that famous tryst took place?" Except that he was too stuffed with crème Chantilly, he'd have taken out his notebook, further to extend the historical **jape.** (From *Saving the Queen,* p. 117, Doubleday & Company, 1976)

jejune (adjective) *Devoid of substance, interest, significance.*
One of Edgar Smith's editorial contributions to the *Times* on prison reform had come out embarrassingly **jejune.** (From *Right Reason,* p. 194, Doubleday & Company, 1985)

jeremiad (noun) *A lamenting and denunciatory complaint: a dolorous tirade.*
Soaring taxes, inadequate police protection, irregular garbage collection, traffic congestion, the scarcity of low-cost housing: Great **jeremiads** can be written on each of these major deprivations which underwrite such a categorical disillusion as Mr. Richard Whalen's. (From *The Unmaking of a Mayor,* p. 30, The Viking Press, 1966)

juridical (adjective) *Of or relating to law in general or to jurisprudence.*
A call by the President for a declaration of war last November would have passed Congress overwhelmingly and, you betcha, with Senator Kennedy voting in favor. The de-

claration having passed, the **juridical** house is now in order. Not only the impounding of funds, which the President managed under an old law, but much more. (From *Right Reason,* p. 74, Doubleday & Company, 1985)

juxtapose (verb) *Place side by side.*

The device was to contrive wisps of frivolous conversation, à la *The Women,* and **juxtapose** them with horror stories from the Vietnamese battlefront (get it?), so as to effect a Stendhalian contrast that would Arouse the Conscience of Versailles. (From *Cruising Speed,* p. 83, G. P. Putnam's Sons, 1971)

kedge (verb) *To dig an anchor in securely.*

Mr. Rockefeller's composure, though temporarily adrift, quickly **kedged** up in that splendid self-assurance of investigating panel chairmen. (From *Saving the Queen,* p. 246, Doubleday & Company, 1976)

kite (verb) *To get money or credit by a kite, a check drawn against uncollected funds in a bank account; to create a false bank balance by manipulating deposit accounts.*

Excepting the fiscal deficit, which presumably cannot be **kited** indefinitely, things could probably stumble along much as before without causing New York City to close down its doors. (From *The Unmaking of a Mayor,* p. 28, The Viking Press, 1966)

languorous (adjective) *Producing or tending to produce a state of the body or mind caused by exhaustion or disease and characterized by a weak, sluggish feeling.*

History adduces now and again a morally **languorous** pope who was awakened from his slumbers (and many more popes who slept through it all) by morally energetic laymen, preferably saints. (From *Cruising Speed,* p. 242, G. P. Putnam's Sons, 1971)

lapidary (adjective) *Having the elegance and precision associated with inscriptions on stone.*

To accept Mr. Simpson's thesis is to suppose that writers (and poets) always feel that the language of the moment is **lapidary,** never mind that, when detoxified, they proceed to make changes. (From Mr. Buckley's syndicated column, "On the Right")

lasciviously (adverb) *Luxuriantly, wantonly.*

I had at the moment the campaign began no personal animus, certainly not a shred of that "personal disdain" which John Lindsay's biographer so **lasciviously** records. (From *The Unmaking of a Mayor,* p. 96, The Viking Press, 1966)

latently (adverb) *Dormantly, but usually capable of being evoked, expressed, or brought to light.*

Why would it make for good politics to endorse the impression that the New York City police force is **latently** sympathetic with the brutality shown under stress by the Selma police force? (From *The Unmaking of a Mayor,* p. 21, The Viking Press, 1966)

leech (verb) *To fasten onto, as a leech; feed on the blood or substance of.*

I once contributed to the impression that Beame was ordinary, or rather **leeched** on it, at a speech where I remarked that Mr. Beame constantly stressed that he was educated by the City of New York, "which fact should be obvious," I said; and I am ashamed of it. (From *The Unmaking of a Mayor,* p. 284, The Viking Press, 1966)

lineaments (noun) *An outline, feature, or contour of a body or figure; the distinguishing or characteristic feature of something immaterial.*

It was terribly clear from the visceral reactions of such people as Jackie Robinson that thousands of people were taking very special, even an acute, pleasure from believing that a sudden flash of light had exposed the **lineaments** of the wolf. (From *The Unmaking of a Mayor,* p. 22, The Viking Press, 1966)

longueur (noun) *An overlong passage, made dull or tedious.*

The **longueurs** in Trudeau's "Doonesbury" are sometimes almost teasingly didactic. (From *Right Reason,* p. 388, Doubleday & Company, 1985)

loquacious (adjective) *Given to excessive talking.*

Sometimes we spend as much as a half hour in conversation. He is, oddly, **loquacious,** and enjoys our intercourse. (From *Saving the Queen,* p. 109, Doubleday & Company, 1976)

lugubrious (adjective) *Mournful, sad, lachrymose.*

Jean-François Revel gave many **lugubrious** examples of the working of the Western mind. (From *On the Firing Line: The Public Life of Our Public Figures,* p. 120, Random House, 1989)

machicolation (noun) *An opening for shooting or dropping missiles upon assailants attacking below.*

"After the next war," the queen said cheerily, "when we shall all have exchanged hydrogen bombs, I should think these archives would be tremendously useful, since whoever is left over will be reduced to defending himself by the use of things like moats and **machicolations** and bows and arrows . . ." (From *Saving the Queen,* p. 171, Doubleday & Company, 1976)

magnanimous (adjective) *Generous, suggesting special inclinations to charity or philanthropy.*

Phil Donahue came up with an alternative suggestion that also commended itself to his audience—the Shah should undertake to return to Iran to face the punishment. (This **magnanimous** willingness to bring martyrdom to someone else recalls the wisecrack of 1939 to the effect that the British were prepared to fight to the last Frenchman.) (From *Right Reason,* p. 77, Doubleday & Company, 1985)

maladroitness (noun) *Lacking in shrewdness of execution, craft, or resourcefulness in coping with difficulty or danger.*

One can have no objections whatever to President Carter's mission, restricting our criticism to the **maladroitness** of its execution and the insufficiency of contingency planning. (From *Right Reason,* p. 79, Doubleday & Company, 1985)

malleable (adjective) *Open to outside forces or influences; urging a change in position, viewpoint.*

The courts are less **malleable** than they were even for Roosevelt. The Supreme Court gave him problems, and he tried to pack it, and eventually, got himself a court that would go along. (From *Right Reason,* p. 81, Doubleday & Company, 1985)

malversation (noun) *Corrupt administration.*

The Seabury disclosures that brought Fusion to the fore are not to be confused with the routine **malversations** of public officials. (From *The Unmaking of a Mayor,* p. 436, The Viking Press, 1966)

manumission (noun) *Formal emancipation from slavery.*

The dutiful Mr. Walter Cronkite closes his broadcast every night by citing the number of days in the infinitely prolonged negotiations having as their objective the hostages' release. The result of this kind of thing over a period of five months is that we are not one step closer to the **manumission** than we were on the fifth of last November. (From *Right Reason,* p. 76, Doubleday & Company, 1985)

mastodonic (adjective) *Something unusually, surrealistically large.*

But when you endeavor to shake the conviction that the **mastodonic** oil deposits that guard growlingly the outskirts of Bridgeport reflect the size of your own financial resources, a student at the University of Bridgeport displays amusement at my suggestion that it was neither factually not symbolically correct that I was there to argue the case for the Buckley oil interest in Bridgeport, *über alles.* (From *Cruising Speed,* p. 95, G. P. Putnam's Sons, 1971)

matriculate (verb) *To become admitted to membership in a body, society, or institution.*

Blackford completed his application for graduate school rather listlessly; convinced, correctly, that he would never **matriculate** during this bellicose season. (From *Saving the Queen,* p. 14, Doubleday & Company, 1976)

mete (verb) *To assign by measure; deal out; allot, apportion.*

Too many judges appear to have forgotten that the primary purpose of courts of justice is to assert the demands of the public order—by **meting** out convincing punishment to those who transgress against it. (From *The Unmaking of a Mayor*, p. 195, The Viking Press, 1966)

mien (noun) *The air or bearing of a person, especially as expressive of mood or personality.*

Black's final instructor had obviously spent much time in England. He was a gray man, his **mien**, hair, face, suit, shirt. (From *Saving the Queen*, p. 45, Doubleday & Company, 1976)

militate (verb) *To have weight or effect.*

The young graduate of Yale, the potential entrepreneur, must remember that money costs do not tally with social costs, and that therefore it is quite possible that the enterprise he is considering, regardless of its financial success, will **militate** against the social welfare. (From *God and Man at Yale*, p. 84, Regnery Books, 1986)

mollifying (adjective) *Making more agreeable; conciliatory; soothing.*

I have seen a variety of official answers to correspondents of Mr. Ober's general persuasion. Replies were **mollifying** in tone, but firm, and abundant in phrases like "freedom of speech" and "the great traditions of academic freedom." (From *God and Man at Yale*, p. 137, Regnery Books, 1986)

mordant (adjective) *Biting or caustic in thought, manner, or style; incisive; keen.*

Through it all, Smith had managed to put forward his case in an almost disinterested perspective. He was by turns **mordant**, judicious, inquisitive, impudent, amused. (From *Right Reason*, p. 190, Doubleday & Company, 1985)

mugwumpery (noun) *The views and practices of a mugwump, one who withdraws his support from a political group or organization: a regular member who bolts a party and adopts an independent position.*

Lindsay's biographer does not know how to handle the problem. On the one hand, Lindsay's transcendence of Republicanism must be presented as a statesmanlike projection of true Republican principle. On the other, a touch of **mugwumpery** is always charming. (From *The Unmaking of a Mayor*, p. 72, The Viking Press, 1966)

mulct (verb) *To leach from, gather up from, drain.*

In order for a nation to guard the common defense or look after the unfortunate, there has to be a certain residue. That residue can be **mulcted** from the masses, as in the Soviet Union, leaving them without the essential freedoms to engage in commerce or to blunt the sharp edges of life, or it can come out of what can reasonably be called a "surplus." (From *Right Reason*, p. 252, Doubleday & Company, 1985)

munificent (adjective) *Very liberal in giving or bestowing; lavish; characterized by great liberality or generosity.*

Many people come to New York because they are deluded, at least momentarily, into believing the myth of New York's **munificent** opportunities. (From *The Unmaking of a Mayor*, p. 37, The Viking Press, 1966)

muse (noun) *The creative spirit of an individual, the source of his inspiration.*

I would sooner risk the displeasure of a voter than I would that of my **muse**, who is more demanding. (From *The Unmaking of a Mayor*, p. 191, The Viking Press, 1966)

nepotistically (adverb) *Characterized by nepotism, favoritism shown to relatives.*

It had already been rumored that Blackford's selection to fly the new fighter had been **nepotistically** contrived. (From *Saving the Queen*, p. 222, Doubleday & Company, 1976)

nescience (noun) *The belief that nothing is establishable, provable.*

How is it that the president of a distinguished and cosmopolitan university tells us that God alone knows when human life begins? If you penetrate this rhetorical formulation, you have a dimly obscured invitation to **nescience**. "God alone knows" is the safest way to say, "That-is-unknowable." Inasmuch as God is not invited to teach a regular course at Yale, Mr. Giamatti is saying in effect that the search for the answer to "When does life begin?" should be abandoned—because no one can tell. (From *Right Reason,* p. 49, Doubleday & Company, 1985)

nexus (noun) *Connection, interconnection, tie, link.*

Reason, conscience, and self-restraint are all that we have to rely upon, the burden resting on those who postulate a **nexus** between a sane position and an insane extension of it to make their demonstration. (From *The Unmaking of a Mayor,* p. 235, The Viking Press, 1966)

non grata (adjective) *Not approved; unwelcome.*

Others convey to the student who majors in sociology the definite impression that at best religion is **non grata** to the department, at worst it is the subject of relentless attack. (From *God and Man at Yale,* p. 18, Regnery Books, 1986)

numinous (adjective) *Divine, magical.*

Rosalyn Tureck sits down and pulls out that talismanic handkerchief, the fondling of which precedes the contact of her **numinous** fingers with the keyboard. (From *Cruising Speed,* p. 143, G. P. Putnam's Sons, 1971)

obduracy (noun) *The quality or state of being hard or resistant.*

I am not talking about someone who has familiarized himself sufficiently with the great scientific impasses that at various stages in the struggle to achieve the bomb have constituted roadblocks of historical **obduracy.** (From *Saving the Queen,* p. 147, Doubleday & Company, 1976)

obeisance (noun) *A movement of the body or other gesture made in token of respect or submission.*

Blackford rose, walked gravely to the lectern, and bowed with the faintly wooden truncation that becomes those ill at ease with the filigreed lengths of native **obeisances,** first to the Queen, then to the Archbishop. (From *Saving the Queen,* p. 242, Doubleday & Company, 1976)

objurgation (noun) *An act of decrying vehemently; castigation with harsh or violent language; harsh or violent reproof.*

Mrs. Gunning had, as chief organizer of the Parents and Taxpayers Association, been widely denounced, that being the cant **objurgation,** as an enemy of the Public Schools. (From *The Unmaking of a Mayor,* p. 261, The Viking Press, 1966)

oblation (noun) *Something offered or presented in worship or sacred service.*

I tell about the monk—the ex–circus hand—who, having no relevant skills, and having observed the artful **oblations** rendered by his brothers on the Feast Day of the Virgin, was spotted late that night, standing before her statue juggling his five weatherbeaten circus balls. (From *Cruising Speed,* p. 144, G. P. Putnam's Sons, 1971)

obverse (noun) *A counterpart necessarily involved in or answering to a fact or truth.*

The (conservative) Americans for Constitutional Action have their own poll—the **obverse** of the ADA's—which revealed that the median Republican voted with his party 86 percent of the time on issues of importance to conservatives. (From *The Unmaking of a Mayor,* p. 70, The Viking Press, 1966)

ochlocracy (noun) *Government by the mob; mob rule.*

She found it increasingly easy to achieve informality—to the dismay of her impossibly punctilious husband who desired **ochlocracy** abroad but, at home, to be paid homage even by the baboons at the zoo. (From *Saving the Queen,* p. 130, Doubleday & Company, 1976)

oenophile (noun) *A lover or connoisseur of wine.*

Blackford wondered where the **oenophiles'** journals were and thought Ellison must be a real sport to pass himself off as a winetaster, working in the sunkissed vineyards of Washington, D.C. (From *Saving the Queen,* p. 29, Doubleday & Company, 1976)

omnibus (adjective) *Of, relating to, or providing for many things at once.*

What we have is a great blur, an **omnibus** bill that goes everywhere from collecting taxes on tips at hamburger stands, to one that clips you extra on a phone call, to one that immobilizes one or another business merger because of changes in tax scheduling. (From *Right Reason,* p. 91, Doubleday & Company, 1985)

onus (noun) *Something (as a task, duty, responsibility) that involves considerable difficulty or annoyance; a burden.*

The probabilities are small that the cost of any modern government will reduce: which puts the **onus** back on the private sector to generate additional revenues, and ends us back with the question: Is the scarcity of public funds the major problem? (From *The Unmaking of a Mayor,* p. 32, The Viking Press, 1966)

opéra-bouffe (adjective) *Fit for a light comic opera characterized by parody or burlesque.*

"I persuaded a friend of mine from M.I.T. to go see the old gentleman. They hit it off and my friend is now hired," said Blackford with a feigned air of **opéra-bouffe** secretiveness. (From *Saving the Queen,* p. 171, Doubleday & Company, 1976)

opine (verb) *To give a formal opinion about.*

Pundits need to **opine** on developments in China while fearing that what we write on Monday will be obsolete on Tuesday. (From Mr. Buckley's syndicated column, "On the Right")

orotund (adjective) *Unduly strong in delivery or style.*

"You and your goddam . . . continence. I guess after graduation you'll go into training for the Graduate Engineering School lacrosse team and inflict on the next guy the necessity to go out into the wild night, in search of a normal room, with normal people, and normal supplies of the normal vices of this world."

Johnny got **orotund** when he was tight, and Blackford smiled at the familiar chiding. (From *Saving the Queen,* p. 7, Doubleday & Company, 1976)

ostracism (noun) *The exclusion by general consent from common privilege or social acceptance.*

What should happen is what should have happened when martial law was declared in Poland: a total economic, social, and cultural **ostracism** of the Soviet Union. (From *Right Reason,* p. 89, Doubleday & Company, 1985)

oxymoronic (adjective) *Relating to a combination for epigrammatic effect of contradictory or incongruous words.*

Michael Harrington's **oxymoronic** formulation—"coercion in favor of capitalists"—reminds us of the fashionable jargon in the commodity markets of the left (alas, not greatly changed). (From *God and Man at Yale,* p. xxxiv, Regnery Books, 1986)

palliative (noun) *Something that moderates the intensity of.*

Bowman and Bach's **palliatives** are mild by comparison with some of their brethren textbook writers who have molded the attitudes of so many students. (From *God and Man at Yale,* p. 52, Regnery Books, 1986)

pallid (adjective) *Lacking brightness or intensity.*

The truly extraordinary feature of our time isn't the faithlessness of the Western people; it is their utter, total ignorance of the Christian religion. They travel to Rishikesh to listen to **pallid** seventh-hand imitations of thoughts and words they never knew existed. (From *Cruising Speed,* p. 162, G. P. Putnam's Sons, 1971)

parabolically (adverb) *Expressed in the manner of a parable or figure; allegorically.*

It was easy to deny the rumor, that I had flown to Phoenix, Arizona, a few weeks earlier, there to meet with Barry Goldwater and Mrs. Clare Boothe Luce, since it was not true, not even **parabolically**. (From *The Unmaking of a Mayor,* p. 100, The Viking Press, 1966)

paradigm (noun) *An idealistic model.*

But Lenin had working for him not only the excitement of throwing over a dynasty, but of remaking a state around an ideological **paradigm** that excited everyone by its call to equality. (From *Right Reason,* p. 72, Doubleday & Company, 1985)

paralogist (noun) *One who uses reasoning that begs the question; one who uses a reasoning contrary to logical rules or formulas.*

A good debater is not necessarily an effective vote-getter: you can find a hole in your opponent's argument and thrill at the crystallization of a truth wrung out from a bloody dialogue—which may warm only you and your muse, while the smiling **paralogist** has made votes by the tens of thousands. (From *The Unmaking of a Mayor,* p. 272, The Viking Press, 1966)

parsimonious (adjective) *Excessively frugal.*

Eisenhower, as a young lieutenant, had had to train American soldiers using brooms as facsimiles for rifles, so **parsimonious** had the American isolationist Congress been toward the army. (From *Saving the Queen,* p. 184, Doubleday & Company, 1976)

partita (noun) *A set of musical variations.*

Rosalyn Tureck tells me that the note I sent her, likening Bach's E-minor **Partita** to *King Lear* was right on, that she had played the **partita** a thousand times, but always treated it with awe because she could not know what it would say to her this time around, even as *Lear* cannot be tuned by stroboscope. (From *Cruising Speed,* p. 142, G. P. Putnam's Sons, 1971)

paternalistic (adjective) *Relating to the practices of a government that undertakes to supply the needs or regulate the conduct of the governed in matters affecting them as individuals as well as in their relations to the state and to each other.*

The inflation that comes inevitably with government pump-priming soon catches up with the laborer, setting off a new deflationary spiral which can in turn only be counteracted by more coercive and **paternalistic** government policies. (From *God and Man at Yale,* p. 68, Regnery Books, 1986)

paucity (noun) *Smallness of quantity; dearth, scarcity.*

His subordinates complained with good and ill humor about everything, about the weather, the food, the hygienic facilities, the **paucity** of air cover, the stubbornness of Montgomery, the tenacity of the Germans. (From *Saving the Queen,* p. 140, Doubleday & Company, 1976)

pedagogical (adjective) *Characteristic of teaching.*

BORGES: I tried to teach my students not literature but the *love* of literature. I have taught many people the love of Old English.

WFB: And so there is a **pedagogical** art? It isn't simply a matter of—of exposure— you are indoctrinating your students? (From *On the Firing Line: The Public Life of Our Public Figures,* p. 275, Random House, 1989)

pejorative (noun) *Negative in inclination; critical.*

The term appeaser is used here not merely as a lazy **pejorative**. The appeaser tends to oppose a national draft, to oppose any increase in defense spending, to oppose economic boycotts, cultural boycotts, boycotts of athletic events. (From *Right Reason,* p. 101, Doubleday & Company, 1985)

penchant (noun) *A strong leaning or attraction; strong and continued inclination.*
Henry Regnery has passed along the principal executive responsibilities to his son-in-law, who is apolitical and resists, as financially unproductive, the **penchant** of his father-in-law for conservative-oriented books. (From *Cruising Speed,* p. 117, G. P. Putnam's Sons, 1971)

penury (noun) *Extreme poverty.*
In some measure, the educator is fortified by the knowledge that despite the trials and **penury** of his existence, he is shaping, more directly than members of any other profession, the destiny of the world. (From *God and Man at Yale,* p. 192, Regnery Books, 1986)

pertinacity (noun) *Unyielding persistence, often annoyingly perverse; stubborn inflexibility.*
Blackford muttered something about the **pertinacity** of the press. (From *Saving the Queen,* p. 230, Doubleday & Company, 1976)

phlegmatic (adjective) *Slow, stolid, unexcitable.*
"Frankly," said Black at dinner, to his aunt and her **phlegmatic** ever-silent husband, "the idea of going to school in England gives me the creeps." (From *Saving the Queen,* p. 55, Doubleday & Company, 1976)

pianissimo (adverb) *Very softly.*
Rufus's intensest emotions, like J. S. Bach's, were rendered **pianissimo.** (From *Saving the Queen,* p. 204, Doubleday & Company, 1976)

plenipotentiary (noun) *A person invested with full power to transact any business.*
Caroline drew closer to Perry. "I wish you were my minister **plenipotentiary.** I would trust you to do all these things for me, and then if anything at all went wrong, all I would have to do is simply behead you." (From *Saving the Queen,* p. 145, Doubleday & Company, 1976)

polyglot (noun) *Someone who speaks or writes several languages.*
If you can speak Spanish that easily, he persists, surely you can run through my book in French? **Polyglots** are that way, I find. They reach a point where every language silts up into a more or less recognizable vernacular. (From *Cruising Speed,* p. 49, G. P. Putnam's Sons, 1971)

pomposity (noun) *Ornately showy or pretentiously dignified demeanor, speech, or action.*
Anthony, though formal of speech, was incapable of **pomposity.** He cared more about effective relief for those who suffered than about bombastic relief for those who formed committees. (From *Saving the Queen,* p. 10, Doubleday & Company, 1976)

porcine (adjective) *Suggestive of swine.*
He talked about the necessity of replenishing his supply of French silk shirts, which heretofore were available only in America and other **porcine** countries. (From *Saving the Queen,* p. 156, Doubleday & Company, 1976)

portentous (adjective) *Exhibiting gravity or ponderousness; self-consciously weighty.*
"What matters is the nature of the Commonwealth."
"I have ideas about that," Caroline said. This sounded **portentous** so she added, "Everybody does . . ." (From *Saving the Queen,* p. 144, Doubleday & Company, 1976)

positivist (adjective) *Relating to the theory that rejects theology and metaphysics as being merely earlier imperfect modes of knowledge and instead holds that positive knowledge is based on natural phenomena and their properties and relations as verified by the empirical sciences.*
How much harm does *Playboy* do in fact, I have often asked myself, never getting much further than the presumptive disapproval of it, which I extend to any publica-

tion that declines to accept extra-personal or extra-**positivist** norms. (From *Cruising Speed*, p. 65, G. P. Putnam's Sons, 1971)

postprandial (adjective) *Occurring after a meal, especially after dinner.*

Sitting in the little drawing room of the Moscow apartment, Boris explained to his wife why they must retreat here for any intimate discussions, and routinely after dinner, when, he knew, the **postprandial** relaxation loosens the tongue. (From *Saving the Queen*, p. 106, Doubleday & Company, 1976)

postulate (noun) *A proposition advanced as axiomatic; an essential presupposition, condition, or premise; an underlying hypothesis or assumption.*

When scholars and statesmen disagreed on how to reconcile the **postulates** of America with the survival of slavery, it was to the Declaration of Independence that the abolitionists ideally repaired for guidance. Because the Declaration of Independence spoke of "self-evident" truths. Among them that men are born equal. (From *Cruising Speed*, p. 199, G. P. Putnam's Sons, 1971)

Potemkin (adjective) *(Referring to the Russian statesman who built fake villages along a route taken by Catherine the Great) Relating to creating an imposing façade or display designed to obscure or shield an unimposing or undesirable fact or condition.*

There is a little bit too much of the **Potemkin**-tour in the visit of some of the committees to the university. Appointments are set up for them, and they are put in touch with administration and faculty stalwarts. (From *God and Man at Yale*, p. 128, Regnery Books, 1986)

pragmatism (noun) *An American movement in philosophy founded by Peirce and James and marked by the doctrines that the meaning of conceptions is to be sought in their practical bearings, that the function of thought is as a guide to action, and that the truth is preeminently to be tested by the practical consequences of belief.*

Brief reference should be made to the substantial contribution to secularism that is being made at Yale and elsewhere by widespread academic reliance on relativism, **pragmatism**, and utilitarianism. (From *God and Man at Yale*, p. 25, Regnery Books, 1986)

prefecture (noun) *The office, position, jurisdiction, or term of office of a prefect.*

Though a prefect, Anthony was never a member of the **prefecture**. (From *Saving the Queen*, p. 11, Doubleday & Company, 1976)

prehensile (adjective) *Clutching greedily.*

Later that night, in Sally's car, they made love for the last time under the shadow of the West Rock. She was silent, but **prehensile**. (From *Saving the Queen*, p. 27, Doubleday & Company, 1976)

presumptive (adjective) *Apparent, presumed; based on inference.*

"This is a pretty good job," the Queen remarked. "I have inherited a lot of money, and a lot of junk, and a lot of perquisites, but there is something in it for everybody because of the **presumptive** necessity to worship something—somebody—worldly." (From *Saving the Queen*, p. 185, Doubleday & Company, 1976)

prevarication (noun) *A statement that deviates from or perverts the truth.*

Schlesinger dismissed the **prevarication** as part of the cover story, and confessed that he had not formulated an absolutely satisfactory ethic on the matter of lying to the press. (From *The Unmaking of a Mayor*, p. 101, The Viking Press, 1966)

probative (adjective) *Serving to prove; substantiating.*

With Presidents one proceeds more cautiously, because it is not the business of friends, let alone subordinates, to quiz the President. In the first place, one simply doesn't. In the second, a skillful politician could turn away the question easily; and the interrogator gets no **probative** satisfaction. (From *Cruising Speed*, p. 94, G. P. Putnam's Sons, 1971)

probity (noun) *Uncompromising adherence to the highest principles and ideals; unimpeachable integrity.*

If the educational overseer is interested in the activity of scholarship, let him endow a research center (and let him not, as a man of intelligence and **probity,** stipulate what shall be the findings of research not yet undertaken). (From *God and Man at Yale,* p. 186, Regnery Books, 1986)

prodigy (noun) *An extraordinary, marvelous, or unusual accomplishment, deed, instance, or person.*

Crosstown traffic is bad, but a new traffic commissioner who performed **prodigies** in Baltimore is now in charge. (From *The Unmaking of a Mayor,* p. 31, The Viking Press, 1966)

profanation (noun) *Debasement or vulgarization, especially by misuse or disclosure.*

It is a **profanation** to advance on Kempton's thought with compass, scissors, and tape measure, and it is a sign of his special genius that he inevitably leaves his critics feeling like Philistines. (From *The Unmaking of a Mayor,* p. 199, The Viking Press, 1966)

propensity (noun) *Natural inclination; innate or inherent tendency.*

An economic justification for a redistribution of income is the Keynesian insistence that more money go to that group which has a higher **propensity** to consume, that is, the lower and middle income groups. (From *God and Man at Yale,* p. 54, Regnery Books, 1986)

prosaic (adjective) *Having a dull, flat, unimaginative quality of style or expression.*

I gathered from my own representative that Lindsay's press conferences tended to be **prosaic** affairs, repetitious, formalistic, called for purely personal exposure. (From *The Unmaking of a Mayor,* p. 266, The Viking Press, 1966)

proselytize (verb) *To convert from one religion, opinion, or party to another; to evangelize.*

Mr. Lovett teaches the Historical and Literary Aspects of the Old Testament, but he does not **proselytize** the Christian faith or teach religion at all. (From *God and Man at Yale,* p. 6, Regnery Books, 1986)

prosody (noun) *A method or style of versification.*

To pray during the gymnastic exercise of the modern mass, athwart a vernacular **prosody** that belongs in the Chamber of Literary Horrors, is an exercise in self-discipline achieved most easily by the blind and the deaf. (From *Right Reason,* p. 373, Doubleday & Company, 1985)

pro tanto (Latin) *To a certain extent; proportionately; commensurately.*

Communities blockwide or greater will be given ***pro tanto*** relief in their property taxes, sufficient to pay the local police bills. (From *The Unmaking of a Mayor,* p. 91, The Viking Press, 1966)

provenance (noun) *Place of origin.*

There was just the trace of an accent there, and Blackford could not guess its **provenance,** and of course would not have presumed to inquire. (From *Saving the Queen,* p. 33, Doubleday & Company, 1976)

psephologist (noun) *Someone who pursues the scientific study of elections.*

I announce that the **psephologists** have just completed a study that reveals that the participation of Princeton volunteers was the very thing that brought brother Jim [newly elected junior senator for New York] over the edge of victory. (From *Cruising Speed,* p. 76, G. P. Putnam's Sons, 1971)

purposive (adjective) *Tending to fulfill a conscious purpose or design.*

Individual rights of the sort that for generations were never supposed to be prey to government actions are cheerily disposed of as unjustifiable impedimenta in the way of **purposive** and enlightened state policies. (From *God and Man at Yale,* p. 79, Regnery Books, 1986)

putsch (noun) *A secretly plotted and suddenly executed attempt to overthrow a government or governing body.*

Mr. Adam Clayton Powell, Jr., would be objectionable as a leader whether he became leader following a city-wide **putsch,** or whether he became leader having got one hundred percent of the vote of his constituency. (From *The Unmaking of a Mayor,* p. 253, The Viking Press, 1966)

qua (preposition) *In the character, role, or capacity of; as.*

The Republicans were increasingly maneuvered into the position of believing in John Lindsay *qua* John Lindsay, as their shriveled justification for their original enthusiasm gave way under the weight of one after another entanglement with the same old crowd. (From *The Unmaking of a Mayor,* p. 44, The Viking Press, 1966)

querencia (noun) *An area in the arena taken by the bull because he feels safe there.*

Dulles stared at him silently, then turned to talk with Griswold. Black eased away toward Sally—his *querencia,* his love—to lick his wounds. (From *Saving the Queen,* p. 44, Doubleday & Company, 1976)

Rabelaisian (adjective) *Marked by gross, robust humor, extravagance of caricature, or bold naturalism.*

I remember the old "Truth or Consequences" game they used to play over the radio, which towards the end was coming up with consequences so extravagant as to satisfy **Rabelaisian** appetites for the absurd. (From *Cruising Speed,* p. 59, G. P. Putnam's Sons, 1971)

raffish (adjective) *Vulgar; showy.*

Maria wandered over to the entertainment district and was not entirely surprised to find herself talking with a **raffish** man who in his plushily upholstered office looked at her carefully, asked her matter-of-factly to disrobe, examined her again, focused lights on her from various angles, and agreed to employ her. (From *Mongoose, R.I.P.,* p. 122, Random House, 1987)

recondite (adjective) *Very difficult to understand and beyond the reach of ordinary comprehension and knowledge.*

There is a luxurious offering at Yale of courses in the **recondite** byways of human knowledge, wonderful to behold. (From *God and Man at Yale,* p. xlviii, Regnery Books, 1986)

redoubt (noun) *A small, defensive, secure place; stronghold.*

At places like Harvard, Yale, and Princeton lecturers run into difficulty, because these colleges are not accustomed to paying their speakers the commercial rates; and speakers tend to indulge them, in part out of tradition, in part out of a curiosity to have a look at what used to be the **redoubts** of social and intellectual patricians. (From *Cruising Speed,* p. 67, G. P. Putnam's Sons, 1971)

regicide (noun) *The killing or murder of a king.*

After the original *World-Telegram* story charging vandalism, rape, and **regicide,** the Conservative Party took the precaution of instructing its captains to telephone to inquire whether any complaints had actually been lodged. (From *The Unmaking of a Mayor,* p. 234, The Viking Press, 1966)

reification (noun) *The conversion of something abstract into something concrete.*

A gesture of recognition—of Martin Luther King's courage, of the galvanizing quality of a rhetoric that sought out a **reification** of the dream of brotherhood—is consistent with the ideals of the country, and a salute to a race of people greatly oppressed during much of U.S. history. (From *Right Reason,* pp. 375–76, Doubleday & Company, 1985)

rescind (verb) *To take back; annul, cancel.*

"I've a terrific idea!" said Blackford. "Why don't you kidnap the Queen, hypnotize her, then send her back and have her **rescind** her invitation to me to do the eulogy?" (From *Saving the Queen,* p. 234, Doubleday & Company, 1976)

res manet (Latin) *"There the matter rests."*

School dropouts under the age of fourteen will be sent to special vocational schools, whose administrators will be especially trained. Successful graduates of one year's experience will be qualified to reenter public schools. [***Res manet***] (From *The Unmaking of a Mayor,* p. 93, The Viking Press, 1966)

reticulation (noun) *A network; an arrangement of lines resembling a net.*

When a number of colleges and universities were given over to the thousand blooms of the youth revolution, many of the same people who sharpened their teeth on *God and Man at Yale* were preternaturally silent. They feasted on ideological **reticulation.** (From *God and Man at Yale,* p. xxxii, Regnery Books, 1986)

ribaldry (noun) *Language characterized by broad, indecent humor.*

Before we knew it, FBI chief J. Edgar Hoover was bugging motels in which Martin Luther King spent the night, which tapes resulted in vocal **ribaldry** not suitable for family cassettes. (From Mr. Buckley's syndicated column, "On the Right")

rodomontade (noun) *A vain, exaggerated boast; a bragging speech; empty bluster.*

I teased my brother Jim by sending him, framed, the headline in the *New York Post* the day after the election, "Buckley: 'I AM THE NEW POLITICS,' " getting back from him a winced note of pain at this lapidary record of what looked like a lapse into **rodomontade.** (From *Cruising Speed,* p. 121, G. P. Putnam's Sons, 1971)

rump (adjective) *Relating to a fragment or remainder; as (a) a parliament, committee, or other group carrying on in the name of the original body after the departure or expulsion of a large number of its members; (b) a small group usually claiming to be representative of a larger whole that arises independently or breaks off from a parent body.*

Mr. Lindsay's Republican Party is a **rump** affair, captive in his and others' hands, no more representative of the body of Republican thought than the Democratic Party in Mississippi is representative of the Democratic Party nationally. (From *The Unmaking of a Mayor,* p. 105, The Viking Press, 1966)

sacrosanct (adjective) *Most holy or sacred; inviolable.*

Here in England, three thousand miles away from America, Blackford found it a corporate affront that a **sacrosanct** master should feel free to belittle so great a man as Lindbergh. (From *Saving the Queen,* p. 65, Doubleday & Company, 1976)

salacious (adjective) *Marked by lecherousness or lewdness; lustful.*

The television reporters ask their own questions and always gravitate to the most **salacious** issues of the day, preferably personal. (From *The Unmaking of a Mayor,* p. 267, The Viking Press, 1966)

salutary (adjective) *Effecting or designed to effect an improvement; remedial.*

By age fifteen Rolando had decided he wished to go into an entirely different kind of life—bloody, yes, but bloody-**salutary**, not bloody-destructive. (From *Mongoose, R.I.P.,* p. 17, Random House, 1987)

salvific (adjective) *Having the intent to save or admit to salvation.*

If we undertake a systematic, devoted, evangelical effort to instruct the people of the world that the Soviet Union is animated not by a **salvific** ideology, but by a reactionary desire to kill and torture, intimidate and exploit others, for the benefit of its own recidivist national appetites for imperialism, we will have done, by peaceful means, what is so long overdue. (From *Right Reason,* p. 230, Doubleday & Company, 1985)

sanguinary (adjective) *Bloodthirsty, murderous.*

Let us concede that the death squads of San Salvador are composed primarily of sadistic opportunists who, taking cover in the civil war, pursue their acquisitive and **sanguinary** interests relatively unmolested because of the preoccupation of civil authority with that civil war. (From *Right Reason,* p. 305, Doubleday & Company, 1985)

saprophytic (adjective) *Obtaining nourishment osmotically from dead matter.*
> If the modern politician's invocation of Lincoln is to be taken as other than oppor-
> tunistic and **saprophytic,** the invoker must describe what it is about Lincoln that he
> understands to be the quintessential Lincoln. (From *The Unmaking of a Mayor,* p. 78,
> The Viking Press, 1966)

saraband (noun) *The music of the saraband, a stately court dance of the seventeenth and eighteenth centuries resembling the minuet and evolved from a quick Spanish dance of oriental
origin.*
> Rosalyn [Tureck] giggles her aristocratic warm giggle, leans over, and whispers that she
> will play me the **saraband** she knows I love. (From *Cruising Speed,* p. 143, G. P. Put-
> nam's Sons, 1971)

schuss (noun) *A straight, high-speed run on skis.*
> Ah, the ideological coda, how it afflicts us all! And how paralyzingly sad that someone
> who can muse over the desirability of converting New York into an independent state
> should, having climbed to such a peak, **schuss** down the same old slope, when the
> mountains beckon him on to new, exhilarating runs. (From *The Unmaking of a Mayor,*
> p. 39, The Viking Press, 1966)

scintilla (noun) *A barely perceptible manifestation; the slightest particle or trace.*
> In the two years he had known her, Blackford had never seen in Sally a **scintilla** of cu-
> riosity about anything scientific. (From *Saving the Queen,* p. 26, Doubleday & Com-
> pany, 1976)

sciolism (noun) *Superficial knowledge; a show of learning without substantial foundation.*
> I wasn't sure enough of myself on the facts of Roger Bacon's life, so I didn't note down to
> challenge Clark on the point; and anyway, he who lives off the exposure of **sciolism** will
> die from the exposure of **sciolism.** (From *Cruising Speed,* p. 122, G. P. Putnam's Sons, 1971)

scurrility (noun) *Abusive language usually marked by coarse or indecent wording or innu-
endo, unjust denigration, or clownish jesting.*
> I have seen libelers try to excuse their own **scurrilities** (what a wonderful word!)
> against me by pleading that I am a public figure, leaving open the question whether
> what was said about me was said with actual malice. (From *Cruising Speed,* p. 185,
> G. P. Putnam's Sons, 1971)

secularist (noun) *One who advocates a view of life or of any particular matter based on the
premise that religion and religious considerations should be ignored or purposely excluded.*
> Best equipped to challenge the **secularists** in the Department of Philosophy is Profes-
> sor Robert L. Calhoun, an ordained minister vastly respected as a scholar, as a lecturer,
> and as a man. (From *God and Man at Yale,* p. 19, Regnery Books, 1986)

seemliness (noun) *The quality or state of conforming to accepted standards of good form or
taste; propriety.*
> Such Republican judges as there are, are there simply because judicial **seemliness** re-
> quires that a second party should be seen, if not heard—if only to provide those com-
> fortable democratic delusions which are formally satisfying. (From *The Unmaking of a
> Mayor,* p. 40, The Viking Press, 1966)

seine (verb) *To fish out or pluck from the sea.*
> The arraignment and the trial were conducted with the care and precision of an Apollo
> moon launch, and it is questionable whether even Edgar Smith will succeed in **seining**
> out of the experience reversible error. (From *Right Reason,* p. 210, Doubleday & Com-
> pany, 1985)

sequester (verb) *To set apart; separate for a special purpose; remove, segregate.*
> One can be compassionate for the president of the New York Stock Exchange who
> goes to jail for his greed, and for the rapist who is unable to control his lust. But it is

necessary to **sequester** the transgressors, whatever the genealogy of the aberrations. (From *The Unmaking of a Mayor,* p. 98, The Viking Press, 1966)

seriatim (adverb) *In a series; serially.*

A short, bright, engaging review of the day-in-the-life of each of the candidates appeared **seriatim** in *The New Yorker* during October. (From *The Unmaking of a Mayor,* p. 236, The Viking Press, 1966)

shibboleth (noun) *(1) A word or saying characteristically used by the adherents of a party, sect, or belief and usually regarded as empty of real meaning; (2) a commonplace saying or idea; platitude, truism.*

I appear before you as the only candidate for Mayor of New York who has not a word to say in defense of the proposition that New York ought to stay as big as it is, let alone grow bigger. Is there an argument in defense of this **shibboleth**? (From *The Unmaking of a Mayor,* p. 37, The Viking Press, 1966)

sloth (noun) *Disinclination to action or labor; sluggishness, laziness, idleness, indolence.*

Those who rail against the [microcomputer] chip do so for the most practical reason: They have not mastered its use. They strive for metaphysical formulations to justify their hidden little secret (**sloth** and fear). (From Mr. Buckley's syndicated column, "On the Right")

sonorous (adjective) *Marked by excessively heavy, high-flown, grandiloquent, or self-assured effect or style.*

I maintain that **sonorous** pretensions notwithstanding, Yale does subscribe to an orthodoxy: there are limits within which its faculty members must keep their opinions if they wish to be "tolerated." (From *God and Man at Yale,* p. 151, Regnery Books, 1986)

sophistry (noun) *Reasoning that is superficially plausible but actually fallacious.*

The guardians of this sustaining core of civilization have abdicated their responsibility to mankind. And what is more depressing, they have painted their surrender with flamboyant words and systematic **sophistry** in their efforts to persuade us that far better things are really in store for the world by virtue of their inactivity. (From *God and Man at Yale,* p. 193, Regnery Books, 1986)

soritical (adjective) *Of or relating to an abridged form of stating a series of syllogisms in a series of propositions so arranged that the predicate of each one that precedes forms the subject of each one that follows and the conclusion unites the subject of the first proposition with the predicate of the last proposition. For instance: A = B, B = C, C = D, D = E. Therefore, A = E.*

I remember suggesting to Dan Mahoney that I make the **soritical** leap and announce quite frankly that the defeat of Lindsay was an objective of the Conservative Party. (From *The Unmaking of a Mayor,* p. 301, The Viking Press, 1966)

sotto voce (adverb) *Under the breath; in an undertone.*

"Mr. Oakes, this is Mr. Allen Dulles, deputy director of the Central Intelligence Agency." Black shook hands, and then winked mysteriously and asked *sotto voce:* "How's tricks?" (From *Saving the Queen,* p. 44, Doubleday & Company, 1976)

specious (adjective) *Superficially beautiful or attractive or coveted, but not so in reality; apparently right and proper; superficially fair, just, or correct.*

Note well that Professor Kirkland raised no objection to the fact that what later was demonstrated to be a **specious** biological generalization was taught to several generations of students. (From *God and Man at Yale,* p. 153, Regnery Books, 1986)

splenetic (adjective) *Characterized by morose bad temper, sullen malevolence, or spiteful, peevish anger.*

The war engaged all the **splenetic** instincts of Khomeini, and he urged all Iran's young people to die in the ecstasy of a mission that transcribed God's will. (From Mr. Buckley's syndicated column, "On the Right")

stricture (noun) *Something that closely restrains or limits.*

I am confident that the scholar who holds her in esteem and the scholar who does not could both make their way into Yale. Does this mean that Yale, true to the **strictures** of academic freedom, is unconcerned about the teacher's values? (From *God and Man at Yale*, p. 147, Regnery Books, 1986)

suasion (noun) *The act or an instance of urging, convincing, or persuading.*

It is important that the college student's choice be his own, for it is all the more valuable to him if there has been no exterior **suasion** on behalf of one or the other protagonist. (From *God and Man at Yale*, p. 145, Regnery Books, 1986)

sub specie aeternitatis (adverb) (Latin) *Viewed under the aspects of the heavens; in its essential or universal form or nature.*

Political speculation is necessarily framed by the values that contemporary history composes. So that any distinction-making, however relevant **sub specie aeternitatis**, simply ought not to be attempted in addressing, for instance, six thousand policemen three weeks after the horrors of Selma, Alabama. (From *The Unmaking of a Mayor*, p. 26, The Viking Press, 1966)

succubus (noun) *An evil spirit, but the victim, or supine partner of, the aggressive incubus.*

Blackford thought back on the agonies of the Bruderschaft, and for a moment said, reverently, nothing by way of riposte. This quickly communicated a hint of resistance to her. He got back into his customary role, the **succubus** of her taunts. (From *Mongoose, R.I.P.*, p. 31, Random House, 1987)

sunder (verb) *To break or force apart, in two, or off from a whole; separate, usually by rending, cutting, or breaking, or by intervening time or space; sever.*

David Lindsay and Jim Buckley became fast friends at Yale, and of all the personal dislodgements of the campaign I am most grievously concerned over the possibility that it may have **sundered** that friendship. (From *The Unmaking of a Mayor*, p. 95, The Viking Press, 1966)

supererogatory (adjective) *Verbally redundant, superfluous.*

[On having been requested to send a seconding letter by the sponsor of Franklin Delano Roosevelt, Jr., to the New York Yacht Club] I would have thought that my own inclinations on the matter of his proposed membership would have been (a) **supererogatory**; or (b) ideologically suspect. (From *Cruising Speed*, p. 38, G. P. Putnam's Sons, 1971)

supernal (adjective) *Being or coming from above; that which emanates from heaven.*

On the main highway he stopped, sticking up his thumb with that **supernal** confidence of the young that he would not be kept waiting. (From *Saving the Queen*, p. 51, Doubleday & Company, 1976)

supine (adjective) *Lying, so to speak helplessly, on one's back; manifesting mental or moral lethargy; indifferent to one's duty or welfare or others' needs.*

No one not apathetic to the value issues of the day can in good conscience contribute to the ascendancy of ideas he considers destructive of the best in civilization. To do so is to be guilty of **supine** and unthinking fatalism of the sort that is the surest poison of democracy and the final abnegation of man's autonomy. (From *God and Man at Yale*, p. 196, Regnery Books, 1986)

surcease (noun) *Cessation; especially a temporary suspension, intermission, or respite.*

Having got the votes of men and women who, in this city, are unemployable, the politicians let them institutionalize themselves as social derelicts, at liberty to breed children who, suffering from inherited disadvantages, alternatively seek **surcease** in hyperstimulation and in indolence. (From *The Unmaking of a Mayor*, p. 38, The Viking Press, 1966)

synoptic (adjective) *Affording a general view of a whole, of what came before.*

In the creation of comic strips, there is the nagging mechanical—and therefore artistic—problem of reintroducing the reader to the **synoptic** point at which he was dropped the day before. (From *Right Reason,* p. 385, Doubleday & Company, 1985)

tacit (adjective) *Implied or indicated but not actually expressed.*

One must hope that the President's **tacit** approval of Dole's Bill was wrung from him in the middle of a coughing fit, during which Mr. Reagan could not collect his senses. (From *Right Reason,* p. 89, Doubleday & Company, 1985)

tangential (adjective) *Deviating widely and sometimes erratically; divergent; touching lightly or in the most tenuous way; incidental.*

Why did Wagner subtly underwrite the distorted newspaper accounts? The necessary answer, barring **tangential** motives of unscientific bearing, is—because to do so made good politics. (From *The Unmaking of a Mayor,* p. 21, The Viking Press, 1966)

tantamount (adjective) *Equivalent in value, significance, or effect.*

In most situations only penny-wise thinking and inherent dishonesty would lead to a prescription by the subsidizer as to the outcome of research. This would be **tantamount** to a cigarette company's granting money for research into cancer, with the stipulation that it shall not be discovered that tobacco is in any way conducive to the spread of the disease. (From *God and Man at Yale,* p. 190, Regnery Books, 1986)

tenet (noun) *A principle, dogma, belief, or doctrine generally held to be true; especially one held in common by members of an organization, group, movement, or profession.*

It seems unjust to employ pernicious techniques to undermine the **tenets** of Christianity. Most students are unaffected, but some, impressionable and malleable, lose faith in God. (From *God and Man at Yale,* p. 16, Regnery Books, 1986)

theocracy (noun) *Government of a state by theological doctrine.*

But the state (under the Shah) was not run as a **theocracy,** and one wonders therefore exactly what it is that the Ayatollah has in mind when he speaks of an Islamic republic. (From *Right Reason,* p. 72, Doubleday & Company, 1985)

tort-feasor (noun) *One who is guilty of a wrongful act; a wrongdoer; a trespasser.*

The relevant questions, after the shooting down of the Korean airliner, were: (1) How does one punish a punishable act? (Answer: By demanding reparations.) (2) How does one take reasonable steps to see to it that such an act is not committed again? (Answer: By getting assurances from the **tort-feasor.**) (From *Right Reason,* p. 102, Doubleday & Company, 1985)

traduce (verb) *To lower or disgrace the reputation of; expose to shame or blame by utterance of falsehood or misrepresentation.*

A hundred organizations would lash out against Yale. They would accuse her of **traducing** education, of violating freedom. (From *God and Man at Yale,* p. 226, Regnery Books, 1986)

troglodytic (adjective) *Relating to cave dwellers; dwelling in or involving residence in caves.*

His light suntan belied the **troglodytic** life spent plumbing the mysteries of spooks. (From *Saving the Queen,* p. 41, Doubleday & Company, 1976)

truncated (adjective) *Cut short.*

I try a **truncated** version of the talk I gave the night before, wondering whether I might just discover, in this new version, that it is better communicated short than long. (From *Cruising Speed,* p. 98, G. P. Putnam's Sons, 1971)

tumbril (noun) *A vehicle for carrying condemned persons (as, political prisoners during the French Revolution) to a place of execution.*

We're worried as hell over what Stalin is up to. A purge, maybe of classic proportions, is under way. The **tumbrils** are full and, as usual, full of his own past intimates. (From *Saving the Queen,* p. 122, Doubleday & Company, 1976)

tu quoque (adjective) *Referring to a retort charging an adversary with being or doing what he criticizes in others, as in: "So's your old man."*

At a meeting with the distinguished editors of a distinguished newspaper, the dark point was explicitly raised, and I knew there was no easy answer, save the old **tu quoque** argument. (From *The Unmaking of a Mayor,* p. 236, The Viking Press, 1966)

tutoyer (verb) *To address familiarly, from the French* tu *as distinguished from the more formal* vous.

I am, in public situations, disposed to formality. On *Firing Line,* even if I have **tutoyed** them for decades, I always refer to my guests as Mr., Mrs., or Miss So-and-So. (From *Cruising Speed,* p. 184, G. P. Putnam's Sons, 1971)

ultramontanist (noun) *One who favors greater supremacy of papal over national or diocesan authority in the Roman Catholic Church.*

Sister Elizabeth did not want Manhattanville to be referred to as a "Catholic college." Call Sister Elizabeth, I had asked Aggie Schmidt, an **ultramontanist** graduate of Manhattanville, and tell her we are going to have to discuss the question of Manhattanville's Catholicism on the program, because after all that's the kind of thing the program is about. (From *Cruising Speed,* p. 13, G. P. Putnam's Sons, 1971)

ululation (noun) *Howls or wails; cries of lamentation.*

The original idea [Kemp-Roth] was to reduce taxes evenhandedly. Since everyone knows that 10 percent of $100,000.00 is more than 10 percent of $10,000.00, the Reaganites should have been prepared for all that rhetoric about favoring the rich. But not having stressed the risks of excessive progressivity, they proved unready for it. Came then the big media **ululations** about the rich. (From *Right Reason,* p. 89, Doubleday & Company, 1985)

unctuous (adjective) *Revealing or marked by a smug, ingratiating, and false appearance or spirituality.*

I maintain that if you put every politician in New York who appears before you groveling and **unctuous** and prepared to turn the entire apparatus of New York and put it at your disposal on a silver tray—you will not substantially augment the happiness, the security, the sense of accomplishment of your own people. (From *The Unmaking of a Mayor,* p. 147, The Viking Press, 1966)

unmeeching (adjective) *Not cringing, sneaky, or whining in tone.*

Sometimes the politician will want to identify the demon, in which case the accusations are direct in reference and **unmeeching** in tone. (From *The Unmaking of a Mayor,* p. 21, The Viking Press, 1966)

untenable (adjective) *Unable to be defended or maintained.*

Opposition to the brand of collectivism espoused by Morgan or Tarshis or Samuelson is simply **untenable,** and what little recognition is given to that barely noticeable corps of economists who repudiate the collectivists' program is sometimes forthrightly savage. (From *God and Man at Yale,* p. 81, Regnery Books, 1986)

usurious (adjective) *Involving charging an unconscionable or exorbitant rate or amount of interest.*

A tricky diplomatic business, but the CAB recognized a responsibility to protect American consumers, and therefore acted favorably on a suit the effect of which could be to deny landing rights to foreign carriers that continued to extort from passengers the **usurious** rate. (From *Right Reason,* p. 46, Doubleday & Company, 1985)

vainglorious (adjective) *Marked by ostentation or excessive pride in one's achievements.*

To have mentioned in this book that I had been the co-chairman of an Inter-Faith Conference would have been irrelevant, perhaps even **vainglorious**. (From *God and Man at Yale*, p. xxiii, Regnery Books, 1986)

vapid (adjective) *Lacking flavor, zest, animation, or spirit.*

All the questions were the obvious ones, and it gave me a chance to formulate some of those **vapid** responses that are indispensable to the success of a constitutional monarch. (From *Saving the Queen*, p. 185, Doubleday & Company, 1976)

vestigial (adjective) *Remaining or surviving, however degenerate, atrophied, or imperfect.*

When the Poles declared martial law and a country of forty million people found itself without the **vestigial** liberties it had been exercising, there was an outcry. (From *Right Reason*, p. 97, Doubleday & Company, 1985)

viscous (adjective) *Having a ropy or glutinous consistency and the quality of sticking or adhering.*

I cannot think as the crow flies for very long, unless I am wrestling with somebody, or something, more **viscous** than my own runny thoughts. (From *Cruising Speed*, p. 183, G. P. Putnam's Sons, 1971)

vitiate (verb) *To impair the value or quality of.*

I asked Chiang Ching-kuo, the son of Chiang Kai-shek, whether there was any possibility that Taiwan might make an alliance with the Soviet Union at some point in the future, if necessary to substitute for **vitiating** Western support (President Carter had recently booted CCK's ambassador out of Washington, replacing him with China's). (From *On the Firing Line: The Public Life of Our Public Figures*, p. 334, Random House, 1989)

volatile (adjective) *Characterized by quick or unexpected changes; not steady or predictable.*

Pyotr Ivanovich was a **volatile** man who felt that genuine emotion cannot be communicated except by totalist vocal measures. (From *Saving the Queen*, p. 107, Doubleday & Company, 1976)

voluminous (adjective) *Filling or capable of filling a large volume or several volumes; profuse, exorbitant.*

We should face it that understanding the Russians isn't something we are ever likely to master. James Reston struggles valiantly in his column and says perhaps they shot down the Korean airliner because they were invaded by Napoleon. That's as good a guess as any. Even concentrated Soviet-watchers are surprised by the **voluminous** lies being told about the downing of KA flight 007. (From *Right Reason*, p. 99, Doubleday & Company, 1985)

votary (noun) *A sworn adherent; an ardent enthusiast; a devoted admirer; a disciple, fan.*

A senator might say, "We are going to do everything we can to help the Red Cross," by which he means he, his administrative assistants, his uncles and aunts, friends and **votaries** will jointly do what they all can for the Red Cross. (From *The Unmaking of a Mayor*, p. 85, The Viking Press, 1966)

vox populi (noun) *Popular sentiment.*

The Inquiring Photographer, a New York City institution which delivers the **vox populi** for the *New York Daily News*, asks questions of the people it interviews, the answers to which are often superficial or wrong-headed. (From *The Unmaking of a Mayor*, p. 238, The Viking Press, 1966)

warrant (verb) *To declare or maintain with little or no fear of being contradicted or belied; be certain; be sure that.*

"The collegers at Eton," said Mr. Alex-Hiller, "there on scholarships are selected from the poorer classes. This is not to say that there are brighter boys among the poor than among the rich."

"No, that doesn't say it, but I **warrant** it's true," said the queen. (From *Saving the Queen*, p. 168, Doubleday & Company, 1976)

Weltanschauungen (noun) *Philosophies of life; ideology; the plural form of* Weltanschauung. The answers to The Inquiring Photographer, in twenty-five words or less, are not intended to be taken as conclusive transcriptions of the interviewee's **Weltanschauungen.** (From *The Unmaking of a Mayor*, p. 238, The Viking Press, 1966)

whimsical (adjective) *Characterized by a capricious or eccentric idea.*

Smith's prison mates administered a thorough beating to the child-killer. Sure, Smith's companions thought the murder of a fifteen-year-old a repellent form of crime; but these nice discriminations, among men who mug and rape and kill, are **whimsical.** In their eyes, Edgar Smith's crime was that he had confessed guilt to a murder after maintaining his innocence for twenty years. (From *Right Reason*, p. 200, Doubleday & Company, 1985)

wreak (verb) *To bring about (harm); cause, inflict.*

Most of the analysts reasoned that here was a hard-planned, nationally subsidized, highly organized campaign to **wreak** vengeance on John Lindsay. (From *The Unmaking of a Mayor*, p. 100, The Viking Press, 1966)

LEXICON III—1993

abjure (verb) *To disclaim formally or disclaim upon oath.*

An insurrectionary movement dominated by men committed to Communist doctrine and methods who refused to **abjure** the use of force and terrorism to achieve their goals. (From "On the Right")

absolutized (verb) *Made absolute; converted to an absolute.*

Joyce's *Ulysses* was okayed by a federal court after a long struggle, and pretty soon so was *Lady Chatterley's Lover,* and since then, such a book as *American Psycho,* the First Amendment having been **absolutized** in its application. (From "On the Right")

accelerability (noun) *The capacity to speed up; potential for quickening.*

The **accelerability** of economic development by force of will (a premise of the Point Four Program) is an article of faith for leading liberal spokesmen. (From *Up from Liberalism*, p. 168, Stein & Day, 1984)

acumen (noun) *Acuteness of mind; keenness of perception; discernment or discrimination.*

I bet his students did, all right—if they called Mr. Root a fascist-by-association, they might well have earned a reward for showing high critical **acumen.** (From *Up from Liberalism*, p. 99, Stein & Day, 1984)

adamantine (adjective) *Unyielding, inflexible.*

He gave the relevant details of the life of Bertram Heath. He stressed the central role of Alistair Fleetwood as the formative influence in Bertram Heath's life. He underlined the **adamantine** refusal of Fleetwood to any interview concerning Bertram Heath. (From *High Jinx*, p. 153, Doubleday & Company, 1986)

adducing (verb) *Bringing forward (as an example, reason, proof) for consideration in a discussion, analysis, or contention; offering, presenting, citing. [Used in 1991 calendar in a different form, namely,* **adduce** *(v.)]*

How mischievous is the habit of **adducing** reasons behind everything that is done! I can unassailably delight in lobster and despise crabmeat so long as I refrain from giving reasons. (From *Rumbles Left and Right*, p. 33, G. P. Putnam's Sons, 1963)

ad rem (adjective) *Pertinent to the matter or person at issue; directed at the specific thing.*

Ad rem depersonalizations are necessary to social life, and are not any more inhumane intrinsically than the motions of the mother counting noses before deciding how much dinner to cook. (From *Rumbles Left and Right,* p. 132, G. P. Putnam's Sons, 1963)

adulator (noun) *One who praises effusively and slavishly, flatters excessively, fawns upon.*
Edward Bennett Williams introduced to the jury a man who happens to be a Communist Party-liner in international affairs and an **adulator** of Nikita Khrushchev. (From *Rumbles Left and Right,* p. 88, G. P. Putnam's Sons, 1963)

adumbrate (verb) *To foreshadow, symbolize, or prefigure in a not altogether conclusive or not immediately evident way; to give a sketchy representation of; to outline broadly, omitting details.*
What Richard Rovere resists so fiercely, for reasons he has not thought through, is the insinuation that what one might call the Liberal Establishment holds to a definable orthodoxy (his going on to **adumbrate** that orthodoxy was sheer brinksmanship). (From *Rumbles Left and Right,* p. 20, G. P. Putnam's Sons, 1963)

adventitious (adjective) *Coming from another source; added or appended extrinsically and not sharing original, essential, or intrinsic nature.*
You cannot accomplish the elimination of twenty-five million Xs by so simple an arrangement as multiplying by twenty-five million the **adventitious** elimination of a single X, effected in spontaneous circumstances. (From *Gratitude,* p. 80, Random House, 1990)

Aesopian (adjective) *Conveying an innocent meaning to an outsider but a concealed meaning to an informed member of a conspiracy or underground movement.*
A great deal depends on the question whether Saddam Hussein can think straight, because much of what has come from him, and goes out to him, is rendered in the **Aesopian** mode: stuff that says one thing but implies or seeks to imply another. (From "On the Right")

aggrandize (verb) *To make great or greater (as in power, honor, or wealth).*
We turned over to their Communist oppressors tens of millions not only by defaulting on our moral obligations and diminishing our identification with justice, but also by **aggrandizing** greatly the enemy's power. (From *Rumbles Left and Right,* p. 116, G. P. Putnam's Sons, 1963)

agnosticism (noun) *The doctrine that the existence or nature of any ultimate reality is unknown and probably unknowable or that any knowledge about matters of ultimate concern is impossible or improbable.*
The rhetorical impulses of the day are sluggish in the extreme; they place an immoderate emphasis on moderation, and promote a philosophical gentility, deriving from **agnosticism,** that permeates our moral intellectual life to its distinct disadvantage. (From *Up from Liberalism,* p. 55, Stein & Day, 1984)

allurement (noun) *Something that attracts or entices.*
A great arsenal of rights and perquisites and **allurements** and toys has been organized for the benefit of youth, and it has been questioned whether it does young people the good Americans wish for them to continue in the direction we have taken with respect to their growing years. (From *Gratitude,* p. 122, Random House, 1990)

ambient (adjective) *Surrounding on all sides; encompassing, enveloping.*
Here are some **ambient** data by which we gain perspective. It costs $35,000 per year to maintain a soldier in the army. It costs $30,000 per year to keep an inmate in jail. It costs $13,000 per year for each VISTA volunteer. It costs $20,000 per student for four years of ROTC. (From *Gratitude,* p. 128, Random House, 1990)

amenities (noun) *Social courtesies; pleasantries; civilities.*
They didn't exchange even routine goodbyes. The Director and his principal spymaster were not, really, friends. When there were **amenities** exchanged they tended to be formalistic. (From *High Jinx,* p. 34, Doubleday & Company, 1986)

amorphous (adjective) *(a) Without clearly drawn limits; not precisely indicated or established; (b) without definite nature or character; not allowing clear classification or analysis.*

The National Center for Policy Analysis, based in Dallas, has issued a report called "Tax Fairness: Myths and Reality" . . . which is as lucid and pointed as Goreism is convoluted and **amorphous**. (From "On the Right")

amulet (noun) *Charm often inscribed with a spell, magic incantation, or symbol and believed to protect the wearer against evil.*

The President should be given a line-item veto, sure, but those who think the budget deficit is as easy to solve as by giving the Chief Executive this **amulet** will have to think again. (From "On the Right")

anfractuous (adjective) *Full of twists and turns; winding; tortuous.*

Alistair Fleetwood had several reactions to what he had been told. Triumph, clearly: Unless he had drastically misunderstood the **anfractuous** message of Alice Goodyear Corbett, the Great God Beria had backed down and agreed to see him. (From *High Jinx*, p. 190, Doubleday & Company, 1986)

anthropomorphize (verb) *To attribute a human form or personality to forces or things greater than human.*

But it's also true that his was a critical as well as a symbolic (and telegenic) role, and that the American habit is to **anthropomorphize**—Napoleon, not his footsoldiers, is lionized. (From "On the Right")

antimacassar (noun) *A cover thrown over the backs or arms of chairs to protect them from Macassar hair oil or other soilage; thus, tidily, fussily old-fashioned.*

To the argument that in combat conditions it is a burden to provide two sets of washroom facilities, the pleaders for what they call women's rights argue to the effect that in combat situations, **antimacassar** niceties become simply irrelevant, and that, after all, even in the narrow confines of a foxhole, it is possible to make token adjustments. (From "On the Right")

antiquarian (adjective) *Of or belonging to the antiquities, the study of antiquities, or old times.*

The direction we must travel requires a broadmindedness that strikes us as **antiquarian** and callous. (From *Up from Liberalism*, p. 224, Stein & Day, 1984)

aphoristic (adjective) *Characterized by concise, artful, quotable statements or principles; terse and often ingenious formulations of truth or sentiment.*

As it happens, the camera in Hanover is zooming in on a disaffected young staffer, a Chinese-American who had twice been reprimanded by the staff of *The Dartmouth Review* for seeking to insert bawdy quotations into the page given over to reproducing **aphoristic** or amusing quotes. (From "On the Right")

apogee (noun) *The farthest or highest point.*

Clive Bell observed that the grandeur and nobility of the Allied cause [during World War I] "swelled in ever vaster proportions every time it was restated"—reaching its **apogee** in our explicitly formulated determination to make the world safe for democracy. (From *Up from Liberalism*, p. 148, Stein & Day, 1984)

arrogation (noun) *To claim or seize without right; appropriate to oneself arrogantly; ascribe or attribute without reason.*

In the long view of it, conservatives have tended to be suspicious of the **arrogation** of power by the Executive. (From "On the Right")

arterial (adjective) *Of or designating a route of transportation carrying a main flow with many branches.*

The street outside was a heavily used **arterial** road running into London. (From *High Jinx*, p. 50, Doubleday & Company, 1986)

artifact (noun) *A usually simple object showing human workmanship or modification, as distinguished from a natural object.*

It is encouraging when Professor Galbraith is struck rather by his craftsmanship than by the **artifact.** Michelangelo would have been entitled to admire anything he had sculpted, even gallows. (From *Up from Liberalism,* p. xi, Stein & Day, 1984)

asperity (noun) *Roughness of manner or temper.*

Brother Hildred asked "Leo" if he would like to visit the school's physics laboratory that afternoon. Tucker replied that he would not like to visit it this afternoon, tomorrow, next month, or next year. But quickly he recoiled from his apparent **asperity,** and simply said he did not wish to revisit any aspect of his past professional life. (From *Tucker's Last Stand,* p. 31, Random House, 1990)

atavistic (adjective) *The reappearance, after a considerable interval, of an organism or cultural habit. [Used in 1991 calendar in a different form, namely,* **atavist** *(noun)]*

When it becomes self-evident that biological, intellectual, cultural, and psychic similarities among races render social separation capricious and **atavistic,** then the myths will begin to fade, as they have done in respect of the Irish, the Italians, the Jews. (From *Rumbles Left and Right,* p. 96, G. P. Putnam's Sons, 1963)

athwart (preposition) *Across; from one side to another; against; in opposition to.*

Sometimes one is tempted to take a bucketful of that clayey mud resembling creamy peanut butter and drip it over the heads of the Luddite lobby that stands **athwart** progress yelling Stop! (From "On the Right")

atomistic (adjective) *An object or concept viewed as particles of the whole.*

I do not believe it is undignified to confess to having been critically influenced by a teacher, or a faculty, or a book; but the accent these days is so strong on **atomistic** intellectual independence that to suggest such a thing is highly inflammatory. (From *Up from Liberalism,* Stein & Day, 1984, p. 96.)

aught (noun) *One iota, zero, cipher.*

One irrepressible senior, who did not care **aught** for ideology, but was bent on cashing in on those political impulses, announced that after graduation he would launch a firm to take over the foreign policy of sovereign states. (From *Up from Liberalism,* p. 138, Stein & Day, 1984)

augur (verb) *To predict or foretell, especially from signs or omens.*

Every delegate found a copy of that letter under his door the next morning; this generated wild rumors, huge resentments, a divided convention, a divided Republican Party, and **augured** a defeat in November. (From *Tucker's Last Stand,* p. 126, Random House, 1990)

becket (noun) *A simple device for holding something in place, as a small grommet or a loop of rope with a knot at one end to catch in an eye at the other.*

Racing to Bermuda in 1956, we would wear out a helmsman every half hour, even with the aid of a **becket** made out of several strands of shock cord. (From *Rumbles Left and Right,* p. 174, G. P. Putnam's Sons, 1963)

belletrism (noun) *An interest in belles lettres to the neglect of more practical or informative literature; literary aestheticism. [Used in 1992 calendar in a different form, namely,* **belletristic** *(adjective)]*

Though Chambers was a passionately literary man, always the intellectual, insatiably and relentlessly curious, in the last analysis it was action, not **belletrism,** that moved him most deeply. (From *Rumbles Left and Right,* p. 148, G. P. Putnam's Sons, 1963)

beneficence (noun) *Active goodness or kindness. [Used in 1991 calendar in a different form, namely,* **beneficently** *(adverb)]*

It is prudent to take reasonable precautions against the abuse of a **beneficence;** but it is not correct to evaluate a beneficence on its abuse-potential. (From *Up from Liberalism*, p. 203, Stein & Day, 1984)

bereft (adjective) *Deprived, especially by death; stripped; dispossessed.*

Miss Sayers contends that the faculty for logical thought is a skill of which the entire contemporary generation has been **bereft;** I note, but do not press the point. (From *Up from Liberalism*, p. 37, Stein & Day, 1984)

billingsgate (noun) *Foul, vulgar, abusive talk (named after a fish market in London where such talk was routine).*

The student was drunk, it was way past midnight, he had descended into the campus yard and there began a racist **billingsgate** at the expense of blacks, Jews, and Catholics. (From "On the Right")

blighted (adjective) *Withered or destroyed; disappointed or frustrated.*

That and the obdurate superstition, more widespread than anything since the number thirteen was **blighted** as unlucky, that the rich are not paying their share of taxes. (From "On the Right")

bugbear (noun) *An object of irritation or source of dread or abhorrence; especially a continuing source of annoyance.*

[William Safire's] **bugbear** is the statement made last week jointly by Secretary of State James Baker and Soviet Foreign Minister Alexander Bessmertnykh, "The ministers continue to believe that a cessation of hostilities would be possible if Iraq would make an unequivocal commitment to withdraw from Kuwait." (From "On the Right")

buncombe (noun) *Talk that is empty, insincere, or merely for effect; humbug.*

Arafat's approach to a fresh plan in the Mideast was scorned by the government of Israel as so much diplomatic **buncombe.** (From "On the Right")

burin (noun) *An engraver's tool having a tempered steel shaft ground obliquely to a sharp point at one end and inserted into a handle at the other.*

Not so much in the service itself, then, as in the recall of service, engraved and re-engraved gently but insistently by a dozen **burins,** decade after decade, will the idea of rendering service become lodged in the moral memory. (From *Gratitude,* p. 154, Random House, 1990)

cadre (noun) *A nucleus or core group, especially of trained personnel or active members of an organization who are capable of assuming leadership or of training and indoctrinating others.*

Arafat, who looks like a gangster, often acted as one, and surrounded himself with a terrorist-minded **cadre** pleading the excuse that the Israelis deploy terrorists who need to be coped with. (From "On the Right")

caeteris paribus (adverbial phrase) (Latin) *"If all other relevant things remain unaltered."*

Life for the average citizen, *caeteris paribus,* is about the same, except that in Venezuela any dissenting political activity was forbidden, whereas in Mexico only meaningful political activity is forbidden. (From *Up from Liberalism,* p. 151, Stein & Day, 1984)

calumny (noun) *False charge or misrepresentation intended to blacken one's reputation; slander.*

The **calumny** Mr. Harriman attempted to pin on Mr. Rockefeller was that he would permit the Transit Authority to do the only thing the Transit Authority is permitted by law to do, namely, raise the fares. (From *Up from Liberalism,* p. 162, Stein & Day, 1984)

canard (noun) *A false or unfounded report or story; a groundless rumor or belief.*

There exists an obdurate superstition that the rich are not paying their share of taxes. This **canard** is spread by the Congressional Budget Office, which is a propaganda arm of the Democratic Party that ought to be indicted by the Food and Drug Administration for feeding the general population dangerous stimulants. (From "On the Right")

canon (noun) *A basic general principle or rule commonly accepted as true, valid, and fundamental.*

The **canon** of academic freedom is very clear: no one idea is to find corporate favor in educational institutions over another. (From *Up from Liberalism*, p. 93, Stein & Day, 1984)

capricious (adjective) *Given to changes of interest or attitude according to whims or passing fancies; not guided by steady judgment, intent, or purpose.*

What can be proved between competing crews on different boats? Not very much. There is a feature of ocean racing that can make a shambles of the whole thing. The poorest judgment can, under **capricious** circumstances, pay the handsomest rewards. (From *Rumbles Left and Right*, p. 171, G. P. Putnam's Sons, 1963)

carapace (noun) *A protective covering similar to a hard bony or chitinous outer covering such as the fused dorsal plates of a turtle.*

They sat around a table in a soundproofed, bug-proof room situated within a **carapace** especially designed to frustrate any efforts at electronic intrusion. (From *High Jinx*, p. 152, Doubleday & Company, 1986)

cartelization (noun) *The organization of an industry or commodity in one or more countries so as to dominate commerce.*

The refusal of the principal European nations to defy their farm blocs has suggested the possible **cartelization** of the European economy in the next year or two. (From "On the Right")

Carthaginian (adjective) *Totalist, as in the Roman destruction of Carthage in 146 B.C.*

And one has therefore to pause before proceeding to hold every Iraqi responsible for the crimes of Saddam Hussein and those front-line sadists who disgraced the irreducible maxims of human decency. To consign them all to perpetual poverty is **Carthaginian** in moral architecture, and we must desist from doing this. (From "On the Right")

Carthusian (adjective) *Austerely self-disciplined, self-denying; relating to the Carthusians, members of an austere religious order founded by St. Bruno in 1084.*

Since anyone who chooses to do anything other than become a **Carthusian** monk is almost certain to pay taxes, the prospect of relief from ten thousand dollars in taxes is both real and appropriate. (From *Gratitude*, p. 142, Random House, 1990)

catechetical (adjective) *Relying on questions and answers to inculcate orthodoxy.*

A sane man might seek to designate whatever figurative edifice shelters the household gods of American Liberalism, its high priests, its incense makers, and its **catechetical** press. (From *Rumbles Left and Right*, p. 21, G. P. Putnam's Sons, 1963)

caterwauling (verb) *Complaining loudly; screeching. [Used in 1991 calendar in a different form, namely, *caterwaul* (verb)]*

It is a story that has to do with all the **caterwauling** about nuclear waste and what to do with it. (From "On the Right")

cede (verb) *To give up, give over, grant, or concede, typically by treaty or negotiated pact.*

It is very dangerous to **cede** to a society the right to declare what are and what are not the freedoms worth exercising. (From *Up from Liberalism*, p. 210, Stein & Day, 1984)

centripetal (adjective) *Moving, proceeding, or acting in a direction toward a center or axis. [Used in 1992 calendar in a different form, namely, *centripetalization* (noun)]*

When stopped and everyone turns his eyes on me, I experience that mortification I always feel when I am the center of **centripetal** shafts of curiosity, resentment, perplexity. (From *Rumbles Left and Right*, p. 190, G. P. Putnam's Sons, 1963)

chattel (noun) *Movable item of personal property, such as a piece of furniture, an automobile, a head of livestock.*

It was for this reason, said Mr. Thomas, that he could speak so eloquently on the subject of the Dred Scott decision, which reduced human beings—Negroes—to **chattels.** (From "On the Right")

circumlocution (noun) *Indirect or roundabout expression. [Used in 1992 calendar in a different form, namely, circumlocutory (adjective)]*

She wanted to know what I was up to, and I told her about Vietnam, with the usual **circumlocutions.** (From *Tucker's Last Stand,* p. 88, Random House, 1990)

climacteric (adjective) *A decisive or critical period or stage in any course, career, or developmental process.*

The steel companies irked Murray Kempton by putting on a statistical passion play whose **climacteric** shows that if next summer the steel unions should go after and get higher wages, the American companies will no longer be able to compete with foreign steel companies. (From *Rumbles Left and Right,* p. 132, G. P. Putnam's Sons, 1963)

concert (verb) *To play or arrange by mutual agreement; to contrive or devise.*

I expect you will share your information with your superior. And if it becomes necessary, of course, the Prime Minister and the President will need to **concert** the postponements. (From *High Jinx,* p. 205, Doubleday & Company, 1986)

conduce (verb) *To lead or tend, especially with reference to a desirable result.*

I sense intuitively that while friendship does not necessarily grow out of experience shared, experience shared **conduces** to a bond from which friendship can grow. (From *Gratitude,* p. 161, Random House, 1990)

conflate (verb) *To bring together; collect, merge, fuse.*

Now, nobody is going to be able definitely to establish what happens for every million dollars a state spends on a national service program. Too many questions have to be **conflated** to permit a responsible prediction. (From *Gratitude,* p. 129, Random House, 1990)

confute (verb) *To overwhelm by argument. [Used in 1992 calendar in a different form, namely, confutation (noun)]*

Listening to Marshal Zhukov elaborate the virtues of communism, President Eisenhower found himself "very hard put to it" to **confute** him. (From *Up from Liberalism,* p. 192, Stein & Day, 1984)

contemporaneity (noun) *The quality or state of existing or occurring during the same time.*

They suffer, for one thing, from **contemporaneity.** What was allegedly done by the Democratic team is extremely current, whereas the Republicans came up with events some of which were three to eleven years old. (From "On the Right")

contraband (noun) *Goods or merchandise the importation, exportation, or sometimes possession of which is forbidden; also, smuggled goods.*

The trouble is, the Viets know that however much of the **contraband** they succeed in stopping at sea, the stuff is getting through. (From *Tucker's Last Stand,* p. 169, Random House, 1990)

convention (noun) *General agreement on or acceptance of certain practices or attitudes.*

Alice Goodyear Corbett (the **convention** had always been to use her full name, dating back to when, at age five, asked by a visiting Russian what her name was, she had answered, "*Moye imya* Alice Goodyear Corbett") had attended schools in Moscow from kindergarten. . . . (From *High Jinx,* p. 66, Doubleday & Company, 1986)

cooptation (noun) *Election or selection, usually to a body or group by vote of its own members.*

The **cooptation** of the unions by the bureaucracy forwarded fascism of various kinds, including the militant and ideological fascism of Mussolini's Italy in which the state became precisely that object so correctly feared: the central unit of undifferentiated loyalty. (From *Gratitude,* p. 57, Random House, 1990)

cornucopia (noun) *An inexhaustible supply, variety.*
"*Petit déjeuner, simple,*" she smiled at him, expressing admiration over the **cornucopia** he had ordered and was proceeding, with such wholesome pleasure, to devour. (From *Tucker's Last Stand,* p. 179, Random House, 1990)

cosmopolitanism (noun) *An excessive admiration and imitation of the cultural traits or achievement of others at the expense of the cultural identity or integrity of one's own land or region.*
Olga turned her head to one side and began to cry. She confessed that her parents had become afraid of having foreigners coming to their home, Comrade Stalin having pronounced recently on the dangers of **cosmopolitanism.** (From *High Jinx,* p. 67, Doubleday & Company, 1986)

Couéism (noun) *A system of psychotherapy based on optimistic autosuggestion; the founder is best remembered for his adage "Every day, and in every way, I am becoming better and better."*
The wreckage of two world wars fought for democracy is made up of the collapsed surrealisms of the ideologues, who succeeded finally in pushing **Couéism** right over the cliff. (From *Up from Liberalism,* p. 160, Stein & Day, 1984)

cryptographer (noun) *One adept in the art or process of writing in or deciphering secret code.*
Blackford Oakes reappeared at James Street early in the afternoon, and said to Trust that he would like to consult with an Agency **cryptographer.** (From *High Jinx,* p. 39, Doubleday & Company, 1986)

curio (noun) *Something arousing interest as being novel, rare, or bizarre.*
Why reissue the book? I think the reason for doing so is that it is a historical **curio,** and historical curios are often worth looking at, especially if they are unfamiliar to you. (From *Up from Liberalism,* p. xiii, Stein & Day, 1984)

declamation (noun) *A rhetorical speech; harangue.*
He is fiercely loyal to his family, while firm in insisting that he will not leave his fortune to the second generation as he doesn't believe in inherited wealth. That **declamation** drew a discreet wink from his devoted wife of forty-six years. (From "On the Right")

decrepitude (noun) *A state of ruin, dilapidation, or disrepair; lack of power; decay.*
If indeed the nation is united behind Mr. Eisenhower in this invitation to Mr. Khrushchev, then the nation is united behind an act of diplomatic sentimentality which can only confirm Khrushchev in the contempt he feels for the dissipated morale of a nation far gone, as the theorists of Marxism have all along contended, in **decrepitude.** (From *Rumbles Left and Right,* p. 35, G. P. Putnam's Sons, 1963)

démarche (noun) *A course of action; maneuver; a diplomatic representation or protest.*
He could not now report that his diplomatic initiative had worked in such a way as to give the Soviet Union the opportunity to use its great resources to stall the German **démarche** planned by the Western powers. (From *High Jinx,* p. 213, Doubleday & Company, 1986)

denature (verb) *To change the nature of; take natural qualities away from.*
What the Pope does say with such heartening fidelity is that socialism is an extravagant historical failure and—more—that socialism has a way of **denaturing** human beings by giving power to a central government which tends to use that power to suppress the individual and to come up with false gods for him to worship, like nationalized railroads (the example is mine, not His Holiness's). (From "On the Right")

denominate (verb) *To give a name to; call by a name; designate.*
"The Cold War is a part of the human condition for so long as you have two social phenomena which we can pretty safely **denominate** as constants." (From *Tucker's Last Stand,* p. 79, Random House, 1990)

deprecate (verb) *To disapprove of, often with mildness.*
It is a part of the Japanese tradition to exhibit great modesty, to disparage one's accomplishments, to **deprecate**, even, one's most sacred opinions. (From *Up from Liberalism*, p. 118, Stein & Day, 1984)

depreciate (verb) *To make to seem less valuable or important; to diminish in value.*
Sir Alistair said to Queen Caroline, "Ma'am, I cannot believe that you **depreciate** natural curiosity, even if you don't exhibit it." (From *High Jinx*, p. 61, Doubleday & Company, 1986)

deracinate (verb) *To separate from one's environment. [Used in 1991 calendar in a different form, namely,* **deracination** *(noun)]*
Randall Jarrell was saying Serious Things. He was describing a morally and intellectually **deracinated** environment in which students are encouraged to cut their ties to the world of standards and norms. (From *Up from Liberalism*, p. 124, Stein & Day, 1984)

desiccate (verb) *To drain of vitality, especially to divest of vigor, spirit, passion, or a capability of evoking mental or emotional excitement.*
I have suggested that the principal difficulties of the beginning ocean sailor are (1) the mystifying lack of expertise in much of what goes into ocean sailing; and (2) the tendency in some experts to **desiccate** the entire experience by stripping it of spontaneity, or wonder. (From *Rumbles Left and Right*, p. 173, G. P. Putnam's Sons, 1963)

determinism (noun) *The doctrine that all acts of the will result from causes which determine them in such a manner that man has no alternative modes of action.*
One needs to remind oneself that under Marxism-Leninism it is the people who are supposed to be the vehicle of historical **determinism.** It fits nowhere in Soviet doctrine for the people to assert themselves in favor of reforms which the Kremlin opposes. (From "On the Right")

detritus (noun) *Products of disintegration or wearing away; fragments or fragmentary materials.*
The experience would touch the young, temperamentally impatient with any thought of the other end of the life cycle, with the reality of old age; with the human side of the **detritus** whose ecological counterparts have almost exclusively occupied fashionable attention in recent years. (From *Gratitude*, p. 110, Random House, 1990)

detumesce (verb) *To subside from a state of swelling; to diminish in size. [Used in 1992 calendar in a different form, namely,* **detumescence** *(noun)]*
Brother Leo in his monastic cell consulted the diary he kept of his activities, and counted nine visits to the Alargo mansion to see Josefina Delafuente. He went to the chapel, and on his knees prayed most earnestly. He tried to distract himself, but the daemon would not **detumesce.** (From *Tucker's Last Stand*, p. 34, Random House, 1990)

deviationist (adjective) *Depart from the principles of an organization (as a political party) with which one is affiliated.*
One can say, "disciples of Communism, en bloc, follow the Moscow line." That is a responsible generalization, unaffected by the fact of schismatic flare-ups or **deviationist** sallies. (From *Up from Liberalism*, p. 38, Stein & Day, 1984)

devolution (noun) *Passing down from stage to stage; the passing of property, rights, authority, etc., from one person to another. [Used in 1992 calendar in a different form, namely,* **devolve** *(verb)]*
It is jarring to recall that as recently as during this century, Wales and even Scotland were discussing the kind of "**devolution**" that would have meant, in effect, self-rule. (From "On the Right")

dialectic (noun) *Any systematic reasoning, exposition, or argument that juxtaposes opposed or contradictory ideas and usually seeks to resolve their conflict; play of ideas; cunning or hair-splitting disputation.*

During those months, a fascinating **dialectic** went on. Herbert Matthews would write that American prestige was sinking in Cuba—on account of the aid the U.S. Government was giving to Batista. Our Ambassador in Havana meanwhile complained to the State Department of the demoralization of the Batista government—on account of our failure to provide aid. (From *Rumbles Left and Right*, p. 49, G. P. Putnam's Sons, 1963)

diaphanous (adjective) *Of such fine texture as to be transparent or translucent.*

Three hours later they were in the suite Hilda shared with Minerva: two bedrooms, the living room between them dimly lit by lamps covered in only barely **diaphanous** pink. (From *High Jinx*, p. 102, Doubleday & Company, 1986)

diminution (noun) *Diminishing; lessening; decrease.*

Ask then, would we be better off chucking the opposition to federalized medicine? If we did this, there would be, assuming the validity of the findings above, an instant **diminution** in costs. (From "On the Right")

discursive (adjective) *Wandering from one topic to another; rambling; desultory; digressive.*

[He is] a very old friend about whom I wrote in a **discursive** book that I think of him as the most wholesome young man I have ever known. (From "On the Right")

disestablishmentarian (noun) *An advocate of disestablishing or altering the existent state or national institution.*

The English Establishment rests on deeply embedded institutional commitments against which the Socialists, the angry young men, the **disestablishmentarians,** have railed and howled and wept altogether in vain. (From *Rumbles Left and Right*, p. 16, G. P. Putnam's Sons, 1963)

disfranchisement (noun) *The deprivation of a statutory or constitutional right, especially of the right to vote.*

To deprive him of his vote it becomes necessary to deprive others like him of their vote, hence what amounts to the virtual **disfranchisement** of the race in Southern communities that fear rule by a Negro majority. (From *Up from Liberalism*, p. 156, Stein & Day, 1984)

dislocative (adjective) *Causing confusion; causing to deviate from a normal or predicted course, situation, or relationship.*

Many people shrink from arguments over facts because facts are tedious, because they require a formal familiarity with the subject under discussion, and because they can be ideologically **dislocative.** (From *Up from Liberalism*, p. 61, Stein & Day, 1984)

dispossess (verb) *To remove from someone the possession especially of property or land; put out of occupancy; eject, oust.*

What we deplore is what Saddam Hussein went on to do. Where is the Democrat who was urging all along that we consummate Desert Storm by marching into Baghdad and **dispossessing** Saddam? (From "On the Right")

disquisition (noun) *A formal or systematic inquiry into or discussion of a subject; an elaborate analytical or explanatory essay or discussion.*

Bui Tin began one of his rambling, historical **disquisitions** on the history and culture of the region. (From *Tucker's Last Stand*, p. 239, Random House, 1990)

dissolute (noun) *A person lacking in moral restraint.*

One of the two technicians added that Heath seemed very bored with the work at hand, that he tended to arrive late for work in the morning, and that he had acquired a reputation for being something of a **dissolute,** patronizing the local bars, often with a girl. (From *High Jinx*, p. 117, Doubleday & Company, 1986)

dissonant (adjective) *Marked by a lack of agreement; incongruous, dissident, discrepant.*

Why has the same nation that implicitly endorsed the social boycott of Soviet leaders changed its mind so abruptly—to harmonize with so **dissonant** a change in position by our lackadaisical President? (From *Rumbles Left and Right,* p. 36, G. P. Putnam's Sons, 1963)

doyen (noun) *The senior male member of a body or group; one specifically or tacitly allowed to speak for the body or group.*

So well known is Herbert Matthews as **doyen** of utopian activists that when in June of 1959 a Nicaraguan rebel launched a revolt, he wired the news of it direct to Mr. Matthews at the *New York Times*—much as, a few years ago, a debutante-on-the-make might have wired the news of her engagement to Walter Winchell. (From *Rumbles Left and Right,* p. 51, G. P. Putnam's Sons, 1963)

dramaturgical (adjective) *Pertaining to the art of writing plays or producing them.*

It is somewhere recorded that, reciting a speech written for him by one of his entourage, which speech he had not even read over before delivering it, [Huey Long] reached a line in which he thought the trace of a tear theatrically appropriate, engineered that tear without any difficulty, and later on casually commented on his proficiency in these **dramaturgical** matters. (From "On the Right")

edify (verb) *To instruct and improve, especially in moral and religious knowledge; enlighten, elevate, uplift.*

Transform the Peace Corps into a body of evangelists for freedom, young men and women highly trained in the ways of Communist psychological warfare who could in behalf of freedom, analyze, argue, explain, and **edify**. (From *Rumbles Left and Right,* p. 116, G. P. Putnam's Sons, 1963)

effete (adjective) *Soft or decadent as a result of overrefinement of living conditions or laxity of mental or moral discipline.*

Etiquette is the first value only of the society that has no values, the **effete** society. An occasional disregard for the niceties may bring us face to face with certain facts from which man labors to shield himself. (From *Up from Liberalism,* p. 129, Stein & Day, 1984)

effulgence (noun) *Strong, radiant light; glorious splendor.*

Kenneth Tynan is not a reasoner and his story about appearing before the Senate Internal Security Subcommittee goes on with its poetic **effulgence**. (From *Rumbles Left and Right,* p. 73, G. P. Putnam's Sons, 1963)

effusion (noun) *Unrestrained expression of feelings; something that is poured out with little or no restraint, used especially of self-expression.*

Kenneth Tynan is a young man of letters well enough known among the literati in England because of his precocious **effusions** against the established order. (From *Rumbles Left and Right,* p. 69, G. P. Putnam's Sons, 1963)

élan (noun) (French: "spirit") *Enthusiastic vigor and liveliness.*

The aide pondered the communication, its rather special **élan,** and made the decision to put the whole dossier into the Director's In box. (From *High Jinx,* p. 177, Doubleday & Company, 1986)

elegy (noun) *A poem or song of lament for the dead.*

Milton wrote an **elegy** to a young man dead, and Bach wrote music searingly beautiful, his own tribute to a departed brother. One must suppose that Milton wept over his poetry, and Bach over his music. (From "On the Right")

emanation (noun) *A flowing forth; a quality or property issuing from a source.*

Although Harriet Pilpel was as sharp in debate as any Oxford Union killer, she managed a benevolent **emanation** that, I like to think, after twenty years of carpet-bombing exchanges with her, genuinely reflected her character. (From "On the Right")

emendation (noun) *The word or the matter substituted for incorrect or unsuitable matter.*

The new conservatives, many of whom go by the name of Modern Republicans, have not been very helpful. Their sin consists in permitting so many accretions, modifications, **emendations,** maculations, and qualifications that the original thing quite recedes from view. (From *Up from Liberalism,* p. 189, Stein & Day, 1984)

emplace (verb) *To put into position.*

The Israelis **emplaced** their nuclear-capable Jericho-2 missiles in hardened silos and in September 1988 mounted their first satellite launch. (From "On the Right")

encysted (adjective) *Enclosed in a cyst, capsule, or sac.*

Do we need to describe how bad the scene is in Detroit? It is the **encysted** home of unemployment and unrest, on account of unemployment plus the racial tensions that are engendered in communities in which whites and blacks vie for desperately needed jobs. (From "On the Right")

endemic (adjective) *Widespread; taking hold throughout a community or society.*

A great, indeed a massive, change was under way in America in the late fifties, the beginning of an **endemic** disenchantment with American liberalism. (From *Up from Liberalism,* p. xiii, Stein & Day, 1984)

engender (verb) *To bring into existence; give rise to.*

They spent a relaxed hour talking about this and that, with that odd sense of total relaxation **engendered** by the knowledge of great tension directly ahead. (From *High Jinx,* p. 13, Doubleday & Company, 1986)

ennobling (adjective) *Tending to elevate in degree or excellence.*

Whatever byways, on the road to this final Third Act, George Bush may have missed, this is the time to adjourn any complaints about them and to concentrate on an **ennobling** performance. (From "On the Right")

epicurean (adjective) *Suited to a person with refined taste, especially in food and wine.*

Blackford laughed. "This dinner is **epicurean** by comparison with what you poor English boys have to eat at your fashionable schools, and how do I know that? You guessed it, I was indentured in one." (From *High Jinx,* p. 14, Doubleday & Company, 1986)

epistemology (noun) *The study of the method and grounds of knowledge, especially with reference to its limits and validity. [Used in 1991 calendar in a different form, namely, epistemological (adjective)]*

In an age of relativism one tends to look for flexible devices for measuring this morning's truth. Such a device is democracy; and indeed, democracy becomes **epistemology:** democracy will render reliable political truths just as surely as the marketplace sets negotiable economic values. (From *Up from Liberalism,* p. 149, Stein & Day, 1984)

equanimity (noun) *Evenness of mental disposition; emotional balance, especially under stress.*

Those of us who do not go year after year wondering whether tomorrow will bring yet another war threatening our survival will perhaps find it difficult to understand the relative **equanimity** of the Israeli people. (From "On the Right")

errantry (noun) *A roving in quest of knightly adventure.*

The liberals' mania is their ideology. Deal lightly with any precept of knight-**errantry,** and you might find, as so many innocent Spaniards did, the Terror of La Mancha hurtling toward you. (From *Up from Liberalism,* p. 38, Stein & Day, 1984)

eschatologically (adverb) *Dealing with the ultimate destiny of mankind and the world. [Used in 1991 calendar in a different form, namely, eschatological (adjective)]*

The Communists' program is capable (at least for a period of time, until the illusion wears off) of being wholly satisfactory, emotionally and intellectually, to large numbers of people. The reason for this is that Communist dogma is **eschatologically** conceived. (From *Up from Liberalism,* p. 145, Stein & Day, 1984)

esoterica (noun) *Items intended for or understood by only a few.*
Fleetwood had been designated to give the first toast. After that, he turned his **esoterica** into a single metaphor that suggested the preeminent concern all civilized persons must have for peace. (From *High Jinx*, p. 123, Doubleday & Company, 1986)

essay (verb) *To make an attempt at.*
The operator evidently knew only a single word of English, which sounded like, "Outzide, outzide." He **essayed** first French and then German, to no better end, and then the cinders of his Russian. (From *High Jinx*, p. 170, Doubleday & Company, 1986)

establishmentarian (adjective) *Allied to the dominant institutional forces.*
The most hotly contested primary of the postwar season was that of New Hampshire, when in 1964 the grass roots forces of challenger Barry Goldwater did a pitched battle with the **establishmentarian** forces of Nelson Rockefeller. (From "On the Right")

ethnocentrism (noun) *The belief that one's own ethnic group, nation, or culture is superior to all others.*
I had in mind journalism and the academy, though perhaps most conspicuous at the time I wrote (1965) was the entrenched **ethnocentrism** of certain unions, in which a job is something you deed to your son or son-in-law, if he is faithful. (From "On the Right")

euphonious (adjective) *Pleasing in sound.*
The forces of fascism were not quite ready to give up, but that would come. Meanwhile, if he had to serve as a lord—Lord Fleetwood? Rather **euphonious**—why, he would simply have to do so. (From *High Jinx*, p. 236, Doubleday & Company, 1986)

Eurocentric (adjective) *The disposition to regard Europe as the central historical, intellectual, and cultural concern for American students.*
Ten lashes is about what some of us had in mind as appropriate for those in Stanford who succeeded in abolishing the theretofore compulsory courses in Western culture, deemed too "**Eurocentric**." It has yielded to a required course called Cultures, Ideas, and Values. (From "On the Right")

evanescent (adjective) *Tending to vanish or pass away like vapor. [Used in 1991 calendar in a different form, namely, evanesce (verb)]*
I and the *Panic* have a way of provoking the unreasoned and impulsive resentment of sailors whose view of ocean racing tends to be a little different from my own. That resentment is wholly spontaneous and, I like to feel, **evanescent.** (From *Rumbles Left and Right*, p. 172, G. P. Putnam's Sons, 1963)

eventuate (verb) *To come out finally or in conclusion; come to pass.*
His fluent French and schoolboy knowledge of English and Japanese suggested a clerical career, which never **eventuated** because a few months after his seventeenth birthday the Japanese surrendered. (From *Tucker's Last Stand*, p. 40, Random House, 1990)

execrable (adjective) *Deserving to be declared evil or detestable.*
Crew A, out of an egregious ignorance and showing **execrable** judgment, elects to go around Block Island north to south. (From *Rumbles Left and Right*, p. 171, G. P. Putnam's Sons, 1963)

exegetical (adjective) *Critical explanation or analysis. [Used in 1992 calendar in a different form, namely, exegete (noun)]*
"I understand Bolshevik theory and do not need your **exegetical** help in this matter." (From *High Jinx*, p. 174, Doubleday & Company, 1986)

exhibitionistic (adjective) *Behaving so as to attract attention to oneself; extravagant or willfully conspicuous behavior.*

In the Gulf, notwithstanding the **exhibitionistic** can-can by Gorbachev during the final hours, it was never conceivable that a nuclear power would stand in the way of our military strategy. (From "On the Right")

exogamous (adjective) *Of or relating to or characterized by marriage outside a specific group, especially as required by custom or law.*

I am allergic to **exogamous** comparative dollar figures, so widely used in workaday polemical chitchat, such as, "For the cost of landing a man on the moon, we might have built one million one hundred and thirty-seven thousand and eight low-middle class dwelling units." (From *Gratitude,* p. 134, Random House, 1990)

expertise (noun) *An operative body of knowledge.*

For those on the radical Left and for so many on the moderate Left, the true meaning of our time is the loss of an operative set of values—what one might call an **expertise** in living. (From *Rumbles Left and Right,* p. 63, G. P. Putnam's Sons, 1963)

expostulation (noun) *Strong demand; remonstrance. [Used in 1991 calendar in a different form, namely, expostulate (verb)]*

With no further attention paid to his **expostulations,** his arms were strapped to his sides with the stretcher's harness and he was lifted into the ambulance and deposited alongside the cab driver. (From *High Jinx,* p. 246, Doubleday & Company, 1986)

extortionate (adjective) *Characterized by, or having the nature of, extortion; excessive; exorbitant.*

This requires negotiating with the Saudis to peg the oil price at a reasonable level for, say, twenty years. Without the cooperation of the Saudis, OPEC can never reassemble its **extortionate** cartel. (From "On the Right")

extravasate (verb) *To force out (as blood) or cause to escape from a proper vessel or channel (blood vessel).*

Can the revolutionary essence be **extravasated** and be made to diffuse harmlessly in the network of capillaries that rushes forward to accommodate its explosive force? (From *Up from Liberalism,* p. 221, Stein & Day, 1984)

exult (verb) *To be extremely joyful, often with an outward display of triumph or exuberant self-satisfaction.*

Most recently the Dartmouth administration's mills ran overtime to **exult** over the appearance, alongside the weekly's logo, of an anti-Semitic remark taken from Hitler's *Mein Kampf.* (From "On the Right")

factionalism (noun) *The process of splitting into parties, combinations, or cliques.*

Boris Andreyvich Bolgin could hardly help hearing—experiencing—vibrations of—a mounting division. There was **factionalism,** spying on one another, the sense that no leader without the strength of Stalin was truly a leader. (From *High Jinx,* p. 43, Doubleday & Company, 1986)

fallow (adjective) *Marked by inactivity.*

It had been more than an entire college generation since he had mingled with the hard left community, either students or faculty. Even the Russian he had learned, he was encouraged to let lie **fallow.** (From *High Jinx,* p. 81, Doubleday & Company, 1986)

fervent (adjective) *Having or showing great emotion or warmth; ardent.*

He greatly missed those **fervent** evenings with the select few, the brainy idealists who recognized that the Soviet revolution was the twentieth century's way of saying no to more world wars, to imperialism, to the class system. (From *High Jinx,* p. 81, Doubleday & Company, 1986)

fiduciary (adjective) *Of, having to do with, or involving a confidence or trust; of the nature of a trust.*

In its administration of the funds, the government does not meet orthodox **fiduciary** standards of the kind stipulated by the laws of most of the states for private insurance companies. (From *Up from Liberalism*, p. 197, Stein & Day, 1984)

fillip (noun) *Something added that tends to arouse or excite; a stimulating or rousing agent.*

When Lord Keynes brushed aside the demurrals of a critic concerned with the long-run effect of his program by saying "In the long run we are all dead," he originated a verbal **fillip** that made its way quickly into the annals of definitive retort. (From *Up from Liberalism*, p. 187, Stein & Day, 1984)

fissiparous (adjective) *Reproducing by fission.*

The tribulations of the **fissiparous** Soviet empire will almost certainly guarantee, at least for the short run, a huge number of refugees. (From "On the Right")

fleeted (adjective) *Felicitious; starry; piquant.*

Blackford wondered whether his path and the Queen's would even cross. He half hoped they would not; half hoped they would, three years having passed since their fleeting, **fleeted** encounter. (From *High Jinx*, p. 208, Doubleday & Company, 1986)

flotsam and jetsam (nouns) *These terms usually appear together to refer to that part of the wreckage of a ship and its cargo found floating on the water or washed ashore. The phrase "flotsam and jetsam" now has an extended meaning of "useless trifles," "odds and ends."*

The **flotsam and jetsam** of Edward Bennett Williams's arguments wash up on the shores of reason in irreconcilable pieces, but on he goes, unperturbed. (From *Rumbles Left and Right*, p. 88, G. P. Putnam's Sons, 1963)

foppish (adjective) *Pertaining to or characteristic of a man who is preoccupied with and often vain about his clothes and manners.*

Mr. Mussolini was in his mid-forties, tall and angular. He was well dressed; the Director thought him even rather **foppish**. (From *High Jinx*, p. 178, Doubleday & Company, 1986)

forswear (verb) *To renounce earnestly, determinedly, or with protestations.*

In other words, the South African government was slipping some money (a relatively modest one hundred thousand dollars, one is told) to that domestic force which **forswore** violence, Communism, and boycotts—over against its opposition. What it did was illegal. But hardly evil. (From "On the Right")

fulmination (noun) *Vehement menace or censure; something that is thundered forth. [Used in 1992 calendar in a different form, namely, fulminator (noun)]*

Rubirosa has come to town. **Fulminations,** of course, are in order, but how pleasant **fulminations** can be at the hands of a master. (From *Rumbles Left and Right*, p. 137, G. P. Putnam's Sons, 1963)

gibbet (noun) *An upright post with a projecting arm for hanging the bodies of executed criminals in chains or irons; gallows.*

Now everybody knows you shouldn't talk about **gibbets** to executioners, especially not when they happen also to be head of state. (From *Up from Liberalism*, p. 129, Stein & Day, 1984)

gird (verb) *To prepare (oneself) for a struggle, test of strength, or other action.*

I cannot complain softly. My blood gets hot, my brow wet, I become unbearably and unconscionably sarcastic and bellicose; I am **girded** for a total showdown. (From *Rumbles Left and Right*, p. 189, G. P. Putnam's Sons, 1963)

granitic (adjective) *Very hard; granite-like.*

Now if you think this is because there is **granitic** resistance within Vassar to students of non-white background, how do we account for it that the presidents-elect of the senior class and the student government are black, and the junior class president-elect is Asian-American, and the president-elect of the sophomore class is Hispanic? (From "On the Right")

gravometer (noun) *A geological instrument designed to detect deposits of oil.*
This morning Murray Kempton speaks of the emergence of Romney as a presidential contender. Like a **gravometer,** he is attracted to the irony of the situation. (From *Rumbles Left and Right,* p. 140, G. P. Putnam's Sons, 1963)

grotesquerie (noun) *Something suggestive or resembling grotesque decorative art or the figures or designs of such art; something grotesque.*
There originated in this Couéism the reckless stampede to inflate the electoral lists, culminating in the **grotesquerie** of the state of Georgia, which voted in 1943 to give the vote to every eighteen-year-old. (From *Up from Liberalism,* p. 148, Stein & Day, 1984)

gull (verb) *To make a dupe of; cheat, deceive.*
Dr. J. B. Matthews painstakingly listed the names of dozens upon dozens of the unfortunate clergymen who had collaborated with the Communist movement, and finally reckoned that, percentagewise, more ministers had been **gulled** into supporting Communist fronts than teachers and lawyers. (From *Up from Liberalism,* p. 52, Stein & Day, 1984)

habituate (verb) *To make familiar through use or experience; to make acceptable or desirable through use or experience.*
They had walked almost eight miles that day, the fifth day of Blackford's exploration, and he was **habituated** now to the redundancy of the Trail's surrounding features. (From *Tucker's Last Stand,* p. 6, Random House, 1990)

hagiography (noun) *The writing or study of lives of the saints. [Used in 1992 calendar in a different form, namely, hagiographer (noun)]*
But Lenin, himself as close as any man could be to heartlessness, understood intellectually the need for icons. And as a political matter, he'd have approved the **hagiography** of communism, not because he believed in the elevation of ideological saints, but because he'd have found it useful to accelerate the revolution. (From "On the Right")

hedonism (noun) *An ethical doctrine taught by the ancient Epicureans and Cyrenaics and by the modern utilitarians that asserts that pleasure or happiness is the sole or chief good in life.*
Less conspicuous problems must be thought of as having an economic impact: the instability of family life, listlessness at school, a growing national tendency to corruption, or **hedonism;** and insensitivity to suffering; a callousness that breeds ugliness of behavior. (From *Gratitude,* p. 36, Random House, 1990)

hemidemisemiquaver (noun) *A sixty-fourth note; i.e., thoughts or frustrations lasting for only passing seconds.*
As, wearily, he slid into bed at three in the morning for the second successive night, he blanked out what his musical colleague at Trinity liked to call the **hemidemisemiquavers.**" (From *High Jinx,* p. 196, Doubleday & Company, 1986)

hermetically (adverb) *So as to be impervious to outside interference or influence.*
His brown eyes were either sound asleep (that was when Rufus was given over to analysis, parting company with his surroundings as though **hermetically** insulated from them) or fiercely active. (From *High Jinx,* p. 31, Doubleday & Company, 1986)

hierarchical (adjective) *Of or relating to a classification of people according to artistic, social, economic, or other criteria.*
I note a kind of **hierarchical** polarization going on. When I was at college, it would have been unprecedented to refer to the President of the University other than as "Mr. Seymour." Today, the president is "President Schmidt." Back then, a professor was—"Mr.

Whitehead," which is also what he'd have been called by his students. Today he would be "Dr. Whitehead," and his students would call him Chuck. (From "On the Right")

homophobe (noun) *One who dislikes, disapproves of, or has an irrational hatred of homosexuals or homosexuality.*

If a student these days opposes some of the demands of the Gay Liberation types, he might be branded as a **homophobe,** when all that can verifiably be said about him is that he is opposed to homosexual practices, which is still, though perhaps only just still, a permissible position. (From "On the Right")

hubris (noun) *Overweening pride or self-confidence; arrogance.*

The only autonomy liberalism appears to encourage is moral and intellectual autonomy; solipsism. And that is the autonomy of deracination; the philosophy that has peopled the earth with atomized and presumptuous social careerists diseased with **hubris.** (From *Up from Liberalism*, p. 177, Stein & Day, 1984)

humbuggery (noun) *An attitude or spirit of pretense and deception or self-deception.*

There were those who are free of the superstition of liberalism who joined in denouncing Pérez Jiménez's "election"; for his offense was one of **humbuggery.** (From *Up from Liberalism*, p. 149, Stein & Day, 1984)

hydra-headed (adjective) *Having many centers or branches (from the Hydra, a mythical many-headed serpent).*

The imperative that worldwide attention be given to stop the traffic in **hydra-headed** arms beckons as never before. (From "On the Right")

hypermammiferous (adjective) *Having extremely large breasts.*

The late Congressman Adam Clayton Powell, Jr., once took a highly publicized trip to Greece with a **hypermammiferous** blonde. He was investigating Greek affairs. Congressman Powell, contemplating the bust of Homer. (From "On the Right")

icon (noun) *Object or person attracting worshipful attention.*

Sally was slightly withdrawn, indomitably independent in spirit, dazzling to look at if you began by discarding as irrelevant most of the competition in **icons** of the day—she didn't look like Rita Hayworth or Marilyn Monroe. (From *Tucker's Last Stand*, p. 77, Random House, 1990)

ignominy (noun) *Deep, personal disgrace.*

I am perfectly at home in a small boat, and would, in a small boat race, more often than not come in if not on the side of glory, perhaps this side of **ignominy.** (From *Rumbles Left and Right*, p. 166, G. P. Putnam's Sons, 1963)

impenitent (adjective) *Not repenting of sin; not contrite.*

Norman Mailer and a dozen others signed an advertisement in papers throughout the country under the sponsorship of a group called the Fair Play for Cuba Committee. The episode was less farce than an act of tragedy, though without dire consequence for the players—they are strikingly **impenitent** and insouciant. (From *Rumbles Left and Right*, p. 56, G. P. Putnam's Sons, 1963)

imperturbability (noun) *The quality or state of being extremely calm, impassive, assured, and steady. [Used in 1991 calendar in a different form, namely, **imperturbable** (adjective)]*

I have seen consternation on the faces of more experienced members of my crew at such evidences of inexperience or even ignorance, and I do not myself pretend to **imperturbability** when they occur. (From *Rumbles Left and Right*, p. 170, G. P. Putnam's Sons, 1963)

imposture (noun) *The act or practice of imposing on or deceiving someone by means of an assumed character or name.*

Will Khrushchev respect us more as, by our deeds, we proclaim and proclaim again and again our hallucination, in the grinding teeth of the evidence, that we and the Soviet Union can work together for a better world? It is this **imposture** of irrationality in the guise of rationality that frightens. (From *Rumbles Left and Right*, p. 35, G. P. Putnam's Sons, 1963)

indite (verb) *To write, compose; to set down in writing.*

Fleetwood had been designated to give the first toast, and he had gone out of his way to **indite** a few sentences the meaning of which he knew would be understood by not more than a dozen of the hundred guests there. (From *High Jinx*, p. 123, Doubleday & Company, 1986)

ineradicable (adjective) *Incapable of being gotten rid of completely.*

His scientific intelligence taught him that facts, among them those that had to do with (**ineradicable?** Was this defective loyalty to Marx-Lenin?) human appetites cannot be denied by ideological asseverations. (From *High Jinx*, p. 75, Doubleday & Company, 1986)

ingratiation (noun) *The act of winning favor; the process of insinuating oneself in the good graces of another.*

Mrs. Thatcher's speech was a tribute to her natural eloquence and to her formidable powers of **ingratiation.** Mostly it was a Special Relations speech about the enduring friendship of the two great English-speaking powers. (From "On the Right")

iniquitously (adverb) *Wickedly; sinfully. [Used in 1991 calendar in a different form, namely, iniquitous (adjective)]*

Molotov delivered a speech on the subject of the **iniquitously** close relationship between the U.S. and Japan. (From *High Jinx*, p. 180, Doubleday & Company, 1986)

insularity (noun) *Narrow-mindedness; detachment; isolation; provincialism.*

But Mr. Salinas has gradually eased Mexico away from a protectionism that represented at once socialist **insularity** and yanqui xenophobia. (From "On the Right")

insurrectionary (adjective) *Relating to or constituting an act or instance of revolting against civil authority or against an established government.*

But there was another movement, not properly **insurrectionary** but totally hostile to apartheid. The Inkatha movement is as large as that of the African National Congress, but its leaders were different. (From "On the Right")

intellection (noun) *Exercise of the intellect; reasoning, cognition, apprehension; a specific act of the intellect.*

We believe that millenniums of **intellection** have served an objective purpose. Certain problems have been disposed of. (From *Up from Liberalism*, p. 182, Stein & Day, 1984)

intercredal (adjective) *Conversations or exchanges between members of different faiths.*

The liberals' implicit premise is that **intercredal** dialogues are what one has with Communists, not conservatives, in relationship with whom normal laws of civilized discourse are suspended. (From *Up from Liberalism*, p. 55, Stein & Day, 1984)

intransigence (noun) *Refusal to compromise, to come to an agreement or a reconciliation.*

Mr. Bush having asked Congress for a resolution backing a military response in the Gulf should Saddam Hussein persevere in **intransigence,** a distinction crystallizes. A very important distinction. (From "On the Right")

intrinsic (adjective) *Belonging to the inmost constitution or essential nature of a thing. [Used in 1992 calendar in a different form, namely, intrinsically (adverb)]*

The fact of discrimination in America against the Negro is of no more **intrinsic** concern to the Communists than the fact of discrimination against the Jews in Soviet Russia is of concern to them. (From *Rumbles Left and Right*, p. 114, G. P. Putnam's Sons, 1963)

inure (verb) *To come into operation; flow to; become operative; accrue.*

Those who do not enroll in the program do not make the payments, but neither do the benefits **inure** to them. (From *Up from Liberalism*, p. 205, Stein & Day, 1984)

invective (noun) *Denunciatory or abusive language; vituperation.*

"You, by not using your donkey brain—excuse me donkey," Beria spoke now in a voice of exaggerated deference,—"excuse me, donkey, for insulting your brain by comparing it with Bolgin's!" The **invective** lasted a full ten minutes before Beria sat down. (From *High Jinx*, p. 46, Doubleday & Company, 1986)

irredentism (noun) *A claim by a nation to land that formerly belonged to it. [Used in 1991 calendar in a different form, namely,* **irredentist** *(adjective)]*

A few miles to the west, the disorder and the killings go on in Ulster and Ireland, over the dogged question of self-rule: Ulster wants to hold on to its independence as a part of Great Britain, substantial elements within Ireland want **irredentism**. (From "On the Right")

irreducible (adjective) *Impossible to simplify or make easier or clearer; impossible to make less or smaller.*

And one has therefore to pause before proceeding to hold every Iraqi responsible for the crimes of Saddam Hussein and those front-line sadists who disgraced the **irreducible** maxims of human decency. (From "On the Right")

irruption (noun) *A sudden, violent, or forcible entry; a rushing or bursting in; a sudden or violent invasion.*

The question the white community faces, then, is whether the claims of civilization supersede those of universal suffrage. The British clearly believed they did when they acted to suppress the **irruption** in Kenya in 1952. (From *Up from Liberalism*, p. 157, Stein & Day, 1984)

janissary (noun) *A member of a group of loyal or subservient troops, officials, or supporters.*

When it was finally clear that Carmine DeSapio had been thrown out by the ideological **janissaries** and the playboy reformers, there were still the conventional and highly poignant rituals to go through. (From *Rumbles Left and Right*, p. 134, G. P. Putnam's Sons, 1963)

kinetic (adjective) *Supplying motive force; energizing, dynamic.*

The conclusions of Professor Louis Hartz of Harvard are both historical and philosophical. There never was a sure-enough conservatism in America, he maintains, the American experience having been dynamic, revolutionary, pragmatic, **kinetic**. (From *Up from Liberalism*, p. 90, Stein & Day, 1984)

knell (noun) *A death signal or passing bell; a warning of or a sound indicating the passing away of something.*

If we become identified with the point of view that the social security laws toll the **knell** of our departed freedoms, we will lose our credit at the bar of public opinion, or be dismissed as cultists of a terrestrial mystique. (From *Up from Liberalism*, p. 189, Stein & Day, 1984)

lachrymal (adjective) *Marked by tears.*

Mrs. Chamorro, while making all the appropriate **lachrymal** sounds over the death of Enrique, has not overridden her Sandinista authorities to take charge of the investigation. (From "On the Right")

laconic (adjective) *Using or marked by the use of few words; terse, precise. [Used in 1991 calendar in a different form, namely,* **laconically** *(adverb)]*

Bertram Heath was a quiet, determined young man with the even-featured straight face and the steady brown eyes that signaled what was coming before the **laconic** twenty-year-old got out what was on his mind. (From *High Jinx*, p. 86, Doubleday & Company, 1986)

largesse (noun) *Liberality in giving, especially when attended by condescension.*

He felt positively ennobled by the proposed act of generosity, but also tender in the knowledge of whom he stood now to patronize with his **largesse**. (From *High Jinx*, p. 79, Doubleday & Company, 1986)

levity (noun) *Lacking in seriousness; a frivolity.*

"Not even you can talk that way about Comrade Beria. And this business of going to the British Embassy . . . I mean, Alistair, don't ever say such a thing, not even in **levity**." (From *High Jinx*, p. 175, Doubleday & Company, 1986)

licentious (adjective) *Marked by the absence of legal or moral restraints; by lewdness; by neglect. [Used in 1991 calendar in a different form, namely, licentiousness (noun)]*

Such discrepancies as the bigoted churchman, the protectionist free enterpriser, the provincial internationalist, the **licentious** moralist are all well-known anomalies. (From *Up from Liberalism*, p. 35, Stein & Day, 1984)

licit (adjective) *Legally or otherwise allowable; condonable.*

It is easy to imagine (and frightening to do so) the result of a refusal by the minority to abide by the **licit** authority of the majority. (From *Gratitude*, p. 54, Random House, 1990)

locus classicus (noun) (Latin) *A standard passage important for the elucidation of a word or subject.*

It can be argued by orthodox theologians that God prefers the sinner to the saint, always provided it is understood that overnight the sinner can, and in the past often has, become a saint. Augustine is the **locus classicus**. (From *Gratitude*, p. 63, Random House, 1990)

logorrhea (noun) *Pathologically excessive and often incoherent talkativeness.*

That bit of **logorrhea** is a way of saying that the Founding Fathers were incompetent when they gave individual states, instead of just the federal government, the taxing power, because this federalist invitation to centrifugal disruption adds up to people being able to look Mario Cuomo in the face and say, "Raise taxes one more time, and we'll give you a forwarding address in Pennsylvania." (From "On the Right")

lucidity (noun) *The quality or state of being clear to the understanding; readily intelligible; lacking ambiguity.*

"You have, sometimes, a terribly obscure way of expressing yourself, a difficulty you may have noticed that never afflicted my mentor, Jane Austen, who had no problem in expressing thoughts no matter how subtle, with unambiguous **lucidity**." (From *Tucker's Last Stand*, p. 136, Random House, 1990)

lucubrate (verb) *To discourse learnedly in writing.*

Under the Eisenhower program, one could **lucubrate** over constitutional rights and freedoms and forever abandon captured American soldiers. (From *Up from Liberalism*, p. 128, Stein & Day, 1984)

lumpen (adjective) *An amorphous group of dispossessed and uprooted individuals set off by their inferior status from the economic and social class with which they are identified; a geographical area backward and undistinguished.*

Several years ago I wrote in this space that the Soviet Union, were it deprived of its strategic nuclear weapons, would become nothing much more than a vast **lumpen** territorial mass, something on the order of a north India. (From "On the Right")

Machiavellian (adjective) *Crafty, deceitful; of, like, or characterized by the political principles and methods of expediency, craftiness, and duplicity advocated in Niccolò Machiavelli's book* The Prince.

The **Machiavellian** principle that you do not fool with the prince unless you are prepared to kill him was never more clearly vindicated than in the current exercise. (From "On the Right")

maculation (noun) *Spot, stain, blemish.*

The new conservatives, many of whom go by the name of Modern Republicans, have not been very helpful. Their sin consists in permitting so many accretions, modifications, emendations, **maculations,** and qualifications that the original thing quite recedes from view. (From *Up from Liberalism*, p. 189, Stein & Day, 1984)

malefactor (noun) *One who does ill toward another; evildoer.*

Whatever good they accomplished it can't be denied that they also did great harm, and that the principal **malefactor** was Senator Frank Church, who treated the hearings as a confessional. (From "On the Right")

malfeasance (noun) *The doing by a public officer under cover of authority of his office of something that is unwarranted, that he has contracted not to do, and that is legally unjustified and positively wrongful or contrary to law.*

Edward Bennett Williams pleads for action to deprive the Congress of the right to exercise its traditional power to expose crime and **malfeasance,** to forbid the police from tapping the telephones of putative criminals, to restrain detectives from interrogating suspects. (From *Rumbles Left and Right*, p. 86, G. P. Putnam's Sons, 1963)

malum in se (noun) (Latin) *An act that is evil or wrong from its own nature or by the natural law irrespective of statute.*

What the government of South Africa did is a nice example of the distinction between a *malum prohibitum* and a **malum in se.** It is legally wrong for a government to subsidize one particular political movement at the expense of another. It is not always morally wrong to do so. (From "On the Right")

manifesto (noun) *A public demonstration of intentions, motives, or views; a public statement of policy or opinion.*

Because liberalism has no definitive **manifesto,** one cannot say, prepared to back up the statement with unimpeachable authority, that such-and-such a man or measure is "liberal." (From *Up from Liberalism*, p. 36, Stein & Day, 1984)

matrix (noun) *A situation or surrounding substance within which something originates, develops, or is contained.*

She was to keep a sharp eye out for any student who inclined sufficiently toward the great Communist experiment, of which Russia was the **matrix**, to qualify for possible recruitment. (From *High Jinx*, p. 70, Doubleday & Company, 1986)

meliorative (adjective) *Resulting in or leading toward betterment.*

There is no guarantee behind the value of the policy taken out with a private insurance company, which is subject to the depredations of inflation unmitigated by **meliorative** political pressure. (From *Up from Liberalism*, p. 197, Stein & Day, 1984)

metastasize (verb) *To spread to other parts of the body by metastasis; to change form or matter; to transform.*

And the possibility was also there to be considered that what happened between the judge and his associate wasn't seductive flirtation but something misinterpreted as such, growing grotesque in the imagination, sufficient to **metastasize** as an inclination to bestiality. (From "On the Right")

meticulist (noun) *One who is extremely careful in his use of language, diction; a precise measurer.*

It hurt Governor Sununu, who is a **meticulist** in expression, to use a term inappropriate to his conduct. (From "On the Right") *mille-feuilles* (noun) (French: "one thousand leaves") *A light, layered pastry commonly called a Napoleon.*

The braised chicken and petits pois were fine, the claret excellent, the **mille-feuilles** sensational. (From *High Jinx,* p. 99, Doubleday & Company, 1986)

mirabile dictu (adverb) (Latin) *"Wonder to relate"; incredible.*

Here is a question for which, **mirabile dictu,** I do not have the answer. It is: How much freedom should a college student be given to say or to write what he wishes? (From "On the Right")

miscible (adjective) *Capable of mixing in any ratio without separation of two phases.*

It is a pity that the useless word "equality" ever got into the act, because one cannot in the nature of things make "equal" that which is not the same. You can play around with other words if you wish—fungible? No, the sexes aren't fungible. **Miscible?** Yes: but **miscible** elements retain their identity. (From "On the Right")

miscreant (noun) *One who behaves criminally or viciously.*

That spirit looks upon a nuclear missile not only as a ferule with which to beat the enemy and native **miscreants,** but as a badge of high office. (From "On the Right")

misogynist (noun) *One who hates women.*

Those who believe that a case for differences between the two can be plausibly made might have no trouble suppressing or expelling the student pornographer, but would pause over taking action against the student racist or homophobe or **misogynist** or whatever. (From "On the Right")

monetize (verb) *To coin into money.*

There is a tale (I think it was Ring Lardner's) of an old prospector who shrinks from the attendant complexities and unpleasantness of mining and **monetizing** a rich deposit of gold he has come upon. (From *Up from Liberalism,* p. 181, Stein & Day, 1984)

morphological (adjective) *Of, relating to, or concerned with form or structure. [Used in 1991 calendar in a different form, namely, morphology (noun)]*

The state can rule, but it cannot command loyalty, let alone effect **morphological** changes in human nature. (From *Gratitude,* p. 48, Random House, 1990)

mortification (noun) *The subjection and denial of bodily passions and appetites by abstinence or self-inflicted pain or discomfort.*

When he decided to enter the monastery, he decided, as a novitiate, to impose upon himself the intellectual **mortification** of learning physics. (From *Tucker's Last Stand,* p. 32, Random House, 1990)

multicentrist (noun) *Those who hold that attachments to many positions, political, social, cultural, are educationally advanced.*

Having dealt with Islamic codes on women, the pilgrims in search of better ideas than those of our own culture can study the attitudes of others toward homosexuality, since homophobia is one of the central targets of the **multicentrists.** (From "On the Right")

munificently (adverb) *Liberally, with lavish generosity. [Used in 1992 calendar in a different form, namely, munificent (adjective)]*

Big social thinkers assume that any proposal is emasculated that doesn't call for federal funding on a very large scale. What the Bennet school of criticism wishes to see in national service is a full-scale war against poverty. Again; federal programs **munificently** funded. (From *Gratitude,* p. 80, Random House, 1990)

mutatis mutandis (adverb) (Latin) *The necessary changes having been made.*

How many Americans, reflecting on the misuse of a government limousine, have asked themselves whether they should be fired by their employers because every now and again they use a postage stamp from the office supply to mail a personal letter?

Mutatis mutandis, they might say to themselves, that is the equivalent of misusing a government limousine, if you are chief of staff of the White House. (From "On the Right")

mycology (noun) *The properties and life phenomena exhibited by a fungus, fungus type, or fungus group—the study of mushrooms.*

How many things Whittaker Chambers wanted to write about! Mushrooms, for one thing. Some gentleman had recently published a ten-dollar book on **mycology,** heaping scorn on one of Chambers's most beloved species of toadstools. (From *Rumbles Left and Right,* p. 153, G. P. Putnam's Sons, 1963)

naïf (noun) *A naïve person.*

Within ten minutes Tucker knew he was dealing, in the case of the gook, with a total **naïf.** The Russian's background, on the other hand, was considerable. (From *Tucker's Last Stand,* p. 238, Random House, 1990)

necromancy (noun) *Black magic; sorcery; the practice of claiming to foretell the future by alleged communication with the dead.*

When you raise taxes, you raise taxes. When you forecast spending decreases, you are engaged in **necromancy.** (From "On the Right")

nescient (adjective) *From nescience, the doctine that nothing is truly knowable.*

I intended to call my little book "The Revolt Against the Masses," because I thought I saw on the social horizon in America signs of a disposition to reject the **nescient** aimlessness Ortega y Gasset had diagnosed. (From *Gratitude,* p. 15, Random House, 1990)

nether (adjective) *Situated down or below; lying beneath or in the lower part.*

The conservative should shake loose from his disposition to reject out of hand any gesture in the direction of acknowledging different orders of citizenship. That line of demarcation should exist, among other reasons, in order to prompt those on the **nether** side to traverse it. (From *Gratitude,* p. 67, Random House, 1990)

noblesse oblige (noun) (French) *The inferred obligation of people of high rank or social position to behave nobly or kindly toward others.*

But individual employers, acting on an impulse of **noblesse oblige,** aren't to be confused with the government, which must never discriminate in its own hiring practices. (From "On the Right")

nomenklatura (noun) *The elite within the Soviet bureaucracy.*

A. Well there is no doubt they have considerable influence—the **nomenklatura,** the KGB, the military—but I ask you to imagine how much worse off the Soviet Union would be without Gorbachev. (From "On the Right")

nonplussed (adjective) *At a loss as to what to say, think, or do.*

I put the question to the biographer of Mr. Hoover, Dr. George Nash the distinguished historian. He **nonplussed** me by telling me that he was himself **nonplussed.** So much so that he went to the archives and dug up the first one hundred communications sent to President Hoover after he left the White House. (From "On the Right")

nuance (noun) *A subtle or slight degree of difference as in meaning, color, or tone. [Used in 1991 calendar in a different form, namely, **nuanced** (adjective)]*

She discovered that in his subtle way, the slim young man with no trace of beard, a light sprinkle of faded freckles reaching from his nose to his hair, was quick to grasp **nuance** and to expand and improvise on subjects only tangentially touched upon. (From *High Jinx,* p. 72, Doubleday & Company, 1986)

obloquy (noun) *A strongly and often intemperately condemnatory utterance; defamatory or calumnious language; abusive or slanderous reprehension.*

After an elaborate exposition of the problem, he would pronounce sentence. This ranged from disqualification, on the lenient days, to a terrible warning to which, of course, was attached public **obloquy.** (From *Rumbles Left and Right,* p. 165, G. P. Putnam's Sons, 1963)

obsequy (noun) *Gesture of reverence, or piety, or deference, usually toward the dead.*

And poor Senator Gore! He was accused by properly indignant New York Jews of "pandering" to the Jewish vote by his near-sacramental **obsequies** to whatever Tel Aviv's policy was five minutes ago. (From "On the Right")

obstreperous (adjective) *Stubbornly defiant; resisting control or restraint, often with a show of noisy disorder.*

Mike Wallace introduces Randolph Churchill as an "irascible snob." Now for all I know, that is just what Mr. Churchill is; but this is not the way to introduce one's guests, not even **obstreperous** conservative guests. (From *Up from Liberalism,* p. 61, Stein & Day, 1984)

oeuvre (noun) (French: "a work") *Usually, the sum of an artist's lifework.*

Blackford was showing off here, as he wished Sally to know that he knew where Mr. Knightley and Miss Woodhouse had figured in Miss Austen's **oeuvre.** (From *High Jinx,* p. 18, Doubleday & Company, 1986)

oligarchs (noun) *The controlling members of a party or state.*

Being able to vote is no more to have realized freedom than being able to read is to have realized wisdom. Reasonable limitations upon the vote are not recommended exclusively by tyrants or **oligarchs** (was Jefferson either?). (From *Up from Liberalism,* p. 158, Stein & Day, 1984)

ombudsman (noun) *One who investigates complaints, as from consumers, reports findings, and assists in achieving fair settlements.*

Should the federal government pay **ombudsmen** who would stand at the door of the public library, prepared to extract from the mainframe the information desired by the curious citizen? (From "On the Right")

omnicompetent (adjective) *Well qualified in all respects.*

That morning Rufus had arrived at the safe house in London looking old, but not for that reason less than **omnicompetent.** (From *High Jinx,* p. 54, Doubleday & Company, 1986)

ontological (adjective) *Of or relating to being or existence.*

The persistent misuse of the word democracy reflects either an ignorance of its **ontological** emptiness; or (and is this not the logical derivative of the ignorance?), the pathetic attempt to endow it with substantive meaning. (From *Up from Liberalism,* p. 146, Stein & Day, 1984)

opera (noun) *Plural of opus, a set of compositions usually numbered in order of issue.*

Arthur Schlesinger, Jr., for a decade or so was more or less ex officio in charge of disdaining my **opera** and writing the score for others on just how this was to be done. (From *Up from Liberalism,* p. xxi, Stein & Day, 1984)

opprobrium (noun) *Public or known disgrace or ill fame that ordinarily follows from conduct considered grossly wrong or vicious.*

There are circumstances when the minority can lay claim to preeminent political authority, without bringing down upon its head the moral **opprobrium** of just men. (From *Up from Liberalism,* p. 157, Stein & Day, 1984)

organon (noun) *An instrument for acquiring knowledge, specifically a body of methodological doctrine comprising principles for scientific or philosophic procedure or investigations.*

Those liberating perceptions Norman Mailer has been wrestling to formulate for lo these many years are like the purloined letter, lying about loose in the principles and premises, the **organon,** of the movement the Left finds it so fashionable to ridicule. (From *Rumbles Left and Right,* p. 62, G. P. Putnam's Sons, 1963)

paean (noun) *A fervent expression of joy or praise.*
  Alice wrote poetry, and her poetry included **paeans** to the Soviet state and its leaders, though she had had on more than one occasion to face the metrical choice either of substituting the name of a new leader in the place of the name that figured in her original lines but was now exposed as having been treasonable, or toss the poem away. (From *High Jinx,* p. 69, Doubleday & Company, 1986)

paralogism (noun) *Reasoning contrary to the rules of logic; a faulty argument. [Used in 1992 calendar in a different form, namely, **paralogist** (noun)]*
  This is the critical **paralogism** in the Choicers' line of argument. What they should be saying is that the woman's right to abort is superior to the right of the fetus to live. (From "On the Right")

parlous (adjective) *Characterized by uncertainty; fraught with danger or risk; attended with peril.*
  The situation in South Africa during the past, **parlous** years isn't as vivid seen through the serene eyes of a lecturer at the Kennedy School at Harvard as it has been, and continues to be, for the white South African. (From "On the Right")

parricide (noun) *The act of killing one's father.*
  Now, "fraternity" is a word one needs to pause over, inasmuch as the French Revolution, in enshrining that word, in effect committed **parricide.** (From *Gratitude,* p. 55, Random House, 1990)

perdurable (adjective) *Lasting a long time or indefinitely.*
  It tends to be true that in England the Establishment prevails. The English Establishment mediates the popular political will through **perdurable** English institutions. (From *Rumbles Left and Right,* p. 17, G. P. Putnam's Sons, 1963)

peremptory (adjective) *(1) Expressive of urgency or command; (2) of an arrogant or imperious nature.*
  Mayday moved forward and put her lips on Blackford's—and lingered. Before she was done, Alice felt contrition over her **peremptory** handling of Anthony, and now used lips and hands to express her feeling for him. (From *Tucker's Last Stand,* p. 92, Random House, 1990)

perfidious (adjective) *Characterized by a deliberate breach of faith, a calculated violation of trust, or treachery. [Used in 1991 calendar in a different form, namely, **perfidy** (noun)]*
  "It's your call, Boris. What did bring you out tonight? We have not spoken once in the three years—"
  "In the three years in which I have kept pace with your **perfidious** activities, Mr. Chestnut," replied Bolgin. (From *High Jinx,* p. 204, Doubleday & Company, 1986)

philistinism (noun) *The attitudes, beliefs, and conduct characteristic of a crass, prosaic, often priggish individual guided by material rather than intellectual values.*
  To paraphrase Mr. Tynan, over here we have the impression that in America everybody thinks alike, that the country is in the grip of an iron **philistinism.** (From *Rumbles Left and Right,* p. 69, G. P. Putnam's Sons, 1963)

plainspoken (adjective) *Frank, straightforward, unadorned.*
  Normally, when recruiting someone into the Party, the seniority of the recruiter is utterly **plainspoken.** Her authority rested in her established status as a party member; as a graduate of the University of Moscow; as a linguist; as a longtime resident of the Soviet Union. (From *High Jinx,* p. 77, Doubleday & Company, 1986)

plight (verb) *To put or give in pledge.*
  One eulogist said that as a young woman, graduated from Vassar College and the Columbia Law School, she had **plighted** her professional troth to two causes: the first, her

own individual freedom to do as she chose; the second, her absolute commitment to women's "reproductive rights." (From "On the Right")

plutocratic (adjective) *Relating to government by the wealthy; of the rule or dominion of wealth or of the rich.*

I very much wish that the meaning of the word "masses" was not so fixed in the Anglo-Saxon world because the word as we use it has either Marxist or **plutocratic** connotations. (From *Gratitude,* p. 16, Random House, 1990)

polarization (noun) *Division (as of groups, ideologies, systems, or forces) into two opposites.*

The occasion drove home the infinitely sad **polarization** between the Choicers and the Lifers. (From "On the Right")

polemicize (verb) *To engage in controversy; dispute aggressively. [Used in 1991 calendar in a different form, namely, polemical (adjective)]*

Give me the right to spend my dollars as I see fit—to devote them to learning, to taking pleasure, to **polemicizing,** and if I must make the choice, I will surrender you my political franchise in trade. (From *Up from Liberalism,* p. 208, Stein & Day, 1984)

polity (noun) *Political organization.*

Some libertarians will never agree that a responsibility of the **polity** is to encourage virtue directly, through such disciplines as service in the militia, reverence for religious values, and jury service. (From *Gratitude,* p. 50, Random House, 1990)

posit (verb) *To set in place or position; situate; to set down or assume as fact; postulate.*

I **posit** in this case that he is absolutely ignorant of malfeasance. I do this as a matter of character judgment. (From "On the Right")

praepostor (noun) *A monitor at an English public school.*

As **praepostor** at the British public school it had fallen to Anthony Trust to help hold down young Blackford, age fifteen, over one end of a sofa as he received a serious flogging from the headmaster. (From *Tucker's Last Stand,* p. 86, Random House, 1990)

pre-infanticide (noun) *Killing of a child prior to its birth.*

But to defend the reproductive rights, so-called, of women, it is absolutely necessary to celebrate the act of **pre-infanticide,** and this is not easy for fellow Americans to do. (From "On the Right")

preponderant (adjective) *Having superior weight, force, or influence; having greater prevalence.*

This means many things, among them that no economic reform that would get in the way of channeling the **preponderant** economic machinery of the country can be tolerated. (From "On the Right")

preponderate (verb) *To exceed in power, influence, or importance.*

It is well known that in certain quarters in the South where blacks heavily **preponderate,** the marginal black voter (the man whose vote would tip the scales in favor of the Negro block) is, by one evasion or another, deprived of the vote. (From *Up from Liberalism,* p. 156, Stein & Day, 1984)

prepossession (noun) *An attitude, belief, or impression formed beforehand; a preconceived opinion.*

In the hands of a skillful indoctrinator, the average student not only thinks what the indoctrinator wants him to think (assuming no **prepossession** in the way), but is altogether positive that he has arrived at his position by independent intellectual exertion. (From *Up from Liberalism,* p. 83, Stein & Day, 1984)

priapic (adjective) *Preoccupied with or employing the phallus symbolically; featuring or stressing the phallus.*

"At first I thought that his rushing off to see her so often was simply the **priapic** imperative at work." (From *Tucker's Last Stand,* p. 210, Random House, 1990)

primogenitive (adjective) *Of or pertaining to the firstborn.*
The English Establishment is more frozen than our own, primarily because theirs is a society based on class. Their Establishment has rites and honorifics and **primogenitive** continuities. (From *Rumbles Left and Right*, p. 16, G. P. Putnam's Sons, 1963)

pro bono publico (adverb) (Latin) *For the public good.*
Paul Hughes was prepared, ***pro bono publico***, to report secretly to the editors of the *Democratic Digest* the secret doings of the Sub-Committee on Investigations. (From *Up from Liberalism*, p. 103, Stein & Day, 1984)

proffer (verb) *To offer; tender.*
"You are the most exciting, and the most handsome, young physicist in the world. Everybody knows that. What they don't know is that you are also the greatest lover in—in—"
"The spy world?" Alistair Fleetwood **proffered**, laughing. (From *High Jinx*, p. 127, Doubleday & Company, 1986)

progenitive (adjective) *Pertaining to those who beget; as in parents, founders, discoverers.*
The proposition that American citizens owe something to the community that formulated and fought to establish their **progenitive** rights was proffered in 1910 by William James, "The Moral Equivalent of War." (From *Gratitude*, p. xvii, Random House, 1990)

propitious (adjective) *Presenting favorable circumstances; auspicious.*
With great solemnity, Alistair had been presented the Order of Lenin. Beria explained, "We left out your name—the space is there for it. Security. When the climate is **propitious**, you may take it to a jeweler and have your name inscribed." (From *High Jinx*, p. 235, Doubleday & Company, 1986)

proprietary (adjective) *Having to do with the owner; befitting an owner.*
My gal Sal, he had referred to her a few letters back, intending to be affectionate. She had replied, "My gal Sal is entirely too **proprietary** for my taste, Blacky my boy (and how do you like 'Blacky my boy'?")." (From *High Jinx*, p. 17, Doubleday & Company, 1986)

proscriptively (adverb) *The adverbial form of "proscriptive"—prohibiting or interdicting; proscribing.*
The persecution in Harvard of Professor Stephan Thernstrom, for the sin of talking about Jim Crow and about slavery in the South descriptively, rather than **proscriptively**. (From "On the Right")

protégé (noun) *A person whose welfare, training, or career is promoted by someone, usually influential or efficient or both.*
By the time Alice Goodyear Corbett had graduated from secondary school she had achieved a minor eminence in the student world of Moscow: the perfectly trained Soviet **protégée**. (From *High Jinx*, p. 68, Doubleday & Company, 1986)

proto- (prefix) *First in time; beginning; giving rise to.*
In "corporatism," the state would have the bureaucracy, and, together with the labor union, would work in harmony, creating something on the order of the syndicalism that later excited the **proto**-fascists. (From *Gratitude*, p. 57, Random House, 1990)

provincial (adjective) *Limited in scope; narrow, sectional.*
Mr. John Crosby writes: "How do you get on a blacklist? Well, some actors have got on by having foreign names." Tacit premise: blacklisters are reckless, **provincial**, xenophobic. (From *Up from Liberalism*, p. 73, Stein & Day, 1984)

pulchritude (noun) *Physical comeliness; beauty.*
"Why Baltimore indeed! First, some of the best beer on the East Coast is made here. Second, much of the best seafood in the East is found here. Third, there is **pulchritude** at hand here." (From *Tucker's Last Stand*, p. 86, Random House, 1990)

pullulate (verb) *To sprout out; germinate; breed quickly; spring up in abundance.*
But only 1.5 percent of black police officers pass the New York sergeants' test: and the result is a failure of effective social integration, and a them-and-us attitude which now and again **pullulates** into such incidents as we saw in Los Angeles. (From "On the Right")

quizzically (adverb) *In a slightly and amusingly eccentric manner; questioningly; curiously.*
Alphonse smiled, and bowed his head. "I feel in a bargaining mood, Mr. Oakes."
Blackford looked up sharply, **quizzically.**
"I will do as you say," said Alphonse, "provided you give me another drink of vodka." (From *Tucker's Last Stand,* p. 160, Random House, 1990)

raillery (noun) *Good-natured ridicule; pleasantry touched with satire; banter, chaffing, mockery.*
I note that the Eighties are held up for scorn and **raillery** by trendy opinion-makers. Everything that came out of the Eighties is held to be somehow contaminated, the grand contaminator being, of course, Ronald Reagan. (From "On the Right")

recision (noun) *The act of rescinding or canceling.*
Former Secretary of Defense Caspar Weinberger was in favor of **recision,** but somehow President Reagan never got around to it, in part because it had become a kind of liberal sanctuary, to which disarmament fetishists took pilgrimages every few days, sowing seeds of alarm that suggested that to amend the ABM Treaty was to say goodbye to disarmament. (From "On the Right")

rectilinear (adjective) *Moving in a straight line; having an undeviating direction; forming a straight line.*
What gets in the way of **rectilinear** moral reasoning is our insistence on dressing up the moral arguments in opportunistic ways. (From "On the Right")

reductio ad absurdum (noun) (Latin) *Reduction of an argument to the absurd.*
But perhaps the example is a *reductio ad absurdum:* If the United States had a first-strike force, the Soviet Union would presumably fear that it might be used, never mind that during the twenty-odd years when we did have a first-strike force we did not use it. (From "On the Right")

refractory (adjective) *Resisting control or authority.*
It is easier to deal with **refractory** twelve-year-olds than with eighteen-year-olds. Young children are not consulted on the question of whether they should take instruction. (From *Gratitude,* p. 113, Random House, 1990)

reifiable (adjective) *Convertible into something concrete.*
It is in the nature of natural law that it is not fully comprehensible, let alone **reifiable.** What a belief in the natural law actually amounts to is a propensity to do the right thing. (From "On the Right")

reinstitutionalize (verb) *To incorporate again into a system of organized and often highly formalized belief, practice, or acceptance.*
Gorbachev, who only a year ago declared that the Communist Party's monopoly on political power had to end, is now reaching out for means of **reinstitutionalizing** a Communist hegemony. (From "On the Right")

replete (adjective) *Well filled or plentifully supplied; gorged.*
As is almost always the case, special pleaders will find in a 25,000-word document **replete** with qualifications, favorite phrases or clauses designed to make their point. (From "On the Right")

repristinate (verb) *To restore to an original state or condition.*
Wearily he began to undress, first removing the beard in front of the mirror and staring fondly at his **repristinated** face. (From *High Jinx,* p. 170, Doubleday & Company, 1986)

requital (noun) *Return or repayment for something; something given in return or compensation.*
By asking our eighteen-year-olds to make sacrifices we are reminding them that they owe a debt. And reminding them that **requital** of a debt is the purest form of acknowledging that debt. (From *Gratitude*, p. xiv, Random House, 1990)

resonant (adjective) *Having an effect; being heard; being acted on.*
And, finally, that little boot, quiet but **resonant,** that he finally gave to Mikhail Gorbachev was done adroitly, efficiently, with just the right touch of hauteur: "Gorby, you are getting in the way." Mr. Bush is rightly the man of the hour. (From "On the Right")

restive (adjective) *Inquisitive; tempted to inquiry, defiance.*
The intellectuals of Spain, in hindsight, recognize the inappropriateness of the republic most of them once supported; but they are **restive,** anxious to get on with the job of crafting organic and responsive and durable political mechanisms. (From *Rumbles Left and Right*, p. 39, G. P. Putnam's Sons, 1963)

roistering (noun) *Characterized by or associated with noisy revelry.*
What ensues is an uproar, in part because the tradition of gentility at the University of Virginia is pronounced, and although a certain amount of alcoholic **roistering** is known to go on, the general protocols are that utter discretion is in order. (From "On the Right")

rotarian (adjective) *Of or relating to Rotarian societies; hail-fellow-well-met; concerned with social, civic, and workaday matters.*
People continue to tolerate and to patronize schools and colleges and universities which treat their children like half-rational biological mechanisms, whose highest ambition in life is to develop in such fashion as to render glad the **Rotarian** heart in Anywhere, U.S.A. (From *Rumbles Left and Right*, p. 99, G. P. Putnam's Sons, 1963)

rotund (adjective) *Rounded, plump.*
Dr. Callard, the retired headmaster of Winchester, invited in to tea the pleasant young solicitor. Dr. Callard, silver-haired, **rotund,** and genial, served the tea and reminisced. (From *High Jinx*, p. 115, Doubleday & Company, 1986)

routinization (noun) *Reduction to a prescribed and detailed course of action to be followed regularly.*
She was amusing herself, draining the meeting of the kind of **routinization** which so many of her predecessors had invested it with. (From *High Jinx*, p. 135, Doubleday & Company, 1986)

sacerdotal (adjective) *Of or relating to priests or priesthood.*
A half hour into the walk, Brother Hildred asked "Leo"—the monks called themselves by their **sacerdotal** names—if he would like to visit the school's physics laboratory. (From *Tucker's Last Stand*, p. 31, Random House, 1990)

sass (verb) *To talk impudently or disrespectfully to (an elder or superior).*
Senator McCarthy is dead, but the mania he illuminated lives on, and even now asserts control over sensible men whenever their ideology is threatened, questioned, or **sassed.** (From *Up from Liberalism*, p. 54, Stein & Day, 1984)

satyriasis (noun) *Abnormal or uncontrollable desire by a man for sexual intercourse.*
But Henry VIII enters the history books as an effective monarch, never mind his **satyriasis,** and his inclination to dispose of unsatisfactory wives on the scaffold. (From "On the Right")

sciolist (noun) *One whose knowledge or learning is superficial; a pretender to scholarship. [Used in 1992 calendar in a different form, namely, sciolism (noun)]*
"I don't believe you. You are an unaccomplished fake. An academic **sciolist.**" (From *Tucker's Last Stand*, p. 48, Random House, 1990)

scrupulosity (noun) *The quality or state of carefully adhering to ethical standards; overstrict in applying the strictest standards to oneself.*

He would work at home. I begged him to desist from what I had denounced as his sin of **scrupulosity**. (From *Rumbles Left and Right,* p. 153, G. P. Putnam's Sons, 1963)

seminal (adjective) *Having the character of an originative power, or source; containing or contributing the seeds of later development.*

In order to penetrate the public mind, it was necessary not only to do such **seminal** thinking as was being done by such as Eric Voegelin, it was necessary also to photograph the ideological father figure in just the right light. (From *Up from Liberalism,* p. xiii, Stein & Day, 1984)

sentimentalization (noun) *The act or process of analyzing a problem with exclusive concern for the sentimental dimension.*

The attempt to answer military questions by asking the question, How much do you love the kid over there who just got married, the youngest son of proud and devoted parents, is a **sentimentalization** of important calculations that are necessarily made, so to speak, in cold blood. (From "On the Right")

skein (noun) *Something suggesting the twistings and contortions of a loosely coiled length of yarn or thread.*

J. William Fulbright is renowned as a leading American liberal, and as the author of a vast **skein** of international scholarships whose aim is to foster world understanding and tolerance. (From *Up from Liberalism,* p. 58, Stein & Day, 1984)

slavish (adjective) *Resembling or characteristic of a slave; spineless, submissive.*

Some companies are moving in that direction, but most of them are **slavish** in meeting the demands of executives they want to stick around. (From "On the Right")

slovenly (adjective) *Lazily slipshod.*

There is indeed a fusion of justice and anti-Communist activity; the redemptions of the tens of millions whom, because of a **slovenly,** cowardly, and unimaginative diplomacy, we turned over to their Communist oppressors. (From *Rumbles Left and Right,* p. 116, G. P. Putnam's Sons, 1963)

sojourn (verb) *To stay as a temporary resident.*

In the spring of 1958, shortly before Mr. Truman was due to **sojourn** at Yale University, I wrote to a professor there whose lot it was to spend hours in close quarters with Mr. Truman. (From *Up from Liberalism,* p. 50, Stein & Day, 1984)

Solomonic (adjective) *Marked by notable wisdom, reasonableness, or discretion, especially under trying circumstances.*

Primakov returned to Moscow and foreign ministry spokesman Vitaly Churkin has given us the **Solomonic** judgment of his superiors. (From "On the Right")

sommelier (noun) *A waiter in a restaurant who has charge of wines and their service; a wine steward.*

At La Tambourine, the recessed little table was reserved and Toi, the grandfatherly **sommelier,** had their champagne waiting. (From *Tucker's Last Stand,* p. 55, Random House, 1990)

sophism (noun) *An argument that is correct in form or appearance but is actually invalid. [Used in 1992 calendar in a different form, namely, **sophistry** (noun)]*

At the moment the nation is very much attracted by the **sophism** of Professor Galbraith, namely that we are not as consumers really free, inasmuch as we are pawns of the advertising agencies. (From *Up from Liberalism,* p. 207, Stein & Day, 1984)

sostenuto (noun) *A movement or passage whose notes are markedly sustained or prolonged.*

They made for a wonderful dialectic, James Burnham's **sostenutos** and Whittaker Chambers's enigmatic descants. (From *Rumbles Left and Right,* p. 157, G. P. Putnam's Sons, 1963)

Stakhanovite (noun) *A worker, especially in the U.S.S.R., whose production is consistently above average and who is therefore awarded recognition and special privileges (after Aleksei Stakhanov, Soviet miner whose efforts inspired it in 1935).*

It is now a solid plank of American history that John F. Kennedy, in respect of American mores, was something of a mess: so to speak, a **Stakhanovite** adulterer. (From "On the Right")

stasis (noun) *A state of static equilibrium among opposing tendencies or forces; quiescence, stagnation.*

No one doubted that he, nineteen-year-old Tucker Montana, had done some heavy rowing against that current of physical **stasis** that kept saying No, you can't get there from here, nature won't permit it. (From *Tucker's Last Stand,* p. 28, Random House, 1990)

stentorian (adjective) *Loud, resonant.*

Alistair said, "Why not your stateroom?"

She hesitated, and said, in a voice now entirely feminine, so different from the lightly **stentorian** voice of Alice Goodyear Corbett, tour leader, "If you like." (From *High Jinx,* p. 78, Doubleday & Company, 1986)

strophe (noun) *Any arrangement of lines together as a unit; stanza.*

Almost every Sunday afternoon I would call him and we would talk, at length, discursively, and laugh together, between the **strophes** of his melancholy. (From *Rumbles Left and Right,* p. 144, G. P. Putnam's Sons, 1963)

stultifying (adjective) *Rendering useless or ineffectual; causing to appear stupid, inconsistent, or ridiculous. [Used in 1991 calendar in a different form, namely,* **stultification** *(noun)]*

The relative independence of adjacent Yugoslavia and the relative geographical isolation from Bulgaria argued the military plausibility and the geopolitical excitement of a genuine Western salient in the cold war, instead of the tiresome, enervating, **stultifying** countersalients to which the West had become accustomed. (From *High Jinx,* p. 16, Doubleday & Company, New York, 1986)

subsume (verb) *To view, list, or rate as a component in an overall or more comprehensive classification, summation, or synthesis.*

The geopolitical argument in favor of withdrawal is **subsumed** in the moral argument in favor of liberating Iraq from Saddam Hussein. (From "On the Right")

succinct (adjective) *Marked by brief and compact expression or by extreme compression and lack of unnecessary words and details.*

The basic story is uncomplicated, though the account of it by Kenneth Tynan in the current *Harper's* is not. That is too bad, in a man who knows how to be **succinct.** (From *Rumbles Left and Right,* p. 69, G. P. Putnam's Sons, 1963)

summum bonum (noun) (Latin) *The supreme or highest good, usually in which all other goods are included or from which they are derived.*

Self-rule continues to tyrannize over the liberal ideology, secure in its place as the **summum bonum.** (From *Up from Liberalism,* p. 148, Stein & Day, 1984)

sundry (adjective) *Various; miscellaneous; divers.*

We do not know what would be the cost of rebuilding Kuwait City, and it is of course hard to calculate the damages done by torturers, murderers, rapists, and **sundry** sadists. (From "On the Right")

supernumerary (noun) *Exceeding what is necessary, required, or desired; superfluous.*

Did that auxiliary go on to unemployment? Or might it be that he went on to a higher-paying job? An unanswerable question which challenges the dynamic of a free society to decline to hire someone at a lower wage because by doing so someone being paid a higher wage becomes **supernumerary**. (From *Gratitude*, p. 130, Random House, 1990)

syllabus (noun) *A compendium or summary outline of a discourse, treatise, course of study, or examination requirements.*

The final point in Hart's **syllabus** is the most intriguing. He suggests that abusive language can be and often is a form by which general frustrations get expressed by younger people. (From "On the Right")

syllogism (noun) *An argument or form of reasoning in which two statements or premises are made and a logical conclusion drawn from them; reasoning from the general to the particular; deductive logic.*

What is curious about the proposed reform is that its unwritten language is suggesting: Our senators are for sale for speaking fees. Therefore, we shan't have speaking fees. Therefore our senators will no longer be for sale. The **syllogism** is very leaky. (From "On the Right")

synaesthetic (adjective) *Experiencing a subjective sensation or image that appeals to all the senses. [Used in 1991 calendar in a different form, namely, **synaesthetically** (adverb)]*

All I need do to repay everyone from Bach to the piccolo player is to shell out fifteen or twenty dollars for the music that can realize sublimity for the ear and the mind, if the experience, appealing at once to all the senses, is **synaesthetic**. (From *Gratitude*, p. 12, Random House, 1990)

synergistic (adjective) *Having the capacity to act in cooperative action of discrete agencies such that the total effect is greater than the sum of the two or more effects taken independently.*

Moskos believes we are ready to march together under a **synergistic** banner enjoining us to do everything we can for our country, while our country does everything it can for us. (From *Gratitude*, p. 72, Random House, 1990)

syntactical (adjective) *Relating to the rules of syntax, a connected system of order; orderly arrangement; harmonious adjustment of parts or elements.*

It is a highly regarded national secret that Mr. Eisenhower has a way of easing virtually every subject he touches into a **syntactical** jungle in which every ray of light, every breath of air, is choked out. (From *Up from Liberalism*, p. 194, Stein & Day, 1984)

taciturn (adjective) *Temperamentally disinclined or reluctant to talk or converse.*

The reporter talked on and on, but my **taciturn** answers finally discouraged him; we shook hands and he left. (From *Rumbles Left and Right*, p. 145, G. P. Putnam's Sons, 1963)

talismanic (adjective) *Having the properties of something that produces extraordinary or apparently magical or miraculous effects.*

It is a pity that there has developed the **talismanic** view of democracy, as the indispensable and unassailable solvent of the free and virtuous society. (From *Up from Liberalism*, p. 159, Stein & Day, 1984)

taxonomize (verb) *Systematically to distinguish, order, and name type groups within a subject field.*

Now there is of course no set rule by which pork is **taxonomized** as exactly that. (From "On the Right")

temporize (verb) *To act to suit the time; adapt to a situation; bow to practical necessities.*

We are therefore at one and the same time taking, against Saddam Hussein, a principled line with moral appeal; while, with Gorbachev, we **temporize**. (From "On the Right")

thither (adverb) *To or toward that place; in that direction; there.*
Alistair Fleetwood, for the moment confused, pointed vaguely at a corner of the room. **Thither** the porter went. (From *High Jinx*, p. 189, Doubleday & Company, 1986)

toothsome (adjective) *Agreeable, pleasant; abundant.*
He had lived, up until just after his fortieth year, a robust sensual life, in America and in Europe, using up most of the **toothsome** legacy he had been left by his parents. (From *Tucker's Last Stand*, p. 32, Random House, 1990)

torpor (noun) *Mental or spiritual sluggishness; apathy; lethargy.*
If the nation is constantly at war, or subject to plagues and starvation, national **torpor** threatens to set in. (From *Gratitude*, p. 36, Random House, 1990)

totalism (noun) *Exercising total autocratic powers: tending toward monopoly.*
The thoroughly non-Ideological Man is usually designated as steward of the American political community. This is partly a good thing, because everyone knows that ideological **totalism** can bring whole societies down. (From *Up from Liberalism*, p. xxi, Stein & Day, 1984)

totemism (noun) *A system of social organizations based on emblematic affiliations.*
Not a week goes by that we at *National Review* do not need to call a point of order; or fit together the parts to show a current piece of humbuggery; or scrub down someone's shiny new proposal to expose the structure for what it is—usually Liberal **totemism**. (From *Rumbles Left and Right*, p. 66, G. P. Putnam's Sons, 1963)

transcendent (adjective) *Going beyond or exceeding usual limits; surpassing; being above material existence or apart from the universe.*
The dissipation of the moral satisfaction earned by Mr. Bush merits careful examination: because it teaches us that rigid geopolitical formulae have to yield, in special circumstances, to moral considerations, when these achieve **transcendent** importance. (From "On the Right")

transliterate (verb) *To represent or spell (words, letters, or characters of one language) in the letters or characters of another language or alphabet.*
The Japanese use many self-effacing conventions which, **transliterated** into English, are startling to say the least. (From *Up from Liberalism*, p. 119, Stein & Day, 1984)

travesty (noun) *A debased distortion or imitation or representation; sham, mockery.*
In Venezuela, Pérez Jiménez was boss. He decided to hold an "election" at which all the people, of course, would have the option of "approving" the government of Pérez Jiménez or—well, no one was exactly sure, or what. Indeed, here was a palpable **travesty** on democracy. (From *Up from Liberalism*, p. 149, Stein & Day, 1984)

treacle (noun) *Something (as a tone of voice, manner, or compliment) resembling treacle, a blend of molasses, invert sugar, and corn syrup, being heavily sweet and cloying.*
Shall we attempt to mulct some meaning out of that **treacle**? He is suggesting that President Reagan was not "determined." And that he was not a "leader." That will not be very easy to establish about a man who when he ran for reelection, garnered the vote of forty-nine states. (From "On the Right")

tremulous (adjective) *Trembling; quivering; palpitating; timid.*
Never having heard Kirsten Flagstad speak, I can say only that her singing voice was a **tremulous** experience. (From "On the Right")

trenchantly (adverb) *In a keenly articulate or sharply perceptive manner; cogently. [Used in 1991 calendar in a different form, namely, trenchant (adjective)]*
The educated man, Russell Kirk has **trenchantly** said, is the man who has come to learn how to apprehend ethical norms by intellectual means. (From *Rumbles Left and Right*, p. 105, G. P. Putnam's Sons, 1963)

tripartite (adjective) *Divided into or being in three parts; composed of three parts or kinds.*

Yes, [the Israeli people] have lined up for gas masks and are practicing civil defense, as who would not at this moment. But the great drama is **tripartite.** (From "On the Right")

tropism (noun) *An innate tendency to react in a definite manner to stimuli; a natural born inclination.*

Because we know that women should be educated and should vote and should exercise their capacity to lead does not dissipate that **tropism** that assigns to the woman primary responsibility for the care of the child, and to the man, primarily responsibility for the care of the woman. (From "On the Right")

truculently (adverb) *Belligerently, pugnaciously. [Used in 1991 calendar in a different form, namely,* **truculent** *(adjective)]*

"What's the matter with that?" Baroody's pipe tilted up **truculently.** (From *Tucker's Last Stand,* p. 14, Random House, 1990)

uncongruous (adjective) *Not conforming to the circumstances or requirements of a situation; unreasonable, unsuitable.*

A teacher who devotes himself to undermining the premises of the school at which he teaches, or the society in which he lives, may properly be deemed **uncongruous.** (From *Rumbles Left and Right,* p. 104, G. P. Putnam's Sons, 1963)

urbane (adjective) *Having or showing the refined manners of polite society; elegant, cosmopolitan.*

The aide wrote back to the box number designated. That letter got back an **urbane** letter advising the aide that if the Director was not interested in knowing what the internal fighting within the Kremlin was all about, perhaps the Director should resign his position as head of CIA and become Baseball Commissioner? (From *High Jinx,* p. 177, Doubleday & Company, 1986)

utilitarian (adjective) *Stressing the value of practical over aesthetic qualities; characterized by or aiming at utility as distinguished from beauty or ornament.*

The apartment was appropriately **utilitarian,** as though quickly furnished for a transient client. (From *Tucker's Last Stand,* p. 258, Random House, 1990)

vacuity (noun) *Emptiness of mind; lack of intelligence, interest, or thought; an inane or senseless thing, remark, or quality.*

Six weeks before he was inaugurated, I lunched privately with Senator Quayle, taking the opportunity to search out that highly advertised **vacuity.** I didn't find it. (From "On the Right")

varicose (adjective) *Abnormally swollen or dilated.*

He was habituated now to the redundancy of the Trail's surrounding features—the hanging Spanish moss–like vegetation, the sprouts of sharp underbrush, the **varicose** little ditches engraved by the spring floods. (From *Tucker's Last Stand,* p. 6, Random House, 1990)

variegated (adjective) *Varied; especially marked with different colors or tints in spots, streaks, or stripes.*

At twelve I persuaded my indulgent father to give me a boat. The boat was a sixteen-foot Barracuda (a class since extinct), and I joined the **variegated** seven-boat fleet in Lakeville, Connecticut. (From *Rumbles Left and Right,* p. 165, G. P. Putnam's Sons, 1963)

venial (adjective) *That may be forgiven; pardonable; excused; overlooked.*

It is proper to raise the question whether this is an indication of the dulled morality of the public, or whether the misuse of public transportation is merely a **venial** offense. (From "On the Right")

vexatious (adjective) *Annoying, troublesome.*

On the other hand, to suppose that the latter won't get into **vexatious** troubles is to guess wrong, as witness the matter of Edwin Meese. (From "On the Right")

vinous (adjective) *Caused by or resulting from drinking wine or spirits; showing the effects of the use of wine.*

Bui Tin once said to him, after a long and **vinous** meal, that Le Duc Sy's mutinous inclinations were really undifferentiated; he had not got on with the Reverend Mother, nor with the principal at their primary school; nor had he really got on with his father. (From *Tucker's Last Stand,* p. 118, Random House, 1990)

vitriol (noun) *Virulence of feeling or speech.*

Lyndon Baines Johnson was morose. When that happened, the **vitriol** reigned for the initial period, and then he would focus his powerful mind on the vexation, the irritant, the goddam son of a bitch creating the problem! (From *Tucker's Last Stand,* p. 184, Random House, 1990)

voluptuously (adverb) *Full and appealing in form.*

"Sir Alistair!" He allowed the syllable to pass **voluptuously** through his lips. Until exactly 12:44 that afternoon he had been simply Mr. Alistair Fleetwood. (From *High Jinx,* p. 57, Doubleday & Company, 1986)

vulgar (adjective) *Deficient in taste, delicacy, or refinement. [Used in 1991 calendar in a different form, namely, **vulgarian** (noun and adjective)]*

The four of them shared the living room for a few minutes, after which they separated. And in due course, in that charmingly **vulgar** room, Minerva was soon giggling as "Charles" expressed his affection for her. (From *High Jinx,* p. 103, Doubleday & Company, 1986)

Wykehamist (noun) *A student or graduate of Winchester College, England.*

Fleetwood had been attracted to the tall, rangy **Wykehamist** who devoted himself equally to physics, soccer, and politics. (From *High Jinx,* p. 86, Doubleday & Company, 1986)

Index

ABOUT THE AUTHOR

A biographical sketch of WILLIAM F. BUCKLEY's life
and works appears in the preface to the *Paris Review*
interview, in the chapter "On Fiction."

ABOUT THE TYPE

This book was set in Garamond, a typeface originally designed by the Parisian type cutter Claude
Garamond (1480–1561). This version of Garamond
was modeled on a 1592 specimen sheet from the
Egenolff-Berher foundry, which was produced from
types assumed to have been brought to Frankfurt by
the punch cutter Jacques Sabon (d. 1580).

Claude Garamond's distinguished romans and
italics first appeared in *Opera Ciceronis* in 1543–44.
The Garamond types are clear, open, and elegant.